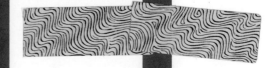

Medicinal Herbs in Primary Care

Medicinal Herbs in Primary Care

AN EVIDENCE-GUIDED REFERENCE FOR HEALTHCARE PROVIDERS

JEAN M. BOKELMANN, MD

Department of Family Medicine
Idaho State University
United States

ELSEVIER

Elsevier
1600 John F. Kennedy Blvd.
Ste 1800
Philadelphia, PA 19103-2899

MEDICINAL HERBS IN PRIMARY CARE, FIRST EDITION

ISBN: 978-0-323-84676-9

Copyright © 2022 by Elsevier, Inc. All rights reserved.

Notice

Library of Congress Control Number : 2021937500

Content Strategist: Charlotta Kryhl
Editorial Project Manager: Mona Zahir
Production Project Manager: Poulouse Joseph
Cover Designer: Christian Bilbow

  Working together to grow libraries in developing countries

Last digit is the print number: 9   8   7   6   5   4   3   2   1

www.elsevier.com • www.bookaid.org

CONTENTS

PART 3

Herbal Monographs with References

PREFACE

Books and apps on medicinal herbs are plentiful. Yet, in my experience as a family physician and teacher of integrative medicine, medical providers remain unfamiliar and uncomfortable with herbal options for their patients. Although this lack of herbal familiarity and alacrity has in the past been due to a conventional medical bias against herbal medicine, the field of phytotherapy has gained adequate credibility in the past 20 years to foster an open mind to medicinal herbs and other forms of alternative medicine, particularly in younger healthcare providers. While the available literature in the form of books and apps provides thorough and scientific information on individual herbs, it generally leaves busy healthcare providers without a quick reference for particular diseases. In today's medical climate, providers need a quick download without taking dangerous shortcuts. They need to know what might be recommended for a particular patient with diagnoses X, Y, and Z; they need to know what the safest application with the least side effects and drug interactions might be; and they need to know what formulation, dosage, and frequency to recommend. Healthcare providers also need the reassurance of original data including details such as the statistical significance and number needed to treat.

As a faculty member and integrative medicine coordinator for the Idaho State University Department of Family Medicine, I was frequently asked for advice on herbs and natural supplements when a resident's or colleague's patient refused pharmaceuticals but was agreeable to "something natural." When I announced my decision in November 2017 to retire in July 2018, one of the residents asked me who would advise them about medicinal herbs after my retirement. My response was, "Don't worry, I'll just make you up a table of my favorites."

Shortly thereafter I began creating such a table (Part 2), or as it turned out, a set of 60 system-based disease tables. Each table lists the herbs alphabetically according to the herbs' common names in the United States, with the Latin names identified secondarily for specificity. As the extent of the tables grew, it became apparent that I would need to provide more information on general herbalism and on each herb in the table. So, I created Part 1 to describe medical herbalism in its alternative medicine niche, to dispel some common misconceptions about herbs, to address the challenges in herbal research, and to explain herbal chemistry and formulations. I also decided the tables would need to be backed up by medically oriented monographs for each herb (Part 3). The monographs are also alphabetized according to their common names. Each monograph provides information on the uses of the herb, the supporting research, the chemical make-up of the herb ("Active Constituents"), commonly available preparations and dosage, and safety concerns. Well aware of the thirst for clinical evidence that has been instilled in every healthcare provider, for every herbal monograph I included a representative selection of clinical trial summaries to convey whatever level of confidence would be appropriate for each herb. I refrained from weighing in on the strength of the evidence, as the quality of each trial would be apparent to any reader who had been trained in an evidence-based healthcare field. For the handful of herbs that had sparse clinical evidence I presented more details from preclinical research.

I selected the herbs to include in the monographs based on three factors: First, the herbs with which I was most familiar; second, the herbs that were backed by good evidence; and third, the herbs that tended to be popular with herbalists and patients. While some of the included herbs lack clinical evidence, their preclinical evidence is compelling, and inclusion is intended to stimulate further research. I recognize that many extremely useful herbs did not make the cut for this first edition, leaving open the possibility of adding more herbs in a second edition.

Even though the United States has provided increased funding for herbal research since 1998, the vast majority of clinical trials have taken place outside the United States. Countries with strong herbal traditions, including China, India, Iran, and Russia, lead the field in herbal research. Given this heterogeneous source of information, I made every attempt to homogenize the study summaries into a more predictable formula, starting with the duration of the trial, the type of trial (mostly RCTs), the size of the patient sample, the nature of the patient sample, and descriptions of the treatment and control groups. Unless otherwise specified, the duration of the trial indicates the duration of the actual observation of the patients, which in most cases was also the duration of the intervention. Limitations in evidence were routinely encountered. On several occasions, details of the herbal intervention dosing or formulation were

not available. Because medical herbalism commonly uses herbal blends, many of the clinical trials utilized combinations of herbs, often proprietary blends. These combination formulas create uncertainty as to the efficacy of the single herb in question, but the information is nevertheless useful for clinical application. While I tried to avoid any appearance of commercial bias, I included the names of the studied proprietary blends, when available, for clarity.

In keeping with the "quick reference" concept I utilized some shorthand and shortcuts. I made extensive use of accepted medical and research abbreviations (the abbreviations are clarified in Appendix I). I eliminated confidence intervals and a few other statistical details, knowing that the reader could look up the original citation if interested in further analysis. I reduced the number of digits behind decimal points, such as with P-values, unless it seemed to make a meaningful difference. For the list of references at the end of each monograph, I left out the preclinical references if the herb in question had a large volume of clinical research. For herbs with sparse clinical research, the references from preclinical research are listed.

ACKNOWLEDGMENTS

■ ■

I would like to give special thanks to those who have contributed to or supported my path in medical herbalism:

- My hands-on herbal teachers, specifically, Darcy Williamson, Annette Davis CN, Jean Claude Lapraz MD, and my patients.
- The 2004 Idaho State University Family Medicine faculty, especially its director Jonathan Cree MD, who supported my creation of an integrative medicine track.
- My family for their advice and patience.
- The American Botanical Council, an organization that has prioritized evidence, safety, and reliability in the herbal industry since 1988.
- Researchers and research subjects for leading us to the evidence.

INTRODUCTION

■ ■

What do our patients want from us? They want guidance to restore and maintain wellness, and they want affordable and effective options to achieve that wellness. If our conventional methods fall short in this endeavor, we might consider alternatives. We might think about medicinal herbs. Our patients also want fast answers. These are the reasons you opened this book.

This book was written with the intention of putting more tools in your medical toolbox without your having to spend an inordinate amount of time and money. While I would certainly be honored if you read this book from cover to cover, I understand the time pressures of primary care and the need to efficiently help patients who wish to pursue herbal alternatives for their medical conundrums or for prevention of disease. If your approach to medical information is more in line with mine, you want the fastest and most direct way to get the information needed to proceed effectively and safely.

To efficiently use this book, consider the example of a hypothetical patient. Say you have a patient with a particular problem, be it a clear-cut diagnosis or a strange constellation of undiagnosable symptoms. And this patient is not a candidate for conventional pharmaceutical intervention because of one or more of the following:

(a) a preference for a nature-derived remedy
(b) a history of adverse effects from pharmaceuticals
(c) a lack of pharmaceutical options to address the issue safely and effectively
(d) an inability to afford prescription medication
(e) a lack of clear-cut diagnosis and yet a desire on your part to help ease this patient's suffering

Step I: The first time you use this book I recommend that you read Part I at least once to have an overview of the history, research, formulations, safety generalizations, and applications of medicinal herbs and to understand how medicinal herbs differ from other forms of natural healing and from pharmaceuticals. It would be ideal if you read Part I right now before you actually need it as a case-based reference.

Step II: Go to the appropriate disease table for the case at hand. The tables are organized according to either organ system (such as "Ears, Nose, and Throat Disorders" or "Dermatological Disorders," etc.) or to systemic issues (such as "Endocrine Disorders," "Disorders of Vitality," or "Autoimmune Disorders"). Refer to the book's table of contents to find the appropriate table. The disease tables frequently lump together several related disorders, so the particular issue you would like to address may be grouped with other issues. You might need to scan down through the column labeled "Scope of Potential Benefits" to find the particular disorder you are seeking. Since the herbs in the table are listed alphabetically rather than by significance, I have bolded the medical indications that have the strongest evidence for any given herb to catch your eye. If a medical indication is in regular text, this indicates that there is clinical evidence. If the herb has only preclinical evidence, the medical indication is in smaller text and italics.

Step III: Once you find the herb or herbs that might be most beneficial for the medical disorder in question, look again at the "Scope of Potential Benefits" column for the selected herbs to see what other disorders can be helped by that herb. Does your patient have any of the other disorders mentioned in that column? If so, might they derive a bigger bang for their buck with that herb? This two-for-one approach might earn you some extra stars in online reviews.

Step IV: Now that you have selected one or more herbal options to recommend, you can look up the monograph for those herbs in Part III. The monographs are also in alphabetical order based on their common names. Each monograph gives you a brief general overview and summaries of the evidence for that herb. It provides a list of the main chemical constituents that are thought to be the active ingredients in that herb. It provides information on how to best administer the herb based on tradition or evidence. And it goes over safety issues. If you are in a hurry, at the very least read the "Commonly Used Preparations and Dosage" and the "Safety and Precaution" sections of the monograph. I also recommend that you read the clinical trial summaries specific for the disorder in question (the summaries are grouped according to disorders) so that you may derive an appropriate level of confidence or uncertainty about efficacy. This is important information to convey to the patient in shared decision-making. The "In Vitro and Animal Research" and "Active Chemical Constituents" sections provide further understanding of mechanisms of action for each herb. If you need further details about the research, you can look up the original literature from the list of references at the end of each monograph.

Step V: If you are not clear on herbal terminology, you may refer to Chapter 3 on herbal preparations and Chapter 7 on common herbal terms.

Step VI: Once you have discussed your findings and agreed upon an herbal remedy through shared decision-making with your patient, you may either write out an herbal prescription based on how it was used in the research so that the patient may to take it to the local herb store, or, based on the information in the "Commonly Used Preparations and Dosage" section you may simply advise your patient to find a reputable brand of that particular herb at a local pharmacy or supermarket and follow the directions on the label. Under "Commonly Used Preparations and Dosage" you should make note of whether the capsule (the form that is available in most pharmacies and supermarkets) is simply a powdered herb, an extract, a concentrated extract, or standardized extract. As is occasionally noted in a comment beneath the list of commonly used preparations and dosage, some herbs work better if they are in a standardized preparation, while others are more effective when not standardized. If you want to prescribe an herbal tincture or a tincture blend of more than one herb, you will have to find a reliable herbal company to provide these. I have been fortunate enough to have access to a local company Time Labs for high-quality individualized polyherbal prescriptions.

PART 1

Herbal Basics—The History, Terminology, and Unique Characteristics of Medicinal Herbs

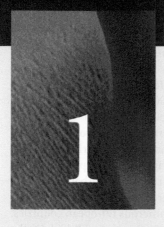

THE ANCIENT HISTORY AND MODERN REGULATION OF MEDICINAL HERBS

ANCIENT HERBAL HISTORY

Herbal medicine predates written history. Otzi the Iceman was discovered in 1991 on a mountaintop in the Ötztal Alps with a satchel full of medicinal herbs. He was carrying birch fungus 5300 years ago, which is now known to have antiinflammatory, antiparasitic, and antibacterial properties. The remains of Otzi suggest he had arthritis and intestinal parasites. Was this mere coincidence?

Modern civilization has inherited a wealth of herbal literature from past centuries. The Sumerians wrote lists of herbs on clay tablets as far back as 3000 BCE. Further east around the same time, Shen Nung wrote *Pen Ts'ao* or *Shennong Ben Cao Jing*, a list of herbs that is most likely a compilation of an even older oral tradition of Chinese herbalism. A more comprehensive Chinese book of medicine, the *Huangdi Neijing*, was written around 250 BCE. The *Kahoun Papyrus* on gynecological disease and the *Papyrus Ebers*, both from ancient Egypt, date back to 1950 BCE and 1500 BCE, respectively. The latter included a broad range of remedies, one example being the use of elderberry for treating diabetes, an application that is now supported by scientific research.

Greeks and Romans have records of using herbs a millennium or two later through the work of Dioscorides (40–90 CE) and Claudius Galen (131–200 CE), from whom the herbal term "galenicals" is derived and who formulated the *materia medica* texts that continued to be referenced for the next 1500 years. Iranian physician Ibn Sina aka Avicenna (980–1037 CE) compiled *The Canon of Medicine*, which was widely used in Europe during the 11th and 12th centuries. Herbal knowledge was preserved in monasteries during the Middle Ages of Europe. Perhaps best known from this time is Hildegard von Bingen, a 12th-century Benedictine nun and polymath who wrote on medicinal herbs, among other things. All these works became more widely distributed with the invention of the printing press in 1439, and herbal healing entered into widespread use by lay practitioners. Meanwhile, over in the New World, the Aztecs were found by the conquering Spanish to be expert herbalists. In 1552, the Badianus Manuscript entitled *Libellus de Medicinalibus Indorum Herbis* ("Little Book of the Medicinal Herbs of the Indians") was compiled as a list of herbs that had been used by the Aztecs as medicines for centuries.

With such extensive herbal literature surviving the millennia and continuing to be applied currently, and with modern scientific research verifying the efficacy of a vast number of traditional herbal usages, the big question is, "How did they know?" Was it just trial and error over hundreds of years or was it something more mysterious? Medicinal herbs are known to have come into use through a few different approaches. Initially, there was a recognition that adding culinary herbs to foods bestowed upon the foods an increase in safety margin largely due to the antimicrobial effects of the essential oil constituents of the herbs. Another herbal application theory is called "the doctrine of signatures." According to this theory, every herb has its own "sign." The appearance of the plant and its color, scent, or living environment indicate its medicinal use. Walnuts that look like the brain are good for the brain.

Herbs used to cure jaundice such as marigold and dandelion have yellow flowers. Hard-barked trees are good for bones. Willow, with its flexibility, was identified as being good for joints. Astrology was another means for deciphering the applications of herbs. Then, in the late 16th century came experimental science. A rift evolved between the more scientifically inclined medical practitioners and those who continued to look at plants or the stars. The scientific method was born and continues to be the guiding light for the field of medicine. It is fascinating that the scientific method appears to be increasingly validating many of the practices derived through the more ancient methods of gaining knowledge.

LEGITIMIZATION OF MEDICINAL HERBS IN THE 20TH CENTURY

Although medical herbalism has retained strong thread of continuity in many regions of the world, Western civilization took a time-out from herbalism with the introduction of pharmaceuticals in the late 19th and early 20th centuries. It was later in the 20th century that ancient history and modern science began to find common ground, and with this common ground came the need to proceed cautiously and systematically. In both Europe and the United States, collective agencies arose to address this need.

European Authentication of Herbal Therapy: German Commission E, ESCOP, and BHP

The German Commission E is a scientific advisory board of the "Bundesinstitut für Arzneimittel und Medizinprodukte" formed in 1978. The commission provides scientific expertise for the approval of substances and products previously used in traditional, folk, and herbal medicine. The commission became known beyond Germany in the 1990s for compiling and publishing monographs evaluating the safety and efficacy of 380 herbs for licensed medical prescribing in Germany. The monographs were published between 1984 and 1994 and have not been updated since then; however, they are still considered to hold validity. In 1998, Mark Blumenthal translated the monographs into English and published

The Complete German Commission E Monographs: Therapeutic Guide to Herbal Medicines.

The European Scientific Cooperative on Phytotherapy (ESCOP) was founded in 1989 as an umbrella organization over the national European phytotherapy associations. Like the Commission E in Germany, a working group is assigned to ESCOP for the development of consistent assessment criteria for herbal medicines. Its members come from universities and professional societies of numerous European countries. The collected information is published in the *ESCOP Monographs*.

British Herbal Pharmacopoeia was developed in 1983 by the British Herbal Medical Association. The second edition was published in 1996 and provides quality standards for 169 different herbs. The *British Herbal Compendium* consists of Volumes 1 and 2 that were published by the British Herbal Medical Association in 1992 and 2006, respectively. Volume 1 offers scientific information on medicinal herbs for which quality standards are defined in the revised *British Herbal Pharmacopoeia*. It covers about half of the plant drugs in BHP 1996 and the others are covered in Volume 2. Volume 2 provides concise monographs that summarize and review the evidence for many medicinal herbs.

Authentication of Medicinal Herbs in the United States

United States Pharmacopoeia (USP): The original attempt in the United States to systemize and authenticate medicinal herbs was through monographs written in 1820 to improve the safety of the available drugs of the time. The USP was developed originally by 11 physicians to protect patients from poor-quality medicines. Since then, the USP has developed monograph standards for more than 900 nutritional and dietary supplement products. When the USP was formed in the early 19th century, many new plants were being discovered and used to produce drug components for patient treatment. Until publication of the first USP, there was no standardized information regarding plant processing, such as which part of the plant or which method of extraction of plant material should be used. The first edition of the USP mainly focused on drugs of plant origin, many of which were native to the United States. In 1975, the USP combined with the **National Formulary** to become the **USP-NF**. By 2020, the USP-NF had evolved into more than 5000 monographs for finished drug products. As modern pharmacotherapeutics took over, medicinal herbs fell into the background and were consequently given their own platform in the *Herbal Medicines Compendium* (*HMC*). Between 2014 and 2020, 57 monographs were finalized and made freely available online, with numerous other monographs in the works (See Appendix II). The *HMC* monographs provide standards for ingredients used in herbal medicines. Each monograph contains general information including the definition of the herbal ingredient relative to the monograph title and specifications of tests for critical quality attributes of the herbal ingredient and analytical test procedures.

American Herbal Pharmacopoeia (AHP): The AHP began developing qualitative and therapeutic monographs in 1994, with the intention of providing the most comprehensive and critically reviewed body of information on herbal medicines in the English language. As of 2020, there are 40 completed monographs, with the goal of 300 monographs on botanicals, including many of the Ayurvedic, Chinese, and Western herbs most frequently used in the United States. In 2020 a complete set of colorful hard-copy monographs could be purchased from AHP for $1278.40.

Federal Regulation of Medicinal Herbs in the United States

DSHEA and CGMP Legislation: In the late 1980s and early 1990s, Congress was considering several bills that would tighten regulations regarding dietary supplement labeling. After backlash from the dietary supplement industry, US senators Orrin Hatch (R-Utah) and Tom Harkin (D-Iowa) introduced the "Dietary Supplement Health and Education Act" (DSHEA) in 1994, which was subsequently signed into law by President Bill Clinton. The act defined the term "dietary supplement" to mean a product intended to supplement the diet that bears or contains one or more

dietary ingredients, including "a vitamin, a mineral, an herb or other botanical, an amino acid, a dietary substance for use by man to supplement the diet by increasing the total dietary intake, or a concentrate, metabolite, constituent, extract, or combination of any of the aforementioned ingredients." Under the act, any supplements that were marketed in the United States before 1994 did not require FDA approval. Those marketed after 1994 were designated New Dietary Ingredients and required review by the FDA prior to their marketing. The act stipulated that all dietary supplements be labeled as such, and that they could not be approved or authorized for investigation as new drugs, antibiotics, or biologics, unless they were marketed as food or dietary supplements before such approval or authorization. The act stipulated that each supplement be labeled with quantity of contents, serving size, percent daily value if appropriate, list of ingredients in descending order, plant parts used, safety information, and most importantly a disclaimer if the supplement bore a claim to affect the structure or function of the body, a claim of general well-being, or a claim of a benefit related to a classical nutrient deficiency disease. The disclaimer was to state, "This statement has not been investigated by the Food and Drug Administration. This product is not intended to diagnose, treat, cure, or prevent any disease." DSHEA allowed the option for manufacturers to add information regarding quality assurance to the label.

After the passage of DSHEA, the dietary supplement market grew rapidly, and access to these products expanded to supermarkets and online shopping. Alarm bells started to sound that the natural supplement industry was making huge profits without reasonable safety oversight. To address this concern, the FDA created a new set of current good manufacturing practices (CGMP) in 2007 that applied to the manufacturers of dietary supplements. The CGMP was phased in over 3 years and backed by regular inspections. The CGMP requires manufacturers to demonstrate clean hygienic manufacturing areas with controlled environmental conditions; avoidance of cross-contamination from adulterants and allergens; clearly defined, validated, and documented manufacturing processes; product verification including quality and quantity; adequate training; tracking of batches; safe and reliable distribution methods; the existence of a recall system; and investigation and follow-up on any complaints received. Health care practitioners who directly provided supplements to their patients were excluded from CGMP requirements due to presumption of adequate training in the professional practice and their individualized patient-provider relationship.

NCCAM and NCCIH: Coincident with the legislation of the US Congress to better regulate the dietary supplement industry, Congress passed legislation in October 1992 to establish an office in the National Institutes of Health (NIH) to investigate and evaluate promising unconventional medical practices. This office was originally named the Office of Alternative Medicine (OAM). Six years later the National Center for Complementary and Alternative Medicine (NCCAM) was established in its place, allowing it independent status within the NIH.

In 1999 the Consortium for Advancing Research on Botanical and Other Natural Products (CARBON) Program was initiated, establishing two Botanical Dietary Supplement Research Centers (BDSRC). The purpose of the CARBON Program has been to promote research on the safety, effectiveness, and mechanisms of action of botanical dietary supplements that have a high potential to benefit human health, and to support the development of methods and resources to enhance the progress of this research. Part of the work of CARBON has been the establishment of a Natural Products Nuclear Magnetic Resonance Open Data Exchange to create open access to natural product chemical structure data.

NCCAM awarded its first research grant in 1999 and established *CAM* on *PubMed* in 2001. In May 2004 NCCAM announced its findings from a comprehensive survey on American adults' use of complementary health approaches: 36% of US adults aged 18 years and older were using some form of CAM. In 2007, a survey showed that US adults had spent $33.9 billion out-of-pocket on visits to complementary health practitioners and on purchases of complementary health products, classes, and materials. In 2014 the NCCAM was renamed the National Center for Complementary and Integrative Health (NCCIH). It maintains the research-based website noted in Appendix II. In 2018 NCCIH released its first mobile app, HerbList, which provides science-based information on herbs and herbal products.

RISING DEMAND FOR MEDICINAL HERBS IN THE UNITED STATES: IMPACT OF DRUG PRICES ON HERBAL POPULARITY

In 1997, during roughly the same timeframe as the enactment of DSHEA and development of the NCCAM, the FDA eased up on a rule obliging pharmaceutical companies to offer a detailed list of side effects in their advertisements. This rule was followed by a proliferation of direct-to-consumer pharmaceutical advertisements. Coincidentally, drug price increases began to outpace inflation shortly thereafter. From 2000 through 2019 the AARP Public Policy Institute reported that drug price increases had consistently exceeded inflation (Schondelmeyer and Purvis). In 2006 the AARP reported that the cost of brand-name prescription drugs had outpaced the rate of inflation for the sixth year in a row. Prices had risen 40% on average over the preceding 6-year period, compared to a 17% rise through inflation over the same period. The report noted that the average price that drug makers charged wholesalers and other direct purchasers had increased 6% in 2005. Inflation over the same time had risen 3.4%. That same year, the FDA launched the Unapproved Drugs Initiative (UDI), which took many older "grandfathered" drugs off the market, giving exclusive rights for sales of those drugs to pharmaceutical companies that were willing to jump through the FDA hoops for approval. Using the high costs of obtaining approval for these older drugs as justification, the participating companies increased the prices of the revamped drugs by as much as 100-fold. As for the high costs of obtaining approval, nearly 90% of drugs that received FDA approval through the UDI were supported by literature reviews or bioequivalence studies rather than through new clinical trial evidence (Gupta et al.).

By 2019, even as the US government had begun investigating ways to slow rising drug prices, CBS News reported that manufacturers had hiked prices on 3400 drugs at an average increase of five times that of inflation. The report noted that four out of five Americans believed the cost of prescription drugs was unreasonable and about one in three patients indicated they were skipping prescription medicine because of the cost (CBS News).

Such are the forces that drive the need for increasing knowledge and safety in the natural supplement industry. For a patient looking at adding a new medication to his or her diabetes regimen, the $500–$1000 per month price tag on a newer drug becomes a figuratively bitter pill to swallow when there is an equally effective and reliable herbal product or natural supplement available online for consistently less than $20 per month. Considering the widespread availability, scientific evidence, improved quality, and basic affordability of natural supplements, it is not surprising that the 2019 Council for Responsible Nutrition Consumer Survey on Dietary Supplements revealed the highest overall dietary supplement usage to date, with 77% of Americans reporting they consume dietary supplements and 81% of adults aged 35–54 years reporting usage of dietary supplements. According to the American Botanical Council's 2019 *Herb Market Report*, consumers in the United States spent an estimated $9.602 billion on herbal dietary supplements in 2019, an 8.6% increase in total US sales from 2018. It appears that the economics of health care in the United States are driving an increasing interest in and use of dietary supplements, a trend that is likely to continue into the foreseeable future.

REFERENCES

https://www.cbsnews.com/news/drug-prices-in-2019-are-surging-with-hikes-at-5-times-inflation/.

Gupta R, Dhruva SS, Fox ER, Ross JS. The FDA Unapproved Drugs Initiative: An Observational Study of the Consequences for Drug Prices and Shortages in the United States. J Manag Care Spec Pharm. 2017 Oct;23(10):1066–76.

Schondelmeyer S and Purvis L.: Brand Name Drug Prices Increase More than Twice as Fast as Inflation in 2018. Rx Price Watch 2019-20, November 2019:1–3.

2 THE HERBAL NICHE IN THE SPECTRUM OF INTEGRATIVE MEDICINE

Although integrative medicine has grown rapidly over the past 20 years, common misunderstandings persist with respect to integrative terminology as it relates to medicinal herbs. This chapter intends to clarify integrative medicine terms and concepts for both general healing approaches and botanical healing terms.

HEALING APPROACHES

Conventional Medicine: This is modern medicine as taught in allopathic and osteopathic medical schools, nursing schools, physician assistant schools, colleges of pharmacy, and other allied health profession schools. It is based on Western scientific understanding of anatomy, physiology, and pathophysiology and addresses most disease processes through lifestyle modification, diet, exercise, pharmaceutical prescriptions, and surgical interventions. This is sometimes referred to as "Traditional Medicine," although the latter is used more appropriately to describe traditional indigenous practices such as those performed by medicine men or shamanic healers.

Traditional Medicine (aka Indigenous Medicine): This is the form of medicine that predates the age of "modern medicine" and includes indigenous practices such as those performed by medicine men, shamans, and other community healers. Ayurveda and traditional Chinese medicine (TCM) are two schools of traditional medicine dating back more than 3000–5000 years, with roots in India and China, respectively. Many highly trained practitioners in the United States practice Ayurveda or TCM. When traditional medicine is examined with respect to the regional applica-

tion of plant medicine the term for this is **ethnobotany or indigenous plant medicine**.

Complementary and Alternative Medicine (CAM): This is a term that became popular in the 1990s to describe the spectrum of alternative healing modalities that may be used in combination with or as a substitute for conventional medicine. CAM modalities include herbal medicine, natural supplements, acupuncture, mind-body modalities, energy healing modalities, homeopathic remedies, nutritional therapy, shamanic healing, and others. This term also is used to encompass different healing systems such as **Ayurvedic medicine, traditional Chinese medicine (or, Oriental medicine), naturopathic medicine**, and **homeopathic medicine** that apply CAM modalities through different paradigms of human health and disease.

Integrative Medicine: Integrative medicine is a term developed to describe an area of medicine in which the health care provider offers both conventional medical modalities and CAM modalities, essentially *integrating* the CAM modalities with conventional medical practice.

Holistic Healing or Holistic Medicine: This is a form of healing embraced by a wide range of healers including those who practice conventional medicine. It is based on the premise that the whole is greater than the sum of its parts. Healing efforts are directed at the entire body and mind (mental, emotional, and spiritual) rather than just one target organ or system of the body. According to the holistic medicine philosophy, one can achieve optimal health by gaining proper balance in life through a multiplicity of approaches including pharmaceuticals, medicinal herbs, dietary supplements, diet, acupuncture, manual therapy, energy work, mind-body therapies, spiritual work, and other methods.

Mind-body methods: This is a group of CAM methods that includes hypnosis, meditation, tai chi, qi gong, and even the placebo effect. It recognizes the intricate and bidirectional communication between the brain (both conscious and subconscious processes) and the body that comes about through hormones, neurotransmitters, cytokines, and other substances that remain to be elucidated.

Energy healing: This is the laying on or laying "near" of hands, crystals, stones, colored gems, tuning forks, vocal toning, singing bowls, drumming, and other practices or general intention such as prayer and distance healing. Some of these methods use quantum physics, some use vibrational effects, and some use spiritual effects as a means of explaining the beneficial results. Examples are healing touch, therapeutic touch, reiki, craniosacral therapy, crystals, magnets, electromagnetic machines, shamanic ceremonies, vision quests, sound healing, prayer, blessings, and most anything that appears either "woo-woo" or miraculous to the Western observer.

Nutritional healing: This is the scientifically based application of foods, natural supplements, and herbs to prevent, treat, and cure health problems. Reducing inflammation and oxidation, balancing hormones, detoxification, digestive optimization, and resiliency are some of the goals of nutritional healing.

BOTANICAL HEALING TERMS

Medicinal herb: This is any part of a plant (such as flowers, leaves, or root) that has been prepared and applied in a number of different ways (see Chapter 3) to bring about healing of disease or balancing of physiological equilibrium. In contrast to a pharmaceutical drug, an herb contains hundreds of different chemicals, a few of which provide the main beneficial effects attributed to the herb.

Botanical (the noun): This is plant-based medicine.

Ethnobotany: This is the use of medicinal herbs in traditional medicine.

Phytotherapy: "Phyto" is Latin for "Plant." Phytotherapy is any application of medicinal herbs to promote wellness and healing. This term is more accurate than "herbal therapy," as "herb" is actually the leafy part of the plant, while medical herbalism often uses other parts of the plant, not just the leaves (see Chapter 3).

Gemmotherapy: This is also known as phytoembryotherapy, which is the use of tree and shrub embryonic tissues such as the buds, shoots, seeds, and rootlets. It is thought to provide high concentrations of active constituents, minerals, vitamins, and plant hormones.

Aromatherapy: This is the use of essential oils for maintaining wellness or bringing about healing. Essential oils are produced by plants to attract pollinators or to defend against pathogens and predators (hence their lovely or pungent aromas). These special oils are extracted from plants through distillation with steam or through other processes including expression, solvent extraction (CO_2 or hexane), resin tapping, wax embedding, and cold pressing. The process separates the water-soluble and other components from the highly volatile components that make up the essential oil. A typical distillation will produce gallons of hydrosol (the water-soluble component) and a few ounces of essential oil. Both the hydrosol and the essential oil have healing potential, with different, sometimes overlapping, chemical constituents. Essential oils are very concentrated and therefore potentially harmful if not used appropriately. The oils can be inhaled through a diffuser, applied to the skin usually diluted in a carrier oil like grapeseed or olive oil, or taken orally in very diluted amounts (such as 0.01 mL per dose). The latter use is controversial in the field of aromatherapy due to the postulation that essential oil efficacy occurs through the olfactory system and due to concerns about the human propensity for overdosing. Certified aromatherapists have had extensive training in the safe and appropriate application of essential oils.

Phyto-aromatherapy: This is a combination of medicinal herbs and essential oils, either in a liquid blend, a capsule, or a topical formulation.

Dietary Supplement: This is a term defined by the USFDA as a product added to the diet but not replacing the diet. Dietary supplements include one or more vitamins, minerals, herbals and botanicals, amino acids, enzymes, and other ingredients. This group of products is covered under the Dietary Supplement and Health Education Act (DSHEA).

Natural Supplement: (See *Dietary Supplement*). Occasionally this term is applied to a single-chemical substance found in a natural source and shown to have beneficial physiological effects. This chemical substance may be extracted from the source or produced synthetically but identically to the natural source. Examples of popular and well-studied natural supplements are co-enzyme Q10 (CoQ10), glucosamine, berberine, and curcumin.

Functional Food: This is any food product that can be eaten for its desired therapeutic benefits beyond simple nourishment. Black seed, licorice, and fennel are examples of functional foods.

Medical Food: A medical food is defined by the Orphan Drug Act of 1988 as a food that is formulated to be consumed or administered enterally under the supervision of a physician. It is intended for specific dietary management of a disease that has distinctive nutritional needs. These diseases include phenylketonuria, maple syrup urine disease, tyro-sinemia, and glycogen storage disease. The USFDA does not require formal approval of a medical food, but it must be designated "generally recognized as safe" (GRAS) and manufacturers must follow current good manufacturing practices (CGMP; see Chapter 5).

Homeopathic remedy: This is a highly diluted material from a natural source including animals, vegetables, and minerals. Homeopathic remedies are produced according to the USFDA-recognized *Homeopathic Pharmacopoeia of the United States*. The remedies are derived through a method that involves a series of 1:10 dilutions of the source material in a liquid, each dilution followed by "succussion," which produces agitation of the liquid. This "potentization" process is repeated over and over to the point that there may not be a single molecule of the original substance remaining in the final product. The more dilute the product, the more "potent" the product is thought to be. It is thought to have the energetic essence of the original molecule, and it is the essence that affects the target condition through a "like treats like" mechanism. This principle is often compared to a vaccination, although an evidence-based explanation of the true mechanism remains elusive. Nevertheless, there have been clinical trials indicating efficacy, some of which are included in this book.

3

MEDICINAL HERB PREPARATIONS

Over the years our brilliant botanical ancestors figured out not only which plants help heal which afflictions but also what part of the plant worked the best and how it should be prepared and applied. Beneficial effects have been found in all plant parts including roots, leaves, flowers (petals and stamens), buds, shoots, bark, bark lining, and pollen. Plant byproducts such as gums, waxes, and resins are also considered a part of herbal medicine.

Plants can be prepared in a variety of ways, often referred to as "Galenical" formulations, named after the highly esteemed Dr. Galen (see Chapter 1). The following entries describe the most common formulations used in the herbal industry today.

Infusion (Tea): This refers to an herb that has been added to hot water and steeped longer than your average beverage tea (typically 15 min). It is also referred to as a tisane or a tea. Sometimes the plant matter is pre-soaked in cold water. The infusion is a good preparation for plant parts that have easily macerated tissues such as leafy and floral plant parts, and from which the desired active constituents are mostly water-soluble. Depending on the plant and the method of preparation, the dose ranges from one tablespoonful of infused liquid (three times the dose of chamomile tea given to Peter Rabbit by his mother) to the more common dose of one full cup. There are numerous herbal tea blends at the grocery store that offer symptomatic relief for a variety of ailments, as implied through the clever names of the blends.

Decoction: This is the result of plant parts boiled in water. Decocting entails actively boiling the plant material in water for roughly 15 min. Decoctions are used for roots, stems, bark, and other tougher plant parts

that need to have the active constituents more or less beaten out of them. As with infusions, the desired constituents must be somewhat water-soluble. Cinchona bark is often prepared this way in South America to treat malaria.

Tincture (hydro-alcoholic extract): Tincturing involves soaking and intermittently agitating the selected plant material in a specified ratio of alcohol and water for several days or weeks. Occasionally the term "tincture" is applied to a process using vinegar or glycerin as the solvent. Depending on how water-soluble/polar or fat-soluble/nonpolar the desired constituents are, the solvent might contain more or less water (e.g., 25%–40% alcohol for more water-soluble constituents; 70%–100% alcohol for highly fat-soluble or resinous constituents). Typically, one part (by weight) of dried plant material is soaked in 4–5 parts (by weight or volume) of the liquid (designated 1:4 or 1:5). If fresh plant material is used (which is preferable if desired constituents are highly water-soluble), the ratio of plant to liquid is 1:2. Herbal tinctures allow for easy blending of several different herbs that might be applied uniquely to each patient. A typical dose of a tincture is 1–3 mL (or roughly 30–90 drops), which delivers about the same amount of alcohol that you may find occurring naturally in many foods. When a tincture is specified, it is noted as the ratio of plant matter to liquid and the percent alcohol. For example, the recommended chamomile tincture in this book is "(1:5, 45%) 1-2 ml TID, or 2-5 ml hs for insomnia." That means that one part of dried chamomile is soaked in five parts of liquid and the liquid used is 45% alcohol (roughly your standard vodka). Tinctures have the advantage of allowing the prescriber to individualize the blend of herbs (by mixing tinctures) and titrating the dosage (which generally ranges from 0.25 to 10 mL per dose). Tinctures also have a long shelf life of 5–7 years, provided they are kept away from UV light (which is why they come in brown or blue bottles).

Mother Tincture: A mother tincture most often uses fresh rather than dried plant material. It forms the basic fluid that is subsequently sequentially diluted for homeopathic remedies (hence the "mother" of the diluted offspring).

Glycerite: This is an herbal extract that uses glycerin instead of alcohol as the primary solvent. Water is usually added to reduce the viscosity of the glycerin thereby enhancing the extraction process. Most fresh herbs with their higher water content may be extracted with 100% glycerin. For fresh herbs with lower water content and dried herbs, typically 60%–75% glycerin is blended with 25%–40% water for herbal extraction. Glycerites are useful for patients in whom alcohol is contraindicated. They are also used in the preparation of gemmotherapy formulas. Macerated gemmotherapy glycerin is prepared using glycerin, water, and a small amount of alcohol. Glycerites have a shorter shelf life than alcohol-based tinctures.

Gemmotherapy: This refers to the use of material derived through maceration and extraction of the fresh buds, shoots, seeds, or rootlets of a plant in glycerin and alcohol. The extract contains hormones, nucleic acids, and all the chemicals found in the entire plant.

Fluid extract (aka liquid extract): This is similar to a tincture but uses equal parts of plant material and liquid, so it is more concentrated and requires smaller doses.

Powdered preparations: Powdered herbal preparations may be crude herb, herbal extract, concentrated extract, or standardized extract. All powder forms generally store well and quickly dissolve in water and other beverages. The advantages of powdered extracts are portability, ease of shipping, avoidance of the taste of the herb (if in capsule or tablet form), and avoidance of alcohol if that is an issue (such as if your patient is taking disulfiram). Most patients taking herbal remedies are using powdered extracts in capsules or tablets purchased either at the local grocery store or online. Powdered extracts can be purchased as a single

herb preparation or as herbal blends. The disadvantage to encapsulation is that herbal blends cannot be individualized for the patient in the same way that tincture blends can be. Also, in herbal theory and backed by some evidence, the taste of the herb often imparts therapeutic activity, so this aspect would be lost with encapsulation. A powdered extract may be a hot water extract or an ethanolic extract, depending on the polarity of the desired constituents.

Powdered herb (crude herb):
In powdered herbs the plant part is dried and ground to a fine powder for encapsulation or addition to a beverage. It has the same concentration and chemical composition as the original herb, including any fiber that may alter absorption.

Powdered extract and concentrated extract (dry extract):
An extract that percolates the original herb in water or alcohol; the duration of percolation affecting the concentration. The liquid may then be then further concentrated using a vacuum pump to achieve the proper extraction ratio (5:1, 10:1, 50:1, etc.). Then, the liquid is spray dried and crushed into powder. The concentration ratio, usually either 5:1 or 10:1, indicates how many parts of the original plant went into producing just one part of the final extract. Thus, the volume of a dose of a 5:1 concentrated powdered extract would be one-fifth the volume of the same dose of a crude powdered herb. This powder formulation is often called "full spectrum" in reference to the maintenance of the natural balance of all of the herb's constituents.

Standardized powdered extract:
This is a powdered extract that has a guaranteed minimum amount of what is understood to be the most active constituent or constituents in the herb. The standardized extract is prepared through a similar method as the concentrated extract, except the concentration achieved is based on the desired percent of a target constituent rather than a fixed concentration of the whole herb. Standardized extracts are often utilized in herbal studies to control for the variability in the chemical makeup of herbs due to variations in climate, soil, time of day harvested, time of year harvested, and so on.

For example, studies done on St. John's Wort often cite use of the herb standardized to contain 0.3% of hypericin. The problem with standardizing an herb to one constituent is that it ignores the other constituents that likely play a synergistic role in the herb's efficacy. This may account for some of the variability in outcomes of different studies for a given herb. Herbal companies often address this concern by combining both a standardized extract powder with a nonstandardized "full spectrum" powder into a single capsule.

Essential oil: This is a product of distillation of the plant material. Typically, steam is used to pass through the plant matter and then through a cooling coil where the extracted components are separated into a more water-soluble product (hydrosol) and a much smaller quantity of a highly volatile product (essential oil). The essential oil portion is very concentrated and is thus used in tiny quantities. This product can be potentially toxic in inexperienced hands.

Miscellaneous formulations: Herbs can also be prepared into salves (usually made with beeswax and oil), syrups (usually made with sugar or honey), elixirs (sugar or alcohol), lozenges, lotions, sprays, gels, poultices, suppositories, and other lesser-used forms.

4

THE CHEMISTRY OF MEDICINAL HERBS

It should come as no surprise to hear that plants are chock-full of chemicals, usually several hundreds of them. As plants or plant parts are ingested or applied topically in the form of an herbal preparation, the "active constituents" are accompanied by a host of other often unidentified chemicals that tag along in the more water- or fat-soluble extraction method. In Part III of this book, each herbal monograph contains a section on the *Active Constituents* that are thought to play a role in the effects of the herb as well as some of the other chemicals that are thought to be of significance due to quantity or risk. Plant chemicals are usually grouped according to the following categories.

Carbohydrates: monosaccharides, disaccharides, oligosaccharides, polysaccharides, organic acids.

Lipids: fatty acids, oils, waxes, alkamides, polyalkynes and polyalkenes, phospholipids.

Amino acid derivatives: amino acids, sulfur compounds, glucosinolates, cyanogenic glycosides, amines, enzymes.

Phenolic compounds: simple phenols, phenolic acids, phenylpropanoids, coumarins, lignans, stibenoids, xanthones, styrylpyrones, flavonoids, isoflavones, benzofurans, chromones, quinones, phloroglucinol.

Terpenes: monoterpenes, sesquiterpenes, diterpenes, triterpenes, triterpenoid saponins, tetraterpenes (carotenoids).

Steroids: steroidal saponins, phytosterols, cardiac glycosides.

Alkaloids: betalain alkaloids, diterpenoid alkaloids, imidazole alkaloids, indole alkaloids, isoquinolone alkaloids, piperidine alkaloids, pyridine alkaloids, pyrrolidine alkaloids, pyrrolizidine alkaloids, quinolizidine alkaloids, steroidal alkaloids, tropane alkaloids.

GLOSSARY OF COMMON AND IMPORTANT PLANT CHEMICAL GROUPS

Alkaloids: Many plants contain nitrogen-bearing molecules that make them particularly effective as medicines. Some chemists consider alkaloids to be a subcategory of amines. Alkaloids are commonly used pharmacologically, and they are also known for their toxic effects. Morphine was the first alkaloid to be isolated from a plant, the poppy. Other examples of plant-derived pharmaceutical alkaloids include codeine, quinine, quinidine, ephedrine, atropine, ergotamine, pilocarpine, colchicine, cocaine, vinblastine, and vincristine. Several hallucinogenic drugs or entheogens (used in religious rituals) are based on alkaloids such as lysergic acid, harman, psylocibin, ibogaine, lophophorine, and mescaline (a proto alkaloid). Pyrrolizidine alkaloids, a potentially toxic group, are discussed further below. A clue that a chemical may be an alkaloid is when it ends in "-ine." Alkaloids impart a bitter taste to the plant, which serves as a clue of potential toxicity for the herbivore.

Examples of plants that contain alkaloids include:
Barberry: berberine (improves the glucose and lipid profiles of patients with hypercholesterolemia, metabolic syndrome, and T2DM)
Comfrey: allantoin (wound healing)

17

Fenugreek: trigonelline (hypoglycemic, hypolip-idemic, hypotensive, neuroprotective, antimigraine, sedative, memory-improving, antipyretic, antibacterial, antiviral, antitumor)

Hawthorn: tyramine (inotropic)

Horse Chestnut: quinine (antiprotazoal, spasmolytic, antiarthritic)

Motherwort: leonurine (uterotonic, CNS sedative, oxytocic, uterotonic, vascular relaxant, hypotensive), betonicine (hemostatic, antibacterial), stachydrine (anticancer, provascular, hypoglycemic), betaine (gastric acidification), trigonelline (hypoglycemic, hypolipidemic, hypotensive, neuroprotective, antimigraine, sedative, memory-improving, antipyretic, antibacterial, antiviral, antitumor)

Passionflower: harmaline (reversible MAO-A inhibition, muscle relaxant, sedative)

Yarrow: achilletin (hemostatic, antispasmodic, choleretic, antimicrobial, tonifying), betonicine (hemostatic, antibacterial), stachydrine (anticancer, provascular, hypoglycemic), trigonelline (hypoglycemic, hypolipidemic, hypotensive, neuroprotective, antimigraine, sedative, memory improving, antipyretic, antibacterial, antiviral, antitumor)

Anthocyanins: Anthocyanins are water-soluble pigments that give the plant or berry source its red, purple, or blue color. They are a subclass of flavonoids produced from anthocyanidins via addition of a sugar. They have antioxidant properties in vitro and are thought to enhance vascular stability. There have been more than 500 different anthocyanins identified.

Examples of plants that contain anthocyanins include:

Bilberry: delphinidins, cyanidins, petunidins, malvidins, peonidins, proanthocyanidins B1–B4, neomyrtillin (general and retinal antioxidants, hepatoprotective, antiulcer, antispasmodic, collagen-stabilizing, antiplatelet, antineoplastic)

Cranberry: proanthocyanidins (antioxidant, antineoplastic)

Dandelion: anthocyanins (antioxidant, antiinflammatory, antineoplastic)

Elderberry: cyanidin-3-glucoside and cyanidin-3-sambubioside (antioxidant, antiviral)

Schisandra: cyanidin-3-O-xylosylrutinoside (antioxidant)

Umckaloabo: pelargondin (antioxidant, antiinflammatory, antineoplastic)

Anthraquinones: These are aromatic organic compounds that are insoluble in water and cold solvents. They confer a yellow color to plants. In humans, anthraquinones stimulate the large intestine causing contractions and bowel movements, thus they are used in laxative preparations. They are found in plants like aloe, senna, rhubarb, cascara, and buckthorn. Some anthraquinones (anthracyclines) have antimalarial or antineoplastic properties. Additionally, some anthraquinones including emodin have been shown to inhibit the formation of tau aggregates and to dissolve paired helical filaments thought to be critical for AD progression in vitro and in mice, with no studies to date in humans. *Cautionary note: chronic ingestion of anthraquinones as laxatives results in melanosis coli. Some anthraquinones have demonstrated carcinogenic activity.*

Examples of plants that contain anthraquinones include:

Aloe: aloin A and B, aloresin A and B (laxative, uterotonic), aloe emodin (antineoplastic, apoptotic, antiangiogenic, carcinogenic), isoaloin, 7-hydroxyaloin A, 5-hydroxyaloin A

Gymnema: anthroquinones NOS

Saint John's Wort: hypericin (a naphthodianthrone; antimicrobial, kinase inhibition, dopamine β-hydroxylase inhibition)

Aromatic compounds: *See Volatile oils.*

Bitter principles: Bitter principles include an array of chemicals that give a plant a disagreeable, astringent, or acrid taste. Bitter principles stimulate the flow of saliva and digestive juices and gastric motility, thereby improving appetite and digestive function. The chemicals of particularly bitter herbs are different in each plant. Amarogentin and gentiopicrin are the bitter chemicals in gentian, both secoiridoid glycosides. In hops, the bitter flavor comes from humulone, cohumulone, adhumulone, posthumulone, and prehumulone, which are phloroglucinol derivatives. "Bitters" is also a term used to refer to a tincture of bitter plants such as gentian and cinchona that is commonly ingested in water at the end of a meal in Europe and South America, respectively. In the United States, tonic water with its small amounts of quinine (from cinchona bark) is a more popular bitter.

Examples of plants that contain bitter principles include:

Andrographis: andrographolides (antiinflammatory, antiviral, anti-HIV, neuroprotective, antidepressant, anticancer), neoandrographolides, andrographosides, andrographic acid (diterpenoid lactones)

Burdock: bitter compounds NOS

Dandelion: terpenoids (promote gastric and digestive enzyme secretions, gastric motility, biliary drainage, antiinflammatory, diuretic); eudesmanolides (sesquiterpene lactones; diuretic, antiinflammatory, increase gastric acid), taraxacin

Hops: isohumulones (phloroglucinol derivatives; activate PPAR-α and -γ)

Saffron: pirocrocin (monoterpene glycoside; antioxidant, antineoplastic, bitter principle)

Turmeric: curcuminoids (phenylpropanoids)

Yarrow: achillein (amino acid derivative; choleretic, digestive stimulant)

Cardiac Glycosides: Foxglove is the best-known example of this class of chemicals, being the source of the cardiac glycoside digitalis. As the name implies, the chemical has cardiac activity through action on the Na-K-ATP pump, increasing cardiac contractility. Similar to the standard cautious approach in prescribing digoxin, caution should likewise be used with any plants containing this chemical class, including foxglove, lily of the valley, oleander, milkweed, and others (generally categorized as potentially toxic). Motherwort contains a small amount of a cardiac glycoside of a different family (bufadienolide/bufanolide) and is considered safe and nontoxic.

Coumarins: Coumarins are aromatic compounds that give that fresh-mown hay aroma. They are found in many plants, but unmodified coumarins do not have any anticoagulant effects on the vitamin K system or on the action of warfarin-type drugs (which are 4-hydroxylations of coumarin). Plant coumarins reduce edema by increasing macrophage degradation of extracellular albumin.

Examples of plants that contain coumarins include:

German chamomile: umbelliferone (antiinflammatory, venotonic, lymphatotonic, possibly anticoagulant, antispasmodic, antigenotoxic, hepatoprotective, antifungal), herniarin (antispasmodic, antigenotoxic, antimicrobial in presence of UV light)

Dong quai: low levels of angelol, angelicone, bergapten (antiinflammatory, neuroprotective, dermatoprotective, photosensitizing, anticancer), oxypeucedanin (anticancer), osthole (antiproliferative, antiinflammatory, hepatoprotective, neuroprotective, antiosteoporotic, anticonvulsant, antiplatelet, antiallergic, anticancer), and 7-desmethylsuberosin

Eleuthero: isofraxidin (venotonic, lymphatotonic, inhibits cell invasion and the expression of MMP-7 by human hepatoma cell lines)

Goji berry: scopoletin, AKA chrysatropic acid (antiinflammatory, α-glucosidase inhibitor, AChE inhibitor, neuroprotective, antipsychotic, melanogenic, anticancer), escopoletin (anticancer), gelseminic acid, and scopoletol (AChE inhibitor, Th2 inhibitor, anticancer, α-glucosidase inhibitor, antipsychotic activity)

Holy basil/Tulsi: ocimarin (antistress)

Horse chestnut: scopeletin glucoside, aesculetin (anticancer), fraxin (antiinflammatory, antioxidant, vascular integrity, hepatoprotective), aesculin (venotonic, lymphatotonic). *Aesculin (a coumarin glycoside) found on the bark, leaves, and seeds needs to be removed from extracts because it is toxic.*

Licorice: liqcoumarin, glabrocoumarone A and B, herniarin (antispasmodic, antigenotoxic, antimicrobial in presence of UV light), umbelliferone (antiinflammatory, venotonic, lymphatotonic, possibly anticoagulant, antispasmodic, antigenotoxic, hepatoprotective, antifungal), glycyrin (PPARγ activity), glycocoumarin, licofuranocoumarin, licopyranocoumarin and glabrocoumarin

Passionflower: scopoletin (antiinflammatory, α-glucosidase inhibitor, AChE inhibitor, neuroprotective, antipsychotic, melanogenic, anticancer), gamma-pyrone derivatives (activation of GABA receptors)

Skullcap: scuteflorin A, scuteflorin B (dihydropyranocoumarins)

Stinging nettle: scopoletin (antiinflammatory, α-glucosidase inhibitor, AChE inhibitor, neuroprotective, antipsychotic, melanogenic, anticancer)

Umckaloabo: umckalin (antibacterial), fraxetin (anticancer, hepatoprotective, antifibrotic, antiosteoporotic), artelin (antiviral, antibacterial); coumarin glycosides: magnolioside, isofraxoside, umckalin-7-β-D-glucoside

Cyanogenic Glycosides: These are the glycosides of cyanohydrin (related to cyanide). The best-known cyanogenic glycoside is amygdalin, the source of Laetrile, which has been put to controversial use in alternative cancer treatment. The biggest sources of cyanogenic glycosides are seeds and pits (apple seeds, apricot pits, etc.). Casava also contains a significant amount, but poisonings are rare despite widespread consumption in some regions. In small doses these chemicals can relax smooth muscle and are thought to be responsible for the antitussive effects of cherry bark and elder leaves. Obviously, dosing is critical, and given the human tendency of "more is better," caution should be used when plants contain this chemical group. Sambunigrin, the cyanogenic glycoside in elderberry, is present in raw and unripe berries, so the berries must be harvested and processed accordingly to avoid this toxic chemical.

Essential oils: *See Volatile oils.*

Flavonoids (aka bioflavonoids): Flavonoids comprise a large class of beneficial polyphenolic chemicals that have the general structure of a fifteen-carbon skeleton, with two phenyl rings and a heterocyclic ring. More than 5000 flavonoids have been characterized. The subclasses of flavonoids include anthoxanthins, flavanones, flavanonols, flavans, ellagitannins, gallotannins, proanthocyanidins, and anthocyanidins. Flavonoids have demonstrated a variety of activities including antiallergic, antiinflammatory, antioxidant, antimicrobial, anticancer, antidiarrheal antithrombotic, antihypertensive, antiaging, lipid-lowering, and glucose-lowering activities. Some better-known chemicals in this group include catechins (e.g., EGCG of green tea fame), quercetin, and rutin.

Examples of the most prevalent flavonoids include:

Apigenin (antiinflammatory, antioxidant, antihistamine, hypotensive, antiserotonin release, GABA agonism, antispasmodic, antibacterial, chemopreventive, antineoplastic, ERB): found in bacopa, chamomile, chasteberry, coleus, holy basil, lemon balm, milk thistle, motherwort, skullcap, valerian, and yarrow.

Hyperoside (antioxidant, antiinflammatory, antiproliferative, apoptotic, hepatoprotective, nephroprotective, antiosteoporotic): found in elderberry, hawthorn, motherwort, St. John's wort, and uva ursi.

Isovitexin (hepatoprotective, anticarcinogenic, apoptotic, antistapyholcoccal): found in chasteberry, dandelion, hawthorn, and passionflower.

Kaempferol (antiinflammatory, antidepressant, strengthens capillaries): found in ginkgo, gynostemma, horse chestnut, horsetail, milk thistle, motherwort, saffron, saw palmetto, stinging nettle, tribulus, and yarrow.

Luteolin (antiinflammatory, antispasmodic, antibacterial, antiviral, hepatoprotective, antiestrogenic, antiproliferative): found in bacopa, chamomile, coleus, dandelion, horsetail, lemon balm, peppermint, skullcap, and yarrow.

Quercetin (antiinflammatory, antioxidant, hypotensive, antidiabetic, antispasmodic, neuroprotective, XO inhibition, antibacterial, anticancer): found in astragalus, bacopa, bilberry, chamomile, elderberry, gynostemma, hawthorn, milk thistle, St. John's wort, tribulus, and uva ursi.

Rutin (antioxidant, antiinflammatory, antidiabetic, nephroprotective, antiosteoporotic, antispasmodic, neuroprotective, antianxiety): found in astragalus, elderberry, gynostemma, hawthorn, horse chestnut, motherwort, passionflower, St. John's wort, saw palmetto, and yarrow.

Vitexin (antioxidant, antiinflammatory, hepatoprotective, estrogen-β agonism, antihyperalgesic, antiarthritis, neuroprotective, antidepressant, dopaminergic, serotonergic, anticancer): found in chasteberry, dandelion, gynostemma, hawthorn, passionflower, and motherwort.

Examples of plants that contain uniquely active flavonoids (additional details of activity may be found in respective monographs) include:

Andrographis: andrographidine A

Astragalus: isoliquiritigenin, liquiritigenin

Bacopa: glucuronyl-7-apigenin, glucuronyl-7-luteolin, luteolin-7-glucoside

Bilberry: catechins (inhibit prostacyclin synthesis, reduce capillary permeability and fragility, scavenge free radicals, antiplatelet, antineoplastic)

Black seed: comferol diglucside, comferol digalactoside

Calendula: patulitrin, patuletin

Chamomile: isohamnetin (antimicrobial); chamaemeloside (roman chamomile—hypoglycemic)

Chasteberry: casticin (dopaminergic, opioid through the activation of mu- and delta-opioid receptor subtypes), orientin, penduletin, quercetagetin

Coleus: acacetin, scullarein, acacetin

Gynostemma: ombuoside, ombuin, isorhamnetin

Hawthorn: vitexin 2'-O-rhamnoside, vitexin 4'-O-rhamnoside, acetyl-2-vutexin 2'-O-rhamnoside, 2'-O-rhamnoside

Holy basil/Tulsi: orientin, vicenin, cirsilineol, cirsimaritin, isothymusin, isothymonin

Hops: prenyl-flavonoids (antiproliferative, antineoplastic, antiinflammatory): xanthohumol (antiangioigenic via inhibition of NF-kB and Akt pathway, antineoplastic), isoxanthohumol, 8-prenylaringen (8-PN; most estrogenic; low quantities, requires certain intestinal bacteria to metabolize xanthohumol to 8-PN, antiinflammatory). *Prenyl flavonoids from hops inhibit aromatase activity*

HCSE: tamarixetin

Horsetail: gendwanin, kaempferol glycosides

Lemon balm: luteolin 7-O-β-D-glucopyranoside, apigenin 7-O-β-D-glucopyranoside, luteolin 3'-O-β-D-gluconopuranoside

Licorice: liquiritin, liquiritigenin, rhamnoliquiritin, neoliquiritin, isoliquiritin, isoliquiritigenin, neoisoliquiritin, licuraside, glabrolide, licoflavonol, glabridin, galbrene, glabrone, shinpterocarpin, licoisoflavones A and B, glyzarin, kumatakenin, hispaglabridin A, hispaglabridin B

Motherwort: orientin

Passionflower: chrysin, isoshaftoside, shaftoside, isorientin, swertisin

Rhodiola: rodiolin, rodionin, rodiosin, acetylrodalgin, tricin, catechins, proanthocyanidins (antioxidant, antilipemic)

St. John's Wort: EGCG, isoquercetin

Skullcap: scutellarin (esp. Chinese), scutellarein, baicalin, baicalein, wogonin, lateriflorin (American), oroxylin A, dihydrochrysin (American), dihydrooroxylin A, chrysin, decursin (American), neobaicalein (Chinese), viscidulins (Chinese), carthamidin (Chinese)

Tribulus: kaempferol-3-glucoside, kaempferol-3-rutinoside, tribuloside caffeoyl derivatives, quercetin glycosides

Umckaloabo: gallocatechin, epigallocatechin

Uva ursi: myricetin (ERB), hyperin, myricitrin, isoquercitrin

Valerian: 6-methylapigenin, hesperidin, linarin

Yarrow: artemetin (hypotensive), cynaroside I and cosmosiin II (antispasmodic)

Glucosinolates: These valuable chemicals are responsible for the pungency of plants like horse radish, mustard, cabbage, and other plants in the *Brassica* family. They are the reason people are reluctant to cook up a big pot of brussels sprouts before company arrives. They are derived from sugar and amino acids and contain both sulfur and nitrogen. Beneficial effects of glucosinolates include regulatory functions in inflammation, the stress response, phase I metabolism, and antioxidant activities as well as direct antimicrobial properties. In high doses they have antithyroid effects (goitrogenic). When ingested, gut bacteria convert glucosinolates into isothiocyanates, which are potent inducers of phase II enzymes in vitro. Isothiocyanates also inhibit mitosis and stimulate apoptosis in human tumor cells, in vitro and in vivo.

Examples of plants that contain glucosinolates include:

Maca: glucoalyssin, glucosinalbin, glucoaubrietin, benzyl glucosinolate (red maca- suppresses prostatic hyperplasia), glucotropaeolin, *m*-methoxyglucotropaeolin, and *p*-methoxyglucotropaeolin

Turmeric: *p*-tolymethylcarbinol (increases gastrin, secretin, bicarbonate, pancreatic enzyme secretion)

Isoflavonoids: These are closely related to flavonoids and best known for their phytoestrogenic molecules such as genistein. They are most commonly found in legumes such as soybeans, which contain genistein and daidzein. Isoflavones bind to estrogen receptors and display the antioxidant, antiinflammatory, antimicrobial, and anticancer properties of the general flavonoid class.

Examples of plants that contain isoflavonoids include:

Astragalus: calycosin (antimelanin), formononetin, op, calycosin-7-Obeta-D-glucoside, trigonosides

I–III, biochanin A (hypoglycemiant, stimulate NK cell activity, antioxidant, apoptotic, antiviral), ononin (isoflavone glycoside; apoptotic, anticancer, phytoestrogen)

Black cohosh: formononetin

Licorice: formononetin, licoisoflavones A and B, glycyrrhisoflavone (tyrosinase inhitibor, MAO-I, α-glucosidase inhibitor)

Minerals: Mineral-rich herbs like nettle and dandelion can act as mineral supplements in their own right. Nettle contains iron, potassium, phosphorous, silica, magnesium, manganese, cobalt, selenium, chromium, and sodium. Oat straw is rich in calcium, chromium, iron, magnesium, phosphorus, selenium, silicon, and sodium. Horsetail is particularly high in silica, a bone-loving mineral.

Mucilage (think "mucus"): This is a polar glycoprotein made by most plants, but the famously demulcent plants like aloe, licorice, slippery elm, and mullein are particularly adept at mucilage production. Mucilage soothes inflammation and stops irritation and acidity by lining the mucous membranes with a protective film. It is also immune stimulating.

Phenolic compounds: The phenolic compounds that occur commonly in plants may be classified into two major groups, namely, simple phenols and polyphenols. Simple phenols are mono-phenols and diphenols such as hydroquinone, the derivatives of which have strong antioxidant activity. Simple phenols, being fairly acidic, can be both antimicrobial and irritative. Polyphenols are the most widely distributed group of bioactive molecules. Gallic acid, a tri-phenol, is a phenolic acid. Phenylpropanoids are another important subcategory of polyphenols (see "phenylpropanoids"). Flavonoids are the single most important group of phenolics in plants and consist mainly of catechins, proanthocyanins, anthocyanidins, flavons, flavonols, and their glycosides (see "Flavonoids" above). Various bioactivities of phenolic compounds are responsible for their chemopreventive properties (e.g., antioxidant, anticarcinogenic, antimutagenic and antiinflammatory effects). These bioactivities contribute to phenolic induction of apoptosis through numerous mechanisms.

Phenylpropanoids: These comprise one of the subclasses of polyphenols and are a subcategory of phenolic acids. They are also known as cinnamic acid derivatives, cinnamates, or hydroxicinamates. They

tend to have general antioxidant, antiinflammatory, cardioprotective, antimutagenic, antitumor, immunomodulatory, and antimicrobial properties.

Examples of common phenylpropanoids and their parent compounds include:

Cinnamic acid and hydroxycinnamic acid (PPAR-α activity, stimulation of insulin secretion, improvement of pancreatic β-cell functionality, inhibition of hepatic gluconeogenesis, enhanced glucose uptake, increased insulin signaling pathway, delay of carbohydrate digestion and glucose absorption, inhibition of protein glycation, inhibition of insulin fibrillation, neuroprotective, antipseudamonal): found in black cohosh, cranberry, gymnema, and rhodiola.

Caffeic acid (antioxidant, hepatoprotective, neuroprotective, antimelanin, antiviral): found in black cohosh, coleus, dandelion, echinacea, gynostemma, hawthorn, horsetail, lemon balm, peppermint, St. John's wort, stinging nettle, and yarrow.

Cichoric acid/Chicoric acid (antioxidant, antiinflammatory, antiatherogenic, antidiabetic, hepatoprotective, antihylauronidase activity, immunomodulatory, anti-HIV, antitumor, apoptotic): found in dandelion and echinacea.

Chlorogenic acid (antioxidant, antiinflammatory, antiglycation, antihypertensive, cardioprotective, antidiabetic, antiobesity, hepatoprotective, attenuates UC and BPH, pro-probiotic): found in bilberry, dandelion, echinacea, eleuthero, hawthorn, lemon balm, motherwort, peppermint, rhodiola, St. John's wort, stinging nettle, and valerain.

Ferulic acid (antioxidant, cardioprotective, antidiabetic, neuroprotective, antimelanin, antitumor): found in black cohosh, dong quai, and St. John's wort.

Rosmarinic acid (antioxidant, antiinflammatory, antihypertensive, antidiabetic, hepatoprotective, neuroprotective, antiallergic, anticancer, antiviral): found in coleus, lemon balm, and peppermint.

Rosavins (antioxidant, adaptogenic): found in rhodiola. *Rosavins (rosavin, rosin, rosarin) are phenylpropanoid glycosides.*

Polyphenols: The second major subcategory of phenols along with phenolic acids, polyphenols comprise a vast and diverse category of important medicinal molecules. This category includes 18 important subclasses: phenolic acids, phenylpropanoids, coumarins, furanocoumarins, lignans, phenylpropanoid derivatives, stilbenoids, xanthones, styrylpyrones, flavonoids, hydrolysable tannins, proanthocyanidins and condensed tannins, isoflavones, benzofurans, chromones, quinones, phloroglucinol derivatives, and phenolic resins.

Examples of plants that contain polyphenols include:
Ginger: gingerenone A (antiobesity, antiinflammatory, antistaphylococcal)
HCSE: proanthocyanidin A2 (antioxidant)
Licorice: glabridin (antioxidant, antiinflammatory, antilipemic, antidiabetic, neuroprotective, SERM)

Pyrrolizidine alkaloids (PAs): This is a class of alkaloids that warrants caution. PAs exhibit a wide range of toxicity from the nontoxic saturated PAs to the potentially hepatotoxic macrocyclic unsaturated PAs. Long-term, low-dose exposures to the latter group can result in hepatic veno-occlusive disease. Acute toxicity from high doses can result in cardiac, pulmonary, and hepatic complications and related deaths. Butterbur and comfrey are two examples of herbs that contain potentially toxic unsaturated PAs and may increase risk for veno-occulsive disease. Butterbur may be used safely when the preparation has guaranteed the removal of PAs, a common practice. Although there is an argument in the herbal community about the actual risks posed by ingestion of comfrey, a cautious approach would be to restrict its use to topical applications.

Saponins: These are amphipathic glycosides of which there are two types, namely, steroidal saponins and triterpenoid saponins. Steroidal saponins such as those found in licorice, gynostemma, and ginseng have effects on hormonal activity. Diosgenin from wild yam is a steroidal saponin used in the pharmaceutical synthesis of cortisone and progesterone. In addition to their hormonal activities, steroidal saponins have antilipemic and immunomodulating activities. Triterpenoid saponins are strong expectorants, increasing bronchial secretions and promoting their expulsion. They also reduce GI absorption of cholesterol, decrease tissue swelling, increase capillary perfusion, and have an-

ticarcinogenic, cytotoxic, antimicrobial, antiinflammatory, immune-modulating, hypoglycemiant, and gastroprotective properties. They tend to be poorly absorbed unless modified by intestinal flora.

Examples of plants that contain steroidal saponins include:
Fenugreek: fenusides, diosgenin (antineoplastic), trigofaenoside A, glycoside D, protodioscin (aphrodisiac, antineoplastic)
Ginseng, Asian and American: 40 distinct ginsenosides that vary in quantity between white and red ginseng, notoginsenoside-Fe, notoginsenoside R1, ginpanaxosides (corticosteroid-like; antiallergic; bronchorelaxant; coronary vasodilating; hepatoprotective; GABA, NE, dopamine, glutamate, and serotonin reuptake inhibition; CNS depressant; neuroregenerative; analgesic; increase cellular and humoral immunity; hematopoietic; angiogenic; antineoplastic. Some vasoconstrict and others vasodilate, some increase cardiac contractility and others decrease cardiac contractility; some are hemostatic and others are anticoagulant, some are CNS stimulant and others are CNS depressant)
Gynostemma: ginsenosides Rb1, Rb3, Rd., F2 (antineovascular; anticonvulsant; analgesic; tranquilizing; hypotensive; antiulcer; vulnerary; antiinflammatory; stimulates humoral and cell-mediated immunity; increases T helper cells, T lymphocytes, and NK cells)
Horsetail: equisitonin (diuretic)
Tribulus fruit/root: protodioscin (up to 45% of dry extract), pseudoprotodioscin, protogracillin, diosgenin, chlorogenin, ruscogenin, sarsasapogenin, protodibestin, tribestin (aphrodisiac), terrestroside A and B, terrestrinin B, terrestroneoside A, chloromaloside, hecogenin

Examples of plants that contain triterpenoid saponins include:
Astragalus: astragalosides I–IV (hypoglycemiant, antiischemic, increase GH)
Bacopa: D-mannitol, hersaponin acid A, monnierin, bacogenins, bacosides, bacopasides I and II (antidepressant), bacopasaponins (antidepressant), bacoside A and B5–9 (neuroprotective, antibacterial, antiinflammatory)

Bilberry: oleanolic acid (chemoprotective, hepatoprotective), ursolic acid (anti-HIV, anti-EBV, antiviral, androgenic, AChEI, pro-collagen, pro-ceramide, antitumor)

Black seed: α-hederin (apoptotic)

Calendula: oleanolic acid (chemoprotective, hepatoprotective), ursolic acid (anti-HIV, anti-EBV, antiviral, AChEI, pro-collagen, pro-ceramide, antitumor), calendasaponins A–D

Fenugreek: yamogenin

Eleuthero: eleutheroside A, ciwujianosides A1–4, B, C1–4, D1–3, E, sessiloside, hederasaponin B, chiisanoside, gypsogenin

Gymnema: gymnema saponins III–V (antisweet), gymnemasins A–D, saponin I (antisweet), saponin glycosides (antiarthritic)

Gynostemma: gypenosides actiponin, phanoside, damulens, and others (AMPK activation, PTP1B inhibition, cytotoxicity against hepatic adenocarcinoma cell lines, inducer of p53 tumor suppressor gene)

Hawthorn: ursolic acid (anti-HIV, anti-EBV, antiviral, androgenic, AChEI, pro-collagen, pro-ceramide, antitumor)

Holy Basil/Tulsi: ursolic acid (anti-HIV, anti-EBV, antiviral, androgenic, AChEI, pro-collagen, pro-ceramide, antitumor)

HCSE: β-escins and α-escins Ia, Ib, IIa, IIb, IIIa, IIIb, IV, V, VI and isoescins Ia, Ib and V (antiinflammatory, venotonic)

Lemon balm: carnosic acid, ursolic acid (anti-HIV, anti-EBV, antiviral, androgenic, AChEI, pro-collagen, pro-ceramide, antitumor), oleanolic acid (chemoprotective, hepatoprotective)

Licorice: glycyrrhizin, glycyrrhizic acid, 18-β glycyrrhetinic acid, liquiritic acid, glycyrretol, glabrolide, isoglaborlide, licorice acid

Motherwort: ursolic acid (anti-HIV, anti-EBV, antiviral, androgenic, AChEI, pro-collagen, pro-ceramide, antitumor)

Skullcap: pomolic acid, ursolic acid (anti-HIV, anti-EBV, antiviral, androgenic, AChEI, pro-collagen, pro-ceramide, antitumor)

Tribulus: tigogenin, neotigogenin, gitogenin, neogitogenin, hecogenin, neohecogenin

Uva ursi: ursolic acid (anti-HIV, anti-EBV, antiviral, androgenic, AChEI, pro-collagen, pro-ceramide, antitumor)

Tannins: These are polyphenolic molecules, members of the flavonoid family of chemicals. They have a long history of use for tanning leather, an ability that well demonstrates their activity. They are astringent, binding to and precipitating proteins, amino acids, and alkaloids. The astringency from the tannins is what causes the dry and puckery feeling in the mouth following the consumption of unripened fruit, dry red wine, or tea. Tannins, being polyphenols, are antioxidant, antimicrobial, anticarcinogenic, and antimutagenic. Tannins can be particularly useful for treating diarrhea and reducing bleeding.

Examples of plants that contain tannins include:
Burdock: phlobaphone
Bilberry
Butterbur
Cranberry
Elderberry
Gymnema
HCSE
Horsetail
Lemon balm
Motherwort
Peppermint
Tribulus
Stinging nettle/Nettle/Nettles
Umcklaobo
Uva ursi: ellagic and gallic tannins, corilagin (potentiates β-lactam efficacy against MRSA)

Vitamins: A variety of herbs contain high concentrations of vitamins A, C, and B (all types). Vitamin D is present in alfalfa and watercress. Vitamin E is present in alfalfa, dandelion, kelp, raspberry, rose hip, and watercress.

Volatile oils (essential oils): These oils are the hydrophobic liquids that impart the characteristic odors of plants. They contain **aromatic compounds**. As the name implies, these oils evaporate easily and thus are often used to that advantage through inhalation, where much of their effects are attributed to activation of receptors in the rhinencephalon. Essential oils are also used for food flavoring and perfumery. The two main groups of chemicals in essential oils include hydrocarbons (monoterpenes, sesquiterpenes, and diterpenes) and oxygenated compounds (esters, aldehydes, ketones, alcohols, phenols, and oxides). Depending on the oil, the effects are wide-ranging from the anxiolytic effects of lavender essential oil to the antimicrobial effects of tea tree essential oil. As they are highly concentrated, they can also be topically irritating when used undiluted (neat), so caution is advised.

Examples of plants that contain aromatic compounds include:

Black seed: thymoquinone (antioxidant, hepatoprotective, antitumor, antibacterial), nigellone (through in vivo dimerization, antihistamine), *t*-anethole, thymol (strong antimicrobial)

Butterbur: petasin, exopetasin, isopetasin

Chamomile: alpha bisabolol (antimicrobial, antiinflammatory, antiulcer, antispasmodic), alpha bisabololoxide A–C (antiinflammatory, augments 5-fluorouracil in leukemic cells), chamazulene (only present after distillation, increases cortisol release, reduces histamine, antiinflammatory, hepatoregenerative, antifungal, antineoplastic), matricin (antiinflammatory), nobilin (antineoplastic), cis-spiroethers (antispasmodic), α-pinene, anthemic acid, *n*-butyl angelate, isoamyl angelate (roman chamomile)

Chasteberry: bornyl acetate, limonene (antineoplastic, detoxifying, antifungal, antibacterial, insect-repellent), pinene, cineole (antispasmodic, carminative, antimicrobial), sabinene

Dong quai: asligustilide, butylidenephthalide (anticancer), butylphthalide (antispasmodic), *n*-butylidenephthalide, ligustilide (neuroprotective), *n*-butylphthalide, senkyunolide A

Fennel: anethole (dopaminergic, antineoplastic, antiinflammatory, antispasmodic), fenchone, estragole, alpha-pinene, beta-pinene, alpha-phellandrene, β-phellandrene, alpha-terpineol, beta-myrcene, camphene, *p*-cymene, safrole, limonene (antineoplastic, detoxifying) (generally hypoglycemic)

Fenugreek: neryl acetate, camphor, β-Pinene, β-caryophyllene, 2,5-dimethylpyrazine, geranial

Frankincense: alpha-thujene, pinene, dipentene, phellandrene, sclarene, *p*-cymene

Ginger: zingiberene, bisabolene (both antilipid, vasodilating, antispasmodic, antioxidant)

Holy basil/Tulsi: eugenol (chief constituent), methyl eugenol, cinnamyl acetate, β-elemene, caryophyllene

Hops: myrcene, α-humulene, β-caryophyllene, farnesene (generally sedative-hypnotic, antimicrobial)

Lemon balm: citronellal, citral b (neral), citral a/geranial (anxiolytic, antiviral), eugenol (antispasmodic, anesthetic, antibacterial), sabinene, β-pinene, limonene (antineoplastic, detoxifying), phellandrene, methyl citronellate, ocimene, citronellol, geraniol, nerol, β-caryophyllene, β-caryophyllene oxide, linalool (sedative, antispasmodic), ethric oil (generally anti-HSV, antiviral, antibacterial, antiprotozoal)

Licorice: β-caryophyllene oxide, decadienol, 1α, 10α-epoxyamorpha-4-ene, β-dihydroionone, thymol (strong antimicrobial), carvacrol

Maca: phenyl acetonitrile, benzaldehyde, 3-methoxyphenylacetonitrile

Peppermint: menthol (up to 50% of the oil content, carminative, antispasmodic), menthone (20%–30%), cineole (2%–13%), pulegone (1%–11%), menthyl acetate, menthofuran, limonene

Saffron: safranal (antioxidant, hypotensive, anticonvulsant, antineoplastic, antidepressant), safranol, hydroxysafranol

Turmeric: zingiberene, turmerones (increase absorption of curcumin), atlantone, elemene, furanodiene, curdione, bisacurone, curcumenone, curcumenol, germacrone (generally antiinflammatory, anticancer)

Uva ursi: linalool (sedative, antispasmodic), α-terpineol

Valerian: valeranone, valerenal, valerenic acids (generally sedative, antispasmodic)

Yarrow: borneol (antimicrobial), camphor, thujone (antifungal, antimicrobial, emmenagogue and immuno-stimulant), chamazulene (only present after distillation, increases cortisol release, reduces histamine, antiinflammatory, hepatoregenerative, antifungal, antineoplastic), azulene, linalool (sedative, antispasmodic), limonene (antineoplastic, detoxifying), cineole (antispasmodic, carminative and antiseptic, antimicrobial), sesquiterpene lactones (antiinflammatory, antimicrobial, cytotoxic), caryophyllene (antiallergic, antiinflammatory, and hepatic)

5 MEDICINAL HERB SAFETY

GENERAL SAFETY CONSIDERATIONS WHEN PRESCRIBING MEDICINAL HERBS

Concern about herb safety has been one of the greatest obstacles to integration of botanical medicine into primary care. Yet, in clinical trials, the most widely used medicinal herbs have been found to be generally safer and better tolerated than pharmaceuticals. The reason for this is a simple matter of chemistry. A pharmaceutical has a single chemical, the dose of which ranges from micrograms to grams. A medicinal herb contains tens to hundreds of chemicals in varying quantities, all adding up to roughly the quantity of the single chemical in a pharmaceutical. A 500 mg capsule of any herb is going to contain considerably less than 500 mg of its chief constituent, even when (see *Standardized powdered extract* in chapter 3) to that constituent. For many herbs, regular consumption may be likened to eating a bowl of oatmeal or drinking a cup of green tea, natural products that contain hundreds of unique chemicals, with each product offering benefits even when consumed on a regular basis for years.

Nevertheless, the existence of highly toxic plants such as poison hemlock is common knowledge, and many of the constituents present in commonly used medicinal herbs are potentially toxic in high doses or with chronic use. The most common adverse effects that have been reported with medicinal herbs are hepatotoxicity and excess bleeding from antiplatelet effects. In addition to direct adverse effects, many medicinal herbs may augment or inhibit the effects of pharmaceuticals if given concurrently. Thus, herbal safety is a legitimate concern.

A prospective, multicenter, observational study of integrative physicians who participated in the Evaluation of Anthroposophical Medicine (EvaMed) Pharmacovigilance Network compared the adverse drug reaction (ADR) reports on complementary and alternative medicine (CAM) and conventional drugs. The study period was January 2004 through June 2009. There were 1,018,626 drugs, 54.8% of which were CAM, prescribed by 38 anthroposophical physicians for 88,431 patients. In 389 patients there were 412 ADRs reported, and 30% of the ADRs were for CAM drugs. The majority were reported in children and females. There were 4.4 and 13.0 ADRs per 10,000 prescriptions for CAM prescriptions and conventional drugs, respectively. The CAM drug with the highest frequency of ADRs was *Pelargonium sidoides* root (Umckaloabo) at a rate of 0.21%. The most frequently reported ingredient in CAM preparations was ivy leaf with an ADR frequency of 0.17%. The most reported conventional drug connected with ADRs was amoxicillin (1.3%). Of the four ADRs rated as being serious, all were associated with conventional drugs. The authors concluded that there were no serious ADRs reported for CAM drugs and there was a higher rate of ADRs with conventional drugs (Tabali et al., 2012).

Case reports: Most case reports available about adverse consequences of medicinal herbs involve overuse by the patient, misidentification of the plant, mislabeling of the product, or inadvertent or intentional adulteration. Given reasonable precautions and moderation in use, medicinal herbs may be used safely and effectively. If a primary care provider does nothing else in this regard, taking an herbal history without an adversarial attitude and advising patients against excesses in herbal regimens would go a long way in preventing cases of liver failure and adverse drug-herb interactions.

RELIABLE COMMERCIAL SOURCES FOR MEDICINAL HERBS

It is important to advise patients about sourcing their herbs from reliable companies. Herbal products that have been manufactured in the United States are subject to the current Good Manufacturing Practices (cGMP) and are more reliable for quality and safety. Imported products are at risk of containing adulterants or being mislabeled altogether. Providing patients with guidance on a safe and reliable selection of commercial herbal products may follow some basic principles:

Quality Guarantees on the Label

A supplement manufacturer displays a cGMP seal on its label if, at the time of inspection, the equipment was up to code and all testing documentation was provided (See *Governmental Regulation of Herb Safety* in this chapter.).

Company Size

Larger natural product companies are generally preferred as they have been held more accountable for a longer period of time by the FDA. Larger companies have more quality control resources, and their herbal sourcing is more reliable due to the risk to of losing large accounts if the product is found to be substandard or adulterated.

Consumer Reports

Several third-party private companies regularly test dietary supplements to verify quality, purity, potency, and composition. These may be found through an online search and include Banned Substances Control Group, ConsumerLab, Informed Choice, Labdoor, NSF International, and United States Pharmacopeia.

MEDICINAL HERB PRECAUTION GENERAL GUIDELINES

In the herbal monographs of Section III, you will notice under *Safety and Precaution* that there are two common general precautions. The first pertains to pregnancy and lactation. The second pertains to drug interactions including antiplatelet activity and effects on drug metabolism through CYP and other pathways.

Pregnancy and Lactation

Under this section, "insufficient human safety data" is almost universally noted and should be translated as "do not use in pregnancy or during lactation." This general principle applies even to herbs that have been widely used during pregnancy, unless there is good evidence of safety. The rationale for this extreme prudence is due to recognition that, over the years, different pharmaceuticals that were once thought to be safe in smaller and shorter clinical trials were later found to have potential for teratogenicity or adverse effects on the fetus or the gestation (e.g., neurobehavioral development or preterm labor). True safety of a product during pregnancy requires demonstration of a lack of even subtle adverse physical and neurobehavioral effects in large populations with follow-up over several years. Such a high level of reassurance is not practically feasible with herbal research. Therefore, it makes sense to be extremely cautious when it comes to herbs and pregnancy. *Primum non nocere*. There are a few exceptions to a general policy of herbal avoidance during pregnancy. Herbs such as ginger, when taken as a food rather than as a supplement, have a long history of effective and safe use in pregnancy.

Drug Interactions

Most herbs have an impact on at least one CYP enzyme if not a whole host of enzymes including UGT and P-glycoprotein. It is a reasonable assumption that any given herb will have some interactions with drugs as well as other herbs. The practical question is how critical is this interaction? This is the same approach you take when looking at the potential drug interactions from a given patient's list of medications. Interactions happen. They happen quite commonly. The question is, can you monitor for effects of these interactions (such as measuring blood pressure, checking blood sugar, or monitoring symptoms)? Of more concern, could these interactions lead to a failure in a life-saving drug such as chemotherapy, nitroglycerin, or asthma medicine? Could they cause life-threatening bleeding if added to an anticoagulant (see below)? As the pharmaceutical guidelines recommend on potential interactions, "use caution" if monitorable, or do not use at all if there is potential for life-threatening interactions. It is a reasonable caution to advise patients against using herbs if they are taking life-saving drugs or potentially toxic drugs the effects of which cannot be closely monitored.

Antiplatelet Effects and Interactions with Anticoagulants

According to Natural Medicines Comprehensive Database, nearly 180 dietary supplements and medicinal herbs are likely to interact with warfarin. Many herbs have in vitro and in vivo antiplatelet effects, an understanding that leads to the conventional recommendation that all herbs be held for 7–14 days prior to major surgery. Furthermore, patients on antiplatelet drugs and anticoagulants are routinely advised against taking herbal supplements while on such pharmaceuticals. As is indicated in the research below, many of the herbs with antiplatelet activity do not have a clinically meaningful impact on bleeding times or hemorrhage. However, a handful of herbs such as ginseng have demonstrated an increased risk for bleeding or an adverse interaction with warfarin. As a practical general rule for patients on pharmaceutical anticoagulants, ongoing precaution is advised unless the patient is taking an herb that has demonstrated a lack of risk.

A 2015 systematic review looked at the effects of the most commonly used natural products on blood coagulation and platelet function. Eleven herbal medicines were included (echinacea, ephedra, garlic, ginger, ginkgo, ginseng, green tea, kava, saw palmetto, St John's wort, and valerian) as well as four other dietary supplements (coenzyme Q_{10}, glucosamine and chondroitin sulfate, fish oil, and vitamins). Increased bleeding risks in six of the herbs (garlic, ginkgo, ginseng, green tea, saw palmetto, St John's wort) and fish oil were reported. Cardiovascular instability was observed with ephedra, ginseng, and kava (Wang et al., 2015).

A 2011 metaanalysis of 18 randomized controlled trials (RCTs) ($n = 1985$) looked at effects of

ginkgo on blood flow, blood viscosity, ADP-induced platelet aggregation, fibrinogen concentration, aPTT, and PT. Random-effects models of effects on baseline change or mean difference showed a positive effect of ginkgo on blood perfusion, as shown by a significant reduction in blood viscosity (WMD = −1.03 mPa s), but no evidence of any significant effect on ADP-induced platelet aggregation (WMD = −0.35%), fibrinogen concentration (GIV = −2.45 mg/dL), aPTT (GIV = −0.42 s), and PT (SMD = 0.00). Subgroup analyses revealed a statistically significant reduction in aPTT for subgroups receiving high-dose ginkgo (240 mg/day or more) (GIV = −0.47 s) and for studies including only patients, not healthy volunteers (GIV = −0.61 s); however, both findings were not clinically relevant. The authors concluded that the research did not indicate a greater bleeding risk associated with standardized ginkgo (Kellermann and Kloft, 2011).

A 1-day RCT in healthy male volunteers ($n = 8$) compared ginger 2 g with placebo for effects on platelet function at 3 and 24 h post ingestion. There were no differences between ginger and placebo in bleeding time, platelet count, thromboelastography, and whole blood platelet aggregometry. It was concluded that the effect of ginger on thromboxane synthetase activity is dose dependent, or only occurs with fresh ginger, and that up to 2 g of dried ginger is unlikely to cause platelet dysfunction when used therapeutically (Lumb, 1994).

GOVERNMENTAL REGULATION OF HERB SAFETY: UNITED STATES FEDERAL DRUG ADMINISTRATION

In the United States, the Federal Drug Administration (USFDA or FDA) oversees the marketing, safety, and efficacy of medicinal herbs. According to the FDA, botanical products are classified as a drug, food, or a dietary supplement on the basis of the claims or end use. A product that is used to prevent, diagnose, mitigate, treat, or cure a disease would fall under the category of drug. If the intended use of a botanical product is to affect the structure or function of the human body (e.g., immune support, cardiovascular health), it may be classified as either a drug or a dietary supplement. If classified as a drug, it must be marketed under an approved New

Drug Application. If classified as a dietary supplement, it is regulated under the Dietary Supplement Health and Education Act (DSHEA) of 1994 (see Chapter 1: *DSHEA and CGMP Legislation*). Dietary supplements do not require premarket approval. It is the responsibility of the company to ensure the safety and labeling compliance of its products as per cGMP.

Current Good Manufacturing Practices (cGMP)

cGMP are FDA regulations that promote a quality approach to manufacturing, thereby reducing contamination, misidentification, and errors in production. The regulations require certain activities in manufacturing, packaging, labeling, and holding of dietary supplements to ensure that a dietary supplement contains what it is labeled to contain and is not contaminated with harmful or undesirable substances such as pesticides, heavy metals, or other impurities. It also requires assurance of the identity, purity, quality, strength, and composition of the dietary supplement.

Different countries and the World Health Organization (WHO) have their own Good Manufacturing Practices guidelines, so the source of the herbal material and product is important with regard to quality assurance.

Generally Recognized as Safe/Generally Recognized as Safe and Effective (GRAS/GRASE)

About half the herbs sold by the herb industry are on the GRAS list. GRAS is an FDA term used for any substance that is intentionally added to food. It is given to any food substance that has been shown to be safe either through scientific procedures or through experience based on common use of the food. Many plant products are used in the food industry for flavoring, consistency, and preservation. However, this term does not accurately apply to herbs when they are given medicinally in larger quantities and with greater frequency. Oregano in your pasta sauce, for example, is not the same as oregano capsules taken daily. Thus, the designation as GRAS should not be interpreted as reassurance that a medicinal herb will not cause harm. Rather, confidence in the safety of a medicinal herb should be derived from appropriate studies, preferably human studies, that show lack of harm.

A GRASE designation provides more reassurance regarding a medicinal herb. To qualify for GRASE designation, an herb (or older drug) must have been subjected to adequate, well-controlled clinical investigations to establish the product as safe and effective, the results of which have been subjected to peer review and publication. In addition, experts must agree based on published studies that the product is safe and effective for its intended use. At this time very few botanicals have been granted this designation due to lack of applications for such designation from FDA. Witch hazel and psyllium are two examples that have the GRASE designation.

Reporting Adverse Events: MedWatch

What do you do if you believe your patient has experienced an adverse event from an herbal product? MedWatch is the FDA's program for reporting serious reactions, product quality problems, therapeutic inequivalence/failure, and product use errors with human medical products, including drugs, biologic products, medical devices, dietary supplements, infant formula, and cosmetics. You may contact the FDA at the following link: https://www.fda.gov/Food/DietarySupplements/ReportAdverseEvent/default.htm

AMERICAN NONPROFIT ORGANIZATIONS THAT PROMOTE HERB SAFETY

Promotion of Safety in the Herbal Industry

The American Herbal Products Association published *American Herbal Products Association's Botanical Safety Handbook*, which features the latest evidence-based research and clinical data on nearly 600 species of herbs and other herbal products. The book highlights data on safety, pharmacological, and toxicity studies, medical case reports, and historical texts. Further, a classification system of each herb, including a safety rating and a drug interaction rating, is provided.

Identification of Adulteration in the Herbal Industry

Adulteration is the presence of unexpected or undesired chemicals that are not part of the natural constituents of the herbal product in question.

Adulteration comes about either accidentally through plant misidentification, or through sloppy harvesting or processing management. It may also occur through intentional addition or substitution of pharmaceuticals, herbs, and other chemicals during processing, such as the addition of small amounts of sildenafil to an herbal formula for enhancement of male sexual function. Responsible parties in the herbal and dietary supplement industry have become increasingly concerned about the suspected and confirmed practice of adulteration of numerous ingredients. The existence of adulteration raises questions about the identity and quality of some popular herbal ingredients sold in dietary supplements and other herbal products in the United States and in global markets.

Three leading herbal nonprofit organizations—the American Botanical Council (ABC), the American Herbal Pharmacopoeia (AHP), and the University of Mississippi's National Center for Natural Products Research (NCNPR)—have initiated a large-scale program to educate members of the herbal and dietary supplement industry about ingredient and product adulteration. A quarterly publication, "Botanical Adulterants Monitor," has been made available to the herbal industry and subscribers since 2014.

Education About Misleading Claims in the Media

With the global use and abuse of social media, exaggerated or false claims of benefit for various natural products have been spread widely, with clear potential for harm. The COVID-19 pandemic provided numerous examples of misleading claims about protection from infection, morbidity, and mortality. For example, oleandrin, a constituent of the cardiotoxic plant oleander, received controversial publicity. One organization that quickly responds to inaccuracies and misrepresentations in the media is the American Botanical Council (ABC). The ABC provides proactive, science-based information about herbal medicine through press releases, articles, and media interviews.

REFERENCES

Kellermann A, Kloft C. Is there a risk of bleeding associated with standardized Ginkgo biloba extract therapy? A systematic review and meta-analysis. Pharmacotherapy 2011;31(5):490–502.

Lumb AB. Effect of dried ginger on human platelet function. Thromb Haemost 1994;71(1):110–1.

Tabali M, et al. Adverse drug reactions for CAM and conventional drugs detected in a network of physicians certified to prescribe CAM drugs. J Manag Care Pharm 2012;18(6):427–38.

Wang C-Z, et al. Commonly used dietary supplements on coagulation function during surgery. Medicines (Basel) 2015;2(3):157–85.

6 MEDICINAL HERB RESEARCH

BUILDING A DATA PYRAMID

Due to several factors that will be discussed, research on medicinal herbs lags considerably behind that of pharmaceuticals. To appreciate the current status of research for medicinal herbs, it may be an instructive exercise to briefly recreate the evolution of evidence gathering.

When humans go about trying to identify cause-and-effect relationships, the endeavor begins with a hypothetical observer noticing a single anecdote—**a case report**. That observer starts paying attention to the co-occurrence of the factors in question and notices a cluster of similar anecdotes—**a case series**. Layered upon the case series, the observer reviews past records of a larger number of humans looking for this co-occurrence of factors and finds several similar episodes—**a retrospective cohort**. Recognizing that a review of routine records is an unreliable source of data due to confounding factors, the observer formulates a hypothesis about what is happening and gathers data in a more consistent format from that point going forward for a defined period—**a prospective cohort**. Each of these forms of evidence has drawbacks, but with each new level of evidence there is more reliability, reproducibility, and applicability.

In recognition that **observational studies** are unable to control for a number of variables, experimental intervention is the next step in analyzing a particular cause-and-effect relationship. The observer decides to perform an intervention for which the underlying mechanism or safety is uncertain, and the research process moves into the lab where preclinical (in vitro and in vivo) research is performed. With a base of pathophysiological information and confirmation on the safety and efficacy of the intervention, the observer next studies the intervention in humans, often through a series of phases (see section on *Phases of Trials*). As a first step in humans, all the subjects in the trial are given the same intervention in the same format in an **open-label trial.** The humans have a positive response to the intervention, but perhaps they were going to spontaneously improve even without the intervention. Therefore, some subjects are given the intervention, while others are left to their normal devices in **a controlled** study that is implemented to rule out spontaneous improvement. The study demonstrates a difference between intervention and control groups, but perhaps the difference in outcome was due to a difference between the groups due to the participant selection and group allocation process. So, the participants are randomized to intervention or control groups in a **randomized controlled** study. Then the observer begins to wonder if there was a placebo effect in the intervention group, so a sham intervention is performed on one group and compared with the studied intervention, requiring that subjects in both groups be blinded to their group status (a **blinded placebo-controlled trial**). To ensure that the observer was not accidentally conveying through unconscious mechanisms such as gestures or tone of voice an expectation of effect, the observer also needs to be blinded to the real and sham interventions through a **double-blinded placebo-controlled trial**. Voila, a classic RCT (randomized, placebo-controlled, double-blinded clinical trial) emerges as the best form of basic research.

Next, statistics are applied (*P*-values, Cohen's D, confidence intervals, etc.), at which point it is apparent that studies with smaller numbers of subjects do not create as much confidence in the findings as do studies with huge numbers of subjects. **Large trials or multicenter trials**, Phase III and Phase IV clinical trials, are needed to achieve a high level of confidence in the findings. An alternative to large numbers of subjects in one trial, the analysis of several smaller studies may be performed using the same intervention to determine the range of statistical outcomes. Better studies are given more weight in this analysis. A **systematic review** is thus performed. If the reviewed studies have enough similarity, a **meta-analysis** may be performed, pooling the data and calculating mean differences between intervention and placebo. This is the top of the data pyramid and is the level of evidence that healthcare providers rely upon for clinical decisions in the 21st century.

Phases of Trials: Research in conventional medicine is further categorized into phases of trials, particularly in cancer research. The phases tend to reflect the clinical trial portion of the evolutionary pyramid just described.

> Phase 0: These are the first clinical trials performed in human subjects. They aim to learn the pharmacokinetics and pharmacodynamics of the intervention. A low dose of the intervention and a small number of subjects are involved in Phase 0.
>
> Phase I: The objective of a Phase I trial is to find the ideal dose with the greatest efficacy and fewest side effects. The dose is titrated as effects are monitored in a small number of test subjects.
>
> Phase II: These trials further assess safety and efficacy for a larger group of patients ($n \leq 100$) with a specific disease.
>
> Phase III: These trials compare a new drug to the standard-of-care drug or placebo, for both efficacy and adverse effects, in at least 100 randomized patients.
>
> Phase IV: These trials test new drugs approved by the FDA in several hundreds or thousands of patients, looking for low-signal side effects.

The medicinal herb research presented in this book runs the entire gamut from case reports to systematic reviews with meta-analyses and from Phase I to Phase III clinical trials. The research presented here consists predominantly of smaller RCTs and to a lesser degree open-label trials. Even the systematic reviews presented in this book vary in strength, depending on whether the review was more qualitative or strictly followed standard methodological procedures recommended by the Cochrane Intervention Reviews or use of other criteria such as Jadad scales and the Consolidated Standards of Reporting (CONSORT) checklist.

EXPERT ANALYSIS AND GUIDELINES: EVIDENCE RATING SCALES

Conventional medical providers have come to rely upon the guidance of various agencies and medical societies to analyze the available evidence and make practice recommendations based on the strength of this evidence. The multiplicity of expert agencies has resulted in a confusing array of grading systems.

Levels of Evidence: Conventional medicine has not always relied on large multicenter trials or systematic reviews and meta-analyses to guide practice standards. Medical research has evolved dramatically in the past 40 years. In 1979, Level I (the best) evidence was defined as at least one RCT with proper randomization. Level II.1 evidence was a well-designed cohort or case-control study. Level II.2 evidence came from time series comparisons or dramatic results from uncontrolled studies. Level III evidence was expert opinion.

Currently, by contrast, Level I evidence is defined as a systematic review and/or meta-analysis of all relevant RCTs, evidence-based clinical practice guidelines based on systematic reviews of RCTs, or three or more RCTs of good quality that have similar results. Level II evidence is obtained from at least one well-designed RCT (e.g., a multicenter RCT). Level III evidence is obtained from well-designed controlled trials without randomization. Level IV evidence is from well-designed case-control or cohort studies. Level V evidence is from systematic reviews of descriptive and qualitative studies (meta-synthesis). Level VI is evidence from a single descriptive or qualitative study. Level VII evidence is from the opinion of authorities and/or reports of expert committees.

While Level I evidence serves as the foundation for the strongest recommendations in treatment guidelines in conventional medicine today, it is noteworthy that new drug approval by the FDA generally requires only two adequate well-controlled trials to establish effectiveness.

The various agencies and medical societies that provide guidelines to healthcare providers utilize a variety of grading systems. The following are some examples.

Strength of Recommendation Taxonomy (SORT)

A: Consistent, good-quality patient-oriented evidence
B: Inconsistent or limited-quality patient-oriented evidence
C: Consensus, disease-oriented evidence, usual practice, expert opinion, or case series for studies of diagnosis, treatment, prevention, or screening

Grades of Recommendations

Examples of the grades for the Agency for Healthcare Research and Quality (AHRCQ), the University of Michigan practice guidelines, and the United States Preventive Services Task Force (USPSTF) are shown below.

AHRCQ

A: There is good research-based evidence to support the recommendation
B: There is fair research-based evidence to support the recommendation
C: The recommendation is based on expert opinion and panel consensus
X: There is evidence of harm from this intervention

University of Michigan Practice Guideline

A: Randomized controlled trials
B: Controlled trials; no randomization
C: Observational trials
D: Opinion of an expert panel

USPSTF Guide to Clinical Preventive Services

A: There is good evidence to support the recommendation that the condition be specifically considered in a periodic health examination.
B: There is fair evidence to support the recommendation that the condition be specifically considered in the periodic health examination.
C: There is insufficient evidence to recommend for or against the inclusion of the condition in a periodic health examination, but the recommendations may be made on other grounds.
D: There is fair evidence to support the recommendation that the condition be excluded from consideration in a periodic health examination.
E: There is good evidence to support the recommendation that the condition be excluded from consideration in a periodic health examination.

A small number of medicinal herbs in this book qualify for SORT level A (good evidence) rating or a level A recommendation in the AHRCQ rating system. Most of the herbs presented here, however, would receive a Level B (fair evidence) or C (expert opinion) rating in either system. The purpose of providing such a wide spectrum of quality of evidence in the herbal monographs is to foster an appreciation for the difficulty of obtaining evidence, to shed some appropriate caution with respect to efficacy claims, and to stimulate further research. The research details provided also demonstrate the difficulty of studying various herbal formulations and variations in herbal species. It must be emphasized that the lower quality research does not reflect an herb's inefficacy, but rather reflects the 30-plus-year lag of herbal research behind pharmaceutical research. This lag has been primarily due to a 20th century lack of scientific interest in medicinal herbs by the medical field and by an ongoing lack of funding for research. There has been a vicious cycle of lack of interest leading to lack of funding leading to lack of evidence leading back to lack of interest. All these factors took a turn for the better in the 1990s, but there is still room for improvement as herbal research rises above several challenges.

CHALLENGES IN EVIDENCE BUILDING FOR HERBS

Bottom of the Pyramid: Suffice it to say that the healthcare field needs more evidence for efficacy of medicinal herbs. The standard platitude is "but there is no evidence that Herb X can help alleviate Symptom Y." However, it is important to recognize that "No Evidence" is not the same as "Evidence of No." The former implies that no satisfactory research has been performed to convincingly show benefit. Benefit has not been ruled out. The latter implies that good research has been done and that it showed there was no benefit. A lack of high-level clinical trials should not lead to the conclusion that a particular herb is not effective, particularly if thousands of years of traditional practice indicate otherwise. In fact, traditional practice is a form of evidence in and of itself, upon which further evidence should be built.

Herbal constituent variability: One of the quirkier challenges in herbal medicine is suggested by the definition of **standardized extract**. This challenge is due to herbs being just as individual and unpredictable as human beings are. Herbs respond to their environment by producing varying amounts of one type or another of chemical depending on the plant's needs for water, nutrients, protection from pests, and so on. Also, some plants closely resemble other plants that are of an entirely different class, genus, or species. As such, proper identification of the intended plant is essential. If research is performed one time with a source from the wrong plant, or a batch of plants from depleted soil, the research would likely be skewed. Thus, many studies employ the use of a standardized extract of a plant to ensure that the presumed most active constituent is present in a specified amount. However, standardization is only controlling for a single chemical in the plant's list of active constituents and might be disrupting the beneficial balance of constituents built into the whole plant extract. Thus, complicated uncertainty envelops the outcome of many herbal studies. The American Botanical Council (ABC) is very adept at interpreting research results based on the added challenges inherent in herbal research. (See Index for ABC).

Polyherbal formulas: Another major challenge to herbal research is the use of polyherbal formulas. The culinary-like nature of herbal medicine lends to blending herbs. Therefore, many of the trials presented in this book involve polyherbal blends, leaving uncertainty as to the contribution of the herb in question. Furthermore, most of the healing paradigms that utilize polyherbal formulas such as Endobiogeny, traditional Chinese medicine and Ayurvedic medicine are highly individualized. For example, a person with chronic bronchitis would be treated with one herbal blend if they are prone to diarrhea and a different herbal blend if they are prone to constipation. Conventional research with its homogenizing nature readily overlooks the heterogeneous complexities of these alternative paradigms, so well-designed RCTs can be used to neither validate nor refute such approaches.

Taste and Aroma: Several medicinal herbs, especially those that are high in essential oils, have characteristic odors that are difficult to mask. Valerian, for example, smells like an old pair of sneakers or dirty socks. Herbs with such identifiable odors are difficult to administer in a blinded fashion. Even when they take capsules or tablets, study subjects are often able to taste the herb on their breath or in their burps.

Financing the Evidence: Conventional healthcare providers rely on good evidence. It guides nearly every decision made in clinical practice. Unfortunately, the evidence industry has become an exacting and expensive behemoth. The amount of financial resources behind any phase III clinical trial, considered pivotal in the field of evidence, has become astronomical, forming the basis of the pharmaceutical industry's justification for the assigned prices of new drugs. A study in the September 2018 issue of *JAMA* reported that clinical trials that supported FDA approvals of new drugs had a median cost of $19 million (Moore et al.). This is problematic for any field of healing that does not have vast financial resources. So, when it comes to a medicinal herb, something that can be grown in one's private garden, there will seldom be enough corporate or private investment to fund research at this level. While several of the trials presented in this book were actually funded by the herbal industry, a more unbiased source of funding would be through grants from government agencies or disease-based societies and foundations.

Despite the challenges inherent in medicinal herb research, there is still a great deal to be learned from existing research that may be applied in a conventional symptom-oriented or disease-oriented therapeutic regimen. As the focus of this book is the disease-oriented model for use of medicinal herbs, all these evidence-gathering challenges are on full display in the research presented in the herbal monographs in Part III. Much of the presented research will reasonably assure the healthcare provider of the safety and efficacy of a particular herb. Based on the available evidence, the decision to recommend a medicinal herb will be highly individualized to the prescriber and the patient.

REFERENCES

Moore TJ, Zhang H, Anderson G, Alexander GC. Estimated costs of pivotal trials for novel therapeutic agents approved by the US Food and Drug Administration, 2015-2016. JAMA Intern Med 2018;178(11):1451–7.

THE PRACTICAL USE OF HERBS FOR COMMON PRIMARY CARE CONDITIONS—THE GOOD, THE BAD, AND THE DRUGLESS

THE GOOD: ADVANTAGES OF HERBAL MEDICINE

Polychemistry: Just like the food you eat, medicinal herbs are chock-full of a variety of chemicals in varying but small quantities, whereas pharmaceuticals have varying milligrams to grams of a single chemical. The effects of an herb's numerous chemicals on the body are more like a little nudge here and there rather than a strong kick in the buttocks provided by a larger quantity of a single chemical. Sometimes the body truly needs a strong kick to set things right, but often a little nudging is both more effective and less likely to disrupt equilibrium or cause side effects.

Supporting the advantage of multiple chemicals in lower doses, recent medical research addresses the concept that small doses of multiple chemicals might be a better way to go. Take, for example, the study reported in *JAMA* in 2018 that showed patients taking an antihypertensive pill made up of low doses of three different antihypertensive agents achieved target blood pressures more readily than patients in the usual care group (Webster et al., 2018).

Multitude of prescriptive alternatives: Herbs can be applied through dozens of different formulations including crude herb preparations, extracts, concentrated extracts, standardized extracts, and distillations packaged in the form of liquids, oils, powders, capsules, tablets, lozenges, salves, suppositories, syrups, compresses, poultices, and other forms. A well-trained herbalist can skillfully navigate these options to select the most appropriate formulation for

a given patient to achieve optimal benefit. However, this advantage for herbalists is may be a confusing and overwhelming disadvantage for conventional healthcare providers who are the target audience of this book. To compound the confusion, depending on the guiding agency (e.g., *British Herbal Pharmacopeia* (BHP), *United States Pharmacopeia* (USP), or German Commission E), recommended dosing can vary widely. To ameliorate this challenge, the "Common Usage" section of each monograph attempts to familiarize the conventional medical provider with the common formulations for each herb, also redirecting to Part III "Introduction to the Monographs" where a less sophisticated but more practical approach to prescribing herbs is outlined.

Internal synergism: For many medicinal herbs, the whole is greater than the sum of the parts. This is because the chemical constituents in some herbs support each other through improved absorption or complementary activity. For example, Oregon grape root contains isoquinolone alkaloids such as berberine that have bactericidal activity. It also contains 5′-methoxyhydnocarpin (5′-MHC), an efflux pump inhibitor that prevents bacteria from exporting the alkaloids. Turmeric contains the essential oil turmerone, which enhances absorption of the chief constituent curcumin.

Internal compensation: While some chemicals in herbs can be a little problematic for a certain body part, often that same herb contains another chemical that buffers the effect of the first chemical. For example, meadowsweet contains salicylates that may be erosive to the stomach, but the mucilage portion of meadowsweet, through its demulcent activity, protects against and heals gastric ulcerations.

The entourage effect: Internal synergism and internal compensation, when applied to cannabis, are referred to as the *entourage effect*, whereby cannabis compounds other than THC act synergistically to modulate the overall psychoactive effects of the plant, mitigating the negative effects of THC.

Versatility: Because individual herbs contain tens to hundreds of different chemicals, they exert **pleiotropic effects** on the physiology of the patient. This can be useful when attempting to address more than one disorder, as is often the task with patients. Frequently, a single herb will achieve several desired effects in a patient. This versatility of herbs has the same multiuse advantage as using an ACE inhibitor in a patient with diabetes, high blood pressure, microalbuminuria, and heart failure. The disease tables in Part II of this book demonstrate the pleiotropic effects of each herb under the column "Scope of Potential Benefits."

Stability over time: Herbs generally have a good shelf life. Tinctures are particularly stable for years if kept in a UV-resistant (usually brown or blue) bottle. One example of stability comes from a sample of black cohosh collected in 1919 and recently identified in the collections of the New York Botanical Garden. It was analyzed and compared with the triterpene glycosidic and phenolic constituents of a modern collection of black cohosh. The two samples showed similarity in their constituents and both extracts showed similar antioxidant activity.

Basis for pharmaceutical research: The constituents in medicinal herbs provide infinite opportunities to find answers to some of medicine's more pressing needs. Antibiotic resistance, for example, may be addressed through plant constituent research. A group of researchers at Emory University performed a review of nearly 200 papers published between 2012 and 2019 that met strict standardization criteria for authenticating plant-derived compounds that significantly inhibited antibacterial activity. It found 459 compounds that met rigorous criteria for antibacterial activity. These compounds came from a diverse range of plant species. Roughly half of the compounds were phenolic derivatives, a quarter were terpenoids, and nearly

6% were alkaloids (https://www.sciencedaily.com/releases/2020/11/201111122846.htm).

THE BAD: DISADVANTAGES OF HERBAL MEDICINE

Frequent dosing: It is not unusual for medicinal herbs to require thrice-daily dosing due to the standard metabolism and excretion intervals of human physiology. If the herb is to have a sustained level in the body, frequent dosing is advised. However, herbs such as adaptogens are applied chronotherapeutically where their effect is exerted according to circadian rhythms, in which case once-daily dosing might be preferred.

Polychemistry: Herbal strength may also be herbal weakness. In seeking a desired outcome, it is important to consider the totality of effects that the various chemicals have on the physiological process and to avoid unintended consequences. Additionally, one must consider drug-herb and drug-drug interactions. A guideline for dealing with this polychemistry is as follows:

- If the patient has several underlying medical conditions, proceed with great caution.
- If the patient is on numerous pharmaceutical agents, herbs are best avoided due to exponentially increasing risk for interactions. But if the patient insists on adding medicinal herbs to his or her regimen, proceed with caution, informed consent, and an agreement by the patient to intensify his or her own monitoring for adverse effects.
- With cancer patients, unless in the hands of an integrative oncologist in an established research center, patients should not take herbs while on a chemotherapeutic regimen due to risks for increasing toxicity or decreasing efficacy of the chemotherapy.
- With HIV and hepatitis C patients, although numerous herbs show reductions of viral activity for these two viruses, the newer pharmaceuticals are highly effective. Providing a patient has access to them, the antiviral pharmaceuticals are preferable to the herbs. Additionally, as there are several medicinal herbs that alter the efficacy of the antiretroviral pharmaceuticals, vigilance is necessary for detecting interactions if using herbs for other issues in patients with HIV.

Multitude of prescriptive alternatives: (See above "The Good: Advantages of Herbal Medicine" section).

THE DRUGLESS: THINKING LIKE AN HERBALIST

Before diving into the nuts and bolts of using herbs in one's medical practice, it is important to understand some fundamental differences between conventional and herbal prescribing.

First, most herbalists use blends of herbs rather than single herb preparations. This practice helps maximize the desired effects while minimizing possible side effects from the noncontributory chemicals in a particular herb. Herbal blends can address the target symptom through multiple mechanisms similar to the practice of using lower doses of multiple drugs rather than high doses of a single drug to treat hypertension.

Second, under the Dietary Supplement Health and Education Act (DSHEA) (see DSHEA in Chapter 1), herbs may be labeled to support bodily processes, but cannot be labeled to treat specified medical conditions. Therefore, to replace diagnostic terms, an expanded vocabulary is needed to identify the physiological processes that herbs may address. The following terms have been around for eons before the *International Classification of Diseases* (ICD). They are not unique to herbalism, as these terms are presented in most pharmacology courses and many of them are familiar to the conventional medicine provider. For the sake of clarity and review, the more common herbal actions that will be mentioned in the Part III monographs include:

- Adaptogen: Helps the body physiologically respond to stress (physical and mental) by restoring and maintaining homeostatic mechanisms. Adaptogens are nontoxic metabolic regulators that nonspecifically increase the resistance of the organism through pleiotropic effects. Adaptogens have potential for broad applications in this highly driven and stressed-out society (For further discussion of the adaptogenic concept see Panossian et al., 2020)
- Alterative: Gradually restores a healthy body
- Bathmotropic: Modifies the degree of excitability of muscles (positive or negative bathmotrope)

- Bitter: One of numerous chemicals that stimulate digestive secretions and contribute to the herb's bitter taste
- Carminative: Relieves flatulence
- Cholagogue: Promotes the discharge of bile from the biliary system, enhancing gallbladder contractility
- Choleretic: Increases the volume of bile produced by the liver
- Chronotropic: Affects the heart rate (positive or negative chronotrope)
- Cicatrisant: Regenerates cells and heals wounds
- Cytophylactic: Stimulates the generation of new cells, which aid in preserving the health of the skin and healing burns
- Demulcent: Forms a protective and soothing film over a mucus membrane
- Depurative: Creates a purifying or detoxifying effect; a "blood cleanser"
- Dromotropic: Affects speed of conduction in the AV node (positive or negative dromotrope)
- Emunctory: An organ of secretion; includes skin, liver, kidneys, lungs, and intestine
- Eupeptic: Promotes good digestion
- Inotropic: Affects the contraction of the heart muscle (positive or negative inotrope)
- Nervine: Calms the nerves or has a beneficial effect on the nervous system; either a nervine relaxant, a nervine stimulant, or a nervine tonic
- Relaxant: Used in reference to both muscle relaxation and psychological relaxation
- Stimulant: Used in reference to both muscle stimulation and psychological stimulation
- Tonic: Herbs that help restore constitutional tone and vitality; not to be confused with tonic water, which is water with a low dose of quinine. An herbal tonic is typically a blend of herbs
- Vulnerary: Promotes the healing of wounds

REFERENCES

Panossian AG, et al. Evolution of the adaptogenic concept from traditional use to medical systems: pharmacology of stress- and aging-related diseases. Med Res Rev 2020;40(6):1–74.

Webster R, Abdul S, Asita de Silva H, et al. Fixed low-dose triple combination antihypertensive medication vs usual care for blood pressure control in patients with mild to moderate hypertension in Sri Lanka: a randomized clinical trial. JAMA 2018;320(6):566–79.

PART 2

Disease Tables
Introduction to the Disease Tables

The following tables are organized in a conventional disease-oriented format with two major divisions: organ-system diseases and systemic disorders. Several disorders or diseases are grouped together in a given table, based on organ groups, underlying pathophysiology, or frequent co-occurrence. For example, asthma and allergies are grouped together in a table. Diabetes, metabolic syndrome, and obesity are grouped together in a table. Premenstrual syndrome and premenstrual dysphoric disorder are in a table along with dysmenorrhea.

The herbs are identified in the first column of each table by both common names and Latin names, with the latter italicized. The herbs are organized to descend alphabetically according to their common names, as it is the common name that is used on herbal product labels and the name with which patients are most familiar. The Latin botanical name is included for clarity and specificity, as a common name may refer to several different species and Latin names may have been given several different common names. For example, bergamot the flower (*Monarda fistulosa*) is altogether a different plant than bergamot used in making the essential oil (*Citrus bergamia*). For patients outside the United States, the common names are completely different from those used in the United States.

The second column of the disease tables is labeled "Scope of Potential Benefits." This column is intended to be useful when a patient has more than one issue to address, as is often the case. This is where the pleiotropic effects of an herb, or "herbal versatility" (see Chapter 7) may be applied by selecting the herb that will best address more than one issue. Different fonts are utilized in this column to allow the reader at a quick glance to understand the level of evidence for each potential benefit. The potential benefits that are backed by systematic reviews are indicated by bold font, and those backed only by preclinical research are indicated by smaller italic font. Normal font indicates the activity is backed by clinical research.

The third column labeled "Comments" provides brief comments about the research or about special applications or precautions for the herb. On occasion an herb for which there is not an associated monograph will be included in a table due to strong evidence for benefit with the disease in question. When there is no associated monograph, the reference for the supporting research will be listed under the "Comments" column. The reader is invited to read the references and do further research (see Appendix II for resources) to determine appropriate precautions and dosing.

Section I

SYSTEM-BASED DISEASES

EENT NONINFECTIOUS DISORDERS

8

	TABLE 8.A	
	Ophthalmologic Disorders.	
Common Name/ Latin Name	**Scope of Potential Benefits**	**Comments**

Astragalus
*Astragalus
  membranaceus*
	Herpes keratitis, recurrent tonsillitis, allergic rhinitis, atopy,
	  asthma, **viral myocarditis**, CHF, CAD, viral hepatitis, **diabetic
	  nephropathy**, IgA nephropathy, nephrotic syndrome, lupus
	  nephritis, *renal fibrosis, sperm quality*, hemorrhagic stroke, burns,
	  wound healing, age spots, leukopenia, **immune function**, *antiviral*, HBV,
	  TB, **NSCLC**, cancer
		Human research: improves immune
		  imbalance in herpes keratitis, allergic
		  rhinitis; improves immune function in
		  recurrent tonsillitis

Bilberry
Vaccinium myrtillus
	Normal pressure glaucoma, cataracts, night vision, eye fatigue,
	  gingivitis, *HTN*, **dyslipidemia**, T2DM, NAFLD, ulcerative colitis,
	  AD, psoriasis, *wounds*, inflammation, *S. pneumonia, MRSA*,
	  colorectal cancer, *other cancers*
		Human research: reduces IOP; improves
		  visual field in glaucoma; prevents
		  cataract progression; may improve
		  night vision (conflicting); improves
		  eye fatigue

Coleus
Coleus forskohlii
	Glaucoma, *allergy*, asthma, HTN, CHF, *insulin resistance*, obesity,
	  *pancreatic exocrine insufficiency, diarrhea, UTI, urge incontinence,
	  dysmenorrhea, male infertility*, male hypogonadism, subarachnoid
	  hemorrhage, *seizure, neurodegenerative disorders, alcohol abuse,*
	  psoriasis, *photoprotection, hyperthyroidism, cancer*
		*Preclinical research: topical forskolin
		  reduces IOP*
		Human research: orally and topically
		  reduces IOP

Echinacea
*Echinacea
  purpurea,
  angustifolia*
	Anterior uveitis, *candida vaginitis*, genital condylomas, OA, **anxiety**,
	  eczema, athletic performance, immune function, inflammation,
	  URIs, influenza, *Coronavirus*, HPV, *colorectal cancer*
		Human research: reduces flares in
		  autoimmune idiopathic anterior
		  uveitis

Fennel
Foeniculum vulgare
	Glaucoma, dyspepsia, gastroprotection, gastroparesis, **infant colic**,
	  IBS, constipation, *overactive bladder, lactation*, dysmenorrhea,
	  oligomenorrhea, **menopausal disorders**, *dementia*, hirsutism,
	  inflammation
		*Preclinical research: fennel eye drops
		  decreased IOP 31% in rabbits*

Ginkgo
Ginkgo biloba
	Cataracts, ARMD, glaucoma, periodontal dz., **vertigo, tinnitus**,
	  cardiovascular health, dyslipidemia, diabetes, obesity,
	  claudication, hepatic fibrosis, **diabetic nephropathy**, menopausal
	  sexual desire, **acute mountain sickness**, migraines with aura,
	  stroke, MCI, dementias, post-operative delirium, depression,
	  ADHD, **schizophrenia, tardive dyskinesia**, aging skin,
	  inflammation, cancer
		*Preclinical research: delays progression of lens
		  opacification in cataract model*
		**Systematic review: benefits in ARMD
		  inconclusive**
		Human research: improves field damage
		  in glaucoma

Continued on following page

TABLE 8.A
Ophthalmologic Disorders. *(Continued)*

Common Name/ Latin Name	Scope of Potential Benefits	Comments
Ginseng, Asian/ Korean/ Chinese *Panax ginseng*	Dry eyes, **hearing loss**, **HTN**, CHF, **DM**, obesity, **menopause**, **ED**, male infertility, *osteoporosis*, AD, cognitive function, aging skin, alopecia areata, stamina, **chronic fatigue**, **hangover**, immune function, inflammation, influenza, HIV, **cancer**	Human research: reduces dry eyes from glaucoma meds
Goji berry/ wolfberry *Lycium barbarum*	Macular degeneration, *glaucoma*, dyslipidemia, **diabetes**, obesity, *hepatoprotection*, *male infertility*, *male sexual dysfunction*, stroke, AD, insomnia, anxiety, ADD, *dermatitis*, cognition, stress, fatigue, athletic performance, hangover, immunity function, influenza, cancer	*Preclinical research: prevents retinal macular degeneration and damage from glaucoma* Human research: prevents macular pathology
Saffron *Crocus sativus*	ARMD, *cataracts*, diabetic maculopathy, glaucoma, gingivitis, burning mouth syndrome, *allergy*, asthma, HTN, **dyslipidemia**, DM, **obesity**, *hepatotoxicity*, *DM nephropathy*, PMS, menopause, **female and male sexual dysfunction**, male infertility, chronic pain, fibromyalgia, stroke, AD, **anxiety**, insomnia, OCD, **depression**, ADHD, drug and ETOH addiction, *photodamage*, stamina, immune function, inflammation, RA, *bacterial infection*, cancer	*Preclinical research: protects retina and lens against UV* Human research: modestly improves ARMD; improves diabetic maculopathy; reduces IOP in primary open-angle glaucoma
Turmeric (or curcumin) *Curcuma longa*	Anterior uveitis, **oral lichen planus**, **gingivitis**, dental surgery, submucous fibrosis, asthma, **diastolic HTN**, **dyslipidemia**, CAD, endothelial dysfunction, **DM**, obesity, **NAFLD**, hepatoprotective, gallbladder dyskinesia, *GERD*, PUD, dyspepsia, **UC**, DM nephropathy, lupus nephritis, lactational mastitis, LSIL, chronic non-bacterial prostatitis, post-operative pain, **OA**, RA, migraine HA, *neurodegeneration*, **anxiety**, **depression**, **skin disease**, psoriasis, fatigue, **systemic inflammation**, *HIV*, **chemo-related oral mucositis**, cancer prevention, cancer treatment	Human research: reduces relapses in anterior uveitis; comparable response to corticosteroids

TABLE 8.B
Oral and Dental Disorders.

Common Name/ Latin Name	Scope of Potential Benefits	Comments
Aloe *Aloe vera*, *barbadensis*	**Gingivitis**, **submucous fibrosis**, **dyslipidemia**, **diabetes**, insulin resistance, hepatic fibrosis, GERD, **IBS**, IBD, anal fissures, radiation proctitis, AD, *PD*, acne, **psoriasis**, **lichen planus**, **burns**, wounds, pressure ulcers, diabetic foot ulcers, wrinkle and striae reduction, Hashimoto's thyroiditis, inflammation, HIV, cancer	**Systematic reviews and meta-analyses: beneficial for oral diseases**
Astragalus *Astragalus membranaceus*	Herpes keratitis, recurrent tonsillitis, allergic rhinitis, atopy, asthma, **viral myocarditis**, CHF, CAD, viral hepatitis, **diabetic nephropathy**, IgA nephropathy, nephrotic syndrome, lupus nephritis, *renal fibrosis*, *sperm quality*, hemorrhagic stroke, burns, *wound healing*, *age spots*, *leukopenia*, **immune function**, *antiviral*, HBV, TB, **NSCLC**, cancer	Human research: improves immune imbalance in herpes keratitis, allergic rhinitis; improves immune function in recurrent tonsillitis

TABLE 8.B
Oral and Dental Disorders. *(Continued)*

Common Name/ Latin Name	Scope of Potential Benefits	Comments
Bilberry *Vaccinium myrtillus*	Normal pressure glaucoma, cataracts, night vision, eye fatigue, gingivitis, *HTN*, **dyslipidemia**, T2DM, NAFLD, ulcerative colitis, *AD*, psoriasis, *wounds*, inflammation, *S. pneumonia*, *MRSA*, colorectal cancer, *other cancers*	Human research: improves gingivitis; prevents gingival hypertrophy
Black seed/ nigella/black cumin *Nigella sativa*	Periodontal dz., oral submucous fibrosis, chronic rhinosinusitis, nasal dryness, **allergy**, **asthma**, COPD, chemical pneumonitis, **HTN**, *CAD*, CHF, **dyslipidemia**, **DM**, **obesity**, NAFLD, dyspepsia, PUD, diabetic nephropathy, mastalgia, menopause, male infertility, OA, *stroke*, seizure disorder, memory impairment, cognition, anxiety, *depression*, acne, eczema, vitiligo, immune function, Hashimoto's thyroiditis, RA, inflammation, *H. pylori*, *Staph* pustules, HCV, cancer	Human research: thymoquinone gel improves periodontal dz.; reduces oral submucous fibrosis
Calendula *Calendula officinalis*	Gingivitis, dental plaque, radiation mucositis, venous ulcers, lactational cracked nipples, vaginal candidiasis, episiotomy healing, nonbacterial prostatitis, diaper dermatitis, **wound healing**, diabetic foot ulcers, *antibacterial*, *anti-HIV*, radiation dermatitis	Human research: oral rinse reduces gingivitis, dental plaque; attenuates radiation mucositis
Chamomile *Matricaria chamomilla/ recutita*	Gingivitis, mucositis, chronic rhinosinusitis, *allergies*, dyslipidemia, diabetes, *PUD*, colic, IBS, diarrhea, dyspepsia, UC, *candida vaginitis*, menopause, carpal tunnel syndrome, anxiety, insomnia, depression, ADHD, eczema, wounds, radiation or chemotherapy dermatitis, cortisol dysregulation, *inflammation, broadly antimicrobial (bacteria, yeast, fungus), cancer*	Human research: combination with pomegranate reduces gingival bleeding comparable to chlorhexidine; reduces mucositis
Cranberry *Vaccinium macrocarpon*	Gingivitis, dyslipidemia, **DM**, PUD, gut dysbiosis, overactive bladder, **UTI**, post-radiation UTI, BPH, chronic prostatitis, RA, *inflammation, influenza*, prostate CA	*Preclinical research: inhibits oral acid production, attachment, and biofilm formation by S. mutans; inhibits gingival inflammation* Human research: improves gingivitis; reduces *S. mutans*, comparable to chlorhexidine
Elder (berry, flower) *Sambucus nigra*	Gingival recession, ASCVD, *dyslipidemia*, *DM*, obesity, constipation, stroke, *immune function*, **URI**, rhinosinusitis, influenza, *HIV*, *HSV*, Strep, *cancer*	Human research: polyherbal patch plus rinse reduces gingival index and plaque index, increases gingival thickness
Frankincense/ Boswellia *Boswellia serrata, sacra, carterii*	Gingivitis, **asthma**, COPD, UC, **Crohn's**, **collagenous colitis**, IBS, UTI, SUI, benign breast disease, menorrhagia, **OA**, stroke, memory impairment, psoriasis, eczema, aging skin, athletic performance, **RA**, **IBD**, *inflammation*, glioma radiation, chemo-related neuropathy, *cancer*	Human research: comparable to and synergistic with scaling and root planing for gingivitis
Ginkgo *Ginkgo biloba*	*Cataracts*, ARMD, glaucoma, periodontal dz., **vertigo**, **tinnitus**, **cardiovascular health**, **dyslipidemia**, **diabetes**, obesity, claudication, hepatic fibrosis, **diabetic nephropathy**, menopausal sexual desire, **acute mountain sickness**, migraines with aura, **stroke**, **MCI**, **dementias**, post-operative delirium, depression, ADHD, **schizophrenia**, **tardive dyskinesia**, aging skin, *inflammation, cancer*	Human research: reduces periodontal pathogens comparably to minocycline

Continued on following page

	TABLE 8.B
	Oral and Dental Disorders. *(Continued)*

Common Name/ Latin Name	Scope of Potential Benefits	Comments
Gymnema/ Gurmar *Gymnema sylvestre*	*Dental caries*, dyslipidemia, T1DM, **T2DM**, obesity, *arthritis, immune function, cancer*	*Preclinical research: activity against cariogenic bacteria*
Holy basil/Tulsi *Ocimum tenuiflorum/ sanctum*	Gingivitis, asthma, *CAD*, **dyslipidemia**, **diabetes**, obesity, *hepatotoxicity, PUD, male hypogonadism, pain, seizures*, anxiety, depression, memory and concentration, stress and fatigue, immune function, viral encephalitis	Human research: improves gingivitis comparably to chlorhexidine
Hops/Hop *Humulus lupulus*	Dental plaque, allergic rhinitis, ASCVD, dyslipidemia, T2DM, obesity, *NAFLD, dyspepsia*, osteoporosis, OA, RA, atrophic vaginitis, menopause, cognitive decline, **insomnia**, anxiety, depression, cognitive performance, acne, aging skin, body odor, antibacterial, *TB, cancer*	*Preclinical research: reduces S. mutans; reduces oral lactic acid production* Human research: reduces *S. mutans* and plaque formation
Peppermint *Mentha × piperita*	Oral health, weight reduction, nausea, dyspepsia, **IBS**, GI endoscopy, cracked nipples, PCOS, neck pain, tension headaches, postherpetic neuralgia, cognition, nicotine withdrawal, pressure ulcers, pruritis gravidarum, hirsutism, athletic performance, URI, *cancer*	Human research: combination with aloe improves oral moisture, reduces plaque
Saffron *Crocus sativus*	ARMD, *cataracts*, diabetic maculopathy, glaucoma, gingivitis, burning mouth syndrome, *allergy*, asthma, HTN, **dyslipidemia**, DM, **obesity**, *hepatotoxicity, DM nephropathy*, PMS, menopause, **female and male sexual dysfunction**, male infertility, chronic pain, fibromyalgia, stroke, AD, **anxiety**, insomnia, OCD, **depression**, ADHD, drug and ETOH addiction, *photodamage*, stamina, immune function, inflammation, RA, *bacterial infection*, cancer	Human research: modestly improves gingivitis; improves burning mouth syndrome.
Turmeric (or curcumin) *Curcuma longa*	Anterior uveitis, **oral lichen planus**, **gingivitis**, dental surgery, submucous fibrosis, asthma, **diastolic HTN**, **dyslipidemia**, CAD, endothelial dysfunction, **DM**, obesity, **NAFLD**, hepatoprotective, gallbladder dyskinesia, *GERD*, PUD, dyspepsia, **UC**, DM nephropathy, lupus nephritis, lactational mastitis, LSIL, chronic non-bacterial prostatitis, post-operative pain, **OA**, RA, migraine HA, *neurodegeneration*, **anxiety**, **depression**, **skin disease**, psoriasis, fatigue, **systemic inflammation**, *HIV*, **chemo-related oral mucositis**, cancer prevention, cancer treatment	**Systematic review: beneficial for oral lichen planus, comparable to corticosteroids; beneficial for gingivitis, comparable to chlorhexidine** Human research: in dental surgery better than mefenamic acid for pain, comparable to ZOE and formocresol for endodontic response; improves submucous fibrosis; antimicrobial comparable to sodium hypochlorite

TABLE 8.C

Ears, Nose, and Throat Disorders (See Table 9.A for allergic disorders; Table 22.A for infectious ENT disorders.)

Common Name/ Latin Name	Scope of Potential Benefits	Comments
Astragalus *Astragalus membranaceus*	Herpes keratitis, recurrent tonsillitis, allergic rhinitis, atopy, asthma, **viral myocarditis**, CHF, CAD, viral hepatitis, **diabetic nephropathy**, IgA nephropathy, nephrotic syndrome, lupus nephritis, *renal fibrosis, sperm quality,* hemorrhagic stroke, burns, *wound healing, age spots, leukopenia,* **immune function**, *antiviral,* HBV, TB, **NSCLC**, cancer	Human research: improves immune imbalance in herpes keratitis, allergic rhinitis; improves immune function in recurrent tonsillitis
Black seed/ nigella/black cumin *Nigella sativa*	Periodontal dz., oral submucous fibrosis, chronic rhinosinusitis, nasal dryness, **allergy**, **asthma**, COPD, chemical pneumonitis, **HTN**, *CAD*, CHF, **dyslipidemia**, **DM**, **obesity**, NAFLD, dyspepsia, PUD, diabetic nephropathy, mastalgia, menopause, male infertility, OA, *stroke,* seizure disorder, memory impairment, cognition, anxiety, *depression,* acne, eczema, vitiligo, immune function, Hashimoto's thyroiditis, RA, inflammation, *H. pylori, Staph* pustules, HCV, cancer	Human research: nasal spray improves chronic rhinosinusitis, nasal dryness
Butterbur *Petasites hybridus*	**Allergic rhinitis**, asthma, *HTN, GI ulceration,* bladder spasms, **migraine headache**, *neurodegenerative dementias,* somatoform disorder anxiety and depression, *CNS inflammation*	Human research: reduces allergic rhinitis on par with non-sedating antihistamines
Chamomile *Matricaria chamomilla/ recutita*	Gingivitis, mucositis, chronic rhinosinusitis, *allergies,* dyslipidemia, diabetes, *PUD,* colic, IBS, diarrhea, dyspepsia, UC, *candida vaginitis,* menopause, carpal tunnel syndrome, anxiety, insomnia, depression, ADHD, eczema, wounds, radiation or chemotherapy dermatitis, cortisol dysregulation, *inflammation, broadly antimicrobial (bacteria, yeast, fungus), cancer*	Human research: nasal drops improve QOL and endoscopic findings in patients with chronic rhinosinusitis *CAUTION in atopic patients with ragweed or Compositae family allergies*
Ginger *Zingiber officinale*	**Motion sickness**, *HTN,* dyslipidemia, fibrinolysis, diabetes, **nausea**, **vomiting**, *dyspepsia,* gastroparesis, *PUD,* ulcerative colitis, *diabetic nephropathy,* **dysmenorrhea**, *Candida vaginitis,* male infertility, OA, muscle injury, migraine HA, *AD,* **inflammation**, RA, *H. pylori, antibacterial,* **CINV**, cancer	**Systematic review: beneficial for motion sickness** Human research: reduces motion sickness
Ginkgo *Ginkgo biloba*	*Cataracts,* ARMD, glaucoma, periodontal dz., **vertigo**, **tinnitus**, **cardiovascular health**, **dyslipidemia**, **diabetes**, obesity, claudication, hepatic fibrosis, **diabetic nephropathy**, menopausal sexual desire, **acute mountain sickness**, migraines with aura, **stroke**, **MCI**, **dementias**, post-operative delirium, depression, ADHD, **schizophrenia**, **tardive dyskinesia**, aging skin, *inflammation, cancer*	**Systematic review: improves tinnitus and dizziness in patients with dementia** Human research: reduces tinnitus comparably to pentoxifylline; reduces vertigo comparably to betahistine; improves vestibular neuritis with or without steroids
Ginseng, Asian/ Korean/ Chinese *Panax ginseng*	Dry eyes, **hearing loss**, **HTN**, CHF, **DM**, obesity, **menopause**, ED, male infertility, *osteoporosis,* AD, cognitive function, aging skin, alopecia areata, stamina, **chronic fatigue**, **hangover**, immune function, inflammation, influenza, HIV, **cancer**	**Systematic review: prevents sensorineural hearing loss at 4 kHz**
Horse Chestnut *Aesculus hippocastanum*	Hearing loss, *allergy,* **chronic venous insufficiency**, venous ulcers, varicocele-induced infertility, *hemorrhoids,* aging skin, *easy bruising; cancer*	Human research: improves hearing when combined with troxerutin
Lemon Balm *Melissa officinalis*	**Bruxism**, dyslipidemia, DM, palpitations, dyspepsia, IBS, **colic**, PMS, dysmenorrhea, female sexual dysfunction, **AD**, dementia, agitation, *diabetic neuropathy,* insomnia, **anxiety**, depression, **ADHD**, *hyperthyroidism, Graves' disease,* herpes simplex, *cancer, glioblastoma multiforme*	**Systematic review: reduces nocturnal bruxism in children** Human research: homeopathic preparation reduces bruxism in children

Continued on following page

TABLE 8.C

Ears, Nose, and Throat Disorders (See Table 9.A for allergic disorders; Table 22.A for infectious ENT disorders.) *(Continued)*

Common Name/ Latin Name	Scope of Potential Benefits	Comments
Licorice *Glycyrrhiza glabra*	**Postoperative sore throat**, xerostomia, radiation-induced mucositis, aphthous ulcers, *allergy*, **asthma**, **dyslipidemia**, *CAD*, *diabetes*, **obesity**, hepatoprotection, heartburn, PUD, functional dyspepsia, **antipsychotic-induced hyperprolactinemia**, **menopause**, atrophic vaginitis, PCOS, female hirsutism, BPH, *stroke*, *dementia*, PD, *anxiety*, *insomnia*, *depression*, *substance addiction*, **hyperpigmentation**, **atopic eczema**, Addison's disease, *stamina*, *multiple sclerosis*, *inflammation*, H. Pylori, cancer, *breast cancer*	**Systematic review: topically prevents postoperative sore throat** Human research: reduces postoperative sore throat (RR: 0.3); reduces xerostomia; reduces radiation-induced mucositis comparably to TAC; reduces aphthous ulcer pain and size *(**Caution: use deglycyrrhizinated formulations in patients at risk for HTN and hypokalemia**)*
Skullcap (American, Chinese) *Scutellaria lateriflora, baicalensis*	*Noise induced hearing loss*, allergy, *asthma*, *COPD*, *preterm RDS*, *pneumonia*, *PAH*, *CAD*, *dyslipidemia*, *DM*, *obesity*, *NAFLD*, *ETOH-induced gastritis*, *seizures*, *dementias*, **anxiety**, *depression*, *ADHD*, cognition, *photoprotection*, *autoimmunity*, *inflammation*, *MS*, *influenza*, *pneumonia*, *HIV*, cancer-related anemia, *cancer*	*Preclinical research: baicalin, baicalein, and Chinese skullcap reduce noise-induced hearing loss in mice*
Yarrow *Achillea millefolium*	*Epistaxis*, *asthma*, HTN, **dyslipidemia**, *T1DM*, cirrhosis, *gastritis*, *PUD*, *anorexia*, *IBS*, *IBD*, nipple fissures, candida vaginitis, dysmenorrhea, *menorrhagia*, *menopause*, *anxiety*, *neurodegenerative disorders*, multiple sclerosis, *inflammation*	*Preclinical research: anti-hemorrhagic* Traditional use to stop nose bleeds Human research: reduces bleeding propensity in patients with CKD

9

PULMONARY DISORDERS

	TABLE 9.A	
	Allergic Disorders and Asthma.	
Common Name/ Latin Name	**Scope of Potential Benefits**	**Comments**
Astragalus *Astragalus membranaceus*	Herpes keratitis, recurrent tonsillitis, allergic rhinitis, atopy, asthma, **viral myocarditis**, CHF, CAD, viral hepatitis, **diabetic nephropathy**, IgA nephropathy, nephrotic syndrome, lupus nephritis, *renal fibrosis, sperm quality,* hemorrhagic stroke, burns, *wound healing, age spots, leukopenia,* **immune function,** *antiviral,* HBV, TB, **NSCLC,** cancer	Human research: improves allergic rhinitis sx; balances Th1/Th2 (allergic aspect of asthma)
Black seed/ nigella/black cumin *Nigella sativa*	Periodontal dz., oral submucous fibrosis, chronic rhinosinusitis, nasal dryness, **allergy, asthma,** COPD, chemical pneumonitis, **HTN,** *CAD,* CHF, **dyslipidemia, DM, obesity,** NAFLD, dyspepsia, PUD, diabetic nephropathy, mastalgia, menopause, male infertility, OA, *stroke,* seizure disorder, memory impairment, cognition, anxiety, *depression,* acne, eczema, vitiligo, immune function, Hashimoto's thyroiditis, RA, inflammation, *H. pylori,* Staph pustules, HCV, cancer	*Preclinical research: antihistaminic, anti-asthma, bronchorelaxation comparable to theophylline* **Systematic review: beneficial for asthma** **Review: Beneficial for allergic diseases** Human research: improves asthma control, but less so than theophylline; reduces inflammation; reduces prn asthma med use; reduces nasal IgE and congestion in allergic rhinitis; augments immunotherapy
Butterbur *Petasites hybridus*	**Allergic rhinitis,** asthma, *HTN, GI ulceration,* bladder spasms, **migraine headache,** *neurodegenerative dementias,* somatoform disorder anxiety and depression, *CNS inflammation*	*Preclinical research: reduces airway inflammation* **Systematic review: May be effective for allergic rhinitis** Human research: reduces allergic rhinitis (on par with non-sedating antihistamines); reduces asthma activity
Coleus *Coleus forskohlii*	Glaucoma, *allergy,* asthma, HTN, CHF, *insulin resistance,* obesity, *pancreatic exocrine insufficiency, diarrhea, UTI, urge incontinence, dysmenorrhea, male infertility,* male hypogonadism, subarachnoid hemorrhage, *seizure, neurodegenerative disorders, alcohol abuse,* psoriasis, *photoprotection, hyperthyroidism, cancer*	*Preclinical research: reduces histamine, relaxes airway smooth muscle* Human research: inhaled form comparable to SABA; prophylaxis better than cromoglycate

Continued on following page

53

TABLE 9.A
Allergic Disorders and Asthma. *(Continued)*

Common Name/ Latin Name	Scope of Potential Benefits	Comments
Chamomile *Matricaria chamomilla/ recutita*	Gingivitis, mucositis, chronic rhinosinusitis, *allergies*, dyslipidemia, diabetes, *PUD*, colic, IBS, diarrhea, dyspepsia, UC, *candida vaginitis*, menopause, carpal tunnel syndrome, anxiety, insomnia, depression, ADHD, eczema, wounds, radiation or chemotherapy dermatitis, cortisol dysregulation, *inflammation, broadly antimicrobial (bacteria, yeast, fungus), cancer*	*Preclinical research: raises cortisol and lowers histamine release* *CAUTION in atopic patients with ragweed or Compositae family allergies*
Eleuthero/Siberian Ginseng *Eleutherococcus senticosus/ Acanthopanax senticosus*	*Allergic rhinitis*, dyslipidemia, CHF, edema, *male infertility*, osteoporosis, **stroke recovery**, *AD, insomnia*, **depression**, bipolar disorder, attention, vitality, athletic stamina, **hangover**, immune function, FMF, **URI**, *antiviral, ovarian cancer*	Human ex vivo: reduces nasal allergic and inflammatory response in combination with and additive to skullcap
Frankincense/Boswellia *Boswellia serrata, sacra, carterii*	Gingivitis, **asthma**, *COPD*, UC, **Crohn's, collagenous colitis**, IBS, UTI, SUI, benign breast disease, menorrhagia, **OA**, stroke, memory impairment, psoriasis, eczema, aging skin, athletic performance, **RA, IBD**, *inflammation*, glioma radiation, chemo-related neuropathy, *cancer*	**Systematic review: beneficial in asthma** Human research: improves all symptom parameters; additive benefit with inhaled LABA + ICS.
Gynostemma/Jiaogulan *Gynostemma pentaphyllum*	*Asthma, CAD,* dyslipidemia, DM, obesity, *arrhythmia,* NAFLD, *PUD,* PCOS, *PD, white matter disease,* dementia, *stamina,* immune function, cancer	*Preclinical research: reduced airway reactivity and eosinophil infiltration following challenge*
Holy basil/Tulsi *Ocimum tenuiflorum/ sanctum*	Gingivitis, asthma, *CAD,* **dyslipidemia, diabetes**, obesity, *hepatotoxicity, PUD, male hypogonadism, pain, seizures,* anxiety, depression, memory and concentration, stress and fatigue, immune function, viral encephalitis	Human research: improvement in asthma after 3 days
Hops/Hop *Humulus lupulus*	Dental plaque, allergic rhinitis, ASCVD, dyslipidemia, T2DM, obesity, *NAFLD, dyspepsia,* osteoporosis, OA, RA, atrophic vaginitis, menopause, cognitive decline, **insomnia**, anxiety, depression, cognitive performance, acne, aging skin, body odor, antibacterial, *TB, cancer*	Human research: water extract benefits Japanese cedar allergic rhinitis
Horse Chestnut *Aesculus hippocastanum*	Hearing loss, *allergy,* **chronic venous insufficiency**, venous ulcers, varicocele-induced infertility, *hemorrhoids,* aging skin, *easy bruising, cancer*	*Preclinical research: inhibits early and late phases of allergic response*
Licorice *Glycyrrhiza glabra*	**Postoperative sore throat**, xerostomia, radiation-induced mucositis, aphthous ulcers, *allergy,* **asthma, dyslipidemia**, *CAD,* diabetes, **obesity**, *hepatoprotection,* heartburn, PUD, functional dyspepsia, **antipsychotic-induced hyperprolactinemia, menopause**, atrophic vaginitis, PCOS, female hirsutism, BPH, *stroke, dementia, PD, anxiety, insomnia, depression, substance addiction,* **hyperpigmentation, atopic eczema**, Addison's disease, *stamina, multiple sclerosis, inflammation, H. pylori,* cancer, *breast cancer*	*Preclinical research: balances TH1/Th2, stabilizes mast cells, attenuates IgE production* **Systematic review: in combination formulas augments efficacy of asthma meds; beneficial for allergic eczema** Human research: improves asthma, better than frankincense *(Caution: use deglycyrrhizinated formulations in patients at risk for HTN and hypokalemia)*

TABLE 9.A
Allergic Disorders and Asthma. (Continued)

Common Name/ Latin Name	Scope of Potential Benefits	Comments
Passionflower *Passiflora incarnata* (*Passiflora edulis*)	*Asthma, diabetes,* **menopause**, OA (fruit peel), *seizure disorder,* **anxiety**, somatoform disorder, *depression,* insomnia, **ADHD**, opiate withdrawal	*Preclinical research: anti-asthmatic*
Saffron *Crocus sativus*	ARMD, *cataracts*, diabetic maculopathy, glaucoma, gingivitis, burning mouth syndrome, *allergy,* asthma, HTN, **dyslipidemia**, DM, **obesity**, *hepatotoxicity, DM nephropathy,* PMS, menopause, **female and male sexual dysfunction**, male infertility, chronic pain, fibromyalgia, stroke, AD, **anxiety**, insomnia, OCD, **depression**, ADHD, drug and ETOH addiction, *photodamage,* stamina, immune function, inflammation, RA, *bacterial infection,* cancer	*Preclinical research: reduces histamine and tracheal* *constriction* Human research: improves asthma symptoms and PFTs; reduces rescue med use and inflammation in asthma; reduces anti-HSP and hs-CRP
Skullcap (Chinese, American) *Scutellaria baicalensis,* *lateriflora*	*Noise-induced hearing loss,* allergy, *asthma,* COPD, *preterm RDS, pneumonia, PAH, CAD, dyslipidemia,* DM, obesity, NAFLD, ETOH-induced gastritis, *seizures, dementias,* **anxiety**, depression, *ADHD,* cognition, *photoprotection, autoimmunity,* *inflammation, MS, influenza, pneumonia, HIV,* cancer-related anemia, *cancer*	*Preclinical research: attenuates asthma; maternal* *administration improves fetal surfactant* Human ex vivo: reduces nasal allergic and inflammatory response in combination with eleuthero
Stinging Nettle *Urtica dioica*	Allergic rhinitis, HTN, dyslipidemia, **DM**, NAFLD, *colitis, nephrotoxicity,* menopause, **BPH**, prostatitis, OA, inflammation, *prostate cancer,* *cisplatin toxicity*	*Preclinical research: H-1 receptor reverse agonist* Human research: antihistaminic comparable to pharmaceutical antihistamines
Turmeric or curcumin *Curcuma longa*	Anterior uveitis, **oral lichen planus**, **gingivitis**, dental surgery, submucous fibrosis, asthma, **diastolic HTN**, **dyslipidemia**, CAD, endothelial dysfunction, **DM**, obesity, **NAFLD**, hepatoprotective, gallbladder dyskinesia, *GERD,* PUD, dyspepsia, **UC**, DM nephropathy, lupus nephritis, lactational mastitis, LSIL, chronic non-bacterial prostatitis, post-operative pain, **OA**, RA, migraine HA, *neurodegeneration,* **anxiety**, **depression**, **skin disease**, psoriasis, fatigue, **systemic inflammation**, *HIV,* **chemo-related** **oral mucositis**, cancer prevention, cancer treatment	Human research: in children with chronic persistent asthma, reduced disease severity, nocturnal awakenings, rescue medication
Umckaloabo/South African Geranium *Pelargonium sidoides*	Asthma, COPD, *PUD,* immune function, inflammation, **bronchitis**, **URI**, pharyngitis, rhinosinusitis, *influenza, Coronavirus, pneumonia,* *HIV, HSV 1&2, TB*	Human research: reduces infection-related asthma exacerbations
Yarrow *Achillea millefolium*	*Epistaxis, asthma,* HTN, **dyslipidemia**, *T1DM,* cirrhosis, *gastritis, PUD, anorexia, IBS, IBD,* nipple fissures, candida vaginitis, dysmenorrhea, *menorrhagia, menopause, anxiety, neurodegenerative* *disorders,* multiple sclerosis, *inflammation*	*Preclinical research: bronchodilating activity ex vivo*

TABLE 9.B

Chronic Obstructive Pulmonary Disease, Chronic Bronchitis, and Pulmonary Artery Hypertension.

Common Name/ Latin Name	Scope of Potential Benefits	Comments
Black seed/nigella/ black cumin *Nigella sativa*	Periodontal dz., oral submucous fibrosis, chronic rhinosinusitis, nasal dryness, **allergy**, **asthma**, COPD, chemical pneumonitis, **HTN**, *CAD*, CHF, **dyslipidemia**, **DM**, **obesity**, NAFLD, dyspepsia, PUD, diabetic nephropathy, mastalgia, menopause, male infertility, OA, *stroke*, seizure disorder, memory impairment, cognition, anxiety, *depression*, acne, eczema, vitiligo, immune function, Hashimoto's thyroiditis, RA, inflammation, *H. pylori*, *Staph* pustules, HCV, cancer	Human research: improves chemical war pneumonitis; improves PFTs in COPD with reduced inflammation and oxidation
Dang shen *Codonopsis pilosula*	**COPD**	Shergis et al. (2015)
Dong quai *Angelica sinensis*	Pulmonary HTN, *HTN*, CAD, *atrial fibrillation*, cirrhosis, portal HTN, abd pain, UC, *renal fibrosis, dysmenorrhea,* menopausal symptoms, *osteoporosis*, OA, stroke, *cerebrovascular insufficiency, neurodegenerative disorders, wound healing, aging skin, alopecia, stamina, inflammation,* anemia of chronic disease, cancer	Human research: reduces pulmonary artery pressure and pulmonary vascular resistance; augments nifedipine in pulmonary HTN
Frankincense/ Boswellia *Boswellia serrata, sacra, carterii*	Gingivitis, **asthma**, COPD, UC, **Crohn's**, **collagenous colitis**, IBS, UTI, SUI, benign breast disease, menorrhagia, **OA**, stroke, memory impairment, psoriasis, eczema, aging skin, athletic performance, **RA**, **IBD**, *inflammation*, glioma radiation, chemo-related neuropathy, *cancer*	*Preclinical research: blocks human leukocyte elastase (thereby reducing emphysema and cystic fibrosis lung damage)*
Skullcap (Chinese, American) *Scutellaria baicalensis, lateriflora*	*Noise induced hearing loss*, allergy, *asthma, COPD, preterm RDS, pneumonia, PAH, CAD, dyslipidemia, DM, obesity, NAFLD, ETOH-induced gastritis, seizures, dementias,* **anxiety**, depression, *ADHD*, cognition, *photoprotection, autoimmunity, inflammation, MS, influenza, pneumonia, HIV,* cancer-related anemia, *cancer*	*Preclinical research: prevents damage from tobacco smoke, reduces inflammation, prevents pulmonary artery smooth muscle cell proliferation*
Umckaloabo/South African Geranium *Pelargonium sidoides*	Asthma, COPD, *PUD*, immune function, inflammation, **bronchitis**, **URI**, pharyngitis, rhinosinusitis, *influenza, Coronavirus, pneumonia, HIV, HSV 1&2, TB*	Human research: reduces COPD exacerbations

REFERENCE

Shergis JL, Liu S, Chen X, et al. Dang shen [*Codonopsis pilosula* (Franch.) Nannf] herbal formulae for chronic obstructive pulmonary disease: a systematic review and meta-analysis. Phytother Res 2015;29(2):167–86.

10

CARDIOVASCULAR DISORDERS

| | **TABLE 10.A** | |
| | **Hypertension.** | |
Common Name/ **Latin Name**	**Scope of Potential Benefits**	**Comments**
Andrographis *Andrographis* *paniculata*	*HTN, hepatoprotection,* ulcerative colitis, *dysmenorrhea,* OA, RA, FMF, *inflammation,* **URI prevention and treatment**, *cancer*	*Preclinical research: hypotensive, smooth* *muscle relaxant through beta-blocking* *activity*
Bilberry *Vaccinium myrtillus*	Normal pressure glaucoma, cataracts, night vision, eye fatigue, gingivitis, *HTN,* **dyslipidemia**, T2DM, NAFLD, ulcerative colitis, AD, psoriasis, *wounds,* inflammation, *S. pneumonia, MRSA,* colorectal cancer, *other cancers*	*Preclinical research: ACE-I activity*
Black seed/ **nigella/black** **cumin** *Nigella sativa*	Periodontal dz, oral submucous fibrosis, chronic rhinosinusitis, nasal dryness, **allergy, asthma**, COPD, chemical pneumonitis, **HTN**, *CAD,* CHF, **dyslipidemia, DM, obesity**, NAFLD, dyspepsia, PUD, diabetic nephropathy, mastalgia, menopause, male infertility, OA, *stroke,* seizure disorder, memory impairment, cognition, anxiety, *depression,* acne, eczema, vitiligo, immune function, Hashimoto's thyroiditis, RA, inflammation, *H. pylori, Staph* pustules, HCV, cancer	*Preclinical research: diuretic, CCB* *properties; lowers BP, HR* **Systematic review: lowered SBP and** **DBP in 4 of 9 trials**
Butterbur *Petasites hybridus*	**Allergic rhinitis**, asthma, *HTN, GI ulceration,* bladder spasms, **migraine headache**, neurodegenerative dementias, somatoform disorder anxiety and depression, *CNS inflammation*	*Preclinical research: S-petasin shows* $Ca^{2}+$ *antagonism in vascular muscle;* *hypotensive in rats*
Coleus *Coleus forskohlii*	Glaucoma, *allergy,* asthma, HTN, CHF, *insulin resistance,* obesity, *pancreatic exocrine insufficiency, diarrhea, UTI, urge incontinence,* *dysmenorrhea, male infertility,* male hypogonadism, subarachnoid hemorrhage, *seizure, neurodegenerative disorders, alcohol abuse,* psoriasis, *photoprotection, hyperthyroidism, cancer*	Human research: mildly improves HTN in elderly
Dandelion *Taraxacum officinale*	HTN, dyslipidemia, DM, *obesity, edema,* liver toxicity, NAFLD, *gastroparesis,* dyspepsia, *neurodegenerative disorders, depression,* *stamina, inflammation, endotoxic shock, cancer*	*Preclinical research: potassium-sparing* *diuretic in vivo* Human research: increases urinary output

Continued on following page

TABLE 10.A
Hypertension. *(Continued)*

Common Name/ Latin Name	Scope of Potential Benefits	Comments
Dong quai *Angelica sinensis*	Pulmonary HTN, *HTN*, CAD, *atrial fibrillation*, cirrhosis, portal HTN, abd pain, UC, *renal fibrosis, dysmenorrhea*, menopausal symptoms, osteoporosis, OA, stroke, *cerebrovascular insufficiency, neurodegenerative disorders, wound healing, aging skin, alopecia, stamina, inflammation*, anemia of chronic disease, cancer	*Preclinical research: reduces blood pressure; reduces endothelin and angiotensin II*
Ginger *Zingiber officinale*	**Motion sickness**, *HTN*, dyslipidemia, fibrinolysis, diabetes, **nausea, vomiting**, *dyspepsia*, gastroparesis, *PUD*, ulcerative colitis, *diabetic nephropathy*, **dysmenorrhea**, *Candida vaginitis*, male infertility, OA, muscle injury, migraine HA, *AD*, **inflammation**, RA, *H. pylori*, antibacterial, **CINV**, cancer	*Preclinical research: hypotensive effects*
Ginseng, American *Panax quinquefolius*	HTN, dyslipidemia, DM, PVD, cognition, ADHD, schizophrenia, immune function, **URIs**, influenza, cancer	Human research: improves vascular elasticity, lowers SBP 12%
Ginseng, Asian/ Korean/Chinese *Panax ginseng*	Dry eyes, **hearing loss**, **HTN,** CHF, **DM**, obesity, **menopause**, ED, male infertility, *osteoporosis*, AD, cognitive function, aging skin, alopecia areata, stamina, **chronic fatigue**, **hangover,** immune function, inflammation, influenza, HIV, **cancer**	**Systematic review: KRG produces small reductions in SBP and DBP acutely and chronically** Human research (mixed): vasodilating, small reductions in SBP and DBP
Hawthorn *Crataegus* spp.	HTN, CAD, **CHF** (HrEF and HpEF), arrhythmia, **orthostatic hypotension**, *NAFLD*, anxiety, *inflammation*	*Preclinical research: negative chronotropic, vasodilating; ACE-inhibiting; improves endothelial function* Human research: decrease in diastolic BP; increase in nitric oxide; studies conflicting
Maca *Lepidium meyenii, peruvianum*	HTN, DM, weight reduction, perimenopause, **menopause**, **sexual dysfunction**, antidepressant-induced sexual dysfunction, **male sexual dysfunction**, **male infertility**, *BPH*, osteoporosis, *memory impairment*, anxiety, depression, fatigue, inflammation	Human research: lowers blood pressure while reducing depression in postmenopausal women; observational research shows reduced systolic BP
Motherwort *Leonurus cardiaca*	*HTN 2/2 anxiety or hyperthyroidism, dyslipidemia, CAD, arrhythmia, nausea, IBS, AKI, lactation, postpartum bleeding, menorrhagia, amenorrhea, menopause, pain, stroke, anxiety, insomnia, hyperthyroidism; inflammation; breast tumors*	*Preclinical research: lowers BP* Traditional use: especially with anxiety-induced or hyperthyroid-related HTN
Saffron *Crocus sativus*	ARMD, *cataracts*, diabetic maculopathy, glaucoma, gingivitis, burning mouth syndrome, *allergy*, asthma, HTN, **dyslipidemia**, DM, **obesity**, *hepatotoxicity, DM nephropathy*, PMS, menopause, **female and male sexual dysfunction**, male infertility, chronic pain, fibromyalgia, stroke, AD, **anxiety**, insomnia, OCD, **depression**, ADHD, drug and ETOH addiction, *photodamage*, stamina, immune function, inflammation, RA, *bacterial infection*, cancer	*Preclinical research: decreases peripheral resistance and BP* Human research: decreases SBP and DBP in asthma patients
Stinging Nettle *Urtica dioica*	Allergic rhinitis, HTN, dyslipidemia, **DM**, NAFLD, *colitis, nephrotoxicity*, menopause, **BPH**, prostatitis, OA, inflammation, *prostate cancer, cisplatin toxicity*	*Preclinical research: diuretic properties* Human research: reduces mild HTN
Tribulus/Puncture vine/Goathead *Tribulus terrestris*	HTN, CAD, dyslipidemia, DM, *hepatotoxicity, IBS, nephrolithiasis*, **sexual dysfunction,** hypoactive sexual desire, *pain, anxiety, depression, inflammation*, cancer	*Preclinical research: ACE-I and K+-sparing diuretic activity; lowers BP in rats* Human research: BP lowered by 18/9 mmHg

TABLE 10.A
Hypertension. *(Continued)*

Common Name/ Latin Name	Scope of Potential Benefits	Comments
Turmeric *Curcuma longa*	Anterior uveitis, **oral lichen planus, gingivitis,** dental surgery, submucous fibrosis, asthma, **diastolic HTN, dyslipidemia,** CAD, endothelial dysfunction, **DM,** obesity, **NAFLD,** hepatoprotective, gallbladder dyskinesia, *GERD,* PUD, dyspepsia, **UC,** DM nephropathy, lupus nephritis, lactational mastitis, LSIL, chronic nonbacterial prostatitis, postoperative pain, **OA,** RA, migraine HA, *neurodegeneration,* **anxiety, depression, skin disease,** psoriasis, fatigue, **systemic inflammation,** *HIV,* **chemo-related oral mucositis,** cancer prevention, cancer treatment	**Systematic review: reduces DBP in patients with metabolic syndrome**
Valerian *Valeriana officinalis*	*HTN, CAD, IBS,* PMS, dysmenorrhea, **menopause,** tension HA, RLS, cognitive, anxiety, insomnia, OCD, *cancer*	*Preclinical research: hypotensive via potassium channel activation*
Yarrow *Achillea millefolium*	*Epistaxis, asthma,* HTN, **dyslipidemia,** *T1DM,* cirrhosis, *gastritis, PUD, anorexia, IBS, IBD,* nipple fissures, candida vaginitis, dysmenorrhea, *menorrhagia, menopause, anxiety, neurodegenerative disorders,* multiple sclerosis, *inflammation*	*Preclinical research: demonstrates CCB and ACE-I properties; reduces SBP in normotensive mice* Human research: reduces SBP and DBP

TABLE 10.B
Atherosclerotic Cardiovascular Disease and Coronary Artery Disease/Ischemic Heart Disease.

Common Name/ Latin Name	Scope of Potential Benefits	Comments
Astragalus *Astragalus membranaceus*	Herpes keratitis, recurrent tonsillitis, allergic rhinitis, atopy, asthma, **viral myocarditis,** CHF, CAD, viral hepatitis, **diabetic nephropathy,** IgA nephropathy, nephrotic syndrome, lupus nephritis, *renal fibrosis, sperm quality,* hemorrhagic stroke, burns, *wound healing, age spots, leukopenia,* **immune function,** *antiviral,* HBV, TB, **NSCLC,** cancer	**Systematic review: positive benefit for viral myocarditis, but bias noted** Human research: protects against ischemia and reperfusion; improves recovery from viral myocarditis
Black seed/nigella/ black cumin *Nigella sativa*	Periodontal dz, oral submucous fibrosis, chronic rhinosinusitis, nasal dryness, **allergy, asthma,** COPD, chemical pneumonitis, **HTN,** *CAD,* CHF, **dyslipidemia, DM, obesity,** NAFLD, dyspepsia, PUD, diabetic nephropathy, mastalgia, menopause, male infertility, OA, *stroke,* seizure disorder, memory impairment, cognition, anxiety, *depression,* acne, eczema, vitiligo, immune function, Hashimoto's thyroiditis, RA, inflammation, *H. pylori, Staph* pustules, HCV, cancer	*Preclinical research: inhibits foam cells; protects against ischemia-reperfusion injury*
Dong quai *Angelica sinensis*	Pulmonary HTN, *HTN,* CAD, *atrial fibrillation,* cirrhosis, portal HTN, abd pain, UC, *renal fibrosis, dysmenorrhea,* menopausal symptoms, *osteoporosis, OA,* stroke, *cerebrovascular insufficiency, neurodegenerative disorders, wound healing, aging skin, alopecia, stamina, inflammation,* anemia of chronic disease, cancer	*Preclinical research: reduces ischemic myocardial injury; improves coronary artery flow; quinidine-like effect* Human research: in combination with astragalus and Korean ginseng reduces angina, normalizes ST-T, improves LV function; in combination with goji reduces adverse CV outcomes over 1 year

Continued on following page

TABLE 10.B

Atherosclerotic Cardiovascular Disease and Coronary Artery Disease/Ischemic Heart Disease. *(Continued)*

Common Name/ Latin Name	Scope of Potential Benefits	Comments
Elder (berry, flower) *Sambucus nigra*	Gingival recession, ASCVD, *dyslipidemia, DM*, obesity, constipation, stroke, *immune function*, **URI**, rhinosinusitis, influenza, *HIV, HSV, Strep, cancer*	*Preclinical research: endothelial antioxidant* Human research: polyherbal product decreases carotid intimal thickness
Gynostemma/ Jiaogulan *Gynostemma pentaphyllum*	*Asthma, CAD, dyslipidemia*, DM, obesity, *arrhythmia*, NAFLD, *PUD*, PCOS, *PD, white matter disease*, dementia, *stamina*, immune function, cancer	*Preclinical research: improves lipids; protective against coronary spasm and arrhythmia*
Hawthorn *Crataegus* spp.	HTN, CAD, **CHF** (HrEF and HpEF), arrhythmia, **orthostatic hypotension**, *NAFLD*, anxiety, *inflammation*	*Preclinical research: improves endothelial function, protects myocardium against ischemia and reperfusion* Human research: reduces endothelial inflammation; reduces lipids; decreases sudden cardiac death with CHF and EF ≥25%; noninferior to captopril; improves HFpEF and HFrEF
Holy basil/Tulsi *Ocimum tenuiflorum/ sanctum*	Gingivitis, asthma, *CAD*, **dyslipidemia**, **diabetes**, obesity, *hepatotoxicity, PUD, male hypogonadism, pain, seizures*, anxiety, depression, memory and concentration, stress and fatigue, immune function, viral encephalitis	*Preclinical research: cardioprotective in MI, lowers TC and lipid peroxidation*
Licorice *Glycyrrhiza glabra*	**Postoperative sore throat,** xerostomia, radiation-induced mucositis, aphthous ulcers, *allergy*, **asthma, dyslipidemia,** *CAD*, *diabetes*, **obesity,** hepatoprotection, heartburn, PUD, functional dyspepsia, **antipsychotic-induced hyperprolactinemia, menopause,** atrophic vaginitis, PCOS, female hirsutism, **BPH, stroke,** *dementia*, PD, *anxiety, insomnia, depression*, **substance addiction, hyperpigmentation, atopic eczema,** Addison's disease, *stamina, multiple sclerosis, inflammation, H. pylori*, cancer, *breast cancer*	*Preclinical research: reduces atherosclerotic area; protects against ischemia/reperfusion* Human research: reduces LDL oxidation ***(Caution: use deglycyrrhizinated formulations in patients at risk for HTN and hypokalemia)***
Motherwort *Leonurus cardiaca*	*HTN 2/2 anxiety or hyperthyroidism, dyslipidemia, CAD, arrhythmia, nausea, IBS, AKI, lactation, postpartum bleeding, menorrhagia, amenorrhea*, menopause, *pain*, stroke, anxiety, *insomnia, hyperthyroidism, inflammation, breast tumors*	*Preclinical research: slows atherosclerotic progression; antiplatelet; cardioprotective against ischemia; vasorelaxant; decreases lipid peroxidation* Human research: decreases blood viscosity and fibrinogen volume
Rhodiola *Rhodiola rosea*	**CAD,** *menorrhagia, amenorrhea, female infertility*, menopause, *male hypogonadism*, premature ejaculation, **anxiety, depression, cognition,** eczema, burnout, fatigue, **athletic stamina,** cancer	*Preclinical research: reduces reperfusion arrhythmias via beta endorphin and enkephalin increase and blunting of catecholamines; reduces CRP* **Systematic reviews: beneficial alone or with conventional treatment for IHD and chronic stable angina**
Schisandra *Schisandra chinensis*	*CAD*, **CHF**, DM, NAFLD, viral hepatitis, menopause, FMF, *stroke, AD, anxiety*, cognition, physical stress, stamina, pneumonia, *HCV, fungal infections*, cancer	*Preclinical research: protects post-MI myocardium via NOS*
Skullcap (Chinese, American) *Scutellaria baicalensis, lateriflora*	*Noise-induced hearing loss*, allergy, *asthma, COPD, preterm RDS, pneumonia, PAH, CAD, dyslipidemia, DM, obesity, NAFLD, ETOH-induced gastritis, seizures, dementias,* **anxiety,** depression, *ADHD*, cognition, *photoprotection, autoimmunity, inflammation, MS, influenza, pneumonia, HIV*, cancer-related anemia, *cancer*	*Preclinical research: Chinese skullcap reduces myocardial infarct size*

TABLE 10.B
Atherosclerotic Cardiovascular Disease and Coronary Artery Disease/Ischemic Heart Disease. *(Continued)*

Common Name/ Latin Name	Scope of Potential Benefits	Comments
Tribulus/Puncture vine/Goathead *Tribulus terrestris*	HTN, CAD, dyslipidemia, DM, *hepatotoxicity, IBS, nephrolithiasis,* **sexual dysfunction,** hypoactive sexual desire, *pain, anxiety, depression, inflammation, cancer*	*Preclinical research: cardioprotective against ischemia, dilates coronary arteries, stabilizes endothelium* Human research: remits angina
Turmeric (or curcumin) *Curcuma longa*	Anterior uveitis, **oral lichen planus, gingivitis,** dental surgery, submucous fibrosis, asthma, **diastolic HTN, dyslipidemia,** CAD, endothelial dysfunction, **DM,** obesity, **NAFLD,** hepatoprotective, gallbladder dyskinesia, *GERD,* PUD, dyspepsia, **UC,** DM nephropathy, lupus nephritis, lactational mastitis, LSIL, chronic nonbacterial prostatitis, postoperative pain, **OA,** RA, migraine HA, *neurodegeneration,* **anxiety, depression, skin disease,** psoriasis, fatigue, **systemic inflammation,** *HIV,* **chemo-related oral mucositis,** cancer prevention, cancer treatment	Human research: improves endothelial function; reduces post-CABG MI incidence
Valerian *Valeriana officinalis*	*HTN, CAD, IBS,* PMS, dysmenorrhea, **menopause,** tension HA, RLS, cognitive, anxiety, insomnia, OCD, *cancer*	*Preclinical research: protective effect against vasopressin-induced coronary spasm and pressor response*

TABLE 10.C
Congestive Heart Failure.

Common Name/ Latin Name	Scope of Potential Benefits	Comments
Astragalus *Astragalus membranaceus*	Herpes keratitis, recurrent tonsillitis, allergic rhinitis, atopy, asthma, **viral myocarditis,** CHF, CAD, viral hepatitis, **diabetic nephropathy,** IgA nephropathy, nephrotic syndrome, lupus nephritis, *renal fibrosis, sperm quality,* hemorrhagic stroke, burns, *wound healing, age spots, leukopenia,* **immune function,** *antiviral,* HBV, TB, **NSCLC,** cancer	**Systematic review: positive benefit for viral myocarditis, but bias noted** Human research: improves LV function, protects against ischemia and reperfusion; improves recovery from viral myocarditis
Black seed/nigella/ black cumin *Nigella sativa*	Periodontal dz, oral submucous fibrosis, chronic rhinosinusitis, nasal dryness, **allergy, asthma,** COPD, chemical pneumonitis, **HTN,** *CAD,* CHF, **dyslipidemia, DM, obesity,** NAFLD, dyspepsia, PUD, diabetic nephropathy, mastalgia, menopause, male infertility, OA, *stroke,* seizure disorder, memory impairment, cognition, anxiety, *depression,* acne, eczema, vitiligo, immune function, Hashimoto's thyroiditis, RA, inflammation, *H. pylori, Staph* pustules, HCV, cancer	Human research: reduces diastolic and systolic dysfunction in DM patients
Coleus *Coleus forskohlii*	Glaucoma, *allergy,* asthma, HTN, CHF, *insulin resistance,* obesity, *pancreatic exocrine insufficiency, diarrhea, UTI, urge incontinence, dysmenorrhea, male infertility,* male hypogonadism, subarachnoid hemorrhage, *seizure, neurodegenerative disorders, alcohol abuse,* psoriasis, *photoprotection, hyperthyroidism, cancer*	*Preclinical research: vasodilates myocardium, increases myocardial contractility* Human research: reduces preload and afterload; reduces PCWP; increases stroke volume

Continued on following page

TABLE 10.C

Congestive Heart Failure. *(Continued)*

Common Name/ Latin Name	Scope of Potential Benefits	Comments
Eleuthero/Siberian Ginseng *Eleutherococcus senticosus/ Acanthopanax senticosus*	*Allergic rhinitis*, dyslipidemia, CHF, edema, *male infertility*, osteoporosis, **stroke recovery**, *AD*, *insomnia*, **depression**, bipolar disorder, attention, vitality, athletic stamina, **hangover,** immune function, FMF, **URI,** *antiviral*, ovarian cancer	Human research: improves feeling of well-being in elderly with CHF
Ginseng, Asian/ Korean/Chinese *Panax ginseng*	Dry eyes, **hearing loss**, **HTN,** CHF, **DM**, obesity, **menopause, ED**, male infertility, *osteoporosis*, AD, cognitive function, aging skin, alopecia areata, stamina, **chronic fatigue**, **hangover,** immune function, inflammation, influenza, HIV, **cancer**	Human research: improves CHF alone or additive with digoxin; comparable to digoxin
Hawthorn *Crataegus* spp.	HTN, CAD, **CHF** (HrEF and HpEF), arrhythmia, **orthostatic hypotension**, *NAFLD*, anxiety, *inflammation*	**Systematic reviews: beneficial in CHF** Human research: decreases sudden cardiac death with CHF and EF ≥ 25%; noninferior to captopril; improves HFpEF and HFrEF
Schisandra *Schisandra chinensis*	*MI*, **CHF**, DM, NAFLD, viral hepatitis, menopause, FMF, *stroke*, *AD*, *anxiety*, cognition, physical stress, stamina, pneumonia, *HCV*, *fungal infections*, cancer	**Systematic review: in TCM polyherbal formula, improves NYHA classification, myocardial performance**

TABLE 10.D

Arrhythmia and Palpitation.

Common Name/Latin Name	Scope of Potential Benefits	Comments
Dong quai *Angelica sinensis*	Pulmonary HTN, *HTN*, CAD, *atrial fibrillation*, cirrhosis, portal HTN, abd pain, UC, *renal fibrosis*, *dysmenorrhea*, menopausal symptoms, *osteoporosis*, *OA*, stroke, *cerebrovascular insufficiency*, *neurodegenerative disorders*, *wound healing*, *aging skin*, *alopecia*, *stamina*, *inflammation*, anemia of chronic disease, cancer	*Preclinical research: prevents a-fib (quinidine-like)*
Gynostemma/Jiaogulan *Gynostemma pentaphyllum*	*Asthma*, *CAD*, dyslipidemia, DM, obesity, *arrhythmia*, NAFLD, *PUD*, PCOS, *PD*, *white matter disease*, dementia, *stamina*, immune function, cancer	*Preclinical research: protective against arrhythmia*
Hawthorn *Crataegus* spp.	HTN, CAD, **CHF** (HrEF and HpEF), arrhythmia, **orthostatic hypotension**, *NAFLD*, anxiety, *inflammation*	*Preclinical research: antiarrhythmic* Human research: reduces arrhythmias
Lemon balm *Melissa officinalis*	**Bruxism**, dyslipidemia, DM, palpitations, dyspepsia, IBS, **colic**, PMS, dysmenorrhea, female sexual dysfunction, **AD,** dementia, agitation, *diabetic neuropathy*, insomnia, **anxiety**, depression, **ADHD,** *hyperthyroidism*, *Graves' disease*, herpes simplex, *cancer*, *glioblastoma multiforme*	Human research: reduces benign palpitations
Motherwort *Leonurus cardiaca*	HTN 2/2 anxiety or hyperthyroidism, dyslipidemia, CAD, *arrhythmia*, *nausea*, *IBS*, *AKI*, *lactation*, *postpartum bleeding*, *menorrhagia*, *amenorrhea*, menopause, *pain*, stroke, anxiety, *insomnia*, hyperthyroidism; *inflammation*; breast tumors	*Preclinical research: antiarrhythmic, negative chronotropic activity* Traditional use: arrhythmia, palpitations with hyperthyroidism

TABLE 10.E
Vascular Disorders: Arterial insufficiency, Endothelial Dysfunction, Venous Insufficiency, Varicose Veins, Hemorrhoids and Peripheral Edema.

Common Name/ Latin Name	Scope of Potential Benefits	Comments
Calendula *Calendula officinalis*	Gingivitis, dental plaque, radiation mucositis, venous ulcers, lactational cracked nipples, vaginal candidiasis, episiotomy healing, nonbacterial prostatitis, diaper dermatitis, **wound healing**, diabetic foot ulcers, *antibacterial, anti-HIV*, radiation dermatitis	Human research: heals venous ulcers
Dandelion *Taraxacum officinale*	HTN, dyslipidemia, *DM, obesity, edema,* liver toxicity, NAFLD, *gastroparesis,* dyspepsia, *neurodegenerative disorders, depression, stamina, inflammation, endotoxic shock, cancer*	Human research: leaf extract has diuretic effect
Eleuthero/Siberian Ginseng *Eleutherococcus senticosus/ Acanthopanax senticosus*	*Allergic rhinitis,* dyslipidemia, CHF, edema, *male infertility,* osteoporosis, **stroke recovery**, *AD, insomnia,* **depression**, bipolar disorder, attention, vitality, athletic stamina, **hangover,** immune function, FMF, **URI**, *antiviral,* ovarian cancer	Human research: reduces leg edema via stabilization of lymphatic endothelial cells
Ginkgo *Ginkgo biloba*	*Cataracts,* ARMD, glaucoma, periodontal dz, **vertigo, tinnitus, cardiovascular health, dyslipidemia, diabetes,** obesity, claudication, hepatic fibrosis, **diabetic nephropathy,** menopausal sexual desire, **acute mountain sickness,** migraines with aura, **stroke, MCI, dementias,** postoperative delirium, depression, ADHD, **schizophrenia, tardive dyskinesia,** aging skin, *inflammation, cancer*	Human research: small improvements in walking distance in claudication
Ginseng, American *Panax quinquefolius*	HTN, dyslipidemia, DM, PVD, cognition, ADHD, schizophrenia, immune function, **URIs**, influenza, cancer	Human research: reduces vascular stiffness by 5%
Gotu kola *Centella asiatica*	**Chronic Venous Insufficiency**	Chong et al. (2013)
Hawthorn *Crataegus* spp.	HTN, CAD, **CHF** (HrEF and HpEF), arrhythmia, **orthostatic hypotension,** *NAFLD,* anxiety, *inflammation*	*Preclinical research: flavonoids improve integrity of blood vessels* **Systematic review: fixed combination formula with camphor improves hypotension** Human research: reduces endothelial inflammation
Horse Chestnut *Aesculus hippocastanum*	Hearing loss, *allergy,* **chronic venous insufficiency**, venous ulcers, varicocele-induced infertility, *hemorrhoids,* aging skin, *easy bruising; cancer*	**Systematic reviews: improves leg pain, edema, itching in CVI** Human research: improves capillary fragility; reduces wound care costs Traditional use: hemorrhoids

Continued on following page

TABLE 10.E

Vascular Disorders: Arterial insufficiency, Endothelial Dysfunction, Venous Insufficiency, Varicose Veins, Hemorrhoids and Peripheral Edema. *(Continued)*

Common Name/ Latin Name	Scope of Potential Benefits	Comments
Turmeric (or curcumin) *Curcuma longa*	Anterior uveitis, **oral lichen planus, gingivitis,** dental surgery, submucous fibrosis, asthma, **diastolic HTN, dyslipidemia,** CAD, endothelial dysfunction, **DM,** obesity, **NAFLD,** hepatoprotective, gallbladder dyskinesia, *GERD,* PUD, dyspepsia, **UC,** DM nephropathy, lupus nephritis, lactational mastitis, LSIL, chronic nonbacterial prostatitis, postoperative pain, **OA,** RA, migraine HA, *neurodegeneration,* **anxiety, depression, skin disease,** psoriasis, fatigue, **systemic inflammation,** *HIV,* **chemo-related oral mucositis,** cancer prevention, cancer treatment	Human research: improves endothelial function in several studies

TABLE 10.F

Cardiometabolic Disorders: Hyperlipidemia and Dyslipidemia.

Common Name/ Latin Name	Scope of Potential Benefits	Comments
Aloe *Aloe vera, barbadensis*	**Gingivitis, submucous fibrosis, dyslipidemia, diabetes,** insulin resistance, hepatic fibrosis, GERD, **IBS,** IBD, anal fissures, radiation proctitis, AD, *PD,* acne, **psoriasis, lichen planus, burns,** wounds, pressure ulcers, diabetic foot ulcers, wrinkle and striae reduction, Hashimoto's thyroiditis, inflammation, HIV, cancer	**Systematic review: beneficial for all lipids** Human research: normalizes lipids
Ashwagandha *Withania somnifera*	Dyslipidemia, DM, **sexual dysfunction, infertility,** *osteoporosis,* gout, OA, *AD, PD,* MCI, **anxiety,** insomnia, OCD, *depression,* schizophrenia, hypothyroidism, stress, endurance, *fatigue,* immune function, TB, *cancer*	Human research: one small trial reduced BG and normalized lipids
Bilberry *Vaccinium myrtillus*	Normal pressure glaucoma, cataracts, night vision, eye fatigue, gingivitis, *HTN,* **dyslipidemia,** T2DM, NAFLD, ulcerative colitis, *AD,* psoriasis, *wounds,* inflammation, *S. pneumonia, MRSA,* colorectal cancer, *other cancers*	**Systematic review: beneficial for LDL-C and HDL-C** Human research: improves lipids, enhances cellular cholesterol efflux; lowers hs-CRP and other inflammatory markers
Black seed/nigella/ black cumin *Nigella sativa*	Periodontal dz, oral submucous fibrosis, chronic rhinosinusitis, nasal dryness, **allergy, asthma,** COPD, chemical pneumonitis, **HTN,** *CAD,* CHF, **dyslipidemia, DM, obesity,** NAFLD, dyspepsia, PUD, diabetic nephropathy, mastalgia, menopause, male infertility, OA, *stroke,* seizure disorder, memory impairment, cognition, anxiety, *depression,* acne, eczema, vitiligo, immune function, Hashimoto's thyroiditis, RA, inflammation, *H. pylori, Staph* pustules, HCV, cancer	*Preclinical research: inhibits foam cells* Human research: Normalizes lipids esp. at 2 g/day; reduces TNF-α and hs-CRP
Burdock *Arctium lappa*	*Dyslipidemia,* diabetes, *hepatic function and protection, gastroparesis, dyspepsia,* diverticulitis, diabetic nephropathy, OA, wrinkles, acne, cough, *inflammation, influenza A, cancer*	*Preclinical research: normalizes lipids in diabetic mice*

TABLE 10.F

Cardiometabolic Disorders: Hyperlipidemia and Dyslipidemia. *(Continued)*

Common Name/ Latin Name	Scope of Potential Benefits	Comments
Cranberry *Vaccinium macrocarpon*	Gingivitis, dyslipidemia, **DM**, PUD, gut dysbiosis, overactive bladder, **UTI**, postradiation UTI, BPH, chronic prostatitis, RA, *inflammation, influenza,* prostate CA	*Preclinical research: blocks LPS-induced inflammation* Human research: increases HDL, decreases oxidized LDL
Dandelion *Taraxacum officinale*	HTN, dyslipidemia, DM, *obesity, edema,* liver toxicity, NAFLD, *gastroparesis,* dyspepsia, *neurodegenerative disorders, depression, stamina, inflammation, endotoxic shock, cancer*	*Preclinical research: leaf extract lowers TC, TGs* Human research: small reduction in TC, LDL-C, and TG
Chamomile *Matricaria chamomilla/ recutita*	Gingivitis, mucositis, chronic rhinosinusitis, *allergies,* dyslipidemia, diabetes, *PUD,* colic, IBS, diarrhea, dyspepsia, UC, *candida vaginitis,* menopause, carpal tunnel syndrome, anxiety, insomnia, depression, ADHD, eczema, wounds, radiation or chemotherapy dermatitis, cortisol dysregulation, *inflammation, broadly antimicrobial (bacteria, yeast, fungus), cancer*	Human research: lowers TC, LDL-C, and TG
Elder (berry, flower) *Sambucus nigra*	Gingival recession, ASCVD, *dyslipidemia, DM,* obesity, constipation, stroke, *immune function,* **URI**, rhinosinusitis, influenza, *HIV, HSV, Strep, cancer*	*Preclinical research: endothelial antioxidant; decreases TC, LDL-C, and TG* Human research: multiberry drink decreases lipids
Eleuthero/Siberian Ginseng *Eleutherococcus senticosus/ Acanthopanax senticosus*	*Allergic rhinitis,* dyslipidemia, CHF, edema, *male infertility,* osteoporosis, **stroke recovery**, *AD, insomnia,* **depression**, bipolar disorder, attention, vitality, athletic stamina, **hangover**, immune function, FMF, **URI**, *antiviral,* ovarian cancer	Human research: reduces LDL/HDL and lipid peroxidation
Fenugreek *Trigonella foenum-graecum*	Dyslipidemia, **DM**, prediabetes, *diabetic nephropathy, urolithiasis,* lactation, dysmenorrhea, PCOS, menopause, male sexual dysfunction, hypogonadism, PD, *peripheral neuropathy, thyroid T3/T4 balance,* stamina, cancer	*Preclinical research: hypolipidemic, antioxidant* Human research: lowers TC, LDL-C, and TGs
Ginger *Zingiber officinale*	**Motion sickness**, *HTN,* dyslipidemia, fibrinolysis, diabetes, **nausea, vomiting**, *dyspepsia,* gastroparesis, PUD, ulcerative colitis, *diabetic nephropathy,* **dysmenorrhea**, *Candida vaginitis,* male infertility, OA, muscle injury, migraine HA, *AD,* **inflammation**, RA, *H. pylori, antibacterial,* **CINV**, cancer	Human research: improves lipid profile (conflicting); increases fibrinolytic activity
Ginkgo *Ginkgo biloba*	*Cataracts,* ARMD, glaucoma, periodontal dz, **vertigo, tinnitus, cardiovascular health, dyslipidemia, diabetes**, obesity, claudication, hepatic fibrosis, **diabetic nephropathy**, menopausal sexual desire, **acute mountain sickness**, migraines with aura, **stroke, MCI, dementias**, postoperative delirium, depression, ADHD, **schizophrenia, tardive dyskinesia**, aging skin, *inflammation, cancer*	**Systematic reviews: additive to statin for lipids** Human research: augments statin effects
Ginseng, American *Panax quinquefolius*	HTN, dyslipidemia, DM, PVD, cognition, ADHD, schizophrenia, immune function, **URIs**, influenza, cancer	Human research: lowers TC in DM patients with CAD

Continued on following page

TABLE 10.F
Cardiometabolic Disorders: Hyperlipidemia and Dyslipidemia. *(Continued)*

Common Name/ Latin Name	Scope of Potential Benefits	Comments
Goji berry/ wolfberry *Lycium barbarum*	Macular degeneration, *glaucoma*, dyslipidemia, **diabetes**, obesity, *hepatoprotection, male infertility, male sexual dysfunction, stroke, AD,* insomnia, anxiety, ADD, *dermatitis,* cognition, stress, fatigue, athletic performance, hangover, immunity function, influenza, cancer	**Systematic review: beneficial for blood glucose, marginally improves TC and TG** Human research: raises HDL-C, reduces blood glucose; reduces lipid peroxidation
Gymnema/Gurmar *Gymnema sylvestre*	*Dental caries,* dyslipidemia, T1DM, **T2DM**, obesity, *arthritis, immune function, cancer*	*Preclinical research: reduces lipid peroxidation* Human research: normalizes lipids across the board
Gynostemma/ Jiaogulan *Gynostemma pentaphyllum*	*Asthma, CAD,* dyslipidemia, *DM,* obesity, *arrhythmia,* NAFLD, *PUD, PCOS, PD, white matter disease,* dementia, *stamina,* immune function, cancer	*Preclinical research: improves lipids*
Holy basil/Tulsi *Ocimum tenuiflorum/ sanctum*	Gingivitis, asthma, *CAD,* **dyslipidemia**, **diabetes**, obesity, *hepatotoxicity, PUD, male hypogonadism, pain, seizures,* anxiety, depression, memory and concentration, stress and fatigue, immune function, viral encephalitis	*Preclinical research: lowers TC and lipid peroxidation* **Systematic review: beneficial effect on lipids** Human research: normalizes lipids in overweight individuals
Hops/Hop *Humulus lupulus*	Dental plaque, allergic rhinitis, ASCVD, dyslipidemia, T2DM, obesity, *NAFLD, dyspepsia,* osteoporosis, OA, RA, atrophic vaginitis, menopause, cognitive decline, **insomnia**, anxiety, depression, cognitive performance, acne, aging skin, body odor, antibacterial, *TB,* cancer	Human research: improves lipids
Lemon balm *Melissa officinalis*	**Bruxism**, dyslipidemia, DM, palpitations, dyspepsia, IBS, **colic**, PMS, dysmenorrhea, female sexual dysfunction, **AD**, dementia, agitation, *diabetic neuropathy,* insomnia, **anxiety**, depression, **ADHD**, hyperthyroidism, *Graves' disease,* herpes simplex, *cancer, glioblastoma multiforme*	Human research: lowers TGs and BP in DM; Lowers AST, LDL/HDL, LDL-C, MDA, hs-CRP; raises ApoA-1, HDL, paraoxonase; reduces vascular glycation
Licorice *Glycyrrhiza glabra*	**Postoperative sore throat**, xerostomia, radiation-induced mucositis, aphthous ulcers, *allergy,* **asthma, dyslipidemia**, *CAD,* diabetes, **obesity**, hepatoprotection, heartburn, PUD, functional dyspepsia, **antipsychotic-induced hyperprolactinemia, menopause,** atrophic vaginitis, PCOS, female hirsutism, BPH, *stroke, dementia, PD, anxiety, insomnia, depression,* substance addiction, **hyperpigmentation, atopic eczema,** Addison's disease, *stamina,* multiple sclerosis, inflammation, H. Pylori, cancer, *breast cancer*	**Systematic review: lowers TC and LDL-C** Human research: reduces LDL oxidation *(Caution: use deglycyrrhizinated formulations in patients at risk for HTN and hypokalemia)*
Milk thistle *Silybum marianum*	**Dyslipidemia, DM, liver disease**, diabetic nephropathy, lactation, *PCOS,* BPH, *gout, AD, diabetic neuropathy,* **OCD**, acne, *psoriasis,* vitiligo, radio-dermatitis, aging skin, RA, inflammation, hepatitis viruses, **iron-overload**, chemotherapy and radiotherapy toxicity, *hepatocellular carcinoma*	*Preclinical research: decreases TC, increases HDL-C* **Systematic review: one of several TCM herbs that decreases TC and LDL-C** Human research: decreases TC, LDL-C, and TG, increases HDL-C; reduces lipid peroxidation
Motherwort *Leonurus cardiaca*	*HTN 2/2 anxiety or hyperthyroidism, dyslipidemia, CAD, arrhythmia, nausea, IBS, AKI, lactation, postpartum bleeding, menorrhagia, amenorrhea,* menopause, *pain, stroke,* anxiety, *insomnia, hyperthyroidism; inflammation; breast tumors*	*Preclinical research: lipid effects comparable to atorvastatin; slows atherosclerotic progression; decreases lipid peroxidation*

TABLE 10.F
Cardiometabolic Disorders: Hyperlipidemia and Dyslipidemia. *(Continued)*

Common Name/ Latin Name	Scope of Potential Benefits	Comments
Saffron *Crocus sativus*	ARMD, *cataracts*, diabetic maculopathy, glaucoma, gingivitis, burning mouth syndrome, *allergy*, asthma, HTN, **dyslipidemia**, DM, **obesity**, *hepatotoxicity*, DM nephropathy, PMS, menopause, **female and male sexual dysfunction**, male infertility, chronic pain, fibromyalgia, stroke, AD, **anxiety**, insomnia, OCD, **depression**, ADHD, drug and ETOH addiction, *photodamage*, stamina, immune function, inflammation, RA, *bacterial infection*, cancer	*Preclinical research: normalizes lipids* **Systematic review: beneficial for reducing TG and TC, increasing HDL-C** Human research: decreases lipid peroxidation; increases SIRT1 and AMPK, decreases LOX1 and NF-κB; reduces anti-HSP in metabolic syndrome
Sage *Salvia officinalis, lavandulifolia*	**Dyslipidemia, dementia, cognitive performance**	Alasvand et al. (2019)
Sea buckthorn *Hippophae rhamnoides*	**Dyslipidemia**	Xiao-Fei et al. (2017)
Skullcap (Chinese, American) *Scutellaria baicalensis, lateriflora*	*Noise-induced hearing loss*, allergy, *asthma, COPD, preterm RDS, pneumonia, PAH, CAD, dyslipidemia, DM, obesity, NAFLD, ETOH-induced gastritis, seizures, dementias,* **anxiety**, depression, *ADHD,* cognition, *photoprotection, autoimmunity, inflammation, MS, influenza, pneumonia, HIV,* cancer-related anemia, *cancer*	*Preclinical research: Chinese skullcap and baicalin reduce TC*
Stinging nettle *Urtica dioica*	Allergic rhinitis, HTN, dyslipidemia, **DM**, NAFLD, *colitis, nephrotoxicity,* menopause, **BPH**, prostatitis, OA, inflammation, *prostate cancer, cisplatin toxicity*	*Preclinical research: lowers lipids* Human research: lowers TG, inflammation, and IR; raises HDL-C, antioxidant, and insulin levels in T2DM
Tribulus/Puncture vine/Goathead *Tribulus terrestris*	HTN, CAD, dyslipidemia, DM, *hepatotoxicity, IBS, nephrolithiasis,* **sexual dysfunction**, hypoactive sexual desire, *pain, anxiety, depression, inflammation, cancer*	*Preclinical research: lowers TGs and TC, stabilizes endothelium* Human research: lowers TC and LDL-C
Turmeric (or curcumin) *Curcuma longa*	Anterior uveitis, **oral lichen planus, gingivitis,** dental surgery, submucous fibrosis, asthma, **diastolic HTN, dyslipidemia**, CAD, endothelial dysfunction, **DM,** obesity, **NAFLD**, hepatoprotective, gallbladder dyskinesia, *GERD,* PUD, dyspepsia, **UC,** DM nephropathy, lupus nephritis, lactational mastitis, LSIL, chronic nonbacterial prostatitis, postoperative pain, **OA,** RA, migraine HA, *neurodegeneration,* **anxiety, depression, skin disease,** psoriasis, fatigue, **systemic inflammation,** *HIV,* **chemo-related oral mucositis,** cancer prevention, cancer treatment	**Systematic review: variably beneficial (depending on patient co-morbidities) for normalizing TG, TC, LDL-C, and HDL-C** Human research: improves endothelial function
Yarrow *Achillea millefolium*	*Epistaxis, asthma,* HTN, **dyslipidemia,** *T1DM,* cirrhosis, *gastritis,* PUD, anorexia, IBS, IBD, nipple fissures, candida vaginitis, dysmenorrhea, *menorrhagia, menopause, anxiety, neurodegenerative disorders,* multiple sclerosis, *inflammation*	**Systematic review: one of several TCM herbs that decreases TC and LDL-C** Human research: *Achillea wilhelmsii* lowers TG, TC, and LDL-C; raises HDL-C

TABLE 10.G
Cardiometabolic Disorders: Diabetes, Prediabetes, Metabolic Syndrome, and Obesity.

Common Name/ Latin Name	Scope of Potential Benefits	Comments
Aloe *Aloe vera, barbadensis*	**Gingivitis, submucous fibrosis, dyslipidemia, diabetes**, insulin resistance, hepatic fibrosis, GERD, **IBS**, IBD, anal fissures, radiation proctitis, AD, *PD*, acne, **psoriasis, lichen planus, burns**, wounds, pressure ulcers, diabetic foot ulcers, wrinkle and striae reduction, Hashimoto's thyroiditis, inflammation, HIV, cancer	**Systematic reviews: improves FBG, A1C, and lipids in prediabetics and diabetics**
Bilberry *Vaccinium myrtillus*	Normal pressure glaucoma, cataracts, night vision, eye fatigue, gingivitis, HTN, **dyslipidemia**, T2DM, NAFLD, ulcerative colitis, *AD*, psoriasis, *wounds, inflammation, S. pneumonia, MRSA*, colorectal cancer, *other cancers*	*Preclinical research: reduces weight* Human research: improves glycemia, NAFLD, and lipids
Black seed/ nigella/black cumin *Nigella sativa*	Periodontal dz, oral submucous fibrosis, chronic rhinosinusitis, nasal dryness, **allergy, asthma**, COPD, chemical pneumonitis, **HTN**, *CAD*, CHF, **dyslipidemia, DM, obesity**, NAFLD, dyspepsia, PUD, diabetic nephropathy, mastalgia, menopause, male infertility, OA, *stroke*, seizure disorder, memory impairment, cognition, anxiety, *depression*, acne, eczema, vitiligo, immune function, Hashimoto's thyroiditis, RA, inflammation, *H. pylori, Staph* pustules, HCV, cancer	*Preclinical research: AMPK activation and PPARγ activity; increases GLUT 4; decreases appetite; weight loss* **Systematic reviews: reduces body weight and BMI, possibly WC; reduces glycemia and lipids** Human research: reduces weight, IR, β-cell function; reduces A1C by 0.6%–1.5% at 12 weeks; reduces inflammation, normalizes lipids, increases insulin sensitivity, reduces NAFLD
Burdock *Arctium lappa*	*Dyslipidemia*, diabetes, *hepatic function and protection, gastroparesis, dyspepsia*, diverticulitis, diabetic nephropathy, OA, wrinkles, acne, cough, *inflammation, influenza A, cancer*	*Preclinical research: reduces BG and increases insulin levels in diabetic rats* Human research: fruit extract plus astragalus reduces lipids, postprandial BG, and urinary albumin
Chamomile *Matricaria chamomilla/ recutita*	Gingivitis, mucositis, chronic rhinosinusitis, *allergies*, dyslipidemia, diabetes, *PUD*, colic, IBS, diarrhea, dyspepsia, UC, *candida vaginitis*, menopause, carpal tunnel syndrome, anxiety, insomnia, depression, ADHD, eczema, wounds, radiation or chemotherapy dermatitis, cortisol dysregulation, *inflammation, broadly antimicrobial (bacteria, yeast, fungus), cancer*	Human research: reduces A1C and lipids
Coleus *Coleus forskohlii*	Glaucoma, *allergy*, asthma, HTN, CHF, *insulin resistance*, obesity, *pancreatic exocrine insufficiency, diarrhea, UTI, urge incontinence, dysmenorrhea, male infertility*, male hypogonadism, subarachnoid hemorrhage, *seizure, neurodegenerative disorders, alcohol abuse*, psoriasis, *photoprotection, hyperthyroidism, cancer*	*Preclinical research: lowers insulin resistance, promotes insulin and glucagon secretion; reduces weight* Human research: reduces fat mass; increases lean mass; increases testosterone in men, mixed results in women

TABLE 10.G
Cardiometabolic Disorders: Diabetes, Prediabetes, Metabolic Syndrome, and Obesity. *(Continued)*

Common Name/ Latin Name	Scope of Potential Benefits	Comments
Cranberry *Vaccinium* *macrocarpon*	Gingivitis, dyslipidemia, **DM**, PUD, gut dysbiosis, overactive bladder, **UTI**, postradiation UTI, BPH, chronic prostatitis, RA, *inflammation, influenza,* prostate CA	**Systematic review: lowers blood glucose** Human research: lowers insulin resistance, glucose, TG, CRP, and MDA; increases HDL-C
Dandelion *Taraxacum officinale*	HTN, dyslipidemia, DM, *obesity, edema,* liver toxicity, NAFLD, *gastroparesis,* dyspepsia, *neurodegenerative disorders, depression, stamina, inflammation, endotoxic shock, cancer*	*Preclinical research: leaf extract lowers IR, glucose; activates AMPK; inhibits α-glucosidase; reduces fat absorption* Human research: in combination formula reduced A1C by 2%
Elder (berry, flower) *Sambucus nigra*	Gingival recession, ASCVD, *dyslipidemia, DM,* obesity, constipation, stroke, *immune function,* **URI,** rhinosinusitis, influenza, *HIV, HSV, Strep, cancer*	*Preclinical research: increases insulin secretion and glucose uptake, PPAR-γ activity* Human research: reduces weight in combination with asparagus
Fenugreek *Trigonella* *foenum-graecum*	Dyslipidemia, **DM,** prediabetes, *diabetic nephropathy, urolithiasis,* lactation, dysmenorrhea, PCOS, menopause, male sexual dysfunction, hypogonadism, PD, *peripheral neuropathy, thyroid T3/ T4 balance,* stamina, *cancer*	*Preclinical research: reduces glucose through multiple mechanisms* **Systematic review: supportive evidence for glycemic control in DM** Human research: improves blood glucose, A1C, insulin sensitivity, and prediabetes
Ginger *Zingiber officinale*	**Motion sickness**, *HTN,* dyslipidemia, fibrinolysis, diabetes, **nausea, vomiting**, *dyspepsia,* gastroparesis, *PUD,* ulcerative colitis, *diabetic nephropathy,* **dysmenorrhea**, *Candida vaginitis,* male infertility, OA, muscle injury, migraine HA, *AD,* **inflammation**, RA, *H. pylori, antibacterial,* **CINV**, cancer	*Preclinical research: improves insulin resistance, lowers glucose and TGs* **Systematic review: reduces A1C but not FBS** Human research: single trial shows some benefit as add-on therapy for FBS
Ginkgo *Ginkgo biloba*	*Cataracts,* ARMD, glaucoma, periodontal dz, **vertigo, tinnitus, cardiovascular health, dyslipidemia, diabetes,** obesity, claudication, hepatic fibrosis, **diabetic nephropathy**, menopausal sexual desire, **acute mountain sickness**, migraines with aura, **stroke, MCI, dementias,** postoperative delirium, depression, ADHD, **schizophrenia, tardive dyskinesia,** aging skin, *inflammation, cancer*	**Systematic review: reduces FBS and albumin excretion in early diabetic nephropathy; improves A1C and HDL-C** Human research: effective adjuvant to metformin for glycemia, IR, and weight in patients with DM or metabolic syndrome
Ginseng, American *Panax quinquefolius*	HTN, dyslipidemia, DM, PVD, cognition, ADHD, schizophrenia, immune function, **URIs**, influenza, cancer	Human research: reduces PPG, increases insulin output
Ginseng, Asian/ Korean/Chinese *Panax ginseng*	Dry eyes, **hearing loss, HTN,** CHF, **DM**, obesity, **menopause, ED,** male infertility, *osteoporosis,* AD, cognitive function, aging skin, alopecia areata, stamina, **chronic fatigue, hangover,** immune function, inflammation, influenza, HIV, **cancer**	**Systematic review: beneficial for reducing FBS and A1C** Human research: reduces blood glucose and body weight; mixed effects on IR
Goji berry/ wolfberry *Lycium barbarum*	Macular degeneration, *glaucoma,* dyslipidemia, **diabetes**, obesity, *hepatoprotection, male infertility, male sexual dysfunction, stroke, AD,* insomnia, anxiety, ADD, *dermatitis,* cognition, stress, fatigue, athletic performance, hangover, immunity function, influenza, cancer	**Systematic review: beneficial for glycemic control** Human studies: increases metabolic rate and HDL-C; reduces WC and BG

Continued on following page

	TABLE 10.G	
Cardiometabolic Disorders: Diabetes, Prediabetes, Metabolic Syndrome, and Obesity. *(Continued)*		
Common Name/ Latin Name	**Scope of Potential Benefits**	**Comments**
Gymnema/Gurmar *Gymnema sylvestre*	*Dental caries,* dyslipidemia, T1DM, **T2DM**, obesity, *arthritis, immune function, cancer*	*Preclinical research: regenerates islet cells, promotes insulin secretion; reduces absorption, decreases gluconeogenesis* **Systematic review: possibly beneficial for T2DM** Human research: improves T1DM and T2DM, decreases caloric intake
Gynostemma/ Jiaogulan *Gynostemma pentaphyllum*	*Asthma, CAD, dyslipidemia,* DM, obesity, *arrhythmia,* NAFLD, *PUD,* PCOS, *PD, white matter disease,* dementia, *stamina, immune function, cancer*	*Preclinical research: AMPK activator, increases insulin secretion; reduces obesity* Human research: 2% decrease in A1C at 12 wks; improves glycemia alone or as adjuvant; reduces BMI, visceral fat, and total fat
Holy basil/Tulsi *Ocimum tenuiflorum/ sanctum*	Gingivitis, asthma, *CAD,* **dyslipidemia**, **diabetes**, obesity, *hepatotoxicity, PUD, male hypogonadism, pain, seizures,* anxiety, depression, memory and concentration, stress and fatigue, immune function, viral encephalitis	*Preclinical research: lowers BG, increases insulin secretion* **Systematic review: additive to diabetic medication; requires several weeks** Human research: reduces BG, A1C, and IR in T2DM; reduces weight
Hops/Hop *Humulus lupulus*	Dental plaque, allergic rhinitis, ASCVD, dyslipidemia, T2DM, obesity, *NAFLD, dyspepsia,* osteoporosis, OA, RA, atrophic vaginitis, menopause, cognitive decline, **insomnia**, anxiety, depression, cognitive performance, acne, aging skin, body odor, antibacterial, Licorice *TB, cancer*	*Preclinical research: increases PPAR-α and -γ; reduces glucose and IR; decreases adipocyte size* Human research: improves glycemia, reduces visceral fat and total fat; reduces BG and A1C; reduces IR combined with *Acacia*
Horsetail *Equisetum arvense*	*Diabetes,* nephrolithiasis, *UTI, interstitial cystitis,* BPH, osteoporosis, *OA,* RA, *chronic pain, anxiety, cognition,* psoriatic nails, wound healing, aging skin, alopecia, inflammation	*Preclinical research: improves BG and heals pancreas in streptozotocin mouse model*
Lemon balm *Melissa officinalis*	**Bruxism**, dyslipidemia, DM, palpitations, dyspepsia, IBS, **colic**, PMS, dysmenorrhea, female sexual dysfunction, **AD**, dementia, agitation, *diabetic neuropathy,* insomnia, **anxiety**, depression, **ADHD**, *hyperthyroidism, Graves' disease,* herpes simplex, *cancer, glioblastoma multiforme*	*Preclinical research: essential oil normalizes blood glucose in rats* Human research: lowers FBS and A1C, improves beta cell activity; reduces vascular and dermal glycation
Licorice *Glycyrrhiza glabra*	**Postoperative sore throat**, xerostomia, radiation-induced mucositis, aphthous ulcers, *allergy,* **asthma, dyslipidemia,** *CAD,* diabetes, **obesity**, hepatoprotection, heartburn, PUD, functional dyspepsia, **antipsychotic-induced hyperprolactinemia, menopause,** atrophic vaginitis, PCOS, female hirsutism, BPH, *stroke, dementia, PD, anxiety, insomnia,* depression, *substance addiction,* **hyperpigmentation, atopic eczema,** Addison's disease, *stamina, multiple sclerosis, inflammation, H. pylori,* cancer, *breast cancer*	*Preclinical research: increases insulin sensitivity; reduces BG in rats* **Systematic review: reduces BW -0.43 kg** Human research: in combination formula reduces IR and BMI in PCOS *(Caution: use deglycyrrhizinated formulations in patients at risk for HTN and hypokalemia)*
Maca *Lepidium meyenii, peruvianum*	HTN, DM, weight reduction, perimenopause, **menopause, sexual dysfunction**, antidepressant- induced sexual dysfunction, **male sexual dysfunction, male infertility**, *BPH,* osteoporosis, *memory impairment,* anxiety, depression, fatigue, inflammation	Human research: reduces BMI in perimenopausal women; black maca reduces blood glucose

TABLE 10.G

Cardiometabolic Disorders: Diabetes, Prediabetes, Metabolic Syndrome, and Obesity. *(Continued)*

Common Name/Latin Name	Scope of Potential Benefits	Comments
Milk thistle *Silybum marianum*	**Dyslipidemia, DM, liver disease**, diabetic nephropathy, lactation, *PCOS*, BPH, *gout, AD, diabetic neuropathy*, **OCD**, acne, *psoriasis*, vitiligo, radio-dermatitis, aging skin, RA, inflammation, hepatitis viruses, **iron-overload**, chemotherapy and radiotherapy toxicity, *hepatocellular carcinoma*	*Preclinical research: reduces liver fibrosis, weight, visceral fat; inhibits aldose reductase; protects pancreatic beta cells; activates PPAR γ, inhibits GLUT-4 uptake; reduces A1C; normalizes insulin* **Systematic reviews: beneficial in T2DM** Human research: reduces A1C by 0.5%–1%; reduces IR; reduces macroalbuminuria, improves NAFLD; reduces insulin dose in T1DM in a combination formula; reduces oxidation status; augments berberine via enhanced absorption
Passionflower *Passiflora incarnata*	*Asthma, diabetes*, **menopause**, OA *(fruit peel), seizure disorder*, **anxiety**, somatoform disorder, *depression,* insomnia, **ADHD**, opiate withdrawal	*Preclinical research: reduces blood glucose and lipids in STZ-treated mice*
Peppermint *Mentha x piperita*	Oral health, weight reduction, nausea, dyspepsia, **IBS**, GI endoscopy, cracked nipples, PCOS, neck pain, tension headaches, postherpetic neuralgia, cognition, nicotine withdrawal, pressure ulcers, pruritis gravidarum, hirsutism, athletic performance, URI, *cancer*	Human research: reduces appetite and gastric motility
Saffron *Crocus sativus*	ARMD, *cataracts*, diabetic maculopathy, glaucoma, gingivitis, burning mouth syndrome, *allergy,* asthma, HTN, **dyslipidemia**, DM, **obesity**, *hepatotoxicity, DM nephropathy*, PMS, menopause, **female and male sexual dysfunction**, male infertility, chronic pain, fibromyalgia, stroke, AD, **anxiety**, insomnia, OCD, **depression**, ADHD, drug and ETOH addiction, *photodamage*, stamina, immune function, inflammation, RA, *bacterial infection*, cancer	*Preclinical research: reduces leptin, insulin resistance, BG, and STZ-induced damage* **Systematic reviews and metaanalysis: conflicting findings on FBS and BMI benefits; reduces body weight and WC** Human research: decreases FPG and A1C; prevents metabolic syndrome associated with olanzapine; reduces antiheat-shock protein 27 and 70 in metabolic syndrome; decreases appetite
Schisandra *Schisandra chinensis*	*MI*, **CHF**, DM, NAFLD, viral hepatitis, menopause, FMF, *stroke, AD, anxiety*, cognition, physical stress, stamina, pneumonia, *HCV, fungal infections*, cancer	*Preclinical research: lowers insulin resistance* Human research: alters fat-producing gut flora; trend toward reducing BMI, waistline, FBG, AST, ALT, and TG
Skullcap (Chinese, American) *Scutellaria baicalensis, lateriflora*	*Noise-induced hearing loss, allergy, asthma, COPD, preterm RDS, pneumonia, PAH, CAD, dyslipidemia, DM, obesity, NAFLD, ETOH-induced gastritis, seizures, dementias,* **anxiety**, depression, *ADHD*, cognition, *photoprotection, autoimmunity, inflammation, MS, influenza, pneumonia, HIV, cancer-related anemia, cancer*	*Preclinical research: activates PPAR-γ and AMPK; prevents weight gain, reduces visceral fat, lowers insulin, lowers glucose after 2 weeks*
Stinging Nettle (leaf) *Urtica dioica*	Allergic rhinitis, HTN, dyslipidemia, **DM**, NAFLD, *colitis, nephrotoxicity*, menopause, **BPH**, prostatitis, OA, inflammation, *prostate cancer, cisplatin toxicity*	*Preclinical research: insulin secretagogue, PPAR-γ agonistic, α-glucosidase inhibitory effects* **Systematic reviews: nettle leaf reduces FBS, not insulin or IR** Human research: augments glycemic control of drugs; raises insulin; lowers IR; reduces inflammatory cytokines, oxidation, lipids (combination formula)

Continued on following page

TABLE 10.G
Cardiometabolic Disorders: Diabetes, Prediabetes, Metabolic Syndrome, and Obesity. *(Continued)*

Common Name/ Latin Name	Scope of Potential Benefits	Comments
Tribulus/Puncture vine/Goathead *Tribulus terrestris*	HTN, CAD, dyslipidemia, DM, *hepatotoxicity, IBS, nephrolithiasis,* **sexual dysfunction,** hypoactive sexual desire, *pain, anxiety, depression, inflammation, cancer*	*Preclinical research: reduces glucose, TGs, glucosidase, gluconeogenesis* Human research: lowers blood glucose, TC, and LDL-C
Turmeric (or curcumin) *Curcuma longa*	Anterior uveitis, **oral lichen planus, gingivitis,** dental surgery, submucous fibrosis, asthma, **diastolic HTN, dyslipidemia,** CAD, endothelial dysfunction, **DM,** obesity, **NAFLD,** hepatoprotective, gallbladder dyskinesia, *GERD,* PUD, dyspepsia, **UC,** DM nephropathy, lupus nephritis, lactational mastitis, LSIL, chronic nonbacterial prostatitis, postoperative pain, **OA,** RA, migraine HA, *neurodegeneration,* **anxiety, depression, skin disease,** psoriasis, fatigue, **systemic inflammation,** *HIV,* **chemo-related oral mucositis,** cancer prevention, cancer treatment	**Systematic review: reduces FBG and A1C in dysglycemic patients; reduces leptin levels** Human research: lowers FBG, TG, diastolic BP; decreases A1C -0.5%, decreases leptin levels, increases adiponectin levels; decreases hs-CRP, decreases TNF-α; augments metformin Variable evidence for benefits on WC, BW, BMI, and insulin resistance
Yarrow *Achillea millefolium*	*Epistaxis, asthma,* HTN, **dyslipidemia,** *T1DM,* cirrhosis, *gastritis, PUD, anorexia, IBS, IBD,* nipple fissures, candida vaginitis, dysmenorrhea, *menorrhagia, menopause, anxiety, neurodegenerative disorders, multiple sclerosis, inflammation*	*Preclinical research: spares streptozotocin destruction of pancreas, spares β cells*

REFERENCES

Alasvand S, et al. Effectiveness of salvia officinalis on mediation of serum lipid in clinical trials: systematic review and metaanalysis. Curr Dev Nutr 2019;3(Suppl. 1).

Chong NJ, et al. A systematic review of the efficacy of centella asiatica for improvement of the signs and symptoms of chronic venous insufficiency. Evid Based Complement Alternat Med 2013;627182.

Xiao-Fei G, et al. Effect of sea buckthorn (*Hippophae rhamnoides L.*) on blood lipid profiles: a systematic review and metaanalysis from 11 independent randomized controlled trials. Trends Food Sci Technol 2017;61:1–10.

GASTROINTESTINAL DISORDERS

■ ■ ■ ■ ■ ■ ■ ■ ■ ■ ■ ■ ■ ■

TABLE 11.A		
Hepatobiliary Disorders: Liver Disease, Nonalcoholic Fatty Liver Disease, Hepatitis B Virus, Hepatitis C Virus, Biliary Disorders.		
Common Name/ Latin Name	**Scope of Potential Benefits**	**Comments**
Aloe *Aloe vera, barbadensis*	**Gingivitis, submucous fibrosis**, **dyslipidemia, diabetes**, insulin resistance, hepatic fibrosis, GERD, **IBS**, IBD, anal fissures, radiation proctitis, AD, *PD*, acne, **psoriasis, lichen planus, burns,** wounds, pressure ulcers, diabetic foot ulcers, wrinkle and striae reduction, Hashimoto's thyroiditis, inflammation, HIV, cancer	Human research: improves liver fibrosis
Astragalus *Astragalus membranaceus*	Herpes keratitis, recurrent tonsillitis, allergic rhinitis, atopy, asthma, **viral myocarditis**, CHF, CAD, viral hepatitis, **diabetic nephropathy**, IgA nephropathy, nephrotic syndrome, lupus nephritis, *renal fibrosis, sperm quality*, hemorrhagic stroke, burns, *wound healing, age spots, leukopenia*, **immune function**, *antiviral*, HBV, TB, **NSCLC**, cancer	*Preclinical research: activity against hepatitis B* Human research: improves HBV treatment response and disease activity; improves fibrosis in chronic viral hepatitis
Bilberry *Vaccinium myrtillus*	Normal pressure glaucoma, cataracts, night vision, eye fatigue, gingivitis, *HTN*, **dyslipidemia**, T2DM, NAFLD, ulcerative colitis, *AD*, psoriasis, *wounds,* inflammation, *S. pneumonia, MRSA,* colorectal cancer, *other cancers*	Human research: improves NAFLD
Black seed/nigella/ black cumin *Nigella sativa*	Periodontal dz, oral submucous fibrosis, chronic rhinosinusitis, nasal dryness, **allergy, asthma**, COPD, chemical pneumonitis, **HTN**, *CAD*, CHF, **dyslipidemia, DM, obesity**, NAFLD, dyspepsia, PUD, diabetic nephropathy, mastalgia, menopause, male infertility, OA, *stroke,* seizure disorder, memory impairment, cognition, anxiety, *depression*, acne, eczema, vitiligo, immune function, Hashimoto's thyroiditis, RA, inflammation, *H. pylori, Staph* pustules, HCV, cancer	Human research: improves NAFLD; reduces HCV viral load 50% and normalizes hematologic changes in HCV infection
Burdock *Arctium lappa*	*Dyslipidemia*, diabetes, *hepatic function and protection, gastroparesis,* dyspepsia, diverticulitis, diabetic nephropathy, OA, wrinkles, acne, cough, *inflammation, influenza A, cancer*	*Preclinical research: promotes hepatic detoxification, protects against liver toxins*
Andrographis *Andrographis paniculata*	HTN, hepatoprotection, ulcerative colitis, *dysmenorrhea*, OA, RA, FMF, *inflammation*, **URI prevention and treatment**, *cancer*	*Preclinical research: hepatoprotective comparable to silymarin from milk thistle*
Bacopa *Bacopa monnieri*	*Gastric ulcer*, hepatic encephalopathy, IBS-D, *seizures,* memory impairment, **dementia-related anxiety**, test anxiety, **cognitive performance**, ADHD, inflammation	Human research: improves hepatic encephalopathy

Continued on following page

TABLE 11.A

Hepatobiliary Disorders: Liver Disease, Nonalcoholic Fatty Liver Disease, Hepatitis B Virus, Hepatitis C Virus, Biliary Disorders. *(Continued)*

Common Name/ Latin Name	Scope of Potential Benefits	Comments
Dandelion *Taraxacum officinale*	HTN, dyslipidemia, DM, *obesity, edema,* liver toxicity, NAFLD, *gastroparesis,* dyspepsia, *neurodegenerative disorders, depression, stamina, inflammation, endotoxic shock, cancer*	*Preclinical research: leaf extract lowers ALT, AST, and GGT; promotes bile drainage; prevents hepatotoxicity* Human research: combination formula lowers ALT, AST, and GGT in dyspeptic patients
Dong quai *Angelica sinensis*	Pulmonary HTN, *HTN,* CAD, *atrial fibrillation,* cirrhosis, portal HTN, abd pain, UC, *renal fibrosis, dysmenorrhea,* menopausal symptoms, *osteoporosis,* OA, stroke, *cerebrovascular insufficiency, neurodegenerative disorders, wound healing, aging skin, alopecia, stamina, inflammation,* anemia of chronic disease, cancer	Human research: reduces serum gastrin levels to normal in patients with cirrhosis (may reduce portal HTN)
Ginkgo *Ginkgo biloba*	*Cataracts,* ARMD, glaucoma, periodontal dz, **vertigo, tinnitus, cardiovascular health, dyslipidemia, diabetes,** obesity, claudication, hepatic fibrosis, **diabetic nephropathy,** menopausal sexual desire, **acute mountain sickness,** migraines with aura, **stroke, MCI, dementias,** postoperative delirium, depression, ADHD, **schizophrenia, tardive dyskinesia,** aging skin, *inflammation, cancer*	Human research: reduces fibrosis and improves microcirculation in chronic HBV
Goji berry/wolfberry *Lycium barbarum*	Macular degeneration, *glaucoma,* dyslipidemia, **diabetes,** obesity, *hepatoprotection, male infertility, male sexual dysfunction,* stroke, AD, insomnia, anxiety, ADD, *dermatitis,* cognition, stress, fatigue, athletic performance, hangover, immunity function, influenza, cancer	*Preclinical research: hepatoprotective against toxins*
Gynostemma/ Jiaogulan *Gynostemma pentaphyllum*	*Asthma, CAD, dyslipidemia,* DM, obesity, *arrhythmia,* NAFLD, *PUD,* PCOS, *PD, white matter disease,* dementia, *stamina,* immune function, cancer	Human research: reduces transaminases and fatty liver score
Hawthorn *Crataegus* spp.	HTN, CAD, **CHF** (HrEF and HpEF), arrhythmia, **orthostatic hypotension,** *NAFLD,* anxiety, *inflammation*	Traditional use: review found most frequently used herb in TCM combinations for effective treatment of NAFLD
Holy basil/Tulsi *Ocimum tenuiflorum/ sanctum*	Gingivitis, asthma, *CAD,* **dyslipidemia, diabetes,** obesity, *hepatotoxicity, PUD, male hypogonadism, pain, seizures,* anxiety, depression, memory and concentration, stress and fatigue, immune function, viral encephalitis	*Preclinical research: hepatoprotective, eliminates cadmium*
Hops/Hop *Humulus lupulus*	Dental plaque, allergic rhinitis, ASCVD, dyslipidemia, T2DM, obesity, *NAFLD, dyspepsia,* osteoporosis, OA, RA, atrophic vaginitis, menopause, cognitive decline, **insomnia,** anxiety, depression, cognitive performance, acne, aging skin, body odor, antibacterial, *TB, cancer*	*Preclinical research: prevents liver fibrosis, toxic hepatitis*
Licorice *Glycyrrhiza glabra*	**Postoperative sore throat,** xerostomia, radiation-induced mucositis, aphthous ulcers, *allergy,* **asthma, dyslipidemia,** *CAD,* diabetes, **obesity,** hepatoprotection, heartburn, PUD, functional dyspepsia, **antipsychotic-induced hyperprolactinemia, menopause,** atrophic vaginitis, PCOS, female hirsutism, BPH, *stroke, dementia,* PD, anxiety, insomnia, depression, substance addiction, **hyperpigmentation, atopic eczema,** Addison's disease, *stamina, multiple sclerosis, inflammation, H. pylori, cancer, breast cancer*	Human research: protects liver against alcohol toxicity ***(Caution: use deglycyrrhizinated formulations in patients at risk for HTN and hypokalemia)***

TABLE 11.A

Hepatobiliary Disorders: Liver Disease, Nonalcoholic Fatty Liver Disease, Hepatitis B Virus, Hepatitis C Virus, Biliary Disorders. *(Continued)*

Common Name/ Latin Name	Scope of Potential Benefits	Comments
Milk thistle *Silybum marianum*	**Dyslipidemia, DM, liver disease**, diabetic nephropathy, lactation, PCOS, BPH, *gout*, *AD*, *diabetic neuropathy*, **OCD**, acne, *psoriasis*, vitiligo, radio-dermatitis, aging skin, RA, inflammation, hepatitis viruses, **iron-overload**, chemotherapy and radiotherapy toxicity, *hepatocellular carcinoma*	*Preclinical research: silymarin hepatoprotective at level of cell membrane; choleretic; promotes hepatocyte regeneration* **Systematic review: beneficial for anti-TB drug prophylaxis; beneficial in NAFLD; not beneficial for HCV** Human research: IV silybin decreases HCV viral load in nonresponders; silymarin reduces HCV and transaminases; silymarin improves histology and survival in alcoholic liver disease; silymarin improves NAFLD; reduces drug-induced hepatotoxicity; reduces bile cholesterol concentrations
Saffron *Crocus sativus*	ARMD, *cataracts*, diabetic maculopathy, glaucoma, gingivitis, burning mouth syndrome, *allergy*, asthma, HTN, **dyslipidemia**, DM, **obesity**, *hepatotoxicity*, *DM nephropathy*, PMS, menopause, **female and male sexual dysfunction**, male infertility, chronic pain, fibromyalgia, stroke, AD, **anxiety**, insomnia, OCD, **depression**, ADHD, drug and ETOH addiction, *photodamage*, stamina, immune function, inflammation, RA, *bacterial infection*, cancer	*Preclinical research: reduces drug-induced liver toxicity*
Schisandra *Schisandra chinensis*	MI, **CHF**, DM, NAFLD, viral hepatitis, menopause, FMF, *stroke*, AD, *anxiety*, cognition, physical stress, stamina, pneumonia, HCV, *fungal infections*, cancer	*Preclinical research: hepatoprotective against toxins; prevents HCV entry into hepatocytes* Human research: reduces ALT and AST in combination with sesamin; may reduce host-immune hepatocyte damage in HBV
Skullcap (Chinese, American) *Scutellaria baicalensis, lateriflora*	*Noise induced hearing loss*, allergy, *asthma*, *COPD*, *preterm RDS*, pneumonia, *PAH*, *CAD*, dyslipidemia, DM, obesity, NAFLD, *ETOH-induced gastritis*, seizures, dementias, **anxiety**, depression, *ADHD*, cognition, *photoprotection*, autoimmunity, inflammation, MS, influenza, pneumonia, HIV, cancer-related anemia, *cancer*	*Preclinical research: increases hepatic antioxidants; reduces fatty liver*
Stinging Nettle *Urtica dioica*	Allergic rhinitis, HTN, dyslipidemia, **DM**, NAFLD, *colitis*, *nephrotoxicity*, menopause, **BPH**, prostatitis, OA, inflammation, *prostate cancer*, *cisplatin toxicity*	*Preclinical research: hepatoprotective* Human research: reduces ALT in patients with T2DM
Tribulus/Puncture vine/Goathead *Tribulus terrestris*	HTN, CAD, dyslipidemia, DM, *hepatotoxicity*, *IBS*, nephrolithiasis, **sexual dysfunction**, hypoactive sexual desire, *pain*, *anxiety*, *depression*, *inflammation*, cancer	*Preclinical research: hepatoprotective against APAP toxicity*

Continued on following page

TABLE 11.A

Hepatobiliary Disorders: Liver Disease, Nonalcoholic Fatty Liver Disease, Hepatitis B Virus, Hepatitis C Virus, Biliary Disorders. *(Continued)*

Common Name/ Latin Name	Scope of Potential Benefits	Comments
Turmeric (or **curcumin**) *Curcuma longa*	Anterior uveitis, **oral lichen planus, gingivitis,** dental surgery, submucous fibrosis, asthma, **diastolic HTN, dyslipidemia,** CAD, endothelial dysfunction, **DM,** obesity, **NAFLD,** hepatoprotective, gallbladder dyskinesia, *GERD,* PUD, dyspepsia, **UC,** DM nephropathy, lupus nephritis, lactational mastitis, LSIL, chronic nonbacterial prostatitis, postoperative pain, **OA,** RA, migraine HA, *neurodegeneration,* **anxiety, depression, skin disease,** psoriasis, fatigue, **systemic inflammation,** *HIV,* **chemo-related oral mucositis,** cancer prevention, cancer treatment	*Preclinical research: hepatoprotective comparable to silymarin (from milk thistle), choleretic (gall bladder support)* **Systematic review: curcumin but not turmeric beneficial for NAFLD in shorter trials and higher doses** Human research: hepatoprotective in antitubercular treatment; enhances gallbladder contractility, improves biliary dyskinesia; reduces hepatic iron burden in thalassemia
Yarrow *Achillea millefolium*	*Epistaxis, asthma,* HTN, **dyslipidemia,** *T1DM,* cirrhosis, *gastritis, PUD, anorexia, IBS, IBD,* nipple fissures, candida vaginitis, dysmenorrhea, *menorrhagia, menopause, anxiety, neurodegenerative disorders,* multiple sclerosis, *inflammation*	Human research: reduces cirrhosis progression in polyherbal formula

TABLE 11.B

Upper Gastrointestinal Disorders: Gastro-esophageal Reflux Disorder, Peptic Ulcer Disease, *H. pylori* infection.

Common Name/ Latin Name	Scope of Potential Benefits	Comments
Aloe *Aloe vera, barbadensis*	**Gingivitis, submucous fibrosis, dyslipidemia, diabetes,** insulin resistance, hepatic fibrosis, GERD, **IBS,** IBD, anal fissures, radiation proctitis, AD, *PD,* acne, **psoriasis, lichen planus, burns,** wounds, pressure ulcers, diabetic foot ulcers, wrinkle and striae reduction, Hashimoto's thyroiditis, inflammation, HIV, cancer	Human research: improves GERD
Bacopa *Bacopa monnieri*	*Gastric ulcer,* hepatic encephalopathy, IBS-D, *seizures,* memory impairment, **dementia-related anxiety,** test anxiety, **cognitive performance,** ADHD, inflammation	*Preclinical research: heals gastric ulcers through PGE, prostacyclin, anti-H. pylori*
Black seed/nigella/ black cumin *Nigella sativa*	Periodontal dz, oral submucous fibrosis, chronic rhinosinusitis, nasal dryness, **allergy, asthma,** COPD, chemical pneumonitis, **HTN,** *CAD,* CHF, **dyslipidemia, DM, obesity,** NAFLD, dyspepsia, PUD, diabetic nephropathy, mastalgia, menopause, male infertility, OA, *stroke,* seizure disorder, memory impairment, cognition, anxiety, *depression,* acne, eczema, vitiligo, immune function, Hashimoto's thyroiditis, RA, inflammation, *H. pylori, Staph* pustules, HCV, cancer	Human research: improves *H. pylori* and dyspepsia; noninferior to triple therapy for *H. pylori*
Butterbur *Petasites hybridus*	**Allergic rhinitis,** asthma, *HTN, GI ulceration,* bladder spasms, **migraine headache,** *neurodegenerative dementias,* somatoform disorder anxiety and depression, *CNS inflammation*	*Preclinical research: protective against gastric and intestinal ulcers from ethanol and indomethacin*

TABLE 11.B

Upper Gastrointestinal Disorders: Gastro-esophageal Reflux Disorder, Peptic Ulcer Disease, H. pylori infection. *(Continued)*

Common Name/ Latin Name	Scope of Potential Benefits	Comments
Chamomile *Matricaria chamomilla/recutita*	Gingivitis, mucositis, chronic rhinosinusitis, *allergies,* dyslipidemia, diabetes, *PUD,* colic, IBS, diarrhea, dyspepsia, UC, *candida vaginitis,* menopause, carpal tunnel syndrome, anxiety, insomnia, depression, ADHD, eczema, wounds, radiation or chemotherapy dermatitis, cortisol dysregulation, *inflammation, broadly antimicrobial (bacteria, yeast, fungus), cancer*	*Preclinical research: reduced H. pylori aggregation; heals gastric ulcers*
Cranberry *Vaccinium macrocarpon*	Gingivitis, dyslipidemia, **DM**, PUD, gut dysbiosis, overactive bladder, **UTI**, postradiation UTI, BPH, chronic prostatitis, RA, *inflammation, influenza,* prostate CA	Human research: improves efficacy of triple therapy
Fennel *Foeniculum vulgare*	*Glaucoma, dyspepsia, gastroprotection, gastroparesis,* **infant colic**, IBS, constipation, *overactive bladder, lactation,* dysmenorrhea, oligomenorrhea, **menopausal disorders**, *dementia, hirsutism, inflammation*	*Preclinical research: gastroprotective*
Ginger *Zingiber officinale*	**Motion sickness**, *HTN,* dyslipidemia, fibrinolysis, diabetes, **nausea, vomiting**, *dyspepsia,* gastroparesis, *PUD,* ulcerative colitis, *diabetic nephropathy,* **dysmenorrhea**, *Candida vaginitis,* male infertility, OA, muscle injury, migraine HA, *AD,* **inflammation**, RA, *H. pylori, antibacterial,* **CINV**, cancer	*Preclinical research: inhibits H. pylori; prevents gastric ulcers*
Gynostemma/ Jiaogulan *Gynostemma pentaphyllum*	*Asthma, CAD, dyslipidemia,* DM, obesity, *arrhythmia,* NAFLD, PUD, PCOS, *PD, white matter disease,* dementia, *stamina,* immune function, cancer	*Preclinical research: gastroprotective against H. pylori, alcohol, stress*
Holy basil/Tulsi *Ocimum tenuiflorum/ sanctum*	Gingivitis, asthma, *CAD,* **dyslipidemia, diabetes**, obesity, *hepatotoxicity, PUD, male hypogonadism, pain, seizures,* anxiety, depression, memory and concentration, stress and fatigue, immune function, viral encephalitis	*Preclinical research: gastroprotective against ASA*
Licorice *Glycyrrhiza glabra*	**Postoperative sore throat**, xerostomia, radiation-induced mucositis, aphthous ulcers, *allergy,* **asthma, dyslipidemia**, *CAD, diabetes,* **obesity**, hepatoprotection, heartburn, PUD, functional dyspepsia, **antipsychotic-induced hyperprolactinemia, menopause**, atrophic vaginitis, PCOS, female hirsutism, BPH, *stroke, dementia, PD,* anxiety, insomnia, depression, substance addiction, **hyperpigmentation, atopic eczema**, Addison's disease, *stamina, multiple sclerosis, inflammation, H. pylori, cancer, breast cancer*	Human research: reduces *H. pylori;* augments efficacy of triple therapy for PUD; improves PUD symptoms; no benefit from DGL, however *(Caution: use deglycyrrhizinated formulations in patients at risk for HTN and hypokalemia)*
Skullcap (Chinese, American) *Scutellaria baicalensis, lateriflora*	*Noise induced hearing loss,* allergy, *asthma, COPD, preterm RDS, pneumonia, PAH, CAD, dyslipidemia, DM, obesity, NAFLD, ETOH-induced gastritis, seizures, dementias,* **anxiety,** depression, *ADHD,* cognition, *photoprotection, autoimmunity, inflammation, MS, influenza, pneumonia, HIV, cancer-related anemia, cancer*	*Preclinical research: protects against alcohol-induced gastritis*

Continued on following page

TABLE 11.B

Upper Gastrointestinal Disorders: Gastro-esophageal Reflux Disorder, Peptic Ulcer Disease, H. pylori infection. *(Continued)*

Common Name/ Latin Name	Scope of Potential Benefits	Comments
Turmeric *Curcuma longa*	Anterior uveitis, **oral lichen planus, gingivitis,** dental surgery, submucous fibrosis, asthma, **diastolic HTN, dyslipidemia,** CAD, endothelial dysfunction, **DM,** obesity, **NAFLD,** hepatoprotective, gallbladder dyskinesia, *GERD,* PUD, dyspepsia, **UC,** DM nephropathy, lupus nephritis, lactational mastitis, LSIL, chronic nonbacterial prostatitis, postoperative pain, **OA,** RA, migraine HA, *neurodegeneration,* **anxiety, depression, skin disease,** psoriasis, fatigue, **systemic inflammation,** *HIV,* **chemo-related oral mucositis,** cancer prevention, cancer treatment	*Preclinical research: prevents mucosal damage from gastroesophageal reflux; better than lansoprazole for bile-acid reflux* Human research: improves symptoms of *H. pylori* with triple therapy better than triple therapy alone; promotes healing of peptic ulcers and reduces symptoms of nonulcer dyspepsia
Umckaloabo/South African Geranium *Pelargonium sidoides*	Asthma, COPD, *PUD,* immune function, inflammation, **bronchitis, URI,** pharyngitis, rhinosinusitis, *influenza, Coronavirus, pneumonia, HIV, HSV 1&2, TB*	*Preclinical research: prevents adhesion of H. pylori to gastric mucosa*
Yarrow *Achillea millefolium*	*Epistaxis, asthma,* HTN, **dyslipidemia,** *T1DM,* cirrhosis, *gastritis, PUD, anorexia, IBS, IBD,* nipple fissures, candida vaginitis, dysmenorrhea, *menorrhagia, menopause, anxiety, neurodegenerative disorders,* multiple sclerosis, *inflammation*	*Preclinical research: gastroprotective against ETOH and acid, heals gastric erosions; promotes appetite*

TABLE 11.C

Functional Upper GI Disorders: Gastroparesis, Nausea, Dyspepsia, Exocrine Pancreatic Insufficiency, and Infantile Colic.

Common Name/ Latin Name	Scope of Potential Benefits	Comments
Black seed/nigella/ black cumin *Nigella sativa*	Periodontal dz, oral submucous fibrosis, chronic rhinosinusitis, nasal dryness, **allergy, asthma,** COPD, chemical pneumonitis, **HTN,** *CAD,* CHF, **dyslipidemia, DM, obesity,** NAFLD, dyspepsia, PUD, diabetic nephropathy, mastalgia, menopause, male infertility, OA, *stroke,* seizure disorder, memory impairment, cognition, anxiety, *depression,* acne, eczema, vitiligo, immune function, Hashimoto's thyroiditis, RA, inflammation, *H. pylori, Staph* pustules, HCV, cancer	Human research: improves functional dyspepsia
Burdock *Arctium lappa*	*Dyslipidemia, diabetes, hepatic function and protection, gastroparesis, dyspepsia,* diverticulitis, diabetic nephropathy, OA, wrinkles, acne, cough, *inflammation, influenza A, cancer*	*Preclinical research: promotes gastric motility and digestive enzyme secretion (bitter principles)*
Chamomile *Matricaria chamomilla/ recutita*	Gingivitis, mucositis, chronic rhinosinusitis, *allergies,* dyslipidemia, diabetes, *PUD,* colic, IBS, diarrhea, dyspepsia, UC, *candida vaginitis,* menopause, carpal tunnel syndrome, anxiety, insomnia, depression, ADHD, eczema, wounds, radiation or chemotherapy dermatitis, cortisol dysregulation, *inflammation, broadly antimicrobial (bacteria, yeast, fungus), cancer*	Human research: improves colic in combination formula; improves functional dyspepsia in combination formula Traditional use: indigestion and gastroenteritis

TABLE 11.C
Functional Upper GI Disorders: Gastroparesis, Nausea, Dyspepsia, Exocrine Pancreatic Insufficiency, and Infantile Colic. *(Continued)*

Common Name/ Latin Name	Scope of Potential Benefits	Comments
Coleus *Coleus forskohlii*	Glaucoma, *allergy*, asthma, HTN, CHF, *insulin resistance*, obesity, *pancreatic exocrine insufficiency, diarrhea, UTI, urge incontinence, dysmenorrhea, male infertility*, male hypogonadism, subarachnoid hemorrhage, *seizure, neurodegenerative disorders, alcohol abuse*, psoriasis, *photoprotection, hyperthyroidism, cancer*	*Preclinical research: promotes pancreatic exocrine output*
Dandelion *Taraxacum officinale*	HTN, dyslipidemia, DM, *obesity, edema*, liver toxicity, NAFLD, *gastroparesis*, dyspepsia, *neurodegenerative disorders, depression, stamina, inflammation, endotoxic shock, cancer*	*Preclinical research: bitters promote gastric acid and gastric motility, digestive enzyme secretion* Human research: improves dyspepsia in combination formula
Dong quai *Angelica sinensis*	Pulmonary HTN, *HTN*, CAD, *atrial fibrillation*, cirrhosis, portal HTN, abd pain, UC, *renal fibrosis, dysmenorrhea*, menopausal symptoms, *osteoporosis, OA*, stroke, *cerebrovascular insufficiency, neurodegenerative disorders, wound healing, aging skin, alopecia, stamina, inflammation*, anemia of chronic disease, cancer	Human research: reduces chronic abdominal pain comparable to atropine
Fennel *Foeniculum vulgare*	*Glaucoma, dyspepsia, gastroprotection, gastroparesis*, **infant colic**, IBS, constipation, *overactive bladder, lactation, dysmenorrhea, oligomenorrhea*, **menopausal disorders**, *dementia*, hirsutism, *inflammation*	*Preclinical research: gastric motility and acid stimulant; gastroprotective; antispasmodic* **Systematic review: beneficial for infantile colic** Human research: improves IBS in combination formulas Traditional use: dyspepsia
Ginger *Zingiber officinale*	**Motion sickness**, *HTN*, dyslipidemia, fibrinolysis, diabetes, **nausea, vomiting**, *dyspepsia*, gastroparesis, *PUD*, ulcerative colitis, *diabetic nephropathy*, **dysmenorrhea**, *Candida vaginitis*, male infertility, OA, muscle injury, migraine HA, *AD*, **inflammation**, RA, *H. pylori, antibacterial*, **CINV**, cancer	*Preclinical research: promotes digestive enzymes and bile* **Systematic review: beneficial for post-op N/V; N/V of pregnancy; seasickness; chemo-related N/V** Human research: reduces gastroparesis
Hops/Hop *Humulus lupulus*	Dental plaque, allergic rhinitis, ASCVD, dyslipidemia, T2DM, obesity, *NAFLD, dyspepsia*, osteoporosis, OA, RA, atrophic vaginitis, menopause, cognitive decline, **insomnia**, anxiety, depression, cognitive performance, acne, aging skin, body odor, antibacterial, *TB, cancer*	*Preclinical research: increases gastric secretions (bitter principles)*
Lemon balm *Melissa officinalis*	**Bruxism**, dyslipidemia, DM, palpitations, dyspepsia, IBS, **colic**, PMS, dysmenorrhea, female sexual dysfunction, **AD,** dementia, agitation, *diabetic neuropathy*, insomnia, **anxiety**, depression, **ADHD**, *hyperthyroidism, Graves' disease*, herpes simplex, *cancer, glioblastoma multiforme*	**Systematic review: reduces infantile colic in combination formula** Human research: reduces dyspepsia in combination formula
Licorice *Glycyrrhiza glabra*	**Postoperative sore throat**, xerostomia, radiation-induced mucositis, aphthous ulcers, *allergy*, **asthma, dyslipidemia**, *CAD, diabetes*, **obesity**, hepatoprotection, heartburn, PUD, functional dyspepsia, **antipsychotic-induced hyperprolactinemia, menopause**, atrophic vaginitis, PCOS, female hirsutism, BPH, *stroke, dementia, PD, anxiety, insomnia, depression, substance addiction*, **hyperpigmentation, atopic eczema**, Addison's disease, *stamina, multiple sclerosis, inflammation, H. pylori*, cancer, breast cancer	Human research: reduces heartburn and dyspepsia ***(Caution: use deglycyrrhizinated formulations in patients at risk for HTN and hypokalemia)***

Continued on following page

TABLE 11.C

Functional Upper GI Disorders: Gastroparesis, Nausea, Dyspepsia, Exocrine Pancreatic Insufficiency, and Infantile Colic. *(Continued)*

Common Name/ Latin Name	Scope of Potential Benefits	Comments
Motherwort *Leonurus cardiaca*	*HTN 2/2 anxiety or hyperthyroidism, dyslipidemia, CAD, arrhythmia, nausea, IBS, AKI, lactation, postpartum bleeding, menorrhagia, amenorrhea,* menopause, *pain, stroke,* anxiety, insomnia, hyperthyroidism; inflammation; breast tumors	*Preclinical research: antagonizes 5HT-3A receptors*
Peppermint *Mentha x piperita*	Oral health, weight reduction, nausea, dyspepsia, **IBS**, GI endoscopy, cracked nipples, PCOS, neck pain, tension headaches, postherpetic neuralgia, cognition, nicotine withdrawal, pressure ulcers, pruritis gravidarum, hirsutism, athletic performance, URI, *cancer*	Human research: reduces spasms with EGD; improves symptoms of functional dyspepsia combined with caraway oil comparably to cisapride; enteric coated best tolerated; reduces nausea of many etiologies
Turmeric *Curcuma longa*	Anterior uveitis, **oral lichen planus, gingivitis,** dental surgery, submucous fibrosis, asthma, **diastolic HTN, dyslipidemia,** CAD, endothelial dysfunction, **DM,** obesity, **NAFLD,** hepatoprotective, gallbladder dyskinesia, *GERD,* PUD, dyspepsia, **UC,** DM nephropathy, lupus nephritis, lactational mastitis, LSIL, chronic nonbacterial prostatitis, postoperative pain, **OA,** RA, migraine HA, *neurodegeneration,* **anxiety, depression, skin disease,** psoriasis, fatigue, **systemic inflammation,** *HIV,* **chemo- related oral mucositis,** cancer prevention, cancer treatment	Human research: reduces symptoms of nonulcer dyspepsia

TABLE 11.D

Inflammatory Bowel Disorders: Crohn's Disease, Ulcerative Colitis, Collagenous Colitis, and Diverticulitis.

Common Name/ Latin Name	Scope of Potential Benefits	Comments
Aloe *Aloe vera, barbadensis*	**Gingivitis, submucous fibrosis, dyslipidemia, diabetes,** insulin resistance, hepatic fibrosis, GERD, **IBS,** IBD, anal fissures, radiation proctitis, AD, *PD,* acne, **psoriasis, lichen planus, burns,** wounds, pressure ulcers, diabetic foot ulcers, wrinkle and striae reduction, Hashimoto's thyroiditis, inflammation, HIV, cancer	Human research: improves UC, radiation proctitis, and chronic anal fissures
Andrographis *Andrographis paniculata*	*HTN, hepatoprotection,* ulcerative colitis, *dysmenorrhea,* OA, RA, FMF, *inflammation,* **URI prevention and treatment,** *cancer*	*Preclinical research: promotes resolution of colitis* Human research: beneficial for UC
Bilberry *Vaccinium myrtillus*	Normal pressure glaucoma, cataracts, night vision, eye fatigue, gingivitis, *HTN,* **dyslipidemia,** T2DM, NAFLD, ulcerative colitis, *AD,* psoriasis, *wounds,* inflammation, *S. pneumonia, MRSA,* colorectal cancer, *other cancers*	Human research: improves UC
Burdock *Arctium lappa*	*Dyslipidemia,* diabetes, *hepatic function and protection, gastroparesis, dyspepsia,* diverticulitis, diabetic nephropathy, OA, wrinkles, acne, cough, *inflammation, influenza A, cancer*	Human research: delays recurrence of diverticulitis

TABLE 11.D

Inflammatory Bowel Disorders: Crohn's Disease, Ulcerative Colitis, Collagenous Colitis, and Diverticulitis. *(Continued)*

Common Name/ Latin Name	Scope of Potential Benefits	Comments
Chamomile *Matricaria chamomilla/ recutita*	Gingivitis, mucositis, chronic rhinosinusitis, *allergies*, dyslipidemia, diabetes, *PUD*, colic, IBS, diarrhea, dyspepsia, UC, *candida vaginitis*, menopause, carpal tunnel syndrome, anxiety, insomnia, depression, ADHD, eczema, wounds, radiation or chemotherapy dermatitis, cortisol dysregulation, *inflammation, broadly antimicrobial (bacteria, yeast, fungus), cancer*	Human research: improves UC in combination formula
Dong quai *Angelica sinensis*	Pulmonary HTN, *HTN*, CAD, *atrial fibrillation*, cirrhosis, portal HTN, abd pain, UC, *renal fibrosis, dysmenorrhea*, menopausal symptoms, *osteoporosis, OA*, stroke, *cerebrovascular insufficiency, neurodegenerative disorders, wound healing, aging skin, alopecia, stamina, inflammation*, anemia of chronic disease, cancer	Human research: in patients with UC, normalizes platelet aggregation, improves microcirculation, reduces endothelial injury
Frankincense/ Boswellia *Boswellia serrata, sacra, carterii*	Gingivitis, **asthma**, *COPD*, UC, **Crohn's**, **collagenous colitis**, IBS, UTI, SUI, benign breast disease, menorrhagia, **OA**, stroke, memory impairment, psoriasis, eczema, aging skin, athletic performance, **RA, IBD**, *inflammation*, glioma radiation, chemo-related neuropathy, *cancer*	**Systematic review: beneficial in Crohn's and collagenous colitis** Human research: improves UC comparable to sulfasalazine; improves Crohn's comparable to mesalamine
Ginger *Zingiber officinalis*	**Motion sickness**, *HTN*, dyslipidemia, fibrinolysis, diabetes, **nausea, vomiting**, *dyspepsia*, gastroparesis, *PUD*, ulcerative colitis, *diabetic nephropathy*, **dysmenorrhea**, *Candida vaginitis*, male infertility, OA, muscle injury, migraine HA, *AD*, **inflammation**, RA, *H. pylori, antibacterial*, **CINV**, cancer	Human research: reduces clinical disease activity and MDA levels in patients with UC
Stinging nettle *Urtica dioica*	Allergic rhinitis, HTN, dyslipidemia, **DM**, NAFLD, *colitis, nephrotoxicity*, menopause, **BPH**, prostatitis, OA, inflammation, *prostate cancer, cisplatin toxicity*	*Preclinical research: reduces colitis*
Turmeric (or curcumin) *Curcuma longa*	Anterior uveitis, **oral lichen planus, gingivitis,** dental surgery, submucous fibrosis, asthma, **diastolic HTN, dyslipidemia**, CAD, endothelial dysfunction, **DM**, obesity, **NAFLD**, hepatoprotective, gallbladder dyskinesia, *GERD*, PUD, dyspepsia, **UC**, DM nephropathy, lupus nephritis, lactational mastitis, LSIL, chronic non-bacterial prostatitis, postoperative pain, **OA**, RA, migraine HA, *neurodegeneration*, **anxiety, depression, skin disease**, psoriasis, fatigue, **systemic inflammation**, *HIV*, **chemo-related oral mucosis**, cancer prevention, cancer treatment	**Systematic reviews: beneficial for UC in conjunction with mesalamine** Human research: adjunctively improves remission status in UC (oral or enema administration)
Yarrow *Achillea millefolium*	*Epistaxis, asthma*, HTN, **dyslipidemia**, *T1DM*, cirrhosis, *gastritis, PUD, anorexia, IBS, IBD*, nipple fissures, candida vaginitis, dysmenorrhea, *menorrhagia, menopause, anxiety, neurodegenerative disorders*, multiple sclerosis, *inflammation*	*Preclinical research: antispasmodic, antiinflammatory properties* Traditional use: Crohn's disease and UC

TABLE 11.E
Functional Bowel Disorders: Constipation, Diarrhea, and Irritable Bowel Syndrome.

Common Name/ Latin Name	Scope of Potential Benefits	Comments
Aloe *Aloe vera, barbadensis*	**Gingivitis, submucous fibrosis, dyslipidemia, diabetes,** insulin resistance, hepatic fibrosis, GERD, **IBS**, IBD, anal fissures, radiation proctitis, AD, *PD,* acne, **psoriasis, lichen planus, burns,** wounds, pressure ulcers, diabetic foot ulcers, wrinkle and striae reduction, Hashimoto's thyroiditis, inflammation, HIV, cancer	**Systematic review: beneficial for IBS**
Bacopa *Bacopa monnieri*	*Gastric ulcer,* hepatic encephalopathy, IBS-D, *seizures,* memory impairment, **dementia-related anxiety,** test anxiety, **cognitive performance,** ADHD, inflammation	Human research: improves IBS-D in combination formula
Chamomile *Matricaria chamomilla/ recutita*	Gingivitis, mucositis, chronic rhinosinusitis, *allergies,* dyslipidemia, diabetes, *PUD,* colic, IBS, diarrhea, dyspepsia, UC, *candida vaginitis,* menopause, carpal tunnel syndrome, anxiety, insomnia, depression, ADHD, eczema, wounds, radiation or chemotherapy dermatitis, cortisol dysregulation, *inflammation, broadly antimicrobial (bacteria, yeast, fungus), cancer*	Human research: improves diarrhea in combination formula
Coleus *Coleus forskohlii*	Glaucoma, *allergy,* asthma, HTN, CHF, *insulin resistance,* obesity, *pancreatic exocrine insufficiency, diarrhea, UTI, urge incontinence, dysmenorrhea, male infertility,* male hypogonadism, subarachnoid hemorrhage, *seizure, neurodegenerative disorders, alcohol abuse,* psoriasis, *photoprotection, hyperthyroidism, cancer*	*Preclinical research: improves diarrhea better than loperamide*
Cranberry *Vaccinium macrocarpon*	Gingivitis, dyslipidemia, **DM,** PUD, gut dysbiosis, overactive bladder, **UTI,** postradiation UTI, BPH, chronic prostatitis, RA, *inflammation, influenza,* prostate CA	Human research: reverses gut flora imbalance from a meat diet
Elder (berry, flower) *Sambucus nigra*	Gingival recession, ASCVD, *dyslipidemia, DM,* obesity, constipation, stroke, *immune function,* **URI,** rhinosinusitis, influenza, *HIV, HSV, Strep, cancer*	*Preclinical research: has laxative effects* Human research: laxative effects in combination formula
Fennel *Foeniculum vulgare*	*Glaucoma, dyspepsia, gastroprotection, gastroparesis,* **infant colic,** IBS, constipation, *overactive bladder, lactation,* dysmenorrhea, oligomenorrhea, **menopausal disorders,** dementia, hirsutism, *inflammation*	*Preclinical research: antispasmodic activity* Human research: improves constipation in combination formulas
Frankincense/ Boswellia *Boswellia serrata, sacra, carterii*	Gingivitis, **asthma,** *COPD,* UC, **Crohn's, collagenous colitis,** IBS, UTI, SUI, benign breast disease, menorrhagia, **OA,** stroke, memory impairment, psoriasis, eczema, aging skin, athletic performance, **RA, IBD,** *inflammation,* glioma radiation, chemo-related neuropathy, *cancer*	Human research: improves IBS with less SEs
Lemon balm *Melissa officinalis*	**Bruxism,** dyslipidemia, DM, palpitations, dyspepsia, IBS, **colic,** PMS, dysmenorrhea, female sexual dysfunction, **AD,** dementia, agitation, *diabetic neuropathy,* insomnia, **anxiety,** depression, **ADHD,** *hyperthyroidism, Graves' disease,* herpes simplex, *cancer, glioblastoma multiforme*	Human research: reduces IBS in combination formula

	TABLE 11.E	
Functional Bowel Disorders: Constipation, Diarrhea, and Irritable Bowel Syndrome. *(Continued)*		
Common Name/ Latin Name	**Scope of Potential Benefits**	**Comments**
Motherwort *Leonurus cardiaca*	*HTN 2/2 anxiety or hyperthyroidism, dyslipidemia, CAD, arrhythmia, nausea, IBS, AKI, lactation, postpartum bleeding, menorrhagia, amenorrhea,* menopause, *pain, stroke,* anxiety, insomnia, hyperthyroidism; inflammation; breast tumors*	*Preclinical research: antagonizes 5HT-3A receptors*
Peppermint *Mentha x piperita*	Oral health, weight reduction, nausea, dyspepsia, **IBS**, GI endoscopy, cracked nipples, PCOS, neck pain, tension headaches, postherpetic neuralgia, cognition, nicotine withdrawal, pressure ulcers, pruritis gravidarum, hirsutism, athletic performance, URI, *cancer*	**Systematic reviews: beneficial for IBS, better than antispasmodics; NNT 3-4** Human research: improves functional abdominal pain, IBS, colic; reduces colonoscopic spasms; enteric coated better tolerated
Tribulus/Puncture vine/Goathead *Tribulus terrestris*	HTN, CAD, dyslipidemia, DM, *hepatotoxicity, IBS, nephrolithiasis,* **sexual dysfunction**, hypoactive sexual desire, *pain, anxiety, depression, inflammation, cancer*	*Preclinical research: antispasmodic in rabbit jejunum*
Valerian *Valeriana officinalis*	*HTN, CAD, IBS,* PMS, dysmenorrhea, **menopause,** tension HA, RLS, cognitive, anxiety, insomnia, OCD, *cancer*	*Preclinical research: direct musculotropic GI antispasmodic*
Yarrow *Achillea millefolium*	*Epistaxis, asthma,* HTN, **dyslipidemia,** *T1DM, cirrhosis, gastritis, PUD, anorexia, IBS, IBD,* nipple fissures, candida vaginitis, dysmenorrhea, *menorrhagia, menopause, anxiety, neurodegenerative disorders,* multiple sclerosis, *inflammation*	*Preclinical research: antispasmodic, antiinflammatory properties*

12

NEPHROLOGICAL AND UROLOGICAL DISORDERS

▪ ▪ ▪ ▪ ▪ ▪ ▪ ▪ ▪ ▪ ▪ ▪ ▪ ▪ ▪ ▪ ▪

TABLE 12.A		
Renal Disorders: Nephropathy, Nephrosis, Nephritis, Renal Fibrosis, and Acute Kidney Injury.		
Common Name/Latin Name	**Scope of Potential Benefits**	**Comments**
Astragalus *Astragalus membranaceus*	Herpes keratitis, recurrent tonsillitis, allergic rhinitis, atopy, asthma, **viral myocarditis**, CHF, CAD, viral hepatitis, **diabetic nephropathy**, IgA nephropathy, nephrotic syndrome, lupus nephritis, *renal fibrosis, sperm quality*, hemorrhagic stroke, burns, *wound healing, age spots, leukopenia,* **immune function**, *antiviral*, HBV, TB, **NSCLC,** cancer	*Preclinical research: prevents renal fibrosis in combination with dong quai* **Systematic reviews: beneficial in diabetic nephropathy** Human research: improves diabetic nephropathy, IgA nephropathy, nephrotic syndrome, and lupus nephritis
Black seed/nigella/black cumin *Nigella sativa*	Periodontal dz, oral submucous fibrosis, chronic rhinosinusitis, nasal dryness, **allergy, asthma**, COPD, chemical pneumonitis, **HTN**, *CAD*, CHF, **dyslipidemia, DM, obesity**, NAFLD, dyspepsia, PUD, diabetic nephropathy, mastalgia, menopause, male infertility, OA, *stroke*, seizure disorder, memory impairment, cognition, anxiety, *depression*, acne, eczema, vitiligo, immune function, Hashimoto's thyroiditis, RA, inflammation, *H. pylori, Staph* pustules, HCV, cancer	Human research: improves creatinine, urinary albumin, and GFR in T2DM
Burdock *Arctium lappa*	*Dyslipidemia*, diabetes, *hepatic function and protection, gastroparesis, dyspepsia*, diverticulitis, diabetic nephropathy, OA, wrinkles, acne, cough, *inflammation, influenza A, cancer*	Human research: burdock fruit extract plus astragalus reduced urinary protein and albumin
Dong quai *Angelica sinensis*	Pulmonary HTN, *HTN*, CAD, *atrial fibrillation*, cirrhosis, portal HTN, abd pain, UC, *renal fibrosis, dysmenorrhea*, menopausal symptoms, *osteoporosis, OA*, stroke, *cerebrovascular insufficiency, neurodegenerative disorders, wound healing, aging skin, alopecia, stamina, inflammation*, anemia of chronic disease, cancer	*Preclinical research: prevents renal fibrosis in combination with astragalus* Human case report: improved recombinant human erythropoietin-resistant anemia of chronic disease
Fenugreek *Trigonella foenum-graecum*	Dyslipidemia, **DM,** prediabetes, *diabetic nephropathy, urolithiasis*, lactation, dysmenorrhea, PCOS, menopause, male sexual dysfunction, hypogonadism, PD, *peripheral neuropathy, thyroid T3/T4 balance*, stamina, *cancer*	*Preclinical research: protective against diabetic nephropathy*

Continued on following page

TABLE 12.A
Renal Disorders: Nephropathy, Nephrosis, Nephritis, Renal Fibrosis, and Acute Kidney Injury. *(Continued)*

Common Name/Latin Name	Scope of Potential Benefits	Comments
Ginkgo *Ginkgo biloba*	*Cataracts*, ARMD, glaucoma, periodontal dz, **vertigo, tinnitus, cardiovascular health, dyslipidemia, diabetes,** obesity, claudication, hepatic fibrosis, **diabetic nephropathy**, menopausal sexual desire, **acute mountain sickness**, migraines with aura, **stroke, MCI, dementias,** postoperative delirium, depression, ADHD, **schizophrenia, tardive dyskinesia,** aging skin, *inflammation, cancer*	**Systematic review: improves early diabetic nephropathy**
Horsetail *Equisetum arvense*	*Diabetes*, nephrolithiasis, *UTI, interstitial cystitis*, BPH, osteoporosis, *OA*, RA, *chronic pain, anxiety, cognition,* psoriatic nails, wound healing, aging skin, alopecia, inflammation	*Preclinical research: reduces microcalcifications and renal fibrosis*
Milk thistle *Silybum marianum*	**Dyslipidemia, DM, liver disease**, diabetic nephropathy, lactation, *PCOS*, BPH, *gout, AD, diabetic neuropathy*, **OCD**, acne, *psoriasis*, vitiligo, radio-dermatitis, aging skin, RA, inflammation, hepatitis viruses, **iron-overload**, chemotherapy and radiotherapy toxicity, *hepatocellular carcinoma*	*Preclinical research: protects against diabetic nephropathy* Human research: reduces urinary excretion of albumin, TNF-α, and MDA
Motherwort *Leonurus cardiaca*	*HTN 2/2 anxiety or hyperthyroidism, dyslipidemia, CAD, arrhythmia, nausea, IBS, AKI, lactation, postpartum bleeding, menorrhagia, amenorrhea,* menopause, *pain, stroke,* anxiety, *insomnia, hyperthyroidism; inflammation; breast tumors*	*Preclinical research: protects against AKI via antiinflammatory and antioxidant mechanisms*
Saffron *Crocus sativus*	ARMD, *cataracts*, diabetic maculopathy, glaucoma, gingivitis, burning mouth syndrome, *allergy*, asthma, HTN, **dyslipidemia**, DM, **obesity**, *hepatotoxicity, DM nephropathy*, PMS, menopause, **female and male sexual dysfunction**, male infertility, chronic pain, fibromyalgia, stroke, AD, **anxiety**, insomnia, OCD, **depression**, ADHD, drug and ETOH addiction, *photodamage*, stamina, immune function, inflammation, RA, *bacterial infection*, cancer	*Preclinical research: reduces urine volume and BUN in diabetic model*
Stinging nettle *Urtica dioica*	Allergic rhinitis, HTN, dyslipidemia, **DM**, NAFLD, *colitis, nephrotoxicity*, menopause, **BPH**, prostatitis, OA, inflammation, *prostate cancer, cisplatin toxicity*	*Preclinical research: renal sparing*
Turmeric (or curcumin) *Curcuma longa*	Anterior uveitis, **oral lichen planus, gingivitis,** dental surgery, submucous fibrosis, asthma, **diastolic HTN, dyslipidemia,** CAD, endothelial dysfunction, **DM,** obesity, **NAFLD,** hepatoprotective, gallbladder dyskinesia, *GERD*, PUD, dyspepsia, **UC**, DM nephropathy, lupus nephritis, lactational mastitis, LSIL, chronic nonbacterial prostatitis, postoperative pain, **OA,** RA, migraine HA, *neurodegeneration*, **anxiety, depression, skin disease**, psoriasis, fatigue, **systemic inflammation,** *HIV,* **chemo-related oral mucositis,** cancer prevention, cancer treatment	Human research: reduces posttransplant rejection; improves diabetic nephropathy; reduces proteinuria and hematuria in lupus nephritis; reduces SBP in lupus nephritis

	TABLE 12.B	
	Nephrolithiasis.	
Common Name/Latin Name	**Scope of Potential Benefits**	**Comments**
Fenugreek *Trigonella foenum-graecum*	Dyslipidemia, **DM,** prediabetes, *diabetic nephropathy, urolithiasis,* lactation, dysmenorrhea, PCOS, menopause, male sexual dysfunction, hypogonadism, PD, *peripheral neuropathy, thyroid T3/T4 balance,* stamina, *cancer*	*Preclinical research: protective against urolithiasis*
Horsetail *Equisetum arvense*	*Diabetes,* nephrolithiasis, *UTI, interstitial cystitis,* BPH, osteoporosis, *OA, RA, chronic pain, anxiety, cognition,* psoriatic nails, wound healing, aging skin, alopecia, inflammation	*Preclinical research: combination formula lowers Ca-oxalate excretion and reduces microcalcifications and renal fibrosis* Human research: diuretic properties on par with HCTZ; reduces urinary uric acid crystals
Tribulus/Puncture vine/Goathead *Tribulus terrestris*	HTN, CAD, dyslipidemia, DM, *hepatotoxicity, IBS, nephrolithiasis,* **sexual dysfunction,** hypoactive sexual desire, *pain, anxiety, depression, inflammation, cancer*	*Preclinical research: reduces stone formation, promotes expulsion*

	TABLE 12.C	
	Bladder Disorders: Overactive Bladder, Urge Incontinence and Stress Urinary Incontinence.	
Common Name/Latin Name	**Scope of Potential Benefits**	**Comments**
Butterbur *Petasites hybridus*	**Allergic rhinitis,** asthma, *HTN, GI ulceration,* bladder spasms, **migraine headache,** *neurodegenerative dementias,* somatoform disorder anxiety and depression, *CNS inflammation*	Human research: in small trial, lengthened voiding intervals in women with overactive bladder
Coleus *Coleus forskohlii*	Glaucoma, *allergy,* asthma, HTN, CHF, *insulin resistance,* obesity, *pancreatic exocrine insufficiency, diarrhea, UTI, urge incontinence, dysmenorrhea, male infertility,* male hypogonadism, subarachnoid hemorrhage, *seizure, neurodegenerative disorders, alcohol abuse,* psoriasis, *photoprotection, hyperthyroidism, cancer*	*Preclinical research: relaxes detrusor muscle*
Cranberry *Vaccinium macrocarpon*	Gingivitis, dyslipidemia, **DM**, PUD, gut dysbiosis, overactive bladder, **UTI**, postradiation UTI, BPH, chronic prostatitis, RA, *inflammation, influenza,* prostate CA	Human research: reduces OAB symptoms in women
Fennel *Foeniculum vulgare*	*Glaucoma, dyspepsia, gastroprotection, gastroparesis,* **infant colic,** IBS, constipation, *overactive bladder, lactation,* dysmenorrhea, oligomenorrhea, **menopausal disorders,** *dementia,* hirsutism, *inflammation*	*Preclinical research: bladder smooth muscle relaxant*
Frankincense/Boswellia *Boswellia serrata, sacra, carterii*	Gingivitis, **asthma,** *COPD,* UC, **Crohn's, collagenous colitis,** IBS, UTI, SUI, benign breast disease, menorrhagia, **OA,** stroke, memory impairment, psoriasis, eczema, aging skin, athletic performance, **RA, IBD,** *inflammation,* glioma radiation, chemo-related neuropathy, *cancer*	Human research: combined with *Cyperus scariosus,* reduces SUI.
Saw palmetto *Serenoa repens*	*Overactive bladder, female hirsutism,* PCOS, **BPH**, chronic inflammatory prostatitis, male pattern alopecia, *inflammation*	*Preclinical research: antispasmodic and antiinflammatory activities in bladder; antimuscarinic* **(Caution: contraindicated in pregnancy due to antiandrogen properties)**

TABLE 12.D

Infection: Urinary Tract Infection and Recurrent Urinary Tract Infection.

Common Name/ Latin Name	Scope of Potential Benefits	Comments
Coleus *Coleus forskohlii*	Glaucoma, *allergy*, asthma, HTN, CHF, *insulin resistance, obesity, pancreatic exocrine insufficiency, diarrhea, UTI, urge incontinence, dysmenorrhea, male infertility,* male hypogonadism, subarachnoid hemorrhage, *seizure, neurodegenerative disorders, alcohol abuse,* psoriasis, *photoprotection, hyperthyroidism, cancer*	*Preclinical research: causes bladder epithelium to eject uropathogenic E. coli*
Cranberry *Vaccinium macrocarpon*	Gingivitis, dyslipidemia, **DM**, PUD, gut dysbiosis, overactive bladder, **UTI**, postradiation UTI, BPH, chronic prostatitis, RA, *inflammation, influenza,* prostate CA	*Preclinical research: antiadhesion activity for uropathogenic E. coli, Proteus, Pseudomonas; reduces adhesion of E. coli to vaginal epithelium* **Systematic reviews: prevents UTI recurrence; variably noninferior to antibiotics for prevention; some inconsistencies** Human research: for recurrent UTI but not bacteriuria; less antibiotic resistance; prevents UTIs associated with BPH or catheters
Frankincense/Boswellia *Boswellia serrata, sacra, carterii*	Gingivitis, **asthma**, *COPD*, UC, **Crohn's, collagenous colitis**, IBS, UTI, SUI, benign breast disease, menorrhagia, **OA**, stroke, memory impairment, psoriasis, eczema, aging skin, athletic performance, **RA, IBD**, *inflammation,* glioma radiation, chemo-related neuropathy, *cancer*	Human research: polyherbal product improves QOL with UTI over antibiotic, but does not clear microbes compared to antibiotic; may be useful as adjunct
Horsetail *Equisetum arvense*	*Diabetes*, nephrolithiasis, *UTI, interstitial cystitis*, BPH, osteoporosis, OA, RA, *chronic pain, anxiety, cognition,* psoriatic nails, wound healing, aging skin, alopecia, inflammation	Traditional use: recurrent UTI, interstitial cystitis
Uva ursi *Arctostaphylos uva-ursi*	*UTI*, recurrent UTI, *dementia, dermatitis, skin hyperpigmentation, cough*	*Preclinical research: antibacterial; prevents bacterial urothelial adhesion* Traditional use: prevention and treatment of UTI Human research: reduces recurrence of UTIs

13 WOMEN'S BREAST AND GENITOURINARY DISORDERS

■ ■ ■ ■ ■ ■ ■ ■ ■ ■ ■ ■ ■ ■ ■ ■ ■

TABLE 13.A		
Breast and Lactation Disorders.		
Common Name/ Latin Name	**Scope of Potential Benefits**	**Comments**
Frankincense/Boswellia *Boswellia serrata, sacra, carterii*	Gingivitis, **asthma**, *COPD*, UC, **Crohn's**, **collagenous colitis**, IBS, UTI, SUI, benign breast disease, menorrhagia, **OA**, stroke, memory impairment, psoriasis, eczema, aging skin, athletic performance, **RA, IBD**, *inflammation*, glioma radiation, chemo-related neuropathy, *cancer*	Human research: reduces fibrocystic changes, fibroadenoma volume and breast density in combination formula
Black cohosh *Actaea racemosa/ Cimicifuga racemosa*	Breast density, uterine fibroids, female infertility, PCOS, **menopausal syndrome**, osteoporosis, breast cancer	Human research: does not increase breast density caused by other SERMs
Black seed/nigella/ black cumin *Nigella sativa*	Periodontal dz, oral submucous fibrosis, chronic rhinosinusitis, nasal dryness, **allergy, asthma**, COPD, chemical pneumonitis, **HTN**, *CAD*, CHF, **dyslipidemia, DM, obesity**, NAFLD, dyspepsia, PUD, diabetic nephropathy, mastalgia, menopause, male infertility, OA, *stroke*, seizure disorder, memory impairment, cognition, anxiety, *depression*, acne, eczema, vitiligo, immune function, Hashimoto's thyroiditis, RA, inflammation, *H. pylori, Staph* pustules, HCV, cancer	Human research: comparable to topical diclofenac for cyclical mastalgia
Calendula *Calendula officinalis*	Gingivitis, dental plaque, radiation mucositis, venous ulcers, lactational cracked nipples, vaginal candidiasis, episiotomy healing, nonbacterial prostatitis, diaper dermatitis, **wound healing**, diabetic foot ulcers, *antibacterial, anti-HIV*, radiation dermatitis	Human research: heals cracked nipples
Chasteberry/Chaste tree/Vitex *Vitex agnus-castus*	**Cyclical mastalgia, PMS, PMDD**, oligomenorrhea, amenorrhea, IUD bleeding, **female infertility**, perimenopause, menstrual migraines, bone healing, insomnia, *inflammation, pain*	**Systematic review: comparable to bromocriptine for cyclical mastalgia** Human research: comparable to flurbiprofen for cyclical mastalgia
Fennel *Foeniculum vulgare*	*Glaucoma, dyspepsia, gastroprotection, gastroparesis,* **infant colic**, IBS, constipation, *overactive bladder, lactation,* dysmenorrhea, oligomenorrhea, **menopausal disorders**, *dementia*, hirsutism, *inflammation*	*Preclinical research: increases lactation* Traditional use: lactation; caution with dosing

Continued on following page

TABLE 13.A
Breast and Lactation Disorders. *(Continued)*

Common Name/ Latin Name	Scope of Potential Benefits	Comments
Fenugreek *Trigonella foenum-graecum*	Dyslipidemia, **DM,** prediabetes, *diabetic nephropathy, urolithiasis,* lactation, dysmenorrhea, PCOS, menopause, male sexual dysfunction, hypogonadism, PD, *peripheral neuropathy, thyroid T3/T4 balance,* stamina, *cancer*	Human research: improves lactational insufficiency
Licorice *Glycyrrhiza glabra*	**Postoperative sore throat,** xerostomia, radiation-induced mucositis, aphthous ulcers, *allergy,* **asthma, dyslipidemia,** CAD, *diabetes,* **obesity,** hepatoprotection, heartburn, PUD, functional dyspepsia, **antipsychotic-induced hyperprolactinemia,** menopause, atrophic vaginitis, PCOS, female hirsutism, BPH, *stroke, dementia,* PD, *anxiety, insomnia, depression, substance addiction,* **hyperpigmentation, atopic eczema,** Addison's disease, *stamina, multiple sclerosis, inflammation, H. pylori,* cancer, *breast cancer*	**Systematic review: reduces antipsychotic-induced hyperprolactinemia in combination with peony *(Caution: use deglycyrrhizinated formulations in patients at risk for HTN and hypokalemia)***
Milk thistle *Silybum marianum*	**Dyslipidemia, DM, liver disease,** diabetic nephropathy, lactation, *PCOS,* BPH, *gout, AD, diabetic neuropathy,* **OCD,** acne, *psoriasis,* vitiligo, radio-dermatitis, aging skin, RA, inflammation, hepatitis viruses, **iron-overload,** chemotherapy and radiotherapy toxicity, *hepatocellular carcinoma*	Human research: increases milk production 85%
Motherwort *Leonurus cardiaca*	*HTN 2/2 anxiety or hyperthyroidism, dyslipidemia, CAD, arrhythmia, nausea, IBS, AKI, lactation, postpartum bleeding, menorrhagia, amenorrhea, menopause, pain, stroke, anxiety, insomnia, hyperthyroidism, inflammation, breast tumors*	Traditional use: lactation promotion
Peppermint *Mentha x piperita*	Oral health, weight reduction, nausea, dyspepsia, **IBS,** GI endoscopy, cracked nipples, PCOS, neck pain, tension headaches, postherpetic neuralgia, cognition, nicotine withdrawal, pressure ulcers, pruritis gravidarum, hirsutism, athletic performance, URI, *cancer*	Human research: topical application reduces pruritis gravidarum; prevents nipple cracks and pain with lactation (better than lanolin or expressed breast milk)
Turmeric (or curcumin) *Curcuma longa*	Anterior uveitis, **oral lichen planus, gingivitis,** dental surgery, submucous fibrosis, asthma, **diastolic HTN, dyslipidemia,** CAD, endothelial dysfunction, **DM,** obesity, **NAFLD,** hepatoprotective, gallbladder dyskinesia, *GERD,* PUD, dyspepsia, **UC,** DM nephropathy, lupus nephritis, lactational mastitis, LSIL, chronic nonbacterial prostatitis, postoperative pain, **OA,** RA, migraine HA, *neurodegeneration,* **anxiety, depression, skin disease,** psoriasis, fatigue, **systemic inflammation,** *HIV,* **chemo-related oral mucositis,** cancer prevention, cancer treatment	Human research: topical formula improves lactational mastitis
Yarrow *Achillea millefolium*	*Epistaxis, asthma,* HTN, **dyslipidemia,** *T1DM,* cirrhosis, *gastritis, PUD, anorexia, IBS, IBD,* nipple fissures, candida vaginitis, dysmenorrhea, *menorrhagia, menopause, anxiety, neurodegenerative disorders,* multiple sclerosis, *inflammation*	Human research: heals breastfeeding nipple fissures comparable to honey or breastmilk

TABLE 13.B		
Premenstrual Syndrome, Premenstrual Dysphoric Disorder, and Dysmenorrhea.		
Common Name/ Latin Name	**Scope of Potential Benefits**	**Comments**
Andrographis *Andrographis paniculata*	*HTN, hepatoprotection,* ulcerative colitis, *dysmenorrhea,* OA, RA, FMF, *inflammation,* **URI prevention and treatment,** *cancer*	*Preclinical research: relaxes uterine muscle*
Chasteberry/Chaste tree/Vitex *Vitex agnus-castus*	**Cyclical mastalgia, PMS, PMDD,** oligomenorrhea, amenorrhea, IUD bleeding, **female infertility,** perimenopause, menstrual migraines, bone healing, insomnia, *inflammation, pain*	**Systematic review: beneficial in PMS and PMDD; comparable to fluoxetine** Human research: optimal dose 20 mg/ day for PMS/PMDD; most effective on physical symptoms of PMS; improves over 3 mos
Coleus *Coleus forskohlii*	Glaucoma, *allergy,* asthma, HTN, CHF, *insulin resistance,* obesity, *pancreatic exocrine insufficiency, diarrhea, UTI, urge incontinence, dysmenorrhea, male infertility,* male hypogonadism, subarachnoid hemorrhage, *seizure, neurodegenerative disorders, alcohol abuse,* psoriasis, *photoprotection, hyperthyroidism, cancer*	*Preclinical research: relaxes uterine muscle*
Dong quai *Angelica sinensis*	Pulmonary HTN, *HTN,* CAD, *atrial fibrillation,* cirrhosis, portal HTN, abd pain, UC, *renal fibrosis, dysmenorrhea,* menopausal symptoms, *osteoporosis, OA,* stroke, *cerebrovascular insufficiency, neurodegenerative disorders, wound healing, aging skin, alopecia, stamina, inflammation,* anemia of chronic disease, cancer	*Preclinical research: relaxes uterine muscle*
Fennel *Foeniculum vulgare*	*Glaucoma, dyspepsia, gastroprotection, gastroparesis,* **infant colic,** IBS, constipation, *overactive bladder, lactation,* dysmenorrhea, oligomenorrhea, **menopausal disorders,** *dementia,* hirsutism, *inflammation*	*Preclinical research: relaxes uterine muscle* Human research: reduces primary dysmenorrhea
Fenugreek *Trigonella foenum-graecum*	Dyslipidemia, **DM,** prediabetes, *diabetic nephropathy, urolithiasis,* lactation, dysmenorrhea, PCOS, menopause, male sexual dysfunction, hypogonadism, PD, *peripheral neuropathy, thyroid T3/T4 balance,* stamina, *cancer*	Human research: reduces dysmenorrhea
Ginger *Zingiber officinale*	**Motion sickness,** *HTN,* dyslipidemia, fibrinolysis, diabetes, **nausea, vomiting,** *dyspepsia,* gastroparesis, *PUD,* ulcerative colitis, *diabetic nephropathy,* **dysmenorrhea,** *Candida vaginitis,* male infertility, OA, muscle injury, migraine HA, *AD,* **inflammation,** RA, *H. pylori, antibacterial,* **CINV,** cancer	**Systematic review: beneficial for primary dysmenorrhea** Human research: reduces menstrual pain comparable to NSAIDs
Lavender *Lavandula* spp.	**Dysmenorrhea, anxiety, insomnia, depression, wound healing**	Mousavi Kani et al. (2019)
Lemon balm *Melissa officinalis*	**Bruxism,** dyslipidemia, DM, palpitations, dyspepsia, IBS, **colic,** PMS, dysmenorrhea, female sexual dysfunction, **AD,** dementia, agitation, *diabetic neuropathy,* insomnia, **anxiety,** depression, **ADHD,** hyperthyroidism, *Graves' disease,* herpes simplex, *cancer, glioblastoma multiforme*	Human research: reduces PMS symptoms; reduces dysmenorrhea better than mefenamic acid

Continued on following page

TABLE 13.B
Premenstrual Syndrome, Premenstrual Dysphoric Disorder, and Dysmenorrhea. *(Continued)*

Common Name/ Latin Name	Scope of Potential Benefits	Comments
Saffron *Crocus sativus*	ARMD, *cataracts*, diabetic maculopathy, glaucoma, gingivitis, burning mouth syndrome, *allergy*, asthma, HTN, **dyslipidemia**, DM, **obesity**, *hepatotoxicity, DM nephropathy*, PMS, menopause, **female and male sexual dysfunction**, male infertility, chronic pain, fibromyalgia, stroke, AD, **anxiety**, insomnia, OCD, **depression**, ADHD, drug and ETOH addiction, *photodamage*, stamina, immune function, inflammation, RA, *bacterial infection*, cancer	Human research: improves PMS (NNT = 1.5); aroma decreases cortisol, increases estradiol
St. John's Wort *Hypericum perforatum*	PMS, **perimenopause or menopause**, *chronic pain*, neuropathy, **depression,** *opiate addiction*, psoriasis, atopic dermatitis, *sunburn*, inflammation, HSV, *cancer*	Human research: improves physical and behavioral symptoms of PMS but not mood ***See St. John's Wort monograph warnings and precautions***
Valerian *Valeriana officinalis*	*HTN, CAD, IBS*, PMS, dysmenorrhea, **menopause**, tension HA, RLS, cognitive, anxiety, insomnia, OCD, *cancer*	Human research: reduces PMS symptoms; reduces dysmenorrhea
Yarrow *Achillea millefolium*	*Epistaxis, asthma*, HTN, **dyslipidemia**, *T1DM*, cirrhosis, *gastritis, PUD, anorexia, IBS, IBD*, dysmenorrhea, *menorrhagia, menopause, anxiety, neurodegenerative disorders,* multiple sclerosis, *inflammation*	*Preclinical research: antiinflammatory properties* Human research: reduces pain intensity and duration in primary dysmenorrhea

TABLE 13.C
Vaginal Disorders: Vaginitis and Vaginosis (See Table 13.F for Atrophic Disorders).

Common Name/ Latin Name	Scope of Potential Benefits	Comments
Calendula *Calendula officinalis*	Gingivitis, dental plaque, radiation mucositis, venous ulcers, lactational cracked nipples, vaginal candidiasis, episiotomy healing, nonbacterial prostatitis, diaper dermatitis, **wound healing**, diabetic foot ulcers, *antibacterial, anti-HIV*, radiation dermatitis	Human research: slower but longer lasting benefit than clotrimazole in vaginal candidiasis; improves menopausal vulvovaginal atrophy (with probiotic and lactic acid); faster healing of episiotomy
Chamomile *Matricaria chamomilla/ recutita*	Gingivitis, mucositis, chronic rhinosinusitis, *allergies*, dyslipidemia, diabetes, *PUD*, colic, IBS, diarrhea, dyspepsia, UC, *candida vaginitis*, menopause, carpal tunnel syndrome, anxiety, insomnia, depression, ADHD, eczema, wounds, radiation or chemotherapy dermatitis, cortisol dysregulation, *inflammation, broadly antimicrobial (bacteria, yeast, fungus), cancer*	*Preclinical research: activity against candida albicans*
Cranberry *Vaccinium macrocarpon*	Gingivitis, dyslipidemia, **DM**, PUD, gut dysbiosis, overactive bladder, **UTI**, postradiation UTI, BPH, chronic prostatitis, RA, *inflammation, influenza,* prostate CA	*Preclinical research: reduces adhesion of E. coli to vaginal epithelium*
Echinacea *Echinacea purpurea, angustifolia*	Anterior uveitis, *candida vaginitis*, genital condylomas, OA, **anxiety**, eczema, athletic performance, immune function, inflammation, **URIs,** influenza, *Coronavirus*, HPV, *colorectal cancer*	*Preclinical research: activity against C. albicans* Human research: reduces recurrence of genital condylomas

TABLE 13.C

Vaginal Disorders: Vaginitis and Vaginosis (See Table 13.F for Atrophic Disorders). *(Continued)*

Common Name/ Latin Name	Scope of Potential Benefits	Comments
Elder (berry, flower) *Sambucus nigra*	Gingival recession, ASCVD, *dyslipidemia, DM,* obesity, constipation, stroke, *immune function,* **URI,** rhinosinusitis, influenza, *HIV, HSV, Strep, cancer*	*Preclinical research: activity against HSV*
Ginger *Zingiber officinale*	**Motion sickness,** HTN, dyslipidemia, fibrinolysis, diabetes, **nausea, vomiting,** *dyspepsia,* gastroparesis, *PUD,* ulcerative colitis, *diabetic nephropathy,* **dysmenorrhea,** *Candida vaginitis,* male infertility, OA, muscle injury, migraine HA, *AD,* **inflammation,** RA, *H. pylori, antibacterial,* **CINV,** cancer	*Preclinical research: activity against C. albicans*
Mullein *Verbascum thapsus*	Otalgia, otitis media, asthma, bronchitis, cough, diarrhea, trichomoniasis, dermatitis, influenza, HSV, TB	Human ex vivo research: Activity against *T. vaginalis*
Yarrow *Achillea millefolium*	*Epistaxis, asthma,* HTN, **dyslipidemia,** *T1DM,* cirrhosis, *gastritis, PUD, anorexia, IBS, IBD,* nipple fissures, candida vaginitis, dysmenorrhea, *menorrhagia, menopause, anxiety, neurodegenerative disorders,* multiple sclerosis, *inflammation*	Human research: reduces symptoms and eliminates *C. albicans*; inferior to clotrimazole

TABLE 13.D

Disorders of Cervix and Uterus: Cervical Neoplasia, Abnormal Uterine Bleeding, and Endometriosis.

Common Name/ Latin Name	Scope of Potential Benefits	Comments
Black cohosh *Actaea racemosa/Cimicifuga racemosa*	Breast density, uterine fibroids, female infertility, PCOS, **menopausal syndrome,** osteoporosis, breast cancer	Human research: reduces uterine fibroma size, comparable to tibolone
Chasteberry/Chaste tree/ Vitex *Vitex agnus-castus*	**Cyclical mastalgia, PMS, PMDD,** oligomenorrhea, amenorrhea, IUD bleeding, **female infertility,** perimenopause, menstrual migraines, bone healing, insomnia, *inflammation, pain*	Human research: comparable to mefenamic acid by month 4 for IUD-induced bleeding; reduces amenorrhea and oligomenorrhea
Echinacea *Echinacea purpurea/ angustifolia*	Anterior uveitis, *candida vaginitis,* genital condylomas, OA, **anxiety,** eczema, athletic performance, immune function, inflammation, **URIs,** influenza, *Coronavirus,* HPV, *colorectal cancer*	Human research: prevents recurrence of genital condylomas
Frankincense/Boswellia *Boswellia serrata, sacra, carterii*	Gingivitis, **asthma,** COPD, UC, **Crohn's, collagenous colitis,** IBS, UTI, SUI, benign breast disease, menorrhagia, **OA,** stroke, memory impairment, psoriasis, eczema, aging skin, athletic performance, **RA, IBD,** *inflammation,* glioma radiation, chemo-related neuropathy, *cancer*	Human research: synergistic with ibuprofen for menorrhagia
Motherwort *Leonurus cardiaca*	HTN 2/2 anxiety or hyperthyroidism, dyslipidemia, CAD, *arrhythmia, nausea, IBS, AKI, lactation, postpartum bleeding, menorrhagia, amenorrhea,* menopause, *pain,* stroke, anxiety, *insomnia, hyperthyroidism, inflammation, breast tumors*	*Preclinical research: contains uterotonic alkaloids; reduces uterine adenomyosis* Human research: increases postpartum uterine tone; enhances oxytocin

Continued on following page

TABLE 13.D

Disorders of Cervix and Uterus: Cervical Neoplasia, Abnormal Uterine Bleeding, and Endometriosis. *(Continued)*

Common Name/ Latin Name	Scope of Potential Benefits	Comments
Rhodiola *Rhodiola rosea*	**CAD,** *menorrhagia, amenorrhea, female infertility,* menopause, *male hypogonadism,* premature ejaculation, **anxiety**, **depression**, **cognition**, eczema, burnout, fatigue, **athletic stamina**, cancer	*Preclinical research: demonstrates antiestrogenic effects via competitive estrogen receptor binding*
Turmeric (or curcumin) *Curcuma longa*	Anterior uveitis, **oral lichen planus, gingivitis,** dental surgery, submucous fibrosis, asthma, **diastolic HTN**, **dyslipidemia**, CAD, endothelial dysfunction, **DM**, obesity, **NAFLD**, hepatoprotective, gallbladder dyskinesia, *GERD*, PUD, dyspepsia, **UC**, DM nephropathy, lupus nephritis, lactational mastitis, LSIL, chronic nonbacterial prostatitis, postoperative pain, **OA**, RA, migraine HA, *neurodegeneration*, **anxiety, depression, skin disease**, psoriasis, fatigue, **systemic inflammation**, *HIV,* **chemo-related oral mucositis**, cancer prevention, cancer treatment	Human research: 12 weeks of oil extract normalizes LSIL, lasting 36 moths; reduces postoperative pain in gyn laparoscopic surgery
Yarrow *Achillea millefolium*	*Epistaxis, asthma,* HTN, **dyslipidemia,** *T1DM,* cirrhosis, *gastritis, PUD, anorexia, IBS, IBD,* dysmenorrhea, *menorrhagia, menopause, anxiety, neurodegenerative disorders,* multiple sclerosis, *inflammation*	*Preclinical research: antihemorrhagic properties* Human research: reduces hemorrhagic propensity in CKD Traditional use: menorrhagia

TABLE 13.E

Ovarian Disorders: Polycystic Ovary Syndrome, Oligomenorrhea, Amenorrhea, and Female Infertility.

Common Name/ Latin Name	Scope of Potential Benefits	Comments
Black cohosh *Actaea racemosa/ Cimicifuga racemosa*	Breast density, uterine fibroids, female infertility, PCOS, **menopausal syndrome**, osteoporosis, breast cancer	Human research: female infertility with PCOS (out-performed clomiphene); improves outcomes with clomiphene
Chasteberry/Chaste tree/Vitex *Vitex agnus-castus*	**Cyclical mastalgia**, **PMS, PMDD,** oligomenorrhea, amenorrhea, IUD bleeding, **female infertility**, perimenopause, menstrual migraines, bone healing, insomnia, *inflammation, pain*	**Systematic review: reduces hyperprolactinemia, improves mid-luteal progesterone and estradiol** Human research: normalizes menses, promotes fertility, resolves luteal defect
Fennel *Foeniculum vulgare*	*Glaucoma, dyspepsia, gastroprotection, gastroparesis,* **infant colic**, IBS, constipation, *overactive bladder, lactation,* dysmenorrhea, oligomenorrhea, **menopausal disorders**, *dementia*, hirsutism, *inflammation*	Human research: combined with dry cupping, improves oligomenorrhea better than metformin
Fenugreek *Trigonella foenum-graecum*	Dyslipidemia, **DM**, prediabetes, *diabetic nephropathy, urolithiasis,* lactation, dysmenorrhea, PCOS, menopause, male sexual dysfunction, hypogonadism, PD, *peripheral neuropathy, thyroid T3/T4 balance,* stamina, *cancer*	Human research: improves PCOS

TABLE 13.E
Ovarian Disorders: Polycystic Ovary Syndrome, Oligomenorrhea, Amenorrhea, and Female Infertility. *(Continued)*

Common Name/ Latin Name	Scope of Potential Benefits	Comments
Gynostemma/Jiaogulan *Gynostemma pentaphyllum*	*Asthma, CAD, dyslipidemia*, DM, obesity, *arrhythmia*, NAFLD, PUD, PCOS, *PD, white matter disease*, dementia, *stamina*, immune function, cancer	Human research: reduces BMI, visceral and total body fat
Licorice *Glycyrrhiza glabra*	**Postoperative sore throat**, xerostomia, radiation-induced mucositis, aphthous ulcers, *allergy*, **asthma, dyslipidemia,** CAD, *diabetes*, **obesity**, hepatoprotection, heartburn, PUD, functional dyspepsia, **antipsychotic-induced hyperprolactinemia, menopause,** atrophic vaginitis, PCOS, female hirsutism, BPH, *stroke, dementia, PD, anxiety, insomnia, depression, substance addiction,* **hyperpigmentation, atopic eczema**, Addison's disease, *stamina, multiple sclerosis, inflammation, H. pylori*, cancer, *breast cancer*	*Preclinical research: reverses PCOS in rats; reduces conversion of androstenedione to testosterone* Human research: reduces PCOS in combination formula; reduces testosterone 30%; augments and balances spironolactone in PCOS **(Caution: use deglycyrrhizinated formulations in patients at risk for HTN and hypokalemia)**
Milk thistle *Silybum marianum*	**Dyslipidemia, DM, liver disease**, diabetic nephropathy, lactation, *PCOS*, BPH, *gout, AD, diabetic neuropathy,* **OCD**, acne, *psoriasis,* vitiligo, radio-dermatitis, aging skin, RA, inflammation, hepatitis viruses, **iron-overload**, chemotherapy and radiotherapy toxicity, *hepatocellular carcinoma*	*Theoretical: beneficial for PCOS via reduction in IR and glycemia*
Motherwort *Leonurus cardiaca*	*HTN 2/2 anxiety or hyperthyroidism, dyslipidemia, CAD, arrhythmia, nausea, IBS, AKI, lactation, postpartum bleeding, menorrhagia, amenorrhea,* menopause, *pain, stroke,* anxiety, insomnia, hyperthyroidism, inflammation, breast tumors*	Traditional use: amenorrhea, lactation promotion
Peppermint *Mentha x piperita*	Oral health, weight reduction, nausea, dyspepsia, **IBS**, GI endoscopy, cracked nipples, PCOS, neck pain, tension headaches, postherpetic neuralgia, cognition, nicotine withdrawal, pressure ulcers, pruritis gravidarum, hirsutism, athletic performance, URI, *cancer*	*Preclinical research: spearmint > peppermint for reducing androgens in rats* Human research: spearmint reduces androgens, decreases subjective perception of hirsutism
Rhodiola *Rhodiola rosea*	**CAD**, *menorrhagia, amenorrhea, female infertility,* menopause, *male hypogonadism,* premature ejaculation, **anxiety, depression, cognition**, eczema, burnout, fatigue, **athletic stamina**, cancer	*Preclinical research: demonstrates antiestrogenic effects through competitive estrogen receptor binding activity* Human research (unpublished clinical trial): reduces amenorrhea and improves fertility
Saw palmetto *Serenoa repens*	*Overactive bladder, female hirsutism, PCOS,* **BPH**, chronic inflammatory prostatitis, male pattern alopecia, *inflammation*	*Preclinical research: 5-α-reductase inhibition and ovarian prolactin receptor antagonism (PCOS imbalances)* **(Caution: contraindicated in pregnancy due to antiandrogen properties)**
Schisandra *Schisandra chinensis*	*MI,* **CHF**, DM, NAFLD, viral hepatitis, menopause, FMF, *stroke, AD, anxiety,* cognition, physical stress, stamina, pneumonia, *HCV, fungal infections,* cancer	Human research: reduces follicular phase androgens

TABLE 13.F

Ovarian Disorders: Perimenopause and Menopause (See also Table 13.G for Female Sexual Dysfunction).

Common Name/ Latin Name	Scope of Potential Benefits	Comments
Black cohosh *Actaea racemosa/ Cimicifuga racemosa*	Breast density, uterine fibroids, female infertility, **menopausal syndrome**, osteoporosis, breast cancer	**Systematic reviews: better than SSRI or SNRI, less than estradiol, gabapentin for menopausal symptoms** Human research: improves menopausal syndrome
Black seed/nigella/ black cumin *Nigella sativa*	Periodontal dz, oral submucous fibrosis, chronic rhinosinusitis, nasal dryness, **allergy, asthma**, COPD, chemical pneumonitis, **HTN**, *CAD*, CHF, **dyslipidemia, DM, obesity**, NAFLD, dyspepsia, PUD, diabetic nephropathy, mastalgia, menopause, male infertility, OA, *stroke,* seizure disorder, memory impairment, cognition, anxiety, *depression,* acne, eczema, vitiligo, immune function, Hashimoto's thyroiditis, RA, inflammation, *H. pylori, Staph* pustules, HCV, cancer	Human research: reduces menopausal symptoms and improves QOL; modifies weight gain and lipid dysfunction; improves efficacy of citalopram when combined with chasteberry
Chamomile *Matricaria chamomilla/ recutita*	Gingivitis, mucositis, chronic rhinosinusitis, *allergies,* dyslipidemia, diabetes, *PUD,* colic, IBS, diarrhea, dyspepsia, UC, *candida vaginitis,* menopause, carpal tunnel syndrome, anxiety, insomnia, depression, ADHD, eczema, wounds, radiation or chemotherapy dermatitis, cortisol dysregulation, *inflammation, broadly antimicrobial (bacteria, yeast, fungus), cancer*	Human research: improves menopausal symptoms in combination with dong quai; vaginal gel improves menopausal dyspareunia and sexual satisfaction
Chasteberry/Chaste tree/Vitex *Vitex agnus- castus*	**Cyclical mastalgia, PMS, PMDD,** oligomenorrhea, amenorrhea, IUD bleeding, **female infertility,** perimenopause, menstrual migraines, bone healing, insomnia, *inflammation, pain*	Human research: reduces menopausal complaints in combination formula
Dong quai *Angelica sinensis*	Pulmonary HTN, *HTN*, CAD, *atrial fibrillation,* cirrhosis, portal HTN, abd pain, UC, *renal fibrosis, dysmenorrhea,* menopausal symptoms, *osteoporosis, OA,* stroke, *cerebrovascular insufficiency, neurodegenerative disorders, wound healing, aging skin, alopecia, stamina, inflammation,* anemia of chronic disease, cancer	*Preclinical research: not estrogenic* **Systematic review: inconclusive evidence for menopause** Human research: not effective alone; effective in combination formula with chamomile
Fennel *Foeniculum vulgare*	*Glaucoma, dyspepsia, gastroprotection, gastroparesis,* **infant colic**, IBS, constipation, *overactive bladder, lactation,* dysmenorrhea, oligomenorrhea, **menopausal disorders**, *dementia,* hirsutism, *inflammation*	*Preclinical research: estrogenic properties* **Systematic review: beneficial for atrophic vaginitis** Human research: improves menopausal hot flashes, sexual dysfunction, vaginal symptoms
Fenugreek *Trigonella foenum-graecum*	Dyslipidemia, **DM,** prediabetes, *diabetic nephropathy, urolithiasis,* lactation, dysmenorrhea, PCOS, menopause, male sexual dysfunction, hypogonadism, PD, *peripheral neuropathy, thyroid T3/T4 balance,* stamina, *cancer*	Human research: improves menopausal symptoms
Ginseng, Asian/ Korean/Chinese *Panax ginseng*	Dry eyes, **hearing loss, HTN**, CHF, **DM**, obesity, **menopause, ED**, male infertility, *osteoporosis,* AD, cognitive function, aging skin, alopecia areata, stamina, **chronic fatigue, hangover,** immune function, inflammation, influenza, HIV, **cancer**	**Systematic review: beneficial for menopausal sexual function and hot flushes; possibly effective for mood disturbances in menopause**

TABLE 13.F

Ovarian Disorders: Perimenopause and Menopause (See also Table 13.G for Female Sexual Dysfunction). *(Continued)*

Common Name/ Latin Name	Scope of Potential Benefits	Comments
Hops/Hop *Humulus lupulus*	Dental plaque, allergic rhinitis, ASCVD, dyslipidemia, T2DM, obesity, *NAFLD, dyspepsia,* osteoporosis, OA, RA, atrophic vaginitis, menopause, cognitive decline, **insomnia,** anxiety, depression, cognitive performance, acne, aging skin, body odor, antibacterial, *TB, cancer*	*Preclinical research: reduces skin temp rises in ovariectomized rats* Human research: vaginal gel reduces atrophy; oral reduces hot flushes and menopausal symptoms
Licorice *Glycyrrhiza glabra*	**Postoperative sore throat,** xerostomia, radiation-induced mucositis, aphthous ulcers, *allergy,* **asthma, dyslipidemia,** *CAD, diabetes,* **obesity,** hepatoprotection, heartburn, PUD, functional dyspepsia, **antipsychotic-induced hyperprolactinemia, menopause,** atrophic vaginitis, PCOS, female hirsutism, BPH, *stroke, dementia,* PD, *anxiety, insomnia, depression, substance addiction,* **hyperpigmentation, atopic eczema,** Addison's disease, *stamina, multiple sclerosis, inflammation,* H. Pylori, cancer, *breast cancer*	**Systematic reviews: beneficial for acute menopausal symptoms** Human research: reduces menopausal hot flushes beyond treatment duration; vaginal cream improves maturation index **(Caution: use deglycyrrhizinated formulations in patients at risk for HTN and hypokalemia)**
Maca *Lepidium meyenii, peruvianum*	HTN, DM, weight reduction, perimenopause, **menopause, sexual dysfunction,** antidepressant-induced sexual dysfunction, **male sexual dysfunction, male infertility,** *BPH,* osteoporosis, *memory impairment,* anxiety, depression, fatigue, inflammation	**Systematic review: limited evidence of benefits for menopausal symptoms** Human research: improves perimenopausal symptoms and may increase estradiol; improves mood
Motherwort *Leonurus cardiaca*	*HTN 2/2 anxiety or hyperthyroidism, dyslipidemia, CAD, arrhythmia, nausea, IBS, AKI, lactation, postpartum bleeding, menorrhagia, amenorrhea,* menopause, *pain, stroke,* anxiety, *insomnia, hyperthyroidism, inflammation, breast tumors*	*Preclinical research: phyto-estrogenic properties* Human research: reduces menopausal symptoms in combination formula
Passionflower *Passiflora incarnata*	*Asthma, diabetes,* **menopause,** OA (fruit peel), *seizure disorder,* **anxiety,** somatoform disorder, *depression,* insomnia, **ADHD,** opiate withdrawal	**Systematic reviews: one of several herbs beneficial for menopausal syndrome**
Pueraria mirifica *Pueraria mirifica*	**Menopause**	Kongkaew et al. (2016)
Red Clover *Trifolium pratense*	**Menopause**	Ghazanfarpour et al. (2016)
Rhodiola *Rhodiola rosea*	**CAD,** *menorrhagia, amenorrhea, female infertility,* menopause, *male hypogonadism,* premature ejaculation, **anxiety, depression, cognition,** eczema, burnout, fatigue, **athletic stamina,** cancer	Human research: Augments black cohosh, esp. psych symptoms
Saffron *Crocus sativus*	ARMD, *cataracts,* diabetic maculopathy, glaucoma, gingivitis, burning mouth syndrome, *allergy,* asthma, HTN, **dyslipidemia,** DM, **obesity,** *hepatotoxicity, DM nephropathy,* PMS, menopause, **female and male sexual dysfunction,** male infertility, chronic pain, fibromyalgia, stroke, AD, **anxiety,** insomnia, OCD, **depression,** ADHD, drug and ETOH addiction, *photodamage,* stamina, immune function, inflammation, RA, *bacterial infection,* cancer	Human research: improves menopausal symptoms

Continued on following page

TABLE 13.F

Ovarian Disorders: Perimenopause and Menopause (See also Table 13.G for Female Sexual Dysfunction). *(Continued)*

Common Name/ Latin Name	Scope of Potential Benefits	Comments
St. John's Wort *Hypericum perforatum*	PMS, **perimenopause or menopause**, *chronic pain*, neuropathy, **depression,** *opiate addiction*, psoriasis, atopic dermatitis, *sunburn*, inflammation, HSV, *cancer*	**Systematic review: beneficial for climacteric complaints in combination with black cohosh** Human research: improves QOL, sleep, hot flushes in perimenopause; reduces menopausal symptoms; requires time to work (8 weeks) **See St. John's Wort monograph warnings and precautions**
Schisandra *Schisandra chinensis*	*MI*, **CHF**, DM, NAFLD, viral hepatitis, menopause, FMF, *stroke, AD*, anxiety, cognition, physical stress, stamina, pneumonia, *HCV, fungal infections*, cancer	Human research: reduces menopausal symptoms; weakly estrogenic; reduces follicular phase androgens; reduces estrone in combination formula
Stinging nettle *Urtica dioica*	Allergic rhinitis, HTN, dyslipidemia, **DM**, NAFLD, *colitis, nephrotoxicity,* menopause, **BPH**, prostatitis, OA, inflammation, *prostate cancer, cisplatin toxicity*	Human research: comparable to acupuncture, better than placebo for hot flushes and QOL in menopausal women
Tribulus/Puncture vine/Goathead *Tribulus terrestris*	HTN, CAD, dyslipidemia, DM, *hepatotoxicity, IBS, nephrolithiasis,* **sexual dysfunction**, hypoactive sexual desire, *pain, anxiety, depression, inflammation, cancer*	Human research: Some increase in testosterone in postmenopausal females
Valerian *Valeriana officinalis*	*HTN, CAD, IBS,* PMS, dysmenorrhea, **menopause,** tension HA, RLS, cognitive, anxiety, insomnia, OCD, *cancer*	**Systematic review: one of 10 herbs found to be beneficial for hot flushes** Human research: reduces menopausal hot flashes and sleep disturbance
Yarrow *Achillea millefolium*	*Epistaxis, asthma,* HTN, **dyslipidemia,** *T1DM,* cirrhosis, *gastritis,* PUD, anorexia, IBS, IBD, dysmenorrhea, *menorrhagia, menopause, anxiety, neurodegenerative disorders,* multiple sclerosis, *inflammation*	*Preclinical research: estrogenic activity*

TABLE 13.G

Female Sexual Dysfunction.

Common Name/ Latin Name	Scope of Potential Benefits	Comments
Ashwagandha *Withania somnifera*	Dyslipidemia, DM, **sexual dysfunction**, **infertility,** *osteoporosis,* gout, OA, *AD, PD,* MCI, **anxiety,** insomnia, OCD, *depression,* schizophrenia, hypothyroidism, stress, endurance, *fatigue,* immune function, TB, *cancer*	Human research: improves desire, orgasm, lubrication, and satisfaction in women
Ginseng, Asian/ Korean/Chinese *Panax ginseng*	Dry eyes, **hearing loss, HTN,** CHF, **DM,** obesity, **menopause, ED,** male infertility, *osteoporosis,* AD, cognitive function, aging skin, alopecia areata, stamina, **chronic fatigue, hangover,** immune function, inflammation, influenza, HIV, **cancer**	**Systematic review: beneficial for menopausal sexual function; possibly effective for mood disturbances in menopause**

TABLE 13.G
Female Sexual Dysfunction. *(Continued)*

Common Name/ Latin Name	Scope of Potential Benefits	Comments
Lemon balm *Melissa officinalis*	**Bruxism**, dyslipidemia, DM, palpitations, dyspepsia, IBS, **colic**, PMS, dysmenorrhea, female sexual dysfunction, **AD,** dementia, agitation, *diabetic neuropathy*, insomnia, **anxiety**, depression, **ADHD**, hyperthyroidism, *Graves' disease*, herpes simplex, *cancer, glioblastoma multiforme*	Human research: improves hypoactive sexual dysfunction disorder
Maca *Lepidium meyenii, peruvianum*	HTN, DM, weight reduction, perimenopause, **menopause**, **sexual dysfunction**, antidepressant-induced sexual dysfunction, **male sexual dysfunction**, **male infertility**, *BPH*, osteoporosis, *memory impairment*, anxiety, depression, fatigue, inflammation	**Systematic review: beneficial for female sexual dysfunction** Human research: improves SSRI/SNRI induced sexual dysfunction
Saffron *Crocus sativus*	ARMD, *cataracts*, diabetic maculopathy, glaucoma, gingivitis, burning mouth syndrome, *allergy*, asthma, HTN, **dyslipidemia**, DM, **obesity**, *hepatotoxicity, DM nephropathy*, PMS, menopause, **female and male sexual dysfunction**, male infertility, chronic pain, fibromyalgia, stroke, AD, **anxiety**, insomnia, OCD, **depression**, ADHD, drug and ETOH addiction, *photodamage*, stamina, immune function, inflammation, RA, *bacterial infection*, cancer	**Systematic review: beneficial for sexual dysfunction in men and women**
Tribulus/Puncture vine/ Goathead *Tribulus terrestris*	HTN, CAD, dyslipidemia, DM, *hepatotoxicity, IBS, nephrolithiasis*, **sexual dysfunction**, hypoactive sexual desire, *pain, anxiety, depression, inflammation, cancer*	*Preclinical research: increased sexual activity; increased NOX* **Systematic review: beneficial for ED and sexual desire** Human research: improves both male and female hypoactive desire; no effect on testosterone in males, some increase in postmenopausal females

REFERENCES

Ghazanfarpour M, et al. Red clover for treatment of hot flashes and menopausal symptoms: a systematic review and metaanalysis. J Obstet Gynaecol 2016;36(3):301–11.

Kongkaew C, et al. Efficacy and safety of *Pueraria candollei* var. mirifica (Airy Shaw & Suvat.) Niyomdham for menopausal women: a systematic review of clinical trials and the way forward. J Ethnopharmacol 2018;2016:162–74.

Mousavi Kani K, et al. The effect of aromatherapy (with lavender) on dysmenorrhea: a systematic review and meta-analysis. Int J Pediatr 2019;9657–66.

14 MEN'S GENITOURINARY DISORDERS

■ ■ ■ ■ ■ ■ ■ ■ ■ ■

TABLE 14.A
Disorders of the Prostate: Benign Prostatic Hyperplasia/Hypertrophy and Chronic Prostatitis.

Common Name/ Latin Name	Scope of Potential Benefits	Comments
Calendula *Calendula officinalis*	Gingivitis, dental plaque, radiation mucositis, venous ulcers, lactational cracked nipples, vaginal candidiasis, episiotomy healing, nonbacterial prostatitis, diaper dermatitis, **wound healing**, diabetic foot ulcers, *antibacterial, anti-HIV*, radiation dermatitis	Human research: combined with turmeric, improves chronic non-bacterial prostatitis (CP-CPPS III)
Cranberry *Vaccinium macrocarpon*	Gingivitis, dyslipidemia, **DM**, PUD, gut dysbiosis, overactive bladder, **UTI**, post-radiation UTI, BPH, chronic prostatitis, RA, *inflammation, influenza*, prostate CA	Human research: reduces LUTS, improves flow; reduces BPH-related UTIs; reduces episodes of chronic bacterial prostatitis in combination with goji and saw palmetto
Horsetail *Equisetum arvense*	*Diabetes*, nephrolithiasis, *UTI, interstitial cystitis*, BPH, osteoporosis, *OA*, RA, *chronic pain, anxiety, cognition*, psoriatic nails, wound healing, aging skin, alopecia, inflammation	*Preclinical research: improves BPH in combination formula* Human research: improves BPH in combination formula Traditional use: BPH
Licorice *Glycyrrhiza glabra*	**Postoperative sore throat**, xerostomia, radiation-induced mucositis, aphthous ulcers, *allergy*, **asthma**, **dyslipidemia**, *CAD, diabetes*, **obesity**, hepatoprotection, heartburn, PUD, functional dyspepsia, **antipsychotic-induced hyperprolactinemia**, **menopause**, atrophic vaginitis, PCOS, female hirsutism, BPH, *stroke, dementia*, PD, *anxiety, insomnia, depression, substance addiction*, **hyperpigmentation**, **atopic eczema**, Addison's disease, *stamina, multiple sclerosis, inflammation*, H. pylori, cancer, *breast cancer*	Human research: conflicting evidence of testosterone reduction, DHEA-S reduction *(Caution: use deglycyrrhizinated formulations in patients at risk for HTN and hypokalemia)*
Maca *Lepidium meyenii, peruvianum*	HTN, DM, weight reduction, perimenopause, **menopause**, **sexual dysfunction**, anti-depressant-induced sexual dysfunction, **male sexual dysfunction**, **male infertility**, *BPH*, osteoporosis, *memory impairment*, anxiety, depression, fatigue, inflammation	*Preclinical research: reduces prostatic hyperplasia*

Continued on following page

TABLE 14.A
Disorders of the Prostate: Benign Prostatic Hyperplasia/Hypertrophy and Chronic Prostatitis. *(Continued)*

Common Name/ Latin Name	Scope of Potential Benefits	Comments
Milk thistle *Silybum marianum*	**Dyslipidemia, DM, liver disease**, diabetic nephropathy, lactation, *PCOS*, BPH, *gout, AD, diabetic neuropathy*, **OCD**, acne, *psoriasis*, vitiligo, radio-dermatitis, aging skin, RA, inflammation, hepatitis viruses, **iron-overload**, chemotherapy and radiotherapy toxicity, *hepatocellular carcinoma*	Human research: with selenium improves all parameters of BPH; reduces PSA
Saw palmetto *Serenoa repens*	*Overactive bladder, female hirsutism, PCOS*, **BPH**, chronic inflammatory prostatitis, male pattern alopecia, *inflammation*	**Systematic reviews: hexanic extracts comparable to α-blockers and 5-α-reductase inhibitors in BPH; greater effects when combined with α-blockers; less side effects** Human research: improves BPH; improves bacterial and nonbacterial prostatitis; especially with hexanic extracts or in combination with drugs or stinging nettle; better with larger prostate volume *(Caution: contraindicated in pregnancy due to anti-androgen properties)*
Stinging nettle (root) *Urtica dioica*	Allergic rhinitis, HTN, dyslipidemia, **DM**, NAFLD, *colitis, nephrotoxicity*, menopause, **BPH**, prostatitis, OA, inflammation, *prostate cancer, cisplatin toxicity*	**Systematic review: beneficial for LUTS in BPH** Human research: improves BPH and prostatitis, especially in combination with saw palmetto, comparable to finasteride and tamsulosin in head-to-head trials; combination better than saw palmetto alone
Turmeric (or curcumin) *Curcuma longa*	Anterior uveitis, **oral lichen planus, gingivitis**, dental surgery, submucous fibrosis, asthma, **diastolic HTN, dyslipidemia**, CAD, endothelial dysfunction, **DM**, obesity, **NAFLD**, hepatoprotective, gallbladder dyskinesia, *GERD*, PUD, dyspepsia, **UC**, DM nephropathy, lupus nephritis, lactational mastitis, LSIL, chronic non-bacterial prostatitis, post-operative pain, **OA**, RA, migraine HA, *neurodegeneration*, **anxiety, depression, skin disease**, psoriasis, fatigue, **systemic inflammation**, *HIV*, **chemo-related oral mucositis**, cancer prevention, cancer treatment	Human research: combined with calendula, improves chronic non-bacterial prostatitis (CP-CPPS III)

TABLE 14.B
Testicular Disorders: Sexual Dysfunction, Male Infertility, and Hypogonadism.

Common Name/Latin Name	Scope of Potential Benefits	Comments
Ashwagandha *Withania somnifera*	Dyslipidemia, DM, **sexual dysfunction, infertility**, *osteoporosis*, gout, OA, *AD, PD*, MCI, **anxiety**, insomnia, OCD, *depression*, schizophrenia, hypothyroidism, stress, endurance, *fatigue*, immune function, TB, *cancer*	**Systematic review and meta-analysis: improves semen quality; raises T and LH**
Astragalus *Astragalus membranaceus*	Herpes keratitis, recurrent tonsillitis, allergic rhinitis, atopy, asthma, **viral myocarditis**, CHF, CAD, viral hepatitis, **diabetic nephropathy**, IgA nephropathy, nephrotic syndrome, lupus nephritis, *renal fibrosis, sperm quality*, hemorrhagic stroke, burns, *wound healing, age spots, leukopenia*, **immune function**, *antiviral*, HBV, TB, **NSCLC**, cancer	*Preclinical research: improves sperm quality*
Black seed/nigella/ black cumin *Nigella sativa*	Periodontal dz., oral submucous fibrosis, chronic rhinosinusitis, nasal dryness, **allergy, asthma**, COPD, chemical pneumonitis, **HTN**, *CAD*, CHF, **dyslipidemia, DM, obesity**, NAFLD, dyspepsia, PUD, diabetic nephropathy, mastalgia, menopause, male infertility, OA, *stroke*, seizure disorder, memory impairment, cognition, anxiety, *depression*, acne, eczema, vitiligo, immune function, Hashimoto's thyroiditis, RA, inflammation, *H. pylori, Staph* pustules, HCV, cancer	Human research: improves abnormal semen quality
Coleus *Coleus forskohlii*	Glaucoma, *allergy*, asthma, HTN, CHF, *insulin resistance*, obesity, *pancreatic exocrine insufficiency, diarrhea, UTI, urge incontinence, dysmenorrhea, male infertility*, male hypogonadism, subarachnoid hemorrhage, *seizure, neurodegenerative disorders, alcohol abuse*, psoriasis, *photoprotection, hyperthyroidism, cancer*	*Preclinical research: improves sperm motility* Human research: increases serum testosterone along with lean body mass
Eleuthero/Siberian Ginseng *Eleutherococcus senticosus/ Acanthopanax senticosus*	*Allergic rhinitis*, dyslipidemia, CHF, edema, *male infertility*, osteoporosis, **stroke recovery**, *AD, insomnia*, **depression**, bipolar disorder, attention, vitality, athletic stamina, **hangover**, immune function, FMF, **URI**, *antiviral*, ovarian cancer	Human research: improves sperm motility in ex vivo application
Fenugreek *Trigonella foenum-graecum*	Dyslipidemia, **DM**, pre-diabetes, *diabetic nephropathy, urolithiasis*, lactation, dysmenorrhea, PCOS, menopause, male sexual dysfunction, hypogonadism, PD, *peripheral neuropathy, thyroid T3/T4 balance*, stamina, *cancer*	*Preclinical research: increases DHEA, testosterone; reduces DHT; raises NO in corpus cavernosum* Human research: improves libido and energy, increases testosterone
Ginger *Zingiber officinale*	**Motion sickness**, *HTN*, dyslipidemia, fibrinolysis, diabetes, **nausea, vomiting**, *dyspepsia*, gastroparesis, PUD, ulcerative colitis, *diabetic nephropathy*, **dysmenorrhea**, *Candida vaginitis*, male infertility, OA, muscle injury, migraine HA, *AD*, **inflammation**, RA, *H. pylori, antibacterial*, **CINV**, cancer	Human research: increases testosterone by 17%; reduces sperm fragmentation; improves sperm count and motility
Ginkgo *Ginkgo biloba*	*Cataracts*, ARMD, glaucoma, periodontal dz., **vertigo, tinnitus, cardiovascular health, dyslipidemia, diabetes**, obesity, claudication, hepatic fibrosis, **diabetic nephropathy**, menopausal sexual desire, **acute mountain sickness**, migraines with aura, **stroke, MCI, dementias**, post-operative delirium, depression, ADHD, **schizophrenia, tardive dyskinesia**, aging skin, *inflammation, cancer*	Human research: improves sexual desire in menopausal women

Continued on following page

TABLE 14.B

Testicular Disorders: Sexual Dysfunction, Male Infertility, and Hypogonadism. *(Continued)*

Common Name/Latin Name	Scope of Potential Benefits	Comments
Ginseng, Asian/ Korean/Chinese *Panax ginseng*	Dry eyes, **hearing loss**, **HTN**, CHF, **DM**, obesity, **menopause**, **ED**, male infertility, *osteoporosis*, AD, cognitive function, aging skin, alopecia areata, stamina, **chronic fatigue**, **hangover**, immune function, inflammation, influenza, HIV, **cancer**	**Systematic review: beneficial for ED** Human research: improves libido and erections; superior to trazodone; improves sperm count and motility; increases T, DHT, FSH, LH
Goji berry/wolfberry *Lycium barbarum*	Macular degeneration, *glaucoma*, dyslipidemia, **diabetes**, obesity, *hepatoprotection, male infertility, male sexual dysfunction, stroke*, AD, insomnia, anxiety, ADD, *dermatitis*, cognition, stress, fatigue, athletic performance, hangover, immunity function, influenza, cancer	*Preclinical research: protects spermatogenesis against toxicity and radiation; improves sexual performance*
Holy basil/Tulsi *Ocimum tenuiflorum/ sanctum*	Gingivitis, asthma, *CAD*, **dyslipidemia**, **diabetes**, obesity, *hepatotoxicity, PUD, male hypogonadism, pain, seizures*, anxiety, depression, memory and concentration, stress and fatigue, immune function, viral encephalitis	*Preclinical research: testosterone agonist, lowers LH, causes sperm dysmorphia and dysmotility*
Horse chestnut *Aesculus hippocastanum*	Hearing loss, *allergy*, **chronic venous insufficiency**, venous ulcers, varicocele-induced infertility, *hemorrhoids*, aging skin, *easy bruising, cancer*	Human research: improves varicocele-induced male infertility
Maca *Lepidium meyenii, peruvianum*	HTN, DM, weight reduction, perimenopause, **menopause**, **sexual dysfunction**, anti-depressant-induced sexual dysfunction, **male sexual dysfunction**, **male infertility**, *BPH*, osteoporosis, *memory impairment*, anxiety, depression, fatigue, inflammation	**Systematic reviews: improves sexual function in healthy males, menopausal females; improves semen quality and quantity** Human research: improves erectile function; improves desire with no effect on hormones; improves sperm concentration and motility; improves SSRI-/SNRI-related sexual dysfunction
Rhodiola *Rhodiola rosea*	**CAD**, *menorrhagia, amenorrhea, female infertility*, menopause, *male hypogonadism*, premature ejaculation, **anxiety**, **depression**, **cognition**, eczema, burnout, fatigue, **athletic stamina**, cancer	*Preclinical research: anti-estrogen effects through competitive estrogen receptor binding activity* Human research: improves premature ejaculation combined with biotin and zinc
Saffron *Crocus sativus*	ARMD, *cataracts*, diabetic maculopathy, glaucoma, gingivitis, burning mouth syndrome, *allergy*, asthma, HTN, **dyslipidemia**, DM, **obesity**, *hepatotoxicity, DM nephropathy*, PMS, menopause, **female and male sexual dysfunction**, male infertility, chronic pain, fibromyalgia, stroke, AD, **anxiety**, insomnia, OCD, **depression**, ADHD, drug and ETOH addiction, *photodamage*, stamina, immune function, inflammation, RA, *bacterial infection*, cancer	**Systematic review: beneficial for sexual dysfunction; conflicting findings for improving semen parameters** Human research: improves ED; improves fluoxetine-induced sexual dysfunction; improves sperm quality
Tribulus/Puncture vine/Goathead *Tribulus terrestris*	HTN, CAD, dyslipidemia, DM, *hepatotoxicity, IBS, nephrolithiasis*, **sexual dysfunction**, hypoactive sexual desire, *pain, anxiety, depression, inflammation, cancer*	*Preclinical research: increased sexual activity; increased NOX* **Systematic review: beneficial for ED and sexual desire** Human research: improves both male and female hypoactive desire, ED (mixed); no effect on testosterone in humans

15 MUSCULOSKELETAL DISORDERS

Common Name/ Latin Name	Scope of Potential Benefits	Comments
	TABLE 15.A	
	Osteopenia and Osteoporosis.	
Ashwagandha *Withania somnifera*	Dyslipidemia, DM, **sexual dysfunction**, **infertility**, *osteoporosis*, gout, OA, *AD*, *PD*, MCI, **anxiety**, insomnia, OCD, *depression*, schizophrenia, hypothyroidism, stress, endurance, *fatigue*, immune function, TB, *cancer*	*Preclinical research: improves bone calcification in ovariectomized rats*
Black cohosh *Actaea racemosa/ Cimicifuga racemosa*	Breast density, uterine fibroids, female infertility, PCOS, **menopausal syndrome**, osteoporosis, breast cancer	Human research: reduces markers of bone turnover, short-term comparable to CEE, but no difference with high impact exercise in BMD over 10 years
Chasteberry/Chaste tree/Vitex *Vitex agnus-castus*	**Cyclical mastalgia**, **PMS**, **PMDD**, oligomenorrhea, amenorrhea, IUD bleeding, **female infertility**, perimenopause, menstrual migraines, bone healing, insomnia, *inflammation*, *pain*	Human research: improves markers of bone healing with and without magnesium
Dong quai *Angelica sinensis*	Pulmonary HTN, *HTN*, CAD, *atrial fibrillation*, cirrhosis, portal HTN, abd pain, UC, *renal fibrosis*, *dysmenorrhea*, menopausal symptoms, *osteoporosis*, OA, stroke, *cerebrovascular insufficiency*, *neurodegenerative disorders*, *wound healing*, *aging skin*, *alopecia*, *stamina*, *inflammation*, anemia of chronic disease, cancer	*Preclinical research: higher dose increases BMD similar to estradiol*
Eleuthero/Siberian Ginseng *Eleutherococcus senticosus/ Acanthopanax senticosus*	*Allergic rhinitis*, dyslipidemia, CHF, edema, *male infertility*, osteoporosis, **stroke recovery**, *AD*, *insomnia*, **depression**, bipolar disorder, attention, vitality, athletic stamina, **hangover**, immune function, FMF, **URI**, *antiviral*, ovarian cancer	Human research: improves bone turnover markers in postmenopausal women
Ginseng, Asian/ Korean/Chinese *Panax ginseng*	Dry eyes, **hearing loss**, **HTN**, CHF, **DM**, obesity, **menopause**, **ED**, male infertility, *osteoporosis*, AD, cognitive function, aging skin, alopecia areata, stamina, **chronic fatigue**, **hangover**, immune function, inflammation, influenza, HIV, **cancer**	*Preclinical research: reduces radiation and steroid-induced bone loss*

Continued on following page

TABLE 15.A
Osteopenia and Osteoporosis. *(Continued)*

Common Name/ Latin Name	Scope of Potential Benefits	Comments
Hops/Hop *Humulus lupulus*	Dental plaque, allergic rhinitis, ASCVD, dyslipidemia, T2DM, obesity, *NAFLD, dyspepsia*, osteoporosis, OA, RA, atrophic vaginitis, menopause, cognitive decline, **insomnia**, anxiety, depression, cognitive performance, acne, aging skin, body odor, antibacterial, *TB, cancer*	*Preclinical research: stimulates bone estrogen receptors; inhibits osteoclasts; high silica* Human research: combination formula reduces osteocalcin, raises IGF-1
Horsetail *Equisetum arvense*	*Diabetes*, nephrolithiasis, *UTI, interstitial cystitis*, BPH, osteoporosis, *OA*, RA, *chronic pain, anxiety, cognition*, psoriatic nails, wound healing, aging skin, alopecia, inflammation	*Preclinical research: combination formula promotes bone density comparable to raloxifene* Human research: 2 years, increased DXA scores
Maca *Lepidium meyenii, peruvianum*	HTN, DM, weight reduction, perimenopause, **menopause, sexual dysfunction**, anti-depressant-induced sexual dysfunction, **male sexual dysfunction**, **male infertility**, *BPH*, osteoporosis, *memory impairment*, anxiety, depression, fatigue, inflammation	*Preclinical research: increases bone density* Human research: reduces fractures

TABLE 15.B
Osteoarthritis, Gout, Myofascial Pain and Miscellaneous Chronic Pain Syndromes (See Table 21.B. for inflammation; 21.C. for RA and SLE; 15.B., 16.E., 117.A., 17.E., and 20.A. for Fibromyalgia Manifestations).

Common Name/ Latin Name	Scope of Potential Benefits	Comments
Andrographis *Andrographis paniculata*	*HTN, hepatoprotection*, ulcerative colitis, *dysmenorrhea*, OA, RA, FMF, *inflammation*, **URI prevention and treatment**, *cancer*	Human research: andrographolide formula reduces pain and improves QOL in OA of knee
Ashwagandha *Withania somnifera*	Dyslipidemia, DM, **sexual dysfunction, infertility**, *osteoporosis*, gout, OA, *AD, PD*, MCI, **anxiety**, insomnia, OCD, *depression*, schizophrenia, hypothyroidism, stress, endurance, *fatigue*, immune function, TB, *cancer*	*Preclinical research: reduces gout pain comparable to indomethacin* Human research: improves OA knee pain
Black seed/nigella/ black cumin *Nigella sativa*	Periodontal dz., oral submucous fibrosis, chronic rhinosinusitis, nasal dryness, **allergy, asthma**, COPD, chemical pneumonitis, **HTN**, *CAD*, CHF, **dyslipidemia, DM, obesity**, NAFLD, dyspepsia, PUD, diabetic nephropathy, mastalgia, menopause, male infertility, OA, *stroke*, seizure disorder, memory impairment, cognition, anxiety, *depression*, acne, eczema, vitiligo, immune function, Hashimoto's thyroiditis, RA, inflammation, *H. pylori*, Staph pustules, HCV, cancer	Human research: topical knee application better than APAP orally for OA; oral consumption trended better than placebo
Burdock *Arctium lappa*	*Dyslipidemia*, diabetes, *hepatic function and protection, gastroparesis, dyspepsia*, diverticulitis, diabetic nephropathy, OA, wrinkles, acne, cough, *inflammation, influenza A, cancer*	Human research: reduces inflammatory and oxidative markers in OA patients
Chasteberry/Chaste tree/Vitex *Vitex agnus-castus*	**Cyclical mastalgia, PMS, PMDD**, oligomenorrhea, amenorrhea, IUD bleeding, **female infertility**, perimenopause, menstrual migraines, bone healing, insomnia, *inflammation, pain*	*Preclinical research: oil reduces inflammation and pain equivalent to diclofenac and morphine*

TABLE 15.B

Osteoarthritis, Gout, Myofascial Pain and Miscellaneous Chronic Pain Syndromes (See Table 21.B. for inflammation; 21.C. for RA and SLE; 15.B, 16.E., 117.A., 17.E., and 20.A. for Fibromyalgia Manifestations). *(Continued)*

Common Name/ Latin Name	Scope of Potential Benefits	Comments
Devil's claw *Harpagophytum procumbens*	**OA, low back pain**	Brendler et al. (2006)
Echinacea *Echinacea purpurea, angustifolia*	Anterior uveitis, *candida vaginitis*, genital condylomas, OA, **anxiety**, eczema, athletic performance, immune function, inflammation, **URIs**, influenza, *Coronavirus*, HPV, *colorectal cancer*	Human research: reduces knee pain and swelling combined with ginger
Frankincense/ Boswellia *Boswellia serrata, sacra, carterii*	Gingivitis, **asthma**, *COPD*, UC, **Crohn's**, **collagenous colitis**, IBS, UTI, SUI, benign breast disease, menorrhagia, **OA**, stroke, memory impairment, psoriasis, eczema, aging skin, athletic performance, **RA**, **IBD**, *inflammation*, glioma radiation, chemo-related neuropathy, *cancer*	**Systematic reviews: beneficial in OA, well tolerated** Human research: slower onset but longer lasting improvement compared to valdecoxib in OA; synergistic with curcuminoids; reduces synovial MMP-3; reduces athletic muscle pain; reduces acute muscle injury pain
Dong quai *Angelica sinensis*	Pulmonary HTN, *HTN*, CAD, *atrial fibrillation*, cirrhosis, portal HTN, abd pain, UC, *renal fibrosis*, *dysmenorrhea*, menopausal symptoms, *osteoporosis*, OA, stroke, *cerebrovascular insufficiency*, *neurodegenerative disorders*, *wound healing*, *aging skin*, *alopecia*, *stamina*, *inflammation*, anemia of chronic disease, cancer	*Preclinical research: anti-inflammatory, pro-GAG, pro-chondrocyte, pro-hyaluronic acid; anti-TNF*
Ginger *Zingiber officinale*	**Motion sickness**, *HTN*, dyslipidemia, fibrinolysis, diabetes, **nausea**, **vomiting**, *dyspepsia*, gastroparesis, *PUD*, ulcerative colitis, *diabetic nephropathy*, **dysmenorrhea**, *Candida vaginitis*, male infertility, OA, muscle injury, migraine HA, *AD*, **inflammation**, RA, *H. pylori, antibacterial*, **CINV**, cancer	Human research: reduces pain with OA; reduces pain with muscle strain; longer studies more impressive for OA
Gymnema/Gurmar *Gymnema sylvestre*	*Dental caries*, dyslipidemia, T1DM, **T2DM**, obesity, *arthritis*, *immune function*, *cancer*	*Preclinical research: reduces inflammatory arthritis*
Holy basil/Tulsi *Ocimum tenuiflorum/ sanctum*	Gingivitis, asthma, *CAD*, **dyslipidemia**, **diabetes**, obesity, *hepatotoxicity*, *PUD*, *male hypogonadism*, *pain*, *seizures*, anxiety, depression, memory and concentration, stress and fatigue, immune function, viral encephalitis	*Preclinical research: anti-inflammatory, analgesic via opioid and serotonergic systems*
Hops/Hop *Humulus lupulus*	Dental plaque, allergic rhinitis, ASCVD, dyslipidemia, T2DM, obesity, *NAFLD*, dyspepsia, osteoporosis, OA, RA, atrophic vaginitis, menopause, cognitive decline, **insomnia**, anxiety, depression, cognitive performance, acne, aging skin, body odor, antibacterial, *TB, cancer*	*Preclinical research: prevents loss of hyaluronan, collagen and proteoglycan* Human research: reduces pain in OA and RA subjects; 54% reduction in WOMAC scores
Horsetail *Equisetum arvense*	*Diabetes*, nephrolithiasis, *UTI, interstitial cystitis*, BPH, osteoporosis, *OA*, RA, *chronic pain, anxiety, cognition*, psoriatic nails, wound healing, aging skin, alopecia, inflammation	*Preclinical research: reduces nociception through non-opiate mechanism* Traditional use: OA Human research: reduces TNF-α, IL-10, ESR, and RF in RA patients

Continued on following page

TABLE 15.B

Osteoarthritis, Gout, Myofascial Pain and Miscellaneous Chronic Pain Syndromes (See Table 21.B. for inflammation; 21.C. for RA and SLE; 15.B, 16.E., 117.A., 17.E., and 20.A. for Fibromyalgia Manifestations). (Continued)

Common Name/ Latin Name	Scope of Potential Benefits	Comments
Milk thistle *Silybum marianum*	**Dyslipidemia**, **DM**, **liver disease**, diabetic nephropathy, lactation, *PCOS*, BPH, *gout*, *AD*, *diabetic neuropathy*, **OCD**, acne, *psoriasis*, vitiligo, radio-dermatitis, aging skin, RA, inflammation, hepatitis viruses, **iron-overload**, chemotherapy and radiotherapy toxicity, *hepatocellular carcinoma*	*Preclinical research: inhibits XO on par with allopurinol*
Motherwort *Leonurus cardiaca*	*HTN 2/2 anxiety or hyperthyroidism, dyslipidemia, CAD, arrhythmia, nausea, IBS, AKI, lactation, post-partum bleeding, menorrhagia, amenorrhea, menopause, pain, stroke, anxiety, insomnia, hyperthyroidism, inflammation, breast tumors*	*Preclinical research: reduces central and peripheral pain response*
Passionflower *Passiflora incarnata (Passiflora edulis)*	*Asthma, diabetes,* **menopause**, OA (fruit peel), *seizure disorder,* **anxiety**, somatoform disorder, *depression,* insomnia, **ADHD**, opiate withdrawal	Human research: passion fruit peel (*Passiflora edulis*) reduces WOMAC scores 18%
Peppermint *Mentha × piperita*	Oral health, weight reduction, nausea, dyspepsia, **IBS**, GI endoscopy, cracked nipples, PCOS, neck pain, tension headaches, postherpetic neuralgia, cognition, nicotine withdrawal, pressure ulcers, pruritis gravidarum, hirsutism, athletic performance, URI, *cancer*	Human research: combination essential oil (4 oils) topically reduces neck pain
Rose hips *Rosa canina*	**OA**	Chrubasik et al. (2006)
Saffron *Crocus sativus*	ARMD, *cataracts*, diabetic maculopathy, glaucoma, gingivitis, burning mouth syndrome, *allergy*, asthma, HTN, **dyslipidemia**, DM, **obesity**, *hepatotoxicity*, DM *nephropathy*, PMS, menopause, **female and male sexual dysfunction**, male infertility, chronic pain, fibromyalgia, stroke, AD, **anxiety**, insomnia, OCD, **depression**, ADHD, drug and ETOH addiction, *photodamage*, stamina, immune function, inflammation, RA, *bacterial infection*, cancer	*Preclinical research: antinociceptive; reduces chronic inflammation* Human research: comparable to duloxetine in FMS
St. John's Wort *Hypericum perforatum*	PMS, **perimenopause or menopause**, *chronic pain,* neuropathy, **depression**, *opiate addiction*, psoriasis, atopic dermatitis, *sunburn*, inflammation, HSV, *cancer*	*Preclinical research: reduces acute and chronic pain; reduces hyperalgesia; augments morphine; effect blocked by naloxone.* **See St. John's Wort monograph warnings and precautions.**
Schisandra *Schisandra chinensis*	*MI,* **CHF**, DM, NAFLD, viral hepatitis, menopause, FMF, *stroke, AD, anxiety,* cognition, physical stress, stamina, pneumonia, *HCV, fungal infections,* cancer	Human research: in combination formula reduces attacks of FMF
Stinging nettle *Urtica dioica*	Allergic rhinitis, HTN, dyslipidemia, **DM**, NAFLD, *colitis, nephrotoxicity,* menopause, **BPH**, prostatitis, OA, inflammation, *prostate cancer, cisplatin toxicity*	*Preclinical research: nonselective COX and PGD2 synthase inhibition* Human Research: reduces OA pain in combination formulas; topically reduces pain in hand OA

TABLE 15.B

Osteoarthritis, Gout, Myofascial Pain and Miscellaneous Chronic Pain Syndromes (See Table 21.B. for inflammation; 21.C. for RA and SLE; 15.B, 16.E., 117.A., 17.E., and 20.A. for Fibromyalgia Manifestations). *(Continued)*

Common Name/ Latin Name	Scope of Potential Benefits	Comments
Tribulus/Puncture vine/Goathead *Tribulus terrestris*	HTN, CAD, dyslipidemia, DM, *hepatotoxicity, IBS, nephrolithiasis*, **sexual dysfunction**, hypoactive sexual desire, *pain, anxiety, depression, inflammation, cancer*	*Preclinical research: COX, TNF inhibition; analgesic activity greater than ASA*
Turmeric (or curcumin) *Curcuma longa*	Anterior uveitis, **oral lichen planus**, **gingivitis**, dental surgery, submucous fibrosis, asthma, **diastolic HTN**, **dyslipidemia**, CAD, endothelial dysfunction, **DM**, obesity, **NAFLD**, hepatoprotective, gallbladder dyskinesia, *GERD*, PUD, dyspepsia, **UC**, DM nephropathy, lupus nephritis, lactational mastitis, LSIL, chronic non-bacterial prostatitis, post-operative pain, **OA**, RA, migraine HA, *neurodegeneration*, **anxiety**, **depression**, **skin disease**, psoriasis, fatigue, **systemic inflammation**, *HIV*, **chemo-related oral mucositis**, cancer prevention, cancer treatment	**Systematic reviews: large and clinically meaningful short-term pain reduction in OA, comparable to analgesics** Human research: reduces pain and stiffness and improves function in OA; reduces inflammatory markers; non-inferior to ibuprofen 1200 mg/day; reduces cartilage degradation at high doses; combination with frankincense superior to celecoxib; reduces inflammatory markers and disease activity in RA; combined with frankincense reduces early post-operative shoulder surgery pain
Yarrow *Achillea millefolium*	*Epistaxis, asthma*, HTN, **dyslipidemia**, *T1DM*, cirrhosis, *gastritis*, PUD, *anorexia, IBS, IBD*, dysmenorrhea, *menorrhagia, menopause, anxiety, neurodegenerative disorders*, multiple sclerosis, *inflammation*	*Preclinical research: anti-inflammatory properties*

REFERENCES

Brendler T, Gruenwald J, Ulbricht C. Devil's Claw (*Harpagophytum procumbens* DC): an evidence-based systematic review by the Natural Standard Research Collaboration. J Herb Pharmacother 2006;6(1):89–126.

Chrubasik C, Duke RK, Chrubasik S. The evidence for clinical efficacy of rose hip and seed: a systematic review. Phytother Res 2006;20:1–3.

16

NEUROLOGICAL DISORDERS

▪ ▪

TABLE 16.A
Migraine Headache, Tension Headache, and Seizures.

Common Name/Latin Name	Scope of Potential Benefits	Comments
Bacopa *Bacopa monnieri*	*Gastric ulcer*, hepatic encephalopathy, IBS-D, *seizures*, memory impairment, **dementia-related anxiety**, test anxiety, **cognitive performance**, ADHD, inflammation	*Preclinical research: anticonvulsant through GABA*
Black seed/nigella/black cumin *Nigella sativa*	Periodontal dz., oral submucous fibrosis, chronic rhinosinusitis, nasal dryness, **allergy**, **asthma**, COPD, chemical pneumonitis, **HTN**, *CAD*, CHF, **dyslipidemia**, **DM**, **obesity**, NAFLD, dyspepsia, PUD, diabetic nephropathy, mastalgia, menopause, male infertility, OA, *stroke*, seizure disorder, memory impairment, cognition, anxiety, *depression*, acne, eczema, vitiligo, immune function, Hashimoto's thyroiditis, RA, inflammation, *H. pylori*, *Staph* pustules, HCV, cancer	*Preclinical research: GABAergic; anticonvulsant superior to valproate* Human research: black seed, thymoquinone reduce seizures in children
Butterbur *Petasites hybridus*	**Allergic rhinitis**, asthma, *HTN*, *GI ulceration*, bladder spasms, **migraine headache**, *neurodegenerative dementias*, somatoform disorder anxiety and depression, *CNS inflammation*	**Systematic review: standardized extract effective in migraine reduction** Human research: reduces migraines
Chasteberry/Chaste tree/Vitex *Vitex agnus-castus*	**Cyclical mastalgia**, **PMS**, **PMDD**, oligomenorrhea, amenorrhea, IUD bleeding, **female infertility**, perimenopause, menstrual migraines, bone healing, insomnia, *inflammation*, *pain*	Human research: (open label) reduces menstrual migraine headaches
Coleus *Coleus forskohlii*	Glaucoma, *allergy*, asthma, HTN, CHF, *insulin resistance*, obesity, *pancreatic exocrine insufficiency*, *diarrhea*, *UTI*, *urge incontinence*, *dysmenorrhea*, *male infertility*, male hypogonadism, subarachnoid hemorrhage, *seizure*, *neurodegenerative disorders*, *alcohol abuse*, psoriasis, *photoprotection*, *hyperthyroidism*, *cancer*	*Preclinical research: reduces seizures*
Feverfew (dried powdered leaf) *Tanacetum parthenium*	**Migraine prevention**	Wider et al. (2015) Saranitzky et al. (2009)

Continued on following page

111

TABLE 16.A
Migraine Headache, Tension Headache, and Seizures. *(Continued)*

Common Name/Latin Name	Scope of Potential Benefits	Comments
Ginger *Zingiber officinale*	**Motion sickness**, *HTN*, dyslipidemia, fibrinolysis, diabetes, **nausea**, **vomiting**, *dyspepsia*, gastroparesis, *PUD*, ulcerative colitis, *diabetic nephropathy*, **dysmenorrhea**, *Candida vaginitis*, male infertility, OA, muscle injury, migraine HA, *AD*, **inflammation**, RA, *H. pylori*, *antibacterial*, **CINV**, cancer	Human research: abortive for migraine headaches comparable to sumatriptan; synergistic with injected NSAID
Ginkgo *Ginkgo biloba*	*Cataracts*, ARMD, glaucoma, periodontal dz., **vertigo**, **tinnitus**, **cardiovascular health**, **dyslipidemia**, **diabetes**, obesity, claudication, hepatic fibrosis, **diabetic nephropathy**, menopausal sexual desire, **acute mountain sickness**, migraines with aura, **stroke**, **MCI**, **dementias**, post-operative delirium, depression, ADHD, **schizophrenia**, **tardive dyskinesia**, aging skin, *inflammation*, *cancer*	**Systematic review: beneficial as prophylaxis for acute mountain sickness** Human research: reduces migraine aura duration when combined with B2, preliminary trial
Holy basil/Tulsi *Ocimum tenuiflorum/sanctum*	Gingivitis, asthma, *CAD*, **dyslipidemia**, **diabetes**, obesity, *hepatotoxicity*, PUD, *male hypogonadism*, *pain, seizures*, anxiety, depression, memory and concentration, stress and fatigue, immune function, viral encephalitis	*Preclinical research: anticonvulsant properties*
Passionflower *Passiflora incarnata*	*Asthma, diabetes*, **menopause**, OA (fruit peel), *seizure disorder*, **anxiety**, somatoform disorder, *depression*, insomnia, **ADHD**, opiate withdrawal	*Preclinical research: stimulates GABA-A currents; reduces seizure frequency and severity in mice*
Peppermint *Mentha × piperita*	Oral health, weight reduction, nausea, dyspepsia, **IBS**, GI endoscopy, cracked nipples, PCOS, neck pain, tension headaches, postherpetic neuralgia, cognition, nicotine withdrawal, pressure ulcers, pruritis gravidarum, hirsutism, athletic performance, URI, *cancer*	Human research: forehead and temple topical application reduces pain sensitivity with tension headaches, additive with acetaminophen
Skullcap (Chinese, American) *Scutellaria baicalensis, lateriflora*	*Noise-induced hearing loss*, allergy, *asthma*, COPD, *preterm RDS, pneumonia, PAH, CAD, dyslipidemia, DM, obesity, NAFLD, ETOH-induced gastritis, seizures, dementias*, **anxiety**, depression, ADHD, cognition, *photoprotection, autoimmunity, inflammation, MS, influenza, pneumonia, HIV, cancer-related anemia, cancer*	*Preclinical research: reduces seizures via GABA activation*
Turmeric (or curcumin) *Curcuma longa*	Anterior uveitis, **oral lichen planus**, **gingivitis**, dental surgery, submucous fibrosis, asthma, **diastolic HTN**, **dyslipidemia**, CAD, endothelial dysfunction, **DM**, obesity, **NAFLD**, hepatoprotective, gallbladder dyskinesia, *GERD*, PUD, dyspepsia, **UC**, DM nephropathy, lupus nephritis, lactational mastitis, LSIL, chronic non-bacterial prostatitis, post-operative pain, **OA**, RA, migraine HA, *neurodegeneration*, **anxiety**, **depression**, **skin disease**, psoriasis, fatigue, **systemic inflammation**, *HIV*, **chemo-related oral mucositis**, cancer prevention, cancer treatment	Human research: reduces COX-2 expression, iNOS expression, and frequency and severity of migraine HA in combination with omega-3FA
Valerian *Valeriana officinalis*	*HTN, CAD, IBS*, PMS, dysmenorrhea, **menopause**, tension HA, RLS, cognitive, anxiety, insomnia, OCD, *cancer*	Human research: reduces tension headache severity and disability

TABLE 16.B
Cerebrovascular Disease and Stroke.

Common Name/Latin Name	Scope of Potential Benefits	Comments
Astragalus *Astragalus membranaceus*	Herpes keratitis, recurrent tonsillitis, allergic rhinitis, atopy, asthma, **viral myocarditis**, CHF, CAD, viral hepatitis, **diabetic nephropathy**, IgA nephropathy, nephrotic syndrome, lupus nephritis, *renal fibrosis*, *sperm quality*, hemorrhagic stroke, burns, *wound healing*, *age spots*, *leukopenia*, **immune function**, *antiviral*, HBV, TB, **NSCLC**, cancer	Human research: improves recovery from hemorrhagic stroke
Black seed/nigella/black cumin *Nigella sativa*	Periodontal dz., oral submucous fibrosis, chronic rhinosinusitis, nasal dryness, **allergy**, **asthma**, COPD, chemical pneumonitis, **HTN**, *CAD*, CHF, **dyslipidemia**, **DM**, **obesity**, NAFLD, dyspepsia, PUD, diabetic nephropathy, mastalgia, menopause, male infertility, OA, *stroke*, seizure disorder, memory impairment, cognition, anxiety, *depression*, acne, eczema, vitiligo, immune function, Hashimoto's thyroiditis, RA, inflammation, *H. pylori*, *Staph* pustules, HCV, cancer	*Preclinical research: improves stroke recovery, reduces infarct size, comparable to ASA*
Coleus *Coleus forskohlii*	Glaucoma, *allergy*, asthma, HTN, CHF, *insulin resistance*, obesity, *pancreatic exocrine insufficiency*, *diarrhea*, *UTI*, *urge incontinence*, *dysmenorrhea*, *male infertility*, male hypogonadism, subarachnoid hemorrhage, *seizure*, *neurodegenerative disorders*, *alcohol abuse*, psoriasis, *photoprotection*, *hyperthyroidism*, *cancer*	Human research: reduces vasospasm following subarachnoid hemorrhage
Dong quai *Angelica sinensis*	Pulmonary HTN, *HTN*, CAD, *atrial fibrillation*, cirrhosis, portal HTN, abd pain, UC, *renal fibrosis*, *dysmenorrhea*, menopausal symptoms, *osteoporosis*, OA, stroke, *cerebrovascular insufficiency*, *neurodegenerative disorders*, *wound healing*, *aging skin*, *alopecia*, *stamina*, *inflammation*, anemia of chronic disease, cancer	*Preclinical research: neuroprotective; improves cerebral blood flow* Human research: decreases infarct volume and improved function in stroke
Elder (berry or flower) *Sambucus nigra*	Gingival recession, ASCVD, *dyslipidemia*, *DM*, obesity, constipation, stroke, *immune function*, **URI**, rhinosinusitis, influenza, *HIV*, *HSV*, *Strep*, *cancer*	Human research: decreases carotid IMT progression in combination formula
Eleuthero/Siberian Ginseng *Eleutherococcus senticosus/* *Acanthopanax senticosus*	*Allergic rhinitis*, dyslipidemia, CHF, edema, *male infertility*, osteoporosis, **stroke recovery**, *AD*, insomnia, **depression**, bipolar disorder, attention, vitality, athletic stamina, **hangover**, immune function, FMF, **URI**, *antiviral*, ovarian cancer	**Cochrane review: beneficial for stroke recovery**
Frankincense/Boswellia *Boswellia serrata, sacra, carterii*	Gingivitis, **asthma**, *COPD*, UC, **Crohn's**, **collagenous colitis**, IBS, UTI, SUI, benign breast disease, menorrhagia, **OA**, stroke, memory impairment, psoriasis, eczema, aging skin, athletic performance, **RA**, **IBD**, *inflammation*, glioma radiation, chemo-related neuropathy, *cancer*	Human research: boswellic acids improve recovery from stroke; reduces inflammation

Continued on following page

TABLE 16.B
Cerebrovascular Disease and Stroke. *(Continued)*

Common Name/Latin Name	Scope of Potential Benefits	Comments
Ginkgo *Ginkgo biloba*	*Cataracts*, ARMD, glaucoma, periodontal dz., **vertigo**, **tinnitus**, **cardiovascular health**, **dyslipidemia**, **diabetes**, obesity, claudication, hepatic fibrosis, **diabetic nephropathy**, menopausal sexual desire, **acute mountain sickness**, migraines with aura, **stroke**, **MCI**, **dementias**, post-operative delirium, depression, ADHD, **schizophrenia**, **tardive dyskinesia**, aging skin, *inflammation, cancer*	*Preclinical research: neuroprotective following brain ischemia* **Systematic review: improves function and reduces dependence in CVA convalescence**
Goji berry/wolfberry *Lycium barbarum*	Macular degeneration, *glaucoma*, dyslipidemia, **diabetes**, obesity, *hepatoprotection, male infertility, male sexual dysfunction*, stroke, AD, insomnia, anxiety, ADD, *dermatitis*, cognition, stress, fatigue, athletic performance, hangover, immunity function, influenza, cancer	*Preclinical research: neuroprotective against ischemia in stroke models*
Licorice *Glycyrrhiza glabra*	**Postoperative sore throat**, xerostomia, radiation-induced mucositis, aphthous ulcers, *allergy*, **asthma**, **dyslipidemia**, *CAD*, *diabetes*, **obesity**, hepatoprotection, heartburn, PUD, functional dyspepsia, **antipsychotic-induced hyperprolactinemia**, **menopause**, atrophic vaginitis, PCOS, female hirsutism, BPH, *stroke, dementia, PD, anxiety, insomnia, depression, substance addiction*, **hyperpigmentation**, **atopic eczema**, Addison's disease, *stamina, multiple sclerosis, inflammation*, H. Pylori, cancer, *breast cancer*	*Preclinical research: attenuates neurological deficit in animal stroke model; inhibits microglial inflammation* **(Caution: use deglycyrrhizinated formulations in patients at risk for HTN and hypokalemia)**
Motherwort *Leonurus cardiaca*	*HTN 2/2 anxiety or hyperthyroidism, dyslipidemia, CAD, arrhythmia, nausea, IBS, AKI, lactation, post-partum bleeding, menorrhagia, amenorrhea*, menopause, *pain*, stroke, anxiety, *insomnia, hyperthyroidism, inflammation, breast tumors*	*Preclinical research: limits size of brain infarct and improves recovery in rat stroke model*
Saffron *Crocus sativus*	ARMD, *cataracts*, diabetic maculopathy, glaucoma, gingivitis, burning mouth syndrome, *allergy*, asthma, HTN, **dyslipidemia**, DM, **obesity**, *hepatotoxicity, DM nephropathy*, PMS, menopause, **female and male sexual dysfunction**, male infertility, chronic pain, fibromyalgia, stroke, AD, **anxiety**, insomnia, OCD, **depression**, ADHD, drug and ETOH addiction, *photodamage*, stamina, immune function, inflammation, RA, *bacterial infection*, cancer	Human research: improves recovery from stroke
Schisandra *Schisandra chinensis*	*MI*, **CHF**, DM, NAFLD, viral hepatitis, menopause, FMF, *stroke, AD, anxiety*, cognition, physical stress, stamina, pneumonia, *HCV, fungal infections*, cancer	*Preclinical research: neuroprotective against stroke via NO pathway*

TABLE 16.C
Age-Related Cognitive Impairment, Dementia, and Alzheimer's Disease.

Common Name/Latin Name	Scope of Potential Benefits	Comments
Aloe *Aloe vera, barbadensis*	**Gingivitis**, **submucous fibrosis**, **dyslipidemia**, **diabetes**, insulin resistance, hepatic fibrosis, GERD, **IBS**, IBD, anal fissures, radiation proctitis, AD, *PD*, acne, **psoriasis**, **lichen planus**, **burns**, wounds, pressure ulcers, diabetic foot ulcers, wrinkle and striae reduction, Hashimoto's thyroiditis, inflammation, HIV, cancer	Human research: aloe polymannose complex beneficial at 12 months in AD
Ashwagandha *Withania somnifera*	Dyslipidemia, DM, **sexual dysfunction**, **infertility**, *osteoporosis*, gout, OA, *AD, PD*, MCI, **anxiety**, insomnia, OCD, *depression*, schizophrenia, hypothyroidism, stress, endurance, *fatigue*, immune function, TB, *cancer*	*Preclinical research: improves cognition in AD model* Human research: improves multiple cognitive domains in MCI
Bacopa *Bacopa monnieri*	*Gastric ulcer*, hepatic encephalopathy, IBS-D, *seizures*, memory impairment, **dementia-related anxiety**, test anxiety, **cognitive performance**, ADHD, inflammation	Human research: improves cognitive performance in elderly with and without dementia in polyherbal combination
Bilberry *Vaccinium myrtillus*	Normal pressure glaucoma, cataracts, night vision, eye fatigue, gingivitis, *HTN*, **dyslipidemia**, T2DM, NAFLD, ulcerative colitis, *AD*, psoriasis, *wounds*, inflammation, *S. pneumonia, MRSA*, colorectal cancer, *other cancers*	*Preclinical research: inhibits Aβ fibril formation and toxic aggregates*
Black seed/nigella/black cumin *Nigella sativa*	Periodontal dz., oral submucous fibrosis, chronic rhinosinusitis, nasal dryness, **allergy**, **asthma**, COPD, chemical pneumonitis, **HTN**, *CAD*, CHF, **dyslipidemia**, **DM**, **obesity**, NAFLD, dyspepsia, PUD, diabetic nephropathy, mastalgia, menopause, male infertility, OA, *stroke*, seizure disorder, memory impairment, cognition, anxiety, *depression*, acne, eczema, vitiligo, immune function, Hashimoto's thyroiditis, RA, inflammation, *H. pylori, Staph* pustules, HCV, cancer	*Preclinical research: improves memory* Human research: improves memory, attention, and cognition in elderly; improves cognition in young volunteers
Butterbur *Petasites hybridus*	**Allergic rhinitis**, asthma, *HTN*, *GI ulceration*, bladder spasms, **migraine headache**, *neurodegenerative dementias*, somatoform disorder anxiety and depression, *CNS inflammation*	*Preclinical research: neuroprotective against Aβ, reduces neurologic inflammation*
Dandelion *Taraxacum officinale*	HTN, dyslipidemia, DM, *obesity, edema*, liver toxicity, NAFLD, *gastroparesis*, dyspepsia, *neurodegenerative disorders, depression, stamina, inflammation, endotoxic shock, cancer*	*Preclinical research: fruit extract antioxidant to brain hippocampus and striatum*
Eleuthero/Siberian Ginseng *Eleutherococcus senticosus/ Acanthopanax senticosus*	*Allergic rhinitis*, dyslipidemia, CHF, edema, *male infertility*, osteoporosis, **stroke recovery**, *AD*, insomnia, **depression**, bipolar disorder, attention, vitality, athletic stamina, **hangover**, immune function, FMF, **URI**, *antiviral*, ovarian cancer	*Preclinical research: protection against Aβ*

Continued on following page

TABLE 16.C

Age-Related Cognitive Impairment, Dementia, and Alzheimer's Disease. *(Continued)*

Common Name/Latin Name	Scope of Potential Benefits	Comments
Fennel *Foeniculum vulgare*	*Glaucoma, dyspepsia, gastroprotection, gastroparesis,* **infant colic**, IBS, constipation, *overactive bladder, lactation,* dysmenorrhea, oligomenorrhea, **menopausal disorders**, *dementia,* hirsutism, *inflammation*	*Preclinical research: AChEI activity; improves cognitive performance*
Frankincense/Boswellia *Boswellia serrata, sacra, carterii*	Gingivitis, **asthma**, *COPD*, UC, **Crohn's, collagenous colitis**, IBS, UTI, SUI, benign breast disease, menorrhagia, **OA**, stroke, memory impairment, psoriasis, eczema, aging skin, athletic performance, **RA, IBD**, *inflammation,* glioma radiation, chemo-related neuropathy, *cancer*	Human research: reduces memory impairment in combination with lemon balm
Ginger *Zingiber officinale*	**Motion sickness**, *HTN*, dyslipidemia, fibrinolysis, diabetes, **nausea**, **vomiting**, *dyspepsia,* gastroparesis, PUD, ulcerative colitis, *diabetic nephropathy,* **dysmenorrhea**, *Candida vaginitis,* male infertility, OA, muscle injury, migraine HA, *AD,* **inflammation**, RA, *H. pylori, antibacterial,* **CINV**, cancer	*Preclinical research: neuroprotective against Aβ toxicity*
Ginkgo *Ginkgo biloba*	*Cataracts,* ARMD, glaucoma, periodontal dz., **vertigo**, **tinnitus, cardiovascular health, dyslipidemia, diabetes**, obesity, claudication, hepatic fibrosis, **diabetic nephropathy**, menopausal sexual desire, **acute mountain sickness**, migraines with aura, **stroke, MCI, dementias**, post-operative delirium, depression, ADHD, **schizophrenia, tardive dyskinesia**, aging skin, *inflammation, cancer*	**Systematic reviews: variably beneficial in MCI and dementia for cognition, ADLs, behavioral and psychological symptoms; standardized extract 240 mg/d** Human Research: minimum dose 200 mg per day, may take 12 months to show full efficacy; additive to AChEI; MCI, AD, and vascular dementia benefit; benefit for behavioral-psychological symptoms and vertigo. Shortens post-operative delirium, improves cerebral O_2 supply
Ginseng, Asian/Korean/ Chinese *Panax ginseng*	Dry eyes, **hearing loss**, HTN, CHF, **DM**, obesity, **menopause, ED**, male infertility, *osteoporosis,* AD, cognitive function, aging skin, alopecia areata, stamina, **chronic fatigue, hangover**, immune function, inflammation, influenza, HIV, **cancer**	**Systematic review: findings inconsistent for dementia** Human research: stabilizes cognitive function in AD over 2-year trial
Goji berry/wolfberry *Lycium barbarum*	Macular degeneration, *glaucoma,* dyslipidemia, **diabetes**, obesity, *hepatoprotection, male infertility, male sexual dysfunction, stroke, AD,* insomnia, anxiety, ADD, *dermatitis,* cognition, stress, fatigue, athletic performance, hangover, immunity function, influenza, cancer	*Preclinical research: neuroprotective against Aβ*
Gynostemma/Jiaogulan *Gynostemma pentaphyllum*	*Asthma, CAD, dyslipidemia,* DM, obesity, *arrhythmia,* NAFLD, *PUD,* PCOS, *PD, white matter disease,* dementia, *stamina,* immune function, cancer	*Preclinical research: prevents scopolamine-induced memory impairment; protective against PD, memory impairment, white matter disease* Human research: improves cognition, antioxidant
Hop/Hops *Humulus lupulus*	Dental plaque, allergic rhinitis, ASCVD, dyslipidemia, T2DM, obesity, *NAFLD, dyspepsia,* osteoporosis, OA, RA, atrophic vaginitis, menopause, cognitive decline, **insomnia**, anxiety, depression, cognitive performance, acne, aging skin, body odor, antibacterial, *TB, cancer*	Human research: improves cognitive performance in subjects with perceived cognitive decline

TABLE 16.C
Age-Related Cognitive Impairment, Dementia, and Alzheimer's Disease. *(Continued)*

Common Name/Latin Name	Scope of Potential Benefits	Comments
Horsetail *Equisetum arvense*	*Diabetes*, nephrolithiasis, *UTI*, *interstitial cystitis*, BPH, osteoporosis, *OA*, RA, *chronic pain*, *anxiety*, *cognition*, psoriatic nails, wound healing, aging skin, alopecia, inflammation	*Preclinical research: improves learning and memory in mice*
Lemon balm *Melissa officinalis*	**Bruxism**, dyslipidemia, DM, palpitations, dyspepsia, IBS, **colic**, PMS, dysmenorrhea, female sexual dysfunction, **AD**, dementia, agitation, *diabetic neuropathy*, insomnia, **anxiety**, depression, **ADHD**, *hyperthyroidism*, *Graves' disease*, herpes simplex, *cancer*, *glioblastoma multiforme*	**Systematic review: beneficial for AD** Human research: improves cognition; EO reduces agitation and improves social engagement
Licorice *Glycyrrhiza glabra*	**Postoperative sore throat**, xerostomia, radiation-induced mucositis, aphthous ulcers, *allergy*, **asthma**, **dyslipidemia**, *CAD*, *diabetes*, **obesity**, hepatoprotection, heartburn, PUD, functional dyspepsia, **antipsychotic-induced hyperprolactinemia**, **menopause**, atrophic vaginitis, PCOS, female hirsutism, BPH, *stroke*, *dementia*, PD, *anxiety*, *insomnia*, *depression*, *substance addiction*, **hyperpigmentation**, **atopic eczema**, Addison's disease, *stamina*, *multiple sclerosis*, *inflammation*, *H. pylori*, cancer, *breast cancer*	*Preclinical research: AChEI properties; prevents cognitive decline in rats; binds NMDA; reduces oligomeric Aβ proteins, inhibits microglial inflammation* Human research: improves symptoms of PD ***(Caution: use deglycyrrhizinated formulations in patients at risk for HTN and hypokalemia)***
Maca *Lepidium meyenii, peruvianum*	HTN, DM, weight reduction, perimenopause, **menopause**, **sexual dysfunction**, anti-depressant-induced sexual dysfunction, **male sexual dysfunction**, **male infertility**, BPH, osteoporosis, *memory impairment*, anxiety, depression, fatigue, inflammation	*Preclinical research: black maca improves memory and learning in memory-impaired mice*
Milk thistle *Silybum marianum*	**Dyslipidemia, DM, liver disease**, diabetic nephropathy, lactation, *PCOS*, BPH, *gout, AD, diabetic neuropathy*, **OCD**, acne, *psoriasis*, vitiligo, radio-dermatitis, aging skin, RA, inflammation, hepatitis viruses, **iron-overload**, chemotherapy and radiotherapy toxicity, *hepatocellular carcinoma*	*Preclinical research: suppresses Aβ protein fibril and oligomer formation and neurotoxicity; improves behavior in mouse model of AD*
Saffron *Crocus sativus*	ARMD, *cataracts*, diabetic maculopathy, glaucoma, gingivitis, burning mouth syndrome, *allergy*, asthma, HTN, **dyslipidemia**, DM, **obesity**, *hepatotoxicity*, *DM nephropathy*, PMS, menopause, **female and male sexual dysfunction**, male infertility, chronic pain, fibromyalgia, stroke, AD, **anxiety**, insomnia, OCD, **depression**, ADHD, drug and ETOH addiction, *photodamage*, stamina, immune function, inflammation, RA, *bacterial infection*, cancer	*Preclinical research: attenuates Aβ protein fibril formation* Human research: comparable to donepezil and memantine in AD with less ADRs than donepezil; improves multidomain cognitive impairment; adjuvant to meds
Sage *Salvia officinalis/ lavandulifolia*	**Dyslipidemia, dementia, cognitive performance**	Miroddi et al. (2014)

Continued on following page

TABLE 16.C

Age-Related Cognitive Impairment, Dementia, and Alzheimer's Disease. *(Continued)*

Common Name/Latin Name	Scope of Potential Benefits	Comments
Schisandra *Schisandra chinensis*	*MI*, **CHF**, DM, NAFLD, viral hepatitis, menopause, FMF, *stroke, AD, anxiety*, cognition, physical stress, stamina, pneumonia, *HCV, fungal infections*, cancer	*Preclinical research: prevents neurodegeneration, preserves cognition in mouse model of AD.* **Blocks beta secretase** *(AD source of Aβ).*
Skullcap (Chinese, American) *Scutellaria baicalensis, lateriflora*	*Noise-induced hearing loss*, allergy, *asthma, COPD, preterm RDS*, pneumonia, *PAH, CAD, dyslipidemia, DM, obesity, NAFLD, ETOH-induced gastritis, seizures, dementias*, **anxiety**, depression, *ADHD*, cognition, *photoprotection, autoimmunity, inflammation, MS, influenza, pneumonia, HIV, cancer-related anemia, cancer*	*Preclinical research: neuroprotective and memory-enhancing; increases cholinergic neurons and NMDA receptors; reduces memory impairment in ischemic model; induces hippocampal proliferation*
Turmeric (or curcumin) *Curcuma longa*	Anterior uveitis, **oral lichen planus**, **gingivitis**, dental surgery, submucous fibrosis, asthma, **diastolic HTN**, **dyslipidemia**, CAD, endothelial dysfunction, **DM**, obesity, **NAFLD**, hepatoprotective, gallbladder dyskinesia, *GERD*, PUD, dyspepsia, **UC**, DM nephropathy, lupus nephritis, lactational mastitis, LSIL, chronic non-bacterial prostatitis, post-operative pain, **OA**, RA, migraine HA, *neurodegeneration*, **anxiety**, **depression**, **skin disease**, psoriasis, fatigue, **systemic inflammation**, *HIV*, **chemo-related oral mucositis**, cancer prevention, cancer treatment	*Preclinical research: increases BDNF levels; reduces Aβ formation, dissolves amyloid plaque; stimulates neural stem cells*
Uva ursi *Arctostaphylos uva-ursi*	*UTI*, recurrent UTI, *dementia, dermatitis, skin hyperpigmentation, cough*	*Preclinical research: AChEI activity*
Valerian *Valeriana officinalis*	*HTN, CAD, IBS*, PMS, dysmenorrhea, **menopause**, RLS, cognitive, anxiety, insomnia, OCD, *cancer*	*Preclinical research: improves memory and learning in rats* Human research: reduces decline in cognition post CABG

TABLE 16.D

Parkinson's Disease and Other Neurodegenerative Disorders (See Table 21.C for Multiple Sclerosis).

Common Name/Latin Name	Scope of Potential Benefits	Comments
Aloe *Aloe vera, barbadensis*	**Gingivitis**, **submucous fibrosis**, **dyslipidemia**, **diabetes**, insulin resistance, hepatic fibrosis, GERD, **IBS**, IBD, anal fissures, radiation proctitis, AD, *PD*, acne, **psoriasis**, **lichen planus**, **burns**, wounds, pressure ulcers, diabetic foot ulcers, wrinkle and striae reduction, Hashimoto's thyroiditis, inflammation, HIV, cancer	*Preclinical research: protects striatal region against damage in PD model*
Ashwagandha *Withania somnifera*	Dyslipidemia, DM, **sexual dysfunction**, **infertility**, *osteoporosis*, gout, OA, *AD, PD*, MCI, **anxiety**, insomnia, OCD, *depression*, schizophrenia, hypothyroidism, stress, endurance, *fatigue*, immune function, TB, *cancer*	*Preclinical research: prevents neurodegeneration in PD model*

TABLE 16.D
Parkinson's Disease and Other Neurodegenerative Disorders (See Table 21.C for Multiple Sclerosis). *(Continued)*

Common Name/Latin Name	Scope of Potential Benefits	Comments
Coleus *Coleus forskohlii*	Glaucoma, *allergy*, asthma, HTN, CHF, *insulin resistance*, obesity, *pancreatic exocrine insufficiency, diarrhea, UTI, urge incontinence, dysmenorrhea, male infertility*, male hypogonadism, subarachnoid hemorrhage, *seizure, neurodegenerative disorders, alcohol abuse*, psoriasis, *photoprotection, hyperthyroidism, cancer*	*Preclinical research: prevents neurodegenerative mechanisms*
Dandelion *Taraxacum officinale*	HTN, dyslipidemia, DM, *obesity, edema*, liver toxicity, NAFLD, *gastroparesis*, dyspepsia, *neurodegenerative disorders, depression, stamina, inflammation, endotoxic shock, cancer*	*Preclinical research: fruit extract antioxidant to brain hippocampus and striatum*
Dong quai *Angelica sinensis*	Pulmonary HTN, *HTN*, CAD, *atrial fibrillation*, cirrhosis, portal HTN, abd pain, UC, *renal fibrosis, dysmenorrhea*, menopausal symptoms, *osteoporosis, OA*, stroke, *cerebrovascular insufficiency, neurodegenerative disorders, wound healing, aging skin, alopecia, stamina, inflammation*, anemia of chronic disease, cancer	*Preclinical research: neuroprotective through anti-oxidation; improves cerebral blood flow*
Fenugreek *Trigonella foenum-graecum*	Dyslipidemia, **DM**, pre-diabetes, *diabetic nephropathy, urolithiasis*, lactation, dysmenorrhea, PCOS, menopause, male sexual dysfunction, hypogonadism, PD, *peripheral neuropathy, thyroid T3/T4 balance*, stamina, *cancer*	Human research: improves Hoehn and Yahr scales in 21% of patients with PD
Gynostemma/Jiaogulan *Gynostemma pentaphyllum*	*Asthma, CAD, dyslipidemia*, DM, obesity, *arrhythmia*, NAFLD, *PUD*, PCOS, *PD, white matter disease*, dementia, *stamina*, immune function, cancer	*Preclinical research: prevents scopolamine-induced memory impairment; protective against PD, memory impairment, white matter disease* Human research: improves cognition, antioxidant effects
Licorice *Glycyrrhiza glabra*	**Postoperative sore throat**, xerostomia, radiation-induced mucositis, aphthous ulcers, *allergy*, **asthma**, **dyslipidemia**, *CAD, diabetes*, **obesity**, hepatoprotection, heartburn, PUD, functional dyspepsia, **antipsychotic-induced hyperprolactinemia**, **menopause**, atrophic vaginitis, PCOS, female hirsutism, BPH, *stroke, dementia*, PD, *anxiety, insomnia, depression, substance addiction*, **hyperpigmentation**, **atopic eczema**, Addison's disease, *stamina, multiple sclerosis, inflammation*, H. Pylori, cancer, *breast cancer*	*Preclinical research: inhibits microglial inflammation* Human research: improves symptoms of PD ***(Caution: use deglycyrrhizinated formulations in patients at risk for HTN and hypokalemia)***
Schisandra *Schisandra chinensis*	*MI*, **CHF**, DM, NAFLD, viral hepatitis, menopause, FMF, *stroke, AD, anxiety*, cognition, physical stress, stamina, pneumonia, *HCV, fungal infections*, cancer	*Preclinical research: prevents neurodegeneration*
Yarrow *Achillea millefolium*	*Epistaxis, asthma*, HTN, **dyslipidemia**, *T1DM*, cirrhosis, *gastritis, PUD, anorexia, IBS, IBD*, dysmenorrhea, *menorrhagia*, menopause, *anxiety, neurodegenerative disorders*, multiple sclerosis, *inflammation*	*Preclinical research: reduces neurodegeneration*

TABLE 16.E
Neuropathy and Restless Legs Syndrome.

Common Name/Latin Name	Scope of Potential Benefits	Comments
Chamomile *Matricaria chamomilla/ recutita*	Gingivitis, mucositis, chronic rhinosinusitis, *allergies*, dyslipidemia, diabetes, *PUD*, colic, IBS, diarrhea, dyspepsia, UC, *candida vaginitis*, menopause, carpal tunnel syndrome, anxiety, insomnia, depression, ADHD, eczema, wounds, radiation or chemotherapy dermatitis, cortisol dysregulation, *inflammation*, *broadly antimicrobial (bacteria, yeast, fungus)*, *cancer*	Human research: topical oil improves CTS symptoms but not electro diagnostics
Fenugreek *Trigonella foenum-graecum*	Dyslipidemia, **DM**, pre-diabetes, *diabetic nephropathy*, *urolithiasis*, lactation, dysmenorrhea, PCOS, menopause, male sexual dysfunction, hypogonadism, PD, *peripheral neuropathy*, *thyroid T3/T4 balance*, stamina, *cancer*	*Preclinical research: peripheral neuropathy reversed*
Horsetail *Equisetum arvense*	*Diabetes*, nephrolithiasis, *UTI*, *interstitial cystitis*, BPH, osteoporosis, *OA*, RA, *chronic pain*, anxiety, *cognition*, psoriatic nails, wound healing, aging skin, alopecia, inflammation	*Preclinical research: reduces nociception in mice, non-opiate mechanism*
Lemon balm *Melissa officinalis*	**Bruxism**, dyslipidemia, DM, palpitations, dyspepsia, IBS, **colic**, PMS, dysmenorrhea, female sexual dysfunction, **AD**, dementia, agitation, *diabetic neuropathy*, insomnia, **anxiety**, depression, **ADHD**, *hyperthyroidism*, *Graves' disease*, herpes simplex, *cancer*, *glioblastoma multiforme*	*Preclinical research: EO reduces diabetic hyperalgesia*
Milk thistle *Silybum marianum*	**Dyslipidemia, DM, liver disease**, diabetic nephropathy, lactation, *PCOS*, BPH, *gout*, *AD*, *diabetic neuropathy*, **OCD**, acne, *psoriasis*, vitiligo, radio-dermatitis, aging skin, RA, inflammation, hepatitis viruses, **iron-overload**, chemotherapy and radiotherapy toxicity, *hepatocellular carcinoma*	*Preclinical research: protective against diabetic neuropathy*
Peppermint *Mentha × piperita*	Oral health, weight reduction, nausea, dyspepsia, **IBS**, GI endoscopy, cracked nipples, PCOS, neck pain, tension headaches, postherpetic neuralgia, cognition, nicotine withdrawal, pressure ulcers, pruritis gravidarum, hirsutism, athletic performance, URI, *cancer*	Human case report: improves postherpetic neuralgia in resistant case
St. John's Wort *Hypericum perforatum*	PMS, **perimenopause or menopause**, *chronic pain*, neuropathy, **depression**, *opiate addiction*, psoriasis, atopic dermatitis, *sunburn*, inflammation, HSV, *cancer*	*Preclinical research: reduces hyperalgesia and nociception; augments morphine; reduces oxycodone levels* Human research: topically antineuralgic ***(See St. John's Wort monograph warnings and precautions)***
Valerian *Valeriana officinalis*	*HTN, CAD, IBS*, PMS, dysmenorrhea, **menopause**, RLS, cognitive, anxiety, insomnia, OCD, *cancer*	Human research: improves RLS in subjects with daytime sleepiness

REFERENCES

Miroddi M, Navarra M, Quattropani MC, Calapai F, Gangemi S, Calapai G. Systematic review of clinical trials assessing pharmacological properties of Salvia species on memory, cognitive impairment and Alzheimer's disease. CNS Neurosci Ther 2014;20(6):485–95.

Saranitzky E, White CM, Baker EL, Baker WL, Coleman CI. Feverfew for migraine prophylaxis: a systematic review. J Diet Suppl 2009;6(2):91–103.

Wider B, Pittler MH, Ernst E. Feverfew for preventing migraine. Cochrane Database Syst Rev 2015;4(4), CD002286.

17

PSYCHIATRIC DISORDERS

	TABLE 17.A	
	Anxiety, Panic Disorder, Insomnia, and Obsessive-Compulsive Disorder.	
Common Name/ Latin Name	**Scope of Potential Benefits**	**Comments**
Ashwagandha *Withania somnifera*	Dyslipidemia, DM, **sexual dysfunction**, **infertility**, *osteoporosis*, gout, OA, *AD*, *PD*, MCI, **anxiety**, insomnia, OCD, *depression*, schizophrenia, hypothyroidism, stress, endurance, *fatigue*, immune function, TB, *cancer*	*Preclinical research: comparable to lorazepam for anxiety* **Systematic review: beneficial for anxiety** Human research: improves sleep, reduces OCD
Bacopa *Bacopa monnieri*	*Gastric ulcer*, hepatic encephalopathy, IBS-D, *seizures*, memory impairment, **dementia-related anxiety**, test anxiety, **cognitive performance**, ADHD, inflammation	**Systematic review: reduces anxiety in patients with dementia** Human research: reduces test-associated anxiety
Black seed/nigella/black cumin *Nigella sativa*	Periodontal dz., oral submucous fibrosis, chronic rhinosinusitis, nasal dryness, **allergy**, **asthma**, COPD, chemical pneumonitis, **HTN**, *CAD*, CHF, **dyslipidemia**, **DM**, **obesity**, NAFLD, dyspepsia, PUD, diabetic nephropathy, mastalgia, menopause, male infertility, OA, *stroke*, seizure disorder, memory impairment, cognition, anxiety, *depression*, acne, eczema, vitiligo, immune function, Hashimoto's thyroiditis, RA, inflammation, *H. pylori*, *Staph* pustules, HCV, cancer	*Preclinical research: GABAergic, anti-anxiety comparable to diazepam* Human research: improves cognition and mood; reduces anxiety in healthy young volunteers
Chamomile (German) *Matricaria chamomilla/ recutita*	Gingivitis, mucositis, chronic rhinosinusitis, *allergies*, dyslipidemia, diabetes, *PUD*, colic, IBS, diarrhea, dyspepsia, UC, *candida vaginitis*, menopause, carpal tunnel syndrome, anxiety, insomnia, depression, ADHD, eczema, wounds, radiation or chemotherapy dermatitis, cortisol dysregulation, *inflammation, broadly antimicrobial (bacteria, yeast, fungus), cancer*	Human research: reduces anxiety; reduces insomnia variably, including in the elderly and transiently in postpartum; normalizes cortisol rhythm in GAD; one small trial also showed some benefit with ADHD
Chasteberry/Chaste tree/Vitex *Vitex agnus-castus*	**Cyclical mastalgia**, **PMS**, **PMDD**, oligomenorrhea, amenorrhea, IUD bleeding, **female infertility**, perimenopause, menstrual migraines, bone healing, insomnia, *inflammation, pain*	Human research: increases nocturnal melatonin release

Continued on following page

TABLE 17.A
Anxiety, Panic Disorder, Insomnia, and Obsessive-Compulsive Disorder. *(Continued)*

Common Name/ Latin Name	Scope of Potential Benefits	Comments
Echinacea *Echinacea purpurea, angustifolia*	Anterior uveitis, *candida vaginitis*, genital condylomas, OA, **anxiety**, eczema, athletic performance, immune function, inflammation, **URIs**, influenza, *Coronavirus*, HPV, *colorectal cancer*	**Systematic review: one of several herbs with evidence for efficacy in anxiety** Human research: 40 mg dose decreases STAI scores
Eleuthero/Siberian Ginseng *Eleutherococcus senticosus/ Acanthopanax senticosus*	*Allergic rhinitis*, dyslipidemia, CHF, edema, *male infertility*, osteoporosis, **stroke recovery**, *AD*, *insomnia*, **depression**, bipolar disorder, attention, vitality, athletic stamina, **hangover**, immune function, FMF, **URI**, *antiviral*, ovarian cancer	*Preclinical research: reduces sleep latency, prolongs sleep duration*
Goji berry/wolfberry *Lycium barbarum*	Macular degeneration, *glaucoma*, dyslipidemia, **diabetes**, obesity, *hepatoprotection*, *male infertility*, *male sexual dysfunction*, *stroke*, *AD*, insomnia, anxiety, ADD, *dermatitis*, cognition, stress, fatigue, athletic performance, hangover, immunity function, influenza, cancer	Human research: improves calmness and sleep quality
Hawthorn *Crataegus* spp.	HTN, CAD, **CHF** (HrEF and HpEF), arrhythmia, **orthostatic hypotension**, *NAFLD*, anxiety, *inflammation*	Human research: trend toward reduced anxiety with HTN; lowers anxiety when combined with California poppy and magnesium
Holy basil/Tulsi *Ocimum tenuiflorum/ sanctum*	Gingivitis, asthma, *CAD*, **dyslipidemia**, **diabetes**, obesity, *hepatotoxicity*, *PUD*, *male hypogonadism*, *pain*, *seizures*, anxiety, depression, memory and concentration, stress and fatigue, immune function, viral encephalitis	Human research: reduces anxiety, improves mood, reduces stress
Hops/Hop *Humulus lupulus*	Dental plaque, allergic rhinitis, ASCVD, dyslipidemia, T2DM, obesity, *NAFLD*, *dyspepsia*, osteoporosis, OA, RA, atrophic vaginitis, menopause, cognitive decline, **insomnia**, anxiety, depression, cognitive performance, acne, aging skin, body odor, antibacterial, *TB*, *cancer*	**Systematic review: beneficial for insomnia in combination with valerian** Human research: reduces NE under mental stress; reductions in depression anxiety stress scale; reduces insomnia in combination with valerian or passionflower (on par with zolpidem, diphenhydramine, benzodiazepine)
Horsetail *Equisetum arvense*	*Diabetes*, nephrolithiasis, *UTI*, *interstitial cystitis*, BPH, osteoporosis, *OA*, RA, *chronic pain*, anxiety, *cognition*, psoriatic nails, wound healing, aging skin, alopecia, inflammation	*Preclinical research: reduces anxious behavior under stress*
Kava *Kava kava*	**Anxiety (short term)**	Smith and Leiras (2018) Pittler and Ernst (2000)
Lavender *Lavandula* spp.	**Dysmenorrhea, anxiety, insomnia, depression, wounds**	Donelli et al. (2019) Fismer and Pilkington (2012)
Lemon balm *Melissa officinalis*	**Bruxism**, dyslipidemia, DM, palpitations, dyspepsia, IBS, **colic**, PMS, dysmenorrhea, female sexual dysfunction, **AD**, dementia, agitation, *diabetic neuropathy*, insomnia, **anxiety**, depression, **ADHD**, *hyperthyroidism*, *Graves' disease*, herpes simplex, *cancer*, *glioblastoma multiforme*	**Systematic review: beneficial for anxiety** Human research: multiple studies show anxiety reduction, stress-response reduction, mood and sleep improvement, several in combination with valerian; larger doses impair select cognitive domains

TABLE 17.A
Anxiety, Panic Disorder, Insomnia, and Obsessive-Compulsive Disorder. *(Continued)*

Common Name/ Latin Name	Scope of Potential Benefits	Comments
Licorice *Glycyrrhiza glabra*	**Postoperative sore throat**, xerostomia, radiation-induced mucositis, aphthous ulcers, *allergy*, **asthma**, **dyslipidemia**, *CAD*, *diabetes*, **obesity**, hepatoprotection, heartburn, PUD, functional dyspepsia, **antipsychotic-induced hyperprolactinemia**, **menopause**, atrophic vaginitis, PCOS, female hirsutism, BPH, *stroke*, *dementia*, PD, *anxiety*, *insomnia*, *depression*, *substance addiction*, **hyperpigmentation**, **atopic eczema**, Addison's disease, *stamina*, *multiple sclerosis*, *inflammation*, *H. pylori*, cancer, *breast cancer*	*Preclinical research: constituent has GABA$_A$ agonism; sedation comparable to zolpidem* **(Caution: use deglycyrrhizinated formulations in patients at risk for HTN and hypokalemia)**
Maca *Lepidium meyenii, peruvianum*	HTN, DM, weight reduction, perimenopause, **menopause**, **sexual dysfunction**, anti-depressant-induced sexual dysfunction, **male sexual dysfunction**, **male infertility**, *BPH*, osteoporosis, *memory impairment*, anxiety, depression, fatigue, inflammation	Human research: reduces anxiety and depression in postmenopausal women
Milk thistle *Silybum marianum*	**Dyslipidemia**, **DM**, **liver disease**, diabetic nephropathy, lactation, *PCOS*, BPH, *gout*, *AD*, *diabetic neuropathy*, **OCD**, acne, *psoriasis*, vitiligo, radio-dermatitis, aging skin, RA, inflammation, hepatitis viruses, **iron-overload**, chemotherapy and radiotherapy toxicity, *hepatocellular carcinoma*	**Systematic review: tentative support for OCD** Human research: similar efficacy to fluoxetine 30 mg/day for OCD
Motherwort *Leonurus cardiaca*	*HTN 2/2 anxiety or hyperthyroidism, dyslipidemia, CAD, arrhythmia, nausea, IBS, AKI, lactation, post-partum bleeding, menorrhagia, amenorrhea, menopause, pain, stroke, anxiety, insomnia, hyperthyroidism, inflammation, breast tumors*	Human research: reduces anxiety in hypertensives
Passionflower *Passiflora incarnata*	*Asthma, diabetes,* **menopause**, OA (fruit peel), *seizure disorder,* **anxiety**, somatoform disorder, *depression,* insomnia, **ADHD**, opiate withdrawal	**Systematic reviews: beneficial acutely and generally for anxiety (strong evidence)** Human research: anxiolytic comparable to oxazepam; preoperative effects comparable to midazolam; less S/E than drugs; herbal combination comparable to zolpidem for insomnia; herbal combination effective for somatoform disorder
Rhodiola *Rhodiola rosea*	**CAD**, *menorrhagia, amenorrhea, female infertility,* menopause, *male hypogonadism,* premature ejaculation, **anxiety**, **depression**, **cognition**, eczema, burnout, fatigue, **athletic stamina**, cancer	**Clinical Review: Rhodiola is one of 13 herbs with supportive evidence for benefit in anxiety** Human research: 340–400 mg per day reduces anxiety
Saffron *Crocus sativus*	ARMD, *cataracts*, diabetic maculopathy, glaucoma, gingivitis, burning mouth syndrome, *allergy*, asthma, HTN, **dyslipidemia**, DM, **obesity**, *hepatotoxicity*, *DM nephropathy*, PMS, menopause, **female and male sexual dysfunction**, male infertility, chronic pain, fibromyalgia, stroke, AD, **anxiety**, insomnia, OCD, **depression**, ADHD, drug and ETOH addiction, *photodamage*, stamina, immune function, inflammation, RA, *bacterial infection*, cancer	*Preclinical research: anxiolytic comparable to diazepam; decreases OCD in rats* **Systematic review: beneficial for anxiety** Human research: numerous studies show benefit especially for mixed anxiety and depression; improves insomnia; comparable to fluvoxamine for OCD

Continued on following page

TABLE 17.A
Anxiety, Panic Disorder, Insomnia, and Obsessive-Compulsive Disorder. *(Continued)*

Common Name/ Latin Name	Scope of Potential Benefits	Comments
Schisandra *Schisandra chinensis*	*MI*, **CHF**, DM, NAFLD, viral hepatitis, menopause, FMF, *stroke, AD, anxiety,* cognition, *physical stress, stamina,* pneumonia, *HCV, fungal infections,* cancer	*Preclinical research: anxiolytic in stressed mice* via *modulation of hyperactive HPA axis*
Skullcap (Chinese, American) *Scutellaria baicalensis, lateriflora*	*Noise induced hearing loss,* allergy, *asthma, COPD, preterm RDS, pneumonia, PAH, CAD, dyslipidemia, DM, obesity, NAFLD, ETOH-induced gastritis, seizures, dementias,* **anxiety**, depression, *ADHD,* cognition, *photoprotection, autoimmunity, inflammation, MS, influenza, pneumonia, HIV, cancer-related anemia, cancer*	**Preclinical research:** *GABA receptor agonist and antagonist; baicalein reduces anxious behavior in mice* **Clinical review: one of 13 herbs with evidence for anxiolytic effect** Human research: American skullcap decreases anxiety in healthy volunteers
Tribulus/Puncture vine/ Goathead *Tribulus terrestris*	HTN, CAD, dyslipidemia, DM, *hepatotoxicity, IBS, nephrolithiasis,* **sexual dysfunction**, hypoactive sexual desire, *pain, anxiety, depression, inflammation, cancer*	*Preclinical research: reduces anxiety and depression in mice; MAO-I activity*
Turmeric (or curcumin) *Curcuma longa*	Anterior uveitis, **oral lichen planus, gingivitis**, dental surgery, submucous fibrosis, asthma, **diastolic HTN, dyslipidemia**, CAD, endothelial dysfunction, **DM**, obesity, **NAFLD**, hepatoprotective, gallbladder dyskinesia, *GERD*, PUD, dyspepsia, **UC**, DM nephropathy, lupus nephritis, lactational mastitis, LSIL, chronic non-bacterial prostatitis, post-operative pain, **OA**, RA, migraine HA, *neurodegeneration*, **anxiety**, **depression**, **skin disease**, psoriasis, fatigue, **systemic inflammation**, *HIV*, **chemo-related oral mucositis**, cancer prevention, cancer treatment	**Systematic review: reduces anxiety with depression** Human research: reduces anxiety states
Valerian *Valeriana officinalis*	*HTN, CAD, IBS, PMS, dysmenorrhea,* **menopause**, *RLS, cognitive, anxiety, insomnia, OCD, cancer*	Human research: reduces anxiety (esp. polyherbal products); reduces perioperative anxiety; reduces HAART anxiety; improves insomnia (esp. polyherbal); comparable to oxazepam, zolpidem (overall mixed evidence for insomnia); reduces OCD symptoms
Yarrow *Achillea millefolium*	*Epistaxis, asthma, HTN,* **dyslipidemia**, *T1DM, cirrhosis, gastritis, PUD, anorexia, IBS, IBD, dysmenorrhea, menorrhagia, menopause, anxiety, neurodegenerative disorders,* multiple sclerosis, *inflammation*	*Preclinical research: anti-anxiety properties*

TABLE 17.B
Depressive Disorders (See Table 20.A for Chronic Fatigue, Burnout, and Stress).

Common Name/Latin Name	Scope of Potential Benefits	Caution/Contraindication
Ashwagandha *Withania somnifera*	Dyslipidemia, DM, **sexual dysfunction**, **infertility**, *osteoporosis*, gout, OA, *AD*, *PD*, MCI, **anxiety**, insomnia, OCD, *depression*, schizophrenia, hypothyroidism, stress, endurance, *fatigue*, immune function, TB, *cancer*	*Preclinical research: comparable to imipramine for depression*
Black seed/nigella/black cumin *Nigella sativa*	Periodontal dz., oral submucous fibrosis, chronic rhinosinusitis, nasal dryness, **allergy**, **asthma**, COPD, chemical pneumonitis, **HTN**, *CAD*, CHF, **dyslipidemia**, **DM**, **obesity**, NAFLD, dyspepsia, PUD, diabetic nephropathy, mastalgia, menopause, male infertility, OA, *stroke*, seizure disorder, memory impairment, cognition, anxiety, *depression*, acne, eczema, vitiligo, immune function, Hashimoto's thyroiditis, RA, inflammation, *H. pylori*, *Staph* pustules, HCV, cancer	*Preclinical research: abolishes LPS-induced (neuroinflammatory) depression*
Chamomile *Matricaria chamomilla/ recutita*	Gingivitis, mucositis, chronic rhinosinusitis, *allergies*, dyslipidemia, diabetes, *PUD*, colic, IBS, diarrhea, dyspepsia, UC, *candida vaginitis*, menopause, carpal tunnel syndrome, anxiety, insomnia, depression, ADHD, eczema, wounds, radiation or chemotherapy dermatitis, cortisol dysregulation, *inflammation*, *broadly antimicrobial (bacteria, yeast, fungus)*, cancer	Human research: improves depressive symptoms concurrently with anxiety reduction
Dandelion *Taraxacum officinale*	HTN, dyslipidemia, DM, *obesity*, *edema*, liver toxicity, NAFLD, *gastroparesis*, dyspepsia, *neurodegenerative disorders*, *depression*, *stamina*, *inflammation*, *endotoxic shock*, *cancer*	*Preclinical research: improves vitality and normalizes HPA axis in stressed mice*
Eleuthero/Siberian Ginseng *Eleutherococcus senticosus/ Acanthopanax senticosus*	*Allergic rhinitis*, dyslipidemia, CHF, edema, *male infertility*, osteoporosis, **stroke recovery**, *AD*, insomnia, **depression**, bipolar disorder, attention, vitality, athletic stamina, **hangover**, immune function, FMF, **URI**, *antiviral*, ovarian cancer	**Systematic review: in combination with SJW improves depression**
Ginkgo *Ginkgo biloba*	*Cataracts*, ARMD, glaucoma, periodontal dz., **vertigo**, **tinnitus**, **cardiovascular health**, **dyslipidemia**, **diabetes**, obesity, claudication, hepatic fibrosis, **diabetic nephropathy**, menopausal sexual desire, **acute mountain sickness**, migraines with aura, **stroke**, **MCI**, **dementias**, post-operative delirium, depression, ADHD, **schizophrenia**, **tardive dyskinesia**, aging skin, *inflammation*, *cancer*	Human research: augments efficacy of SSRI
Holy basil/Tulsi *Ocimum tenuiflorum/ sanctum*	Gingivitis, asthma, *CAD*, **dyslipidemia**, **diabetes**, obesity, *hepatotoxicity*, *PUD*, *male hypogonadism*, *pain*, *seizures*, anxiety, depression, memory and concentration, stress and fatigue, immune function, viral encephalitis	Human research: reduces anxiety; improves mood; reduces stress
Lavender *Lavandula* spp.	**Dysmenorrhea**, **anxiety**, **insomnia**, **depression**	Jafari-Koulaee et al. (2020)

Continued on following page

TABLE 17.B

Depressive Disorders (See Table 20.A for Chronic Fatigue, Burnout, and Stress). *(Continued)*

Common Name/Latin Name	Scope of Potential Benefits	Caution/Contraindication
Lemon balm *Melissa officinalis*	**Bruxism**, dyslipidemia, DM, palpitations, dyspepsia, IBS, **colic**, PMS, dysmenorrhea, female sexual dysfunction, **AD**, dementia, agitation, *diabetic neuropathy*, insomnia, **anxiety**, depression, **ADHD**, hyperthyroidism, *Graves' disease*, herpes simplex, *cancer, glioblastoma multiforme*	*Preclinical research: reduces serotonin turnover* Human research: reduces depression comparable to fluoxetine at 4 wks; reduces depression in patients with chronic stable angina
Licorice *Glycyrrhiza glabra*	**Postoperative sore throat**, xerostomia, radiation-induced mucositis, aphthous ulcers, *allergy*, **asthma**, **dyslipidemia**, *CAD, diabetes*, **obesity**, hepatoprotection, heartburn, PUD, functional dyspepsia, **antipsychotic-induced hyperprolactinemia**, **menopause**, atrophic vaginitis, PCOS, female hirsutism, BPH, *stroke, dementia*, PD, *anxiety, insomnia, depression, substance addiction*, **hyperpigmentation**, **atopic eczema**, Addison's disease, *stamina, multiple sclerosis, inflammation, H. pylori*, cancer, *breast cancer*	*Preclinical research: constituents have MAO-I and SSRI activity* **(Caution: use deglycyrrhizinated formulations in patients at risk for HTN and hypokalemia)**
Maca *Lepidium meyenii, peruvianum*	HTN, DM, weight reduction, perimenopause, **menopause**, **sexual dysfunction**, anti-depressant-induced sexual dysfunction, **male sexual dysfunction**, **male infertility**, *BPH*, osteoporosis, *memory impairment*, anxiety, depression, fatigue, inflammation	Human research: reduces anxiety and depression in postmenopausal women
Passionflower *Passiflora incarnata*	*Asthma, diabetes*, **menopause**, OA (fruit peel), *seizure disorder*, **anxiety**, somatoform disorder, *depression*, insomnia, **ADHD**, opiate withdrawal	*Preclinical research: augments antidepressant effects of St. John's wort in mice.*
Rhodiola *Rhodiola rosea*	**CAD**, *menorrhagia, amenorrhea, female infertility*, menopause, *male hypogonadism*, premature ejaculation, **anxiety**, **depression**, **cognition**, eczema, burnout, fatigue, **athletic stamina**, cancer	**Systematic reviews: beneficial for depression** Human research: not as effective as sertraline for depression, but causes fewer ADRs
Saffron *Crocus sativus*	ARMD, *cataracts*, diabetic maculopathy, glaucoma, gingivitis, burning mouth syndrome, *allergy*, asthma, HTN, **dyslipidemia**, DM, **obesity**, *hepatotoxicity, DM nephropathy*, PMS, menopause, **female and male sexual dysfunction**, male infertility, chronic pain, fibromyalgia, stroke, AD, **anxiety**, insomnia, OCD, **depression**, ADHD, drug and ETOH addiction, *photodamage*, stamina, immune function, inflammation, RA, *bacterial infection*, cancer	*Preclinical research: saffron and several constituents show antidepressant activity through various mechanisms* **Systematic reviews and meta-analyses: beneficial for depression and anxiety, comparable to SSRIs and imipramine; beneficial as adjuvant to antidepressant drugs** Human research: improves depression in postpartum, adolescents, post-methamphetamine addiction; improves dysthymia; reduces homocysteine in depressed patients

TABLE 17.B

Depressive Disorders (See Table 20.A for Chronic Fatigue, Burnout, and Stress). *(Continued)*

Common Name/Latin Name	Scope of Potential Benefits	Caution/Contraindication
St. John's Wort *Hypericum perforatum*	PMS, **perimenopause or menopause**, *chronic pain*, neuropathy, **depression**, *opiate addiction*, psoriasis, atopic dermatitis, *sunburn*, inflammation, HSV, *cancer*	*Preclinical research: inhibits reuptake of DA, serotonin, NE* **Systematic reviews: beneficial for mild-to-moderate depression, comparable to drugs, less ADRs** Human research: 600 and 1200 mg/day similar; reduces relapse; superior to fluoxetine ***See St. John's Wort monograph warnings and precautions***
Skullcap (Chinese, American) *Scutellaria baicalensis, lateriflora*	*Noise induced hearing loss*, allergy, *asthma, COPD, preterm RDS, pneumonia, PAH, CAD, dyslipidemia, DM, obesity, NAFLD, ETOH-induced gastritis, seizures, dementias,* **anxiety**, depression, *ADHD*, cognition, *photoprotection, autoimmunity, inflammation, MS, influenza, pneumonia, HIV,* cancer-related anemia, *cancer*	Human research: American skullcap improves overall mood
Tribulus/Puncture vine/ Goathead *Tribulus terrestris*	HTN, CAD, dyslipidemia, DM, *hepatotoxicity, IBS, nephrolithiasis,* **sexual dysfunction**, hypoactive sexual desire, *pain, anxiety, depression, inflammation, cancer*	*Preclinical research: MAO-I activity*
Turmeric (or curcumin) *Curcuma longa*	Anterior uveitis, **oral lichen planus, gingivitis**, dental surgery, submucous fibrosis, asthma, **diastolic HTN, dyslipidemia**, CAD, endothelial dysfunction, **DM**, obesity, **NAFLD**, hepatoprotective, gallbladder dyskinesia, *GERD*, PUD, dyspepsia, **UC**, DM nephropathy, lupus nephritis, lactational mastitis, LSIL, chronic non-bacterial prostatitis, post-operative pain, **OA**, RA, migraine HA, *neurodegeneration*, **anxiety**, **depression, skin disease**, psoriasis, fatigue, **systemic inflammation**, *HIV*, **chemo-related oral mucositis**, cancer prevention, cancer treatment	**Systematic reviews: beneficial for depression** Human research: reduces depression, especially atypical, especially middle age; comparable to fluoxetine; reduces mood-related fatigue

TABLE 17.C

Bipolar Mood Disorder.

Common Name/Latin Name	Scope of Potential Benefits	Comments
Eleuthero/Siberian Ginseng *Eleutherococcus senticosus/Acanthopanax senticosus*	*Allergic rhinitis*, dyslipidemia, CHF, edema, *male infertility*, osteoporosis, **stroke recovery**, *AD, insomnia*, **depression**, bipolar disorder, attention, vitality, athletic stamina, **hangover**, immune function, FMF, **URI**, *antiviral*, ovarian cancer	Human research: eleuthero plus lithium comparable to lithium plus fluoxetine with less manic episodes in adolescents

TABLE 17.D
Attention-Deficit/Hyperactivity Disorder and Cognitive Performance.

Common Name/Latin Name	Scope of Potential Benefits	Comments
Bacopa *Bacopa monnieri*	*Gastric ulcer*, hepatic encephalopathy, IBS-D, *seizures*, memory impairment, **dementia-related anxiety**, test anxiety, **cognitive performance**, ADHD, inflammation	Systematic reviews: **improves cognition, speed of processing, delayed word recall** Human research: improves cognition in elderly with and without dementia; reduces ADHD scores in children
Black seed/nigella/black cumin *Nigella sativa*	Periodontal dz., oral submucous fibrosis, chronic rhinosinusitis, nasal dryness, **allergy**, **asthma**, COPD, chemical pneumonitis, **HTN**, *CAD*, CHF, **dyslipidemia**, **DM**, **obesity**, NAFLD, dyspepsia, PUD, diabetic nephropathy, mastalgia, menopause, male infertility, OA, *stroke*, seizure disorder, memory impairment, cognition, anxiety, *depression*, acne, eczema, vitiligo, immune function, Hashimoto's thyroiditis, RA, inflammation, *H. pylori*, *Staph* pustules, HCV, cancer	Human research: improves cognition in young healthy volunteers
Chamomile *Matricaria chamomilla/recutita*	Gingivitis, mucositis, chronic rhinosinusitis, *allergies*, dyslipidemia, diabetes, *PUD*, colic, IBS, diarrhea, dyspepsia, UC, *candida vaginitis*, menopause, carpal tunnel syndrome, anxiety, insomnia, depression, ADHD, eczema, wounds, radiation or chemotherapy dermatitis, cortisol dysregulation, *inflammation, broadly antimicrobial (bacteria, yeast, fungus), cancer*	Human research: one small study showed improved ADHD scores
Eleuthero/Siberian Ginseng *Eleutherococcus senticosus/ Acanthopanax senticosus*	*Allergic rhinitis*, dyslipidemia, CHF, edema, *male infertility*, osteoporosis, **stroke recovery**, *AD, insomnia*, **depression**, bipolar disorder, attention, vitality, athletic stamina, **hangover**, immune function, FMF, **URI**, *antiviral*, ovarian cancer	Human research: combination formula improves attention under stress
Ginkgo *Ginkgo biloba*	*Cataracts*, ARMD, glaucoma, periodontal dz., **vertigo**, **tinnitus**, **cardiovascular health**, **dyslipidemia**, **diabetes**, obesity, claudication, hepatic fibrosis, **diabetic nephropathy**, menopausal sexual desire, **acute mountain sickness**, migraines with aura, **stroke**, **MCI**, **dementias**, post-operative delirium, depression, ADHD, **schizophrenia**, **tardive dyskinesia**, aging skin, *inflammation, cancer*	Human research: enhances response to methylphenidate
Ginseng, American *Panax quinquefolius*	HTN, dyslipidemia, DM, PVD, cognition, ADHD, schizophrenia, immune function, **URIs**, influenza, cancer	Human research: improves working memory, accuracy, calmness; improves ADHD in children in combination with ginkgo
Ginseng, Asian/Korean/ Chinese *Panax ginseng*	Dry eyes, **hearing loss**, **HTN**, CHF, **DM**, obesity, **menopause**, **ED**, male infertility, *osteoporosis*, AD, cognitive function, aging skin, alopecia areata, stamina, **chronic fatigue**, **hangover**, immune function, inflammation, influenza, HIV, **cancer**	Human research: enhances speed of attention and memory task performance when acutely dosed

TABLE 17.D

Attention-Deficit/Hyperactivity Disorder and Cognitive Performance. *(Continued)*

Common Name/Latin Name	Scope of Potential Benefits	Comments
Goji berry/wolfberry *Lycium barbarum*	Macular degeneration, *glaucoma*, dyslipidemia, **diabetes**, obesity, *hepatoprotection, male infertility, male sexual dysfunction, stroke, AD,* insomnia, anxiety, ADD, *dermatitis,* cognition, stress, fatigue, athletic performance, hangover, immunity function, influenza, cancer	*Preclinical research: neuroprotective against Aβ, ischemia* Human studies: improves cognitive focus
Holy basil/Tulsi *Ocimum tenuiflorum/sanctum*	Gingivitis, asthma, *CAD,* **dyslipidemia**, **diabetes**, obesity, *hepatotoxicity, PUD, male hypogonadism, pain, seizures,* anxiety, depression, memory and concentration, stress and fatigue, immune function, viral encephalitis	Human research: improves cognitive performance under stress
Hops/Hop *Humulus lupulus*	Dental plaque, allergic rhinitis, ASCVD, dyslipidemia, T2DM, obesity, *NAFLD, dyspepsia,* osteoporosis, OA, RA, atrophic vaginitis, menopause, cognitive decline, **insomnia**, anxiety, depression, cognitive performance, acne, aging skin, body odor, antibacterial, *TB, cancer*	Human research: improves cognition and mood in middle-aged adults
Horsetail *Equisetum arvense*	*Diabetes,* nephrolithiasis, *UTI, interstitial cystitis,* BPH, osteoporosis, OA, RA, *chronic pain,* anxiety, *cognition,* psoriatic nails, wound healing, aging skin, alopecia, inflammation	*Preclinical research: improves learning and memory in mice*
Lemon balm *Melissa officinalis*	**Bruxism**, dyslipidemia, DM, palpitations, dyspepsia, IBS, **colic**, PMS, dysmenorrhea, female sexual dysfunction, **AD**, dementia, agitation, *diabetic neuropathy,* insomnia, **anxiety**, depression, **ADHD**, *hyperthyroidism, Graves' disease,* herpes simplex, *cancer, glioblastoma multiforme*	**Systematic review: low level evidence for benefits in ADHD** Human research: improves ADHD symptoms; improves cognition at lower doses and in combination with other herbs
Maca *Lepidium meyenii, peruvianum*	HTN, DM, weight reduction, perimenopause, **menopause**, **sexual dysfunction**, anti-depressant-induced sexual dysfunction, **male sexual dysfunction**, **male infertility**, *BPH,* osteoporosis, *memory impairment,* anxiety, depression, fatigue, inflammation	*Preclinical research: black maca improves memory and learning in memory-impaired mice*
Passionflower *Passiflora incarnata*	*Asthma, diabetes,* **menopause**, OA (fruit peel), *seizure disorder,* **anxiety**, somatoform disorder, *depression,* insomnia, **ADHD**, opiate withdrawal	**Systematic review: low level evidence for benefits in ADHD** Human research: comparable to methylphenidate with less S/E
Peppermint *Mentha × piperita*	Oral health, weight reduction, nausea, dyspepsia, **IBS**, GI endoscopy, cracked nipples, PCOS, neck pain, tension headaches, postherpetic neuralgia, cognition, nicotine withdrawal, pressure ulcers, pruritis gravidarum, hirsutism, athletic performance, URI, *cancer*	*Preclinical research: improves cognition and attention* Human research: Reduces sleepiness and improves performance on cognitively demanding tests; improves memory
Rhodiola *Rhodiola rosea*	**CAD**, *menorrhagia, amenorrhea, female infertility,* menopause, *male hypogonadism,* premature ejaculation, **anxiety**, **depression**, **cognition**, eczema, burnout, fatigue, **athletic stamina**, cancer	**Systematic review: beneficial for cognitive performance** Human research: improves cognitive performance in stressed and burned-out patients; reduces mental fatigue; enhances attention and memory with acute dosing

Continued on following page

TABLE 17.D

Attention-Deficit/Hyperactivity Disorder and Cognitive Performance. *(Continued)*

Common Name/Latin Name	Scope of Potential Benefits	Comments
Saffron *Crocus sativus*	ARMD, *cataracts*, diabetic maculopathy, glaucoma, gingivitis, burning mouth syndrome, *allergy*, asthma, HTN, **dyslipidemia**, DM, **obesity**, *hepatotoxicity*, *DM nephropathy*, PMS, menopause, **female and male sexual dysfunction**, male infertility, chronic pain, fibromyalgia, stroke, AD, **anxiety**, insomnia, OCD, **depression**, ADHD, drug and ETOH addiction, *photodamage*, stamina, immune function, inflammation, RA, *bacterial infection*, cancer	Human research: comparable to methylphenidate in children with ADHD
Schisandra *Schisandra chinensis*	*MI*, **CHF**, DM, NAFLD, viral hepatitis, menopause, FMF, *stroke*, *AD*, *anxiety*, cognition, physical stress, stamina, pneumonia, *HCV*, *fungal infections*, cancer	Human research: improves cognition in combination with other herbs
Skullcap (Chinese, American) *Scutellaria baicalensis, lateriflora*	*Noise induced hearing loss*, allergy, *asthma*, COPD, *preterm RDS*, *pneumonia*, PAH, *CAD*, *dyslipidemia*, *DM*, *obesity*, *NAFLD*, *ETOH-induced gastritis*, *seizures*, *dementias*, **anxiety**, depression, *ADHD*, cognition, *photoprotection*, *autoimmunity*, *inflammation*, *MS*, *influenza*, *pneumonia*, *HIV*, cancer-related anemia, *cancer*	*Preclinical research: increases NMDA; alleviates ADHD in rats; improves cognition in healthy young rats; selectively inhibits DA reuptake without addictive behavior in rats* Human research: improves cognition in children with minimal brain dysfunction in combination with other herbs

TABLE 17.E

Schizophrenia and Somatoform Disorder.

Common Name/Latin Name	Scope of Potential Benefits	Comments
Ashwagandha *Withania somnifera*	Dyslipidemia, DM, **sexual dysfunction**, **infertility**, *osteoporosis*, gout, OA, *AD*, *PD*, MCI, **anxiety**, insomnia, OCD, *depression*, schizophrenia, hypothyroidism, stress, endurance, *fatigue*, immune function, TB, *cancer*	Human research: improves negative symptoms in schizophrenia
Butterbur *Petasites hybridus*	**Allergic rhinitis**, asthma, *HTN*, *GI ulceration*, bladder spasms, **migraine headache**, *neurodegenerative dementias*, somatoform disorder anxiety and depression, *CNS inflammation*	Human research: improves anxiety and depression in somatoform disorders
Ginkgo *Ginkgo biloba*	*Cataracts*, ARMD, glaucoma, periodontal dz., **vertigo**, **tinnitus**, **cardiovascular health**, **dyslipidemia**, **diabetes**, obesity, claudication, hepatic fibrosis, **diabetic nephropathy**, menopausal sexual desire, **acute mountain sickness**, migraines with aura, **stroke**, **MCI**, **dementias**, post-operative delirium, depression, ADHD, **schizophrenia**, **tardive dyskinesia**, aging skin, *inflammation*, *cancer*	**Systematic review: beneficial adjuvant to antipsychotics in schizophrenia; reduces tardive dyskinesia** Human research: reduces tardive dyskinesia
Ginseng, American *Panax quinquefolius*	HTN, dyslipidemia, DM, PVD, cognition, ADHD, schizophrenia, immune function, **URIs**, influenza, cancer	Human research: improves working memory and reduces EPS in schizophrenic subjects
Licorice *Glycyrrhiza glabra*	**Postoperative sore throat**, xerostomia, radiation-induced mucositis, aphthous ulcers, *allergy*, **asthma**, **dyslipidemia**, *CAD*, *diabetes*, **obesity**, hepatoprotection, heartburn, PUD, functional dyspepsia, **antipsychotic-induced hyperprolactinemia**, **menopause**, atrophic vaginitis, PCOS, female hirsutism, BPH, *stroke*, *dementia*, PD, *anxiety*, insomnia, depression, *substance addiction*, **hyperpigmentation**, **atopic eczema**, Addison's disease, *stamina*, *multiple sclerosis*, inflammation, *H. pylori*, cancer, *breast cancer*	**Systematic review: beneficial for antipsychotic-induced hyperprolactinemia** *(Caution: use deglycyrrhizinated formulations in patients at risk for HTN and hypokalemia)*

	TABLE 17.F	
	Addiction Disorders.	
Common Name/Latin Name	Scope of Potential Benefits	Comments
Coleus *Coleus forskohlii*	Glaucoma, *allergy*, asthma, HTN, CHF, *insulin resistance*, obesity, *pancreatic exocrine insufficiency, diarrhea, UTI, urge incontinence, dysmenorrhea, male infertility*, male hypogonadism, subarachnoid hemorrhage, *seizure, neurodegenerative disorders, alcohol abuse*, psoriasis, *photoprotection, hyperthyroidism, cancer*	*Preclinical research: reduces alcohol consumption and neurotoxicity*
Licorice *Glycyrrhiza glabra*	**Postoperative sore throat**, xerostomia, radiation-induced mucositis, aphthous ulcers, *allergy*, **asthma**, **dyslipidemia**, *CAD, diabetes,* **obesity**, hepatoprotection, heartburn, PUD, functional dyspepsia, **antipsychotic-induced hyperprolactinemia**, **menopause**, atrophic vaginitis, PCOS, female hirsutism, BPH, *stroke, dementia, PD, anxiety, insomnia, depression, substance addiction*, **hyperpigmentation**, **atopic eczema**, Addison's disease, *stamina, multiple sclerosis, inflammation, H. pylori*, cancer, *breast cancer*	*Preclinical research: suppresses cocaine-induced dopamine release; reduces cocaine-induced locomotion* **(Caution: use deglycyrrhizinated formulations in patients at risk for HTN and hypokalemia)**
Passionflower *Passiflora incarnata*	*Asthma, diabetes*, **menopause**, OA (fruit peel), *seizure disorder*, **anxiety**, somatoform disorder, *depression*, insomnia, **ADHD**, opiate withdrawal	Human research: enhances efficacy of clonidine for opiate withdrawal
Peppermint *Mentha × piperita*	Oral health, weight reduction, nausea, dyspepsia, **IBS**, GI endoscopy, cracked nipples, PCOS, neck pain, tension headaches, postherpetic neuralgia, cognition, nicotine withdrawal, pressure ulcers, pruritis gravidarum, hirsutism, athletic performance, URI, *cancer*	Human research: menthol reduces metabolism of nicotine (may increase addiction potential of products such as menthol cigarettes)
Saffron *Crocus sativus*	ARMD, *cataracts*, diabetic maculopathy, glaucoma, gingivitis, burning mouth syndrome, *allergy*, asthma, HTN, **dyslipidemia**, DM, **obesity**, *hepatotoxicity, DM nephropathy*, PMS, menopause, **female and male sexual dysfunction**, male infertility, chronic pain, fibromyalgia, stroke, AD, **anxiety**, insomnia, OCD, **depression**, ADHD, drug and ETOH addiction, *photodamage*, stamina, immune function, inflammation, RA, *bacterial infection*, cancer	*Preclinical research: antinociceptive; reduces chronic inflammation* Human research: attenuates symptoms of opioid withdrawal; reduces depression in former methamphetamine addicts; combination reduces symptoms during alcohol detoxification
St. John's Wort *Hypericum perforatum*	PMS, **perimenopause or menopause**, *chronic pain*, neuropathy, **depression**, *opiate addiction*, psoriasis, atopic dermatitis, *sunburn*, inflammation, HSV, *cancer*	*Preclinical research: reduces nociception, augments morphine, lowers oxycodone levels; antineuralgic* **See St. John's Wort monograph warnings and precautions**

REFERENCES

Donelli D, Antonelli M, Bellinazzi C, Gensini GF, Firenzuoli F. Effects of lavender on anxiety: a systematic review and meta-analysis. Phytomedicine 2019;65:153099. https://doi.org/10.1016/j.phymed.2019.153099.

Fismer KL, Pilkington K. Lavender and sleep: a systematic review of the evidence. Eur J Integr Med 2012;4(4):e436–47.

Jafari-Koulaee A, Elyasi F, Taraghi Z, Ilali ES, Moosazadeh M. A systematic review of the effects of aromatherapy with lavender essential oil on depression. Central Asian J Global Health 2020;9(1). https://doi.org/10.5195/cajgh.2020.442.

Pittler MH, Ernst E. Efficacy of kava extract for treating anxiety: systematic review and meta-analysis. J Clin Psychopharmacol 2000;20(1):84–9.

Smith K, Leiras C. The effectiveness and safety of Kava Kava for treating anxiety symptoms: a systematic review and analysis of randomized clinical trials. Complement Ther Clin Pract 2018;33:107–17.

18 DERMATOLOGICAL DISORDERS

TABLE 18.A		
Acne.		
Common Name/ Latin Name	**Scope of Potential Benefits**	**Comments**
Aloe *Aloe vera, barbadensis*	**Gingivitis**, **submucous fibrosis**, **dyslipidemia**, **diabetes**, insulin resistance, hepatic fibrosis, GERD, **IBS**, IBD, anal fissures, radiation proctitis, AD, *PD*, acne, **psoriasis**, **lichen planus**, **burns**, wounds, pressure ulcers, diabetic foot ulcers, wrinkle and striae reduction, Hashimoto's thyroiditis, inflammation, HIV, cancer	Human research: when added to tretinoin, better than tretinoin alone for acne
Black seed/nigella/ black cumin *Nigella sativa*	Periodontal dz., oral submucous fibrosis, chronic rhinosinusitis, nasal dryness, **allergy**, **asthma**, COPD, chemical pneumonitis, **HTN**, *CAD*, CHF, **dyslipidemia**, **DM**, **obesity**, NAFLD, dyspepsia, PUD, diabetic nephropathy, mastalgia, menopause, male infertility, OA, *stroke*, seizure disorder, memory impairment, cognition, anxiety, *depression*, acne, eczema, vitiligo, immune function, Hashimoto's thyroiditis, RA, inflammation, *H. pylori*, *Staph* pustules, HCV, cancer	Human research: improves acne in topical formulation
Burdock *Arctium lappa*	*Dyslipidemia*, diabetes, *hepatic function and protection*, *gastroparesis*, dyspepsia, diverticulitis, diabetic nephropathy, OA, wrinkles, acne, cough, *inflammation, influenza A, cancer*	Human research: homeopathic preparation reduces acne
Hops/Hop *Humulus lupulus*	Dental plaque, allergic rhinitis, ASCVD, dyslipidemia, T2DM, obesity, *NAFLD*, *dyspepsia*, osteoporosis, OA, RA, atrophic vaginitis, menopause, cognitive decline, **insomnia**, anxiety, depression, cognitive performance, acne, aging skin, body odor, antibacterial, *TB, cancer*	Human research: topical formula reduces sebum production; reduces *Corynebacterium xerosis* and *Staphylococcus epidermidis*
Milk thistle *Silybum marianum*	**Dyslipidemia**, **DM**, **liver disease**, diabetic nephropathy, lactation, PCOS, BPH, *gout*, *AD*, *diabetic neuropathy*, **OCD**, acne, *psoriasis*, vitiligo, radio-dermatitis, aging skin, RA, inflammation, hepatitis viruses, **iron-overload**, chemotherapy and radiotherapy toxicity, *hepatocellular carcinoma*	Human research: reduces inflammatory acne lesions and reduces markers of oxidation

TABLE 18.B
Psoriasis.

Common Name/ Latin Name	Scope of Potential Benefits	Comments
Aloe *Aloe vera, barbadensis*	**Gingivitis**, **submucous fibrosis**, **dyslipidemia**, **diabetes**, insulin resistance, hepatic fibrosis, GERD, **IBS**, IBD, anal fissures, radiation proctitis, AD, *PD*, acne, **psoriasis**, **lichen planus**, **burns**, wounds, pressure ulcers, diabetic foot ulcers, wrinkle and striae reduction, Hashimoto's thyroiditis, inflammation, HIV, cancer	**Systematic reviews and meta-analyses: beneficial for psoriasis; noninferior to topical steroid**
Bilberry *Vaccinium myrtillus*	Normal pressure glaucoma, cataracts, night vision, eye fatigue, gingivitis, *HTN*, **dyslipidemia**, T2DM, NAFLD, ulcerative colitis, *AD*, psoriasis, *wounds*, inflammation, *S. pneumonia*, *MRSA*, colorectal cancer, *other cancers*	Human research: reduces psoriatic scaling and erythema (bilberry seed oil)
Coleus *Coleus forskohlii*	Glaucoma, *allergy*, asthma, HTN, CHF, *insulin resistance*, obesity, *pancreatic exocrine insufficiency, diarrhea, UTI, urge incontinence, dysmenorrhea, male infertility*, male hypogonadism, subarachnoid hemorrhage, *seizure, neurodegenerative disorders, alcohol abuse*, psoriasis, *photoprotection, hyperthyroidism, cancer*	*Preclinical research: increases cAMP/cGMP ratio* Human research: small study (*n* = 4) showed improvement
Frankincense/ Boswellia *Boswellia serrata, sacra, carterii*	Gingivitis, **asthma**, *COPD*, UC, **Crohn's**, **collagenous colitis**, IBS, UTI, SUI, benign breast disease, menorrhagia, **OA**, stroke, memory impairment, psoriasis, eczema, aging skin, athletic performance, **RA**, **IBD**, *inflammation*, glioma radiation, chemo-related neuropathy, *cancer*	Human research: improves scales, itching, and erythema in psoriasis and erythematous eczema
Horsetail *Equisetum arvense*	*Diabetes*, nephrolithiasis, *UTI, interstitial cystitis*, BPH, osteoporosis, OA, RA, *chronic pain, anxiety, cognition*, psoriatic nails, wound healing, aging skin, alopecia, inflammation	Human research: reduces nail psoriasis in combination with nail lacquer
Milk thistle *Silybum marianum*	**Dyslipidemia**, **DM**, **liver disease**, diabetic nephropathy, lactation, PCOS, BPH, *gout*, AD, *diabetic neuropathy*, **OCD**, acne, *psoriasis*, vitiligo, radio-dermatitis, aging skin, RA, inflammation, hepatitis viruses, **iron-overload**, chemotherapy and radiotherapy toxicity, *hepatocellular carcinoma*	*Preclinical research: inhibits cAMP phosphodiesterase and leukotriene synthesis (both overactive in psoriasis)*
Oregon grape *Berberis (Mahonia) aquifolium*	**Psoriasis**, atopic dermatitis	Janeczek et al. (2018)
St. John's Wort *Hypericum perforatum*	PMS, **perimenopause or menopause**, *chronic pain*, neuropathy, **depression**, *opiate addiction*, psoriasis, atopic dermatitis, *sunburn*, inflammation, HSV, *cancer*	Human research: reduces psoriasis applied topically; lowers TNF-α **See St. John's Wort monograph warnings and precautions**
Turmeric (or curcumin) *Curcuma longa*	Anterior uveitis, **oral lichen planus**, **gingivitis**, dental surgery, submucous fibrosis, asthma, **diastolic HTN**, **dyslipidemia**, CAD, endothelial dysfunction, **DM**, obesity, **NAFLD**, hepatoprotective, gallbladder dyskinesia, *GERD*, PUD, dyspepsia, **UC**, DM nephropathy, lupus nephritis, lactational mastitis, LSIL, chronic non-bacterial prostatitis, post-operative pain, **OA**, RA, migraine HA, *neurodegeneration*, **anxiety**, **depression**, **skin disease**, psoriasis, fatigue, **systemic inflammation**, *HIV*, **chemo-related oral mucositis**, cancer prevention, cancer treatment	**Systematic review: improves several skin diseases** Human research: topical formulation reduces psoriatic lesions; oral formulation improves psoriasis when augmented by visible light phototherapy

TABLE 18.C
Dermatitis, Eczema, Lichen Planus, Vitiligo, and Nonspecific Rash.

Common Name/ Latin Name	Scope of Potential Benefits	Comments
Aloe *Aloe vera, barbadensis*	**Gingivitis, submucous fibrosis, dyslipidemia, diabetes,** insulin resistance, hepatic fibrosis, GERD, **IBS**, IBD, anal fissures, radiation proctitis, AD, *PD*, acne, **psoriasis, lichen planus, burns,** wounds, pressure ulcers, diabetic foot ulcers, wrinkle and striae reduction, Hashimoto's thyroiditis, inflammation, HIV, cancer	**Meta-analysis: beneficial for oral lichen planus** Human research: beneficial for non-oral lichen planus
Black seed/nigella/ black cumin *Nigella sativa*	Periodontal dz., oral submucous fibrosis, chronic rhinosinusitis, nasal dryness, **allergy, asthma,** COPD, chemical pneumonitis, **HTN,** *CAD,* CHF, **dyslipidemia, DM, obesity,** NAFLD, dyspepsia, PUD, diabetic nephropathy, mastalgia, menopause, male infertility, OA, *stroke,* seizure disorder, memory impairment, cognition, anxiety, *depression,* acne, eczema, vitiligo, immune function, Hashimoto's thyroiditis, RA, inflammation, *H. pylori, Staph* pustules, HCV, cancer	Human research: ointment comparable to betamethasone for hand eczema; reduces vitiligo
Calendula *Calendula officinalis*	Gingivitis, dental plaque, radiation mucositis, venous ulcers, lactational cracked nipples, vaginal candidiasis, episiotomy healing, nonbacterial prostatitis, diaper dermatitis, **wound healing,** diabetic foot ulcers, *antibacterial, anti-HIV,* radiation dermatitis	Human research: reduces diaper dermatitis; reduces radiation dermatitis
Chamomile *Matricaria chamomilla/ recutita*	Gingivitis, mucositis, chronic rhinosinusitis, *allergies,* dyslipidemia, diabetes, *PUD,* colic, IBS, diarrhea, dyspepsia, UC, *candida vaginitis,* menopause, carpal tunnel syndrome, anxiety, insomnia, depression, ADHD, eczema, wounds, radiation or chemotherapy dermatitis, cortisol dysregulation, *inflammation, broadly antimicrobial (bacteria, yeast, fungus), cancer*	Human research: reduces mucositis; reduces peristomal wounds; promotes wound healing
Echinacea *Echinacea purpurea, angustifolia*	Anterior uveitis, *candida vaginitis,* genital condylomas, OA, **anxiety,** eczema, athletic performance, immune function, inflammation, **URIs,** influenza, *Coronavirus,* HPV, *colorectal cancer*	Human research: topical formulation improves eczema
Frankincense/ Boswellia *Boswellia serrata, sacra, carterii*	Gingivitis, **asthma,** *COPD,* UC, **Crohn's, collagenous colitis,** IBS, UTI, SUI, benign breast disease, menorrhagia, **OA,** stroke, memory impairment, psoriasis, eczema, aging skin, athletic performance, **RA, IBD,** *inflammation,* glioma radiation, chemo-related neuropathy, *cancer*	Human research: improves scales, itching, and erythema in psoriasis and erythematous eczema
Goji berry/wolfberry *Lycium barbarum*	Macular degeneration, *glaucoma,* dyslipidemia, **diabetes,** obesity, *hepatoprotection, male infertility, male sexual dysfunction, stroke, AD,* insomnia, anxiety, ADD, *dermatitis,* cognition, stress, fatigue, athletic performance, hangover, immunity function, influenza, cancer	Traditional Chinese use: dermatitis

Continued on following page

TABLE 18.C
Dermatitis, Eczema, Lichen Planus, Vitiligo, and Nonspecific Rash. *(Continued)*

Common Name/ Latin Name	Scope of Potential Benefits	Comments
Licorice *Glycyrrhiza glabra*	**Postoperative sore throat**, xerostomia, radiation-induced mucositis, aphthous ulcers, *allergy*, **asthma**, **dyslipidemia**, *CAD*, *diabetes*, **obesity**, hepatoprotection, heartburn, PUD, functional dyspepsia, **antipsychotic-induced hyperprolactinemia**, **menopause**, atrophic vaginitis, PCOS, female hirsutism, BPH, *stroke*, *dementia*, *PD*, *anxiety*, *insomnia*, *depression*, *substance addiction*, **hyperpigmentation**, **atopic eczema**, Addison's disease, *stamina*, *multiple sclerosis*, *inflammation*, H. pylori, cancer, *breast cancer*	**Systematic review: beneficial for allergic eczema** *(Caution: use deglycyrrhizinated formulations in patients at risk for HTN and hypokalemia)*
Milk thistle *Silybum marianum*	**Dyslipidemia**, **DM**, **liver disease**, diabetic nephropathy, lactation, *PCOS*, BPH, *gout*, *AD*, *diabetic neuropathy*, **OCD**, acne, *psoriasis*, vitiligo, radio-dermatitis, aging skin, RA, inflammation, hepatitis viruses, **iron-overload**, chemotherapy and radiotherapy toxicity, *hepatocellular carcinoma*	Human research: enhances phototherapy for vitiligo; reduces radio-dermatitis
Peppermint *Mentha × piperita*	Oral health, weight reduction, nausea, dyspepsia, **IBS**, GI endoscopy, cracked nipples, PCOS, neck pain, tension headaches, postherpetic neuralgia, cognition, nicotine withdrawal, pressure ulcers, pruritis gravidarum, hirsutism, athletic performance, URI, *cancer*	Human research: topical application reduces pruritis gravidarum; prevents nipple cracks and pain with lactation (better than lanolin or expressed breast milk)
Rhodiola *Rhodiola rosea*	**CAD**, *menorrhagia*, *amenorrhea*, *female infertility*, menopause, *male hypogonadism*, premature ejaculation, **anxiety**, **depression**, **cognition**, eczema, burnout, fatigue, **athletic stamina**, cancer	Human research: improves skin barrier and reduces sensitivity in combination cream with L-carnosine
Saffron *Crocus sativus*	ARMD, *cataracts*, diabetic maculopathy, glaucoma, gingivitis, burning mouth syndrome, *allergy*, asthma, HTN, **dyslipidemia**, DM, **obesity**, *hepatotoxicity*, DM *nephropathy*, PMS, menopause, **female and male sexual dysfunction**, male infertility, chronic pain, fibromyalgia, stroke, AD, **anxiety**, insomnia, OCD, **depression**, ADHD, drug and ETOH addiction, *photodamage*, stamina, immune function, inflammation, RA, *bacterial infection*, cancer	*Preclinical research: cream has SPF properties; antioxidant properties protect against UV damage*
St. John's Wort *Hypericum perforatum*	PMS, **perimenopause or menopause**, *chronic pain*, neuropathy, **depression**, *opiate addiction*, psoriasis, atopic dermatitis, *sunburn*, inflammation, HSV, *cancer*	*Preclinical research: free-radical scavenging in UV irradiation* Human research: topical formula reduces atopic dermatitis **See St. John's Wort monograph warnings and precautions**
Uva ursi *Arctostaphylos uva-ursi*	*UTI, recurrent UTI, dementia, dermatitis, skin hyperpigmentation, cough*	*Preclinical research: reduces dermatitis, epidermal inflammation; augments topical steroid*

TABLE 18.D
Wounds and Burns.

Common Name/ Latin Name	Scope of Potential Benefits	Comments
Aloe *Aloe vera,* *barbadensis*	**Gingivitis**, **submucous fibrosis**, **dyslipidemia**, **diabetes**, insulin resistance, hepatic fibrosis, GERD, **IBS**, IBD, anal fissures, radiation proctitis, AD, *PD*, acne, **psoriasis**, **lichen planus**, **burns**, wounds, pressure ulcers, diabetic foot ulcers, wrinkle and striae reduction, Hashimoto's thyroiditis, inflammation, HIV, cancer	**Meta-analysis: beneficial for burns** Human research: improves wound healing, ulcer healing
Astragalus *Astragalus* *membranaceus*	Herpes keratitis, recurrent tonsillitis, allergic rhinitis, atopy, asthma, **viral myocarditis**, CHF, CAD, viral hepatitis, **diabetic nephropathy**, IgA nephropathy, nephrotic syndrome, lupus nephritis, *renal fibrosis, sperm quality,* hemorrhagic stroke, burns, *wound healing, age spots, leukopenia,* **immune function**, *antiviral,* HBV, TB, **NSCLC**, cancer	*Preclinical research: triples rate of wound healing.* Human research: protects endothelium; anti-inflammatory effect in burns
Bilberry *Vaccinium myrtillus*	Normal pressure glaucoma, cataracts, night vision, eye fatigue, gingivitis, *HTN,* **dyslipidemia**, T2DM, NAFLD, ulcerative colitis, *AD,* psoriasis, *wounds,* inflammation, *S. pneumonia, MRSA,* colorectal cancer, *other cancers*	*Preclinical research: stabilizes connective tissue*
Calendula *Calendula officinalis*	Gingivitis, dental plaque, radiation mucositis, venous ulcers, lactational cracked nipples, vaginal candidiasis, episiotomy healing, nonbacterial prostatitis, diaper dermatitis, **wound healing**, diabetic foot ulcers, *antibacterial, anti-HIV,* radiation dermatitis	*Preclinical research: improves subepidermal collagen synthesis* **Systematic review: weak evidence for wound healing** Human research: promotes healing of diabetic foot ulcers, neuropathic ulcers, nonhealing venous ulcers, and lactational cracked nipples
Chamomile *Matricaria* *chamomilla/* *recutita*	Gingivitis, mucositis, chronic rhinosinusitis, *allergies,* dyslipidemia, diabetes, *PUD,* colic, IBS, diarrhea, dyspepsia, UC, *candida vaginitis,* menopause, carpal tunnel syndrome, anxiety, insomnia, depression, ADHD, eczema, wounds, radiation or chemotherapy dermatitis, cortisol dysregulation, *inflammation, broadly antimicrobial (bacteria, yeast, fungus), cancer*	Human research: improves wound healing following dermabrasion; reduces peristomal skin lesions with colostomy
Dong quai *Angelica sinensis*	Pulmonary HTN, *HTN,* CAD, *atrial fibrillation,* cirrhosis, portal HTN, abd pain, UC, *renal fibrosis, dysmenorrhea,* menopausal symptoms, *osteoporosis, OA,* stroke, *cerebrovascular insufficiency, neurodegenerative disorders, wound healing, aging skin, alopecia, stamina, inflammation,* anemia of chronic disease, cancer	*Preclinical research: patented extract promotes wound healing; increases collagen production in human dermal fibroblasts*
Hops *Humulus lupulus*	Dental plaque, allergic rhinitis, ASCVD, dyslipidemia, T2DM, obesity, *NAFLD, dyspepsia,* osteoporosis, OA, RA, atrophic vaginitis, menopause, cognitive decline, **insomnia**, anxiety, depression, cognitive performance, acne, aging skin, body odor, antibacterial, *TB,* cancer	*Preclinical research: positive dermal effects on collagen and elastin*
Horse chestnut *Aesculus* *hippocastanum*	Hearing loss, *allergy,* **chronic venous insufficiency**, venous ulcers, varicocele-induced infertility, *hemorrhoids,* aging skin, *easy bruising, cancer*	Human research: venous ulcer healing orally and topically
Horsetail *Equisetum arvense*	*Diabetes,* nephrolithiasis, *UTI, interstitial cystitis,* BPH, osteoporosis, *OA,* RA, *chronic pain, anxiety, cognition,* psoriatic nails, wound healing, aging skin, alopecia, inflammation	*Preclinical research: speeds wound healing in diabetic mice* Human research: improves episiotomy healing

Continued on following page

TABLE 18.D
Wounds and Burns. *(Continued)*

Common Name/ Latin Name	Scope of Potential Benefits	Comments
Lavender *Lavandula* spp.	**Dysmenorrhea, anxiety, insomnia, depression, wounds**	Samuelson et al. (2020)
Peppermint *Mentha × piperita*	Oral health, weight reduction, nausea, dyspepsia, **IBS**, GI endoscopy, cracked nipples, PCOS, neck pain, tension headaches, postherpetic neuralgia, cognition, nicotine withdrawal, pressure ulcers, pruritis gravidarum, hirsutism, athletic performance, URI, *cancer*	Human research: reduces Stage I pressure ulcers in ICU patients
St. John's Wort *Hypericum perforatum*	PMS, **perimenopause or menopause**, *chronic pain*, neuropathy, **depression**, *opiate addiction*, psoriasis, atopic dermatitis, *sunburn*, inflammation, HSV, *cancer*	*Preclinical research: free-radical scavenging in UV irradiation* **See St. John's Wort monograph warnings and precautions**
Skullcap (Chinese, American) *Scutellaria baicalensis, lateriflora*	*Noise induced hearing loss, allergy, asthma, COPD, preterm RDS, pneumonia, PAH, CAD, dyslipidemia, DM, obesity, NAFLD, ETOH-induced gastritis, seizures, dementias,* **anxiety**, *depression, ADHD, cognition, photoprotection, autoimmunity, inflammation, MS, influenza, pneumonia, HIV,* cancer-related anemia, *cancer*	*Preclinical research: protects against UV-B irradiation topically*

TABLE 18.E
Cosmetic Disorders: Wrinkles and Photoaging.

Common Name/ Latin Name	Scope of Potential Benefits	Comments
Aloe *Aloe vera, barbadensis*	**Gingivitis, submucous fibrosis, dyslipidemia, diabetes**, insulin resistance, hepatic fibrosis, GERD, **IBS**, IBD, anal fissures, radiation proctitis, AD, *PD*, acne, **psoriasis, lichen planus, burns**, wounds, pressure ulcers, diabetic foot ulcers, wrinkle and striae reduction, Hashimoto's thyroiditis, inflammation, HIV, cancer	Human research: reduces wrinkles and striae; hydrates skin
Astragalus *Astragalus membranaceus*	Herpes keratitis, recurrent tonsillitis, allergic rhinitis, atopy, asthma, **viral myocarditis**, CHF, CAD, viral hepatitis, **diabetic nephropathy**, IgA nephropathy, nephrotic syndrome, lupus nephritis, *renal fibrosis, sperm quality,* hemorrhagic stroke, burns, *wound healing, age spots, leukopenia,* **immune function**, *antiviral,* HBV, TB, **NSCLC**, cancer	*Preclinical research: blocks melanin (may lighten age spots)*
Bilberry *Vaccinium myrtillus*	Normal pressure glaucoma, cataracts, night vision, eye fatigue, gingivitis, *HTN,* **dyslipidemia**, T2DM, NAFLD, ulcerative colitis, *AD,* psoriasis, *wounds,* inflammation, *S. pneumonia,* MRSA, colorectal cancer, *other cancers*	*Preclinical research: stabilizes connective tissue*
Burdock *Arctium lappa*	*Dyslipidemia, diabetes, hepatic function and protection, gastroparesis, dyspepsia,* diverticulitis, diabetic nephropathy, OA, wrinkles, acne, cough, *inflammation, influenza A, cancer*	*Preclinical research: fruit extract increases collagen and reduces wrinkles* Human research: fruit extract increases collagen and reduces wrinkles

TABLE 18.E
Cosmetic Disorders: Wrinkles and Photoaging. *(Continued)*

Common Name/ Latin Name	Scope of Potential Benefits	Comments
Chamomile *Matricaria chamomilla/ recutita*	Gingivitis, mucositis, chronic rhinosinusitis, *allergies*, dyslipidemia, diabetes, *PUD*, colic, IBS, diarrhea, dyspepsia, UC, *candida vaginitis*, menopause, carpal tunnel syndrome, anxiety, insomnia, depression, ADHD, eczema, wounds, radiation or chemotherapy dermatitis, cortisol dysregulation, *inflammation, broadly antimicrobial (bacteria, yeast, fungus), cancer*	Human research: improves wound healing following dermabrasion
Coleus *Coleus forskohlii*	Glaucoma, *allergy*, asthma, HTN, CHF, *insulin resistance*, obesity, *pancreatic exocrine insufficiency, diarrhea, UTI, urge incontinence, dysmenorrhea, male infertility*, male hypogonadism, subarachnoid hemorrhage, *seizure, neurodegenerative disorders, alcohol abuse*, psoriasis, *photoprotection, hyperthyroidism, cancer*	*Preclinical research: increases tanning with and without UV*
Dong quai *Angelica sinensis*	Pulmonary HTN, *HTN*, CAD, *atrial fibrillation*, cirrhosis, portal HTN, abd pain, UC, *renal fibrosis, dysmenorrhea*, menopausal symptoms, *osteoporosis, OA*, stroke, *cerebrovascular insufficiency, neurodegenerative disorders, wound healing, aging skin, alopecia, stamina, inflammation*, anemia of chronic disease, cancer	*Preclinical research: increases collagen production in human dermal fibroblasts*
Frankincense/ Boswellia *Boswellia serrata, sacra, carterii*	Gingivitis, **asthma**, COPD, UC, **Crohn's**, **collagenous colitis**, IBS, UTI, SUI, benign breast disease, menorrhagia, **OA**, stroke, memory impairment, psoriasis, eczema, aging skin, athletic performance, **RA**, **IBD**, *inflammation*, glioma radiation, chemo-related neuropathy, *cancer*	Human research: topical boswellic acid reduces fine lines and improves smoothness and elasticity in photo-aged skin
Ginkgo *Ginkgo biloba*	*Cataracts*, ARMD, glaucoma, periodontal dz., **vertigo**, **tinnitus**, **cardiovascular health**, **dyslipidemia**, **diabetes**, obesity, claudication, hepatic fibrosis, **diabetic nephropathy**, menopausal sexual desire, **acute mountain sickness**, migraines with aura, **stroke**, **MCI**, **dementias**, post-operative delirium, depression, ADHD, **schizophrenia**, **tardive dyskinesia**, aging skin, *inflammation, cancer*	Human research: topical preparation increases skin moisturization and smoothness
Ginseng, Asian/ Korean/Chinese *Panax ginseng*	Dry eyes, **hearing loss**, **HTN**, CHF, **DM**, obesity, **menopause**, **ED**, male infertility, *osteoporosis*, AD, cognitive function, aging skin, alopecia areata, stamina, **chronic fatigue**, **hangover**, immune function, inflammation, influenza, HIV, **cancer**	Human research: topical product decreases eye region wrinkle development
Hops *Humulus lupulus*	Dental plaque, allergic rhinitis, ASCVD, dyslipidemia, T2DM, obesity, *NAFLD, dyspepsia*, osteoporosis, OA, RA, atrophic vaginitis, menopause, cognitive decline, **insomnia**, anxiety, depression, cognitive performance, acne, aging skin, body odor, antibacterial, *TB, cancer*	*Preclinical research: positive dermal effects on collagen and elastin*
Horse chestnut *Aesculus hippocastanum*	Hearing loss, *allergy*, **chronic venous insufficiency**, venous ulcers, varicocele-induced infertility, *hemorrhoids*, aging skin, *easy bruising, cancer*	Human research: topical formula decreases aging wrinkle scores
Horsetail *Equisetum arvense*	*Diabetes*, nephrolithiasis, *UTI, interstitial cystitis*, BPH, osteoporosis, *OA*, RA, *chronic pain, anxiety, cognition*, psoriatic nails, wound healing, aging skin, alopecia, inflammation	Human research: silica has evidence for improving aging skin

Continued on following page

TABLE 18.E

Cosmetic Disorders: Wrinkles and Photoaging. *(Continued)*

Common Name/ Latin Name	Scope of Potential Benefits	Comments
Licorice *Glycyrrhiza glabra*	**Postoperative sore throat**, xerostomia, radiation-induced mucositis, aphthous ulcers, *allergy*, **asthma**, **dyslipidemia**, *CAD*, *diabetes*, **obesity**, hepatoprotection, heartburn, PUD, functional dyspepsia, **antipsychotic-induced hyperprolactinemia**, **menopause**, atrophic vaginitis, PCOS, female hirsutism, BPH, *stroke*, *dementia*, PD, *anxiety*, *insomnia*, *depression*, *substance addiction*, **hyperpigmentation**, **atopic eczema**, Addison's disease, *stamina*, *multiple sclerosis*, *inflammation*, H. pylori, cancer, *breast cancer*	**Systematic review: beneficial for hyperpigmentation** *(Caution: use deglycyrrhizinated formulations in patients at risk for HTN and hypokalemia)*
Milk thistle *Silybum marianum*	**Dyslipidemia**, **DM**, **liver disease**, diabetic nephropathy, lactation, *PCOS*, BPH, *gout*, *AD*, *diabetic neuropathy*, **OCD**, acne, *psoriasis*, vitiligo, radio-dermatitis, aging skin, RA, inflammation, hepatitis viruses, **iron-overload**, chemotherapy and radiotherapy toxicity, *hepatocellular carcinoma*	Human research: combination cream improves aging skin changes
Uva ursi *Arctostaphylos uva-ursi*	*UTI, recurrent UTI, dementia, dermatitis, skin hyperpigmentation, cough*	*Preclinical research: reduces melanin production in epidermal cells so may benefit age spots*

TABLE 18.F

Cosmetic Disorders: Hirsutism, Alopecia, and Body Odor.

Common Name/ Latin Name	Scope of Potential Benefits	Comments
Dong quai *Angelica sinensis*	Pulmonary HTN, *HTN*, CAD, *atrial fibrillation*, cirrhosis, portal HTN, abd pain, UC, *renal fibrosis*, *dysmenorrhea*, menopausal symptoms, *osteoporosis*, OA, stroke, *cerebrovascular insufficiency*, *neurodegenerative disorders*, *wound healing*, *aging skin*, *alopecia*, *stamina*, *inflammation*, anemia of chronic disease, cancer	*Preclinical research: increases hair growth*
Fennel *Foeniculum vulgare*	*Glaucoma, dyspepsia, gastroprotection, gastroparesis*, **infant colic**, IBS, constipation, *overactive bladder*, lactation, dysmenorrhea, oligomenorrhea, **menopausal disorders**, *dementia*, hirsutism, *inflammation*	*Preclinical research: estrogenic properties* Human research: topical gel reduces hair diameter in hirsute females
Ginseng, Asian/ Korean/Chinese *Panax ginseng*	Dry eyes, **hearing loss**, **HTN**, CHF, **DM**, obesity, **menopause**, **ED**, male infertility, *osteoporosis*, AD, cognitive function, aging skin, alopecia areata, stamina, **chronic fatigue**, **hangover**, immune function, inflammation, influenza, HIV, **cancer**	Human research: orally increases follicle count and hair girth in alopecia areata
Hops *Humulus lupulus*	Dental plaque, allergic rhinitis, ASCVD, dyslipidemia, T2DM, obesity, *NAFLD*, *dyspepsia*, osteoporosis, OA, RA, atrophic vaginitis, menopause, cognitive decline, **insomnia**, anxiety, depression, cognitive performance, acne, aging skin, body odor, antibacterial, *TB*, cancer	Human research: topical formula reduces *Corynebacterium xerosis* and *Staphylococcus epidermidis* and body odor
Horsetail *Equisetum arvense*	*Diabetes*, nephrolithiasis, *UTI*, *interstitial cystitis*, BPH, osteoporosis, OA, RA, *chronic pain*, *anxiety*, *cognition*, psoriatic nails, wound healing, aging skin, alopecia, inflammation	Human research: silica has evidence for improving hair loss
Peppermint *Mentha × piperita*	Oral health, weight reduction, nausea, dyspepsia, **IBS**, GI endoscopy, cracked nipples, PCOS, neck pain, tension headaches, postherpetic neuralgia, cognition, nicotine withdrawal, pressure ulcers, pruritis gravidarum, hirsutism, athletic performance, URI, *cancer*	Human research: reduces testosterone; reduces subjective perception of hirsutism (idiopathic and other causes)
Saw palmetto *Serenoa repens*	*Overactive bladder*, *female hirsutism*, *PCOS*, **BPH**, chronic inflammatory prostatitis, male pattern alopecia, *inflammation*	Human research: improves male-pattern alopecia *(Caution: contraindicated in pregnancy due to anti-androgen properties)*

REFERENCE

Janeczek M, Moy L, Lake EP, Swan J. Review of the efficacy and safety of topical *Mahonia aquifolium* for the treatment of psoriasis and atopic dermatitis. J Clin Aesthet Dermatol 2018;11(12):42–7.

Samuelson R, Lobl M, Higgins S, Clarey D, Wysong A. The effects of lavender essential oil on wound healing: a review of the current evidence. J Altern Complement Med 2020;26(8):680–90.

Section II

GENERALIZED SYSTEMIC DISORDERS

19 ENDOCRINE DISORDERS

	TABLE 19.A	
	Adrenal Disorders (See Table 20.A for Chronic Fatigue, Burnout, and Stress).	
Common Name/ Latin Name	**Scope of Potential Benefits**	**Comments**
Chamomile *Matricaria chamomilla/ recutita*	Gingivitis, mucositis, chronic rhinosinusitis, *allergie*s, dyslipidemia, diabetes, *PUD*, colic, IBS, diarrhea, dyspepsia, UC, *candida vaginitis*, menopause, carpal tunnel syndrome, anxiety, insomnia, depression, ADHD, eczema, wounds, radiation or chemotherapy dermatitis, cortisol dysregulation, *inflammation, broadly antimicrobial (bacteria, yeast, fungus), cancer*	Human research: normalizes cortisol curve, parallels reduction in GAD
Eleuthero/Siberian Ginseng *Eleutherococcus senticosus/ Acanthopanax senticosus*	*Allergic rhinitis*, dyslipidemia, CHF, edema, *male infertility*, osteoporosis, **stroke recovery**, *AD, insomnia*, **depression**, bipolar disorder, attention, vitality, athletic stamina, **hangover**, immune function, FMF, **URI**, *antiviral*, ovarian cancer	*Preclinical research: adrenocorticoid and mineralocorticoid receptor agonism* Human research: improves athletic stamina
Goji berry/ wolfberry *Lycium barbarum*	Macular degeneration, diabetes, liver disease, obesity, dyslipidemia, fatigue, athletic performance, anxiety, ADD, dementia, stroke, insomnia, immune modulation, cancer	Human research: reduces stress-induced rises in cortisol and DHEA
Licorice *Glycyrrhiza glabra*	**Postoperative sore throat**, xerostomia, radiation-induced mucositis, aphthous ulcers, *allergy*, **asthma**, **dyslipidemia**, CAD, *diabetes*, **obesity**, hepatoprotection, heartburn, PUD, functional dyspepsia, **antipsychotic-induced hyperprolactinemia**, **menopause**, atrophic vaginitis, PCOS, female hirsutism, BPH, *stroke, dementia*, PD, *anxiety, insomnia, depression, substance addiction*, **hyperpigmentation**, **atopic eczema**, Addison's disease, *stamina, multiple sclerosis, inflammation, H. pylori, cancer, breast cancer*	Human research: increases the AUC for cortisol in stable Addison's disease (*precautionary drug-herb interaction*) (*Caution: use deglycyrrhizinated formulations in patients at risk for HTN and hypokalemia*)
Schisandra *Schisandra chinensis*	*MI*, **CHF**, DM, NAFLD, viral hepatitis, menopause, FMF, *stroke, AD, anxiety*, cognition, physical stress, stamina, pneumonia, HCV, *fungal infections*, cancer	Human research: stabilizes NO, cortisol, and physical performance under athletic stress in athletes

TABLE 19.B

Thyroid Disorders (see also Table 21.C for autoimmune disorders).

Common Name/ Latin Name	Scope of Potential Benefits	Comments
Aloe *Aloe vera, barbadensis*	**Gingivitis**, **submucous fibrosis**, **dyslipidemia**, **diabetes**, insulin resistance, hepatic fibrosis, GERD, **IBS**, IBD, anal fissures, radiation proctitis, AD, *PD*, acne, **psoriasis**, **lichen planus**, **burns**, wounds, pressure ulcers, diabetic foot ulcers, wrinkle and striae reduction, Hashimoto's thyroiditis, inflammation, HIV, cancer	Human research: improves Hashimoto's thyroiditis
Ashwagandha *Withania somnifera*	Dyslipidemia, DM, **sexual dysfunction**, **infertility**, *osteoporosis*, gout, OA, *AD*, *PD*, MCI, **anxiety**, insomnia, OCD, *depression*, schizophrenia, hypothyroidism, stress, endurance, *fatigue*, immune function, TB, *cancer*	Human research: improves hormone levels in subclinical hypothyroidism
Black seed/nigella/ black cumin *Nigella sativa*	Periodontal dz., oral submucous fibrosis, chronic rhinosinusitis, nasal dryness, **allergy**, **asthma**, COPD, chemical pneumonitis, **HTN**, *CAD*, CHF, **dyslipidemia**, **DM**, **obesity**, NAFLD, dyspepsia, PUD, diabetic nephropathy, mastalgia, menopause, male infertility, OA, *stroke*, seizure disorder, memory impairment, cognition, anxiety, *depression*, acne, eczema, vitiligo, immune function, Hashimoto's thyroiditis, RA, inflammation, *H. pylori*, *Staph* pustules, HCV, cancer	Human research: decreases anti-TPO antibodies in Hashimoto's thyroiditis
Bugleweed/ Gypsywort *Lycopus europaeus*	Hyperthyroidism (mild)	Beer et al. (2008)
Coleus *Coleus forskohlii*	Glaucoma, *allergy*, asthma, HTN, CHF, *insulin resistance*, obesity, *pancreatic exocrine insufficiency*, *diarrhea*, *UTI*, *urge incontinence*, *dysmenorrhea*, *male infertility*, male hypogonadism, subarachnoid hemorrhage, *seizure*, *neurodegenerative disorders*, *alcohol abuse*, psoriasis, *photoprotection*, *hyperthyroidism*, *cancer*	*Preclinical research: mildly reduces thyroid hormones*
Fenugreek *Trigonella foenum-graecum*	Dyslipidemia, **DM**, pre-diabetes, *diabetic nephropathy*, *urolithiasis*, lactation, dysmenorrhea, PCOS, menopause, male sexual dysfunction, hypogonadism, PD, *peripheral neuropathy*, *thyroid T3/T4 balance*, stamina, *cancer*	*Preclinical research: raises T4 and lowers T3*
Lemon balm *Melissa officinalis*	**Bruxism**, dyslipidemia, DM, palpitations, dyspepsia, IBS, **colic**, PMS, dysmenorrhea, female sexual dysfunction, **AD**, dementia, agitation, *diabetic neuropathy*, insomnia, **anxiety**, depression, **ADHD**, *hyperthyroidism*, *Graves' disease*, herpes simplex, *cancer*, *glioblastoma multiforme*	*Preclinical research: anti-thyroid activity at several levels; blocks TSH receptors*
Motherwort *Leonurus cardiaca*	*HTN 2/2 anxiety or hyperthyroidism*, *dyslipidemia*, *CAD*, *arrhythmia*, *nausea*, *IBS*, *AKI*, *lactation*, *post-partum bleeding*, *menorrhagia*, *amenorrhea*, menopause, *pain*, *stroke*, anxiety, *insomnia*, *hyperthyroidism*, *inflammation*, *breast tumors*	*Preclinical research: inhibits TSH, reduces overproduction of T4* Traditional use: hyperthyroidism with palpitations

TABLE 19.C

Diabetes (See Table 10.G for Cardiometabolic: Diabetes, Prediabetes, Metabolic Syndrome, and Obesity).

REFERENCE

Beer AM, Wiebelitz KR, Schmidt-Gayk H. *Lycopus europaeus* (Gypsywort): effects on the thyroidal parameters and symptoms associated with thyroid function. Phytomedicine 2008;15(1–2):16–22.

20 DISORDERS OF VITALITY

TABLE 20.A		
Chronic Fatigue, Burnout, and Stress.		
Common Name/ Latin Name	**Scope of Potential Benefits**	**Comments**
Ashwagandha *Withania somnifera*	Dyslipidemia, DM, **sexual dysfunction**, **infertility**, *osteoporosis*, gout, OA, *AD, PD*, MCI, **anxiety**, insomnia, OCD, *depression*, schizophrenia, hypothyroidism, stress, endurance, *fatigue*, immune function, TB, *cancer*	*Preclinical research: reduces depletion of cortisol* Human research: improves perceived stress and reduces cortisol
Eleuthero/Siberian Ginseng *Eleutherococcus senticosus/ Acanthopanax senticosus*	*Allergic rhinitis*, dyslipidemia, CHF, edema, *male infertility*, osteoporosis, **stroke recovery**, *AD*, insomnia, **depression**, bipolar disorder, attention, vitality, athletic stamina, **hangover**, immune function, FMF, **URI**, *antiviral*, ovarian cancer	**Systematic review: beneficial for hangovers** Human research: reduces hangover; improves short-term vitality in elderly; increases cortisol adaptively
Ginseng, Asian/ Korean/Chinese *Panax ginseng*	Dry eyes, **hearing loss**, **HTN**, CHF, **DM**, obesity, **menopause**, **ED**, male infertility, *osteoporosis*, AD, cognitive function, aging skin, alopecia areata, stamina, **chronic fatigue**, **hangover**, immune function, inflammation, influenza, HIV, **cancer**	**Systematic reviews: beneficial for fatigue; beneficial for hangover effect** Human research: improves fatigue and chronic fatigue; mixed results on stamina with evidence for "responders" and "nonresponders"; reduces oxidative stress
Goji berry/ wolfberry *Lycium barbarum*	Macular degeneration, *glaucoma*, dyslipidemia, **diabetes**, obesity, *hepatoprotection*, *male infertility*, *male sexual dysfunction*, *stroke, AD*, insomnia, anxiety, ADD, *dermatitis*, cognition, stress, fatigue, athletic performance, hangover, immunity function, influenza, cancer	Human research: reduces stress-induced rise in DHEA and cortisol; reduces hangover in combination formula
Holy basil/Tulsi *Ocimum tenuiflorum/ sanctum*	Gingivitis, asthma, *CAD*, **dyslipidemia**, **diabetes**, obesity, *hepatotoxicity, PUD, male hypogonadism, pain, seizures*, anxiety, depression, memory and concentration, stress and fatigue, immune function, viral encephalitis	Human research: reduces stress; improves performance under stress
Maca *Lepidium meyenii, peruvianum*	HTN, DM, weight reduction, perimenopause, **menopause**, **sexual dysfunction**, anti-depressant-induced sexual dysfunction, **male sexual dysfunction**, **male infertility**, BPH, osteoporosis, *memory impairment*, anxiety, depression, fatigue, inflammation	Human research: improves energy and mood

Continued on following page

	TABLE 20.A	
	Chronic Fatigue, Burnout, and Stress. *(Continued)*	
Common Name/ Latin Name	**Scope of Potential Benefits**	**Comments**
Rhodiola *Rhodiola rosea*	**CAD**, *menorrhagia, amenorrhea, female infertility,* menopause, *male hypogonadism,* premature ejaculation, **anxiety, depression, cognition,** eczema, burnout, fatigue, **athletic stamina,** cancer	Human research: reduces chronic fatigue and burnout
Schisandra *Schisandra chinensis*	*MI,* **CHF,** DM, NAFLD, viral hepatitis, menopause, FMF, *stroke, AD, anxiety,* cognition, physical stress, stamina, pneumonia, *HCV, fungal infections,* cancer	Human research: improves energy, stamina, and post-operative recovery in combination with other herbs
Turmeric (or curcumin) *Curcuma longa*	Anterior uveitis, **oral lichen planus, gingivitis,** dental surgery, submucous fibrosis, asthma, **diastolic HTN, dyslipidemia,** CAD, endothelial dysfunction, **DM,** obesity, **NAFLD,** hepatoprotective, gallbladder dyskinesia, *GERD,* PUD, dyspepsia, **UC,** DM nephropathy, lupus nephritis, lactational mastitis, LSIL, chronic non-bacterial prostatitis, post-operative pain, **OA,** RA, migraine HA, *neurodegeneration,* **anxiety, depression, skin disease,** psoriasis, fatigue, **systemic inflammation,** *HIV,* **chemo-related oral mucositis,** cancer prevention, cancer treatment	Human research: improves mood-related fatigue

	TABLE 20.B	
	Stamina and Athletic Performance.	
Common Name/Latin Name	**Scope of Potential Benefits**	**Comments**
Ashwagandha *Withania somnifera*	Dyslipidemia, DM, **sexual dysfunction, infertility,** *osteoporosis,* gout, OA, *AD, PD,* MCI, **anxiety,** insomnia, OCD, *depression,* schizophrenia, hypothyroidism, stress, endurance, *fatigue,* immune function, TB, *cancer*	*Preclinical research: doubles swimming time* Human research: improves athletic performance and muscle growth
Dandelion *Taraxacum officinale*	HTN, dyslipidemia, DM, *obesity, edema,* liver toxicity, NAFLD, *gastroparesis,* dyspepsia, *neurodegenerative disorders, depression, stamina, inflammation, endotoxic shock, cancer*	*Preclinical research: leaf extract improves performance and normalizes adrenal response in swimming and tail suspension*
Dong quai *Angelica sinensis*	Pulmonary HTN, *HTN,* CAD, *atrial fibrillation,* cirrhosis, portal HTN, abd pain, UC, *renal fibrosis, dysmenorrhea,* menopausal symptoms, *osteoporosis,* OA, stroke, *cerebrovascular insufficiency, neurodegenerative disorders, wound healing, aging skin, alopecia, stamina, inflammation,* anemia of chronic disease, cancer	*Preclinical research: improves swimming duration and metabolic parameters*
Echinacea *Echinacea purpurea, angustifolia*	Anterior uveitis, *candida vaginitis,* genital condylomas, OA, **anxiety,** eczema, athletic performance, immune function, inflammation, **URIs,** influenza, *Coronavirus,* HPV, *colorectal cancer*	Human research: improves running performance, increases EPO
Eleuthero/Siberian Ginseng *Eleutherococcus senticosus/ Acanthopanax senticosus*	*Allergic rhinitis,* dyslipidemia, CHF, edema, *male infertility,* osteoporosis, **stroke recovery,** *AD,* insomnia, **depression,** bipolar disorder, attention, vitality, athletic stamina, **hangover,** immune function, FMF, **URI,** *antiviral,* ovarian cancer	Human research: enhances athletic endurance and cardiovascular fitness

TABLE 20.B
Stamina and Athletic Performance. *(Continued)*

Common Name/Latin Name	Scope of Potential Benefits	Comments
Fenugreek *Trigonella foenum-graecum*	Dyslipidemia, **DM**, pre-diabetes, *diabetic nephropathy, urolithiasis,* lactation, dysmenorrhea, PCOS, menopause, male sexual dysfunction, hypogonadism, PD, *peripheral neuropathy, thyroid T3/T4 balance,* stamina, *cancer*	Human research: increases muscle glycogen concentration after exercise; improves exercise performance and lean body mass
Frankincense/ Boswellia *Boswellia serrata, sacra, carterii*	Gingivitis, **asthma**, COPD, UC, **Crohn's**, **collagenous colitis**, IBS, UTI, SUI, benign breast disease, menorrhagia, **OA**, stroke, memory impairment, psoriasis, eczema, aging skin, athletic performance, **RA**, **IBD**, *inflammation,* glioma radiation, chemo-related neuropathy, *cancer*	Human research: reduces synovial MMP-3; reduces athletic muscle pain; reduces acute muscle injury pain
Goji berry/wolfberry *Lycium barbarum*	Macular degeneration, *glaucoma,* dyslipidemia, **diabetes,** obesity, *hepatoprotection, male infertility, male sexual dysfunction, stroke, AD,* insomnia, anxiety, ADD, *dermatitis,* cognition, stress, fatigue, athletic performance, hangover, immunity function, influenza, cancer	Human research: improves energy, focus, athletic performance, and QOL
Gynostemma/Jiaogulan *Gynostemma pentaphyllum*	*Asthma, CAD, dyslipidemia,* DM, obesity, *arrhythmia, NAFLD, PUD, PCOS, PD, white matter disease,* dementia, *stamina,* immune function, cancer	*Preclinical research: improves swimming duration*
Licorice *Glycyrrhiza glabra*	**Postoperative sore throat**, xerostomia, radiation-induced mucositis, aphthous ulcers, *allergy,* **asthma**, **dyslipidemia,** *CAD, diabetes,* **obesity**, hepatoprotection, heartburn, PUD, functional dyspepsia, **antipsychotic-induced hyperprolactinemia**, **menopause**, atrophic vaginitis, PCOS, female hirsutism, BPH, *stroke, dementia, PD, anxiety, insomnia, depression, substance addiction,* **hyperpigmentation**, **atopic eczema**, Addison's disease, *stamina, multiple sclerosis, inflammation, H. pylori,* cancer, *breast cancer*	*Preclinical research: enhances swimming duration in mice* **(Caution: use deglycyrrhizinated formulations in patients at risk for HTN and hypokalemia)**
Peppermint *Mentha × piperita*	Oral health, weight reduction, nausea, dyspepsia, **IBS**, GI endoscopy, cracked nipples, PCOS, neck pain, tension headaches, postherpetic neuralgia, cognition, nicotine withdrawal, pressure ulcers, pruritis gravidarum, hirsutism, athletic performance, URI, *cancer*	Human research: increases strength and improves spirometrics in exercise
Rhodiola *Rhodiola rosea*	CAD, *menorrhagia, amenorrhea, female infertility,* menopause, *male hypogonadism,* premature ejaculation, **anxiety**, **depression**, **cognition**, eczema, burnout, fatigue, **athletic stamina**, cancer	**Systematic review: beneficial for physical performance** Human research: ergogenic; improves attitude, stamina, and athletic performance under stress; reduces muscle damage
Saffron *Crocus sativus*	ARMD, *cataracts,* diabetic maculopathy, glaucoma, gingivitis, burning mouth syndrome, *allergy,* asthma, HTN, **dyslipidemia**, DM, **obesity**, *hepatotoxicity, DM nephropathy,* PMS, menopause, **female and male sexual dysfunction**, male infertility, chronic pain, fibromyalgia, stroke, AD, **anxiety**, insomnia, OCD, **depression**, ADHD, drug and ETOH addiction, *photodamage,* stamina, immune function, inflammation, RA, *bacterial infection,* cancer	*Preclinical research: improves stamina in mice* Human research: prevents exercise-induced muscle soreness better than indomethacin; reduces anti-heat-shock protein 27 and 70 in metabolic syndrome

Continued on following page

TABLE 20.B
Stamina and Athletic Performance. *(Continued)*

Common Name/Latin Name	Scope of Potential Benefits	Comments
Schisandra *Schisandra chinensis*	*MI*, **CHF**, DM, NAFLD, viral hepatitis, menopause, FMF, *stroke, AD, anxiety*, cognition, physical stress, stamina, pneumonia, HCV, *fungal infections*, cancer	*Preclinical research: enhances endurance and cognition* Human research: improves energy and stamina
Turmeric (or curcumin) *Curcuma longa*	Anterior uveitis, **oral lichen planus**, **gingivitis**, dental surgery, submucous fibrosis, asthma, **diastolic HTN**, **dyslipidemia**, CAD, endothelial dysfunction, **DM**, obesity, **NAFLD**, hepatoprotective, gallbladder dyskinesia, *GERD*, PUD, dyspepsia, **UC**, DM nephropathy, lupus nephritis, lactational mastitis, LSIL, chronic non-bacterial prostatitis, post-operative pain, **OA**, RA, migraine HA, *neurodegeneration*, **anxiety**, **depression**, **skin disease**, psoriasis, fatigue, **systemic inflammation**, *HIV*, **chemo-related oral mucositis**, cancer prevention, cancer treatment	Human research: reduces exercise-induced endothelial dysfunction
Umckaloabo/South African Geranium *Pelargonium sidoides*	Asthma, COPD, *PUD*, immune function, inflammation, **bronchitis**, **URI**, pharyngitis, rhinosinusitis, *influenza, Coronavirus, pneumonia, HIV, HSV 1&2, TB*	Human research: prevents exertional depression of immune function in athletes

21

IMMUNE SYSTEM DISORDERS

TABLE 21.A

Immune Function (See Table 9.A for Allergic Disorders and Asthma).

Common Name/ Latin Name	Scope of Potential Benefits	Comments
Ashwagandha *Withania somnifera*	Dyslipidemia, DM, **sexual dysfunction**, **infertility**, *osteoporosis*, gout, OA, *AD*, *PD*, MCI, **anxiety**, insomnia, OCD, *depression*, schizophrenia, hypothyroidism, stress, endurance, *fatigue*, immune function, TB, *cancer*	Human research: increases CD4 expression and NK activation
Astragalus *Astragalus membranaceus*	Herpes keratitis, recurrent tonsillitis, allergic rhinitis, atopy, asthma, **viral myocarditis**, CHF, CAD, viral hepatitis, **diabetic nephropathy**, IgA nephropathy, nephrotic syndrome, lupus nephritis, *renal fibrosis, sperm quality*, hemorrhagic stroke, burns, *wound healing, age spots*, leukopenia, **immune function**, *antiviral*, HBV, TB, **NSCLC**, cancer	*Preclinical research: balances TH1/TH2, reduces allergic component, improves CD4/CD8; improves leukopenia* **Systematic review: activates macrophage production of TNF-α and iNOS**
Black seed/nigella/ black cumin *Nigella sativa*	Periodontal dz., oral submucous fibrosis, chronic rhinosinusitis, nasal dryness, **allergy**, **asthma**, COPD, chemical pneumonitis, **HTN**, *CAD*, CHF, **dyslipidemia**, **DM**, **obesity**, NAFLD, dyspepsia, PUD, diabetic nephropathy, mastalgia, menopause, male infertility, OA, *stroke*, seizure disorder, memory impairment, cognition, anxiety, *depression*, acne, eczema, vitiligo, immune function, Hashimoto's thyroiditis, RA, inflammation, *H. pylori, Staph* pustules, HCV, cancer	Human research: increases phagocytic and intracellular killing action of PMNs
Echinacea *Echinacea purpurea, angustifolia*	Anterior uveitis, *candida vaginitis*, genital condylomas, OA, **anxiety**, eczema, athletic performance, immune function, inflammation, **URIs**, influenza, *Coronavirus*, HPV, *colorectal cancer*	*Preclinical research: upregulates IL-2 and IL-8; downregulates TNF-α and IL-6; stimulates NK cells; stimulates WBC production and phagocytosis; increases antibody-dependent cytotoxicity* Human research: decreases IL-6, TNF-α, and IL-8; increases IL-10

Continued on following page

TABLE 21.A
Immune Function (See Table 9.A for Allergic Disorders and Asthma). *(Continued)*

Common Name/ Latin Name	Scope of Potential Benefits	Comments
Elder (berry, flower) *Sambucus nigra*	Gingival recession, ASCVD, *dyslipidemia*, *DM*, obesity, constipation, stroke, *immune function*, **URI**, rhinosinusitis, influenza, *HIV*, *HSV*, *Strep*, *cancer*	*Preclinical research: increases TNF-α, IL-1β, and IL 8-10, consequently activating and mobilizing phagocytes*
Eleuthero/Siberian Ginseng *Eleutherococcus senticosus/ Acanthopanax senticosus*	*Allergic rhinitis*, dyslipidemia, CHF, edema, *male infertility*, osteoporosis, **stroke recovery**, *AD*, *insomnia*, **depression**, bipolar disorder, attention, vitality, athletic stamina, **hangover**, immune function, FMF, **URI**, *antiviral*, ovarian cancer	Human research: improves T-lymphocyte count and function
Ginseng, American *Panax quinquefolius*	HTN, dyslipidemia, DM, PVD, cognition, ADHD, schizophrenia, immune function, **URIs**, influenza, cancer	**Systematic review: shortens duration of URIs when taken preventively** Human research: preventively reduces episodes, severity, and duration of URIs and influenza
Ginseng, Asian/ Korean/Chinese *Panax ginseng*	Dry eyes, **hearing loss**, **HTN**, CHF, **DM**, obesity, **menopause**, **ED**, male infertility, *osteoporosis*, AD, cognitive function, aging skin, alopecia areata, stamina, **chronic fatigue**, **hangover**, immune function, inflammation, influenza, HIV, **cancer**	*Preclinical research: enhances NK cell activity and phagocytosis* Human research: improves response to influenza vaccine, reduces URIs, polysaccharide increases NK cell and phagocyte activity; increases TNF-α
Goji berry/wolfberry *Lycium barbarum*	Macular degeneration, *glaucoma*, dyslipidemia, **diabetes**, obesity, *hepatoprotection*, *male infertility*, *male sexual dysfunction*, stroke, *AD*, insomnia, anxiety, ADD, *dermatitis*, cognition, stress, fatigue, athletic performance, hangover, immunity function, influenza, cancer	*Preclinical research: increases IL-2 and TNF-α in leukemia cells* Human research: improves response to vaccination, improves response to oncologic immunotherapy
Gymnema/Gurmar *Gymnema sylvestre*	*Dental caries*, dyslipidemia, T1DM, **T2DM**, obesity, *arthritis*, *immune function*, *cancer*	*Preclinical research: increases neutrophil activity*
Gynostemma/Jiaogulan *Gynostemma pentaphyllum*	*Asthma*, CAD, *dyslipidemia*, DM, obesity, *arrhythmia*, NAFLD, PUD, PCOS, PD, *white matter disease*, dementia, *stamina*, immune function, cancer	*Preclinical research: polysaccharides increase TNF-α, IFN-γ, IL-10 and IL-12* Human research: improves T-cell function in cancer patients
Holy basil/Tulsi *Ocimum tenuiflorum/ sanctum*	Gingivitis, asthma, *CAD*, **dyslipidemia**, **diabetes**, obesity, *hepatotoxicity*, *PUD*, *male hypogonadism*, *pain*, *seizures*, anxiety, depression, memory and concentration, stress and fatigue, immune function, viral encephalitis	Human research: increases inflammatory cytokines and T-helper cells
Saffron *Crocus sativus*	ARMD, *cataracts*, diabetic maculopathy, glaucoma, gingivitis, burning mouth syndrome, *allergy*, asthma, HTN, **dyslipidemia**, DM, **obesity**, *hepatotoxicity*, DM *nephropathy*, PMS, menopause, **female and male sexual dysfunction**, male infertility, chronic pain, fibromyalgia, stroke, AD, **anxiety**, insomnia, OCD, **depression**, ADHD, drug and ETOH addiction, *photodamage*, stamina, immune function, inflammation, RA, *bacterial infection*, cancer	Human research: transiently increases IgG and decreases IgM, increases monocyte %, normalizing by 6 weeks
Umckaloabo/South African Geranium *Pelargonium sidoides*	Asthma, COPD, *PUD*, immune function, inflammation, **bronchitis**, **URI**, pharyngitis, rhinosinusitis, *influenza*, *Coronavirus*, *pneumonia*, *HIV*, *HSV 1&2*, *TB*	*Preclinical research: increases TNF-α, IL-1α, IL-12, phagocytosis, and iNOS; blocks adherence and adsorption of pathogens* Human research: prevents exertional depression of immune function in athletes

TABLE 21.B
Inflammation.

Common Name/ Latin Name	Scope of Potential Benefits	Comments
Aloe *Aloe vera, barbadensis*	**Gingivitis**, **submucous fibrosis**, **dyslipidemia**, **diabetes**, insulin resistance, hepatic fibrosis, GERD, **IBS**, IBD, anal fissures, radiation proctitis, AD, *PD*, acne, **psoriasis**, **lichen planus**, **burns**, wounds, pressure ulcers, diabetic foot ulcers, wrinkle and striae reduction, Hashimoto's thyroiditis, inflammation, HIV, cancer	Human research: improves Hashimoto's thyroiditis, ulcerative colitis; reduces TNF-α, VEGF, IL-2, and IL-4 in polymannose complex
Andrographis *Andrographis paniculata*	*HTN, hepatoprotection*, ulcerative colitis, *dysmenorrhea*, OA, RA, FMF, *inflammation*, **URI prevention and treatment**, *cancer*	*Preclinical research: inhibits COX-2, NOX*
Bacopa *Bacopa monnieri*	*Gastric ulcer*, hepatic encephalopathy, IBS-D, *seizures*, memory impairment, **dementia-related anxiety**, test anxiety, **cognitive performance**, ADHD, inflammation	Human research: reduces homocysteine, CRP, TNF-α, SOD, and GSH levels in AD patients in combination formula
Bilberry *Vaccinium myrtillus*	Normal pressure glaucoma, cataracts, night vision, eye fatigue, gingivitis, *HTN*, **dyslipidemia**, T2DM, NAFLD, ulcerative colitis, *AD*, psoriasis, *wounds*, inflammation, *S. pneumonia*, MRSA, colorectal cancer, *other cancers*	Human research: reduces CRP, IL-6, IL-15, LPS, PAI-1, and monokines induced by IFN-γ; reduces p65-NF-κB; enhances IL-22
Black seed/nigella/ black cumin *Nigella sativa*	Periodontal dz., oral submucous fibrosis, chronic rhinosinusitis, nasal dryness, **allergy**, **asthma**, COPD, chemical pneumonitis, **HTN**, *CAD*, CHF, **dyslipidemia**, **DM**, **obesity**, NAFLD, dyspepsia, PUD, diabetic nephropathy, mastalgia, menopause, male infertility, OA, *stroke*, seizure disorder, memory impairment, cognition, anxiety, *depression*, acne, eczema, vitiligo, immune function, Hashimoto's thyroiditis, RA, inflammation, *H. pylori*, *Staph* pustules, HCV, cancer	Human research: modulates CD4+/CD8+ in RA; decreases TNF-α, IL-6, MDA, NO; increases IL-10
Burdock *Arctium lappa*	*Dyslipidemia*, diabetes, *hepatic function and protection*, *gastroparesis, dyspepsia*, diverticulitis, diabetic nephropathy, OA, wrinkles, acne, cough, *inflammation, influenza A, cancer*	*Preclinical research: seeds decrease IL-6 and TNF-α in dermis*
Butterbur *Petasites hybridus*	**Allergic rhinitis**, asthma, *HTN*, *GI ulceration*, bladder spasms, **migraine headache**, *neurodegenerative dementias*, somatoform disorder anxiety and depression, *CNS inflammation*	*Preclinical research: decreases microglial IL-1β, IL-6, IL-12 and TNF-α*
Chamomile *Matricaria chamomilla/ recutita*	Gingivitis, mucositis, chronic rhinosinusitis, *allergies*, dyslipidemia, diabetes, *PUD*, colic, IBS, diarrhea, dyspepsia, UC, *candida vaginitis*, menopause, carpal tunnel syndrome, anxiety, insomnia, depression, ADHD, eczema, wounds, radiation or chemotherapy dermatitis, cortisol dysregulation, *inflammation, broadly antimicrobial (bacteria, yeast, fungus), cancer*	*Preclinical research: inhibits COX2 and LOX; reduces IL-1β and TNF-α*
Cranberry *Vaccinium macrocarpon*	Gingivitis, dyslipidemia, **DM**, PUD, gut dysbiosis, overactive bladder, **UTI**, post-radiation UTI, BPH, chronic prostatitis, RA, *inflammation, influenza*, prostate CA	*Preclinical research: blocks LPS-induced inflammation*
Dandelion *Taraxacum officinale*	HTN, dyslipidemia, DM, *obesity*, edema, liver toxicity, NAFLD, *gastroparesis*, dyspepsia, *neurodegenerative disorders*, depression, *stamina, inflammation, endotoxic shock, cancer*	*Preclinical research: reduces TNF-α, IFN-γ, IL-1β, IL-6, NO and PGE$_2$*

Continued on following page

TABLE 21.B
Inflammation. *(Continued)*

Common Name/ Latin Name	Scope of Potential Benefits	Comments
Dong quai *Angelica sinensis*	Pulmonary HTN, *HTN*, CAD, *atrial fibrillation*, cirrhosis, portal HTN, abd pain, UC, *renal fibrosis, dysmenorrhea*, menopausal symptoms, *osteoporosis, OA*, stroke, *cerebrovascular insufficiency, neurodegenerative disorders, wound healing, aging skin, alopecia, stamina, inflammation*, anemia of chronic disease, cancer	*Preclinical research: inhibits TNF/TNFR signal transduction*
Echinacea *Echinacea purpurea, angustifolia*	Anterior uveitis, *candida vaginitis*, genital condylomas, OA, **anxiety**, eczema, athletic performance, immune function, inflammation, **URIs**, influenza, *Coronavirus*, HPV, *colorectal cancer*	*Preclinical research: decreases TNF-α and IL-6* Human research: decreases IL-6, TNF-α, and IL-8, increases IL-10.
Eleuthero/Siberian Ginseng *Eleutherococcus senticosus/ Acanthopanax senticosus*	*Allergic rhinitis, dyslipidemia*, CHF, edema, *male infertility*, osteoporosis, **stroke recovery**, *AD, insomnia*, **depression**, bipolar disorder, attention, vitality, athletic stamina, **hangover**, immune function, FMF, **URI**, *antiviral*, ovarian cancer	Human research: combination formula improves FMF
Fennel *Foeniculum vulgare*	*Glaucoma, dyspepsia, gastroprotection, gastroparesis*, **infant colic**, IBS, constipation, *overactive bladder, lactation*, dysmenorrhea, oligomenorrhea, **menopausal disorders**, *dementia*, hirsutism, *inflammation*	*Preclinical research: suppresses NF-κB -dependent gene expression induced by TNF*
Frankincense/ Boswellia *Boswellia serrata, sacra, carterii*	Gingivitis, **asthma**, *COPD*, UC, **Crohn's**, **collagenous colitis**, IBS, UTI, SUI, benign breast disease, menorrhagia, **OA**, stroke, memory impairment, psoriasis, eczema, aging skin, athletic performance, **RA**, **IBD**, *inflammation*, glioma radiation, chemo-related neuropathy, *cancer*	*Preclinical research: inhibits NF-κB, TNF-α, and COX-1*
Ginger *Zingiber officinale*	**Motion sickness**, *HTN*, dyslipidemia, fibrinolysis, diabetes, **nausea**, **vomiting**, *dyspepsia*, gastroparesis, *PUD*, ulcerative colitis, *diabetic nephropathy*, **dysmenorrhea**, *Candida vaginitis*, male infertility, OA, muscle injury, migraine HA, *AD*, **inflammation**, RA, *H. pylori, antibacterial*, **CINV**, cancer	*Preclinical research: inhibits COX-1, COX-2, PGI-2, 5-LOX, and thromboxane* **Systematic review: reduces CRP, hs-CRP, and TNF-α** Human research: reduces colonic COX-1 protein levels in high-risk patients
Ginkgo *Ginkgo biloba*	*Cataracts, ARMD, glaucoma*, periodontal dz., **vertigo**, **tinnitus**, **cardiovascular health**, **dyslipidemia**, **diabetes**, obesity, claudication, hepatic fibrosis, **diabetic nephropathy**, menopausal sexual desire, **acute mountain sickness**, migraines with aura, **stroke**, **MCI**, **dementias**, post-operative delirium, depression, ADHD, **schizophrenia**, **tardive dyskinesia**, aging skin, *inflammation, cancer*	*Preclinical research: inhibits IL-6; reduces MDA; increases glutathione*
Ginseng, Asian/ Korean/Chinese *Panax ginseng*	Dry eyes, **hearing loss**, **HTN**, CHF, **DM**, obesity, **menopause**, **ED**, male infertility, *osteoporosis*, AD, cognitive function, aging skin, alopecia areata, stamina, **chronic fatigue**, **hangover**, immune function, inflammation, influenza, HIV, **cancer**	*Preclinical research: inhibits COX-2, iNOS, NF-kB* **Systematic Review: reduces CRP if elevated > 3** Human research: reduces TNF-α in combination formula
Hawthorn *Crataegus* spp.	HTN, CAD, **CHF** (HrEF and HpEF), arrhythmia, **orthostatic hypotension**, *NAFLD*, anxiety, *inflammation*	*Preclinical research: prevents upregulation of arterial COX-1 and COX-2 in aging arteries*

TABLE 21.B

Inflammation. *(Continued)*

Common Name/ Latin Name	Scope of Potential Benefits	Comments
Hops/hop *Humulus lupulus*	Dental plaque, allergic rhinitis, ASCVD, dyslipidemia, T2DM, obesity, *NAFLD, dyspepsia,* osteoporosis, OA, RA, atrophic vaginitis, menopause, cognitive decline, **insomnia**, anxiety, depression, cognitive performance, acne, aging skin, body odor, antibacterial, *TB, cancer*	*Preclinical research: inhibits several TNF-α-induced cytokines in endothelial and monocytic cells; inhibits LPS-stimulated PGE2 and inducible COX-2* Human research: increases adiponectin; decreases TNF-α; reduces pain in OA and RA subjects; 54% reduction in WOMAC scores
Horsetail *Equisetum arvense*	*Diabetes,* nephrolithiasis, *UTI, interstitial cystitis,* BPH, osteoporosis, *OA,* RA, *chronic pain, anxiety, cognition,* psoriatic nails, wound healing, aging skin, alopecia, inflammation	Human research: reduces TNF-α, IL-10, ESR, and RF in RA patients
Licorice *Glycyrrhiza glabra*	**Postoperative sore throat**, xerostomia, radiation-induced mucositis, aphthous ulcers, *allergy,* **asthma**, **dyslipidemia**, *CAD, diabetes,* **obesity**, hepatoprotection, heartburn, PUD, functional dyspepsia, **antipsychotic-induced hyperprolactinemia**, **menopause**, atrophic vaginitis, PCOS, female hirsutism, BPH, *stroke,* dementia, PD, *anxiety, insomnia, depression, substance addiction,* **hyperpigmentation**, **atopic eczema**, Addison's disease, *stamina, multiple sclerosis, inflammation,* H. pylori, cancer, *breast cancer*	*Preclinical research: inhibits PGE2, thromboxane A2, LTB4 COX, LOX and NF-kB activation; inhibits microglial inflammation* **(Caution: use deglycyrrhizinated formulations in patients at risk for HTN and hypokalemia)**
Maca *Lepidium meyenii, peruvianum*	HTN, DM, weight reduction, perimenopause, **menopause**, **sexual dysfunction**, anti-depressant-induced sexual dysfunction, **male sexual dysfunction**, **male infertility**, *BPH,* osteoporosis, *memory impairment,* anxiety, depression, fatigue, inflammation	Human research: reduces IL-6 at high altitudes.
Milk thistle *Silybum marianum*	**Dyslipidemia**, **DM**, **liver disease**, diabetic nephropathy, lactation, *PCOS,* BPH, *gout, AD, diabetic neuropathy,* **OCD**, acne, *psoriasis,* vitiligo, radio-dermatitis, aging skin, RA, inflammation, hepatitis viruses, **iron-overload**, chemotherapy and radiotherapy toxicity, *hepatocellular carcinoma*	Human research: decreases TNF-α and MDA levels in CKD
Motherwort *Leonurus cardiaca*	*HTN 2/2 anxiety or hyperthyroidism, dyslipidemia, CAD, arrhythmia, nausea, IBS, AKI, lactation, post-partum bleeding, menorrhagia, amenorrhea,* menopause, *pain, stroke,* anxiety, *insomnia, hyperthyroidism, inflammation, breast tumors*	*Preclinical research: downregulates expression of TNF-α, IL-1, IL-6, IL-8, KIM-1*
Saffron *Crocus sativus*	ARMD, *cataracts,* diabetic maculopathy, glaucoma, gingivitis, burning mouth syndrome, *allergy,* asthma, HTN, **dyslipidemia**, DM, **obesity**, *hepatotoxicity, DM nephropathy,* PMS, menopause, **female and male sexual dysfunction**, male infertility, chronic pain, fibromyalgia, stroke, AD, **anxiety**, insomnia, OCD, **depression**, ADHD, drug and ETOH addiction, *photodamage,* stamina, immune function, inflammation, RA, *bacterial infection,* cancer	Human research: reduces antibodies to HSP17 and 70 in patients with metabolic syndrome; decreases MDA, IL-6, and EGF
St. John's wort *Hypericum perforatum*	PMS, **perimenopause or menopause**, *chronic pain,* neuropathy, **depression**, *opiate addiction,* psoriasis, atopic dermatitis, *sunburn,* inflammation, HSV, *cancer*	Human research: reduces dermal TNFα in psoriasis **See St. John's Wort monograph warnings and precautions**

Continued on following page

TABLE 21.B
Inflammation. *(Continued)*

Common Name/ Latin Name	Scope of Potential Benefits	Comments
Saw palmetto *Serenoa repens*	*Overactive bladder, female hirsutism, PCOS,* **BPH**, *chronic inflammatory prostatitis, male pattern alopecia, inflammation*	*Preclinical research: decreases prostaglandins, leukotrienes, B lymphocyte infiltrates, IL-1b and TNF-α; inhibits COX and 5-LOX* **(Caution: contraindicated in pregnancy due to anti-androgen properties)**
Skullcap (Chinese, American) *Scutellaria baicalensis, lateriflora*	*Noise induced hearing loss,* allergy, *asthma, COPD, preterm RDS, pneumonia, PAH, CAD, dyslipidemia, DM, obesity, NAFLD, ETOH-induced gastritis, seizures, dementias,* **anxiety**, depression, *ADHD,* cognition, *photoprotection, autoimmunity, inflammation, MS, influenza, pneumonia, HIV,* cancer-related anemia, *cancer*	*Preclinical research: reduces inflammation in auto-immune encephalomyelitis (model for MS); decreases TNF-α; inhibits COX-2 in cancer cells*
Stinging nettle *Urtica dioica*	Allergic rhinitis, HTN, dyslipidemia, **DM**, NAFLD, *colitis, nephrotoxicity,* menopause, **BPH**, prostatitis, OA, inflammation, *prostate cancer, cisplatin toxicity*	*Preclinical research: inhibits COX-1, COX-2, PGD2 synthase* Human research: reduces IL-6 and hs-CRP in patients with T2DM
Tribulus/Puncture vine/Goathead *Tribulus terrestris*	HTN, CAD, dyslipidemia, DM, *hepatotoxicity, IBS, nephrolithiasis,* **sexual dysfunction**, hypoactive sexual desire, *pain, anxiety, depression, inflammation, cancer*	*Preclinical research: inhibits COX-2, iNOS, TNF-α and IL-4*
Turmeric (or curcumin) *Curcuma longa*	Anterior uveitis, **oral lichen planus**, **gingivitis**, dental surgery, submucous fibrosis, asthma, **diastolic HTN**, **dyslipidemia**, CAD, endothelial dysfunction, **DM**, obesity, **NAFLD**, hepatoprotective, gallbladder dyskinesia, *GERD, PUD, dyspepsia,* **UC**, DM nephropathy, lupus nephritis, lactational mastitis, LSIL, chronic non-bacterial prostatitis, post-operative pain, **OA**, RA, migraine HA, *neurodegeneration,* **anxiety**, **depression**, **skin disease**, psoriasis, fatigue, **systemic inflammation**, *HIV,* **chemo-related oral mucositis**, cancer prevention, cancer treatment	*Preclinical research: down-regulates COX-2 via suppression of NF-κB; down-regulates LOX, iNOS, mitogen-activated and Janus kinases; inhibits TNF-α; inhibits IL-1, -2, -6, -8, and -12; inhibits monocyte chemoattractant protein* **Systematic reviews: reduces TNFα and IL-6** Human research: mixed results on reduction of other inflammation markers
Umckaloabo/South African Geranium *Pelargonium sidoides*	Asthma, COPD, *PUD,* immune function, inflammation, **bronchitis**, **URI**, pharyngitis, rhinosinusitis, *influenza, Coronavirus, pneumonia, HIV, HSV 1&2, TB*	Human research: decreases IL-15 and IL-6 in face of intense exercise

TABLE 21.C
Autoimmune Disorders *(see also Table 11.D for inflammatory bowel disorders; Table 19.B for thyroid disorders).*

Common Name/ Latin Name	Scope of Potential Benefits	Comments
Aloe *Aloe vera, barbadensis*	**Gingivitis**, **submucous fibrosis**, **dyslipidemia**, **diabetes**, insulin resistance, hepatic fibrosis, GERD, **IBS**, IBD, anal fissures, radiation proctitis, AD, *PD,* acne, **psoriasis**, **lichen planus**, **burns**, wounds, pressure ulcers, diabetic foot ulcers, wrinkle and striae reduction, Hashimoto's thyroiditis, inflammation, HIV, cancer	Human research: improves Hashimoto's thyroiditis and ulcerative colitis
Astragalus *Astragalus membranaceus*	Herpes keratitis, recurrent tonsillitis, allergic rhinitis, atopy, asthma, **viral myocarditis**, CHF, CAD, viral hepatitis, **diabetic nephropathy**, IgA nephropathy, nephrotic syndrome, lupus nephritis, *renal fibrosis, sperm quality,* hemorrhagic stroke, burns, *wound healing, age spots,* leukopenia, **immune function**, *antiviral,* HBV, TB, **NSCLC**, cancer	Human research: beneficial for lupus nephritis and IgA nephropathy; improves leukopenia

TABLE 21.C

Autoimmune Disorders (see also Table 11.D for inflammatory bowel disorders; Table 19.B for thyroid disorders). *(Continued)*

Common Name/ Latin Name	Scope of Potential Benefits	Comments
Andrographis *Andrographis paniculata*	*HTN, hepatoprotection,* ulcerative colitis, *dysmenorrhea,* OA, RA, FMF, *inflammation,* **URI prevention and treatment,** *cancer*	Human research: beneficial for ulcerative colitis, comparable to mesalamine; beneficial for RA
Bilberry *Vaccinium myrtillus*	Normal pressure glaucoma, cataracts, night vision, eye fatigue, gingivitis, *HTN,* **dyslipidemia,** T2DM, NAFLD, ulcerative colitis, *AD,* psoriasis, *wounds,* inflammation, *S. pneumonia, MRSA,* colorectal cancer, *other cancers*	Human research: improves ulcerative colitis
Black seed/ nigella/black cumin *Nigella sativa*	Periodontal dz., oral submucous fibrosis, chronic rhinosinusitis, nasal dryness, **allergy, asthma,** COPD, chemical pneumonitis, **HTN, CAD,** CHF, **dyslipidemia, DM, obesity,** NAFLD, dyspepsia, PUD, diabetic nephropathy, mastalgia, menopause, male infertility, OA, *stroke,* seizure disorder, memory impairment, cognition, anxiety, *depression,* acne, eczema, vitiligo, immune function, Hashimoto's thyroiditis, RA, inflammation, *H. pylori, Staph* pustules, HCV, cancer	Human research: decreases anti-TPO antibodies in Hashimoto's thyroiditis; improves response to DMARDs in RA; modulates CD4+/CD8+ in RA; more effective than fish oil in vitiligo
Cranberry *Vaccinium macrocarpon*	Gingivitis, dyslipidemia, **DM,** PUD, gut dysbiosis, overactive bladder, **UTI,** post-radiation UTI, BPH, chronic prostatitis, RA, *inflammation, influenza,* prostate CA	Human research: reduces disease activity scores and anti-CCP in women with RA
Echinacea *Echinacea purpurea, angustifolia*	Anterior uveitis, *candida vaginitis,* genital condylomas, OA, **anxiety,** eczema, athletic performance, immune function, inflammation, **URIs,** influenza, *Coronavirus,* HPV, *colorectal cancer*	Human research: improves autoimmune uveitis
Frankincense/ Boswellia *Boswellia serrata, sacra, carterii*	Gingivitis, **asthma,** *COPD,* UC, **Crohn's, collagenous colitis,** IBS, UTI, SUI, benign breast disease, menorrhagia, **OA,** stroke, memory impairment, psoriasis, eczema, aging skin, athletic performance, **RA, IBD,** *inflammation,* glioma radiation, chemo-related neuropathy, *cancer*	**Systematic review: beneficial for RA, Crohn's, and collagenous colitis** Human research: improves UC, Crohn's, and collagenous colitis comparably to drugs
Ginger *Zingiber officinale*	**Motion sickness,** *HTN,* dyslipidemia, fibrinolysis, diabetes, **nausea, vomiting,** *dyspepsia,* gastroparesis, *PUD,* ulcerative colitis, *diabetic nephropathy,* **dysmenorrhea,** *Candida vaginitis,* male infertility, OA, muscle injury, migraine HA, *AD,* **inflammation,** RA, *H. pylori, antibacterial,* **CINV,** cancer	Human research: improves RA; improves UC
Hops/Hop *Humulus lupulus*	Dental plaque, allergic rhinitis, ASCVD, dyslipidemia, T2DM, obesity, *NAFLD, dyspepsia,* osteoporosis, OA, RA, atrophic vaginitis, menopause, cognitive decline, **insomnia,** anxiety, depression, cognitive performance, acne, aging skin, body odor, antibacterial, *TB, cancer*	Human research: reduces pain in OA and RA subjects; 54% reduction in WOMAC scores
Horsetail *Equisetum arvense*	*Diabetes,* nephrolithiasis, *UTI, interstitial cystitis,* BPH, osteoporosis, OA, RA, *chronic pain, anxiety, cognition,* psoriatic nails, wound healing, aging skin, alopecia, inflammation	Human research: reduces TNF-α, IL-10, ESR, and RF in RA patients
Lemon balm *Melissa officinalis*	**Bruxism,** dyslipidemia, DM, palpitations, dyspepsia, IBS, **colic,** PMS, dysmenorrhea, female sexual dysfunction, **AD,** dementia, agitation, *diabetic neuropathy,* insomnia, **anxiety,** depression, **ADHD,** *hyperthyroidism, Graves' disease,* herpes simplex, *cancer,* glioblastoma multiforme	*Preclinical research: blocks TSH receptors*

Continued on following page

TABLE 21.C

Autoimmune Disorders (see also Table 11.D for inflammatory bowel disorders; Table 19.B for thyroid disorders). *(Continued)*

Common Name/ Latin Name	Scope of Potential Benefits	Comments
Milk thistle *Silybum marianum*	**Dyslipidemia**, **DM**, **liver disease**, diabetic nephropathy, lactation, PCOS, BPH, *gout*, *AD*, *diabetic neuropathy*, **OCD**, acne, *psoriasis*, vitiligo, radio-dermatitis, aging skin, RA, inflammation, hepatitis viruses, **iron-overload**, chemotherapy and radiotherapy toxicity, *hepatocellular carcinoma*	Human research: reduces disease activity in RA
Saffron *Crocus sativus*	ARMD, *cataracts*, diabetic maculopathy, glaucoma, gingivitis, burning mouth syndrome, *allergy*, asthma, HTN, **dyslipidemia**, DM, **obesity**, *hepatotoxicity*, *DM nephropathy*, PMS, menopause, **female and male sexual dysfunction**, male infertility, chronic pain, fibromyalgia, stroke, AD, **anxiety**, insomnia, OCD, **depression**, ADHD, drug and ETOH addiction, *photodamage*, stamina, immune function, inflammation, RA, *bacterial infection*, cancer	Human research: reduces joint pain and swelling, inflammatory markers in RA
Skullcap (Chinese, American) *Scutellaria baicalensis, lateriflora*	*Noise induced hearing loss*, allergy, *asthma*, COPD, preterm RDS, pneumonia, PAH, CAD, dyslipidemia, DM, obesity, NAFLD, ETOH-induced gastritis, seizures, dementias, **anxiety**, depression, ADHD, cognition, photoprotection, autoimmunity, inflammation, MS, influenza, pneumonia, HIV, cancer-related anemia, cancer	Preclinical research: reduces inflammation in experimental autoimmune encephalomyelitis (model for MS)
Yarrow *Achillea millefolium*	*Epistaxis, asthma, HTN, **dyslipidemia**, T1DM, cirrhosis, gastritis, PUD, anorexia, IBS, IBD, dysmenorrhea, menorrhagia, menopause, anxiety, neurodegenerative disorders*, multiple sclerosis, *inflammation*	Preclinical research: improves experimental autoimmune encephalomyelitis (model for MS) Human research: reduces recurrences and lesion volume in MS

22

INFECTIOUS DISEASES

■ ■

TABLE 22.A

Upper Respiratory Tract Infections: Rhinitis, Rhinosinusitis, Tonsillopharyngitis, and Acute Bronchitis.

Common Name/ Latin Name	Scope of Potential Benefits	Comments
Astragalus *Astragalus membranaceus*	Herpes keratitis, recurrent tonsillitis, allergic rhinitis, atopy, asthma, **viral myocarditis**, CHF, CAD, viral hepatitis, **diabetic nephropathy**, IgA nephropathy, nephrotic syndrome, lupus nephritis, *renal fibrosis*, *sperm quality*, hemorrhagic stroke, burns, *wound healing*, *age spots*, *leukopenia*, **immune function**, *antiviral*, HBV, TB, **NSCLC**, cancer	Human research: improves immune function in recurrent tonsillitis
Andrographis *Andrographis paniculata*	*HTN, hepatoprotection*, ulcerative colitis, *dysmenorrhea*, OA, RA, FMF, *inflammation*, **URI prevention and treatment**, SARS-CoV-2, *cancer*	**Systematic reviews: beneficial for URI prevention and treatment in combination with eleuthero**
Echinacea *Echinacea purpurea, angustifolia*	Anterior uveitis, *candida vaginitis*, genital condylomas, OA, **anxiety**, eczema, athletic performance, immune function, inflammation, **URIs**, influenza, *coronavirus*, HPV, *colorectal cancer*	**Systematic reviews: positive or mixed for acute URI; reduces recurrences** Human research: prevents URIs; reduces oral microbes
Elder (**berry, flower**) *Sambucus nigra*	Gingival recession, ASCVD, *dyslipidemia*, DM, obesity, constipation, stroke, *immune function*, URI, rhinosinusitis, influenza, *HIV, HSV, Strep, cancer*	*Preclinical research: antiviral, anti-streptococcal* **Systematic review: reduces duration of viral URIs** Human research: reduces duration and severity of URIs; improves rhinosinusitis
Eleuthero/Siberian Ginseng *Eleutherococcus senticosus/ Acanthopanax senticosus*	*Allergic rhinitis*, dyslipidemia, CHF, edema, *male infertility*, osteoporosis, **stroke recovery**, AD, *insomnia*, **depression**, bipolar disorder, attention, vitality, athletic stamina, **hangover**, immune function, FMF, **URI**, *antiviral*, ovarian cancer	**Systematic reviews: shortens duration and severity of URIs in combination with andrographis**
Ginseng, American *Panax quinquefolius*	HTN, dyslipidemia, DM, PVD, cognition, ADHD, schizophrenia, immune function, **URIs**, influenza, cancer	**Systematic review: shortens duration of URIs when taken preventively** Human research: taken preventively reduces episodes, severity, and duration of URIs and influenza

Continued on following page

159

TABLE 22.A
Upper Respiratory Tract Infections: Rhinitis, Rhinosinusitis, Tonsillopharyngitis, and Acute Bronchitis. *(Continued)*

Common Name/ Latin Name	Scope of Potential Benefits	Comments
Peppermint *Mentha × piperita*	Oral health, weight reduction, nausea, dyspepsia, **IBS**, GI endoscopy, cracked nipples, PCOS, neck pain, tension headaches, postherpetic neuralgia, cognition, nicotine withdrawal, pressure ulcers, pruritis gravidarum, hirsutism, athletic performance, URI, *cancer*	Human research: topical spray in combination with three other essential oils provided short-term relief of URI symptoms
Umckaloabo/South African Geranium *Pelargonium sidoides*	Asthma, COPD, *PUD*, immune function, inflammation, **bronchitis**, **URI**, pharyngitis, rhinosinusitis, *influenza, coronavirus, pneumonia, HIV, HSV 1&2, TB*	**Systematic reviews: beneficial for bronchitis, RTIs in children and adults, cough** Human research: reduces duration of bronchitis, rhinosinusitis, pharyngotonsillitis, and URTIs
Uva ursi *Arctostaphylos uva-ursi*	*UTI*, recurrent UTI, *dementia, dermatitis, skin hyperpigmentation, cough*	*Preclinical research: anti-tussive in cats*

TABLE 22.B
Influenza and Pneumonia.

Common Name/ Latin Name	Scope of Potential Benefits	Comments
Burdock *Arctium lappa*	*Dyslipidemia*, diabetes, *hepatic function and protection, gastroparesis, dyspepsia*, diverticulitis, diabetic nephropathy, OA, wrinkles, acne, cough, *inflammation, influenza A, cancer*	*Preclinical research: synergistic with oseltamivir against Influenza A; anti-tussive in cats*
Cranberry *Vaccinium macrocarpon*	Gingivitis, dyslipidemia, **DM**, PUD, gut dysbiosis, overactive bladder, **UTI**, post-radiation UTI, BPH, chronic prostatitis, RA, *inflammation, influenza*, prostate CA	*Preclinical research: reduces hemagglutination and infectivity of influenza A&B*
Echinacea *Echinacea purpurea, angustifolia*	Anterior uveitis, *candida vaginitis*, genital condylomas, OA, **anxiety**, eczema, athletic performance, immune function, inflammation, **URIs**, influenza, *coronavirus*, HPV, *colorectal cancer*	Human research: noninferior to oseltamivir when taken early
Elder (berry, flower) *Sambucus nigra*	Gingival recession, ASCVD, *dyslipidemia, DM*, obesity, constipation, stroke, *immune function*, **URI**, rhinosinusitis, influenza, *HIV, HSV, Strep, cancer*	Human research: reduces duration and severity of influenza when taken early
Ginseng, American *Panax quinquefolius*	HTN, dyslipidemia, DM, PVD, cognition, ADHD, schizophrenia, immune function, **URIs**, influenza, cancer	Human research: reduces influenza and RSV in institutionalized elderly when taken preventively
Ginseng, Asian/ Korean/Chinese *Panax ginseng*	Dry eyes, **hearing loss**, **HTN**, CHF, **DM**, obesity, **menopause**, **ED**, male infertility, *osteoporosis*, AD, cognitive function, aging skin, alopecia areata, stamina, **chronic fatigue**, **hangover**, immune function, inflammation, influenza, HIV, **cancer**	Human research: improves response to influenza vaccine

TABLE 22.B

Influenza and Pneumonia. *(Continued)*

Common Name/ Latin Name	Scope of Potential Benefits	Comments
Goji berry/ wolfberry *Lycium barbarum*	Macular degeneration, *glaucoma*, dyslipidemia, **diabetes**, obesity, *hepatoprotection, male infertility, male sexual dysfunction*, stroke, *AD*, insomnia, anxiety, ADD, *dermatitis*, cognition, stress, fatigue, athletic performance, hangover, immunity function, influenza, cancer	Human research: improves response to influenza vaccine
Skullcap (Chinese, American) *Scutellaria baicalensis, lateriflora*	*Noise induced hearing loss*, allergy, *asthma, COPD, preterm RDS, pneumonia, PAH, CAD, dyslipidemia, DM, obesity, NAFLD, ETOH-induced gastritis, seizures, dementias*, **anxiety**, depression, *ADHD*, cognition, *photoprotection, autoimmunity, inflammation, MS, influenza, pneumonia, HIV*, cancer-related anemia, *cancer*	*Preclinical research: reduces influenza viral titers, prolongs survival, improves recovery from influenza; prevents S. aureus pneumonia*
Schisandra *Schisandra chinensis*	*MI*, **CHF**, DM, NAFLD, viral hepatitis, menopause, FMF, *stroke, AD, anxiety*, cognition, physical stress, stamina, pneumonia, HCV, *fungal infections*, cancer	Human research: speeds recovery from pneumonia in combination formula
Umckaloabo/South African Geranium *Pelargonium sidoides*	Asthma, COPD, *PUD*, immune function, inflammation, **bronchitis**, **URI**, pharyngitis, rhinosinusitis, *influenza, coronavirus, pneumonia, HIV, HSV 1&2, TB*	*Preclinical research: activity against H1N1 and H3N1 influenza, coronavirus, and several bacteria commonly causing pneumonia*

TABLE 22.C

HIV (See footnote).*

Common Name/ Latin Name	Scope of Potential Benefits	Comments
Aloe *Aloe vera, barbadensis*	**Gingivitis**, **submucous fibrosis**, **dyslipidemia**, **diabetes**, insulin resistance, hepatic fibrosis, GERD, **IBS**, IBD, anal fissures, radiation proctitis, AD, *PD*, acne, **psoriasis**, **lichen planus**, **burns**, wounds, pressure ulcers, diabetic foot ulcers, wrinkle and striae reduction, Hashimoto's thyroiditis, inflammation, HIV, cancer	Human research (Nigerian study): improves HIV status. *(No studies on safety with antiretrovirals)*
Calendula *Calendula officinalis*	Gingivitis, dental plaque, radiation mucositis, venous ulcers, lactational cracked nipples, vaginal candidiasis, episiotomy healing, nonbacterial prostatitis, diaper dermatitis, **wound healing**, diabetic foot ulcers, *antibacterial, anti-HIV*, radiation dermatitis	*Preclinical research: activity against HIV (ethanolic extract)*
Elder (berry, flower) *Sambucus nigra*	Gingival recession, ASCVD, *dyslipidemia, DM*, obesity, constipation, stroke, *immune function*, **URI**, rhinosinusitis, influenza, *HIV, HSV, Strep, cancer*	*Preclinical research: activity against HIV* Case reports: reduction of viral loads in HIV patients
Ginseng, Asian/ Korean/Chinese *Panax ginseng*	Dry eyes, **hearing loss**, **HTN**, CHF, **DM**, obesity, **menopause**, **ED**, male infertility, *osteoporosis*, AD, cognitive function, aging skin, alopecia areata, stamina, **chronic fatigue**, **hangover**, immune function, inflammation, influenza, HIV, **cancer**	Human research: alters HIV Nef gene advantageously
Skullcap (Chinese, American) *Scutellaria baicalensis, lateriflora*	*Noise induced hearing loss*, allergy, *asthma, COPD, preterm RDS, pneumonia, PAH, CAD, dyslipidemia, DM, obesity, NAFLD, ETOH-induced gastritis, seizures, dementias*, **anxiety**, depression, *ADHD*, cognition, *photoprotection, autoimmunity, inflammation, MS, influenza, pneumonia, HIV*, cancer-related anemia, *cancer*	*Preclinical: inhibits HIV/RT; reduces HIV infection and replication*

Continued on following page

	TABLE 22.C	
	HIV. *(Continued)*	

Common Name/ Latin Name	Scope of Potential Benefits	Comments
Turmeric *Curcuma longa*	Anterior uveitis, **oral lichen planus**, **gingivitis**, dental surgery, submucous fibrosis, asthma, **diastolic HTN**, **dyslipidemia**, CAD, endothelial dysfunction, **DM**, obesity, **NAFLD**, hepatoprotective, gallbladder dyskinesia, *GERD*, PUD, dyspepsia, **UC**, DM nephropathy, lupus nephritis, lactational mastitis, LSIL, chronic non-bacterial prostatitis, post-operative pain, **OA**, RA, migraine HA, *neurodegeneration*, **anxiety**, **depression**, **skin disease**, psoriasis, fatigue, **systemic inflammation**, *HIV*, coronavirus, **chemo-related oral mucositis**, cancer prevention, cancer treatment	*Preclinical research: inhibits HIV infection and replication*
Umckaloabo/ South African Geranium *Pelargonium sidoides*	Asthma, COPD, *PUD*, immune function, inflammation, **bronchitis**, **URI**, pharyngitis, rhinosinusitis, *influenza*, *coronavirus*, *pneumonia*, HIV, HSV 1&2, TB	*Preclinical research: activity against HIV*
Valerian *Valeriana officinalis*	*HTN*, *CAD*, *IBS*, PMS, dysmenorrhea, **menopause**, RLS, cognitive, anxiety, insomnia, OCD, *cancer*	Human research: reduces anxiety related to HAART

* This table is included primarily for research purposes. Due to established efficacy, HAART is always preferable to herbal therapy for HIV infection.

	TABLE 22.D	
	HSV, Coronavirus, and Miscellaneous Viral and Fungal Infections (See Table 11.A for HBV and HCV; Table 13.C for *C. albicans*; Table 22.C for HIV).	

Common Name/ Latin Name	Scope of Potential Benefits	Comments
Andrographis *Andrographis paniculata*	*HTN*, *hepatoprotection*, ulcerative colitis, *dysmenorrhea*, OA, RA, FMF, *inflammation*, **URI prevention and treatment**, SARS-CoV-2, *cancer*	*Preclinical research: Andrographolide strongly inhibitory of SARS-CoV-2 in vitro* Human research: improvement by 3–5 days in Phase I clinical trial
Astragalus *Astragalus membranaceus*	Herpes keratitis, recurrent tonsillitis, allergic rhinitis, atopy, asthma, **viral myocarditis**, CHF, CAD, viral hepatitis, **diabetic nephropathy**, IgA nephropathy, nephrotic syndrome, lupus nephritis, *renal fibrosis*, *sperm quality*, hemorrhagic stroke, burns, *wound healing*, *age spots*, *leukopenia*, **immune function**, *antiviral*, HBV, TB, **NSCLC**, cancer	*Preclinical research: activity against hepatitis B, Coxsackie B3, parainfluenza type1, and Japanese encephalitis viruses*
Black seed/nigella/ black cumin *Nigella sativa*	Periodontal dz., oral submucous fibrosis, chronic rhinosinusitis, nasal dryness, **allergy**, **asthma**, COPD, chemical pneumonitis, **HTN**, *CAD*, CHF, **dyslipidemia**, **DM**, **obesity**, NAFLD, dyspepsia, PUD, diabetic nephropathy, mastalgia, menopause, male infertility, OA, *stroke*, seizure disorder, memory impairment, cognition, anxiety, *depression*, acne, eczema, vitiligo, immune function, Hashimoto's thyroiditis, RA, inflammation, *H. pylori*, *Staph* pustules, HCV, *SARS-CoV-2*, cancer	*Preclinical research: in silico research shows several constituents with high affinity for SARS-CoV-2 enzymes and proteins*

TABLE 22.D

HSV, Coronavirus, and Miscellaneous Viral and Fungal Infections (See Table 11.A for HBV and HCV; Table 13.C for *C. albicans*; Table 22.C for HIV). *(Continued)*

Common Name/ Latin Name	Scope of Potential Benefits	Comments
Chamomile *Matricaria chamomilla/ recutita*	Gingivitis, mucositis, chronic rhinosinusitis, *allergies*, dyslipidemia, diabetes, *PUD*, colic, IBS, diarrhea, dyspepsia, UC, *candida vaginitis*, menopause, carpal tunnel syndrome, anxiety, insomnia, depression, ADHD, eczema, wounds, radiation or chemotherapy dermatitis, cortisol dysregulation, *inflammation, broadly antimicrobial (bacteria, yeast, fungus), cancer*	*Preclinical research: inhibits Candida albicans, polio virus, herpes virus, trichophytons*
Echinacea *Echinacea purpurea, angustifolia*	Anterior uveitis, *candida vaginitis*, genital condylomas, OA, **anxiety**, eczema, athletic performance, immune function, inflammation, **URIs**, influenza, *coronavirus*, HPV, *colorectal cancer*	*Preclinical research: activity against several strains of coronavirus including MERS and SARS-CoV-2* Human research: prevents recurrence of genital condylomas
Elder (berry, flower) *Sambucus nigra*	Gingival recession, ASCVD, *dyslipidemia, DM*, obesity, constipation, stroke, *immune function*, **URI**, rhinosinusitis, influenza, *HIV, HSV, Strep, cancer*	*Preclinical research: activity against HSV*
Eleuthero/Siberian Ginseng *Eleutherococcus senticosus/ Acanthopanax senticosus*	*Allergic rhinitis*, dyslipidemia, CHF, edema, *male infertility*, osteoporosis, **stroke recovery**, AD, insomnia, **depression**, bipolar disorder, attention, vitality, athletic stamina, **hangover**, immune function, FMF, **URI**, *antiviral*, ovarian cancer	*Preclinical research: activity against RNA viruses*
Ginger *Zingiber officinale*	**Motion sickness**, *HTN*, dyslipidemia, fibrinolysis, diabetes, **nausea**, **vomiting**, *dyspepsia*, gastroparesis, *PUD*, ulcerative colitis, *diabetic nephropathy*, **dysmenorrhea**, *Candida vaginitis*, male infertility, OA, muscle injury, migraine HA, *AD*, **inflammation**, RA, *H. pylori*, *antibacterial*, **CINV**, cancer	*Preclinical research: activity against C. albicans; promotes interferon release*
Holy basil/Tulsi *Ocimum tenuiflorum/ sanctum*	Gingivitis, asthma, *CAD*, **dyslipidemia**, **diabetes**, obesity, *hepatotoxicity, PUD, male hypogonadism, pain, seizures*, anxiety, depression, memory and concentration, stress and fatigue, immune function, viral encephalitis	Human research: report of improved survival in viral encephalitis
Lemon balm *Melissa officinalis*	**Bruxism**, dyslipidemia, DM, palpitations, dyspepsia, IBS, **colic**, PMS, dysmenorrhea, female sexual dysfunction, **AD**, dementia, agitation, *diabetic neuropathy*, insomnia, **anxiety**, depression, **ADHD**, *hyperthyroidism, Graves' disease*, herpes simplex, *cancer, glioblastoma multiforme*	*Preclinical research: activity against HSV* Human research: topical application improves recurrent HSV1
Licorice *Glycyrrhiza glabra*	**Postoperative sore throat**, xerostomia, radiation-induced mucositis, aphthous ulcers, *allergy*, **asthma**, **dyslipidemia**, *CAD, diabetes*, **obesity**, hepatoprotection, heartburn, PUD, functional dyspepsia, **antipsychotic-induced hyperprolactinemia**, **menopause**, atrophic vaginitis, PCOS, female hirsutism, BPH, *stroke, dementia, PD, anxiety, insomnia, depression, substance addiction*, **hyperpigmentation**, **atopic eczema**, Addison's disease, *stamina, multiple sclerosis, inflammation, H. pylori, SARS-CoV-2*, cancer, *breast cancer*	*Preclinical research: in vitro and in silico evidence for activity against SARS-CoV-1, SARS-CoV-2, and several other viruses*
Peppermint *Mentha × piperita*	Oral health, weight reduction, nausea, dyspepsia, **IBS**, GI endoscopy, cracked nipples, PCOS, neck pain, tension headaches, postherpetic neuralgia, cognition, nicotine withdrawal, pressure ulcers, pruritis gravidarum, hirsutism, athletic performance, URI, *cancer*	Case report: reduced pain in resistant postherpetic neuralgia

Continued on following page

TABLE 22.D		
HSV, Coronavirus, and Miscellaneous Viral and Fungal Infections (See Table 11.A for HBV and HCV; Table 13.C for *C. albicans;* Table 22.C for HIV). *(Continued)*		

Common Name/ Latin Name	Scope of Potential Benefits	Comments
St. John's Wort *Hypericum perforatum*	PMS, **perimenopause or menopause**, *chronic pain*, neuropathy, **depression**, *opiate addiction*, psoriasis, atopic dermatitis, *sunburn*, inflammation, HSV, *cancer*	Human research: combination topical application for HSV 1&2 superior to topical acyclovir **See St. John's Wort monograph warnings and precautions**
Schisandra *Schisandra chinensis*	*MI*, **CHF**, DM, NAFLD, viral hepatitis, menopause, FMF, stroke, *AD*, *anxiety*, cognition, physical stress, stamina, pneumonia, *HCV*, *fungal infections*, cancer	*Preclinical research: more antifungal than most other herbs tested in TCM combination*
Turmeric *Curcuma longa*	Anterior uveitis, **oral lichen planus**, **gingivitis**, dental surgery, submucous fibrosis, asthma, **diastolic HTN**, **dyslipidemia**, CAD, endothelial dysfunction, **DM**, obesity, **NAFLD**, hepatoprotective, gallbladder dyskinesia, *GERD*, PUD, dyspepsia, **UC**, DM nephropathy, lupus nephritis, lactational mastitis, LSIL, chronic non-bacterial prostatitis, post-operative pain, **OA**, RA, migraine HA, *neurodegeneration*, **anxiety**, **depression**, **skin disease**, psoriasis, fatigue, **systemic inflammation**, *HIV*, SARS-CoV-2, **chemo-related oral mucositis**, cancer prevention, cancer treatment	*Preclinical research: inhibits numerous viruses including SARS-CoV-2 through numerous mechanisms*
Umckaloabo/South African Geranium *Pelargonium sidoides*	Asthma, COPD, *PUD*, immune function, inflammation, **bronchitis**, **URI**, pharyngitis, rhinosinusitis, *influenza*, coronavirus, pneumonia, HIV, HSV 1&2, TB	*Preclinical research: activity against respiratory viruses (including coronavirus and influenza), HIV, HSV 1&2, and H. pylori*

TABLE 22.E		
Tuberculosis and Miscellaneous Bacterial Infections (See Table 11.B for *H. pylori*).		

Common Name/ Latin Name	Scope of Potential Benefits	Comments
Ashwagandha *Withania somnifera*	Dyslipidemia, DM, **sexual dysfunction**, **infertility**, *osteoporosis*, gout, OA, *AD*, *PD*, MCI, **anxiety**, insomnia, OCD, *depression*, schizophrenia, hypothyroidism, stress, endurance, *fatigue*, immune function, TB, *cancer*	Human research: improves antituberculosis response to anti-tuberculosis drug regimen, reduces hepatotoxicity
Astragalus *Astragalus membranaceus*	Herpes keratitis, recurrent tonsillitis, allergic rhinitis, atopy, asthma, **viral myocarditis**, CHF, CAD, viral hepatitis, **diabetic nephropathy**, IgA nephropathy, nephrotic syndrome, lupus nephritis, *renal fibrosis*, *sperm quality*, hemorrhagic stroke, burns, *wound healing*, *age spots*, *leukopenia*, **immune function**, *antiviral*, HBV, TB, **NSCLC**, cancer	Human research: enhances immune function in TB patients
Bilberry *Vaccinium myrtillus*	Normal pressure glaucoma, cataracts, night vision, eye fatigue, gingivitis, **HTN**, **dyslipidemia**, T2DM, NAFLD, ulcerative colitis, *AD*, psoriasis, *wounds*, inflammation, *S. pneumonia*, MRSA, colorectal cancer, *other cancers*	*Preclinical research: activity against S. pneumonia and MRSA*
Black seed/ nigella/ black cumin *Nigella sativa*	Periodontal dz., oral submucous fibrosis, chronic rhinosinusitis, nasal dryness, **allergy**, **asthma**, COPD, chemical pneumonitis, **HTN**, CAD, CHF, **dyslipidemia**, **DM**, **obesity**, NAFLD, dyspepsia, PUD, diabetic nephropathy, mastalgia, menopause, male infertility, OA, *stroke*, seizure disorder, memory impairment, cognition, anxiety, *depression*, acne, eczema, vitiligo, immune function, Hashimoto's thyroiditis, RA, inflammation, *H. pylori*, *Staph* pustules, HCV, coronavirus, cancer	Human research: noninferior to mupirocin for neonatal *Staph* pustulosis

TABLE 22.E

Tuberculosis and Miscellaneous Bacterial Infections (See Table 11.B for *H. pylori*). *(Continued)*

Common Name/ Latin Name	Scope of Potential Benefits	Comments
Calendula *Calendula officinalis*	Gingivitis, dental plaque, radiation mucositis, venous ulcers, lactational cracked nipples, vaginal candidiasis, episiotomy healing, nonbacterial prostatitis, diaper dermatitis, **wound healing**, diabetic foot ulcers, *antibacterial, anti-HIV*, radiation dermatitis	*Preclinical research: activity against P. aeruginosa, S. aureus, B. subtilis, E. coli, and K. pneumonia*
Chamomile *Matricaria chamomilla/recutita*	Gingivitis, mucositis, chronic rhinosinusitis, *allergies*, dyslipidemia, diabetes, *PUD*, colic, IBS, diarrhea, dyspepsia, UC, *candida vaginitis*, menopause, carpal tunnel syndrome, anxiety, insomnia, depression, ADHD, eczema, wounds, radiation or chemotherapy dermatitis, cortisol dysregulation, *inflammation, broadly antimicrobial (bacteria, yeast, fungus), cancer*	*Preclinical research: reduces E. coli aggregation; inhibits Staph, Strep, Pneumococcus, Mycobacterium (TB and avian)*
Dandelion *Taraxacum officinale*	HTN, dyslipidemia, DM, *obesity, edema*, liver toxicity, NAFLD, *gastroparesis*, dyspepsia, *neurodegenerative disorders, depression, stamina, inflammation, endotoxic shock, cancer*	*Preclinical research: reduces endotoxic shock via reduction in TNF-α, IFN-γ, IL-1β, IL-6, NO and PGE$_2$*
Elder (berry, flower) *Sambucus nigra*	Gingival recession, ASCVD, *dyslipidemia, DM*, obesity, constipation, stroke, *immune function*, **URI**, rhinosinusitis, influenza, *HIV, HSV, Strep, cancer*	*Preclinical research: activity against several bacteria*
Ginger *Zingiber officinale*	**Motion sickness**, HTN, dyslipidemia, fibrinolysis, diabetes, **nausea, vomiting**, *dyspepsia*, gastroparesis, *PUD*, ulcerative colitis, *diabetic nephropathy*, **dysmenorrhea**, *Candida vaginitis*, male infertility, OA, muscle injury, migraine HA, *AD*, **inflammation**, RA, *H. pylori, antibacterial*, **CINV**, cancer	*Preclinical research: activity against S. aureus, P. aeruginosa, S. typhimurium, E. coli, and M. luteus*
Hops/Hop *Humulus lupulus*	Dental plaque, allergic rhinitis, ASCVD, dyslipidemia, T2DM, obesity, *NAFLD, dyspepsia*, osteoporosis, OA, RA, atrophic vaginitis, menopause, cognitive decline, **insomnia**, anxiety, depression, cognitive performance, acne, aging skin, body odor, antibacterial, *TB, cancer*	*Preclinical research: activity against G + and G- bacteria, and M. tuberculosis* Human research: topically reduces *Corynebacterium xerosis* and *Staphylococcus epidermidis*
Saffron *Crocus sativus*	ARMD, *cataracts*, diabetic maculopathy, glaucoma, gingivitis, burning mouth syndrome, *allergy*, asthma, HTN, **dyslipidemia**, DM, **obesity**, *hepatotoxicity, DM nephropathy*, PMS, menopause, **female and male sexual dysfunction**, male infertility, chronic pain, fibromyalgia, stroke, AD, **anxiety**, insomnia, OCD, **depression**, ADHD, drug and ETOH addiction, *photodamage, stamina, immune function, inflammation, RA, bacterial infection*, cancer	*Preclinical research: activity against S. aureus, B cereus, S. typhi, E. coli, and S. dysenteriae*
Skullcap (Chinese, American) *Scutellaria baicalensis, lateriflora*	*Noise induced hearing loss*, allergy, *asthma, COPD, preterm RDS, pneumonia, PAH, CAD, dyslipidemia, DM, obesity, NAFLD, ETOH-induced gastritis, seizures, dementias*, **anxiety**, *depression, ADHD, cognition, photoprotection, autoimmunity, inflammation, MS, influenza, pneumonia, HIV, cancer-related anemia, cancer*	*Preclinical: binds α-hemolysin*
Umckaloabo/South African Geranium *Pelargonium sidoides*	Asthma, COPD, *PUD*, immune function, inflammation, **bronchitis**, **URI**, pharyngitis, rhinosinusitis, *influenza, coronavirus, pneumonia, HIV, HSV 1&2, TB*	*Preclinical research: activity against group A strep, G + and G- bacteria, and M. tuberculosis*

23

HEMATOLOGY AND ONCOLOGY

TABLE 23.A
Hematologic Disorders.

Common Name/ Latin Name	Scope of Potential Benefits	Comments
Dong quai *Angelica sinensis*	Pulmonary HTN, *HTN*, CAD, *atrial fibrillation*, cirrhosis, portal HTN, abd pain, UC, *renal fibrosis, dysmenorrhea*, menopausal symptoms, *osteoporosis, OA*, stroke, *cerebrovascular insufficiency, neurodegenerative disorders, wound healing, aging skin, alopecia, stamina, inflammation*, anemia of chronic disease, cancer	Human case report: improvement in recombinant human erythropoietin resistant anemia of chronic disease
Milk thistle *Silybum marianum*	**Dyslipidemia, DM, liver disease**, diabetic nephropathy, lactation, PCOS, BPH, *gout, AD, diabetic neuropathy*, **OCD**, acne, *psoriasis*, vitiligo, radio-dermatitis, aging skin, RA, inflammation, hepatitis viruses, **iron-overload**, chemotherapy and radiotherapy toxicity, *hepatocellular carcinoma*	**Literature review: beneficial for iron overload in β-thalassemia** Human research: reduces Fe absorption and Fe load in hemochromatosis and β-thalassemia with or without deferoxamine
Skullcap (Chinese, American) *Scutellaria baicalensis, lateriflora*	*Noise induced hearing loss*, allergy, *asthma, COPD, preterm RDS, pneumonia, PAH, CAD, dyslipidemia, DM, obesity, NAFLD, ETOH-induced gastritis, seizures, dementias*, **anxiety**, depression, *ADHD*, cognition, *photoprotection, autoimmunity, inflammation, MS, influenza, pneumonia, HIV*, cancer-related anemia, *cancer*	Human research: hemopoietic with chemotherapy

TABLE 23.B
Oncologic Disorders (see important footnote).*

Common Name/ Latin Name	Scope of Potential Benefits	Comments
Aloe *Aloe vera, barbadensis*	**Gingivitis, submucous fibrosis, dyslipidemia, diabetes**, insulin resistance, hepatic fibrosis, GERD, **IBS**, IBD, anal fissures, radiation proctitis, AD, *PD*, acne, **psoriasis, lichen planus, burns**, wounds, pressure ulcers, diabetic foot ulcers, wrinkle and striae reduction, Hashimoto's thyroiditis, inflammation, HIV, cancer	Human research: improves solid tumor response to chemotherapy

Continued on following page

TABLE 23.B
Oncologic Disorders. *(Continued)*

Common Name/ Latin Name	Scope of Potential Benefits	Comments
Andrographis *Andrographis paniculata*	*HTN, hepatoprotection*, ulcerative colitis, *dysmenorrhea*, OA, RA, FMF, *inflammation*, **URI prevention and treatment**, *cancer*	*Preclinical research: inhibits a number of cancer cell lines and augments several chemotherapeutic drugs*
Ashwagandha *Withania somnifera*	Dyslipidemia, DM, **sexual dysfunction**, **infertility**, *osteoporosis*, gout, OA, *AD, PD*, MCI, **anxiety**, insomnia, OCD, *depression*, schizophrenia, hypothyroidism, stress, endurance, *fatigue*, immune function, TB, *cancer*	*Preclinical research: antitumor in ovarian, lung, and colorectal tumors; enhances paclitaxel cytotoxicity; enhances 5-FU efficacy, and reduces neutropenia*
Astragalus *Astragalus membranaceus*	Herpes keratitis, recurrent tonsillitis, allergic rhinitis, atopy, asthma, **viral myocarditis**, CHF, CAD, viral hepatitis, **diabetic nephropathy**, IgA nephropathy, nephrotic syndrome, lupus nephritis, *renal fibrosis, sperm quality*, hemorrhagic stroke, burns, *wound healing, age spots, leukopenia*, **immune function**, *antiviral*, HBV, TB, **NSCLC**, cancer	**Systematic reviews: enhances survival when added to chemotherapy in NSCLC** Human research: enhances efficacy of some chemotherapy and reduces side effects
Bilberry *Vaccinium myrtillus*	Normal pressure glaucoma, cataracts, night vision, eye fatigue, gingivitis, *HTN*, **dyslipidemia**, T2DM, NAFLD, ulcerative colitis, *AD*, psoriasis, *wounds*, inflammation, *S. pneumonia, MRSA*, colorectal cancer, *other cancers*	*Preclinical research: activity against breast, colon, leukemia, and NSCLC* Small human trial: slows proliferation in colorectal cancer
Black cohosh *Actaea racemosa/Cimicifuga racemosa*	Breast density, uterine fibroids, female infertility, PCOS, **menopausal syndrome**, osteoporosis, breast cancer	*Preclinical research: inhibitory in breast, uterine, and prostate cancer cell lines* Human research: slows recurrence in breast cancer; reduces menopausal sx with tamoxifen
Black seed/nigella/black cumin *Nigella sativa*	Periodontal dz., oral submucous fibrosis, chronic rhinosinusitis, nasal dryness, **allergy**, **asthma**, COPD, chemical pneumonitis, **HTN**, *CAD*, CHF, **dyslipidemia**, **DM**, **obesity**, NAFLD, dyspepsia, PUD, diabetic nephropathy, mastalgia, menopause, male infertility, OA, *stroke*, seizure disorder, memory impairment, cognition, anxiety, *depression*, acne, eczema, vitiligo, immune function, Hashimoto's thyroiditis, RA, inflammation, *H. pylori, Staph* pustules, HCV, cancer	*Preclinical research: activity against hepatocellular carcinoma, cervical SCC* Human research: reduces febrile neutropenia in brain cancer; reduces MTX hepatotoxicity and improves survival in ALL; reduces radiation dermatitis in breast ca
Burdock *Arctium lappa*	*Dyslipidemia, diabetes, hepatic function and protection, gastroparesis, dyspepsia*, diverticulitis, diabetic nephropathy, OA, wrinkles, acne, cough, *inflammation, influenza A, cancer*	*Preclinical research: active against pancreatic and other tumor cells; promotes cell cycle arrest, apoptosis; inhibits proliferation*
Calendula *Calendula officinalis*	Gingivitis, dental plaque, radiation mucositis, venous ulcers, lactational cracked nipples, vaginal candidiasis, episiotomy healing, nonbacterial prostatitis, diaper dermatitis, **wound healing**, diabetic foot ulcers, *antibacterial, anti-HIV*, radiation dermatitis	Human research: reduces radiation dermatitis

TABLE 23.B
Oncologic Disorders. *(Continued)*

Common Name/ Latin Name	Scope of Potential Benefits	Comments
Chamomile *Matricaria chamomilla/recutita*	Gingivitis, mucositis, chronic rhinosinusitis, *allergie*s, dyslipidemia, diabetes, *PUD*, colic, IBS, diarrhea, dyspepsia, UC, *candida vaginitis*, menopause, carpal tunnel syndrome, anxiety, insomnia, depression, ADHD, eczema, wounds, radiation or chemotherapy dermatitis, cortisol dysregulation, *inflammation, broadly antimicrobial (bacteria, yeast, fungus), cancer*	*Preclinical research: reduces mutagenesis, increases apoptosis* Human research: reduces mucositis during radiation and chemotherapy
Coleus *Coleus forskohlii*	Glaucoma, *allergy*, asthma, HTN, CHF, *insulin resistance*, obesity, *pancreatic exocrine insufficiency, diarrhea, UTI, urge incontinence, dysmenorrhea, male infertility*, male hypogonadism, subarachnoid hemorrhage, *seizure, neurodegenerative disorders, alcohol abuse*, psoriasis, *photoprotection, hyperthyroidism, cancer*	*Preclinical research: reduces lung and colon cancer metastasis; inhibits gastric, myeloid, and lymphoid cancer cells; increases doxorubicin efficacy and toxicity*
Cranberry *Vaccinium macrocarpon*	Gingivitis, dyslipidemia, **DM**, PUD, gut dysbiosis, overactive bladder, **UTI**, post-radiation UTI, BPH, chronic prostatitis, RA, *inflammation, influenza*, prostate CA	*Preclinical research: antiproliferative activity against several cancer cell lines; synergistic with cyclophosphamide* Human research: reduces prostate cancer post-radiation UTIs; reduces PSA
Dandelion *Taraxacum officinale*	HTN, dyslipidemia, DM, *obesity, edema*, liver toxicity, NAFLD, *gastroparesis*, dyspepsia, *neurodegenerative disorders, depression, stamina, inflammation, endotoxic shock, cancer*	*Preclinical research: activity against breast cancer, prostate cancer, colon cancer, melanoma, and leukemia cell lines*
Dong quai *Angelica sinensis*	Pulmonary HTN, *HTN*, CAD, *atrial fibrillation*, cirrhosis, portal HTN, abd pain, UC, *renal fibrosis, dysmenorrhea*, menopausal symptoms, *osteoporosis, OA*, stroke, *cerebrovascular insufficiency, neurodegenerative disorders, wound healing, aging skin, alopecia, stamina, inflammation*, anemia of chronic disease, cancer	*Preclinical research: activity against glioblastoma, other cell lines; prolongs survival; antiangiogenic; antiproliferative* Human research: epidemiologic evidence for prevention of uterine cancer in breast cancer survivors on tamoxifen; however, weakly stimulates some breast cancer cells
Echinacea *Echinacea purpurea, angustifolia*	Anterior uveitis, *candida vaginitis*, genital condylomas, OA, **anxiety**, eczema, athletic performance, immune function, inflammation, **URIs**, influenza, *Coronavirus*, HPV, *colorectal cancer*	*Preclinical research: activity against colon cancer cells*
Elder (berry, flower) *Sambucus nigra*	Gingival recession, ASCVD, *dyslipidemia, DM*, obesity, constipation, stroke, *immune function*, **URI**, rhinosinusitis, influenza, *HIV, HSV, Strep, cancer*	*Preclinical research: antagonizes VEGFR*
Eleuthero/Siberian Ginseng *Eleutherococcus senticosus/ Acanthopanax senticosus*	*Allergic rhinitis*, dyslipidemia, CHF, edema, *male infertility*, osteoporosis, **stroke recovery**, *AD*, insomnia, **depression**, bipolar disorder, attention, vitality, athletic stamina, **hangover**, immune function, FMF, **URI**, *antiviral*, ovarian cancer	Human research: combination formula improves immune resilience during chemo for ovarian cancer
Fenugreek *Trigonella foenum-graecum*	Dyslipidemia, **DM**, pre-diabetes, *diabetic nephropathy, urolithiasis*, lactation, dysmenorrhea, PCOS, menopause, male sexual dysfunction, hypogonadism, PD, *peripheral neuropathy, thyroid T3/T4 balance*, stamina, *cancer*	*Preclinical research: activity against breast, ovarian, colorectal, and leukemia cell lines*

Continued on following page

TABLE 23.B
Oncologic Disorders. *(Continued)*

Common Name/ Latin Name	Scope of Potential Benefits	Comments
Frankincense/Boswellia *Boswellia serrata, sacra, carterii*	Gingivitis, **asthma**, *COPD*, UC, **Crohn's**, **collagenous colitis**, IBS, UTI, SUI, benign breast disease, menorrhagia, **OA**, stroke, memory impairment, psoriasis, eczema, aging skin, athletic performance, **RA**, **IBD**, *inflammation*, glioma radiation, chemo-related neuropathy, *cancer*	*Preclinical research: activity against numerous cell lines through several anti-cancer mechanisms* Human research: reduces post-radiation brain swelling; reduces chemo-induced neuropathy
Ginger *Zingiber officinale*	**Motion sickness**, *HTN*, dyslipidemia, fibrinolysis, diabetes, **nausea**, **vomiting**, *dyspepsia*, gastroparesis, PUD, ulcerative colitis, *diabetic nephropathy*, **dysmenorrhea**, *Candida vaginitis*, male infertility, OA, muscle injury, migraine HA, *AD*, **inflammation**, RA, *H. pylori*, *antibacterial*, **CINV**, cancer	*Preclinical research: promotes apoptosis and inhibits cell cycle of gastric cancer cells, inhibits VEGF and IL-I in ovarian cancer cells; damages microtubules, inducing mitotic arrest* **Systematic Review: reduces acute CINV and fatigue** Ex vivo human colonic mucosa: decreases proliferation, increases apoptosis; prevents carcinogenesis Human research: reduces chemo-induced nausea; synergistic with antiemetics
Ginkgo *Ginkgo biloba*	*Cataracts*, ARMD, glaucoma, periodontal dz., **vertigo**, **tinnitus**, **cardiovascular health**, **dyslipidemia**, **diabetes**, obesity, claudication, hepatic fibrosis, **diabetic nephropathy**, menopausal sexual desire, **acute mountain sickness**, migraines with aura, **stroke**, **MCI**, **dementias**, post-operative delirium, depression, ADHD, **schizophrenia**, **tardive dyskinesia**, aging skin, *inflammation*, *cancer*	*Preclinical research: inhibits proliferation and promotes apoptosis in gastric cancer cells; aromatase inhibitor*
Ginseng, American *Panax quinquefolius*	HTN, dyslipidemia, DM, PVD, cognition, ADHD, schizophrenia, immune function, **URIs**, influenza, cancer	Human research: improves chemo-related fatigue
Ginseng, Asian/Korean/ Chinese *Panax ginseng*	Dry eyes, **hearing loss**, **HTN**, CHF, **DM**, obesity, **menopause**, **ED**, male infertility, *osteoporosis*, AD, cognitive function, aging skin, alopecia areata, stamina, **chronic fatigue**, **hangover**, immune function, inflammation, influenza, HIV, **cancer**	**Systematic reviews: injected combination herbal product plus chemo improved response; beneficial for chemo-induced nausea and vomiting** Human research: reduces risk for several types of cancer (retrospective); improves survival and quality of life in breast cancer patients (despite weak estrogenic activity); improves survival in NSCLC; improves QOL but not survival in ovarian cancer
Goji berry/wolfberry *Lycium barbarum*	Macular degeneration, *glaucoma*, dyslipidemia, **diabetes**, obesity, *hepatoprotection*, *male infertility*, *male sexual dysfunction*, *stroke*, *AD*, insomnia, anxiety, ADD, *dermatitis*, cognition, stress, fatigue, athletic performance, hangover, immunity function, influenza, cancer	*Preclinical research: inhibits ER+ breast cancer cells, leukemia HL-60 cells; induces cell cycle arrest in numerous types of cancer cell lines; prevents cardiotoxicity of doxorubicin* Human research: improves response to biotherapy for several cancer types
Gymnema/Gurmar *Gymnema sylvestre*	*Dental caries*, dyslipidemia, T1DM, **T2DM**, obesity, *arthritis*, *immune function*, *cancer*	*Preclinical research: activity against HeLa cell proliferation, increases neutrophil activity*

TABLE 23.B
Oncologic Disorders. *(Continued)*

Common Name/ Latin Name	Scope of Potential Benefits	Comments
Gynostemma/Jiaogulan *Gynostemma pentaphyllum*	*Asthma, CAD, dyslipidemia,* DM, obesity, *arrhythmia,* NAFLD, *PUD,* PCOS, *PD, white matter disease,* dementia, *stamina,* immune function, cancer	Small human studies: improves survival, reduces relapse and metastasis
Hops/Hop *Humulus lupulus*	Dental plaque, allergic rhinitis, ASCVD, dyslipidemia, T2DM, obesity, *NAFLD,* dyspepsia, osteoporosis, OA, RA, atrophic vaginitis, menopause, cognitive decline, **insomnia**, anxiety, depression, cognitive performance, acne, aging skin, body odor, antibacterial, *TB, cancer*	*Preclinical research: activity against breast cancer (conflicting findings, via SERM activity), colon cancer, prostate cancer* Human research: protects against oxidative DNA damage
Horse chestnut *Aesculus hippocastanum*	Hearing loss, *allergy,* **chronic venous insufficiency**, venous ulcers, varicocele-induced infertility, *hemorrhoids,* aging skin, *easy bruising, cancer*	*Preclinical research: activity against leukemia, multiple myeloma; synergistic with fluorouracil in hepatocellular carcinoma; potentiates gemcitabine*
Lemon balm *Melissa officinalis*	**Bruxism**, dyslipidemia, DM, palpitations, dyspepsia, IBS, **colic**, PMS, dysmenorrhea, female sexual dysfunction, **AD**, dementia, agitation, *diabetic neuropathy,* insomnia, **anxiety**, depression, **ADHD**, *hyperthyroidism, Graves' disease,* herpes simplex, *cancer, glioblastoma multiforme*	*Preclinical research: activity against colon, lung, breast, ovarian, and prostate cancer cells; EO constituent citral induces apoptosis of glioblastoma multiforme cells in absence of antioxidants* Human research: prevents DNA damage under low level radiation exposure
Licorice *Glycyrrhiza glabra*	**Postoperative sore throat**, xerostomia, radiation-induced mucositis, aphthous ulcers, *allergy,* **asthma, dyslipidemia**, CAD, *diabetes,* **obesity**, hepatoprotection, heartburn, PUD, functional dyspepsia, **antipsychotic-induced hyperprolactinemia, menopause**, atrophic vaginitis, PCOS, female hirsutism, BPH, *stroke, dementia,* PD, *anxiety, insomnia, depression, substance addiction,* **hyperpigmentation, atopic eczema**, Addison's disease, *stamina, multiple sclerosis, inflammation,* H. pylori, cancer, *breast cancer*	*Preclinical research: aromatase inhibitor; promotes apoptosis and G2/M arrest; enhances cyclophosphamide; protects against cyclophosphamide cardiotoxicity; reduces testosterone-induced breast tumor growth* ***(Caution: use deglycyrrhizinated formulations in patients at risk for HTN and hypokalemia)***
Milk thistle *Silybum marianum*	**Dyslipidemia, DM, liver disease**, diabetic nephropathy, lactation, *PCOS,* BPH, *gout, AD, diabetic neuropathy,* **OCD**, acne, *psoriasis,* vitiligo, radio-dermatitis, aging skin, RA, inflammation, hepatitis viruses, **iron-overload**, chemotherapy and radiotherapy toxicity, *hepatocellular carcinoma*	*Preclinical research: reduces cisplatin-induced nephrotoxicity; slows hepatocellular carcinoma; reduces MMPs* Human research: protects against hepatic, renal, dermal, and mucosal toxicity of various chemotherapeutic agents; reduces brain edema in metastatic NSCLC
Motherwort *Leonurus cardiaca*	*HTN 2/2 anxiety or hyperthyroidism, dyslipidemia, CAD, arrhythmia, nausea, IBS, AKI, lactation, post-partum bleeding, menorrhagia, amenorrhea,* menopause, *pain, stroke,* anxiety, *insomnia, hyperthyroidism, inflammation, breast tumors*	*Preclinical research: reduces formation of hyperplastic alveolar breast nodules and cancer; however, increases pregnancy-related tumors*
Peppermint *Mentha × piperita*	Oral health, weight reduction, nausea, dyspepsia, **IBS**, GI endoscopy, cracked nipples, PCOS, neck pain, tension headaches, postherpetic neuralgia, cognition, nicotine withdrawal, pressure ulcers, pruritis gravidarum, hirsutism, athletic performance, URI, *cancer*	*Preclinical research: induces PC-3 prostate cancer cell death; antitumorigenic against several cancer cell lines*

Continued on following page

TABLE 23.B
Oncologic Disorders. *(Continued)*

Common Name/ Latin Name	Scope of Potential Benefits	Comments
Rhodiola *Rhodiola rosea*	**CAD**, *menorrhagia, amenorrhea, female infertility,* menopause, *male hypogonadism*, premature ejaculation, **anxiety**, **depression**, **cognition**, eczema, burnout, fatigue, **athletic stamina**, cancer	*Preclinical research: anti-estrogenic; reduces metastasis, increases apoptosis; enhances cisplatin; reduces cachexia* Human research: salidroside protects against chemo-induced cardiotoxicity; improves leukocyte integrins and T-cell response in superficial bladder cancer
Saffron *Crocus sativus*	ARMD, *cataracts*, diabetic maculopathy, glaucoma, gingivitis, burning mouth syndrome, *allergy*, asthma, HTN, **dyslipidemia**, DM, **obesity**, *hepatotoxicity, DM nephropathy*, PMS, menopause, **female and male sexual dysfunction**, male infertility, chronic pain, fibromyalgia, stroke, AD, **anxiety**, insomnia, OCD, **depression**, ADHD, drug and ETOH addiction, *photodamage*, stamina, immune function, inflammation, RA, *bacterial infection*, cancer	*Preclinical research: activity against prostate, esophageal, breast, head and neck, lung, ovarian, cervical cancer cells; creates DNA adducts in various cell lines; synergistic with several chemotherapeutic agents* Human research: improves survival in patients with liver metastases
St. John's Wort *Hypericum perforatum*	PMS, **perimenopause or menopause**, *chronic pain,* neuropathy, **depression**, *opiate addiction*, psoriasis, atopic dermatitis, *sunburn*, inflammation, HSV, *cancer*	*Preclinical research: hyperforin reduces neovascularization and number of metastases* **See St. John's Wort monograph warnings and precautions**
Schisandra *Schisandra chinensis*	*MI*, **CHF**, DM, NAFLD, viral hepatitis, menopause, FMF, *stroke, AD, anxiety,* cognition, physical stress, stamina, pneumonia, *HCV, fungal infections,* cancer	*Preclinical research: protects against doxorubicin-induced cardiotoxicity; reverses the P-glycoprotein-mediated multidrug resistance that cancer cells develop to doxorubicin, vincristine, and paclitaxel* Human research: in combination formulas reduces estrogen-related cancer risk; reduces chemo fatigue; boosts immune response
Skullcap (Chinese, American) *Scutellaria baicalensis, lateriflora*	*Noise induced hearing loss*, allergy, *asthma, COPD, preterm RDS, pneumonia, PAH, CAD, dyslipidemia, DM, obesity, NAFLD, ETOH-induced gastritis, seizures, dementias,* **anxiety**, depression, *ADHD*, cognition, *photoprotection, autoimmunity, inflammation, MS, influenza, pneumonia, HIV*, cancer-related anemia, *cancer*	*Preclinical research: activity against many different cancer cell lines at several different points: apoptosis, proliferation, metastasis; anti-angiogenic at high doses (pro-angiogenic at low doses)* Human research: hemopoietic with chemotherapy
Stinging nettle *Urtica dioica*	Allergic rhinitis, HTN, dyslipidemia, **DM**, NAFLD, *colitis, nephrotoxicity*, menopause, **BPH**, prostatitis, OA, inflammation, *prostate cancer, cisplatin toxicity*	*Preclinical research: activity against prostate cancer cells, enhances effect and reduces toxicity of cisplatin*
Tribulus/Puncture vine/ Goathead *Tribulus terrestris*	HTN, CAD, dyslipidemia, DM, *hepatotoxicity, IBS, nephrolithiasis*, **sexual dysfunction**, hypoactive sexual desire, *pain, anxiety, depression, inflammation, cancer*	*Preclinical research: active against liver cancer cells; protects against radiation S/Es*

TABLE 23.B		
Oncologic Disorders. *(Continued)*		

Common Name/ Latin Name	Scope of Potential Benefits	Comments
Turmeric (or curcumin) *Curcuma longa*	Anterior uveitis, **oral lichen planus**, **gingivitis**, dental surgery, submucous fibrosis, asthma, **diastolic HTN**, **dyslipidemia**, CAD, endothelial dysfunction, **DM**, obesity, **NAFLD**, hepatoprotective, gallbladder dyskinesia, *GERD*, PUD, dyspepsia, **UC**, DM nephropathy, lupus nephritis, lactational mastitis, LSIL, chronic non-bacterial prostatitis, post-operative pain, **OA**, RA, migraine HA, *neurodegeneration*, **anxiety**, **depression**, **skin disease**, psoriasis, fatigue, **systemic inflammation**, *HIV*, **chemo-related oral mucositis**, cancer prevention, cancer treatment	*Preclinical research: prevents and inhibits cancer through several mechanisms and for many cancer cell types* **Systematic review: reduces oral mucositis when applied topically** Human research: topical application reduces oral mucositis; safe adjunct to FOLFOX in colon cancer; safe adjunct to gemcitabine in resistant pancreatic cancer; reduces hand-foot syndrome
Valerian *Valeriana officinalis*	*HTN*, *CAD*, *IBS*, PMS, dysmenorrhea, **menopause**, RLS, cognitive, anxiety, insomnia, OCD, *cancer*	*Preclinical research: activity against ovarian, lung, prostate, colon, and liver cancer cell lines*

* This table is included primarily for research purposes. Most of the herbs listed in Table 23.B lack clinical trials for safety and efficacy but are included due to their preclinical evidence for anti-cancer activity, thus warranting further research. It is **not** recommended that the herbs included in this table be used in place of well-studied conventional cancer therapy. Furthermore, very few herbs have been shown in clinical trials to be safe and effective when used in conjunction with chemotherapy, so medicinal herbs should generally be avoided during the course of chemotherapy due to the potential for drug-herb interactions that may reduce efficacy or increase toxicity of chemotherapy. Until adequate clinical trials have established efficacy and safety, use of any medicinal herb in cancer treatment should only be undertaken by comprehensive oncology centers in the course of clinical research.

PART 3 | Herbal Monographs With References

Introduction to the monographs

Each of the following 55 herbal monographs is organized according to general overview, preclinical research, human research, active constituents, commonly used preparations and dosage, safety and precaution, and references. In each monograph, the "Human Research" section is organized according to organ systems and systemic disorders. The stronger evidence (systematic reviews, meta-analyses, and trials with larger numbers of subjects or of longer duration) is presented first, with weaker trials and polyherbal research presented toward the end of each disease section. Because the information is based on research abstracts, and because many full reports are not openly available online, information is often missing such as duration of the trial, the number of subjects, or the dosing of the interventions. Unless otherwise specified, the duration of the trial refers to the duration of observation, which is usually also the duration of the intervention. It should be noted that the systematic reviews vary greatly in quality and confidence. Although not specifically noted with each systematic review, it is almost universal that the review authors recommended that further research was warranted. The list of references at the end of each monograph includes references for the clinical trials described in the monograph. If clinical evidence is sparse for a particular herb, preclinical research is referenced more extensively.

The presentation of clinical trial outcomes in this book does not imply endorsement of the trial or use of the herb for the application under investigation. Several weaker trials are included to stimulate further research or to demonstrate the pitfalls of herbal research. The evidence-based clinician, for whom this book was written, will need to discern when the evidence is adequate for appropriate use. Some evidence is only applicable to the parts of the world where conventional medicines are not available or feasible.

HOW HERBS WERE SELECTED FOR INCLUSION

The herbs in this book were chosen due to one or a combination of factors including popularity with the US population, popularity with US herbalists, strong evidence for efficacy, or broad scope of activity.

Public Popularity

The American Botanical Council published in issue 127 of its publication *HerbalGram* a list of the 40 top-selling herbs in 2019 in mainstream retail outlets (see below table). This list represents what your patients are buying (often what is the latest fad or was recently discussed on popular TV shows for weight loss) or what the industry is including in its over-the-counter formulations (for example, horehound is part of popular or well-advertised cough remedies). Most, but not all, of these herbs will be monographed in Part III.

Top-selling herbal supplements in 2019—US mainstream multioutlet channel.

Rank	Primary ingredient	Latin binomial	Total sales ($)	% change from 2018 (%)
1	Horehound	*Marrubium vulgare*	152,731,013.98	4.2
2	Echinacea[a]	*Echinacea* spp.	120,185,302.86	4.9
3	Elderberry	*Sambucus nigra* and *S. canadensis*	107,574,611.46	110.8
4	Turmeric[b]	*Curcuma longa*	92,432,701.70	2.0
5	Cranberry	*Vaccinium macrocarpon*	88,900,064.38	6.3
6	Ivy leaf	*Hedera helix*	43,122,837.27	14.0
7	Ginger	*Zingiber officinale*	39,455,176.99	6.4
8	Garlic	*Allium sativum*	37,938,646.26	0.7
9	Cannabidiol (CBD)	*Cannabis sativa*	35,899,378.48	872.3
10	Green tea	*Camellia sinensis*	33,754,156.23	−25.3
11	Red yeast rice[c]	*Oryza sativa*	33,648,588.26	8.0
12	Apple cider vinegar	*Malus* spp.	33,644,761.68	10.4
13	Fenugreek	*Trigonella foenum-graecum*	33,238,113.57	2.3
14	Saw palmetto	*Serenoa repens*	30,700,004.93	3.7
15	Black cohosh	*Actaea racemosa*	28,078,996.24	−15.7
16	Wheatgrass/Barley grass	*Triticum aestivum/Hordeum vulgare*	26,259,511.29	25.0
17	Ginkgo	*Ginkgo biloba*	25,543,153.93	18.9
18	Flax seed/Flax oil	*Linum usitatissimum*	23,005,712.31	−11.6
19	Aloe vera	*Aloe vera*	21,074,250.16	−3.7
20	Yohimbe	*Pausinystalia johimbe*	18,366,189.44	−20.7
21	Cinnamon	*Cinnamomum* spp.	16,525,708.00	−6.6
22	Valerian	*Valeriana officinalis*	16,252,463.12	−9.1
23	Milk thistle	*Silybum marianum*	16,244,188.41	−1.8
24	Garcinia	*Garcinia gummi-gutta*	14,991,877.54	−33.5
25	Bioflavonoid complex[d]	—	14,681,912.64	−17.3
26	Horny goat weed	*Epimedium* spp.	14,201,565.49	27.1
27	Coconut oil	*Cocos nucifera*	14,036,848.91	−23.3
28	Goji berry	*Lycium* spp.	13,812,253.72	12.9
29	Green coffee extract	*Coffea arabica*	13,013,379.34	−18.9
30	Ginseng	*Panax* spp.	12,572,733.72	−4.2
31	Senna[e]	*Senna alexandrina*	10,912,381.12	−8.3
32	Plant sterols[f]	—	10,894,757.52	−4.1

	Top-selling herbal supplements in 2019—US mainstream multioutlet channel. *(Continued)*			
Rank	Primary ingredient	Latin binomial	Total sales ($)	% change from 2018 (%)
33	Ashwagandha	*Withania somnifera*	10,835,737.05	45.2
34	Beet root	*Beta vulgaris*	9,827,665.87	18.4
35	Boswellia	*Boswellia serrata*	8,923,628.32	–7.3
36	Açai	*Euterpe oleracea*	8,816,949.58	2.7
37	Rhodiola	*Rhodiola* spp.	8,737,768.32	–9.7
38	Fennel	*Foeniculum vulgare*	8,663,058.49	6.1
39	Maca	*Lepidium meyenii*	8,133,656.61	5.3
40	Grapefruit seed extract	Citrus × paradisi	7,779,003.70	7.8

[a]Includes three *Echinacea* species: *E. angustifolia*, *E. pallida*, and *E. purpurea*.
[b]Includes standardized turmeric extracts with high levels of curcumin.
[c]Red yeast rice is fermented with the yeast *Monascus purpureus*.
[d]Bioflavonoids are phytochemicals that are often extracted from citrus (*Citrus* spp., Rutaceae) fruits.
[e]Excludes OTC laxative drugs containing senna or sennosides.
[f]Not including beta-sitosterol.
Source: Smith, T., May, G., Eckl, V., and Reynolds, C.M. (2020). US Sales of Herbal Supplements Increase by 8.6% in 2019. Retrieved from http://herbalgram.org/media/15608/hg127-hmr.pdf. © 2020 American Botanical Council, www.herbalgram.org. Reprinted with permission.

Herbalist Popularity

Representative herbs that hold the admiration of natural healthcare providers have also been included in this book despite underwhelming clinical evidence. The fact that these herbs have withstood the test of time and have preclinical research that supports their traditional application warrants their inclusion. Examples are burdock, dandelion, and yarrow.

Strength of Evidence

Lesser-known herbs have been included in this book if they have demonstrated relatively good evidence for efficacy. Black seed and umckaloabo are examples of lesser-known herbs that are backed by relatively strong research.

Scope of Potential Activities

Those herbs that appear to be beneficial for multiple disorders deserve attention. Most of these herbs have good clinical evidence for one or two disorders, and preclinical evidence for a host of additional disorders.

Excluded Herbs

Botanical products that are primarily available as food products (e.g., coffee, green tea, cinnamon, flax seed, chia seed, and garlic) were not included in this book, as they better fit the definition of functional foods than of herbal supplements. Mushrooms, while legitimately medicinal botanicals, were not included due to having entirely different taxonomy from plants. Mushrooms deserve their own book, such as that written by Christopher Hobbs (see Appendix II). Also absent from this book are controversial herbs such as marijuana, kratom, *kava kava*, and the herbs that comprise the entheogenic blend in ayahuasca. Due to the current controversies surrounding their legality and use, the evidence for these herbs is insufficient yet rapidly evolving and warrants more focus in the future. Herbs that are over-harvested and on threatened species lists such as goldenseal are left out as well to avoid contributing to their disappearance. With the exceptions of dong quai and peppermint, herbs such as lavender that are primarily used as essential oils have been omitted, as aromatherapy has unique applications outside the scope of this book.

HOW TO PRESCRIBE MEDICINAL HERBS

The "Commonly Used Preparations and Dosage" section of each monograph attempts to provide a ballpark idea of what is typically available for your patients.

While well-trained herbalists may be comfortable prescribing tinctures, glycerites, fluid extracts, and various oral and topical blended formulas, the convolutions and mathematical exigencies of many formulations are beyond the training and time allowance of the conventional medical provider. Furthermore, even the commercially available herbal options for patients can be confusing and overwhelming for both the patient and the provider. Should your patient take a powder, a powdered extract, an encapsulation, a standardized extract, or a concentrated extract? What is the difference in dosing? Fortunately, the numerous reputable companies that comprise the herbal industry have formulated their products according to the available research as to what is safe and effective. As a **general rule**, it is reasonable to identify two to four reputable brands of larger companies (those that have cGMP noted on the label and are found in most pharmacies and grocery stores), advise your patient to find one of these brands locally or online, and recommend that your patient follow the directions on the label using the lower dosage range initially. In all fairness, the herbal products of smaller companies may also be recommended provided they follow cGMP rules (see Chapter 5 "Herb Safety").

HERBAL MONOGRAPHS (LISTED BY COMMON NAMES)

- Aloe
- Andrographis
- Ashwagandha
- Astragalus
- Bacopa
- Bilberry
- Black cohosh
- Black seed/Nigella/Black cumin
- Burdock
- Butterbur
- Calendula
- Chamomile
- Chasteberry/Chaste tree/Vitex
- Coleus
- Cranberry
- Dandelion
- Dong quai
- Echinacea
- Elderberry/Elder flower
- Eleuthero/Siberian ginseng
- Fennel
- Fenugreek
- Frankincense/Boswellia
- Ginger
- Ginkgo
- Ginsengs (Asian/Korean/Chinese Ginseng, American Ginseng)
- Goji berry/Wolfberry
- Gymnema/Gurmar
- Gynostemma/Jiaogulan
- Hawthorn
- Holy basil/Tulsi
- Hops
- Horsetail
- Lemon balm
- Licorice
- Maca
- Milk thistle
- Motherwort
- Passionflower
- Peppermint
- Rhodiola
- Saffron
- Saint John's wort
- Saw palmetto
- Schisandra
- Skullcap
- Stinging nettle/Nettle/Nettles
- Tribulus
- Turmeric
- Umckaloabo/South African geranium
- Uva ursi
- Valerian
- Yarrow

24

ALOE (*ALOE VERA, ALOE BARBARDENSIS*)
Leaf and Leaf Pulp

GENERAL OVERVIEW

Aloe is well known in the medical and cosmetic world as medicine for the skin. Its use dates back 6000 years to early Egypt, where the plant was depicted on stone carvings and presented as a funeral gift to pharaohs. Aloe has been used for a variety of purposes, including treatment of wounds, hair loss, constipation, and hemorrhoids.

The clear thick gel obtained from the pulp of aloe leaves is primarily used topically for healing wounds, ulcers, and burns. It may also be useful for psoriasis and lichen planus. The gel may be used orally for osteoarthritis, irritable bowel syndrome (IBS), ulcerative colitis, dementia, and fever. Aloe latex, derived from the whole leaf, is taken orally for constipation. When taken orally for extended periods of time, it is important to use "decolorized" juice that contains little, if any, of the anthraquinone aloe emodin, as this constituent has been linked to toxicity and carcinogenesis (see Section "Safety and Precaution").

Clinical research indicates that aloe, alone or in combination formulas, may be beneficial for numerous oral diseases, dyslipidemia, diabetes, hepatic fibrosis, gastroesophageal reflux disease (GERD), IBS, ulcerative colitis, radiation proctitis, chronic anal fissures, Alzheimer's disease (AD), acne, striae gravidarum, photoaging, xeroderma, vulvar lichen planus, psoriasis, skin ulcers and wounds, burns, HIV, and cancer survival.

IN VITRO AND ANIMAL RESEARCH

Aloe sterols have been shown in cell culture to stimulate collagen and hyaluronic acid production by human dermal fibroblasts. A polymer fraction of aloe appears to protect mucosa via reduction of NOX and MMP-9 enzymes. Research in a mouse model of Parkinson's disease (PD) showed that aloe had significant antioxidative effects in the striatal region of the brain based on malondialdehyde (MDA) and glutathione (GSH) measurements. Histopathological analysis of brain tissue of aloe-treated groups revealed minimal neuronal destruction compared with N-methyl-4-phenyl-1, 2, 3, 6-tetrahydropyridine (MPTP) and haloperidol groups.

Aloe has demonstrated anticancer effects attributed to several constituents including acemannan and aloeride, both of which are immunomodulating. Aloeride is a potent immunostimulator via increasing NF-κB activities. Another constituent, aloe emodin, inhibits cell proliferation, induces apoptosis in human liver cancer cell lines, and enhances the effects of radiation treatment.

HUMAN RESEARCH

Oral and Dental Disorders

A 2019 systematic review and meta-analysis sought to assess the effectiveness of aloe in alleviating pain and clinical signs of oral submucous fibrosis. Six randomized controlled trials (RCTs) fulfilled the inclusion criteria. The results of meta-analysis showed statistically significant differences between aloe and control groups in alleviating pain/burning sensation at the end of the first and second months, in favor of aloe, but no significant differences were found at the end of the third month (Al-Maweri et al., 2019).

A 2018 systematic review of natural products for gingivitis identified aloe along with pomegranate, green tea, and *Salvadora persica* as having a large body of evidence supporting its effectiveness for gingivitis (Safiaghdam et al., 2018).

A 2016 systematic review of aloe for oral lesions found 15 studies that satisfied the inclusion criteria. These included five on oral lichen planus, two on oral submucous fibrosis, and the remainder on burning mouth syndrome, radiation-induced mucositis, candida-associated denture stomatitis, xerostomic patients, and minor recurrent aphthous stomatitis. Most studies showed statistically significant results demonstrating the effectiveness of aloe in treatment of oral diseases (Nair et al., 2016).

A 2016 systematic review of all clinical trials evaluating aloe compared with placebo or corticosteroids for treatment of oral lichen planus concluded that there was weak evidence that aloe was more efficient than placebo and was comparable to triamcinolone acetonide (Ali and Wahbi, 2016).

An 8-week RCT in patients ($n = 54$) with oral lichen planus compared aloe gel with placebo. A good response to treatment (reduction in ulcerative and erosive lesions) occurred in 81% in the aloe group and 4% in the placebo group ($P < 0.001$). Complete remission occurred in 7% of patients who used aloe. Symptoms improved by at least 50% in 63% with aloe and 7% with placebo ($P < 0.001$). Burning pain completely disappeared in 33% with aloe and 4% with placebo ($P = 0.005$). The authors concluded that aloe gel was a safe alternative for treatment of patients with oral lichen planus (Choonhakarn et al., 2008).

A 5-day RCT in intensive care unit patients ($n = 80$) studied oral care with an oral moisturizing gel containing aloe and peppermint compared with a placebo gel for effects on mouth dryness and plaque development. By the third day, the mean oral health score was significantly better in the treatment group than in the placebo group ($P = 0.0001$), and by the fifth day, the mean score of mouth dryness in the intervention group was significantly lower than the placebo group ($P = 0.0001$). The authors concluded that this combination gel was useful for relieving mouth dryness, preventing dental plaque formation, and improving oral health, and thus may be used for improving oral care outcomes in ICUs (Atashi et al., 2018).

Cardiometabolic Disorders: Dyslipidemia and Diabetes

A 2016 systematic review of studies assessing glycemic effects of aloe found eight trials ($n = 470$) that met search criteria. In prediabetes, aloe significantly improved fasting blood glucose (FBG) (MD $= -0.22$ mmol/L; $P < 0.0001$), with no effect on A1C (MD $= -2$ mmol/mol). In type 2 diabetes mellitus (T2DM) there was a marginal improvement in FBG (MD $= -1.17$ mmol/L; $P = 0.05$) and a significant improvement in A1C (MD $= -11$ mmol/mol; $P = 0.01$). The authors concluded that there was some potential benefit from aloe in improving glycemic control in prediabetes and T2DM; further studies were warranted (Suksomboon et al., 2016).

A 2016 meta-analysis was performed to ascertain the effectiveness of oral aloe consumption on the reduction of fasting blood sugar (FBS) and A1C. Nine studies were included in the FBS parameter ($n = 283$) showing that aloe decreased FBS by 46.6 mg/dL ($P < 0.0001$). There was a mean FBS reduction of 110 mg/dL ($P \leq 0.0001$) in patients with baseline FBS > 200 mg/dL. Five of the included studies also had A1C data ($n = 89$) and showed a reduction in A1C by 1.05% ($P = 0.004$). The authors found that the results supported the use of oral aloe for significantly reducing FBS and A1C, but that further clinical studies were warranted (Dick et al., 2016).

A 2016 systematic review included a total of five RCTs ($n = 415$) and found that, compared with controls, aloe supplementation significantly improved the concentrations of FBG (WMD $= -30.05$ mg/dL; $P = 0.02$), A1C (WMD $= -0.41\%$; $P < 0.00001$); triglycerides (TG) ($P = 0.0001$), total cholesterol (TC), LDL-C ($P < 0.00001$), and HDL-C ($P = 0.04$). The authors concluded that the available evidence, albeit of poor quality, showed that aloe might effectively reduce the levels of FBS, A1C, TG, TC, and LDL-C, and increase the levels of HDL-C in prediabetic and early untreated diabetic patients (Zhang et al., 2016).

A 2013 systematic review to assess the efficacy of glucose-lowering effects of medicinal plants identified 18 human studies that met inclusion criteria. Among the RCTs, the best results in glycemic control were found with milk thistle, aloe, nettle, *Citrullus colocynthus*, *Plantago ovata*, and *Rheum ribes* (Rashidi et al., 2013).

An 8-week RCT in patients ($n=72$) with prediabetes or early diabetes compared aloe leaf gel extract 300 or 500 mg with placebo, each given BID. FBS level in the 300-mg group significantly decreased in the fourth week compared with placebo ($P=0.001$). A1C levels in this group showed a significant decrease by week 8 ($P=0.042$). TC and LDL-C in the 500-mg group decreased by week 8 ($P<0.001$ and $P=0.01$), respectively, and HDL-C increased ($P=0.004$). TG also decreased significantly ($P<0.045$) by 4 weeks. The authors concluded that aloe extract could normalize impaired glucose within 4 weeks in prediabetic patients and could alleviate their abnormal lipid profiles after 8 weeks (Alinejad-Mofrad et al., 2015).

In a 2-month RCT in hyperlipidemic patients ($n=60$) with T2DM that was not controlled on 10 mg of glyburide plus 1000 mg of metformin, the efficacy and safety of taking aloe gel capsules (300 mg every 12 h) combined with the hypoglycemic drugs was investigated and compared with placebo. Compared with placebo, the aloe gel lowered FBG, A1C, TC, and LDL-C significantly ($P=0.036$; $P=0.036$; $P=0.006$, and $P=0.004$, respectively) without any significant effects on other blood lipid levels and liver/kidney function tests ($P>0.05$). The authors concluded that aloe gel may be a safe antihyperglycemic and antihypercholesterolemic agent for hyperlipidemic T2DM patients (Huseini et al., 2012).

A 12-week RCT in diabetic patients ($n=50$) with dyslipidemia despite statin therapy investigated a combination of aloe, black seed, fenugreek, garlic, milk thistle, and psyllium (one sachet BID) plus conventional therapy compared with conventional therapy alone. Each sachet contained 300 mg of aloe leaf gel, 1.8 g of black seed, 300 mg of garlic, 2.5 g of fenugreek seed, 1 g of psyllium seed, and 500 mg of milk thistle seed. The levels of serum TG, TC, LDL-C, and A1C, but not FBS, showed a significant in-group improvement in the intervention group. Renal and hepatic transaminases were unchanged with the herbal compound. The authors concluded that this herbal compound was a safe and effective adjunctive treatment in lowering serum lipids in diabetic patients with uncontrolled dyslipidemia (Ghorbani et al., 2019).

A 40-day Phase I open-label clinical trial in diabetic patients ($n=30$) with uncontrolled hyperglycemia and dyslipidemia despite standard therapy evaluated the effects of a polyherbal formulation containing garlic, aloe, black seed, psyllium, fenugreek, and milk thistle (one sachet BID) in addition to their usual medications. The herbal formula significantly decreased FBG from 162 to 146 mg/dL and A1C from 8.4% to 7.7%. LDL-C decreased significantly from 138 to 108 mg/dL, and TG decreased from 203 to 166 mg/dL. There were no changes in liver function, kidney function, or hematologic parameters. The authors concluded that the formulation was safe and effective in lowering blood glucose and serum lipids in patients with advanced-stage T2DM. After consumption of the herbal combination, two patients complained of mild nausea and two patients reported diarrhea (Zarvandi et al., 2017).

Gastrointestinal Disorders: Liver Fibrosis

A 12-week study in patients with liver fibrosis ($n=40$) and in healthy volunteers ($n=15$) compared aloe high molecular weight fraction (AHM) with placebo. The use of AHM significantly ameliorated fibrosis, inhibited inflammation, and resulted in minimal infiltration and minimal fibrosis compared with the placebo group. The serum levels of the fibrosis markers (HA, TGF-β, and MMP-2) were also reduced significantly after treatment. The authors concluded that oral supplementation with AHM could be helpful in alleviating fibrosis and inflammation in hepatic fibrosis patients (Hegazy et al., 2012).

Gastrointestinal Disorders: Gastroesophageal Reflux Disease

A 4-week pilot RCT in patients ($n=79$) with heartburn compared a standardized aloe syrup 10 mL/d with omeprazole 20 mg/day and with ranitidine 150 mg BID. Based on the modified Disease Reflux Questionnaire, the frequency of all GERD symptoms was decreased significantly in all three groups at 2 and 4 weeks. With aloe, the heartburn score decreased from 17 at baseline to 4 at 2 weeks and to 5 at 4 weeks; the dysphagia score decreased from 12 at baseline to 4 at 2 weeks and to 4 at 4 weeks. However, omeprazole outperformed aloe at both 2 and 4 weeks, and ranitidine outperformed aloe at 4 weeks. The authors concluded that aloe was safe and well tolerated and reduced the frequencies of all the assessed GERD symptoms, with no adverse events requiring withdrawal (Panahi et al., 2015).

Gastrointestinal Disorders: Lower GI Disorders

In a 2018 systematic review, aloe gel was investigated for efficacy and safety in patients with IBS. The analysis included three RCTs ($n = 151$). The primary outcome was standard mean difference of the change in severity of IBS symptoms as measured by patient-rated scales. The meta-analysis showed a significant difference for patients treated with aloe compared with those treated with placebo regarding improvement in IBS symptom score (SMD = 0.41; $P = 0.020$). No adverse events were noted (Hong et al., 2018).

In a study of patients ($n = 44$) with mildly to moderately active ulcerative colitis given 100 mL twice daily of an aloe leaf gel liquid, 30% experienced clinical remission compared with 7% of patients given placebo. Improvement was seen in 37% of the aloe group and in 7% of the placebo group, and minor response was seen in 47% with aloe and 14% with placebo. The authors concluded that 4 weeks of oral aloe produced a clinical response in ulcerative colitis more often than placebo; it also reduced histological disease activity and appeared to be safe (Langmead et al., 2004).

A 4-week RCT of patients ($n = 20$) with acute radiation proctitis after external-beam radiation therapy for pelvic malignancies randomized patients to receive 1 g BID of either 3% topical aloe or placebo ointment. Aloe was associated with significant ($P < 0.05$) improvements from baseline in the symptom indexes for diarrhea (from 0.67 to 0.11), fecal urgency (from 0.89 to 0.11), clinical presentation total (from 4.33 to 1.22), and lifestyle (from 1.1 to 0.33) for baseline and 4-week values, respectively. Aloe demonstrated an advantage over placebo for "clinical presentation total" (OR = 3.97) and Radiation Therapy Oncology Group acute toxicity criteria (OR = 5.9). The authors concluded that a substantial number of patients with radiation proctitis seemed to benefit from therapy with aloe 3% ointment (Sahebnasagh et al., 2017).

A 6-week prospective clinical trial was conducted to evaluate the effects of a topical cream containing 0.5% aloe juice powder applied TID compared with a control group in the treatment of chronic anal fissures. Aloe produced statistically significant differences in chronic anal fissure pain, hemorrhaging upon defection, and wound healing before and at the end of the first week of treatment compared with the control group ($P < 0.0001$). The authors concluded that a topical cream containing aloe juice was an effective treatment for chronic anal fissures and that further comparative studies were justified (Rahmani et al., 2014).

Neurologic Disorders: Alzheimer's Disease

A 12-month open-label pilot study investigated the effect of an aloe polymannose multinutrient complex formula (4 tsp. per day) on cognitive and immune functioning among adults diagnosed with Alzheimer's disease. The mean ADAS-cog scores significantly improved at 9 and 12 months from baseline, and 46% of the sample showed clinically significant improvement ($\geq$ 4-point change) from baseline to 12 months. Significant decreases occurred in TNF-α, VEGF, IL-2, and IL-4. The authors concluded that the study showed improvements in both clinical and physiological outcomes for a disease that otherwise had no standard ameliorative remedy (Lewis et al., 2013).

Dermatological Disorders: Acne

An 8-week RCT in patients ($n = 60$) with mild-to-moderate acne investigated the efficacy and safety of a combination of tretinoin cream (0.05%) plus aloe topical gel (50%) compared with tretinoin plus vehicle (control). The combination therapy was significantly more effective in reducing noninflammatory ($P = 0.001$), inflammatory ($P = 0.011$), and total ($P = 0.003$) lesion scores than the control group, and erythema in the combination group was significantly less severe ($P = 0.046$). The authors concluded that this combination of tretinoin plus aloe gel was well tolerated and significantly more effective than tretinoin plus vehicle for the treatment of mild-to-moderate acne vulgaris (Hajheydari et al., 2014).

Dermatological Disorders: Psoriasis

A 2017 systematic review found a total of 27 controlled and uncontrolled clinical trials addressing the use of topical botanical agents for psoriasis. It found that the most widely studied and efficacious topical botanical therapeutics were aloe, *Mahonia aquifolium,* and *Indigo naturalis.* The most reported adverse effects were local skin irritation, erythema, pruritus, burning, and pain. The authors concluded that while most agents appeared to be safe, further research was necessary before topical botanical agents could be consistently recommended to patients (Farahnik et al., 2017).

An 8-week RCT in patients ($n = 80$) with mild-to-moderate psoriasis compared topical aloe cream with 0.1% triamcinolone cream (TAC). The mean Psoriasis Area Severity Index score decreased from 11.6 to 3.9 (-7.7) in the aloe group and from 10.9 to 4.3 (-6.6) in the TAC group. Between-group difference was 1.1 ($P = 0.0237$). The mean Dermatology Life Quality Index score decreased from 8.6 to 2.5 (-6.1) with aloe and from 8.1 to 2.3 (-5.8) with TAC. Between-group difference was 0.3 ($P = 0.5497$). The authors concluded that aloe cream may be more effective than 0.1% triamcinolone cream in reducing clinical symptoms of psoriasis (Choonhakarn et al., 2010).

A 12-week open-label study followed patients with moderate-to-severe palmoplantar psoriasis ($n = 857$) who were treated with a combination mixture of propolis 50% (from honey) and aloe 3%. Excellent response was seen in 62% of patients and good results were exhibited in 24% of patients treated. The authors concluded that patients with palmoplantar psoriasis had noteworthy improvement with the propolis plus aloe topical formula (El-Gammal et al., 2018).

Dermatological Disorders: Dermatitis and Lichen Planus

A 10-day study of infants ($n = 66$) with diaper dermatitis compared aloe cream with calendula ointment TID. Improvement in the severity of the diaper dermatitis was observed in both groups ($P < 0.001$). The calendula group had significantly fewer rash sites compared with the aloe group ($P = 0.001$). No adverse effect was reported from either of the medications. The authors concluded that topical aloe and in particular calendula could serve as safe and effective treatment of diaper dermatitis in infants (Panahi et al., 2012).

An 8-week RCT of women ($n = 34$) with vulvar lichen planus compared topical application of aloe gel with placebo. After 8 weeks, erosive and ulcerative lesions were present in 17% and 83% of aloe- and placebo-treated patients, respectively. Good response was seen in 82% and 5% of aloe- and placebo-treated patients, respectively ($P < 0.001$). One patient treated with aloe had a complete clinical remission. The authors concluded that aloe gel was a safe and effective treatment for patients with vulvar lichen planus (Rajar et al., 2008).

Dermatological Disorders: Wounds and Burns

A 2019 systematic review evaluating the efficacy of aloe for healing wounds found 23 trials that met inclusion criteria. The results of the studies showed that aloe had been used to prevent skin ulcers and to treat burn wounds, postoperative wounds, cracked nipples, genital herpes, psoriasis, and chronic wounds including pressure ulcers. The authors concluded that aloe and its compounds could be used to retain skin moisture and integrity, prevent ulcers, and improve wound healing (Hekmatpou et al., 2019).

A 2007 systematic review evaluating the efficacy of aloe in treating burns found four trials ($n = 371$) that met inclusion criteria. Based on a meta-analysis using duration of wound healing as an outcome measure, the WMD in healing time of the aloe group was 8.79 days shorter than that in the control group ($P = 0.006$). The authors concluded that despite the variation in products used, cumulative evidence supported that aloe might be effective in burn wound healing for first- to second-degree burns (Maenthaisong et al., 2007).

An RCT looked at patients ($n = 12$) who underwent split-thickness skin graft harvesting from the thigh. Times to complete epithelization for the aloe and placebo groups were 11.5 and 13.7 days, respectively ($P < 0.05$). VAS pain scores after wound dressing for the aloe and placebo groups were 17.18 and 18.63, respectively (N.S.). The authors concluded that topical aloe gel significantly demonstrated accelerated split-thickness skin graft donor-site healing but did not show significant pain relief (Burusapat et al., 2018).

A 5-day study of episiotomy healing in primiparous women ($n = 111$) studied aloe plus calendula ointment every 8 h compared with hospital routine episiotomy care. The researchers concluded that aloe and calendula ointment increased the speed of episiotomy wound healing considerably (Eghdampour et al., 2013).

A 10-day RCT looking at prevention of pressure ulcers in patients ($n = 80$) on an orthopedic ward compared aloe gel with placebo gel applied BID to pressure areas. After 10 days, ulcers occurred in 3 patients with aloe and 12 patients with placebo ($P = 0.047$). The authors concluded that aloe gel should be used preventively in patients at high risk of pressure ulcers (Hekmatpou et al., 2018).

A 4-week RCT in patients ($n = 40$) with diabetic foot ulcers randomly assigned patients to a combination of topical aloe plus *Plantago major* gel or placebo gel BID in addition to routine care. A significant difference was observed between the two groups in terms of total ulcer score ($P < 0.001$) and surface area ($P = 0.039$). Ulcer depth difference did not reach statistical significance ($P = 0.263$). The authors concluded that the studied gel appeared to be an effective, inexpensive, and safe treatment, pending further studies (Najafian et al., 2018).

A 3-month RCT of patients ($n = 60$) with chronic skin ulcers compared usual care with usual care plus the addition of topical aloe gel BID. After 3 months, wound healing occurred in 93% of patients in the aloe group and 47% of patients in the control group ($P < 0.05$). The overall mean time of wound healing was 31 and 63 days in the aloe and control groups, respectively ($P < 0.05$). The authors concluded that aloe gel was a beneficial and cost-effective treatment for patients with chronic ulcers (Avijgan et al., 2016).

Dermatological Disorders: Cosmetic Disorders

A left-right side comparison RCT in patients ($n = 24$) with striae who were treated with fractional CO_2 laser compared topical aloe gel with recombinant human EGF (rhEGF) cream applied BID for 1 month beyond the last laser treatment. Skin biopsy revealed a statistically significant increase in epidermal thickness and decrease in elastic fragmentation in both groups. However, patients tended to be more satisfied with the EGF treatment. The authors concluded that laser plus rhEGF and laser plus aloe both significantly improved striae surface texture (Disphanurat et al., 2019).

An RCT in nulliparous women ($n = 160$) studied 700 g topical aloe gel compared with sweet almond oil, with base cream, and with nothing on abdominal skin for effect on striae gravidarum. The aloe and sweet almond oil creams were more effective than the base cream and the control group at decreasing itching and erythema and preventing the spread of striae on the surface of the abdomen ($P < 0.05$); however, all three creams had a similar effect on the diameter and the number of striae ($P > 0.05$). The authors concluded that aloe and sweet almond oil creams reduced the itching of striae and prevented their progression (Hajhashemi et al., 2018).

An 8-week placebo-controlled trial in Japanese women with dry skin investigated the effect of intake of oral aloe gel powder (AVGP) containing 40 µg aloe sterols on the skin conditions. A nonsignificant increase in arm skin hydration was observed at 8 weeks in the AVGP group, whereas a slight decrease in arm skin hydration was noted in the placebo group. The change in the mean wrinkle depth was significantly lower in the AVGP group than in the control group. Interestingly, the percent body fat after 8 weeks was significantly lower in the AVGP group. No adverse effects were observed during the study period. The authors concluded that daily oral AVGP significantly reduced facial wrinkles in women aged ≥ 40 years, and that aloe sterols stimulated collagen and hyaluronic acid production by human dermal fibroblasts (Tanaka et al., 2015).

In a 90-day wrinkle study, healthy females ($n = 30$) older than 45 years were given two different doses (1200 or 3600 mg/day) of aloe gel oral supplementation for 90 days. Their baseline status was used as a control. The facial wrinkles improved significantly ($P < 0.05$) in both groups, and facial elasticity improved in the lower-dose group. MMP-1 mRNA levels (indicating collagen degradation) were significantly decreased in the higher-dose group. Type I procollagen immunostaining was substantially increased throughout the dermis in both groups. The authors concluded that aloe gel significantly improved wrinkles and elasticity in photoaged human skin, with an increase in collagen production in the photoprotected skin and a decrease in collagen-degrading MMP-1 gene expression. No dose-response relationship was found between the low-dose and high-dose groups (Cho et al., 2009).

Autoimmune Disorders: Hashimoto's Thyroiditis

A 9-month study in women ($n = 30$) with subclinical hypothyroidism due to Hashimoto's thyroiditis looked at the effect of a daily dose of 100 mL of *Aloe barbardensis* juice (a close cousin of, and often considered synonymous with, *Aloe vera*) on thyroid peroxidase antibodies and thyroid function. TSH, FT4, and TPOAb improved significantly by -61%, $+23\%$, and -56%, respectively. FT3 decreased significantly (-16%) so that the FT4:FT3 ratio increased significantly ($+49\%$).

A control group ($n = 15$ untreated women) had no significant changes in any index. The authors concluded that *Aloe barbardensis* juice decreased the burden of thyroid autoimmune inflammation in women with Hashimoto's thyroiditis and improved thyrocyte function, with inhibition of T4 deiodination (Metro et al., 2018).

Infectious Disease: HIV

A preliminary 1-year study in Nigerian women ($n = 10$) with HIV who did not meet national criteria for antiretroviral drugs compared oral aloe gel with a control group of women ($n = 20$) on antiretroviral drugs. The average weight gain was 4.7 and 4.8 kg with aloe and antiretrovirals, respectively ($P = 0.916$), and the average increase in CD4 count was 153.7 and 238.85 cells/µL, respectively ($P = 0.087$). The authors concluded that consumption of aloe may be of help to HIV-infected individuals in the tropics, given its availability and inexpensiveness (Olatunya et al., 2012).

Oncologic Disorders

A study of patients ($n = 240$) undergoing standard treatment for metastatic solid tumors randomized patients to receive chemotherapy with or without *Aloe arborescens*. Aloe was given orally at 10 mL TID. The percentage of both objective tumor regressions and disease control, as well as the percent of 3-year survival patients, was significantly higher in patients concomitantly treated with aloe than with chemotherapy alone. The authors concluded that *Aloe arborescens* could be successfully associated with chemotherapy to increase its efficacy in both tumor regression rate and survival time (Lissoni et al., 2009).

ACTIVE CONSTITUENTS

Whole Leaf

- Carbohydrates
  - Polysaccharides (immunomodulating, immunostimulating): aloeride, acemannan
- Phenolic compounds
  - Latex anthraquinones (laxative and potentially toxic): aloin A and B, aloresin A and B, aloe emodin (antineoplastic, apoptotic, antiangiogenic), isoaloin, 7-hydroxyaloin A, 5-hydroxyaloin A

Aloe Gel (From Leaf Pulp)

- Carbohydrates
  - Polysaccharides: glucomannan (moisturizer); acemannan (immunomodulating, immunostimulating, wound healing, antineoplastic, antiviral, radioprotective); mannose-rich polysaccharide fraction (immunostimulant)
- Phenolic compounds
  - Phenolic acids: salicylic acid (antiinflammatory)
  - Flavonoids: tannins
- Steroids: lophenol, cycloartane (activate PPAR, downregulate MMP)
- Auxins (hydrating, wound healing)
- Giberellins (hydrating, wound healing)
- Bradykininase (antiinflammatory)
- Mannose-6-phosphate (fibroblast stimulating)
- Di (2-ethylhexyl) phthalate (antileukemic, antimutagenic, apoptotic)

ALOE COMMONLY USED PREPARATIONS AND DOSAGE (FOR ADULTS UNLESS OTHERWISE SPECIFIED)

The following are examples of some available formulations and ranges of dosing for commercial herbal products. See Part III Introduction "How to prescribe medicinal herbs" for further guidance on herbal advising and prescribing.

- Aloe inner leaf (gel) juice: 15–30 mL BID-TID (for DM or IBD).
- Aloe inner leaf (gel) capsules: 150–500 mg BID.
- Aloe latex capsules: 50–200 mg/day (*contains anthraquinones, strongly laxative; may be taken for up to 10 days for constipation*).
- Aloe topical gels or creams at various strengths: Topical use is considered to be quite safe.

See Section "Safety and Precaution"; ensure that all oral forms of aloe that are taken for more than 10 days are "decolorized," meaning devoid of carcinogenic latex.

SAFETY AND PRECAUTION

Note: Many of the safety issues with aloe are related to the presence of anthraquinones (aloin) in the juice of the leaves. The anthraquinones impart a yellow color.

The USFDA has ruled that aloe juice is not safe as a stimulant laxative. (Many commercial aloe products have removed the anthraquinones.) A 2-year National Toxicology Program study on *oral* consumption of nondecolorized whole leaf extract of aloe found clear evidence of carcinogenic activity in rats, based on tumors of the large intestine. Another study in rats showed that decolorized whole leaf aloe did not cause harmful effects.

Side Effects

Oral consumption of aloe can cause gastrointestinal upset, cramps, diarrhea, and electrolyte abnormalities. Hypokalemia has been reported. There is also potential for hypoglycemia.

Case Reports

Bleeding with sevoflurane during surgery. Hepatitis in conjunction with interferon treatment in MS. Hepatitis resolved with discontinuation of aloe. Several other case reports of hepatitis. Phytobezoar.

Toxicity

Inappropriate use (high dosage or chronic consumption of juice of leaf) of aloe has been linked to thyroid dysfunction, acute hepatitis, and perioperative bleeding. Long-term exposure to "nondecolorized" aloe can cause cancer in animals. Ingestion of 125 mg/kg aloe for 15 days in rats was associated with a decrease in serum T4 (-12.88%) and T3 (-25.13%).

Pregnancy and Lactation

Internal use not recommended. Anthraquinones are uterotonic.

Disease Interactions

Patients with IBS-D, IBD may have worsened diarrhea with internal consumption, especially of juice containing anthraquinones. Hypokalemia from diarrhea may aggravate arrhythmias.

Drug Interactions

- CYP: inhibits CYP3A4 and CYP2D6.
- May augment effects of hypoglycemic agents.
- Increases absorption of vitamins C and E.
- Synergistic with vancomycin against mycobacterium.
- May potentiate the antitumor effect of 5-fluorouracil and cyclophosphamide.
- May potentiate effects of topical steroids.

REFERENCES

Ali S, Wahbi W. The efficacy of Aloe vera in management of oral lichen planus: a systematic review and meta-analysis. Oral Dis 2017 Oct;23(7):913–18.

Alinejad-Mofrad S, Foadoddini M, Saadatjoo SA, Shayesteh M. Improvement of glucose and lipid profile status with Aloe vera in pre-diabetic subjects: a randomized controlled-trial. J Diabetes Metab Disord 2015 Apr 9;14:22.

Al-Maweri SA, Ashraf S, Lingam AS, et al. Aloe vera in treatment of oral submucous fibrosis: a systematic review and meta-analysis. J Oral Pathol Med 2019 Feb;48(2):99–107.

Atashi V, Yazdannik A, Mahjobipoor H, Ghafari S, Bekhradi R, Yousefi H. The effects of Aloe vera-peppermint (Veramin) moisturizing gel on mouth dryness and Oral health among patients hospitalized in intensive care units: a triple-blind randomized placebo-controlled trial. J Res Pharm Pract 2018 Apr-Jun;7(2):104–10.

Avijgan M, Kamran A, Abedini A. Effectiveness of *Aloe vera* gel in chronic ulcers in comparison with conventional treatments. Iran J Med Sci 2016 May;41(3):S30.

Burusapat C, Supawan M, Pruksapong C, Pitiseree A, Suwantemee C. Topical Aloe vera gel for accelerated wound healing of Split-thickness skin graft donor sites: a double-blind, randomized, controlled trial and systematic review. Plast Reconstr Surg 2018 Jul;142(1):217–26.

Cho S, Lee S, Lee MJ, et al. Dietary Aloe vera supplementation improves facial wrinkles and elasticity and it increases the type I procollagen gene expression in human skin *in vivo*. Ann Dermatol 2009 Feb;21(1):6–11.

Choonhakarn C, Busaracome P, Sripanidkulchai B, Sarakarn P. A prospective, randomized clinical trial comparing topical aloe vera with 0.1% triamcinolone acetonide in mild to moderate plaque psoriasis. J Eur Acad Dermatol Venereol 2010 Feb;24(2):168–72.

Choonhakarn C, Busaracome P, Sripanidkulchai B, Sarakarn P. The efficacy of aloe vera gel in the treatment of oral lichen planus: a randomized controlled trial. Br J Dermatol 2008 Mar;158(3):573–7.

Dick WR, Fletcher EA, Shah SA. Reduction of fasting blood glucose and hemoglobin A1C using oral Aloe vera: a meta-analysis. J Altern Complement Med 2016 Jun;22(6):450–7.

Disphanurat W, Kaewkes A, Suthiwartnarueput W. Comparison between topical recombinant human epidermal growth factor and Aloe vera gel in combination with ablative fractional carbon dioxide laser as treatment for striae alba: a randomized double-blind trial. Lasers Surg Med 2020 Feb;52(2):166–75.

Eghdampour F, Jahdie F, Kheyrkhah M, Taghizadeh M, Naghizadeh S, Hagani H. The impact of *Aloe vera* and calendula on perineal healing after episiotomy in primiparous women: a randomized clinical trial. J Caring Sci 2013 Nov 30;2(4):279–86.

El-Gammal E, Nardo VD, Daaboul F, et al. Apitherapy as a new approach in treatment of palmoplantar psoriasis. Open Access Maced J Med Sci 2018 Jun 10;6(6):1059–61.

Farahnik B, Sharma D, Alban J, Sivamani RK. Topical botanical agents for the treatment of psoriasis: a systematic review. Am J Clin Dermatol 2017 Aug;18(4):451–68.

Ghorbani A, Zarvandi M, Rakhshandeh H. A randomized controlled trial of an herbal compound for improving metabolic parameters in diabetic patients with uncontrolled dyslipidemia. Endocr Metab Immune Disord Drug Targets 2019;19(7):1075–82.

Hajhashemi M, Rafieian M, Rouhi Boroujeni HA, et al. The effect of Aloe vera gel and sweet almond oil on striae gravidarum in nulliparous women. J Matern Fetal Neonatal Med 2018 Jul;31(13):1703–8.

Hajheydari Z, Saeedi M, Morteza-Semnani K, Soltani A. Effect of Aloe vera topical gel combined with tretinoin in treatment of mild and moderate acne vulgaris: a randomized, double-blind, prospective trial. J Dermatolog Treat 2014 Apr;25(2):123–9.

Hegazy SK, El-Bedewy M, Yagi A. Antifibrotic effect of aloe vera in viral infection-induced hepatic periportal fibrosis. World J Gastroenterol 2012 May 7;18(17):2026–34.

Hekmatpou D, Mehrabi F, Rahzani K, Aminiyan A. The effect of Aloe vera clinical trials on prevention and healing of skin wound: a systematic review. Iran J Med Sci 2019 Jan;44(1):1–9.

Hekmatpou D, Mehrabi F, Rahzani K, Aminiyan A. The effect of Aloe vera gel on prevention of pressure ulcers in patients hospitalized in the orthopedic wards: a randomized triple-blind clinical trial. BMC Complement Altern Med 2018 Sep 29;18(1):264.

Hong SW, Chun J, Park S, Lee HJ, Im JP, Kim JS. Aloe vera is effective and safe in short-term treatment of irritable bowel syndrome: a systematic review and meta-analysis. J Neurogastroenterol Motil 2018 Oct 1;24(4):528–35.

Huseini HF, Kianbakht S, Hajiaghaee R, Dabaghian FH. Antihyperglycemic and anti-hypercholesterolemic effects of Aloe vera leaf gel in hyperlipidemic type 2 diabetic patients: a randomized double-blind placebo-controlled clinical trial. Planta Med 2012 Mar;78(4):311–6.

Langmead L, Feakins RM, Goldthorpe S, et al. Randomized, double-blind, placebo-controlled trial of oral aloe vera gel for active ulcerative colitis. Aliment Pharmacol Ther 2004 Apr 1;19(7):739–47.

Lewis JE, McDaniel HR, Agronin ME, et al. The effect of an aloe vera polymannose multinutrient complex on cognitive and immune functioning in Alzheimer's disease. J Alzheimers Dis 2013;33(2):393–406.

Lissoni P, Rovelli F, Brivio F, et al. A randomized study of chemotherapy vs biochemotherapy with chemotherapy plus Aloe arborescens in patients with metastatic cancer. In Vivo 2009 Jan-Feb;23(1):171–5.

Maenthaisong R, Chaiyakunapruk N, Niruntraporn S, Kongkaew C. The efficacy of aloe used for burn wound healing: a systematic review. Burns 2007 Sep;33(6):713–8.

Metro D, Cernaro V, Papa M, Benvenga S. Marked improvement of thyroid function and autoimmunity byAloe barbadensismiller juice in patients with subclinical hypothyroidism. J Clin Transl Endocrinol 2018 Feb 14;11:18–25.

Nair GR, Naidu GS, Jain S, Nagi R, Makkad RS, Jha A. Clinical effectiveness of Aloe vera in the management of oral mucosal diseases—a systematic review. J Clin Diagn Res 2016 Aug;10(8):ZE01–7.

Najafian Y, Mazloum Z, Najaf Najafi M, Hamedi S, Mahjour M, Feyzabadi Z. Efficacy of Aloe vera/Plantago major gel in diabetic foot ulcer: a randomized double-blind clinical trial. Curr Drug Discov Technol 2019;16(2):223–31.

Olatunya OS, Olatunya AM, Anyabolu HC, Adejuyigbe EA, Oyelami OA. Preliminary trial of aloe vera gruel on HIV infection. J Altern Complement Med 2012 Sep;18(9):850–3.

Panahi Y, Khedmat H, Valizadegan G, Mohtashami R, Sahebkar A. Efficacy and safety of Aloe vera syrup for the treatment of gastroesophageal reflux disease: a pilot randomized positive-controlled trial. J Tradit Chin Med 2015 Dec;35(6):632–6.

Panahi Y, Sharif MR, Sharif A, et al. A randomized comparative trial on the therapeutic efficacy of topical Aloe vera and Calendula officinalis in diaper dermatitis in children. ScientificWorldJournal 2012;2012:810234.

Rahmani N, Khademloo M, Vosoughi K, Assadpour S. Effects of Aloe vera cream on chronic anal fissure pain, wound healing and hemorrhaging upon defection: a prospective double-blind clinical trial. Eur Rev Med Pharmacol Sci 2014;18(7):1078–84.

Rajar UD, Majeed R, Parveen N, Sheikh I, Sushel C. Efficacy of aloe vera gel in the treatment of vulval lichen planus. J Coll Physicians Surg Pak 2008 Oct;18(10):612–4.

Rashidi AA, Mirhashemi SM, Taghizadeh M, Sarkhail P. Iranian medicinal plants for diabetes mellitus: a systematic review. Pak J Biol Sci 2013 May 1;16(9):401–11.

Safiaghdam H, Oveissi V, Bahramsoltani R, Farzaei MH, Rahimi R. Medicinal plants for gingivitis: a review of clinical trials. Iran J Basic Med Sci 2018 Oct;21(10):978–91.

Sahebnasagh A, Ghasemi A, Akbari J, et al. Successful treatment of acute radiation proctitis with Aloe Vera: a preliminary randomized controlled clinical trial. J Altern Complement Med 2017 Nov;23(11):858–65.

Suksomboon N, Poolsup N, Punthanitisarn S. Effect of Aloe vera on glycaemic control in prediabetes and type 2 diabetes: a systematic review and meta-analysis. J Clin Pharm Ther 2016 Apr;41(2):180–8.

Tanaka M, Misawa E, Yamauchi K, Abe F, Ishizaki C. Effects of plant sterols derived from Aloe vera gel on human dermal fibroblasts *in vitro* and on skin condition in Japanese women. Clin Cosmet Investig Dermatol 2015 Feb 20;8:95–104.

Zarvandi M, Rakhshandeh H, Abazari M, Shafiee-Nick R, Ghorbani A. Safety and efficacy of a polyherbal formulation for the management of dyslipidemia and hyperglycemia in patients with advanced-stage of type-2 diabetes. Biomed Pharmacother 2017 May;89:69–75.

Zhang Y, Liu W, Liu D, Zhao T, Tian H. Efficacy of Aloe vera supplementation on prediabetes and early non-treated diabetic patients: a systematic review and meta-analysis of randomized controlled trials. Nutrients 2016 Jun 23;8(7):388.

25

ANDROGRAPHIS (*ANDROGRAPHIS PANICULATA*)
Whole Plant

GENERAL OVERVIEW

The root of andrographis is used extensively in Chinese and Ayurvedic medicine. In Ayurvedic medicine, where it is referred to as the "King of Bitters," it is used to treat paresthesia, chronic or intermittent fever, malaria, inflammation, cough, bronchitis, skin diseases, intestinal parasites, dyspepsia, flatulence, colic, diarrhea, and hemorrhoids. In Chinese medicine, andrographis is used for influenza, sore throat, oral ulcers, acute or chronic cough, colitis, dysentery, urinary tract infection, carbuncles, sores, and venomous snake bites. Andrographis has strong evidence for efficacy in upper respiratory infections and immune dysfunction, especially when combined with eleuthero, and has been found to be more efficacious than better-known echinacea for this indication.

Clinical research indicates that andrographis, alone or in combination formulas, may be beneficial for infective hepatitis, male infertility, upper respiratory infection prevention and treatment, sinusitis, pharyngitis, influenza, HIV, rheumatoid arthritis, ulcerative colitis, and Familial Mediterranean Fever (FMF). In December 2020, the government of Thailand approved andrographis for treatment of early COVID-19.

IN VITRO AND ANIMAL RESEARCH

In vitro and animal research has indicated that andrographis has antiplatelet, antipyretic, antiinflammatory, bitter tonic, choleretic, hepatoprotective, antioxidant, euglycemic, immunostimulant, antitumor, antimetastatic, and adaptogenic properties. Animal research has shown that andrographis is as effective as silymarin (from milk thistle) in protecting the liver from toxicity. It has also been shown to bring about resolution of colitis through inhibition of CD4+ T-cell differentiation into Th1 and Th17 cells. In other studies, andrographis extract demonstrated calcium channel inhibition with resultant smooth muscle relaxation thereby lowering blood pressure, heart rate, and uterine tone. Andrographis has been shown to neutralize snake venom.

In 2020, researchers in Thailand found that andrographis extract had moderate inhibitory activity against SARS CoV-2 in human lung cell cultures, while its purified compound andrographolide exhibited 99.9% inhibitory activity against the virus in cell cultures (Sa-ngiamsuntorn et al., 2020) In silico research demonstrated that andrographolide could be docked successfully in the main protease binding site of SARS-CoV-2 (Enmozhi et al., 2020).

In vitro, this herb shows promise for incorporation into cancer prevention and treatment strategies. It has shown various inhibitory effects on human prostate cancer cells and inhibition of invasiveness of colorectal and non-small-cell lung cancer cells. Key constituents called andrographolides were shown to cause apoptosis of human hepatoma cancer cells and to decrease endothelial adhesion of gastric cancer cells as well as inhibit tumor cell growth. The andrographolides were shown to enhance the cytotoxicity of 5-fluorouracil, doxorubicin, and cisplatin when coincubated in multidrug-resistant colorectal cells. They also enhanced doxorubicin-induced cell death in several human cancer cell lines, mainly through JAK-STAT suppression.

HUMAN RESEARCH

Based on clinical trials, andrographis appears to be useful for prevention and abortive treatment of common colds. It may be beneficial for patients with chronic viral hepatitis and HIV. It may also be helpful for patients with dyspepsia and other digestive disturbances. Much of the research on andrographis has been in combination with eleuthero.

Gastrointestinal Disorders: Liver Disease

A clinical trial in patients with infective hepatitis assessed the efficacy of andrographis to normalize clinical and biochemical parameters. A marked symptomatic improvement in the majority of the cases was observed. A decrease was noted in serum bilirubin, turbidity, ALP, AST, ALT, and AG ratio. Total serum protein, globulin, and albumin were all increased. Complete resolution of symptoms and biochemical abnormalities occurred in 80% of patients with improvement in the remaining 20% of patients. The authors concluded that andrographis appeared to be a useful remedy for the treatment of infective hepatitis (Chaturvedi et al., 1983).

Male Genitourinary Disorders: Male Infertility

A Phase I clinical study in healthy males investigated the effects of high doses (three times the human daily dose) of a combination of andrographis plus eleuthero (Kan Jang) compared with separate high doses of Asian ginseng and valerian on semen quality. The results of the study revealed a positive trend toward the number of spermatozoids, percentage of normokinetic forms, and fertility indexes with the andrographis combination. There was also a decrease in percentage of dyskinetic spermatozoids. There were no significant negative effects of the herbal combination on male semen quality and fertility. Asian ginseng also showed no significant negative effects on fertility parameters, and there was a clear decrease in the percentage of dyskinetic forms of spermatozoids. Subjects receiving valerian showed a temporary increase in the percentage of normokinetic spermatozoids and a decrease in dyskinetic forms, but these changes had no effect on fertility indices. The authors concluded that andrographis plus eleuthero, Asian ginseng, and valerian were safe with respect to effects on human male sterility when administered at dose levels corresponding to approximately three times the human daily dose (Mkrtchyan et al., 2005).

Musculoskeletal Disorders: Osteoarthritis

A 12-week randomized controlled trial (RCT) in patients ($n = 103$) with mild-to-moderate knee osteoarthritis (OA) compared standardized andrographis leaf extract (ParActin) 300mg or 600 mg daily with placebo for effects on pain. Western Ontario and McMaster Universities Osteoarthritis Index (WOMAC) stiffness scores, physical function score, and fatigue score showed significant improvements with both 300 and 600 mg of andrographis compared with placebo. Quality of life and Functional Assessment of Chronic Illness Therapy scores showed significant improvements with both strengths of andrographis compared with the placebo. The authors concluded that ParActin in 300 and 600 mg/day dosages was effective and safe in reducing pain in individuals suffering from mild-to-moderate knee OA (Hancke et al., 2019).

Infectious Disease: Upper Respiratory Infection

A 2015 systematic review to assess efficacy of herbal medicines for cough associated with upper respiratory infection (URI) identified six RCTs involving andrographis (they also looked at pelargonium, echinacea, ivy-primrose-thyme, essential oils, and bakumondoto). The meta-analysis revealed strong evidence for andrographis (SMD = − 1.00; $P < 0.001$) and ivy-primrose-thyme (RR = 1.40; $P < 0.001$); moderate evidence for pelargonium (RR = 4.60; $P < 0.001$), and limited evidence for echinacea (SMD = − 0.68; $P = 0.04$) (Wagner et al., 2015).

A 2004 systematic review assessing the efficacy of andrographis in the symptomatic treatment of uncomplicated URIs selected four studies ($n = 433$) that met inclusion criteria. The authors found that andrographis in fixed combination with eleuthero was more effective than placebo (MD = 2.13 points; $P = 0.0002$) on the symptom severity score. The difference in effects between andrographis and placebo was 10.85 points ($P < 0.0001$). The authors concluded that evidence suggested andrographis alone or in combination with eleuthero may be more effective than placebo for uncomplicated acute URI (Poolsup et al., 2004).

A 2004 systematic review on the efficacy of andrographis for URIs selected seven RCTs ($n = 896$) that met inclusion criteria. The authors noted that collectively, the data suggested that andrographis was superior to placebo in alleviating the subjective symptoms of uncomplicated URI and that there was preliminary evidence of a preventative effect. Adverse events were generally mild and infrequent. The authors concluded that andrographis may be a safe and efficacious treatment for the relief of symptoms of uncomplicated URIs (Coon and Ernst, 2004).

A 5-day RCT in patients ($n = 223$) with URIs compared andrographis (KalmCold) 200 mg/day with placebo. In both groups, mean scores of all symptoms showed a decreasing trend from day 1 to day 3 but from day 3 to day 5 most of the symptoms in the placebo group either remained unchanged or worsened. In the andrographis group all symptoms except earache improved significantly compared with placebo ($P < 0.05$). In both placebo and andrographis groups, there were only a few minor adverse effects with no significant difference in occurrence ($P > 0.05$). Andrographis was 53% more effective on VAS scores than placebo. The authors concluded that KalmCold was effective in reducing symptoms of URI (Saxena et al., 2010).

A 5-day RCT in patients ($n = 185$) with acute URIs compared andrographis plus eleuthero (Kan Jang) with placebo. The andrographis group had significant improvement in URI and sinusitis symptoms. Greatest improvements occurred for headache, nasal and throat symptoms, and general malaise. Temperature was moderately reduced with andrographis. The authors concluded that andrographis had a positive effect in the treatment of acute URI and that it also relieved inflammatory symptoms of sinusitis. Andrographis was well tolerated (Gabrielian et al., 2002).

A 5-day RCT in patients ($n = 158$) with URIs compared andrographis 1200 mg/day with placebo with respect to prevalence and intensity of symptoms and signs of URIs. At day 2 of treatment a significant decrease in the intensity of the symptoms of tiredness ($OR = 1.28$), sleeplessness ($OR = 1.71$), sore throat ($OR = 2.3$), and nasal secretion ($OR = 2.51$) was observed with andrographis compared with placebo. At day 4, a significant decrease in the intensity of all symptoms was observed with andrographis over placebo:

sore throat ($OR = 3.59$), nasal secretion ($OR = 3.27$), and earache ($OR = 3.11$). The authors concluded that andrographis had a high degree of efficacy in reducing the prevalence and intensity of symptoms in uncomplicated URIs. No adverse effects were observed or reported (Cáceres et al., 1999).

A 10-day three-arm RCT in children ($n = 130$) with URIs investigated the efficacy of andrographis plus eleuthero compared with echinacea and with standard treatment alone. The andrographis treatment was found to be significantly more effective than echinacea, when started at an early stage of uncomplicated common colds, and the symptoms were less severe in this group. Amount of nasal discharge and nasal congestion showed the greatest impact. Recovery time was also faster with andrographis over echinacea and placebo. Andrographis was well tolerated, and no side effects or adverse reactions were reported (Spasov et al., 2004).

A 7-day RCT in patients ($n = 152$) with pharyngotonsillitis compared andrographis 3 or 6 g/day with paracetamol. Relief of fever and sore throat was significantly greater with paracetamol or high-dose andrographis at 3 days, but by day 7 there was no difference between groups (Thamlikitkul et al., 1991).

A 3-month RCT in teenagers ($n = 107$) compared andrographis 1200 mg/day with placebo for prevention of URIs during the winter months. After the first month, andrographis did not produce any significant difference in URI incidence relative to placebo. However, after the third month of intake the andrographis group demonstrated a significant decrease in the incidence of colds compared with the placebo group. The rate of incidence of colds among the students treated with andrographis was 30% compared with 62% with placebo ($RR = 2.1$). The authors concluded that andrographis may have a preventive effect against common colds during the winter period (Cáceres et al., 1997).

A Phase I study in August 2020 in patients ($n = 6$) with early COVID compared andrographis 60 mg TID with andrographis 100 mg TID. The lower dose of andrographis showed benefits, especially for coughing. Within 3 days, both cough volume and overall symptom severity reportedly decreased significantly. After 5 days, other symptoms improved. Real-time PCR tests were negative for SARS CoV-2 in two patients at 5 days and all patients at 3 weeks. (Trials underway to test efficacy of *Andrographis paniculata* extract for Covid-19. *The Nation Thailand* August 26, 2020. Available at: http://www.nationthailand.com/news/30393547. Accessed January 14, 2021.)

Infectious Disease: Influenza

A pilot study in patients with early influenza compared andrographis 1200 mg TID ($n = 71$) with amantadine ($n = 469$). With andrographis, 30% of subjects developed what they described as lingering or "complicated" influenza, while 68% of the control group developed this condition ($P < 0.01$). The authors concluded that the differences in the duration of sick leave and frequency of post-influenza complications indicated that andrographis not only contributed to quicker recovery, but also reduced the risk of postinfluenza complications (Kulichenko et al., 2003).

Infectious Disease: HIV

A Phase I clinical trial in HIV-positive patients ($n = 13$) and healthy volunteers ($n = 5$) assessed safety, tolerability, and disease efficacy of andrographolide from andrographis 5 mg/kg for 3 weeks then 10 mg/kg for 3 weeks, and then 20 mg/kg for 3 weeks. No subjects used antiretroviral medications during the trial. The trial was interrupted at 6 weeks due to adverse events including an anaphylactic reaction in one patient. All adverse events had resolved by the end of observation. A significant increase in the mean CD4+ lymphocyte level of HIV subjects occurred after administration of 10 mg/kg andrographolide (from a baseline of 405 to 501 cells/mm^3; $P = 0.002$). There were no statistically significant changes in mean plasma HIV-1 RNA levels throughout the trial. The authors postulated that andrographolide may inhibit HIV-induced cell cycle dysregulation, leading to a rise in CD4+ lymphocyte levels in HIV-1 infected individuals (Calabrese et al., 2000).

Autoimmune Disease: Rheumatoid Arthritis and Ulcerative Colitis

A 16-week RCT in patients ($n = 60$) with rheumatoid arthritis (RA) compared a standardized extract of andrographis 170 mg TID with placebo. With andrographis, decreases in scores were significant for tender joints (-0.13; $P = 0.001$), number of swollen joints (-0.15; $P = 0.02$), total grade of swollen joints (-0.27; $P = 0.010$), number of tender joints (-0.25; $P = 0.033$), total grade of tender joints (-0.47; $P = 0.002$), the Health Assessment Questionnaire (-0.52; $P < 0.001$), and the SF36 health questionnaire (0.02; $P < 0.001$). The intensity of joint pain decreased nonsignificantly in the active group compared with the placebo group at the end of treatment. Andrographis was also associated with a reduction of RF, IgA, and C4. The authors concluded that andrographis could be a useful "natural complement" in the treatment of RA (Burgos et al., 2009).

An 8-week RCT in patients ($n = 120$) with mild-to-moderate ulcerative colitis compared andrographis extract 1200 mg/day with slow-release mesalamine 4500 mg/day. The outcome showed a clinical remission in 21% of patients who took andrographis and 16% who took mesalamine. Clinical response occurred in 76% with andrographis and 82% with mesalamine. Colonoscopic remission occurred in 28% with andrographis and 24% with mesalamine. Colonoscopic response occurred in 75% with andrographis and 71% with mesalamine. The differences were not statistically significant. The authors concluded that the studied andrographis extract could be an efficacious alternative to mesalamine in ulcerative colitis (Tang et al., 2011).

An 8-week RCT in patients ($n = 224$) with mild-to-moderate ulcerative colitis who were failing first-line therapy with mesalamine compared andrographis 1200 mg/day, andrographis 1800 mg/day, and placebo. Clinical response occurred by week 8 in 45%, 60%, and 40% of patients receiving 1200, 1800 mg, and placebo, respectively (for difference from placebo, $P = 0.5924$ with 1200 mg and $P = 0.0183$ with 1800 mg, respectively). Clinical remission occurred by week 8 in 34%, 38%, and 25% of patients receiving 1200, 1800 mg, and placebo, respectively (for difference from placebo, $P = 0.258$ with 1200 mg and $P = 0.101$ with 1800 mg vs. placebo). Adverse events developed in 60%, 53%, and 60% of patients receiving 1200, 1800 mg, and placebo, respectively. The authors concluded that patients with mildly-to-moderately active ulcerative colitis treated with 1800 mg/day of andrographis extract were more likely to achieve clinical response than those receiving placebo (Sandborn et al., 2013).

Inflammation: Familial Mediterranean Fever

A 1-month Phase II RCT of young patients ($n = 24$) with FMF compared ImmunoGuard (a standardized fixed combination of eleuthero, andrographis, schisandra, and licorice extracts) four tablets TID with placebo. The patient's self-evaluation was based on symptoms of abdominal pain, chest pain, temperature, arthritis, myalgia, and erysipelas-like erythema. All three features (duration, frequency, and severity of attacks) showed significant improvement in the ImmunoGuard group compared with placebo. In both clinical assessment and self-evaluation, the severity of attacks was most improved in the herbal group. The authors concluded that both the clinical and laboratory results of the study suggested that ImmunoGuard was a safe and efficacious herbal drug for the management of patients with FMF (Amaryan et al., 2003).

ACTIVE CONSTITUENTS

- Carbohydrates
  - Polysaccharides: arabinogalactan (antitussive, hepatoprotective, immunomodulating)
  - Organic acid derivative:14-dehydroandroandrographolide succinic acid monoester (DASM) (protease inhibiting)
- Phenolic compounds
  - Flavonoids (antiinflammatory, antioxidant, cardioprotective, hepatoprotective, renoprotective, immunostimulant, apoptotic, anticancer): andrographidine A
- Terpenes
  - Diterpenoid lactones (antiinflammatory, NOX inhibition, COX-2 inhibition, bitter, immune-stimulating, hepatoprotective, choleretic, vasorelaxant, hypotensive, antineoplastic): andrographolides (antiinflammatory, antiviral, anti-HIV, neuroprotective, antidepressant, anticancer), neoandrographolides, andrographosides, andrographic acid
  - Diterpine dimers

ANDROGRAPHIS COMMONLY USED PREPARATIONS AND DOSAGE (FOR ADULTS UNLESS OTHERWISE SPECIFIED)

The following are examples of some available formulations and ranges of dosing for commercial herbal products. See Part III Introduction "How to prescribe medicinal herbs" for further guidance on herbal advising and prescribing.

Dried Leaf and Underground Stem

- Oral infusion (tea): 1 tsp. of leaves per cup AC (for indigestion).
- Tincture (1:4, 40%–50%): 1–3 mL AC (for indigestion).
- Powdered herb extract: 1/2 tsp. (1232 mg) BID.
- Capsule or tablet of powdered herb extract: 400 mg–3 g BID-TID.
- Capsule or tablet of standardized extract (standardized to ≥ 10% andrographolides): 200–600 mg QD-TID.

SAFETY AND PRECAUTION

Side Effects

Consumption of andrographis can cause GI upset, headache, fatigue, lymphadenopathy, diarrhea, and heartburn. Andrographis also has a bitter/metallic taste.

Case Reports

Acute kidney injury reported with intravenous use.

Toxicity

Some studies have found that prolonged high-dosage standardized extract of andrographis can cause toxicity in the testicles and liver. However, when a standardized extract was investigated in rats for 60 days no testicular toxicity was found with dosages of 20, 200, and 1000 mg/kg.

Pregnancy and Lactation

Insufficient human safety data.

Drug Interactions

- CYP: Inhibits CYP1A2, CYP2C9, and CYP3A4; induces CYP1A1.
- UGT: Inhibits UGT2B7.
- Antiplatelet drugs: use with caution, does not interfere with warfarin.
- Antioxidant effects: may interfere with certain chemotherapeutic drugs.
- Hypotensive effects: may exaggerate effects of antihypertensives.

REFERENCES

Amaryan G, Astvatsatryan V, Gabrielyan E, Panossian A, Panosyan V, Wikman G. Double-blind, placebo-controlled, randomized, pilot clinical trial of ImmunoGuard—a standardized fixed combination of Andrographis paniculata Nees, with Eleutherococcus senticosus maxim, Schisandra chinensis bail. and Glycyrrhiza glabra L. extracts in patients with familial Mediterranean fever. Phytomedicine 2003 May;10(4):271–85.

Burgos RA, Hancke JL, Bertoglio JC, et al. Efficacy of an Andrographis paniculata composition for the relief of rheumatoid arthritis symptoms: a prospective randomized placebo-controlled trial. Clin Rheumatol 2009 Aug;28(8):931–46.

Cáceres DD, Hancke JL, Burgos RA, Sandberg F, Wikman GK. Use of visual analogue scale measurements (VAS) to assess the effectiveness of standardized Andrographis paniculata extract SHA-10 in reducing the symptoms of common cold. A randomized double blind-placebo study. Phytomedicine 1999 Oct;6(4):217–23.

Cáceres DD, Hancke JL, Burgos RA, Wikman GK. Prevention of common colds with Andrographis paniculata dried extract. A pilot double blind trial. Phytomedicine 1997 Jun;4(2):101–4.

Calabrese C, Berman SH, Babish JG, et al. A phase I trial of andrographolide in HIV positive patients and normal volunteers. Phytother Res 2000 Aug;14(5):333–8.

Chaturvedi GN, Tomar GS, Tiwari SK, Singh KP. Clinical studies on kalmegh (Andrographis paniculata) in infective hepatitis. J Int Inst Ayurveda 1983;2:208–11.

Coon JT, Ernst E. Andrographis paniculata in the treatment of upper respiratory tract infections: a systematic review of safety and efficacy. Planta Med 2004 Apr;70(4):293–8.

Enmozhi SK, et al. Andrographolide as a potential inhibitor of SARS-CoV-2 main protease: an in silico approach. J Biomol Struct Dyn 2020 May;5:1–7.

Gabrielian ES, Shukarian AK, Goukasova GI, et al. A double blind, placebo-controlled study of Andrographis paniculata fixed combination Kan Jang in the treatment of acute upper respiratory tract infections including sinusitis. Phytomedicine 2002 Oct;9(7):589–97.

Hancke J, Burgos R, Caceres D, Wikman G. A double-blind study with a new monodrug Kan Jang: decrease of symptoms and improvement in recovery from common colds. Phytother Res 1995;9:559–62.

Hancke JL, Srivastav S, Cáceres DD, Burgos RA. A double-blind, randomized, placebo-controlled study to assess the efficacy of Andrographis paniculata standardized extract (ParActin) on pain reduction in subjects with knee osteoarthritis. Phytother Res 2019 May;33(5):1469–79.

Kulichenko LL, Kireyeva LV, Malyshkina EN, Wikman G. A randomized, controlled study of Kan Jang vs amantadine in the treatment of influenza in Volgograd. J Herb Pharmacother 2003;3:77–93.

Mkrtchyan A, Panosyan V, Panossian A, Wikman G, Wagner H. A phase I clinical study of Andrographis paniculata fixed combination Kan Jang vs ginseng and valerian on the semen quality of healthy male subjects. Phytomedicine 2005 Jun;12(6–7):403–9.

Poolsup N, Suthisisang C, Prathanturarug S, Asawamekin A, Chanchareon U. Andrographis paniculata in the symptomatic treatment of uncomplicated upper respiratory tract infection: systematic review of randomized controlled trials. J Clin Pharm Ther 2004 Feb;29(1):37–45.

Sa-ngiamsuntorn K, et al. Anti-SARS-CoV-2 activity of Andrographis paniculata extract and its major component Andrographolide in human lung epithelial cells and cytotoxicity evaluation in major organ cell representatives. bioRxiv - Microbiology 2020. (in press) https://doi.org/10.1101/2020.12.08.415836.

Sandborn WJ, Targan SR, Byers VS, et al. Andrographis paniculataextract (HMPL-004) for active ulcerative colitis. Am J Gastroenterol 2013;108:90–8.

Saxena RC, Singh R, Kumar P, et al. A randomized double-blind placebo controlled clinical evaluation of extract of Andrographis paniculata (KalmCold) in patients with uncomplicated upper respiratory tract infection. Phytomedicine 2010 Mar;17(3–4):178–85.

Spasov AA, Ostrovskij OV, Chernikov MV, Wikman G. Comparative controlled study of Andrographis paniculata fixed combination, Kan Jang and an Echinacea preparation as adjuvant, in the treatment of uncomplicated respiratory disease in children. Phytother Res 2004 Jan;18(1):47–53.

Tang T, Targan SR, Li Z-S, Xu C, Byers VS, Sandborn WJ. Randomised clinical trial: herbal extract HMPL-004 in active ulcerative colitis—a double-blind comparison with sustained release mesalazine. Aliment Pharmacol Ther January 2011;33(2):194–202.

Thamlikitkul V, Dechatiwongse T, Theerapong S, et al. Efficacy of Andrographis paniculata, Nees for pharyngotonsillitis in adults. J Med Assoc Thai 1991 Oct;74(10):437–42.

Wagner L, Cramer H, Klose P, et al. Herbal medicine for cough: a systematic review and meta-analysis. Forsch Komplementmed 2015;22(6):359–68.

26

ASHWAGANDHA (*WITHANIA SOMNIFERA*)
Root

GENERAL OVERVIEW

Since about 3000 BC, the herb ashwagandha has been a mainstay nervine tonic used in Ayurvedic medicine. Although it is sometimes called "Indian Ginseng," it is not related to Asian or American ginseng but rather is a member of the nightshade family. Its name means "horsey smell" due to the odor of the root, the part of the plant most commonly used. Ashwagandha is primarily an adaptogen, assisting in maintaining homeostasis during stress through its steroidal components.

Clinical research indicates that ashwagandha, alone or in combination formulas, may be beneficial for hyperlipidemia, diabetes, female sexual dysfunction, male infertility, osteoarthritis, cognitive impairment, anxiety, attention-deficit/hyperactivity disorder, schizophrenia, chronic stress, subclinical hypothyroidism, and immune function.

IN VITRO AND ANIMAL RESEARCH

Ashwagandha has antiinflammatory, antiarthritic, and antineuralgic effects. In stressed animal studies, adrenal glands showed reduction in the depletion of vitamin C and cortisol when the animals were pretreated with ashwagandha. It has nearly doubled swimming time in rats, suggesting it can enhance athletic performance. It also shows improved bone calcification in ovariectomized rats.

The glycowithanolide withaferin-A and sitoindosides VII–X isolated from the roots of ashwagandha significantly reversed the cognitive defects in an Alzheimer's disease (AD) model. Other research has shown that chronic oral administration of withanoside

IV from the root attenuated the neurological losses and memory deficits induced by Aβ in mice. The metabolite sominone was shown to induce marked recovery in neurites and synapses and to enhance axonal and dendritic outgrowth and synaptogenesis. Pretreatment with ashwagandha extract was found to prevent all the changes in antioxidant enzyme activities, catecholamine content, dopaminergic D2 receptor binding, and tyrosine hydroxylase expression in an animal model of Parkinson's disease (PD), suggesting the herb may be helpful in protecting the against neuronal injury in PD.

Ashwagandha's calming effect was equivalent to that of lorazepam in one study in rats with the activity thought to be due primarily to effects on the GABA system. Its antidepressant effect in rats was comparable to imipramine in another study. It also reduced stress ulcers in rats. In tests of in vivo efficacy, ginseng was compared with ashwagandha in mice. For swimming endurance, swimming time on average was 163 min with placebo, 536 min with ginseng, and 474 min with ashwagandha. In the anabolic portion of the study both treated groups gained more BW than placebo, more so with ashwagandha. (Grandhi et al., 1994) Ashwagandha has shown antitumor effects in hamster-ovarian cancer cell lines and lung tumors. It has been shown to enhance 5-fluoruracil efficacy in colon cancer cells.

HUMAN RESEARCH

Cardiometabolic Disorders: Diabetes

A small 30-day trial in patients with NIDDM ($n=6$) and hypercholesterolemia ($n=6$) assessed the effects of ashwagandha root powder on metabolic parameters. The authors reported that the decrease in blood glucose was comparable to that of an oral hypoglycemic drug. Significant increases in urine sodium and urine volume, and significant decreases in TC, TG, LD-C, and VLDL-C, were observed (Andallu and Radhika, 2000).

Women's Genitourinary Disorders: Female Sexual Dysfunction

An 8-week RCT in healthy females ($n = 50$) compared ashwagandha root extract 300 mg BID with placebo to assess effects on sexual function. Compared to placebo, the root extract resulted in significant improvements on the Female Sexual Function Index (FSI) Questionnaire and the Female Sexual Distress Scale (FSDS): FSFI Total score ($P < 0.001$), FSFI domain score for "arousal" ($P < 0.001$), "lubrication" ($P < 0.001$), "orgasm" ($P = 0.004$), "satisfaction" ($P < 0.001$), and FSDS score ($P < 0.001$). The number of successful sexual encounters was also improved with ashwagandha ($P < 0.001$). The authors concluded that high-dose ashwagandha root extract may improve sexual function in healthy women (Dongre et al., 2015).

Men's Genitourinary Disorders: Male Infertility

A 2018 systematic review of ashwagandha and male fertility investigated four clinical trials and found significant ($P \leq 0.002$) increases from baseline in sperm concentration (167%), semen volume (59%), and sperm motility (57%) in oligospermic males after 90 days of ashwagandha treatment. Additionally, improvement was noted in levels of serum testosterone (17%) and LH (34%). Meta-analysis of observational studies showed that ashwagandha treatment significantly improved semen parameters over baseline: semen volume (MD = 0.28 mL); sperm concentration (MD = 13.57 million/mL; $P < 0.00001$); and sperm motility (MD = 8.5%; $P < 0.00001$). The authors concluded that, due to the small number of eligible studies, the available data, though promising, were too limited to provide novel and sufficiently robust evidence of the benefits of *Withania somnifera* in male infertility. Further research was recommended (Durg et al., 2018).

A triple-blinded RCT compared the effects of ashwagandha powdered whole root 5 g/day with pentoxifylline 800 mg/day on sperm parameters in men ($n = 100$) with idiopathic infertility. Ashwagandha was associated with improvements in mean sperm count by 12.5% ($P = 0.04$), progressive motility by 21.4% ($P < 0.001$), and sperm morphology by 25.5% ($P = 0.000$) compared with baseline. These results were not significantly different from the improvements seen with pentoxifylline for semen volume ($P = 0.11$), sperm count ($P = 0.09$), morphology ($P = 0.12$), and progressive motility ($P = 0.77$). The authors concluded that ashwagandha improved sperm parameters in idiopathic male infertility without causing adverse effects and could be an alternative to pentoxifylline in this regard (Nasimi Doost Azgomi et al., 2018).

Musculoskeletal Disorders: Osteoarthritis

A 12-week RCT in patients ($n = 60$) with knee joint pain compared two doses of a standardized extract of ashwagandha root plus leaves (250 and 125 mg) BID with placebo. Compared with baseline and placebo, significant reductions were observed in mean WOMAC and KSI scores in both ashwagandha groups: 250 mg ($P < 0.001$) and 125 mg ($P < 0.05$). VAS scores for pain, stiffness, and disability were also significantly reduced with both groups: 250 mg ($P < 0.001$) and 125 mg ($P < 0.01$). The higher dose group showed earliest efficacy (at 4 weeks). All treatments were well tolerated. The authors concluded that both doses of ashwagandha produced significant reduction in outcome variables in a dose-dependent manner and without any significant GI disturbances (Ramakanth et al., 2016).

A 32-week RCT in patients ($n = 90$) with osteoarthritis (OA) compared an Ayurvedic combination containing ashwagandha, frankincense, ginger, and turmeric with placebo. At Week 16, the mean reductions in pain VAS for herb and placebo were 2.7 and 1.3, respectively ($P < 0.05$). At Week 32, the mean reductions in pain VAS for herb and placebo were 2.8 and 1.8, respectively ($P < 0.05$). The improvements in WOMAC scores at Week 16 and Week 32 were also significantly superior to placebo ($P < 0.01$) with the combination herbal product. Both the groups reported mild adverse events without any significant difference between groups. The authors concluded that the study demonstrated the potential efficacy and safety of 32 weeks of treatment with this particular herbal combination in the symptomatic treatment of OA knees (Chopra et al., 2004).

Neurologic Disorders: Cognitive Dysfunction

A 2019 systematic review to evaluate the potential role of ashwagandha in managing cognitive dysfunction found five clinical studies that met eligibility criteria. The studies were heterogeneous. In most instances, ashwagandha extract improved performance on cognitive tasks, executive function, attention, and reaction time. The authors concluded that, overall, there was some early clinical evidence to support the cognitive benefits of ashwagandha. It also appeared to be well tolerated, with good adherence and minimal side effects (Ng et al., 2020).

An 8-week RCT in adults ($n=50$) with mild cognitive impairment (MCI) compared ashwagandha 300 mg BID with placebo. Based on the Wechsler Memory Scale III, ashwagandha demonstrated significant improvements compared with placebo on subtest scores for logical memory I ($P=0.007$), verbal paired associates I ($P=0.042$), faces I ($P=0.020$), family pictures I ($P=0.006$), logical memory II ($P=0.006$), verbal paired associates II ($P=0.031$), faces II ($P=0.014$), and family pictures II ($P=0.006$). Other tests indicated significantly greater improvement with ashwagandha for executive function, sustained attention, and information-processing speed. The authors concluded that ashwagandha may be effective in enhancing both immediate and general memory in people with MCI as well as improving executive function, attention, and information processing speed (Choudhary et al., 2017a).

Psychiatric Disorders: Anxiety, Insomnia, and Obsessive-Compulsive Disorder

A 2014 systematic review of studies on ashwagandha and anxiety found five human trials that met inclusion criteria. Three studies compared several dosage levels of ashwagandha extract with placebo using versions of the HAM-A scale, with two demonstrating significant benefit of ashwagandha compared with placebo, and the third demonstrating beneficial effects that approached but did not achieve significance ($P=0.05$). A fourth study compared ashwagandha with psychotherapy and found that BAI scores decreased by 56.5% in the ashwagandha group and 30.5% in the psychotherapy group ($P<0.0001$). A fifth study that measured changes in Perceived Stress Scale (PSS) scores

in ashwagandha compared with placebo found a 44% reduction in PSS scores in the ashwagandha group and a 5.5% reduction in the placebo group ($P<0.0001$). The authors concluded that ashwagandha resulted in greater score improvements (significantly in most cases) than placebo in outcomes on anxiety or stress scales in all five studies, but that these conclusions were limited by an assortment of study methods and cases of potential bias (Pratte et al., 2014).

A 2013 systematic review looking at plants that had both preclinical and clinical evidence for antianxiety effects found 21 plants with human clinical trial evidence. Support for efficacy identified several herbs with efficacy for anxiety spectrum disorders including ashwagandha, kava, lemon balm, chamomile, ginkgo, skullcap, milk thistle, passionflower, rhodiola, echinacea, *Galphimia glauca, Centella asiatica,* and *Echium amoenum.* Acute anxiolytic activity was found for passionflower, sage, gotu kola, lemon balm, and bergamot. The review also specifically found that bacopa showed anxiolytic effects in people with cognitive decline (Sarris et al., 2013).

A 60-day RCT in healthy adults ($n=60$) compared standardized ashwagandha extract 240 mg/day with placebo for effects on mood and stress. Ashwagandha, compared with placebo, was associated with greater reductions in HAM-A ($P=0.040$) and DASS-21 ($P=0.096$), as well as with greater reductions in morning cortisol ($P<0.001$), and DHEA-S ($P=0.004$). Testosterone levels increased over baseline in males ($P=0.038$) but not in females ($P=0.989$), although this change was not statistically significant compared with the placebo ($P=0.158$). The authors concluded that ashwagandha's stress-relieving effects may occur through effects on the HPA axis and that further studies were warranted (Lopresti et al., 2019).

An 8-week parallel-group RCT in patients with and without insomnia ($n=40$ for each group) compared ashwagandha with placebo for effects on sleep parameters. In patients with and without insomnia, there were significant improvements in sleep parameters with ashwagandha, being more significant in insomnia subjects than in healthy subjects for sleep onset latency ($P<0.0001$), sleep efficiency ($P<0.0001$), total sleep time ($P<0.002$), and wake after sleep onset ($P<0.040$). In healthy subjects, all parameters except for HAM-A and mental alertness improved significantly over baseline ($P < 0.001$). Ashwagandha was well tolerated by all study participants. The authors concluded that ashwagandha root extract could improve sleep quality and could help in managing insomnia (Langade et al., 2020).

A 12-week RCT in older adults ($n = 50$) compared ashwagandha root extract 600 mg/day with placebo for the improvement of general health and sleep. The mean total score of WHOQOL-BREF improved from 140.53 at the baseline to 161.84 at the end of the study, a significant change compared with placebo ($P < 0.0001$). Significant increases in the quality of sleep ($P < 0.0001$) and mental alertness ($P < 0.034$) were observed with ashwagandha compared with placebo. Overall improvement was observed for general well-being, sleep quality, and mental alertness in the study population. Ashwagandha was well tolerated. The authors concluded that ashwagandha root extract was efficient in improving QOL, sleep quality, and mental alertness in elderly participants (Kelgane et al., 2020).

A 6-week RCT in patients ($n = 30$) with obsessive-compulsive disorder (OCD) who were already on selective serotonin reuptake inhibitors (SSRIs) compared adjunctive treatment with ashwagandha 120 mg/day with placebo. Pretreatment to posttreatment change to the Yale-Brown Obsessive-Compulsive Scale score revealed a significantly greater decrease with ashwagandha (26–14) compared with placebo (18–16) ($P < 0.001$). The extract was safe, and no adverse event was reported during the trial. The authors concluded that ashwagandha may be beneficial as a safe and effective adjunct to SSRIs in the treatment of OCD (Jahanbakhsh et al., 2016).

Psychiatric Disorders: Attention-Deficit/Hyperactivity Disorder

A 4-month RCT in children ($n = 120$) newly diagnosed with ADHD studied a polyherbal formula containing ashwagandha, bacopa, lemon balm, *Paeoniae alba*, *Centella asiatica*, and *Spirulina platensis* compared with placebo. The treatment group showed substantial, statistically significant improvement in the four subscales and overall TOVA scores, compared with no improvement in the control group. The authors concluded that the polyherbal formula improved attention, cognition, and impulse control in children with ADHD (Katz et al., 2010).

Psychiatric Disorders: Schizophrenia

In a 12-week RCT, patients ($n = 66$) with schizophrenia who were experiencing an exacerbation of symptoms were given ashwagandha standardized extract 1000 mg/day or placebo in addition to their antipsychotic medication. Beginning at 4 weeks and continuing to the end of treatment, ashwagandha produced significantly greater reductions in the Positive and Negative Syndrome Scale (PANSS) negative, general, and total symptoms (large effect size based on Cohen d), but not positive symptoms, when compared with placebo. Adverse events were mild to moderate and transient; somnolence, epigastric discomfort, and loose stools were more common with ashwagandha. The authors concluded that that adjunctive treatment with a standardized extract of ashwagandha may provide significant benefits with minimal side effects for negative, general, and total symptoms and stress in patients with recent exacerbations of schizophrenia (Chengappa et al., 2018).

Disorders of Vitality: Chronic Stress

An 8-week RCT in subjects ($n = 52$) under chronic stress compared ashwagandha 300 mg BID with placebo. Treatment with ashwagandha resulted in significant improvements in the Perceived Stress Scale and Food Cravings Questionnaire as well as the Oxford Happiness Questionnaire, Three-Factor Eating Questionnaire, serum cortisol, body weight (BW), and BMI. The extract was found to be safe and tolerable. The authors concluded that ashwagandha extract may be useful for BW management in adults under chronic stress (Choudhary et al., 2017b).

A 60-day RCT in patients ($n = 64$) with chronic stress compared ashwagandha 300 mg BID for 45 days with placebo. Ashwagandha was associated with a significant reduction in scores on all the stress-assessment scales on Day 60 compared with placebo ($P < 0.0001$). Serum cortisol levels were reduced with ashwagandha compared with placebo ($P = 0.0006$). The adverse effects were mild in nature and were comparable in both groups. The authors concluded that high-dose ashwagandha safely and effectively improved resistance to stress and self-assessed quality of life (Chandrasekhar et al., 2012).

Disorders of Vitality: Athletic Performance

A 12-week RCT in recreationally active young men ($n = 19$) compared a standardized aqueous extract of ashwagandha 500 mg/day with placebo ($n = 19$) for effects on workouts. Ashwagandha and placebo produced gains in 1-RM squat (+ 19.1 and + 10.0 kg, respectively; $P = 0.009$) and bench press (+ 12.8 and + 8.0 kg, respectively; $P = 0.048$). Ashwagandha was also associated with a change in body mass to a more android composition compared with placebo ($P = 0.03$). The authors concluded that the 500 mg dose of ashwagandha aqueous extract improved upper- and lower-body strength, supported a favorable distribution of body mass, and was well tolerated clinically in recreationally active men over a 12-week period (Ziegenfuss et al., 2018).

An 8-week RCT in young healthy men ($n = 57$) with little experience in resistance training compared ashwagandha root extract 300 mg BID with placebo. After 8 weeks of resistance training, ashwagandha produced greater increases than placebo in muscle strength on the bench-press exercise (46.0 and 26.4 kg, respectively; $P = 0.001$) and the leg-extension exercise (14.5 and 9.8 kg, respectively; $P = 0.04$), and significantly greater muscle size increase at the arms (8.6 and 5.3 cm^2, respectively; $P = 0.01$) and chest (3.3 and 1.4 cm, respectively; $P < 0.001$). Compared with placebo, subjects receiving ashwagandha also had a significantly greater reduction of exercise-induced muscle damage as indicated by the stabilization of serum CK ($P = 0.03$) and a significantly greater increase in testosterone levels (96.2 and 18.0 ng/dL for ashwagandha and placebo, respectively; $P = 0.004$). Decreases in body fat percentage were 3.5% and 1.5% with ashwagandha and placebo, respectively; $P = 0.03$. The authors concluded that ashwagandha was associated with significant increases in muscle mass and strength and may be useful in conjunction with a resistance training program (Wankhede et al., 2015).

Endocrine Disorders: Subclinical Hypothyroidism

An 8-week study of patients ($n = 50$) with subclinical hypothyroidism compared ashwagandha root extract 600 mg/day with placebo. Eight weeks of treatment with ashwagandha improved serum TSH ($P < 0.001$), T3 ($P = 0.0031$), and T4 ($P = 0.0096$) levels significantly compared with placebo, and effectively normalized TSH, T3, and T4 in a significant manner ($P < 0.001$ for all). The authors concluded that ashwagandha may be beneficial for normalizing thyroid indices in subclinical hypothyroid patients (Sharma et al., 2018).

Immune Function

Effects on immune cell activation with use of ashwagandha were assessed in subjects ($n = 5$) who were given 6 mL of ashwagandha root BID for 96 h. Findings showed significant increases in the expression of CD4 on CD3+ T cells and activation of CD56+ NK cells as evidenced by expression of the CD69 receptor. The authors concluded that ashwagandha deserved further study with respect to its effects on immune cell activation (Mikolai et al., 2009).

A 12-week RCT in newly diagnosed tuberculosis (TB) patients ($n = 60$) investigated standard DOT plus ashwagandha compared with standard DOT plus placebo. By 8 weeks, sputum conversion was seen in 87% of patients in the study group and 77% in the placebo group. At the end of 12 weeks a highly significant increase was seen in both CD4 and CD8 counts in the ashwagandha group. ALT and AST levels were increased in 33% and 16% of the ashwagandha group and in 53% and 43% of the placebo group, respectively. Uric acid levels were lower in the ashwagandha group. Average gain in HRQL score was better in patients in the study group. The authors concluded that a favorable effect of ashwagandha as adjuvant to anti-TB drugs was demonstrated for symptoms and immunological parameters in patients with pulmonary TB (Kumar et al., 2018).

ACTIVE CONSTITUENTS

Root

- ■ Steroids
  - ■ Phytosterols
  - ■ Steroid lactones—withanolides: withaferin A (anti-Alzheimer's, antiangiogenic, antimetastatic, reduction NF-kB, proteasomal inhibition, immunomodulating, antiinflammatory), withanone (blocks ACE2 receptor, downregulates P21 in normal cells but upregulates it in cancer cells, delaying cellular aging of normal cells), withanolide D (hormone precursors); sitoindosides: sitoindoside IX, sitoindoside X (antistress, anti-Alzheimer's); withanoside IV (and metabolite sominone) (increase neurogenesis and axonal length, anti-Alzheimer's); acylsterylglucosides (antistress)

ASHWAGANDHA COMMONLY USED PREPARATIONS AND DOSAGE (FOR ADULTS UNLESS OTHERWISE SPECIFIED)

The following are examples of some available formulations and ranges of dosing for commercial herbal products. See Part III Introduction "How to prescribe medicinal herbs" for further guidance on herbal advising and prescribing.

- Oral infusion (tea): Natural Care Tea (contains ashwagandha, licorice, holy basil, cardamom, and ginger) 1 cup TID.
- Tincture (1:5, 60-70%): 0.5-1 mL TID.
- Powdered root extract: 1/5 tsp. (450 mg) QD-BID, traditionally mixed in milk, ghee (clarified butter), or water.
- Capsule or tablet of powdered whole root: 500–2000 mg BID-TID with meals.
- Capsule or tablet of standardized extract (standardized to 1.5%–2.5% withanolides): 240–500 mg QD-TID.

SAFETY AND PRECAUTION

Side Effects

Headaches, gastritis, and nausea were reported in one study. May increase serum testosterone levels.

Case Reports

One confirmed case of burning and itching of distal urethra and discoloration and reddening of penile head and prepuce when taken at high dose (5 g daily) for 10 days. One case of thyrotoxicosis has also been reported.

Toxicity

No toxicity has been identified with recommended doses of ashwagandha, but high doses can have toxic effects including cardiotoxicity and sexual dysfunction. Basic water extract of ashwagandha at 2000 mg/kg to rats failed to exert any clinical or biochemical toxicity over the course of 28 days.

Pregnancy and Lactation

Avoid in pregnancy. May cause abortion.

Drug Interactions

- Avoid with MAO-inhibitors.
- May counteract immunosuppression of cyclosporin.
- May reduce neutropenia with paclitaxel (comparable to GCSF).
- Prolongs effect of morphine via PPARγ-dependent mechanism.
- May potentiate effectiveness of other sedative herbs or pharmaceuticals.
- May cause false elevation in digoxin immunoassay.

REFERENCES

Andallu B, Radhika B. Hypoglycemic, diuretic and hypocholesterolemic effect of winter cherry (Withania somnifera, Dunal) root. Indian J Exp Biol 2000 Jun;38(6):607–9.

Chandrasekhar K, Kapoor J, Anishetty S. A prospective, randomized double-blind, placebo-controlled study of safety and efficacy of a high-concentration full-spectrum extract of ashwagandha root in reducing stress and anxiety in adults. Indian J Psychol Med 2012 Jul;34(3):255–62.

Chengappa KNR, Brar JS, Gannon JM, Schlicht PJ. Adjunctive use of a standardized extract of Withania somnifera (Ashwagandha) to treat symptom exacerbation in schizophrenia: a randomized, double-blind, placebo-controlled study. J Clin Psychiatry 2018 Jul;10:79(5):17m11826.

Chopra A, Lavin P, Patwardhan B, Chitre D. A 32-week randomized, placebo-controlled clinical evaluation of RA-11, an Ayurvedic drug, on osteoarthritis of the knees. J Clin Rheumatol 2004 Oct;10(5):236–45.

Choudhary D, Bhattacharyya S, Bose S. Efficacy and safety of Ashwagandha (Withania somnifera (L.) Dunal) root extract in improving memory and cognitive functions. J Diet Suppl 2017 Nov 2;14(6):599–612.

Choudhary D, Bhattacharyya S, Joshi K. BW management in adults under chronic stress through treatment with Ashwagandha root extract: a double-blind, randomized, placebo-controlled trial. J Evid Based Complementary Altern Med 2017 Jan;22(1):96–106.

Dongre S, Langade D, Bhattacharyya S. Efficacy and safety of Ashwagandha (Withania somnifera) root extract in improving sexual function in women: a pilot study. Biomed Res Int 2015;2015:284154.

Durg S, Shivaram SB, Bavage S. Withania somnifera (Indian ginseng) in male infertility: an evidence-based systematic review and meta-analysis. Phytomedicine 2018 Nov 15;50:247–56.

Grandhi A, Mujumdar AM, Patwardhan B. Pharmacological comparison of activities of Ashwagandha and ginseng. A comparative pharmacological investigation of Ashwagandha and ginseng. J Ethnopharmacol 1994;44:131–5.

Jahanbakhsh SP, Manteghi AA, Emami SA, et al. Evaluation of the efficacy of Withania somnifera (Ashwagandha) root extract in patients with obsessive-compulsive disorder: a randomized double-blind placebo-controlled trial. Complement Ther Med 2016 Aug;27:25–9.

Katz M, et al. A compound herbal preparation (CHP) in the treatment of children with ADHD: a randomized controlled trial. J Atten Disord 2010 Nov;14(3):281–91.

Kelgane S, Salve J, Sampara P, Debnath K. Efficacy and tolerability of Ashwagandha root extract in the elderly for improvement of general well-being and sleep: a prospective, randomized, double-blind, placebo-controlled Study. Cureus 2020 Feb 23;12(2):e7083.

Kumar R, Rai J, Kajal NC, Devi P. Comparative study of effect of Withania somnifera as an adjuvant to DOTS in patients of newly diagnosed sputum smear positive pulmonary tuberculosis. Indian J Tuberc 2018 Jul;65(3):246–51.

Langade D, Thakare V, Kanchi S, Kelgane S. Clinical evaluation of the pharmacological impact of ashwagandha root extract on sleep in healthy volunteers and insomnia patients: a double-blind, randomized, parallel-group, placebo-controlled study. J Ethnopharmacol 2020 Aug;264:113276.

Lopresti AL, Smith SJ, Malvi H, Kodgule R. An investigation into the stress-relieving and pharmacological actions of an ashwagandha (Withaniasomnifera) extract: a randomized, double-blind, placebo-controlled study. Medicine (Baltimore) 2019 Sep;98(37):e17186.

Mikolai J, Erlandsen A, Murison A, et al. *In vivo* effects of Ashwagandha (Withania somnifera) extract on the activation of lymphocytes. J Altern Complement Med 2009 Apr;15(4):423–30.

Nasimi Doost Azgomi R, Nazemiyeh H, Sadeghi Bazargani H, et al. Comparative evaluation of the effects of Withania somnifera with pentoxifylline on the sperm parameters in idiopathic male infertility: a triple-blind randomised clinical trial. Andrologia 2018 Sep;50(7):e13041.

Ng QX, Loke W, Foo NX, et al. A systematic review of the clinicaluse of Withaniasomnifera (Ashwagandha) to ameliorate cognitive dysfunction. Phytother Res 2020 Mar;34(3):583–90.

Pratte MA, Nanavati KB, Young V, Morley CP. An alternative treatment for anxiety: a systematic review of human trial results reported for the Ayurvedic herb ashwagandha (Withania somnifera). J Altern Complement Med 2014 Dec;20(12):901–8.

Ramakanth GS, Uday Kumar C, Kishan PV, Usharani P. A randomized, double blind placebo-controlled study of efficacy and tolerability of Withaina somnifera extracts in knee joint pain. J Ayurveda Integr Med 2016 Jul - Sep;7(3):151–7.

Sarris J, McIntyre E, Camfield DA. Plant-based medicines for anxiety disorders, part 2: a review of clinical studies with supporting preclinical evidence. CNS Drugs 2013 Apr;27(4):301–19.

Sharma AK, Basu I, Singh S. Efficacy and safety of Ashwagandha root extract in subclinical hypothyroid patients: a double-blind, randomized placebo-controlled trial. J Altern Complement Med 2018 Mar;24(3):243–8.

Wankhede S, Langade D, Joshi K, Sinha SR, Bhattacharyya S. Examining the effect of Withania somnifera supplementation on muscle strength and recovery: a randomized controlled trial. J Int Soc Sports Nutr 2015 Nov 25;12:43.

Ziegenfuss TN, Kedia AW, Sandrock JE, Raub BJ, Kerksick CM, Lopez HL. Effects of an aqueous extract of Withania somnifera on strength training adaptations and recovery: the STAR Trial. Nutrients 2018 Nov 20;10(11). pii: E1807.

27 ASTRAGALUS (*ASTRAGALUS MEMBRANACEUS/PROPINQUUS*)
Root

GENERAL OVERVIEW

Astragalus, an increasingly popular herb for immune support, has long been used in traditional Chinese medicine (TCM) for diarrhea, fatigue, anorexia, upper respiratory infections, heart disease, hepatitis, fibromyalgia, and cancer adjunctive treatment. It is usually prepared in combination with one or several other herbs according to TCM syndrome concepts. It is frequently paired with dong quai, as there appears to be a synergism between these two plants, likely related to enhancement of absorption. It is the most frequently used herb in TCM formulas for chronic hepatitis and congestive heart failure. Astragalus is one of the adaptogenic herbs, and it appears to have antiaging effects through preservation of telomere length. This herb is commonly employed to strengthen stress- and age-induced immune senescence. Its other special talent is that it has been shown to be beneficial for kidney disease, including membranous nephropathy.

Clinical research indicates that astragalus, alone or in combination formulas, may be beneficial for herpes keratitis, recurrent tonsillitis, seasonal allergic rhinitis, myocarditis, reperfusion injury, congestive heart failure, hepatic fibrosis, viral hepatitis, diabetic nephropathy, lupus nephritis, membranous nephropathy, recovery from stroke, burns, leukopenia, tuberculosis, nonsquamous cell lung cancer, and cancer survival.

IN VITRO AND ANIMAL RESEARCH

Astragalus has been shown to have antibacterial, antiinflammatory, antioxidant, antiviral, and mild diuretic properties. It appears to balance the immune system, reducing allergic response by normalizing the ratio of Th1 to Th2 cells. The polysaccharides in astragalus markedly enhance humoral and cellular immune responses to the hepatitis B vaccine. Astragalus also appears to have antiviral activity, suppressing proliferation of HBV. It has shown a protective effect in mice against parainfluenza virus type I, Japanese encephalitis virus, and Coxsackie B3.

Astragalus has demonstrated enhancement of the activity and lethality of NK cells in vitro. It has also been shown to potentiate the immune-mediated antitumor activity of IL-2. Astragalus has been shown to play a role in antiinflammatory and fibroblast-proliferating activities and promotes angiogenesis.

Astragalus has been shown to enhance sperm quality in vitro. One constituent inhibits melanin synthesis and may be useful in treating age spots. A 2:1 combination of astragalus and *Rehmannia* 1 g/kg applied to rats in a diabetic foot ulcer rat model resulted in improved wound healing. These two herbs in combination did not individually promote wound healing, so it was concluded that the herbs worked synergistically. The active constituent astragaloside IV has been shown to increase keratinocyte migration and subsequent wound healing, more than doubling the rate of wound healing in rat models.

HUMAN RESEARCH

Several of the human studies, particular those involving myocardial and renal health, have utilized astragalus injections. Studies have demonstrated a renal-sparing effect from diabetes, cardiopulmonary bypass, and postlithotripsy as well as improvements in lupus and IgA nephropathy. Unfortunately, injections would not be considered a practical or approved option for Western medical practitioners.

Ophthalmological Disorders: Herpes Keratitis

An RCT in patients ($n=106$) with herpes keratitis and volunteers ($n=62$) without disease compared astragalus with ribavirin. Levels of serum IL-4 and IL-10 were higher and levels of IL-2 and IFN-γ were lower in patients with keratitis than in healthy controls ($P<0.01$). These parameters were significantly improved with astragalus after treatment but did not change with ribavirin. The authors concluded that astragalus could modulate the imbalance of Th1/Th2 in patients with herpes keratitis and improve their immune function disturbance as part of the management of herpes keratitis (Mao et al., 2004).

Ears, Nose, and Throat Disorders: Recurrent Tonsillitis

A study in children ($n=27$) with recurrent tonsillitis while in remission studied the stimulation of peripheral mononuclear cells with phytohemagglutinin alone compared with phytohemagglutinin plus astragalus. This was compared with phytohemagglutinin-stimulated mononuclear cells from children ($n=21$) without recurrent tonsillitis. The IFN-γ level and the ratio of IFN-γ/IL-4 in the phytohemagglutinin-alone tonsillitis group were statistically lower than those in the nontonsillitis group ($P<0.01$). The level of IFN-γ and the ratio of IFN-γ/IL-4 in the phytohemagglutinin-astragalus tonsillitis group were markedly higher than those in the phytohemagglutinin-alone tonsillitis group ($P<0.01$) but were significantly lower than those in the nontonsillitis group ($P<0.05$). There were no differences in the IL-4 level among the three groups. The authors concluded that a Th1 cell subset dysfunction may play an important role in the pathogenesis of recurrent tonsillitis and that astragalus may improve this dysfunction and be beneficial for recurrent tonsillitis (Yang et al., 2006).

Allergic Disorders: Allergic Rhinitis

A 6-week RCT in patients ($n=48$) with moderate-to-severe seasonal allergic rhinitis compared an astragalus-based herb and mineral complex with placebo for efficacy. The astragalus formula significantly decreased the intensity of rhinorrhea compared with placebo. Blinded investigators and patients equally judged the treatment with the astragalus formula as more efficacious. The analysis of changes from baseline for total symptom score, QOL, and four main symptoms of allergic rhinitis were strikingly in favor of the active treatment. The authors concluded that the study revealed several indicators of therapeutic effectiveness of the studied astragalus formula in patients with seasonal allergic rhinitis (Matkovic et al., 2010).

Cardiovascular Disorders: Congestive Heart Failure, Reperfusion Injury, and Myocarditis

A 2014 systematic review to assess efficacy and safety of astragalus injection combined with conventional therapy in the treatment of viral myocarditis included six RCTs ($n=639$). The methodological quality of the included trials was generally low, and there was high risk of publication bias in the included trials. The total effective rate of astragalus injection combined with conventional treatment was significantly greater than that of conventional treatment alone with faster recovery of cardiac enzymes and ECGs. Two RCTs reported there were no adverse effects from astragalus injection combined with conventional treatment (Piao and Liang, 2014).

A 2013 systematic review to assess the effects and safety of astragalus injection on clinical and indirect outcomes in patients with viral myocarditis selected nine RCTs ($n=894$) that met inclusion criteria. The trials reported ECG results, level of myocardial enzymes, cardiac function, and adverse effects. None of the trials reported outcomes on mortality and quality of life. The authors concluded that the literature suggests that astragalus injection has positive effects in patients with suspected viral myocarditis with respect to abnormal ECG and myocardial enzymes (Liu et al., 2013).

A 4-week RCT in patients ($n=108$) with acute myocardial infarction (AMI) compared injection of astragalus with conventional treatment for effects on LV remodeling. At the fourth week, changes of LV end-diastolic volume index, LV end-systolic volume index, and anterior endocardial segmental length in the astragalus group were not obvious but increased significantly in the control group ($P<0.05$). The LV ejection fraction, the LV peak ejection rate, and the LV peak filling rate were higher with astragalus than with control. The LV time for peak filling rate was shorter, and indications of oxidation were lower with astragalus than control. SOD levels were higher with astragalus ($P < 0.01$ or $P < 0.05$ between groups for all the above). The authors concluded that astragalus was effective in reversal of LV remodeling and improving LV function in patients with AMI (Zhang et al., 2002).

A 6-month RCT in patients ($n = 83$) with NYHA grade II–IV congestive heart failure (CHF) compared astragalus intravenous injection (40 mL, equivalent to 80 g crude drug) in 500 mL D5W with a control group who received nitroglycerin intravenous injection (15 mg in 500 mL D5W) given once daily for 2 weeks. At 1 and 6 months, the clinical heart function improvement rate and the total effective rate were greater in the astragalus group than in the control group ($P < 0.05$ and $P < 0.01$). The levels of LV ejection fraction, the fractional shortening of LV short axis, the ratio of maximum blood flow between the advanced and early atrial systole, stroke volume, cardiac output, and the cardiac index were all improved in both groups ($P < 0.01$ or $P < 0.05$) but showed greater improvement in the astragalus group. By 6 months, the incidence of cardiac events was lower in the treated group than in the control group ($P < 0.05$) (Zhou et al., 2001).

An RCT in patients ($n = 24$) undergoing surgery for either valvular heart diseases or congenital VSD compared astragalus with ligustrazine, either alone or combined, with a control group with respect to reperfusion injury. The treated groups, especially the combination group, showed lower levels of AST, LDH, CK, CK-MB, MDA, and SOD compared with the control group ($P < 0.05$; $P < 0.01$). Astragalus plus ligustrazine demonstrated the greatest NO activity with the astragalus group demonstrating the next greatest activity. The authors concluded that astragalus plus ligustrazine could effectively protect against myocardial reperfusion injury (Zhou et al., 2000).

A 30-day RCT in patients ($n = 90$) with CHF of "qi deficiency and/or yang-deficiency syndromes" (TCM syndromes) compared astragalus granules at three different doses (2.25, 4.5, and 7.5 g) BID plus perindopril 4 mg QD. The heart function grades of all three groups improved compared with baseline, but the improvements in the high-dose group and moderate-dose group were better than in the low-dose group ($P < 0.05$). LV ejection fraction was increased 59% in the high-dose group, 62% in the moderate-dose group, and 51% in the low-dose group, all significant increases, and the differences between the higher two doses and the low-dose groups were also significant ($P < 0.01$). The 6-min walking distance was increased to 420, 387, and 317 m in the high-, medium-, and low-dose groups, respectively, all being significant increases. Minnesota scores decreased to 30, 36, and 43 in the high-, medium-, and low-dose groups, respectively. The difference between the high and low doses was significant for both measures ($P < 0.01$). The authors concluded that astragalus granules had benefit for myocardial contraction at the moderate dose and showed a dose-dependent trend (Yang et al., 2011).

Gastrointestinal Disorders: Chronic Viral Hepatitis

A 2001 systematic review to assess whether Chinese medicinal herbs were effective and safe for treating asymptomatic carriers of hepatitis B (HBV) selected three RCTs ($n = 307$) that met inclusion criteria; however, quality was noted to be poor. The authors noted that *Phyllanthus amarus* and astragalus showed no significant antiviral effect compared with placebo. Analysis of pooling eight RCTs with less than 3 months follow-up (so did not meet inclusion criteria) did not show a significant benefit of Chinese medicinal herbs on viral markers. Data on long-term clinical outcomes and quality of life were noted to be lacking (Liu et al., 2001).

A 48-week RCT in patients ($n = 92$) with liver fibrosis from chronic HBV investigated Astragalus-Polygonum Anti-Fibrosis Decoction (in which astragalus polysaccharide is a chief ingredient) compared with Jinshuibao capsule (cordyceps) in treating liver fibrosis of chronic HBV infection. Levels of serum hyaluronic acid, laminin, procollagen III, and collagen-IV declined more with the astragalus decoction than with the cordyceps capsule ($P < 0.01$). Liver functional tests (Tbili, ALT, A/G ratio, ferritin, and prealbumin) were improved more with astragalus than with cordyceps ($P < 0.01$). The authors concluded that Astragalus-Polygonum Anti-Fibrosis Decoction was more effective than the cordyceps preparation in treating liver fibrosis of chronic HBV infection and liver inflammation (Chen and Weng, 2000).

Renal Disorders: Diabetic Nephropathy, Lupus Nephritis, Nephrotic Syndrome

A 2019 updated systematic review to evaluate the efficacy and safety of astragalus as adjunctive therapy to conventional therapies for diabetic nephropathy found 66 studies ($n = 4785$) that met inclusion criteria. The quality of the included studies was low due to methodological shortfalls. Meta-analysis showed that additional use of astragalus injection was associated with a reduction in albuminuria (SMD: 2.05, $I^2 = 94\%$), proteinuria (SMD: 1.85, $I^2 = 95\%$), and serum creatinine levels ($-14.78\,\mu mol/L$, $I^2 = 97\%$) compared with conventional therapies alone. An antialbuminuria effect was also observed with oral astragalus in four RCTs (SMD: 1.27, $I^2 = 73\%$). The treatment effect of astragalus injection correlated with the baseline serum creatinine level. Astragalus and control groups did not differ in AEs. The authors concluded that low-quality evidence suggested that adjunctive astragalus when added to conventional therapies may be effective and tolerated for short-term reduction of albuminuria, proteinuria, and serum creatinine in patients with diabetic nephropathy, but that further research was indicated (Zhang et al., 2019).

A 2018 meta-analysis investigated the efficacy and safety of Chinese herbal medicine (with either astragalus or *Rehmannia*, both or neither) combined with ACE inhibitors or ARBs for treatment of incipient diabetic nephropathy. A total of 28 RCTs ($n = 2017$) were included. The results showed the urinary albumin excretion rate (UAER) was reduced significantly using Chinese herbal medicine with ACEI or ARB for treatment of diabetic nephropathy compared with ACEI or ARB alone, and reduction of the UAER was greatest with a combination of astragalus and *Rehmannia*. Serum creatinine levels were reduced significantly using Chinese herbal medicine combined with ACEI or ARB, and reduction of creatinine was greater with astragalus or *Rehmannia* than when neither herb was used. The authors recommended that use of astragalus and *Rehmannia* be utilized in stage III of diabetic nephropathy (Liu et al., 2013).

A 2017 systematic review assessed the correlation between astragalus and the different stages of diabetic nephropathy and the effect of astragalus on iNOS. Meta-analysis of astragalus injections on stages III and III–IV diabetic nephropathy and RCTs on other stages showed that astragalus had therapeutic effects on different stages of diabetic nephropathy. It also showed that astragalus had therapeutic effects on macrophages in different states by inducing normal macrophages in a resting state to generate NO and TNF-α via iNOS activation; inhibiting NO generation by normal lipopolysaccharide-activated macrophages; and enhancing NO generation by LPS-induced macrophages from patients with renal failure. The authors concluded that astragalus could regulate iNOS activity of macrophages in different states in vitro and the biphasic or antagonistic effects may explain why astragalus could be used to treat different stages of diabetic nephropathy (Li et al., 2011).

A 3-month RCT in patients ($n = 43$) with lupus nephritis and qi-deficiency syndrome (a TCM diagnosis) investigated IV infusion of 20 mL of astragalus QD for 12 days per month for 3 months plus cyclophosphamide 0.8 g/day for 3 months compared with cyclophosphamide alone. The decrease of active clinical symptom scores after the treatment in the astragalus group was greater than that in the control group ($P < 0.05$). Infections occurred in 4.35% of the astragalus group and 25% of the control group. The decrease of 24-h urine protein and CD8, and the increase of RBC count and serum albumin in the astragalus group were greater than those in the control group ($P < 0.05$). WBC count decreased less with astragalus than with control ($p < 0.05$). The authors concluded that high-dose astragalus injection used in conjunction with cyclophosphamide was more effective than cyclophosphamide alone in decreasing infection rate and urine protein and improving immune function in patients with lupus nephritis (Su et al., 2007).

A case report of a 77-year-old woman with nephrotic syndrome secondary to idiopathic membranous nephropathy was published. The patient had been treated with ACEI, ARB, cyclosporine A, and mycophenolate mofetil, without response. After more than 2 years of unremitting nephrosis, she began therapy with astragalus 15 g/day and there was a marked decrease in proteinuria. Nephrotic syndrome recurred after temporary cessation of astragalus. There was complete remission of nephrosis observed after reintroduction of astragalus. The case report author concluded that the clinical course of this patient suggested that astragalus may have beneficial effects in patients with idiopathic membranous nephropathy (Ahmed et al., 2007).

A 3-month open-label RCT in patients ($n = 32$) with chronic kidney disease (CKD) assessed efficacy of astragalus plus dong quai 30 g each QD plus their standard CKD treatment. Serum creatinine decreased 12%, eGFR increased 21%, and albumin increased 2.8% ($P < 0.05$ for all). TCM syndrome factor integrals also improved across the board. Serum creatinine decreased 5.2% and 20% in patients with and without qi-blood deficiency syndrome, respectively ($P < 0.05$). The authors concluded that this combination of astragalus and dong quai could improve the renal function of CKD patients, elevate their albumin levels, and ameliorate associated qi deficiency syndrome, blood deficiency syndrome, and yin deficiency syndrome, especially for CKD patients of qi blood deficiency syndrome (Li et al., 2014).

An RCT in patients ($n = 100$) with chronic nephritis compared a combination of astragalus plus *Rehmannia* with control (no treatment). The effective rate was 91% and 66.7% in the herbal and control groups, respectively ($P < 0.001$). The herbal combination was deemed most effective for proteinuria, hematuria, improvement and recovery of renal function edema, anemia, and anorexia. It showed no adverse effects on functions of liver, kidney, heart, and GI tract (Su et al., 1993).

Neurological Disorders: Stroke

A 12-week RCT in patients ($n = 78$) with acute hemorrhagic stroke compared astragalus 3 g TID for 14 days with placebo. With astragalus and placebo, respectively, the increases of Functional Independence Measure Scale scores from baseline were 24.5 and 11.9 by Week 4 and 34.7 and 23.9 by Week 12, respectively (both $P \leq 0.05$). In the astragalus group and placebo group, the increase of Glasgow Outcome Scale Score between baseline and Week 12 was 0.75 and 0.41, respectively ($P < 0.05$). The authors concluded that astragalus safely provided an advantage for acute hemorrhagic stroke patients, particularly for functional recovery of grooming and toileting, if treatment was started within 24 h of stroke onset (Chen et al., 2012).

Dermatological Disorders: Burns

A 3-week RCT in patients ($n = 80$) with burns compared astragalus saponin with standard burn treatment alone. Blood level of circulatory endothelial cells,

endothelin, NO, LDH and ALT were all significantly higher in the astragalus group than in the control group. The authors concluded that astragalus saponin had a protective effect on vascular endothelial cells from burn injuries and could improve the function of myocardial and liver cells and alleviate the general inflammatory response (Shi et al., 2001).

Immune Function

An 8-week RCT in patients ($n = 115$) with leukopenia compared astragalus 15 g BID with astragalus 5 g BID. Improvement in leukopenia occurred in 83% of the higher-dose group and 47% of the lower-dose groups, with a total effective rate of 65%, ($P < 0.01$). Average WBC counts after treatment were greater with the 15-g dose of astragalus ($P < 0.05$). The author concluded that astragalus was an effective drug in treating leukopenia in a dose-dependent manner (Weng, 1995).

A study in children ($n = 27$) with recurrent tonsillitis while in remission investigated the stimulation of peripheral mononuclear cells with phytohemagglutinin alone compared withs phytohemagglutinin plus astragalus. This was compared with phytohemagglutinin-stimulated mononuclear cells from children ($n = 21$) without recurrent tonsillitis. The IFN-γ level and the ratio of IFN-γ/IL-4 in the phytohemagglutinin-alone tonsillitis group were statistically lower than those in the nontonsillitis group ($P < 0.01$). The level of IFN-γ and the ratio of IFN-γ/IL-4 in the phytohemagglutinin-astragalus tonsillitis group were markedly higher than those in the phytohemagglutinin-alone tonsillitis group ($P < 0.01$) but were significantly lower than those in the nontonsillitis group ($P < 0.05$). There were no differences in the IL-4 level among the three groups. The authors concluded that a Th1 cell subset dysfunction may play an important role in the pathogenesis of recurrent tonsillitis and that astragalus may improve this dysfunction and be beneficial for recurrent tonsillitis. (Yang et al., 2006).

Infectious Disease: Tuberculosis

A 2-month RCT in older patients ($n = 76$) with pulmonary TB compared astragalus injection (20 mL in 500 mL D5W QD) with a control group while both groups underwent a standard antituberculosis regimen (for first treatment or for retreatment). Erythrocyte immune function in patients of both groups was lower than that in healthy subjects ($P < 0.01$). Rosette rate of RBC-C3b receptor in both groups was increased after treatment, but the increment was higher in the astragalus group than that in the control group ($P < 0.01$). With astragalus, the effective rate of focal absorption on X-ray was 85% and the sputum became negative in 80%. The authors concluded that astragalus elevated immunity in elderly pulmonary TB patients, thereby enhancing the therapeutic effect of treatment (Niu et al., 2001).

Oncologic Disorders

A 2019 systematic review to assess whether Aidi injection (a combination of astragalus, ginseng, eleuthero, and cantharidin) when added to paclitaxel-based chemotherapy in patients with NSCLC could safely improve tumor response and survival found 31 RCTs ($n = 2058$) that met inclusion criteria. The risk ratios were as follows: objective response ratio ($RR = 1.32$), disease control rate ($RR = 1.14$), QOL ($RR = 1.89$), neutropenia ($RR = 0.61$), thrombocytopenia ($RR = 0.62$), gastrointestinal toxicity ($RR = 0.59$), and liver injury ($RR = 0.52$). Compared with chemotherapy alone, all differences were statistically significant. Subgroup analysis showed that only with the paclitaxel-cisplatin therapy did Aidi injection increase the objective response rate and disease control rate. The results were found to be robust. None of the trials reported the overall survival or progression-free survival. The quality of evidence was moderate. The authors concluded that Aidi injection plus paclitaxel-based chemotherapy, particularly paclitaxel-cisplatin therapy, could significantly improve clinical efficacy and QOL for patients with stage III/IV NSCLC, reducing the risk of hematotoxicity, gastrointestinal toxicity, and liver injury (Xiao et al., 2019).

A 2016 systematic review again looked at studies of various astragalus-based Chinese medicines combined with platinum-based chemotherapy in the treatment of lung cancer in Asia, with and without prescription based on syndrome differentiation, as first-line treatment for advanced NSCLC. The authors included 17 RCTs ($n = 1552$) that met inclusion criteria. Compared with platinum-based chemotherapy alone, the addition of astragalus-based TCM to chemotherapy was associated with an increased overall survival (HR = 0.61; $P = 0.011$); 1-year (RR = 0.73; $P < 0.001$); 2-year (RR = 0.334; $P < 0.001$); and 3-year survival rates (RR = 0.30; $P < 0.001$); performance status (RR = 0.43; $P < 0.001$); and tumor overall response rate (RR = 0.7982; $P < 0.001$). Subgroup analyses indicated that astragalus herbal formulae given based on syndrome differentiation were more effective than astragalus-based oral and injection patent medicines (supporting the individualization of therapy). Side effects including anemia, neutropenia, thrombocytopenia, fatigue, poor appetite, nausea, and vomiting were significantly more frequent with platinum-based chemotherapy alone than when platinum-based chemotherapy was combined with astragalus-based TCM. The authors concluded that astragalus-based Chinese herbal therapy, especially when based on syndrome differentiation, was associated with increased efficacy of platinum-based chemotherapy and decreased platinum-derived toxicities for patients with advanced NSCLC (Wang et al., 2016).

A 2010 systematic review to assess the efficacy of astragalus-based herbal preparations in treatment of NSCLC included 65 RCTs ($n = 4751$). All trials included the herbal preparations plus platinum-based chemotherapy compared with chemotherapy alone. The authors found from pooling seven studies ($n = 529$), that the RR was 0.54 ($P \leq 0.0001$) for survival at 6 months with astragalus. Pooling 20 trials ($n = 1520$) on survival at 12 months, the authors found a RR of 0.65 ($P \leq 0.0001$) and noted that the effect was consistent at 24 and 36 months. Pooling data from 57 trials for composite endpoint of any tumor treatment response revealed a RR of 1.35 in favor of addition of herb ($P \leq 0.0001$). The authors concluded that there was a large treatment effect of adding astragalus-based herbal treatment to standard chemotherapy regimens (Dugoua et al., 2010).

A four-cycle RCT in patients ($n = 120$) with malignant tumors studied chemotherapy alone compared with chemotherapy plus astragalus injection 20 mL in 250 mL NS QD for 21 days per course over four successive courses. Compared with the control group, the astragalus group showed a lower incidence of progression and a lesser decrease of WBC and platelet counts ($P < 0.05$). CD8 was lowered ($P < 0.05$), CD4/CD8 ratio was increased ($P < 0.01$), IgG and IgM levels were increased ($P < 0.05$), and Karnofsky scores rose more with astragalus than with control. The authors concluded that astragalus injection added to chemotherapy could inhibit tumor development, decrease toxic-adverse effects of chemotherapy, elevate immune function, and improve quality of life in cancer patients (Duan and Wang, 2002).

A concurrent chemoradiotherapy (CCRT) phase II RCT in patients ($n=17$) with advanced head and neck squamous cell carcinoma (HNSCC) compared injection of astragalus polysaccharides (PG2) with placebo, each given three times per week in parallel with CCRT injection to assess impact on cancer therapy. The chemotherapy regimen included 50 mg/m^2 cisplatin every 2 weeks with daily tegafur-uracil (300 mg/m^2) and leucovorin (60 mg/day). During CCRT, severe treatment-associated AEs were less frequent in the astragalus group than in the placebo group. QOL had fewer fluctuations from baseline during CCRT in the astragalus group with a significant difference in pain, appetite loss, and social eating behavior as compared with the placebo group. The tumor response, disease-specific survival, and overall survival did not differ between the two groups. The authors concluded that PG2 injection had an excellent safety profile and potential to improve the deterioration in QOL and AEs associated with active anticancer treatment among patients with advanced pharyngeal or laryngeal HNSCC under CCRT. Further research was recommended (Hsieh et al., 2020).

ACTIVE CONSTITUENTS

Root

- Carbohydrates
  - Polysaccharides: (hypoglycemiant, immunostimulant, antibone loss)
- Phenolic compounds
  - Flavonoids (antiinflammatory, antioxidant, cardioprotective, hepatoprotective, renoprotective, immunostimulant, apoptotic, anticancer): isoliquiritigenin, liquiritigenin, rutin (antioxidant, antiinflammatory, antidiabetic, nephroprotective, antiosteoporotic, antispasmodic, neuroprotective, antianxiety), quercetin (antiinflammatory, antioxidant, hypotensive, antidiabetic, antispasmodic, neuroprotective, XO inhibition, antibacterial, anticancer)
  - Isoflavonoids (phytoestrogenic): calycosin (antimelanin), formononetin, op, calycosin-

7-Obeta-D-glucoside, trigonosides I–III, biochanin A (hypoglycemiant, stimulate NK cell activity, antioxidant, apoptotic, antiviral)
  - Isoflavone glycosides: ononin (apoptotic, anticancer, phytoestrogen)
- Terpenes
  - Triterpenoid saponins: astragalosides I–IV (hypoglycemiant, antiischemic, increase GH)
- Telomerase activator 65: (lengthens telomeres)

ASTRAGALUS COMMONLY USED PREPARATIONS AND DOSAGE (FOR ADULTS UNLESS OTHERWISE SPECIFIED)

The following are examples of some available formulations and ranges of dosing for commercial herbal products. See Part III Introduction "How to prescribe medicinal herbs" for further guidance on herbal advising and prescribing.

Dried Root

- Decoction: 2–4 tsp. per cup TID.
- Liquid extract: (1:1.5, 40-50%) 1-2 mL TID
- Tincture: (1:5, 30%–40%) 2–8 mL TID.
- Capsule or tablet of powdered root extract: 1–5 g BID-TID.
- Capsule or tablet of standardized root extract (standardized for polysaccharides or to 0.5% astragalosides): 500 mg QD-TID.
- Injectable forms available in Asia.

SAFETY AND PRECAUTION

Side Effects

At low-to-moderate doses, astragalus has few side effects.

Toxicity

No toxicity at normally recommended doses. However, it is a known toxic plant (primarily the seeds) for livestock. Up to 100 g/kg of astragalus produced no serious side effects in rats.

Pregnancy and Lactation

Insufficient human safety data (although animal studies failed to show teratogenicity at toxic doses).

Disease Interactions

Uncertain effect on autoimmune diseases; use with caution. One study showed it helped with an RA model in rats.

Drug Interactions

- CYP: Inhibits CYP3A4.
- Use with caution with lithium due to diuretic effects.
- Use with caution with immunosuppressants (may reverse efficacy).

REFERENCES

Ahmed MS, Hou SH, Battaglia MC, Picken MM, Leehey DJ. Treatment of idiopathic membranous nephropathy with the herb Astragalus membranaceus. Am J Kidney Dis 2007 Dec;50(6):1028–32.

Chen H, Weng L. Comparison on efficacy in treating liver fibrosis of chronic hepatitis B between Astragalus Polygonum anti-fibrosis decoction and jinshuibao capsule. Zhongguo Zhong Xi Yi Jie He Za Zhi 2000 Apr;20(4):255–7.

Chen CC, Lee HC, Chang J, et al. Chinese herb Astragalus membranaceus enhances recovery of hemorrhagic stroke: double-blind, placebo-controlled, randomized study. Evid Based Complement Alternat Med 2012;2012:708452.

Duan P, Wang ZM. Clinical study on effect of Astragalus in efficacy enhancing and toxicity reducing of chemotherapy in patients of malignant tumor. Zhongguo Zhong Xi Yi Jie He Za Zhi 2002;22(7):515–7.

Dugoua JJ, Wu P, Seely D, Eyawo O, Mills E. Astragalus-containing Chinese herbal combinations for advanced non-small-cell lung cancer: a meta-analysis of 65 clinical trials enrolling 4751 patients. Lung Cancer (Auckl). 2010 Jul 8;1:85–100.

Jacques DJ, Wu P, Seely D, Eyawo O, Mills E. Astragalus-containing Chinese herbal combinations for advanced non-small-cell lung cancer: a meta-analysis of 65 clinical trials enrolling 4751 patients. Lung Cancer (Auckl) 2010;1:85–100.

Hsieh C, Lin C, Hsu C, et al. Incorporation of Astragalus polysaccharides injection during concurrent chemoradiotherapy in advanced pharyngeal or laryngeal squamous cell carcinoma: preliminary experience of a phase II double-blind, randomized trial. J Cancer Res Clin Oncol 2020 Jan;146(1):33–41.

Li S, Yin XX, Su T, et al. Therapeutic effect of Astragalus and Angelica mixture on the renal function and TCM syndrome factors in treating stage 3 and 4 chronic kidney disease patients. Zhongguo Zhong Xi Yi Jie He Za Zhi 2014 Jul;34(7):780–5.

Li M, Wang W, Xue J, Gu Y, Lin S. Meta-analysis of the clinical value of Astragalus membranaceus in diabetic nephropathy. J Ethnopharmacol 2011;133(2):412–9.

Liu JP, McIntosh H, Lin H. Chinese medicinal herbs for asymptomatic carriers of hepatitis B virus infection. Cochrane Database Syst Rev 2001;2001(2), CD002231.

Liu Y, Zhou L, Xiao Y, Luo R, Zhao XS. The efficacy of ACEI or ARB combination with Astragalus injection on early-stage diabetic nephropathy: a meta-analysis. J Trop Med 2013;13(5):611–5.

Mao SP, Cheng KL, Zhou YF. Modulatory effect of Astragalus membranaceus on Th1/Th2 cytokine in patients with herpes simplex keratitis. Zhongguo Zhong Xi Yi Jie He Za Zhi 2004;24(2):121–3.

Matkovic Z, Zivkovic V, Korica M, et al. Efficacy and safety of Astragalus membranaceus in the treatment of patients with seasonal allergic rhinitis. Phytother Res 2010;24:175–81.

Niu HR, Lai ZH, Yuan L. Observation on effect of supplementary treatment by Astragalus injection in treating senile pulmonary tuberculosis patients. Zhongguo Zhong Xi Yi Jie He Za Zhi 2001 May;21(5):349–50.

Piao YL, Liang XC. Astragalus membranaceus injection combined with conventional treatment for viral myocarditis: a systematic review of randomized controlled trials. Chin J Integr Med 2014 Oct;20(10):787–91.

Shi FS, Yang ZG, Di GP. Effect of Astragalus saponin on vascular endothelial cell and its function in burn patients. Zhongguo Zhong Xi Yi Jie He Za Zhi 2001 Oct;21(10):750–1.

Su L, Mao JC, Gu JH. Effect of intravenous drip infusion of cyclophosphamide with high-dose Astragalus injection in treating lupus nephritis. Zhong Xi Yi Jie He Xue Bao 2007 May;5(3):272–5.

Su ZZ, He YY, Chen G. Clinical and experimentalstudyon effects of man-shen-ling oral liquid in the treatment of 100 cases of chronic nephritis. Zhongguo Zhong Xi Yi Jie He Za Zhi 1993 May;13(5):269–72 [259-60].

Wang SF, Wang Q, Jiao LJ, Huang YL, Garfield D, Zhang J, Xu L. Astragalus-containing traditional chinese medicine, with and without prescription based on syndrome differentiation, combined with chemotherapy for advanced non-small-cell lung cancer: a systemic review and meta-analysis. Curr Oncol. 2016;23(3): e188–95.

Weng XS. Treatmentof leucopenia with pure Astragalus preparation- -an analysis of 115 leucopenic cases. Zhongguo Zhong Xi Yi Jie He Za Zhi 1995 Aug;15(8):462–4.

Xiao Z, Wang C, Zhou M, et al. Clinical efficacy and safety of Aidi injection plus paclitaxel-based chemotherapy for advanced non-small cell lung cancer: a meta-analysis of 31 randomized controlledtrialsfollowing the PRISMA guidelines. J Ethnopharmacol 2019 Jan 10;228:110–22.

Yang Y, Wang LD, Chen ZB. Effects of astragalus membranaceus on TH cell subset function in children with recurrent tonsillitis. Zhongguo Dang Dai Er Ke Za Zhi 2006 Oct;8(5):376–8.

Yang QY, Lu S, Sun HR. Clinical effect of Astragalus granule of different dosages on quality of life in patients with chronic heart failure. Chin J Integr Med 2011;17(2):146–9.

Zhang JG, Gao DS, Wei GH. Clinical study on effect of Astragalus injection on left ventricular remodeling and left ventricular function in patients with acute myocardial infarction. Zhongguo Zhong Xi Yi Jie He Za Zhi 2002 May;22(5):346–8.

Zhang L, Shergis J, Yang L, et al. Astragalus membranaceus (Huang Qi) as adjunctive therapy for diabetic kidney disease: an updated systematic review and meta-analysis. J Ethnopharmacol 2019 Jul 15;239:111921.

Zhou S, Shao W, Zhang W. Clinical study of Astragalus injection plus ligustrazine in protecting myocardial ischemia reperfusion injury. Zhongguo Zhong Xi Yi Jie He Za Zhi 2000 Jul;20(7):504–7.

Zhou ZL, Yu P, Lin D. Studyon effect of Astragalus injection in treating congestive heart failure. Zhongguo Zhong Xi Yi Jie He Za Zhi 2001 Oct;21(10):747–9.

28

BACOPA (*BACOPA MONNIERI*)
Leaf

GENERAL OVERVIEW

Bacopa is one of the many useful herbs from India where it is known as *Brāhmī ghṛtam*. It is best known for its nootropic effects but also has adaptogenic and anti-anxiety properties. Based on its actions identified in preclinical research, bacopa should be protective against neurodegenerative diseases like Alzheimer's disease and Parkinson's disease, but long-term studies are lacking.

Bacopa appears to improve cognition in young and old alike. It has been shown to enhance attention, verbal learning, memory acquisition, and delayed recall. Studies have thus far been small, but systematic reviews have been generally supportive of the benefits. Anxiety and irritable bowel syndrome may also improve with bacopa. Unfortunately, many of the studies have used herbal combinations that contain bacopa as well as other herbs, so clear attribution of efficacy to bacopa is not possible.

Clinical research indicates that bacopa, alone or in combination formulas, may be beneficial for hepatic encephalopathy, diarrhea-predominant irritable bowel syndrome, cognitive impairment, dementia, anxiety, attention-deficit/hyperactivity disorder, and cognitive performance.

IN VITRO AND ANIMAL RESEARCH

Bacopa has been found to have adaptogenic, anticancer, antioxidant, anti-inflammatory, astringent, cardiotonic, diuretic, mildly laxative, anxiolytic, antidepressant, anticonvulsant, sedative, hepatoprotective, antimicrobial,

vasoconstrictive, and vulnerary (ulcer-healing) properties. It is reported to be dopaminergic, serotonergic, GABAergic, cholinergic, nootropic, and neuroprotective. The dopamine effects appear to be amphoteric, preventing dopamine depletion with chronic stress or toxicity, but also preventing dopamine spikes with addictive drugs and caffeine. Its anxiolytic and anticonvulsant activities appear to be both through GABA activity and upregulation of a presynaptic glutamate receptor. A study in rats showed that a standardized extract (bacoside A content $25.5\% \pm 0.8\%$) of bacopa at doses of 10 and 20 mg/kg had comparable anxiolytic effects to lorazepam at a dose of 0.5 mg/kg, without producing any motor deficit (Bhattacharya et al., 1998).

The neuroprotective antioxidant and anti-inflammatory activities are focused on the hippocampus, striatum, and frontal lobe. Its hepatoprotective effect is also due to its antioxidant and anti-inflammatory properties. It has been shown to heal gastric ulcers through increasing prostaglandin E and prostacyclin as well as having antimicrobial effects against *Helicobacter pylori*.

HUMAN RESEARCH

Gastrointestinal Disorders: Liver Disease

A 5-week RCT of patients ($n = 66$) with Child-Pugh B liver cirrhosis and stage 0–2 hepatic encephalopathy investigated standard treatment alone compared with standard treatment plus a multi-herbal cognitive formula containing bacopa (gingko, cat's claw, gotu kola, and rosemary (CognoBlend) 2 capsules BID for effects) on cognition. The group receiving the herbal formula showed significant improvement of clinical signs, psychometric tests, electroencephalography, and serum biochemistry compared with the group receiving standard therapy alone (Kaziulin, 2006).

Gastrointestinal Disorders: Irritable Bowel Syndrome

A 6-week RCT in patients ($n = 169$) with irritable bowel syndrome (IBS) evaluated an Ayurvedic formula containing bacopa and *Aegle marmelos correa* compared with standard therapy (clidinium bromide, chlordiazepoxide, and isaphaghulla) and with placebo. Efficacy with the Ayurvedic preparation was 64.9%, with standard therapy was 78.3%, and with placebo was 32.7%. The Ayurvedic therapy was particularly beneficial in the diarrhea-predominant form of IBS compared with placebo. The standard therapy was more useful in the painful form of IBS compared with placebo and the Ayurvedic preparation. However, long-term followup (longer than 6 months) showed that both forms of therapy were no better than placebo in limiting relapse (Yadav et al., 1989).

Neurological Disorders: Cognitive Impairment and Dementia

A 12-month RCT in healthy patients ($n = 109$) and patients with AD ($n = 123$) aged 60–75 years investigated a polyherbal test formulation (bacopa, sea buckthorn, and *Dioscorea*) 500 mg BID compared with donepezil 10 mg BID. The test formulation was determined to be effective in improving cognitive functions in AD patients when compared with the donepezil-treated group, as determined by the digital symbol substitution (39 vs 36; $P = 0.0001$), immediate word recall (3.6 vs 2.8; $P < 0.0001$), and attention span (4.9 vs 4.4; $P = 0.0208$), FAQ (11.8 vs 9.8; $P < 0.0001$) and depression (16.3 vs 21.0; $P < 0.0001$) scores. No significant differences were observed in MMSE and delayed word recall scores. Homocysteine, CRP, TNF-α, SOD, and GSH levels were also significantly lower in the herbal group ($P < 0.0001$, < 0.0001; < 0.001, $= 0.0013$, < 0.0001, respectively). The authors concluded that there was therapeutic potential for this polyherbal formulation in the management and treatment of AD (Sadhu et al., 2014).

A 16-week RCT in patients with age-associated memory impairment without any evidence of dementia or psychiatric disorder compared bacopa standardized extract 125 mg BID with placebo for 12 weeks followed by 4 weeks of placebo in both groups. Bacopa produced significant improvement in mental control, logical memory, and paired associated learning during the 12-week drug therapy. The authors concluded that bacopa was effective in patients with age-associated memory impairment (Raghav et al., 2006).

A 2-month RCT in elderly patients ($n = 30$) with MMSE scores 20–27 and self-perceived cognitive decline compared a combination of bacopa, L-theanine, saffron, copper, B vitamins, and vitamin D with placebo. MMSE and Perceived Stress Questionnaire Index significantly improved with the herbal combination compared with both baseline and placebo. Both groups experienced a significant improvement in the Self-rating Depression Scale scores. The authors concluded that this herbal combination produced significant improvement in the cognitive functions tested (Cicero et al., 2016).

A 60-day prospective cohort, noncomparative, multicenter trial of older subjects ($n = 104$) aged 71.2 years assessed the effects of one tablet daily of a combination of bacopa, astaxanthin, phosphatidylserine, and vitamin E on pre- and post-supplementation MMSE, ADAS-cog, and clock drawing tests. Total ADAS-cog scores improved from 13.7 at baseline to 9.7 on day 60 with greatest improvements in memory tasks ($P < 0.001$), and the clock drawing test scores improved from 8.5 to 9.1 ($P < 0.001$). Perceived efficacy was rated as excellent or good by 62% of study subjects. The tested compound was well tolerated. The authors concluded that the combination formula showed potential for counteracting cognitive impairment in subjects with mild cognitive impairment and warranted further investigation in adequately controlled, longerterm studies (Zanotta et al., 2014).

Psychiatric Disorders: Anxiety

A 2013 systematic review looking at plants that had both pre-clinical and clinical evidence for anti-anxiety effects found 21 plants with human clinical trial evidence. Support for efficacy identified several herbs with efficacy for anxiety spectrum disorders including kava, lemon balm, chamomile, ginkgo, skullcap, milk thistle, passionflower, ashwagandha, rhiodola, echinacea, *Galphimia glauca, Centella asiatica,* and *Echium amooenum*. Acute anxiolytic activity was found for passionflower, sage, gotu kola, lemon balm, and bergamot. The review also specifically found that bacopa showed anxiolytic effects in people with cognitive decline (Sarris et al., 2013).

A 2006 systematic review looking at plants that had evidence for anti-anxiety effects found seven studies and one systematic review involving eight plants with human clinical trial evidence. Support for efficacy identified kava and bacopa, with only kava having replicated data (Ernst, 2006).

An acutely dosed crossover RCT tested the anti-anxiety effects in normal healthy participants ($n = 17$) given bacopa extract 320 mg, 640 mg, or placebo. The multi-tasking framework test was given at baseline, then 1 h and 2 h after bacopa dosing, separated by a 7-day washout period. Change from baseline scores indicated positive cognitive effects following bacopa consumption on the Letter Search and Stroop tasks. There were also some positive mood effects and reductions in cortisol levels, pointing to a physiological mechanism for stress reduction associated with bacopa consumption. The authors concluded that bacopa given acutely produced some adaptogenic and nootropic effects that needed to be replicated in a larger sample and in isolation from stressful cognitive tests to quantify the magnitude of these effects (Benson et al., 2014).

A 12-week RCT in healthy urban adults ($n = 72$) compared bacopa 450 mg/day with placebo on learning and memory, information processing and anxiety. The study found no significant differences between the two groups on any of the cognitive measures. However, there was a trend for lower state anxiety in the bacopa group compared with the placebo group. The authors concluded that the results of the study did not replicate findings of some of the earlier studies which had found improvement both on cognitive parameters and a reduction of anxiety scores (Sathyanarayanan et al., 2013).

Psychiatric Disorders: Attention-Deficit/Hyperactivity Disorder

A pilot study in children ($n = 10$) with ADHD investigated the effect of bacopa. It showed a 66% decrease in total ADHD score. The pilot study was followed by a therapeutic confirmatory study in children ($n = 27$) with ADHD. Bacopa was compared with methylphe-

nidate. The effect on ADHD symptoms was assessed using primarily the Dupaul ADHD rating scale. The study showed a 16% improvement with bacopa, which was similar to methylphenidate. The authors concluded that the study adequately demonstrated the efficacy and safety of bacopa in ADHD (Bhalerao et al., 2013).

A 6-month open-label study of children ($n = 31$) ages 6–12 years with ADHD investigated the effects of a standardized bacopa extract 225 mg/day. The Parent Rating Scale was used to assess the ADHD symptom scores at baseline and at 6 months. The extract significantly reduced the subtest scores of ADHD symptoms, except for social problems. The attention-deficit symptoms were reduced in 85% of children, the restlessness symptoms were reduced in 93%, and improvement in self-control was observed in 89% of the children. Symptom scores for learning problems, impulsivity, and psychiatric problems were reduced in 78%, 67%, and 52% of children, respectively. It was observed that 74% of the children exhibited up to a 20% reduction, while 26% of children showed between a 21% and a 50% reduction in total subtest scores. The authors concluded that bacopa standardized extract was found to be effective in alleviating the symptoms of ADHD and was well tolerated by the children (Dave et al., 2014).

A 4-month RCT in children ($n = 120$) with newly diagnosed ADHD compared a polyherbal formula containing ashwagandha, bacopa, lemon balm, *Paeoniae alba*, *Centella asiatica*, and *Spirulina platensis* with placebo. The treatment group showed significant improvement in the four subscales and overall TOVA scores, compared with no improvement in the control group. The authors concluded that the polyherbal formula improved attention, cognition, and impulse control in children with ADHD (Katz et al., 2010).

Psychological Disorders: Cognitive Performance

A 2014 systematic review of bacopa for cognitive enhancement found nine RCTs ($n = 518$) that met inclusion criteria. Meta-analysis of 437 eligible subjects showed improved cognition by shortened Trail B test (-17.9 ms; $P < 0.001$) and decreased choice reaction time (10.6 ms; $P < 0.001$). This suggested to the authors that bacopa had the potential to improve cognition, particularly speed of attention (Kongkeaw et al., 2014).

A 2013 systematic review searched to capture clinical studies on the neurocognitive effects of modafinil, ginseng, and bacopa. The highest effect sizes (Cohen's d) for cognitive outcomes were 0.77 for modafinil (visuospatial memory accuracy), 0.86 for ginseng (simple reaction time), and 0.95 for bacopa (delayed word recall). These data indicated to the authors that neurocognitive enhancement from well-characterized nutraceuticals could produce cognition-enhancing effects of similar magnitude to those of pharmaceutical interventions (Neale et al., 2013).

A 2012 systematic review was performed on the cognitive-enhancing effects of bacopa. Subjects studied were adult humans without dementia or significant cognitive impairment. Six studies met the final inclusion criteria and were included in review. Across trials, three different bacopa extracts were used at dosages of 300–450 mg per day. Bacopa improved performance on 9 of 17 tests in the domain of memory-free recall. There was little evidence of enhancement in any other cognitive domains. The authors concluded that there was some evidence to suggest that bacopa improved memory-free recall. Evidence for enhancement in other cognitive abilities was lacking perhaps due to inconsistent measures employed by studies across these cognitive domains. Further research was warranted (Pase et al., 2012)

A 12-week RCT in healthy elderly subjects ($n = 98$) compared bacopa 300 mg/day with placebo for neuropsychologic performance. Bacopa significantly improved verbal learning, memory acquisition, and delayed recall as measured by the Rey Auditory Verbal Learning Test: trial a4 ($P = 0.000$), trial a5 ($P = 0.016$); trial a6 ($P = 0.000$); trial a7 (delayed recall) ($P = 0.001$); total learning ($P = 0.011$); and retroactive interference ($P = 0.048$). Complex Figure Test, Memory Complaint Questionnaire, and Trail Making Test scores improved, but group differences were not significant. Bacopa compared with placebo caused gastrointestinal tract side effects of increased stool frequency, abdominal cramps, and nausea. The authors concluded that bacopa improved memory acquisition and retention in healthy older adults (Morgan and Stevens, 2010).

A 12-week RCT involving healthy elderly subjects ($n = 60$) compared a standardized bacopa extract at 300 or 600 mg with placebo given daily for effects on attention, cognitive processing, working memory, and cholinergic and monoaminergic functions. All assessments were performed before treatment, every four weeks throughout the study period, and at four weeks after the cessation of intervention. The bacopa-treated group showed improved working memory together with a decrease in both N100 and P300 latencies of event-related potential. Suppression of plasma AChE activity was also observed. The authors concluded that bacopa could possibly improve attention, cognitive processing, and working memory partly via the suppression of AChE activity (Peth-Nui et al., 2012).

A 12-week RCT in healthy elderly participants ($n = 54$) compared bacopa 300 mg/day with placebo for cognitive effects. Bacopa resulted in enhanced Rey Auditory Verbal Learning Test delayed word recall memory scores relative to placebo. Stroop results were similarly significant, with bacopa improving and placebo unchanged. Center for Epidemiologic Studies Depression scale scores, combined state plus trait anxiety scores, and heart rate decreased over time with bacopa, but increased with placebo. No effects were found on the Divided Attention Task, Wechsler Adult Intelligence Scale digit task, mood, or blood pressure. The dose was well tolerated, and side effects were similar, occurring in 9 subjects with bacopa and 10 subjects with placebo, primarily GI disturbance. The authors concluded that the study provided further evidence that bacopa had potential for safely enhancing cognitive performance in the elderly (Calabrese et al., 2008).

A 3-month RCT in healthy middle-aged adults ($n = 76$) compared bacopa with placebo for effects on various memory functions and levels of anxiety. The results showed a significant improvement with bacopa on a test for the retention of new information. Six-week post-treatment follow-up tests showed that the rate of learning was unaffected, suggesting that bacopa decreased the rate of forgetting newly acquired information. Tasks assessing attention, verbal and visual short-term memory, and the retrieval of pre-experimental knowledge were unaffected (Roodenrys et al., 2002).

A repeat-dosing crossover RCT in normal healthy volunteers ($n = 24$) who completed a cognitively demanding series of tests compared bacopa 320 mg with bacopa 640 mg for impact on cognitive performance, mood, and cardiovascular parameters. Change from baseline scores improved with the 320-mg dose of bacopa at the first, second, and fourth repetition post-dosing on the Cognitive Demand Battery. The treatments had no effect on cardiovascular activity or attenuation of task-induced ratings of stress and fatigue (Downey et al., 2013).

A 90-day RCT in healthy volunteers ($n = 107$) compared bacopa 150 mg BID with placebo for cognitive effects. The Cognitive Drug Research cognitive assessment system showed a significantly improved performance on the working memory accuracy with bacopa. The number of false positives recorded in the Rapid Visual Information Processing Task was also reduced with bacopa. The authors concluded that the findings supported other studies demonstrating cognitive enhancing effects in healthy humans after 90 days of bacopa (Stough et al., 2008).

A six-week RCT to evaluate the efficacy of bacopa on memory of medical students ($n = 60$) compared bacopa standardized extract 150 mg BID with placebo. Statistically significant improvement was seen in the tests relating to the cognitive functions with use of bacopa. Blood biochemistry also showed a significant increase in serum calcium levels (still within normal range) (Kumar et al., 2016).

A 4-month RCT in children ($n = 300$) studied a supplementation of bacopa extract plus multiple micronutrients compared with an isocaloric equivalent (control) BID. Cognitive function as assessed by the Cambridge Neuropsychological Automated Test Battery showed that the treatment beverage produced a significant improvement in spatial working memory on day 60 but not on day 121 compared with the control beverage ($P < 0.05$). The other cognitive measures did not differ between groups (Mitra-Ganguli et al., 2017).

ACTIVE CONSTITUENTS

- Phenolic compounds
  - Flavonoids: glucuronyl-7-apigenin, glucuronyl-7-luteolin, luteolin-7-glucoside, luteolin
- Terpenes
  - Triterpenes: betulic acid, bacosine, B-sitosterol, stigmastanol, and stigmasterol
  - Saponins: D-mannitol, hersaponin acid A, monnierin, bacogenins, bacosides, bacopasides

I & II (antidepressant), bacopasaponins (antidepressant), bacoside A and B5-9 (neuroprotective, antibacterial, anti-inflammatory)
- Alkaloids: brahmine, herpestine

BACOPA COMMONLY USED PREPARATIONS AND DOSAGE (FOR ADULTS UNLESS OTHERWISE SPECIFIED)

The following are examples of some available formulations and ranges of dosing for commercial herbal products. See Part III Introduction "How to prescribe medicinal herbs" for further guidance on herbal advising and prescribing.
Leaf

- Fluid extract (1:2): 1–3 mL TID
- Powdered leaf: 1 g in ghee (clarified butter) TID
- Standardized powdered leaf extract (standardized to 50% bacosides): 450 mg (1/6 tsp) QD-BID
- Concentrated powdered leaf (10:1) extract: 50 mg QD-TID
- Capsule or tablet of powdered leaf extract: 450 mg QD-TID
- Capsule or tablet of standardized extract (standardized to 20%–55% bacosides): 150–300 mg BID

Bacopa should be taken with a fatty meal to enhance absorption of the fat-soluble bacoside.

As is the case with SSRIs and SNRIs, bacopa needs to be given time to work, typically 6–12 weeks. However, the anti-anxiety effect appears to be rapid and as effective as lorazepam in some research.

SAFETY AND PRECAUTION

Side Effects

Generally, bacopa is well tolerated. However, it may induce nausea and abdominal cramping if taken on an empty stomach. It may adversely affect sperm and increase T4 at excessively high doses.

Toxicity

One study using 250 mg/kg bodyweight in male mice for 56 days noted no significant health effects, but did notice impaired sperm function, which was reversed 56 days after cessation. A single oral administration at 5000 mg/kg did not cause any serious undesirable effects in rats. Bacopa extract at doses of 30, 60, 300, and 1500 mg/kg given for 270 days did not produce any toxicity in rats. An oral dose of 200 mg/kg daily for 15 days resulted in a 42% increase in serum T4 hormone concentration.

Pregnancy and Lactation

Insufficient human safety data.

Disease Interactions

None reported.

Drug Interactions

None reported.

REFERENCES

Benson S, Downey LA, Stough C, Wetherell M, Zangara A, Scholey A. An acute, double-blind, placebo-controlled crossover study of 320 mg and 640 mg doses of Bacopa monnieri (CDRI 08) on multitasking stress reactivity and mood. Phytother Res 2014;28(4):551–9.

Bhalerao S, Munshi R, Nesari T, Shah H. Evaluation of Brāhmī ghṛtam in children suffering from attention deficit hyperactivity disorder. Anc Sci Life 2013;33(2):123–30.

Bhattacharya SK, Ghosal S. Anxiolytic activity of a standardized extract of Bacopa monniera: an experimental study. Phytomedicine 1998;5(2):77–82.

Calabrese C, Gregory WL, Leo M, Kraemer D, Bone K, Oken B. Effects of a standardized Bacopa monnieri extract on cognitive performance, anxiety, and depression in the elderly: a randomized, double-blind, placebo-controlled trial. J Altern Complement Med 2008;14(6):707–13.

Cicero A, Bove M, Colletti A, et al. Short-term impact of a combined nutraceutical on cognitive function, perceived stress and depression in young elderly with cognitive impairment: a pilot, double-blind, randomized clinical trial. J Prev Alz Dis 2016;4:12–5.

Dave UP, Dingankar SR, Saxena VS, et al. An open-label study to elucidate the effects of standardized Bacopa monnieri extract in the management of symptoms of attention-deficit hyperactivity disorder in children. Adv Mind Body Med 2014;28(2):10–5.

Downey LA, et al. An acute, double-blind, placebo-controlled crossover study of 320mg and 640mg doses of a special extract of Bacopa monnieri (CDRI 08) on sustained cognitive performance. Phytother Res 2013;27(9):1407–13.

Ernst E. Herbal remedies for anxiety—a systematic review of controlled clinical trials. Phytomedicine 2006;13(3):205–8.

Katz M, et al. A compound herbal preparation (CHP) in the treatment of children with ADHD: a randomized controlled trial. J Atten Disord 2010;14(3):281–91.

Kaziulin AN, Petukhov AB, Kucheriavyĭ IA. Efficiency of includes of bioactive substances in diet of patient with hepatic encephalopathy. Vopr Pitan 2006;75(2):40–4.

Kongkeaw C, Dilokthornsakul P, Thanarangsarit P, Limpeanchob N, Norman Scholfield C. Meta-analysis of randomized

controlled trials on cognitive effects of Bacopa monnieri extract. J Ethnopharmacol 2014;151(1):528–35.

Kumar N, Abichandani LG, Thawani V, Gharpure KJ, Naidu MU, Venkat RG. Efficacy of standardized extract of Bacopa monnieri (Bacognize®) on cognitive functions of medical students: a six-week, randomized placebo-controlled trial. Evid Based Complement Alternat Med 2016;4103423.

Mitra-Ganguli T, Kalita S, Bhushan S, et al. A randomized, double-blind study assessing changes in cognitive function in Indian school children receiving a combination of Bacopa monnieri and micronutrient supplementation vs placebo. Front Pharmacol 2017;8:678.

Morgan A, Stevens J. Does Bacopa monnieri improve memory performance in older persons? Results of a randomized, placebo-controlled, double-blind trial. J Altern Complement Med 2010 Jul;16(7):753–9.

Neale C, Camfield D, Reay J, Stough C, Scholey A. Cognitive effects of 2 nutraceuticals Ginseng and Bacopa benchmarked against modafinil: a review and comparison of effect sizes. Br J Clin Pharmacol 2013;75(3):728–37.

Pase MP, Kean J, Sarris J, Neale C, Scholey AB, Stough C. The cognitive-enhancing effects of Bacopa monnieri: a systematic review of randomized, controlled human clinical trials. J Altern Complement Med 2012;18(7):647–52.

Peth-Nui T, Wattanathorn J, Muchimapura S, et al. Effects of 12-week Bacopa monnieri consumption on attention, cognitive processing, working memory, and functions of both cholinergic and monoaminergic systems in healthy elderly volunteers. Evid Based Complement Alternat Med 2012;606424.

Raghav S, et al. Randomized controlled trial of standardized Bacopa monniera extract in age-associated memory impairment. Indian J Psychiatry 2006;48(4):238–42.

Roodenrys S, Booth D, Bulzomi S, Phipps A, Micallef C, Smoker J. Chronic effects of Brahmi (Bacopa monnieri) on human memory. Neuropsychopharmacology 2002;27(2):279–81.

Sadhu A, Upadhyay P, Agrawal A, et al. Management of cognitive determinants in senile dementia of Alzheimer's type: therapeutic potential of a novel polyherbal drug product. Clin Drug Investig 2014;34(12):857–69.

Sarris J, McIntyre E, Camfield DA. Plant-based medicines for anxiety disorders, part 2: a review of clinical studies with supporting preclinical evidence. CNS Drugs 2013;27(4):301–19.

Sathyanarayanan V, Thomas T, Einöther SJ, Dobriyal R, Joshi MK, Krishnamachari S. Brahmi for the better? New findings challenging cognition and anti-anxiety effects of Brahmi (Bacopa monniera) in healthy adults. Psychopharmacology (Berl) 2013;227(2):299–306.

Stough C, Downey LA, Lloyd J, et al. Examining the nootropic effects of a special extract of Bacopa monniera on human cognitive functioning: 90 day double-blind placebo-controlled randomized trial. Phytother Res 2008;22(12):1629–34.

Yadav SK, Jain AK, Tripathi SN, Gupta JP. Irritable bowel syndrome: therapeutic evaluation of indigenous drugs. Indian J Med Res 1989;90:496–503.

Zanotta D, Puricelli S, Bonoldi G. Cognitive effects of a dietary supplement made from extract of Bacopa monnieri, astaxanthin, phosphatidylserine, and vitamin E in subjects with mild cognitive impairment: a noncomparative, exploratory clinical study. Neuropsychiatr Dis Treat 2014;10:225–30.

29

BILBERRY (*VACCINIUM MYRTILLUS*)
Fruit

GENERAL OVERVIEW

Bilberry is commonly utilized to improve eyesight and promote overall eye health. This herb represents one of the richest natural sources of anthocyanins. Anthocyanins have been shown to regenerate the rhodopsin present in retinal photoreceptor cells. They are also thought to be responsible for many other reported health benefits including lowering of blood glucose and lipids. The anti-inflammatory and antioxidant effects give bilberry potential value in the prevention and treatment of conditions associated with inflammation, dyslipidemia, hyperglycemia, and increased oxidative stress. Thus, it may be beneficial for cardiovascular disease, cancer, diabetes, dementia, and other age-related diseases. In 2013 bilberry was reported to be the top medicinal herb used in Norway.

Clinical research indicates that bilberry, alone or in combination formulas, may be beneficial for glaucoma, cataracts, asthenopia, gingivitis, gingival hyperplasia, hyperlipidemia, dyslipidemia, diabetes, nonalcoholic fatty liver disease, ulcerative colitis, psoriasis, eczema, inflammation, and colorectal cancer.

IN VITRO AND ANIMAL RESEARCH

Bilberry fruit anthocyanins have been reported to inhibit smooth muscle contraction and platelet aggregation. Possible antihypertensive effects of bilberry are also suggested by the finding of ACE inhibiting activity in vitro. ACE inhibition seems to be dependent on the specific mixture of anthocyanins in bilberry rather than on any one constituent. Anthocyanins from bilberry were reported to protect against ischemia reperfusion, attenuate leukocyte adhesion, and improve blood perfusion. In rats that were fed bilberry anthocyanins for 12 days prior to inducing HTN, permeability of the blood–brain barrier was kept normal and there was limited increase in the vascular permeability of the skin and aorta.

Animal models suggest bilberry extract may help visual functioning and protect against retinal diseases. In an animal model of uveitis and retinal inflammation, pretreatment with a bilberry extract prevented photoreceptor impairment, relieved intracellular ROS elevation, activated retinal NF-κB in the inflamed retina, and suppressed the decrease of rhodopsin via inhibition of IL-6, which activates STAT3, thereby protecting outer-segment length in photoreceptor cells. Studies have shown that bilberry extract may protect against photooxidation of A2E (a pyridinium disretinoid that initiates blue-light-induced apoptosis in retinal pigment epithelial cells), likely through several antioxidant mechanisms. Another study on the effect of bilberry extract on cultured corneal limbal epithelial cells showed that bilberry promoted physiological renewal and homeostasis of these cells.

The suggested mechanisms for the anti-inflammatory effects of bilberry include inhibiting proteasome activity and inhibiting NF-κB activation. Anthocyanins and other phenolics from bilberry upregulate the oxidative stress defense enzymes heme-oxygenase-1 and glutathione S-transferase-p in cultured human retinal pigment epithelial cells. An in vitro study has suggested that anthocyanosides appear to stabilize connective tissue by enhancing collagen synthesis and cross linking and inhibiting collagen degradation.

Anthocyanins and bilberry have also been reported to have anti-obesity and hypoglycemic effects. The hypoglycemic effect of bilberry may be due to α-glucosidase inhibition, increased insulin secretion, decreased hepatic gluconeogenesis, AMPK activation, and an increase in GLUT 4 in white adipose and skeletal tissue. Anthocyanins have been found to stimulate insulin secretion from cultured rodent pancreatic β cells, with cyanidins and delphinidins showing the greatest effect. Cultured human adipocytes that were treated with anthocyanins for 24 h showed an upregulation of adiponectin and a downregulation of IL-6 and PAI-1 as well as activation of AMPK. Cyanidin-3-glucoside has been shown to suppress the development of obesity in mice fed a high-fat diet and to regulate human adipocyte function.

A bilberry extract added to the diet of diabetic mice at an anthocyanin content of 10 g/kg lowered serum glucose and improved insulin sensitivity. In another mouse study with a water-alcohol extract of bilberry leaves (3 g/kg/day for 4 days) given to streptozotocin-induced diabetic mice, a 26% reduction was seen in plasma glucose. In diabetic mice fed 287 mg/g and 595 mg/g of anthocyanin, blood glucose was significantly decreased by 33% and 51%, respectively. Malividin-3-O-glucoside was the anthocyanin thought to be responsible for the hypoglycemic effect in these animals.

In primary cultures of rat hepatocytes, it was found that bilberry extract protected cells against oxidative damage. Additional rat studies have suggested that the antioxidant effects of bilberry may be seen only in cases of elevated oxidative stress. Hepatoprotective activity has also been demonstrated in stressed mice receiving bilberry extract.

Bilberry is reported to promote short-term memory. In vitro, bilberry polyphenols inhibited amyloid fibril formation and dissolved preformed toxic aggregates and mature fibrils, suggesting a role in Alzheimer's disease (AD) and other neurodegenerative diseases. The berries and fruit polyphenols have been reported to be neuroprotective, to enhance dopamine release, and to improve neuronal communication.

Bilberry and other berry fruits have been reported to show direct antimicrobial effects against human pathogens, including *Salmonella* and *Staphylococcus aureus*. Whole berries or whole berry extracts may be more effective as antimicrobials than purified polyphenol extracts. Bilberry juice has been shown to inhibit adhesion of *Streptococcus pneumoniae* to human bronchial (Calu-3) cells and to inhibit growth of *S. pneumoniae*, but to a lesser degree than cranberry. One preliminary study showed that bilberry had a direct effect against MRSA and potentiated the effects of vancomycin against MRSA. In the presence of 0.6-mg/mL bilberry extract, the MIC for vancomycin was decreased from 1.8 to 0.7 mcg/mL.

In vitro work and animal tumorigenic models have demonstrated that berry anthocyanins have cancer-preventive and -suppressive activity via antioxidant, antiproliferative, apoptotic, anti- angiogenic, and anti-inflammatory effects. The antiproliferative effect appears to be mainly through the p21WAF1 pathway. The anti-angiogenesis effect appears to be through inhibition of ERK 1/2 and Akt phosphorylation. Bilberry extract has also shown a protective effect against chemotherapy-induced oral mucositis in an animal model. Anthocyanins have been reported to stabilize DNA via intercalation, forming a DNA copigmentation complex. A commercial anthocyanin-rich extract from bilberry was shown to inhibit growth of colon cancer cells but did not affect growth of normal colon cells. Bilberry was shown to be more effective than nine other berries at induction of apoptosis in HL60 leukemia and HCT116 colon cancer cells. In animal studies, the number of intestinal adenomas decreased significantly in predisposed rats that were fed a dose of bilberry extract supplying approximately 0.5 g anthocyanin per kilogram per day, a dosage equivalent to approximately 740 g of fresh bilberries in terms of human intake. An extract of bilberry was shown to dose-dependently inhibit cell growth and promote induction of apoptosis in MCF7-GFP-tubulin breast cancer cells. At higher doses (0.5–1.0 mg/mL), bilberry extract arrested the cell cycle at the G2/M phase and inhibited microtubule polymerization. Delphinidin and other anthocyanidins synergistically enhanced cell-cycle arrest and apoptotic induction in aggressive non-small-cell lung cancer (NSCLC) cells by modulating Notch, WNT, and NF-κB signaling pathways.

HUMAN RESEARCH

Ophthalmological Disorders

A 2004 systematic review of bilberry for night vision found that only 12 of the 30 studies were placebo controlled, with 11 of 12 studies using subjects with above-average vision. The conclusion was that there was insufficient rigorous evidence to recommend the use of bilberry for improving night vision (Canter and Ernst, 2004).

A 6-month RCT in patients ($n = 38$) with intra-ocular HTN compared a standardized extract of bilberry plus pycnogenol (Mirtogenol) with control (no treatment). After 2 and 3 months, the mean IOP with the herbal formula decreased from a baseline of 25.2 mmHg to 22.2 mmHg and 22.0 mmHg, respectively, with the 3-month value being significantly better than with controls ($P < 0.05$). Decreased IOP occurred in 19/20 subjects after 3 months of the herb, while only marginal effects were seen in the control subjects. No further improvement was found after 6 months. Ocular blood flow (central retinal, ophthalmic, and posterior ciliary arteries) improved both in the systolic and diastolic components as measured by Color Doppler imaging with the herbal product. After 3 months of treatment, the improvement of ocular blood flow was significant compared with both baseline and controls ($P < 0.05$). The authors concluded that the herbal product may contribute to the prevention of glaucoma (Steigerwalt et al., 2008).

A retrospective analysis of eye health parameters was carried out over 12–59 months by chart review of 332 subjects with normal tension glaucoma (209 men and 123 women) who were treated with anthocyanins ($n = 132$), ginkgo biloba extract ($n = 103$), or no medication (control; $n = 97$). After a mean of 23 months of anthocyanin treatment, the mean best corrected visual acuity for all eyes improved from 0.16 to 0.11 logMAR units ($P = 0.008$), and visual field mean deviation improved from $- 6.44$ to $- 5.34$ ($P = 0.001$). With ginkgo treatment, visual field mean deviation improved from $- 5.25$ to $- 4.31$ ($P = 0.002$). The authors concluded that anthocyanins and ginkgo may be helpful in improving visual function in some individuals with normal tension glaucoma (Shim et al., 2012).

A 4-month study of 50 patients with mild senile cataract investigated the effects of bilberry anthocyanins plus vitamin E. Cataract progression was prevented in 97% of subjects (Bravetti et al., 1989).

A 12-week RCT in healthy adults ($n = 109$) compared standardized bilberry extract 240 mg/day with placebo for effects on tonic accommodation of ciliary muscle caused by visual display terminal (VDT) tasks. High-frequency component (HFC)-1 testing was performed before and after VDT tasks at weeks 0, 4, 8, and 12. HFC-1 values at weeks 8 and 12 were significantly improved with bilberry compared with placebo ($P = 0.014$ and 0.017, respectively). The difference between before and after the task load (ΔHFC-1) was significantly better in the bilberry group than in the placebo group at week 4 and 12 ($P = 0.018$ and 0.049, respectively). The authors concluded that standardized bilberry extract 240 mg/day for 12 weeks relieved the tonic accommodation of the ciliary muscle caused by VDT tasks and near-vision tasks (Kosehira et al., 2020).

An RCT of night vision reported that in six subjects who were given bilberry anthocyanins, dark adaptation post-ingestion was faster (6.5 min) compared with six control subjects (9 min) (Zafra-Stone et al., 2007).

A crossover RCT in young males ($n = 15$) with good vision compared bilberry 160 mg TID with placebo for 3 weeks for effects on night vision. Crossover occurred after a 1-month washout. There was no difference in night VA during any of the measurement periods during active and placebo treatments. In addition, there was no difference in night contrast sensitivity during active and placebo treatments. The authors concluded that the study failed to find benefit from bilberry on night vision, casting doubt on bilberry's use for this indication (Muth et al., 2000).

A 4-week open-label trial in patients ($n = 30$) with symptoms of asthenopia and contrast sensitivity investigated the effect of purified anthocyanin. After 4 weeks, symptoms in 73% of the subjects improved significantly (Lee et al., 2005).

A study of middle-aged office workers who used video display terminals and had positive findings of eye fatigue ($n = 88$) randomized patients to bilberry extract 480 mg/day or placebo for 8 weeks. Subjects in the bilberry group showed alleviation of eye fatigue measures (VDT load-induced ocular fatigue sensation, ocular pain, eye heaviness, uncomfortable sensation, and foreign body sensation) ($P = 0.023$) with no change in the placebo group. The authors concluded that bilberry extract improved some of the objective and subjective parameters of eye fatigue induced by VDT loads (Ozawa et al., 2015).

Oral and Dental Disorders

A 7-day RCT in patients with gingivitis compared 250 g/day or 500 g/day of bilberries with placebo (but no standard dental care) and with standard dental care for effects on markers of inflammation, bleeding on probing (BOP), and gingival crevicular fluid (GCF). The mean reduction in BOP before and after consumption of bilberry was 41% and 59% with bilberry 250 g and 500 g, respectively, 31% with placebo, and 58% with standard of care. There was a significant reduction in cytokine levels and in IL-1b ($P = 0.025$), IL-6 ($P = 0.012$), and VEGF ($P = 0.017$) in GCF samples only in the group that consumed 500 g of bilberries per day. The authors concluded that bilberry intake had an ameliorating effect on some markers of gingival inflammation, reducing gingivitis to a similar extent compared to standard of care (Widén et al., 2015)

A 2-month open-label study in adult diabetics ($n = 12$) investigated the effects of anthocyanosides 600 mg/day on gingival connective tissue synthesis. The use of radioactive labeled amino acids showed a significant decrease of biosynthesis of connective tissue, especially polymeric collagen and structure-glycoproteins. The authors concluded that anthocyanosides help to prevent excess connective tissue synthesis in diabetics (Boniface and Robert, 1996).

Cardiovascular Disorders: Coronary Artery Disease

An 8-week open-label trial in patients ($n = 50$) within 24-h post-PCI evaluated the cardiovascular effects of bilberry powder 40 g/day (equivalent to 480 g fresh bilberries) plus standard medical therapy compared with standard medical therapy alone. The mean 6-min walking distance increased more with bilberry than with control, with a mean difference of 38 m ($P = 0.003$). Oxidized LDL was significantly lowered in the bilberry group over control, with a geometric mean ratio of 0.80 ($P = 0.017$). TC, LDL-C, and hs-CRP did not differ between groups. The authors concluded that bilberries may have clinically relevant beneficial effects following acute myocardial infarction (AMI) and that further research was warranted (Arevström).

Cardiometabolic Disorders: Hyperlipidemia and Dyslipidemia

A meta-analysis of the lipid effects of bilberry and whortleberry found 16 studies ($n = 1109$) that met inclusion criteria. The bilberry groups showed significant differences in reducing LDL-C and increasing HDL-C in comparison with other treatments. The authors concluded that the results from this review provided some evidence of the beneficial effects of bilberry and whortleberry on lipid reduction, but recommending bilberry and whortleberry for lowering lipids levels was not justifiable due to limited data (Zhu et al., 2015).

A 12-week RCT in hypercholesterolemic individuals ($n = 150$) compared anthocyanins 320 mg/day with placebo. Anthocyanins and placebo, respectively, showed increases in the flow-mediated dilation (28.4% and 2.2%) and cGMP (12.6% and − 1.2%) ($P < 0.05$ for both). Anthocyanins produced greater increases in HDL-C concentrations and decreases in the serum soluble vascular adhesion molecule-1 and LDL-C concentrations ($P < 0.05$ for all). The authors concluded that anthocyanin supplementation improved endothelium-dependent vasodilation in hypercholesterolemic individuals, an effect that involved activation of the NO–cGMP signaling pathway, improvements in the serum lipid profile, and decreased inflammation (Zhu et al., 2011).

A 12-week RCT in subjects ($n = 120$) with dyslipidemia compared bilberry plus black currant extract 320 mg/day with placebo for impact on lipids. HDL-C concentrations increased by 13.7% and 2.8% in the anthocyanin and placebo groups, respectively ($P < 0.001$). LDL-C decreased by 13.6% and − 0.6% in the anthocyanin and placebo groups, respectively ($P < 0.001$). Cellular cholesterol efflux to serum increased 20.0% and 0.2% in the anthocyanin and placebo groups, respectively ($P < 0.001$). The mass and activity of plasma CETP decreased by 10.4% and 6.3%, respectively, with anthocyanin and by − 3.5% and 1.1%, respectively, with placebo ($P < 0.001$). The authors concluded that anthocyanin supplementation in humans improved LDL-C and HDL-C concentrations and enhanced cellular cholesterol efflux to serum, likely due to the inhibition of CETP (Qin et al., 2009).

A 6-week open-label trial in healthy men and women ($n = 36$) investigated the effects of consumption of 150 g of frozen bilberries three times a week on lipids. The study found that the consumption of bilberries led to a decrease in TC ($P = 0.017$), LDL-C ($P = 0.0347$), TG ($P = 0.001$), glucose ($P = 0.005$), albumin (P = 0.001), and GGT (P = 0.046) as well as increases in HDL-C (P = 0.044). However, the subfraction of men (n = 11) demonstrated an increase in LDL-C (P = 0.007). The authors concluded that the regular intake of bilberries could be important to reduce CVD risk, by decreasing LDL-C and TG and increasing HDL-C (Habanova et al., 2016).

Cardiometabolic Disorders: Diabetes

A study of men with T2DM (n = 8) administered a single oral capsule of either 0.47 g standardized bilberry extract (the equivalent of about 50 g of fresh bilberries) or placebo followed by a 75-g oral glucose challenge in a double-blinded crossover intervention with a 2-week washout period. The ingestion of the bilberry extract resulted in a significant decrease in the incremental AUC for both glucose (P = 0.003) and insulin (P = 0.03) compared with placebo. There was no change in GLP-1, glucagon, amylin, or monocyte chemotactic protein-1. The most likely mechanism for the lower glycemic response was thought to involve reduced rates of carbohydrate digestion and/or absorption (Hoggard et al., 2013).

A 30-day RCT in overweight women (n = 80) compared frozen bilberries with a variety of sea buckthorn preparations for effects on cardiometabolic parameters. All interventions induced a significant (P < 0.001–0.003) effect on overall metabolic profiles. The effect was observed in participants with both elevated and reduced cardiometabolic risk profiles. However, bilberries caused beneficial changes in serum lipids and lipoproteins in high-risk subjects, whereas the opposite was true in low-risk subjects. The authors concluded that berry intake had overall metabolic effects, which depended on the baseline cardiometabolic risk profiles (Larmo et al., 2013).

Gastrointestinal Disorders: Nonalcoholic Fatty Liver Disease

A 12-week RCT in patients with NAFLD (n = 74) compared purified anthocyanin 320 mg/day (from bilberry and black currant) with placebo. The anthocyanin group exhibited significant decreases compared with placebo in plasma ALT (− 19.1% vs 3.1%), cytokeratin-18 M30 fragment (− 8.8% vs 5.6%), and myeloperoxidase (− 75.0% vs − 44.8%) (P < 0.05 for all comparisons). Significant decreases from baseline

in fasting blood glucose and HOMA-IR were also noted in the treatment group, but these differences were not significant relative to placebo. The 2-h glucose on the OGTT decreased significantly with anthocyanin compared with placebo (− 18.7% vs − 3.8%, P=0.02). The authors concluded that purified anthocyanin improved insulin resistance, indicators of liver injury, and clinical evolution in NAFLD patients and that further studies were warranted (Zhang et al., 2015).

Gastrointestinal Disorders: Inflammatory Bowel Disease

A 9-week open pilot trial in patients (n = 13) with mild-to-moderate ulcerative colitis (UC) investigated an anthocyanin-rich bilberry extract for 6 weeks. Symptom improvement occurred in 90% of patients and remission occurred in 63%. Mean Mayo score decreased from 6.5 to 3.6 by week 7 (P < 0.001). Mean fecal calprotectin levels significantly decreased during the treatment phase (from 778 mcg/g to 305 mcg/g; P = 0.049), including four patients achieving undetectable levels at end of treatment. A decrease in endoscopic Mayo score and histologic Riley index confirmed the beneficial effect. These benefits were reversed with cessation of the bilberry extract. No serious adverse events were observed. The authors concluded that a standardized anthocyanin-rich bilberry preparation had therapeutic potential in UC and that further studies were warranted (Biedermann et al., 2013).

A 6-week open pilot study in patients with UC investigated the effects of an anthocyanin rich bilberry extract on inflammatory pathways in colon specimens. The findings showed that bilberry treatment inhibited the expression of IFN-γ-receptor 2 in human THP-1 monocytic cells. Colon biopsies of UC patients who responded to the bilberry treatment revealed reduced amounts of the pro-inflammatory cytokines IFN-γ and TNF-α. Levels of phosphorylated (activated) p65-NF-κB were reduced and there were enhanced levels of Th17-cell-specific cytokine IL-22 and immunoregulatory cytokine IL-10 as well as reduced serum levels of TNF-α and MCP-1. The authors concluded that the anti-inflammatory effect of anthocyanin-rich bilberry in patients with UC is due to modulating T-cell cytokine signaling and inhibiting IFN-γ signal transduction (Roth et al., 2016).

Dermatological Disorders: Psoriasis and Eczema

An RCT in patients with psoriasis or erythematous eczema investigated a bilberry seed oil compared with a lecithin–frankincense formulation and with placebo. In patients with psoriasis, scales and erythema improved with both frankincense and bilberry seed oil treatment compared with placebo. The frankincense formulation improved scales in 70% of cases and erythema in 50% of cases without any case of worsening. In patients with eczema, bilberry, frankincense formulation, and placebo improved itch (66.7% 60%, and 10% of cases, respectively) and erythema (78%, 60%, and 10% of cases, respectively). The authors concluded that the herbal formulations were promising for the treatment of psoriasis and erythematous eczema (Togni et al., 2015).

Inflammation

A 4-week RCT in subjects ($n = 61$) with elevated levels of at least one cardiovascular risk factor studied daily consumption of bilberry juice 330 mL/day compared with water for inflammatory markers. Significant decreases in plasma concentrations of CRP, IL-6, IL-15, and monokine induced by IFN-γ occurred in the bilberry group, while an increase in the plasma concentration TNF-α was also observed in this group. The authors noted that CRP, IL-6, IL-15, MIG, and TNF-α were all target genes of NF-κB, a transcription factor that is crucial in orchestrating inflammatory responses (Karlsen et al., 2010).

An RCT in volunteers ($n = 27$) compared a diet rich in bilberries (400 g/day) with a control diet. Bilberry supplementation tended to decrease hs-CRP, IL-6, IL-12, and LPS. An inflammation score was significantly different between the groups ($P = 0.024$). There were also noted changes in transcription of toll-like receptor signaling, cytoplasmic ribosomal proteins, and B-cell receptor signaling pathways. The authors concluded that regular bilberry consumption may reduce low-grade inflammation, thereby decreasing cardiometabolic risk (Kolehmainen et al., 2012).

Oncologic Disorders

A 7-day pilot study of patients ($n = 25$) with colorectal cancer investigated the effects of an anthocyanin-standardized extract of bilberry supplying between 0.5 and 2 g of anthocyanins per day prior to surgery. After 7 days, bilberry anthocyanins and their glucuronide and methyl metabolites were detected in plasma as well as in tumor tissue. The tumor tissue showed a 7% decrease in proliferation compared with pre-bilberry values, and there was a small but significant decrease in plasma IGF-1 seen with the lowest dose (Thomasset et al., 2009).

ACTIVE CONSTITUENTS

Berries

- Phenolic compounds
  - Stilbenoids (anti-inflammatory, antineoplastic, antioxidant, cardioprotective, phytoestrogenic): resveratrol
  - Phenolic acids
  - Flavonoids: quercetin (anti-inflammatory, antioxidant, hypotensive, antidiabetic, antispasmodic, neuroprotective, XO inhibition, antibacterial, anticancer), catechins (inhibit prostacyclin synthesis, reduce capillary permeability and fragility, scavenge free radicals, antiplatelet, antineoplastic)
    - Anthocyanins (general and retinal antioxidants, hepatoprotective, anti-ulcer, antispasmodic, collagen-stabilizing, antiplatelet, antineoplastic): delphinidins, cyanidins, petunidins, malvidins, peonidins, proanthocyanidins B1-B4, neomyrtillin
  - Tannins, ellagitannins (antidiarrheal)
  - Quinones: hydroquinone
- Terpenes
  - Triterpenoid saponins: oleanolic acid (chemoprotective, hepatoprotective), ursolic acid (anti-HIV, anti-EBV, antiviral, androgenic, AChEI, pro-collagen, pro-ceremide, antitumor)

Leaves

- Phenolic compounds:
  - Phenolic acids and esters
  - Phenylpropanoids (antioxidant, antimutagenic, antitumor, antimicrobial): chlorogenic acid
  - Flavonoids: anthocyanins, procyanidins (antioxidant, anti-inflammatory, antineoplastic)

BILBERRY COMMONLY USED PREPARATIONS AND DOSAGE (FOR ADULTS UNLESS OTHERWISE SPECIFIED)

The following are examples of some available formulations and ranges of dosing for commercial herbal products. See Part III Introduction "How to prescribe medicinal herbs" for further guidance on herbal advising and prescribing.

Berry

- Oral infusion (tea) or decoction: 5–10 g crushed dried berries in 150 mL water (esp. for diarrhea)
- Fresh bilberries: 250–500 g with food
- Dried berries: 20–60 g QD to TID with meals
- Powdered berry extract: 1/5 tsp (500 mg) QD-BID
- Capsule or tablet of powdered berries: 6 g QD-BID
- Capsule or tablet of powdered berry (4:1) extract: 250–500 mg (equivalent to 1–2 g dried berry) QD-BID
- Capsule or tablet of standardized extract (standardized to 25%–36% anthocyanins): 80–160 mg QD-TID with meals

SAFETY AND PRECAUTION

Side Effects

None reported in recommended doses.

Case Reports

A 77-year-old man on warfarin taking excess doses of bilberry was hospitalized twice for hemorrhage.

Pregnancy/Lactation

Dietary consumption of bilberries appears to be safe during pregnancy and lactation but use as a supplement has not been proven to be safe.

Drug Interactions

- Anticoagulants/Antiplatelets: Bilberry in high doses may potentiate the risk of bleeding and may have added or synergistic antiplatelet effects to ASA and NSAIDs.
- Chemotherapy drugs: Bilberry may interfere with the actions of certain chemotherapy drugs and radiation therapy. May antagonize erlotinib.
- May augment effects of hypoglycemic agents.
- Bilberry does *not* appear to have inhibitory effects on UGT isozymes 1A1, 1A4, 1A6, 1A9, and 2B7 in vitro.

REFERENCES

Arevström L, Bergh C, Landberg R, Wu H, Rodriguez-Mateos A, Waldenborg M, Magnuson A, Blanc S, Fröbert O. Freeze-dried bilberry (Vaccinium myrtillus) dietary supplement improves walking distance and lipids after myocardial infarction: an open-label randomized clinical trial. Nutr Res. 2019 Feb;62:13–23.

Biedermann L, Mwinyi J, Scharl M, et al. Bilberry ingestion improves disease activity in mild to moderate ulcerative colitis—an open pilot study. J Crohns Colitis 2013;7(4):271–9.

Boniface R, Robert AM. Effect of anthocyanins on human connective tissue metabolism in the human. Klin Monbl Augenheilkd 1996;209(6):368–72.

Bravetti GO, Fraboni E, Maccolini E. Preventive medical treatment of senile cataract with vitamin E and Vaccinium myrtillus anthocyanosides: Clinical evaluation. Ann Ottalmol Clin Ocul 1989;115:109–16.

Canter PH, Ernst E. Anthocyanosides of Vaccinium myrtillus (bilberry) for night vision—a systematic review of placebo-controlled trials. Surv Ophthalmol 2004;49(1):38–50.

Habanova M, Saraiva JA, Haban M, et al. Intake of bilberries (Vaccinium myrtillus L.) reduced risk factors for cardiovascular disease by inducing favorable changes in lipoprotein profiles. Nutr Res 2016;36(12):1415–22.

Hoggard N, Cruickshank M, Moar KM, et al. A single supplement of a standardised bilberry (Vaccinium myrtillus L.) extract (36 % wet weight anthocyanins) modifies glycaemic response in individuals with type 2 diabetes controlled by diet and lifestyle. J Nutr Sci 2013;2, e22.

Karlsen A, Paur I, Bøhn SK, et al. Bilberry juice modulates plasma concentration of NF-kappaB related inflammatory markers in subjects at increased risk of CVD. Eur J Nutr 2010;49(6):345–55.

Kolehmainen M, Mykkänen O, Kirjavainen PV, et al. Bilberries reduce low-grade inflammation in individuals with features of metabolic syndrome. Mol Nutr Food Res 2012;56(10):1501–10.

Kosehira M, Machida N, Kitaichi N. A 12-week-long intake of Bilberry extract (*Vaccinium myrtillus* L.) improved objective findings of ciliary muscle contraction of the eye: a randomized, double-blind, placebo-controlled, parallel-group comparison trial. Nutrients 2020;12(3):600.

Larmo PS, Kangas AJ, Soininen P, et al. Effects of sea buckthorn and bilberry on serum metabolites differ according to baseline metabolic profiles in overweight women: a randomized crossover trial. Am J Clin Nutr 2013;98(4):941–51.

Lee J, Lee HK, Kim CY, Choe CM, You TW, Seong GJ. Purified high-dose anthocyanoside oligomer administration improves nocturnal vision and clinical symptoms in myopia subjects. Br J Nutr 2005;93:895–9.

Muth ER, Laurent JM, Jasper P. The effect of bilberry nutritional supplementation on night visual acuity and contrast sensitivity. Altern Med Rev 2000;5(2):164–73.

Ozawa Y, Kawashima M, Inoue S, et al. Bilberry extract supplementation for preventing eye fatigue in video display terminal workers. J Nutr Health Aging 2015;19(5):548–54.

Qin Y, Xia M, Ma J, et al. Anthocyanin supplementation improves serum LDL- and HDL-cholesterol concentrations associated with the inhibition of cholesteryl ester transfer protein in dyslipidemic subjects. Am J Clin Nutr 2009;90:485–92.

Roth S, Spalinger MR, Gottier C, et al. Bilberry-derived anthocyanins modulate cytokine expression in the intestine of patients with ulcerative colitis. PLoS One 2016;11(5), e0154817.

Shim SH, Kim JM, Choi CY, Kim CY, Park KH. Ginkgo biloba extract and bilberry anthocyanins improve visual function in patients with normal tension glaucoma. J Med Food 2012;15(9):818–23.

Steigerwalt RD, Gianni B, Paolo M, Bombardelli E, Burki C, Schonlau F. Effects of Mirtogenol on ocular blood flow and intraocular HTN in asymptomatic subjects. Mol Vis 2008;14:1288–92.

Thomasset S, Berry DP, Cai H, et al. Pilot study of oral anthocyanins for colorectal cancer chemoprevention. Cancer Prev Res (Phila) 2009;2(7):625–33.

Togni S, Maramaldi G, Bonetta A, Giacomelli L, Di Pierro F. Clinical evaluation of safety and efficacy of Boswellia-based cream for prevention of adjuvant radiotherapy skin damage in mammary carcinoma: a randomized placebo-controlled trial. Eur Rev Med Pharmacol Sci 2015;19(8):1338–44.

Widén C, Coleman M, Critén S, Karlgren-Andersson P, Renvert S, Persson GR. Consumption of bilberries controls gingival inflammation. Int J Mol Sci 2015;16(5):10665–73.

Zafra-Stone S, Taharat Y, Bagchi M, Chatterjee A, Vinson JA, Bagchi D. Berry anthocyanins as novel antioxidants in human health and disease prevention. Mol Nutr Food Res 2007;51:675–83.

Zhang PW, Chen FX, Li D, Ling WH, Guo HH. A CONSORT-compliant, randomized, double-blind, placebo-controlled pilot trial of purified anthocyanin in patients with NAFLD. Medicine (Baltimore) 2015;94(20):e758.

Zhu Y, Xia M, Yang Y, et al. Purified anthocyanin supplementation improves endothelial function via NO-cGMP activation in hypercholesterolemic individuals. Clin Chem 2011;57(11):1524–33.

Zhu Y, Miao Y, Meng Z, Zhong Y. Effects of Vaccinium berries on serum lipids: a meta-analysis of randomized controlled trials. Evid Based Complement Alternat Med 2015;2015:790329.

30

BLACK COHOSH (*ACTAEA RACEMOSA/CIMICIFUGA RACEMOSA*)
Root

GENERAL OVERVIEW

Following the publication of the initial findings of the Women's Health Initiative in 2002, panic-stricken women and their equally alarmed healthcare providers stopped taking and prescribing hormone replacement therapy, throwing many older women into fierce menopausal syndromes. Enter black cohosh. Originally used for cognitive and inflammatory conditions, it became a household item for women to use in hopes of relieving menopausal misery. In 2008 it was the tenth most commonly sold supplement in the West. Despite its popularity, which would suggest efficacy, research findings have been mixed and confusing. The studies that have shown benefit for vasomotor symptoms were mostly unblinded. Well-done studies equally support and refute the herb's benefits for menopause. So, the bad news is that black cohosh may not be all that effective for hot flushes. The good news is that it appears to be safe and to have other beneficial effects. Its mechanism of action in menopause, if it does have one, is not due to estrogenic activity but more likely due to activity on central neurotransmitters. Dopaminergic, noradrenergic, serotonergic, and GABAergic effects have been demonstrated. It also appears to have some beneficial effects on bone, but human evidence is underwhelming. Evidence points to black cohosh having greater efficacy for menopausal symptoms when an isopropanolic extract is used, when it is standardized to at least 2.5% triterpene content, or when it is used as part of a mixed-herbal product. However, in women with breast cancer, black cohosh by itself may be the safest choice (see "Human Research" and "Safety and Precaution").

Clinical research indicates that black cohosh, alone or in combination formulas, may be beneficial for uterine fibroids, female infertility, menopause, bone density, anxiety in menopause, and breast cancer.

IN VITRO AND ANIMAL RESEARCH

Black cohosh has been shown to have strong binding to serotonin receptors 5-HT(1A), 5-HT(1D), and 5-HT(7) as well as mu opioid receptor agonist activity. One constituent, isoferulic acid, has demonstrated anti-inflammatory and antispasmodic effects. The constituents actaealactone, cimicifugic acid, and fukinolic acid have demonstrated antioxidant activity in vitro. The constituent acteina has been shown to cause vasodilation and elicit hypotension in animals.

The question of estrogenic activity in black cohosh is complicated. It does not increase circulating estrogen levels, breast density, or uterine weight in animal research. Although early studies indicated some estrogenic activity with black cohosh, more recent research has shown no significant estrogen receptor binding activity or other estrogenic activities. Two studies found no effects of black cohosh on estrogen receptors but did show that black cohosh antagonized the proliferative effects of estradiol. Premature estrus could not be precipitated by black cohosh in infant female mice. However, the herb has been shown to bind to some progesterone receptors.

Black cohosh may be beneficial for bone density. An extract of black cohosh has been shown to significantly diminish the urinary content of pyridinoline and deoxypyridinoline in ovariectomized rats. Treated ovariectomized rats have shown slightly stimulated gene expression of osteoblast and osteoclast activation. In one rat study it reduced bone loss from 53% to 39%.

A black cohosh extract has been shown to have antiproliferative and antiestrogenic effects in ER-negative breast cancer cells. A study on estrogen-sensitive breast cancer cells showed black cohosh extract did not stimulate MCF-7 growth but, rather, inhibited cellular proliferation. Low concentrations of the constituent actein have been shown to cause synergistic inhibition of human breast cancer cell proliferation when combined with different chemotherapeutic agents. However, the constituents actaealactone and cimicifugic acid may have a small stimulating effect on the growth of breast cancer cell proliferation. The proliferation-inhibiting effect of tamoxifen has been enhanced by black cohosh extract. The herb has also been shown to induce apoptosis and suppress estradiol-induced cell proliferation in human endometrial adenocarcinoma cells. It has been shown to inhibit liver and prostate cancer cell proliferation through mechanisms that inhibit proliferation and angiogenesis and promote apoptosis. The effect for prostate cancer applies to both hormone-sensitive and hormone-unresponsive cancer cells.

HUMAN RESEARCH

Breast Disorders: Breast Density

A study compared black cohosh with estradiol/norethisterone 2 mg/1 mg and with tibolone 2.5 mg for effects on breast density changes over 6 months. Estradiol/norethisterone increased breast density by 14.3%, tibolone increased it by 2.3%, and black cohosh did not increase it at all. The authors concluded that black cohosh did not influence mammographic breast density after 6 months treatment (Lundström et al., 2011).

Disorders of the Uterus: Uterine Fibromas

A three-month RCT of menopausal women ($n = 244$) compared black cohosh 40 mg/day with tibolone 2.5 mg/day with respect to size change of uterine fibromas. Median fibroid volume decreased with black cohosh by 30% and increased with tibolone by 4.7% ($P = 0.016$). The percentage of change in volume, the mean diameter change, and the geometric mean diameter change were all significantly greater with black cohosh compared with tibolone ($P = 0.016$, 0.021, 0.016,

respectively). The authors concluded that black cohosh was a valid herbal medicinal product for uterine fibroids (Xi et al., 2014).

Ovarian Disorders: Female Infertility

A three-cycle RCT in women with polycystic ovarian syndrome (PCOS) ($n = 100$) investigated the fertility effects of black cohosh 40 mg/day for 10 days compared with clomiphene 100 mg/day for 5 days, repeated for three cycles. Both groups also received HCG injections at the appropriate time. The black cohosh group had significantly greater reductions in LH levels and LH/FSH ratios ($P = 0.007$ and $P = 0.06$, respectively), and greater progesterone levels ($P = 0.0001$) and endometrial thickness ($P = 0.0004$). Pregnancy rates were 7 pregnancies (2 twin pregnancies) in the black cohosh group and four pregnancies (one twin pregnancy) in the clomiphene group. The authors concluded that black cohosh could be used as an alternative to clomiphene citrate for ovulation induction in women with PCOS (Kamel, 2013).

A study in patients ($n = 119$) with unexplained infertility administered black cohosh 120 mg/day on days 1–12 plus clomiphene 150 mg per usual dosing followed by HCG injection and compared this with a standard clomiphene regimen alone. With black cohosh, endometrial thickness, serum progesterone, and clinical pregnancy rates were significantly higher (8.9 vs 7.5 mm; $P < 0.001$; 13.3 ng/mL vs 9.3 ng/mL; $P < 0.01$; 36.7% vs 13.6%; $P < 0.01$, respectively). There was also a non-significant shortening of induction cycle, and estradiol and LH were higher with black cohosh. The authors concluded that adding black cohosh to clomiphene citrate induction could improve the pregnancy rate and cycle outcomes in infertile couples with unexplained infertility (Shahin et al., 2008).

Ovarian Disorders: Menopause

The big question about efficacy of black cohosh for vasomotor symptoms of menopause has been addressed by several reviews and meta-analyses of a large volume of clinical trials. A representative sample is included here. The research using isopropanolic extracts of black cohosh appears to demonstrate greater efficacy for menopausal complaints.

A 2017 systematic review looked at 47 RCTs of 16 treatment classes ($n = 8326$) and investigated estrogen plus progestin, black cohosh, and SSRIs with respect to superiority over placebo for menopausal symptoms. Efficacy ranking was estrogen/progestin (70% relief), followed by black cohosh. SSRIs and SNRIs were found to be ineffective in relieving vasomotor symptoms but caused more side effects (Sarri et al., 2017).

A 2017 review of clinical trials on herbal efficacy in menopausal symptoms used search terms menopause, climacteric, hot flushes, flashes, herb, and phytoestrogens. The authors found that passionflower, sage, lemon balm, valerian, black cohosh, fenugreek, black cumin, chasteberry, fennel, evening primrose, ginkgo, alfalfa, St. John's wort, Asian ginseng, anise, licorice, red clover, and wild soybean were effective in the treatment of acute menopausal syndrome with different mechanisms. The authors concluded that medicinal plants could play a role in the treatment of acute menopausal syndrome and that further studies were warranted (Kargozar et al., 2017).

A 2016 systematic review to assess effectiveness of Iranian herbal medicine for menopausal hot flushes found 19 RCTs that met inclusion criteria. Overall, studies showed that passionflower, anise, licorice, soy, black cohosh, red clover, evening primrose, flaxseed, sage, chasteberry, St. John's wort, valerian, and avocado plus soybean oil could alleviate hot flushes. The authors concluded that herbal medicines had efficacy in alleviating hot flushes (Ghazanfarpour et al., 2016).

A 2015 systematic review of published hormonal and non-hormonal treatments for hot flushes associated with climacteric or with breast and prostate cancer treatment found 147 studies that included alternative non-hormonal treatments in post-menopausal women and in breast and prostate cancer survivors. The most effective hot flush treatment was estrogenic hormones, or a combination of estrogens and progestins, though benefits were noted to be partially outweighed by a significantly increased risk for breast cancer development. Certain non-hormonal treatments, including SSRIs, gabapentin/pregabalin, and black cohosh extracts, showed a positive risk–benefit ratio. The authors concluded that non-hormonal treatments were useful alternatives in patients with a history of or risk for breast cancer (Drewe et al., 2015).

A 2012 Cochrane review investigated 16 RCTs ($n = 2027$) for effectiveness of black cohosh (dosage range 8–160 mg) in reducing menopausal symptoms.

Study durations were 8 to 54 weeks, with a mean duration of 22.8 weeks. The studies were highly heterogeneous with respect to such factors as design, duration, type, and amount of black cohosh used and main findings. The conclusion was that there was insufficient evidence from these trials to either support or oppose the use of black cohosh for menopausal symptoms (Leach and Moore, 2012).

A 2012 systematic review assessed efficacy of black cohosh, St. John's wort, chasteberry, and vitamins as monotherapy or in combination for menopausal symptoms. The combination of black cohosh and St. John's wort was found to show an improvement of climacteric complaints in comparison with placebo. However, the combination of St. John's wort and chasteberry showed no significant difference in the treatment of menopausal symptoms (Laakmann et al., 2012).

A 2012 systematic review looking at various treatments for hot flushes reviewed 51 studies that met inclusion criteria. Only gabapentin demonstrated consistent and statistically significant benefit over placebo in its well-designed RCTs. Desvenlafaxine, soy-derived isoflavones, and black cohosh demonstrated statistically significant benefit over placebo in 75%, 21%, and 17% of the well-designed RCTs for each compound, respectively (Guttuso, 2012).

A 2010 systematic review of black cohosh for menopausal syndrome found nine placebo-controlled studies that met inclusion criteria. A meta-analysis was performed on seven of the studies. Overall, symptoms improved by 26%, but the trials were quite heterogeneous. Studies showed that isopropanolic extracts of black cohosh tended to have more positive outcomes as did extracts that were standardized to at least 2.5% triterpene content (Shams et al., 2010).

A 2007 systematic review looking at herbs and supplements for menopausal mood disorders found that black cohosh significantly reduced depression and anxiety in all studies reviewed. Five of seven trials of St. John's wort showed benefit for mild-to-moderate depression. One RCT of ginseng in postmenopausal women reported improvements in mood and anxiety. Kava significantly reduced anxiety in four of eight RCTs. All three RCTs of ginkgo found no effect on depression. The authors concluded that St. John's wort and black cohosh appeared to be the most useful in alleviating mood and anxiety changes during menopause, that ginseng may be effective but required more research, and that kava held promise for decreasing anxiety in peri- and postmenopausal women (Geller and Studee, 2007).

A 2003 systematic review to assess the efficacy of herbal medicinal products for treatment of menopausal symptoms selected 18 RCTs that met inclusion criteria. The herbs studied included black cohosh, dong quai, red clover, kava, evening primrose oil, ginseng, and combination products. The authors concluded that there was no convincing evidence for any herbal medical product in the treatment of menopausal symptoms. However, the evidence for black cohosh was promising, albeit limited by the poor methodology of the trials. The studies involving red clover suggested it may be of benefit for more severe menopausal symptoms. There was some evidence for the use of kava, but safety concerns were noted. The evidence was inconclusive for the other herbal medicinal products reviewed (Huntley and Ernst, 2003).

A 16-week RCT in women ($n = 301$) with menopausal complaints and psychological symptoms compared a combination of St. John's wort and black cohosh with placebo. The mean Menopause Rating Scale score decreased 50% (from 0.46 to 0.23) with the herbal product and 19.6% (from 0.46 to 0.37) with placebo. The HAM-D total score decreased 41.8% (from 18.9 to 11.0 points) with the herbal product, and 12.7% (from 18.9 to 16.5) with placebo. The treatment was superior to placebo in both measures ($P < 0.001$ for both). The authors concluded that this fixed combination of black cohosh and St. John's wort was superior to placebo in alleviating menopausal complaints including related psychological aspects (Uebelhack et al., 2006).

A 1-year open-label study of postmenopausal women ($n = 400$) investigated the endometrial safety and overall efficacy of black cohosh 40 mg/day. Clinical parameters showed a reduction in hot flushes, while there were no changes in endometrial thickness or hyperplasia on endometrial biopsy. The authors concluded that black cohosh was a safe alternative for menopausal relief (Raus et al., 2006).

A 3-month study in postmenopausal women ($n = 64$) investigated black cohosh 40 mg/day compared with transdermal estradiol 0.025 mg + 10 days progestin (E + P) for symptom reduction and effects on lipids. Both black cohosh and E + P significantly reduced the number of hot flushes and other vasomotor symptoms per day ($P < 0.001$ for both), starting after the first month of treatment and continuing throughout the 3 months of therapy. Anxiety and depression were also reduced to the same degree in both groups at 3 months ($P < 0.001$ for both). A slight but significant increase of HDL-C was found only in women treated with black cohosh ($P < 0.04$), while LDL-C levels were significantly lowered by 3 months with both black cohosh ($P < 0.003$) and E + P ($P < 0.002$). TC was unchanged by black cohosh treatment but significantly reduced by 3 months with E + P. TG was not affected by either treatment. FSH, LH, and cortisol were not significantly affected after 3 months, while PRL ($P < 0.005$) and 17 β-estradiol ($P < 0.001$) were increased only with E + P. Endometrial thickness was not affected by either black cohosh or E + P. The authors concluded that black cohosh may be a valid alternative to low-dose transdermal estradiol plus a progestin in the management of climacteric complaints (Nappi et al., 2005).

A 12-week study of postmenopausal women ($n = 180$) investigated Remifemin, an isopropanolic extract of black cohosh 20 mg BID, compared with tibolone 2.5 mg/day for effects on menopausal symptoms. Total Kupperman score from baseline to 4 weeks to 12 weeks went from 24 to 11 to 7, respectively, with black cohosh ($P < 0.05$); for the same intervals, the total Kupperman score went from 25 to 11 to 6, respectively, with tibolone ($P < 0.05$). The change between groups was similar ($P > 0.05$ for between-group comparison). The tibolone group had significantly greater adverse effects: 19% vs 0% vaginal bleeding, 36% vs 16% breast swelling, and an increase of endometrial thickness in the tibolone group only (Bai et al., 2009).

A 6-month head-to-head study in menopausal women ($n = 120$) investigated black cohosh compared with fluoxetine for effects on menopausal symptoms. Improvements in Kupperman Index and BDI improved in both groups by the end of the third month. At the end of the 6 month black cohosh reduced the hot flush score by 85%, and fluoxetine reduced it by 62%. Conversely, fluoxetine had better improvements on the BDI. By the sixth month, 33% of women had discontinued the study in each group. The authors concluded that compared with fluoxetine, black cohosh was more effective for treating hot flushes and night sweats, while fluoxetine was more effective in improvements shown on the BDI (Oktem et al., 2007).

A 12-week RCT in women ($n = 220$) with menopausal complaints compared two capsules daily of either black cohosh 6.5 mg, black cohosh 500 mg, a combination of black cohosh and rhodiola (Menopause Relief EP), or placebo. The menopause symptom relief effects of the combination formula were significantly superior in all tests to the effects of either dose of black cohosh alone and placebo after 6 and 12 weeks. There was no statistically significant difference between the effects of the two doses of black cohosh. The combination formula significantly improved the QOL index in patients, compared with the other groups, mainly due to the beneficial effects on the emotional and health domains. The authors concluded that black cohosh was more effective in combination with rhodiola for relief of menopausal symptoms, particularly psychological symptoms (Pkhaladze et al., 2020).

An open-label study in postmenopausal women ($n = 6$) who had been treated with 12 weeks of black cohosh 40 mg/day compared the effect of a saline or a naloxone challenge on LH pulsatility and estrogen concentrations. Black cohosh had no effect on spontaneous LH pulsatility or estrogen concentrations. With naloxone blockade, there was a suppression of mean LH pulse frequency (saline vs naloxone = 9.0 vs 6.0 pulses/16 h; $P = 0.056$), especially during sleep when the mean interpulse interval was prolonged by approximately 90 minutes (saline vs naloxone night interpulse interval = 103 vs 191 min; $P = 0.03$). PET imaging identified significant 10% to 16% in mu-opioid receptor binding potential with black cohosh in the posterior and subgenual cingulate, temporal, and orbitofrontal cortex, thalamus, and nucleus accumbens (brain regions involved in emotional and cognitive function). In contrast, binding potential reductions of lesser magnitude were observed in the anterior cingulate and anterior insular cortex regions (involved in the placebo response). The authors concluded that the neuropharmacological action of black cohosh was related to central opioid function (Reame et al., 2008).

A 3-month open-label study in women with either mild or moderate–severe menopausal symptoms investigated the effect of a combination product containing chasteberry, black cohosh, hyaluronic acid,

zinc, and ginger (ElleN) one tablet daily. Results showed a significant reduction in the Kupperman Index in both groups. The treatment was particularly effective against hot flushes associated with night insomnia and anxiety. The product was well tolerated and did not cause any side effects. The authors concluded that this combination product was able to reduce moderate to severe menopause symptoms (Cappelli et al., 2015).

A 3-month RCT in premenopausal and postmenopausal women ($n = 50$) compared Phyto-Female Complex (black cohosh, dong quai, milk thistle, red clover, American ginseng, and chasteberry) with placebo BID for effect on menopausal symptoms. The women receiving Phyto-Female Complex showed a significantly superior mean reduction in menopausal symptoms compared with the placebo group. Improvements in menopausal symptoms increased over time. In the treatment group, by 3 months there was a 73% decrease in hot flushes and a 69% reduction of night sweats as well as a decrease in hot flush intensity and a significant improvement in sleep quality. Hot flushes ceased completely in 47% and 19% of women with the herbal product and placebo, respectively. There were no changes in findings on vaginal ultrasonography or levels of relevant hormones (estradiol, FSH), liver enzymes, or TSH in either group. The authors concluded that Phyto-Female Complex was safe and effective for the relief of hot flushes and sleep disturbances in pre- and postmenopausal women, when used for at least 3 months (Rotem and Kaplan, 2007).

Musculoskeletal Disorders: Osteoporosis

A 10-year RCT in women ($n = 128$) in early menopause investigated black cohosh 40 mg/day plus high-impact exercise compared with exercise alone and with a wellness control group (low-intensity exercise) for effects on BMD and 10-year CHD risk. BMD at the lumbar spine did not decrease significantly from baseline with high-impact exercise with and without black cohosh (-0.4%; $P = 0.40$ and -0.1%; $P = 0.74$, respectively) and did decrease significantly in the control group (-2%; $P < 0.001$). The difference compared with control was significant for both high-impact exercise groups ($P = 0.005$ and 0.001 for exercise with and without black cohosh, respectively). No differences between the exercise groups with and without black cohosh was determined. Of concern, the 10-year CHD risk significantly increased in the exercise plus black cohosh group (12.9%; $P = 0.018$) and in the control group (16.5%; $P = 0.007$). while the exercise-alone group did not show corresponding changes (-2.7% $P = 0.60$). However, no significant between-group differences were observed. The authors concluded that the high-impact exercise program favorably affected bone density and menopausal symptoms as well as lean body mass and, to a lesser extent 10-year CHD risk in early postmenopausal women, and that addition of black cohosh did not enhance the positive effects (Bebenek et al., 2010).

A 3-month RCT in postmenopausal women ($n = 62$) compared black cohosh 40 mg/day with conjugated estrogens 0.6 mg/day and with placebo. Climacteric complaints and bone metabolism were improved equally with black cohosh and conjugated estrogens, both better than placebo. Black cohosh had no effect on endometrial thickness, which was significantly increased by conjugated estrogens. Vaginal superficial cells were increased by both black cohosh and conjugated estrogens. The authors concluded that black cohosh and conjugated estrogens were equipotent for bone metabolism and climacteric complaints and proposed that black cohosh had substances with SERM activity, that is, with desired effects in the hypothalamus, bone, and vagina, but without exerting uterotrophic effects (Wuttke et al., 2003).

A 12-week RCT in postmenopausal women ($n = 62$) compared black cohosh 40 mg/day with conjugated estrogen 0.6 mg/day and with placebo for effects on markers of bone metabolism, hormones, SHBG, lipid metabolism, vaginal maturity, and routine laboratory parameters. The analyses of bone turnover markers indicated beneficial effects for black cohosh and estrogen on bone metabolism. Black cohosh stimulated osteoblast activity, whereas estrogen inhibited osteoclast activity. Estrogen showed strong estrogenic effects on vaginal mucosa, but black cohosh showed weak estrogen-like activity. No significant effects were seen on blood coagulation markers and liver enzymes. Black cohosh was well tolerated. The authors concluded that black cohosh had beneficial bone remodeling effects and weak estrogen-like effects on vaginal mucosa (Wuttke et al., 2006).

Oncologic Disorders

A 2020 systematic review was undertaken to evaluate the benefits of isopropanolic extracts of black cohosh alone or in combination with St. John's wort in breast cancer patients with anti-estrogen induced menopausal symptoms. Most breast cancer survivors receiving anti-estrogen therapy experienced reductions in climacteric symptoms with black cohosh with or without St. John's wort. Some studies indicated that tamoxifen's interference potential could be countered by using higher doses of either herbal regimen. No estrogen-like effects on breast tissue or hormones were seen. Patients using black cohosh alone or combined with St. John's wort had significantly increased recurrence-free survival rates compared with non-users. These results were noted by the authors to have been substantiated by experimental data demonstrating antiproliferative and anti-invasive effects of black cohosh in breast cancer cells and enhancement of the antineoplastic effects of tamoxifen. St. John's wort was noted to exhibit no clinically relevant interaction potential. The authors concluded that isopropanolic extracts of black cohosh with or without St. John's wort may offer a safe non-hormonal therapeutic option for breast cancer survivors receiving endocrine therapy (Ruan et al., 2019).

A 2018 systematic review to identify single-herb medicines that may warrant further study for treatment of anxiety and depression in cancer patients found 100 studies involving 38 botanicals that met inclusion criteria. Among herbs most studied ($\geq$ six randomized controlled trials each), lavender, passionflower, and saffron produced benefits comparable to standard anxiolytics and antidepressants. Black cohosh, chamomile, and chasteberry were also promising. Overall, 45% of studies reported positive findings with fewer adverse effects compared with conventional medications. The authors concluded that saffron, black cohosh, chamomile, chasteberry, lavender, and passionflower appeared useful in mitigating anxiety or depression with favorable risk–benefit profiles compared with standard treatments, and these botanicals may benefit cancer patients by minimizing medication load and accompanying side effects (Yeung et al., 2018).

A retrospective observational study (mean observation time 3.6 years) of breast cancer patients ($n = 18,861$) found that use of black cohosh ($n = 1102$) enhanced disease-free survival. Recurrence occurred in 14% of the subjects after

2 years in the control group and after 6.5 years in the black cohosh group (Henneicke-von Zepelin et al., 2007).

A 6-month open-label trial in survivors of breast cancer ($n=50$) on tamoxifen assessed the menopausal syndrome effects of black cohosh 2.5 mg 1–4 tablets. Menopausal rating scale II total score was reduced significantly from 17.6 to 13.6. Hot flushes, sweating, sleep problems, and anxiety improved, whereas urogenital and musculoskeletal complaints did not change. Adverse events were reported by 22 women, but none of the events were linked to black cohosh. Tolerability of black cohosh was rated as "very good" or "good" in 90% of subjects. The authors concluded that black cohosh extract seemed to be a reasonable treatment approach in tamoxifen-treated breast cancer patients with predominantly psychovegetative symptoms (Rostock et al., 2011).

A 12-week RCT in breast cancer patients ($n=85$) starting on LHRH-agonists compared an isopropanolic extract of black cohosh (Remifemin) plus the LHRH-a with the LHRH-a alone for effects on menopausal symptoms. At weeks 4, 8, and 12, the Kupperman Index scores were all significantly lower with black cohosh ($P<0.01$). Estradiol, FSH, and LH were similar in the two groups. There was no significant difference between groups in endometrial thickness, ovarian cysts, or uterine fibroids ($P>0.05$), but cervical cyst incidence was greater with black cohosh ($P=0.02$). The authors concluded that Remifemin was an effective and oncologically safe and reliable option for treatment of menopausal symptoms induced by LHRH agonists in breast cancer patients (Wang et al., 2019).

ACTIVE CONSTITUENTS

- Phenolic compounds
  - Phenolics: hydroxytyrosol, protocatechualdehyde
  - Phenolic acids: salicylic acid, protocatechuic acid
  - Phenylpropanoids (antioxidant, antimutagenic, antitumor, antimicrobial): cimiracemate A, cimiracemate B, caffeic acid, cimicifugic acids A, B, and D-F, cinnamic acid ester, dehydrocimicifugic A, dehydrocimicifugic acid B, dihydroxyphenyl lactic acid, fukinolic acid, ferulic acid, isoferulic acid, methyl caffeate acid, p-coumaric acid, ferulate-1-methyl ester, 1-isoferuloyl-beta-D-glucopyranoside
- Lignans: actaealactone
- Isoflavonones (phytoestrogenic): formononetin (varies)
- Terpenes
  - Triterpine glycosides (hypothalamic-pituitary function, nucleoside transport inhibition): 23-epi-26-deoxyactein, acteol, actein, 27-deoxyactein, cimicifugoside A, cimicifugoside M, racemoside, cimiracemoside A-H, cimigenol
  - Tetraterpene/Carotenoids: Actaeaeposcide (anti-inflammatory)
- Steroids
  - Phytosterols: Cyclolanostanol xylosides
- Alkaloids
  - N-Ω-methylserotonin, cimipronidine, dopargine
- Aromatics:
  - Salsolinol

BLACK COHOSH COMMONLY USED PREPARATIONS AND DOSAGE (FOR ADULTS UNLESS OTHERWISE SPECIFIED)

The following are examples of some available formulations and ranges of dosing for commercial herbal products. See Part III Introduction "How to prescribe medicinal herbs" for further guidance on herbal advising and prescribing.

Dried Root

- Decoction: 40-200 mg dried root per cup QD-TID
- Fluid extract (1:1, 90%): 0.3–1.8 mL TID
- Tincture (1:5 or 1:10, 60%): 2–4 mL BID-
- Capsule or tablet of powdered root: 300–540 mg BID-TID
- Capsule or tablet of standardized extract (standardized to 2.5%–5% triterpene glycosides): 20–80 mg QD-BID

SAFETY AND PRECAUTION

Side Effects

Possible treatment-related side effects have a low incidence. GI upset occurred most commonly in 0.5%–15% of subjects in one meta-analysis. Breast swelling, edema, arthralgia, rashes, bradycardia, dizziness, headaches, and vivid dreams have been reported, usually at higher doses of several grams per day. Although around 2002 there were at least 50 isolated case reports of hepatotoxicity associated with use of black cohosh, a meta-analysis of five studies (*n* = 1117) using 40–128 mg black cohosh for 3 to 6 months showed no significant effects on liver function tests compared with placebo. Additional studies have focused on this topic as well and have found no evidence for concern. The discrepancy is most convincingly explained by lack of purity of earlier sources of black cohosh.

Case Reports

Several case reports from 2003–2017 of autoimmune hepatitis with possible causality ascribed consumption of black cohosh.

Toxicity

Mice given 1000 mg/kg black cohosh extract for 92 days had elevated MMA and homocysteine levels suggesting B vitamin deficiency.

Pregnancy and Lactation

Avoid due to conflicting evidence for hormonal effects.

Drug Interactions

- CYP: Cytochrome P3A4: Black cohosh may interact with drugs that are metabolized by CYP3A4 enzyme although one study showed no effect on this enzyme and minimal effect on CYP2D6. Pgp: P-glycoprotein does not appear to be affected by black cohosh.
- Tamoxifen: Theoretically, may interfere with action of tamoxifen due to uncertain underlying activity on estrogen receptors. However, clinical research suggests synergism with tamoxifen.
- Chemotherapy drugs: May increase the toxicity of doxorubicin and docetaxel.
- Black cohosh and actein have synergistic effects with simvastatin, resulting in enhanced activity and increased side effects.

REFERENCES

Bai WP, Wang SY, Liu JL, et al. Efficacy and safety of remifemin compared with tibolone for controlling of perimenopausal symptoms. Zhonghua Fu Chan Ke Za Zhi 2009;44(8):597–600.

Bebenek M, Kemmler W, von Stengel S, Engelke K, Kalender WA. Effect of exercise and Cimicifuga racemosa (CR BNO 1055) on bone mineral density, 10-year coronary heart disease risk, and menopausal complaints: the randomized controlled training and Cimicifuga racemosa Erlangen (TRACE) study. Menopause 2010;17(4):791–800.

Cappelli V, Morgante G, Di Sabatino A, Massaro MG, De Leo V. Evaluation of the efficacy of a new nutraceutical product in the treatment of postmenopausal symptoms. Minerva Ginecol 2015;67(6):515–21.

Drewe J, Bucher KA, Zahner C. A systematic review of non-hormonal treatments of vasomotor symptoms in climacteric and cancer patients. Springerplus 2015;4:65.

Geller SE, Studee L. Botanical and dietary supplements for mood and anxiety in menopausal women. Menopause 2007;14(3 Pt 1):541–9.

Ghazanfarpour M, Sadeghi R, Abdolahian S, Latifnejad RR. The efficacy of Iranian herbal medicines in alleviating hot flushes: a systematic review. Int J Reprod Biomed (Yazd) 2016;14(3):155–66.

Guttuso Jr T. Effective and clinically meaningful non-hormonal hot flush therapies. Maturitas 2012;72(1):6–12.

Henneicke-von Zepelin HH, Meden H, Kostev K, Schröder-Bernhardi D, Stammwitz U, Becher H. Isopropanolic black cohosh extract and recurrence-free survival after breast cancer. Int J Clin Pharmacol Ther 2007;45(3):143–54.

Huntley AL, Ernst E. A systematic review of herbal medicinal products for the treatment of menopausal symptoms. Menopause 2003;10(5):465–76.

Kamel HH. Role of phyto-oestrogens in ovulation induction in women with polycystic ovarian syndrome. Eur J Obstet Gynecol Reprod Biol 2013;168(1):60–3.

Kargozar R, Azizi H, Salari R. A review of effective herbal medicines in controlling menopausal symptoms. Electron Phys 2017;9(11):5826–33.

Laakmann E, Grajecki D, Doege K, zu Eulenburg C, Buhling KJ. Efficacy of Cimicifuga racemosa, Hypericum perforatum and Agnus castus in the treatment of climacteric complaints: a systematic review. Gynecol Endocrinol 2012;28(9):703–9.

Leach MJ, Moore V. Black cohosh (Cimicifuga spp.) for menopausal symptoms. Cochrane Database Syst Rev 2012;9. CD007244.

Lundström E, Hirschberg AL, Söderqvist G. Digitized assessment of mammographic breast density-effects of continuous combined hormone therapy, tibolone and black cohosh compared with placebo. Maturitas 2011;70(4):361–4.

Nappi RE, Malavasi B, Brundu B, Facchinetti F. Efficacy of Cimicifuga racemosa on climacteric complaints: a randomized study vs low-dose transdermal estradiol. Gynecol Endocrinol 2005;20(1):30–5.

Oktem M, Eroglu D, Karahan HB, Taskintuna N, Kuscu E, Zeyneloglu HB. Black cohosh and fluoxetine in the treatment of postmenopausal symptoms: a prospective, randomized trial. Adv Ther 2007;24(2):448–61.

Pkhaladze L, Davidova N, Khomasuridze A, Shengelia R, Panossian A. *Actaea racemosa* L. is more effective in combination with *Rhodiola rosea* L. for relief of menopausal symptoms: a randomized, double-blind, placebo-controlled study. Pharmaceuticals (Basel) 2020;13(5):102.

Raus K, Brucker C, Gorkow C, Wuttke W. First-time proof of endometrial safety of the special black cohosh extract (Actaea or Cimicifuga racemosa extract) CR BNO 1055. Menopause 2006;13(4):678–91.

Reame NE, Lukacs JL, Padmanabhan V, Eyvazzadeh AD, Smith YR, Zubieta JK. Black cohosh has central opioid activity in post-menopausal women: evidence from naloxone blockade and positron emission tomography neuroimaging. Menopause 2008;15(5):832–40.

Rostock M, Fischer J, Mumm A, Stammwitz U, Saller R, Bartsch HH. Black cohosh (Cimicifuga racemosa) in tamoxifen-treated breast cancer patients with climacteric complaints—a prospective observational study. Gynecol Endocrinol 2011;27(10):844–8.

Rotem C, Kaplan B. Phyto-Female Complex for the relief of hot flushes, night sweats and quality of sleep: randomized, controlled, double-blind pilot study. Gynecol Endocrinol 2007.

Ruan X, Mueck A, Beer A-M, Naser B, Pickartz S. Benefit-risk profile of black cohosh (isopropanolic *Cimicifuga racemosa* extract) with and without St John's wort in breast cancer patients. Climacteric 2019;22(4):339–47.

Sarri G, Pedder H, Dias S, Guo Y, Lumsden MA. Vasomotor symptoms resulting from natural menopause: a systematic review and network meta-analysis of treatment effects from the National Institute for Health and Care Excellence guideline on menopause. BJOG 2017;124(10):1514–23.

Shahin AY, Ismail AM, Zahran KM, Makhlouf AM. Adding phytoestrogens to clomiphene induction in unexplained infertility patients—a randomized trial. Reprod Biomed Online 2008;16(4):580–8.

Shams T, Setia MS, Hemmings R, McCusker J, Sewitch M, Ciampi A. Efficacy of black cohosh-containing preparations on menopausal symptoms: a meta-analysis. Altern Ther Health Med 2010;16(1):36–44.

Uebelhack R, Blohmer JU, Graubaum HJ, Busch R, Gruenwald J, Wernecke KD. Black cohosh and St. John's wort for climacteric complaints: a randomized trial. Obstet Gynecol 2006;107(2):247–55.

Wang C, Huang Q, Liang C-L, et al. Effect of cimicifugaracemosa on menopausal syndrome caused by LHRH-a in breast cancer. J Ethnopharmacol 2019;238:111840.

Wuttke W, Seidlová-Wuttke D, Gorkow C. The Cimicifuga preparation BNO 1055 vs conjugated estrogens in a double-blind placebo-controlled study: effects on menopause symptoms and bone markers. Maturitas 2003;44(Suppl 1):S67–77.

Wuttke W, Gorkow C, Seidlova-Wuttke D. Effects of black cohosh (Cimicifuga racemosa) on bone turnover, vaginal mucosa, and various blood parameters in postmenopausal women: a double-blind, placebo-controlled, and conjugated estrogens-controlled study. Menopause 2006;13(2):185–96.

Xi S, Liske E, Wang S, et al. Effect of isopropanolic cimicifuga racemosa extract on uterine fibroids in comparison with tibolone among patients of a recent randomized, double blind, parallel-controlled study in chinese women with menopausal symptoms. Evid Based Complement Alternat Med 2014;717686.

Yeung KS, Hernandez M, Mao JJ, Haviland I, Gubili J. Herbal medicine for depression and anxiety: A systematic review with assessment of potential psycho-oncologic relevance. Phytother Res 2018;32(5):865–91.

31

BLACK SEED/NIGELLA/BLACK CUMIN (*NIGELLA SATIVA*)
Seed

GENERAL OVERVIEW

This seed of many names is usually referred to as black seed or nigella in the United States but is also known as "black cumin" and "black caraway" (although unrelated to the latter two spice plants). As the Latin name of black seed indicates, this herb with black (*Nigella*) seeds has been cultivated (*sativa*) for thousands of years. Archeological sites in Egypt provide evidence of human use of black seed from as far back as the 14th century BCE. Cuneiform tablets of ancient Assyria describe various uses for black seed, including for cases of "a ghost lying on the patient," and its seeds were found in the tomb of the renowned Egyptian pharaoh Tutankhamun. It has documentation of use for difficult breathing, headaches, toothaches, skin imperfections, leprosy, cataracts, postnasal drip, corns, roundworms, amenorrhea, and fluid retention. Black seed is commonly used in Ayurvedic medicine and traditional Arabic and Iranian medicine through which a wealth of clinical research has occurred. Modern traditional medicinal indications for use of black seed include asthma, coughs, hypertension, dyslipidemia, obesity, diarrhea, dysentery, abdominal pain, renal calculi, headache, dermatological problems, back pain, and infections.

Black seed appears to be medicinally active in low doses and does not require any particular extraction process, so is considered a functional food (can be eaten for its desired benefits beyond simple nourishment). However, most of the research on the product uses various methods of extraction including distillation into an essential oil.

Clinical research indicates that black seed, alone or in combination formulas, may be beneficial for periodontitis, chronic rhinosinusitis, nasal dryness, oral submucous fibrosis, allergic rhinitis, asthma, chemical war pneumonitis, hypertension, congestive heart failure, hyperlipidemia, dyslipidemia, diabetes, metabolic syndrome, obesity, non-alcoholic fatty liver disease, hepatotoxicity, peptic ulcer disease and *Helicobacter pylori*, functional dyspepsia, diabetic nephropathy, cyclic mastalgia, menopause, male infertility, osteoarthritis, chronic pain, seizure disorders, cognitive impairment, anxiety, depression, eczema, inflammation, Hashimoto's thyroiditis, rheumatoid arthritis, vitiligo, *S. aureus* pustules, hepatitis C virus, febrile neutropenia, and acute lymphoblastic leukemia.

IN VITRO AND ANIMAL RESEARCH

In vivo and in vitro studies have shown black seed powder and oil to have immunomodulatory, anti-inflammatory, antioxidant, antihistaminic, anti-asthmatic, hepatoprotective, hypoglycemic, antioxytocic, and vulnerary properties. It shows antihypertensive effects through inhibition of sympathetic overactivity, stimulation of NO production, and diuretic and calcium channel blocking mechanisms. It demonstrates antiviral, antiparasitic, antibacterial and antifungal, and anticancer properties.

Two main constituents, nigellone and thymoquinone, have been shown to inhibit mast cell histamine release in rats. Thymoquinone was shown in sensitized guinea pigs to reduce tracheal sensitivity to histamine and acetylcholine, suggesting anti-asthmatic effects. Comferol diglucoside and digalactoside from black seed have been shown to relax precontracted bronchial muscles with comparable potency to theophylline. Research indicates this bronchorelaxation effect is via opening potassium channels, with PDE inhibition and anticholinergic mechanisms also possibly contributing.

Black seed has been shown to reduce foam cells in vitro. Rat studies have shown improved recovery of cardiac tissue following ischemia-reperfusion injury and to show dose-dependent reductions in BP and heart rate likely through cholinergic mechanisms.

In vitro black seed extract has been shown to activate AMPK phosphorylation in muscle cells but not adipocytes. It appears to be similar to metformin and berberine in activation of AMPK and uncoupling of mitochondria to preserve cytoplasmic ATP concentrations.

The seed extract given to rodents in a dose equivalent to a human dose of 2 g of seed extract over 4 weeks increased acetyl-CoA carboxylase phosphorylation in skeletal muscle, indicative of increased AMPK activity. Akt phosphorylation in response to insulin was increased by black seed petroleum extract in rat livers and myocytes but not adipocytes. This is the likely mechanism for the increase in GLUT4 content of skeletal muscles noted in animals fed a basic seed extract equivalent to 2 g in humans. In adipocytes, black seed has been shown to increase glucose uptake and proliferation, likely due to activation of PPARγ activity. Other mechanisms that have been affected by black seed include an increase in baseline ERK 1/2 phosphorylation and enhancement of ERK 1/2 phosphorylation in response to insulin treatment in myocytes but not adipocytes. A study in rats demonstrated a 25% reduction in food intake and mild weight loss one week after ingestion of petroleum extract. Extracts of black seed have been shown to attenuate formation of calcium oxalate stones in a rat model of nephrolithiasis at a dose comparable to 3 g in humans.

Black seed has demonstrated positive effects on memory impairment, prevention of hippocampal pyramidal cell loss, and consolidation of recall capability of stored information and spatial memory in aged rats. Black seed has been found to increase brain GABA concentrations in mice and has been shown inhibit picrotoxin (noncompetitive GABA$_A$ antagonist) induced seizures and to counter bicuculline

(competitive GABA$_A$ antagonist), being more protective than 300 mg/kg sodium valproate against picrotoxin. It has been shown to potentiate the effects of sodium valproate. There is indication that the constituent thymoquinone enhances the GABA$_A$ receptor. In rats, intracerebroventricular injections of thymoquinone reduced by half experimentally induced seizures; this was reversed by flumazenil and attenuated by naloxone. Research in rats has also shown that thymoquinone has opioidergic signaling, which increases GABAergic tone. Thymoquinone has also been shown to suppress stress-induced increases in brain nitrite concentrations, which can dysregulate GABAergic signaling via cGMP suppression of GABA$_A$ function. A study of a stroke model in rats showed that black seed fully preserved locomotor activity and grip strength and reduced oxidative changes and infarct size similar to 100 mg/kg aspirin.

Thymoquinone demonstrated anxiolytic properties in mice, more so in the less stressed mice, with a potency comparable to 2 mg/kg of diazepam. In a model of LPS induced depression (an inflammatory model of depression), black seed and thymoquinone injections abolished the depressant effect. Black seed has demonstrated mild analgesic properties in rats.

At least eight in silico studies have shown that some compounds of black seed, including nigelledine, α-hederin, hederagenin, thymohydroquinone, and thymoquinone, had high-to-moderate affinity with SARS-CoV-2 enzymes and proteins. This molecular docking research indicates that several constituents of black seed may potentially inhibit SARS-CoV-2 attachment and replication (Koshak and Koshak, 2020).

Pre-dosing rats with black seed in an experimental model of hepatocellular carcinoma reduced liver growth and liver enzymes by about 50%. Thymoquinone demonstrated cytotoxic activity in cervical squamous cell carcinoma more effectively than cisplatin and with less toxicity on non-cancerous cells. It induced apoptosis, increased p53 expression, and decreased Bcl-2.

HUMAN RESEARCH

General

A 2017 literature review of RCTs investigated the therapeutic effects of black seed and/or thymoquinone in the prevention and the treatment of different diseases and morbidity in humans. The authors found evidence that black seed and thymoquinone had been shown to possess multiple useful applications including inflammatory and autoimmune disorders and metabolic syndrome. Additional effects of black seed included antimicrobial, anti-nociceptive, and anti-epileptic properties, with minor side effects. The authors concluded that black seed had been sufficiently studied and was sufficiently understood to allow for the next phase of clinical trials or drug developments (Tavakkoli et al., 2017).

Oral and Dental Disorders

A 6-week RCT in dental subjects ($n = 20$) with chronic periodontitis investigated intracrevicular thymoquinone 0.2% gel plus scaling and root planing compared with scaling and root planing alone. The thymoquinone group had a significant reduction in the probing pocket depth and gingival crevicular fluid ALP levels and an increase in relative attachment level compared with the scaling-only group. No differences between groups were seen with plaque index and gingival index. Thymoquinone gel was active against *P. gingivalis*, *A. actinomycetemcomitans*, and *P. intermedia*. The authors concluded that thymoquinone dental gel provided significant changes in clinical and biochemical parameters and could be a beneficial adjunct to scaling and root planing in treating chronic periodontitis (Kapil et al., 2018).

Ears, Nose, and Throat Disorders

An 8-week RCT in patients ($n = 65$) with mild-to-moderate chronic rhinosinusitis without nasal polyps compared black seed nasal spray (2 puffs or 1 g/day) with placebo (nasal saline 0.65%). Lund-McKay, Lund Kennedy, and Sino-Nasal Outcome Test-22 scores decreased significantly in both groups but were lower with the black seed spray ($P < 0.001$ for all). The authors concluded that black seed nasal spray was effective for symptomatic relief of chronic rhinosinusitis without nasal polyps (Rezaeian and Amoushahi, 2018).

A 4-week crossover RCT in geriatric patients ($n = 42$) with nasal dryness compared intranasal black seed oil with isotonic saline each given for 2 weeks and then crossed over after a 3-week washout period. Nasal dryness, obstruction, and crusting improved

significantly with black seed oil compared with saline ($P < 0.05$) without any carryover effects. There was no significant difference between groups for nasal burning and itching ($P > 0.05$). There was no change in mucociliary clearance during any of the treatment periods. The authors concluded that black seed oil was better than nasal saline for geriatric nasal dryness (Oysu et al., 2014).

A 3-month RCT in patients ($n = 40$) with oral submucous fibrosis compared turmeric plus black pepper with black seed. Mouth opening improved by 3.85 mm with turmeric and 3.6 mm with black seed ($P < 0.01$ compared with baseline for both). Burning sensation decreased by 88% with turmeric and by 79% with black seed ($P < 0.01$ for both). SOD levels improved by 0.62 U/mL with turmeric and 0.74 U/mL with black seed ($P < 0.05$ for both). Maximum mouth opening was 8 mm with turmeric and 7 mm with black seed. The authors concluded that turmeric plus black pepper and black seed both improved mouth opening, burning sensation, and SOD levels in patients with oral submucous fibrosis (Pipalia et al., 2016).

Pulmonary Disorders: Chemical War Pneumonitis

A 2-month RCT in patients ($n = 40$) who were chemical war victims compared a 50 g% boiled extract of black seed 0.375 mL/kg/day with a placebo solution. All respiratory symptoms, chest wheezing, and PFT values significantly improved at 1 month and 2 months with black seed compared with baseline ($P < 0.05$ and $P < 0.001$, respectively). Further improvement of chest wheezing and in some of the PFT values occurred between the 1-month and 2-month measurements ($P < 0.05–0.001$). By 2 months, all PFT values and most symptoms were significantly better with black seed than with placebo ($P < 0.01–0.001$). The use of inhaler, oral β-agonists, and oral corticosteroids decreased with black seed but not with placebo. The authors concluded that prophylactic use of black seed was beneficial for chemical war victims (Boskabady and Farhadi, 2008).

Pulmonary Disorders: Chronic Obstructive Pulmonary Disease

A 3-month RCT in patients ($n = 100$) with mild-to-moderate COPD compared black seed oil plus standard therapy with standard therapy alone for effects on lung function. With black seed, there were significant decreases from baseline in oxidation and inflammatory markers: TBARS, protein carbonyl content (biomarker of oxidative stress), IL-6, and TNF-α. There were significant increases in antioxidants: SOD, catalase, GSH, glutathione peroxidase, vitamin C, and vitamin E. There was also a significant improvement in PFTs compared with the control group and with baseline levels. The authors concluded that black seed oil may be effective adjunctive therapy to improve pulmonary function, inflammation, and oxidant–antioxidant imbalance in COPD patients (Al-Azzawi et al., 2020).

Pulmonary Disorders: Allergy and Asthma

A 2020 systematic review to evaluate the efficacy of black seed for asthma control found four RCTs that were included for meta-analysis. Overall, compared with control groups black seed was found to be associated with increased ACT scores (SMD = 0.50; $P = 0.01$) and FEV1 (SMD = 1.84; $P = 0.04$). Black seed demonstrated no obvious impact on PEF (SMD = 3.11; $P = 0.17$), IL-4 (SMD = −0.31; $P = 0.50$), or IFN-γ (SMD = 1.11; $P = 0.16$). The authors concluded that black seed may provide additional benefits for the treatment of asthma (He and Xiaohong, 2020).

A 2017 literature review of black seed to assess the studies supporting the medicinal use of black seed for asthma found 14 preclinical studies and 7 clinical studies that showed improvements in different asthma outcomes including symptoms, pulmonary function, and laboratory parameters. The authors noted that often these studies were small and used ill-defined preparations. The authors concluded that black seed could be therapeutically beneficial in alleviating airway inflammation and the control of asthma symptoms, but that well-designed large clinical studies using chemically well-characterized black seed preparations were required (Koshak et al., 2017a).

A review of four studies ($n = 152$) on the clinical efficacy of black seed for allergic disease using black seed oil 40–80 mg/kg/day noted that the score of subjective symptoms decreased consistently over the courses in the studies. A slight decrease in plasma TG and an increase in HDL-C were noted. There were no changes in lymphocyte subpopulations, endogenous cortisol levels, and ACTH. The authors concluded that black

seed oil had been proven to be an effective adjuvant for treatment of allergic diseases (Kalus et al., 2003).

A 30-day RCT in patients ($n = 66$) with allergic rhinitis compared black seed oil nasal wash with placebo on symptoms, nasal IgE, and nasal eosinophil levels. While total serum IgE was unchanged by day 15 there was a significant reduction from baseline in nasal IgE with black seed but not with placebo ($P = 0.0017$ and $P = 0.455$, respectively). The authors noted that black seed resulted in a reduction in the presence of nasal mucosal congestion, nasal itching, runny nose, sneezing attacks, turbinate hypertrophy, and mucosal pallor by day 15. They concluded that the study supported evidence for antiallergic effects of black seed (Nikakhlagh et al., 2011).

A 6-week RCT in patients ($n = 68$) with allergic rhinitis compared intranasal black seed oil with ordinary food oil. All patients with mild symptoms given black seed oil became symptom-free; 69% of patients with moderate symptoms given black seed oil became symptom-free and 25% were improved. In patients with severe symptoms 58% became symptom-free with black seed oil and 25% were improved. In total, 92% and 30% of patients given black seed oil and food oil, respectively, demonstrated improvement in their symptoms or were symptom-free ($P = 0.000$). The improvement in tolerability of allergen exposure was 55% and 20% with black seed and food oil, respectively ($P = 0.006$). The authors concluded that topical nasal application of black seed oil was effective in the treatment of allergic rhinitis, with minimal side effects (Alsamarai et al., 2014).

A 30-day RCT in patients ($n = 12$) with allergic rhinitis and sensitivity to house dust mites treated with immunotherapy for 30 days and healthy volunteers ($n = 8$) investigated oral black seed 2 g/day plus immunotherapy compared with immunotherapy alone and with saline solution subcutaneously. In patients receiving specific immunotherapy there was a statistically significant increase in the phagocytic and intracellular killing activities of PMNs and this was augmented by black seed. CD8 counts in the combination group significantly increased compared with the immunotherapy-only group. In the healthy volunteers the PMN functions also increased significantly. The authors concluded that black seed supplementation during specific immunotherapy for allergic rhinitis may be considered a potential adjuvant therapy (Işik et al., 2010).

A 4-week RCT in patients ($n = 80$) with asthma compared black seed oil capsules 500 mg BID with placebo. The mean Asthma Control Test score improved by 21.1 and 19.6 with black seed and placebo, respectively ($P = 0.044$). Blood eosinophils changed by -50 and $+15$ with black seed and placebo, respectively ($P = 0.013$). FEV1 improved by 4% of predicted value with black seed and 1% with placebo, respectively ($P = 0.170$). The authors concluded that black seed oil supplementation improved asthma control with a trend toward PFT improvement (Koshak et al., 2017b).

A 3-month single-blind RCT in patients ($n = 76$) with asthma on maintenance therapy compared black seed 1 g/day with black seed 2 g/day and with placebo. FEF 25%–75% and FEV1 increased significantly ($P < 0.05$) at both 6 and 12 weeks with black seed 2 g/day. PEF variability significantly improved with both doses of black seed at 6 and 12 weeks compared with placebo ($P < 0.05$). Both doses of black seed resulted in significant decreases over baseline in fractional exhaled nitric oxide and serum IgE ($P < 0.05$) and a significant increase over baseline in the serum IFN-γ ($P < 0.05$). Asthma Control Test score was significantly improved over baseline with both doses at 6 and 12 weeks ($P < 0.001$; $P < 0.01$, respectively). Significantly fewer patients had exacerbations with black seed 1 g/day ($P < 0.05$). The authors concluded that black seed added to inhaled maintenance therapy improved some measures of pulmonary function and inflammation in incompletely controlled asthma (Salem et al., 2017).

An acutely dosed RCT in asthma patients ($n = 15$) compared black seed boiled extract 50 and 100 mg/kg with theophylline 6 mg/kg. Significant increases in all measured PFTs in most time intervals (30, 60, 90 120, 150, and 180 min after administration) occurred with black seed at both doses ($P < 0.05$ to $P < 0.001$). The increases in FEV1, MMEF, and MEF(50) were significantly less with both doses of black seed than with theophylline, and the increases in MEF(75) and MEF(25) were significantly less with the lower dose of black seed than with theophylline ($P < 0.05$ to $P < 0.001$, respectively). The effects of both doses of the extract were also significantly less than that of salbutamol at 30 min post administration ($P < 0.001$). The onset at 30 min and decline at 150 min of the brochodilatory effect was similar between black seed and theophylline. The authors concluded that black seed had a relatively potent anti-asthmatic effect on asthmatic airways, but the effects on most measured PFTs were less than those of theophylline at the concentrations used (Boskabady et al., 2010).

A 3-month RCT in adults ($n = 29$) with asthma compared a 0.1 g % black seed boiled extract 15 mL/kg with placebo. All asthma symptoms, frequency of asthma symptoms/week, chest wheezing, and PFT values improved significantly over baseline with black seed by 45 and 90 days ($P < 0.05$–0.001). In addition, further improvement of wheezing and severity of disease occurred between days 45 and 90 ($P < 0.05$ for both). At 90 days all symptoms were significantly better with black seed than with placebo ($P < 0.01$–0.001). Use of oral and inhaled β-agonists, oral and inhaled corticosteroids, and oral theophylline decreased at 90 days with black seed, while there were no obvious changes in usage of the drugs with placebo. The author concluded that there may be a prophylactic effect of black seed on asthma (Boskabady et al., 2007).

Cardiovascular Disorders: Hypertension

A 2016 systematic review evaluating the effects of black seed on lipid profiles, glycemic control, BP, and some anthropometric indices found 23 studies ($n = 1531$) that met inclusion criteria. In four trials black seed reduced BP, but in five trials it did not. FBS was reduced significantly, and A1C was reduced in 13 studies. BW and WC decreased significantly in two studies but did not decrease in another six trials. Changes in the lipid profile were very inconsistent across trials. The authors concluded that black seed might be effective in glycemic control in humans (Mohtashami and Entezari, 2016).

A 12-month single-blind RCT in patients ($n = 114$) with T2DM on oral hypoglycemic agents compared black seed 2 g/day with placebo for effects on lipids, BP, and BW. The black seed group had significant declines over baseline and over placebo in TC, LDL-C, TC/HDL-C, and LDL-C/HDL-C. HDL-C was significantly increased with black seed. With placebo there was a significant decrease in HDL-C and increases in the TC/HDL-C and LDL-C/HDL-C. Black seed was associated with significant reductions in SBP, DBP, MAP, and HR over baseline and significant decreases in DBP, MAP, and HR over placebo. Placebo was associated with a significant elevation in MAP. The authors concluded that black seed improved TC, MAP, and HR in patients with T2DM on oral hypoglycemic agents (Badar et al., 2017).

An 8-week RCT in patients with mild HTN compared black seed 100 mg or 200 mg BID with placebo. SBP with both doses of black seed was significantly reduced compared with baseline and with placebo ($P < 0.05$–0.01). DBP was also significantly reduced with both doses of black seed compared with baseline and with placebo ($P < 0.01$). The higher dose of black seed had a greater magnitude of effect. TC and LDL-C were reduced with black seed as well. No complications were reported. The authors concluded that black seed extract may have a blood-pressure lowering effect in patients with mild HTN (Dehkordi and Kamkhah, 2008).

A 28-day RCT in elderly patients ($n = 76$) with HTN compared black seed 300 mg BID with placebo. The mean SBP was decreased from 160.4 mmHg to 145.8 mmHg, and from 160.9 mmHg to 147.53 mmHg with black seed and placebo, respectively. Mean DBP was decreased from 78.3 mmHg to 74.4 mmHg, and from 79.0 mmHg to 78.2 mmHg with black seed and placebo, respectively ($P = 0.35$). Reported adverse events included dyspepsia (15.7%), nausea (7.8%), and constipation (5.2%). No electrolyte abnormalities, liver and renal toxicities, or orthostatic hypotension were observed. The authors concluded that black seed was not proven to decrease BP in the elderly with HTN (Rizka et al., 2017).

An 8-week RCT in healthy volunteers ($n = 70$) with normal BP compared black seed oil 2.5 mL with placebo BID for effects on metabolic parameters. SBP and DBP decreased significantly with black seed oil compared with baseline and with placebo after 8 weeks. BMI, ALT, AST, ALP, creatinine, and BUN did not change significantly in either group. No adverse effects were reported. The authors concluded that black seed oil lowered BP in healthy volunteers after 8 weeks (Fallah Huseini et al., 2013).

Cardiovascular Disorders: Congestive Heart Failure

A 1-year RCT in patients ($n = 60$) with T2DM and A1C > 7% and with no known cardiovascular complications compared black seed 2 g/day with activated charcoal as a placebo for glycemic and cardiovascular effects. Black seed was associated with a significant reduction in A1C compared with placebo. Echocardiographic evaluation with placebo showed impairment in diastolic function after 12 months as well as increased LV volume in diastole and systole, LVM, and LVM index. There were no significant changes in FS or EF. With black seed, no significant changes were found in diastolic function or LVM. LV dimension at systole was decreased, while FS and EF were significantly increased after 6 and 12 months. The authors concluded that black seed may improve systolic function and prevent diastolic dysfunction in patients with T2DM (Bamosa et al., 2015).

Cardiometabolic Disorders: Hyperlipidemia and Dyslipidemia

A 2020 systematic review to assess the effects of black seed on glycemia, lipid profiles, and biomarkers of inflammation and oxidation found 50 trials that met inclusion criteria. Significant reductions were found for TC (WMD: − 16.80), TG (WMD: − 15.73), LDL-C (WMD: − 18.45), VLDL-C (WMD: − 3.72), FBG (WMD: − 15.18). and A1C (WMD: − 0.45). Effects of black seed on CRP (WMD: − 3.61), TNF-α (WMD: − 1.18), TAC (WMD: 0.31), and MDA levels (WMD: − 0.95) did not reach statistical significance. The authors concluded that they found beneficial effects of black seed on fasting glucose, A1C, triglycerides, and total-, VLDL-, and LDL-cholesterol levels (Hallajzadeh et al., 2020).

A 2016 systematic review to evaluate the efficacy of black seed for lipid management found 17 RCTs that met inclusion criteria. Meta-analysis suggested a significant association between black seed supplementation and a reduction in TC (WMD = − 15.65 mg/dL; $P = 0.001$), LDL-C (WMD = − 14.10 mg/dL; $P < 0.001$), and TG (WMD = − 20.64 mg/dL; $P < 0.001$). No significant effect on HDL-C (WMD = 0.28 mg/dL; $P = 0.804$) was found. A greater effect of black seed oil compared with black seed powder was observed on TC and LDL-C levels, and an increase in HDL-C levels was found only with black seed powder. The authors concluded that black seed had a significant impact on plasma lipids, leading to lower TC, LDL-C, and TG levels while increased HDL-C was associated with black seed powder only (Sahebkar et al., 2016).

A 12-month single-blind RCT in patients ($n=114$) with T2DM on oral hypoglycemic agents compared black seed 2 g/day with placebo for effects on lipids, BP, and BW. The black seed group had significant declines over baseline and over placebo in TC, LDL-C, TC/HDL-C, and LDL-C/HDL-C. HDL-C was significantly increased with black seed. With placebo there was a significant decrease in HDL-C and increases in TC/HDL-C and LDL-C/HDL-C. Black seed was associated with significant reductions in SBP, DBP, MAP, and HR over baseline and significant decreases in DBP, MAP, and HR over placebo. Placebo was associated with a significant elevation in MAP. The authors concluded that black seed improved TC, MAP, and HR in patients with T2DM on oral hypoglycemic agents (Badar et al., 2017).

A 4-week RCT in adults ($n=88$) with TC > 200 compared black seed 2 g/day with placebo. TC decreased 4.78%, LDL-C decreased 7.6%, and TG decreased 16.65% with black seed. The difference in changes with black seed were significantly greater than with placebo. HDL-C and FBS did not change significantly. The authors concluded that black seed may have some beneficial therapeutic effects for hyperlipidemia (Sabzghabaee et al., 2012).

A 12-week RCT in patients ($n=94$) with T2DM compared black seed 1, 2, and 3 g/day for effect on lipids. Black seed at 1 g/day was associated with nonsignificant changes in all the lipids except for a significant increase in HDL-C after 4 weeks. Black seed at 2 g/day was associated with significant decreases in TC, TG, and LDL-C, and a significant increase in HDL-C/LDL-C, compared with baseline and with the 1 g/day dose. Increasing the dose to 3 g/day failed to show any increase in the hypolipidemic effect produced by the 2 g/day dose. The authors concluded that black seed at 2 g/day may improve dyslipidemia in diabetic patients (Kaatabi et al., 2015).

An 8-week RCT in women ($n=90$) with BMI 30–35 studied a low-calorie diet plus black seed oil 1 g TID compared with a low-calorie diet plus placebo for effects on weight and lipids. With black seed compared with placebo there were significant reductions in weight (-6.0% vs -3.6%; $P<0.01$), WC (-6.9% vs -3.4%; $P<0.01$), TG (-14.0% vs 1.4%; $P=0.02$), and VLDL (-14.0% vs 7%; $P<0.01$). The authors concluded that black seed oil concurrent with a low-calorie diet could reduce cardiometabolic risk factors in obese women (Mahdavi et al., 2015).

An 8-week RCT in overweight women ($n=20$) compared black seed 2 g/day with placebo, each along with aerobic training three times/week for both groups. Black seed was associated with reductions over baseline in TC by 4.8% ($P<0.01$), LDL-C by 5% ($P<0.001$), TG by 7.8% ($P<0.001$), and BMI by 2.76% ($P<0.01$) as well as increases in HDL-C by 5.76% and VO2$_{max}$ by 2.5% ($P<0.01$). There were significant differences between black seed and placebo for LDL-C ($P<0.05$) and HDL-C ($P<-0.05$). The authors concluded that aerobic training plus black seed had synergistic effects in improving the lipid profile in overweight women (Farzaneh et al., 2014).

An 8-week RCT in patients ($n=40$) with Hashimoto's thyroiditis compared black seed with placebo for effects on cardiometabolic parameters. Black seed was associated with significant reductions in BW, BMI, LDL-C, and TG and significant increases in HDL-C ($P<0.05$). None of these changes were observed with placebo. Nesfatin-1 concentrations were in inverse relationship with TG ($r=-0.31$; $P=0.04$). The authors concluded that black seed improved lipid profiles and anthropometric measurements in patients with Hashimoto's thyroiditis and may be beneficial as an adjunct to levothyroxine (Farhangi et al., 2018).

A 12-week RCT in diabetic patients ($n=50$) with dyslipidemia despite statin therapy investigated a combination of aloe, black seed, fenugreek, garlic, milk thistle, and psyllium (one sachet BID) plus conventional therapy compared with conventional therapy alone. Each sachet contained 300 mg of aloe leaf gel, 1.8 g of black seed, 300 mg of garlic, 2.5 g of fenugreek seed, 1 g of psyllium seed, and 500 mg of milk thistle seed. The levels of serum TG, TC, LDL-C, and A1C, but not FBS, showed a significant in-group improvement in the intervention group. Renal and hepatic transaminases were unchanged with the herbal compound. The authors concluded that this herbal compound was a safe and effective adjunctive treatment in lowering serum lipids in diabetic patients with uncontrolled dyslipidemia (Ghorbani et al., 2019).

Cardiometabolic Disorders: Diabetes, Metabolic Syndrome, and Obesity

A 2020 systematic review to assess the effects of black seed on glycemia, lipid profiles, and biomarkers of inflammation and oxidation found 50 trials that met inclusion criteria. Significant reductions were found for TC (WMD: -16.80), TG (WMD: -15.73), LDL-C (WMD: -18.45), VLDL-C (WMD: -3.72), FBG (WMD: -15.18), and A1C (WMD: -0.45). Effects of black seed on CRP (WMD: -3.61), TNF-α (WMD: -1.18), TAC (WMD: 0.31), and MDA levels (WMD: -0.95) did not reach statistical significance. The authors concluded that they found beneficial effects of black seed on fasting glucose, A1C, triglycerides, and total-, VLDL-, and LDL-cholesterol levels (Hallajzadeh et al., 2020).

A 2018 systematic review to assess the effect of black seed on obesity indices found 13 RCTs ($n=875$) that met inclusion criteria. Combining effect sizes from 10 studies, black seed significantly reduced BW compared with placebo (WMD $= -1.76$ kg, $I^2 = 87.4\%$). A significant reduction was seen in BMI with black seed compared with placebo (WMD $= -0.85$ kg/m^2, $I^2 = 70.6\%$). However, in five studies no significant reduction was found in WC comparing black seed with placebo (WMD $= -4.04$ cm, $I^2 = 97.8\%$). The authors concluded that there was a significant effect of black seed on BW and BMI, but not waist circumference, in adults (Mousavi et al., 2018).

A 2018 systematic review of black seed for obesity management found 11 trials that met inclusion criteria. Black seed reduced BW (-2.11 kg, $I^2 = 72.4\%$), BMI (-1.16 kg/m^2, $I^2 = 40.1\%$) and WC (-3.52 cm, $I^2 = 0\%$) significantly compared with the placebo groups. The authors cautiously concluded that black seed exerted a moderate effect on reduction of BW, BMI, and WC (Namazi et al., 2018).

A 2017 systematic review and meta-analysis to investigate the effectiveness of black seed in T2DM found seven trials that met inclusion criteria. Black seed significantly improved FBS (-17.84 mg/dL; $P < 0.001$), A1C (-0.71%; $P < 0.001$), TC (WMD $= -22.99$ mg/dL; $P < 0.001$), and LDL-C (-22.38 mg/dL; $P < 0.001$). The overall effects for TG and HDL-C were not significant. However, subgroup analysis revealed a significant reduction of TG with black seed oil (-14.8 mg/dL; $P < 0.001$), while TG was increased with seed powder (29.4 mg/dL; $P < 0.001$). The authors concluded that black seed had promising effects on glucose homeostasis and serum lipids (Daryabeygi-Khotbehsara et al., 2017).

A 2016 systematic review evaluating the effects of black seed on lipid profiles, glycemic control, BP,

and some anthropometric indices found 23 studies ($n = 1531$) that met inclusion criteria. In four trials black seed reduced BP, but in five trials it did not. FBS was reduced significantly, and A1C was reduced in 13 studies. BW and WC decreased significantly in two studies but did not decrease in another six trials. Changes in the lipid profile were very inconsistent across trials. The authors concluded that black seed might be effective in glycemic control in humans (Mohtashami and Entezari, 2016).

A 1-year RCT in patients ($n = 114$) with T2DM on oral hypoglycemic drugs compared black seed 2 g/day with placebo (activated charcoal) for glycemic control and oxidation. Comparison between the two groups showed significant decreases with black seed in FBS (from 195 to 172 with black seed and from 180 to 180 with placebo), A1C (from 8.6 to 8.2 with black seed and from 8.2 to 8.5 with placebo), and TBARS (from 54.1 to 41.9 with black seed and from 48.3 to 52.9 with placebo). Black seed was associated with significant increases compared with placebo in TAC, SOD, and glutathione. With black seed, insulin resistance was significantly lower, and β-cell activity was significantly higher than the baseline values. The authors concluded that long term supplementation with black seed improved glucose homeostasis and enhanced antioxidant status in patients with T2DM on oral hypoglycemic drugs (Kaatabi et al., 2012).

A 12-week RCT in patients ($n = 94$) with T2DM compared adjuvant black seed at 1, 2, and 3 g/day for 12 weeks for glycemic effects. Black seed at 2 g/day was associated with significant reductions in FBS, 2hPPG, and A1C without significant change in BW. FBS was reduced by an average of 45, 62, and 56 mg/dL at 4, 8, and 12 weeks, respectively with 2 g/day dosing. A1C was reduced by 1.52% at the end of the 12 weeks of treatment ($P < 0.0001$). Insulin resistance calculated by HOMA2 was reduced significantly ($P < 0.01$), and β-cell function was increased ($P < 0.02$) at 12 weeks. With black seed 1 g/day there were trends toward improvement in all the measured parameters, but these were not statistically significant from the baseline. No further increment in the beneficial response was observed with the 3 g/day dose. Renal and hepatic functions were stable throughout the study in all groups. The authors concluded that black seed at 2 g/day may improve glycemic control and insulin sensitivity in diabetic patients without additional benefit from higher doses (Bamosa et al., 2015).

A 2-month RCT in women ($n = 30$) aged 45–60 years compared black seed 1 g/day with placebo for metabolic effects. With black seed there were improvements in TC, TG, LDL-C, HDL-C, and BG ($P < 0.05$). Anthropometric measures were not significantly different. The authors concluded that black seed improved BG and lipid profiles in the menopausal period (Ibrahim et al., 2014).

An 8-week RCT in women ($n = 50$) with BMI 30–35 compared black seed oil 3 g/day with placebo along with a low-calorie diet for impact on lipid peroxidation and oxidative status. Black seed was associated with decreased weight compared with placebo (-4.80 kg vs -1.40 kg; $P < 0.01$). With black seed compared with placebo there were significant changes in SOD (88.98 U/gHb vs -3.30 U/gHb; $P < 0.01$). No significant changes in lipid peroxidation, glutathione peroxidase, and TAC concentrations were observed. The authors concluded that black seed oil concurrent with a low-calorie diet decreased weight and increased SOD levels in obese women (Namazi et al., 2015).

An 8-week RCT in apparently healthy males ($n = 250$) with metabolic syndrome compared black seed 1.5 g/day with turmeric 2.4 g/day, with a combination of black seed 900 mg plus turmeric 1.5 g/day, and with placebo. At 4 weeks, black seed and turmeric given individually showed improvement over baseline in BMI, WC, and percent body fat. At 8 weeks, compared with placebo, black seed reduced lipids and FBS, while turmeric reduced LDL-C and CRP. The combination of herbs at 60% of the dose of the individual herbs showed an improvement in all parameters from baseline. When compared with placebo, the combination reduced percent body fat, FBS, TC, TG, LDL-C, and CRP and raised HDL-C. The authors concluded that concurrent administration of turmeric and black seed showed improvements in all parameters of metabolic syndrome at 60% of doses of individual herbs with enhanced efficacy and negligible adverse effects (Amin et al., 2015).

A 40-day Phase I open-label clinical trial in diabetic patients ($n = 30$) with uncontrolled hyperglycemia and dyslipidemia despite standard therapy compared a polyherbal formulation containing garlic, aloe, black seed, psyllium, fenugreek, and milk thistle one sachet BID in addition to their usual medications. The herbal formula significantly decreased FBG from 162 mg/dL to 146 mg/dL and A1C from 8.4% to 7.7%. LDL-C decreased significantly from 138 mg/dL to 108 mg/dL, and TG decreased from 203 mg/dL to 166 mg/dL. There were no changes in liver function, kidney function, or hematologic parameters. The authors concluded that the formulation was safe and effective in lowering blood glucose and serum lipids in patients with advanced-stage T2DM. After consumption of the herbal combination, two patients complained of mild nausea, and two patients reported diarrhea (Zarvandi et al., 2017).

Gastrointestinal Disorders: Nonalcoholic Fatty Liver Disease

A 3-month RCT in patients ($n = 70$) with NAFLD compared black seed 1 g BID with placebo. BW decreased from 86 kg to 76 kg with black seed and was significantly superior to placebo ($P = 0.041$). BMI also decreased significantly from 29.06 to 26.25, greater than placebo ($P = 0.012$). With black seed and placebo there were reductions in ALT (78.05 to 52.6 and 76.48 to 74.32 IU/L, respectively; $P = 0.036$) and AST (65.54 to 44.56 IU/l and 63.25 to 59.43 IU/L, respectively; $P = 0.021$). Fatty liver reverted to Grade 0 on ultrasound after treatment in 57% of patients with black seed and this was superior to placebo ($P = 0.002$). The authors concluded that black seed improved biochemical and fatty liver changes in NAFLD patients and may have a preventive benefit in this condition (Hussain et al., 2017).

Gastrointestinal Disorders: Peptic Ulcer Disease and *H. pylori*

A 4-week open-label trial in patients ($n = 19$) with a history of peptic or gastric ulcer or bleeding and positivity for *H. pylori* investigated the effect of a mixture of black seed 6 g/day plus honey given TID for 2 weeks. A 4-week follow-up urea breath test was negative in 57% of subjects. The median and interquartile range of total dyspepsia symptoms was significantly reduced from 5.5 to 1 ($P = 0.005$). Treatment was well tolerated, and no serious adverse events were reported. The authors concluded that black seed with honey had efficacy against *H. pylori* and dyspepsia (Hashem-Dabaghian et al., 2016).

A 4-week RCT in patients ($n = 88$) with *H. pylori* and dyspepsia compared triple therapy (clarithromycin, amoxicillin, omeprazole) with omeprazole plus black seed at 1, 2, or 3 g for 2 weeks. *H. pylori* eradication was 82.6%, 47.6%, 66.7%, and 47.8% with triple therapy, 1 g black seed, 2 g black seed, and 3 g black seed, respectively. The difference in eradication rates between 2 g black seed and triple therapy were not statistically significant. Dyspepsia symptoms improved in all groups to a similar extent. The authors concluded that black seed possessed clinically useful anti-*H. pylori* activity at 2 g dose, comparable to triple therapy (Salem et al., 2010).

Gastrointestinal Disorders: Functional Dyspepsia

An 8-week RCT in patients ($n = 70$) with functional dyspepsia studied black seed oil 5 mL in honey compared with placebo. The mean of the Hong Kong index of dyspepsia severity sores and the rate of *H. pylori* infection were significantly lower with black seed compared with placebo after 8 weeks ($P < 0.001$). No serious adverse event was reported. The authors concluded that the black seed honey formula could improve symptoms in patients with functional dyspepsia who received standard anti-secretory therapy (Mohtashami et al., 2015).

Renal Disorders: Diabetic Nephropathy

A 12-week open-label trial in patients ($n = 68$) with diabetic nephropathy stage 3–4 investigated black seed oil 2.5 mL QD orally compared with conservative management alone. With black seed compared with baseline there was a significant decrease in FBS and PPBG ($P < 0.001$), serum creatinine ($P < 0.001$), BUN ($P < 0.001$), and 24 h total urinary protein levels and an increase in GFR, 24 h total urinary volume ($P < 0.001$) and Hgb ($P < 0.001$). The control group demonstrated improvements as well, but these tended to be less significant ($P < 0.05$) or not significant, and the difference in improvements between black seed and control groups also tended to be significant at the $P < 0.01$ level (Ansari et al., 2017).

Breast Disorders: Mastalgia

A 2-month RCT in women ($n = 156$) with cyclical mastalgia compared topical black seed oil 600 mg with topical diclofenac 20 mg and with placebo, each applied BID. The endpoint pain scores of the active treatment groups decreased significantly compared with baseline (both $P < 0.001$). There was no significant difference between the 1- and 2-month pain scores in the active treatment groups ($P > 0.05$). The active treatments did not show a between-group difference at 1 and 2 months ($P > 0.05$), and both groups were superior to placebo at 1 and 2 months ($P < 0.001$ for both). The pain scores of the placebo group at 1 and 2 months were not significantly different from the baseline ($P > 0.05$). No adverse effects were observed. The authors concluded that topical black seed oil was safe and similar in efficacy to topical diclofenac for cyclic mastalgia (Huseini et al., 2016).

Women's Genitourinary Disorders: Menopause

A 2017 review of clinical trials on herbal efficacy in menopausal symptoms used search terms menopause, climacteric, hot flushes, flashes, herb, and phytoestrogens. The authors found that passionflower, sage, lemon balm, valerian, black cohosh, fenugreek, black seed, chasteberry, fennel, evening primrose, ginkgo, alfalfa, St. John's wort, Asian ginseng, anise, licorice, red clover, and wild soybean were effective in the treatment of acute menopausal syndrome with different mechanisms. The authors concluded that medicinal plants could play a role in the treatment of acute menopausal syndrome and that further studies were warranted (Kargozar et al., 2017).

A 26-week crossover RCT in perimenopausal and postmenopausal women ($n = 69$) compared metabolic effects of black seed 1600 mg/day with placebo, each given for 12 weeks with a 2-week washout. Black seed was associated with significant improvements over placebo in LDL-C, and BG ($P < 0.05$). BMI, TC, HDL-C, creatinine, TBili, SBP, and DBP improved significantly from baseline ($P < 0.05$) with black seed but not with placebo. However, the difference between groups was not significant. Black seed was associated with a significant reduction of prevalence and severity of menopausal symptoms. Green Climacteric Scale total scores decreased from 16.3 to 11.8 with black seed and increased from 15.1 to 15.9 with placebo ($P = 0.024$). Several components of QOL scores were significantly better with black seed than with placebo ($P < 0.001$). The authors concluded that black seed exerted a therapeutic and protective effect in women by modifying weight gain and improving lipid profile, BG, and hormones that play a role in the pathogenesis of metabolic syndrome during menopause (Latiff et al., 2014).

An 8-week RCT in healthy menopausal women ($n=46$) with hot flushes investigated a combination of black seed and chasteberry plus citalopram QD compared with placebo plus citalopram for control of hot flushes. The herbal combination demonstrated superiority over placebo for three MENQOL domain scores including vasomotor ($P<0.001$), physical ($P=0.036$), and psychosocial ($P<0.001$). There were no significant differences between groups for sexual function ($P=0.231$). The authors concluded that the addition of a combination of black seed and chasteberry to citalopram may improve menopausal symptoms (Molaie et al., 2019).

Men's Genitourinary Disorders: Male Infertility

A 2-month RCT in men ($n=68$) with abnormal sperm morphology, motility, or counts compared black seed oil 2.5 mL BID with placebo. Sperm count, motility, and morphology and semen volume, pH, and round cells were improved significantly with black seed compared with placebo. The authors concluded that daily intake of black seed oil improved abnormal semen quality in infertile men without any adverse effects (Kolahdooz et al., 2014).

Musculoskeletal Disorders: Osteoarthritis

A crossover RCT in elderly patients ($n=40$) with OA of the knee studied black seed oil 1 mL applied topically to the knee TID compared with acetaminophen 325 mg given orally TID for 3 weeks followed by a 2-month washout before crossing over for another 3 weeks. The topical application of both black seed oil and oral acetaminophen reduced pain as determined by VAS, and the reduction of pain was greater with black seed than with APAP ($P=0.01$). The authors concluded that topical application of black seed oil was effective in reducing pain in patients with knee OA and may be considered as a safe supplement in such patients (Kooshki et al., 2016).

A 12-week RCT in patients ($n=110$) with OA compared black seed 2 g/day with placebo for efficacy. Both cohorts demonstrated statistically significant within-group improvements on some subscales of the Knee injury and Osteoarthritis Outcome Score questionnaire ($P<0.05$), with improvements being of greater magnitude in the black seed group. However, the difference from placebo was not statistically significant. Mean breakthrough acetaminophen use was less with black seed than with placebo (11 doses and 24 doses, respectively, over 12 weeks; $P=0.06$). The authors concluded that future studies with larger samples and longer follow-up periods were warranted (Salimzadeh et al., 2017).

A 1-month RCT in elderly patients ($n=60$) with knee OA investigated black seed oil applied topically three times per week compared with routine prescriptions in the control group. The mean VAS scores of the patients in the experimental group decreased from 7.50 to 6.3 ($P<0.001$). The authors concluded that black seed oil had pain-relieving efficacy in geriatric patients with knee pain (Tuna et al., 2018).

Neurological Disorders: Epilepsy

A 10-week crossover RCT in children ($n=30$) with intractable epilepsy and five healthy children (controls) compared black seed oil 40–80 mg/kg/day with placebo each given adjunctively for 4 weeks with a 2-week washout period. At baseline, both groups had significantly lower serum TAC levels relative to healthy controls ($P=0.007$), while MDA levels did not differ. After the 4-week period of black seed oil administration, there was no significant difference between the two black seed doses and placebo with regard to seizure frequency, severity, or oxidative stress markers ($P>0.05$). Eight patients had >50% reduction in seizure frequency/severity after black seed oil compared with placebo. The authors concluded that children with intractable epilepsy showed evidence of oxidative stress, but that black seed given adjunctively did not alter oxidative stress markers or seizure frequency or severity in intractable epileptic patients (Shawki et al., 2013).

A 10-week crossover pilot RCT in children ($n=22$) with refractory epilepsy compared the active constituent thymoquinone 1 mg/kg with placebo each given adjunctively for 4 weeks with a 2-week washout period between crossovers. The reduction in frequency of seizures from baseline at the end of first period and the second period demonstrated significant differences between thymoquinone and placebo ($P=0.04$ and $P=0.02$, respectively). The parental satisfaction scores showed a significant difference between the two groups at the end of the first period ($P=0.03$). The authors concluded that thymoquinone had anti-epileptic effects in children with refractory seizures (Akhondian et al., 2011).

A 10-week crossover RCT in children ($n = 23$) with refractory epilepsy compared an aqueous extract of black seed 40 mg/kg TID with placebo, each as adjunctive therapy for 4 weeks with a 2-week washout. The mean frequency of seizures decreased significantly during treatment with black seed ($P < 0.05$). The authors concluded that aqueous extract of black seed had antiepileptic effects in children with refractory seizures (Akhondian et al., 2007).

Neurological Disorders: Cognitive Impairment and Dementia

A 9-week RCT in elderly volunteers ($n = 40$) compared black seed 500 mg BID with placebo for effects on memory, attention, and cognition. The logical memory test-I and -II scores, total score of digit span, 30-min delayed-recall, percent score, and time taken for completion on Rey-Osterrieth complex figure test, letter cancellation test, time taken in trail making test-A and test-B, and score in part C of the Stroop test were all significantly improved over baseline in the black seed group ($P < 0.05$). There were no significant changes in any of the biochemical markers of cardiac, liver, or kidney function during this 9-week study period. The authors concluded that black seed had a role in memory enhancement, attention, and cognition and may have use in preventing or slowing AD (Bin Sayeed et al., 2014).

Psychiatric Disorders: Anxiety and Depression

A 4-week RCT in healthy adolescent males ($n = 48$) compared black seed 500 mg/day with placebo for effects on mood, anxiety, and cognition. By the end of the study period there was a statistically significant positive change from baseline in mood with black seed but not a significant difference between groups. Short-term free recall, long-term free recall, and long-term cued recall had significant changes from baseline with black seed. None of the measured parameters changed significantly from baseline in the placebo group. The authors concluded that black seed stabilized mood, decreased anxiety, and modulated cognition positively (Bin Sayeed et al., 2013).

Psychiatric Disorders: Alcohol Withdrawal

A 15-day open-label pilot trial in patients ($n = 32$) hospitalized for alcohol detoxification investigated the effect of an herbal combination (black seed, saffron, passionflower, cocoa seed, and radish) given TID. The herbal combination was associated with a significantly reduced percentage of patients with hyperhidrosis ($r = 0.815$; $P < 0.001$), a reduction in serum liver enzymes by 50%–80% ($P < 0.05$), and a normalization of appetite ($r = 0.777$; $P < 0.001$). Quality of life measured by Befindlichkeits-Skala improved from 28.3 to 15.6 ($P < 0.001$). The product was rated as good to excellent by 84.4% of patients. The authors concluded that there was potential for use of this herbal combination in patients undergoing alcohol withdrawal and that further studies were warranted (Mansoor et al., 2018).

Dermatological Disorders: Acne

A 60-day RCT in patients ($n = 60$) with acne vulgaris compared topical black seed hydrogel with placebo BID. The Investigator's Global Assessment (IGA) grading score and acne disability index (ADI) were measured. The mean reduction in the IGA score was 78% with black seed and 3.3% with placebo. The ADI score was decreased 63.4% with black seed and 4.5% with placebo. Significant reductions in the number of comedones, papules, and pustules were observed with black seed compared with placebo. No AEs were recorded. The authors concluded that black seed hydrogel had significant effects on improving the symptoms of acne vulgaris with acceptable tolerability (Soleymani et al., 2020).

Dermatological Disorders: Eczema

A 4-week RCT in patients ($n = 60$) with hand eczema compared black seed ointment with beta-methasone ointment and with Eucerin BID. Black seed and betamethasone showed significantly more rapid improvement in hand eczema compared with Eucerin ($P = 0.003$ and $P = 0.012$, respectively). Black seed and betamethasone ointments caused significant decreases in Dermatology Life Quality Index (DLQI) scores compared with Eucerin ($P < 0.0001$ and $P = 0.007$, respectively). No significant difference was detected between black seed and betamethasone in mean DLQI and Hand Eczema Severity index over time ($P = 0.38$ and $P = 0.99$, respectively). The authors concluded that black seed may have efficacy comparable to betamethasone in hand eczema (Yousefi et al., 2013).

Inflammation

An 8-week RCT in women (n=90) with BMI 30–35 studied the anti-inflammatory effects of black seed oil 3 g/day plus a low-calorie diet compared with placebo plus a low-calorie diet. Black seed was associated with greater reductions than placebo of TNF-α (-40.8% vs -16.1%; $P=0.04$) and hs-CRP (-54.5% vs -21.4%; $P=0.01$). There were no significant differences in reductions of IL-6 levels (-8.6% vs -2.4%; $P=0.6$). The authors concluded that black seed oil supplementation combined with a calorie-restricted diet may modulate systemic inflammation in obese women (Mahdavi et al., 2016).

Autoimmune Disorders

A 12-month RCT in patients (n=71) with Behcet's disease compared black seed oil 1000 mg/day with placebo. Disease activity decreased in both groups and the difference between the two groups was not significant. No serious adverse events were seen in the treatment and control groups. The authors concluded that black seed oil 1000 mg/day was not effective in controlling Behcet's disease (Kavandi et al., 2018).

An 8-week RCT in patients (n=40) with Hashimoto's thyroiditis compared black seed with placebo. Black seed significantly reduced BW and BMI. VEGF, TSH, and anti-TPO antibodies decreased, while serum T3 concentrations increased with black seed. None of these changes were observed in the placebo treated group. Waist-to-hip ratio and thyroid hormones were significant predictors of changes in serum VEGF and Nesfatin-1 values with black seed ($P<0.05$). The authors concluded that black seed had potential benefit in improving thyroid function and anthropometric variables in patients with Hashimoto's thyroiditis and that black seed ameliorated disease severity (Farhangi et al., 2016).

A 2-month RCT in women (n=40) with RA compared 1 month of placebo with the following month of black seed oil 500 mg BID. The disease activity score significantly decreased from 4.98 at baseline and 4.99 after placebo to 4.55 after black seed. The number of swollen joints and duration of morning stiffness improved after black seed. There was an improvement in disease activity based on ACR20 and EULAR criteria in 42.5% and 30%, respectively, of patients with black seed. The authors concluded that black seed supplementation during DMARD therapy in RA may be an affordable adjuvant (Gheita and Kenawy, 2012).

An 8-week RCT in patients (n=42) with RA compared black seed oil 1000 mg/day with placebo. Black seed resulted in an increase in the serum level of IL-10 ($P<0.01$) and a reduction in serum MDA and NO compared with baseline ($P<0.05$). There were no significant differences in the TNF-α, SOD, catalase, and total TAC values between or within the groups, before and after the intervention ($P>0.05$). The authors concluded that black seed could improve inflammation and reduce oxidative stress in patients with RA (Hadi et al., 2016).

A 2-month RCT in women (n=43) with mild-to-moderate RA compared black seed 1 g BID with placebo for effect on disease activity and immune function. With black seed there was a significant reduction of hs-CRP and Disease Activity Scores of 28 joints as well as an improved number of swollen joints compared with baseline and with placebo. Black seed reduced CD8+, and increased CD4+CD25+ T cell percentage and the CD4+/CD8+ ratio compared with placebo and baseline. Black seed produced a significant negative correlation between CD8+ and changes in CD4+CD25+ T cells and a positive significant correlation between changes in CD4+CD25+ T cells and changes in the CD4+/CD8+ ratio. The changes in CD4+ percentage did not differ between black seed and placebo. The authors concluded that black seed had potential use in the management of RA through modulation of T lymphocytes (Kheirouri et al., 2016).

A 6-month RCT in patients (n=52) with vitiligo compared black seed oil with fish oil applied BID. The mean Vitiligo Area Scoring Index decreased from 4.98 to 3.75 with black seed and from 4.8 to 4.6 with fish oil. No adverse events were reported. The authors concluded that black seed and fish oil were both effective in reducing vitiligo lesion size and that black seed was more effective (Ghorbanibirgani et al., 2014).

Infectious Disease: Staphylococcal Pustules and Hepatitis C Virus

A response-based RCT in neonates (n=40) with pustules due to *Staphylococcus* studied black seed extract 33% compared with mupirocin applied topically. The mean of recovery time was 75 h with black seed and 69 h with mupirocin ($P=0.13$). The authors concluded that black seed had nearly the efficacy of mupirocin for staphylococcal pustules (Rafati et al., 2014).

A 3-month open-label trial in patients ($n = 30$) with HCV who were not eligible for IFN/ribavirin therapy assessed the effects of black seed 450 mg TID on various disease parameters. Black seed was associated with a decrease in HCV viral load from 380,808 to 147,028 ($P = 0.001$); an increase in TAC from 1.35 to 1.61 ($P = 0.001$); an increase in total protein from 7.1 g/dL to 7.5 g/dL ($P = 0.001$); an increase in albumin from 3.5 g/dL to 3.7 g/dL ($P = 0.008$); an increase in RBC count from 4.13 to 4.3 ($P = 0.001$); and an increase in platelet count from 167,000 to 198,000 ($P = 0.004$). FBS decreased from 104 mg/dL to 92 mg/dL ($P = 0.001$) and PPBG decreased from 144 mg/dL to 112 mg/dL ($P = 0.001$) in both diabetic and non-diabetic HCV patients. The number of patients with leg edema decreased significantly from baseline of 53% to 23% ($P = 0.004$). Adverse drug reactions were unremarkable except for a few cases of epigastric pain and hypoglycemia that did not affect patient compliance. The authors concluded that black seed was tolerable and safe in patients with HCV and decreased viral load while improving oxidative stress, clinical condition, and glycemic control (Barakat et al., 2013).

Oncologic Disorders

A 3-to-9-month chemo-connected RCT in children ($n = 80$) with brain tumors undergoing chemotherapy compared the addition of black seed 5 g/day throughout treatment with no supplemental treatment (control) for effect on febrile neutropenia. Febrile neutropenia was experienced by 2.2% of subjects in the black seed group and 19.3% in the control group ($P = 0.001$). Median length of stay was 2.5 days with black seed and 5 days with control ($P = 0.006$). The authors concluded that black seed showed a decrease in incidence of febrile neutropenia and shortened length of stay in children with brain tumors (Mousa et al., 2017).

A chemo-connected RCT in children ($n = 40$) with ALL investigated methotrexate (MTX) plus black seed 80 mg/kg/day given 1 week after each MTX dose compared with MTX plus placebo in same the manner. With MTX plus placebo there were significant increases in total, direct, and indirect serum bilirubin, serum ALT, AST, and ALP and PT, while with MTX plus black seed the increases were lesser and not significant. Between group differences were significant. After 2 years, 65% and 50% of patients treated adjuvantly with black seed and placebo, respectively, were in remission; 25% and 35%, respectively, had relapsed; 10% and 15%, respectively, had died (combined $P = 0.029$). The authors concluded that black seed decreased MTX hepatotoxicity and improved survival in children with ALL and could be recommended as adjuvant treatment in patients undergoing MTX treatment for ALL (Hagag et al., 2015).

A therapy connected RCT in breast cancer patients ($n = 62$) undergoing radiotherapy compared topical black seed 5% gel with placebo BID for effects on radiation dermatitis. Patients who were treated with black seed gel developed acute radiation dermatitis significantly less frequently compared with those who used placebo ($P < 0.05$ for all weeks except week 2 where $P = 0.36$). The incidence time of Grade 2 and 3 of Radiation Therapy Oncology Group was 39 days with black seed gel and 29 days with placebo ($P = 0.00$). The incidence time of grade 2 and 3 of European Organization for Research and Treatment of Cancer toxicity scale was 42 days with black seed gel and 40 days with placebo ($P = 0.01$). The occurrence of moist desquamation was at 37 days with black seed gel and 33 days with placebo ($P = 0.01$). The mean score of the worst pain that patients experienced at week 3 was 1.2 with black seed and 2.5 with placebo ($P < 0.05$). Black seed gel had no significant effect on the skin related QOL for patients at any week. The authors concluded that black seed significantly decreased the severity of acute radiodermatitis and delayed the onset of moist desquamation in breast cancer patients (Rafati et al., 2019).

ACTIVE CONSTITUENTS

There are several different chemotypes of Nigella sativa (Egyptian, Iranian, Syrian, Turkish) creating variation in chemical constituents.

- ■ Lipids
  - ■ Fatty acids (30%–35%): glycerol ester of linoleic, oleic, palmitic acids; aliphatic hydrocarbons, arachidonic acid, γ-linolenic acid, tocopherols

- Phenolic compounds
  - Phenylpropanoids (antioxidant, antimutagenic, antitumor, antimicrobial): *t*-anethole
  - Flavonoids: comferol diglucoside, comferol digalactoside

- Terpenes
  - Monoterpenes: p-cymene, thymoquinone, thymohydroquinone (antitumor),
    α-pinene, carvacrol, 4-terpineol, thymol (strong antimicrobial), carvone, α-terpinene, γ-terpinene, limonene (antineoplastic, detoxifying)
  - Sesquiterpenes: longifolene, longipinene
- Triterpenoid saponins: α hederin

- Steroids
  - Phytosterols: β-sitosterol and stigmasterol

- Alkaloids
  - Nigellin, nigellidine-4-*O*-sulfite, nigellamines A1 to A5, B1, B2, and C, nigellicimine, nigellidine, nigellidine-4-sulfite
  - Isoquinoline alkaloids: nigellicine and nigellimin-N-oxide,

- Aromatic compounds
  - Thymoquinone (antioxidant, hepatoprotective, antitumor, antibacterial), nigellone (through in vivo dimerization; antihistamine), *t*-anethole, thymol (strong antimicrobial)

BLACK SEED COMMONLY USED PREPARATIONS AND DOSAGE (FOR ADULTS UNLESS OTHERWISE SPECIFIED)

The following are examples of some available formulations and ranges of dosing for commercial herbal products. See Part III Introduction "How to prescribe medicinal herbs" for further guidance on herbal advising and prescribing.

Seeds

- Powdered seeds: 1–3 g per day
- Powdered seed extract: 200 mg QD
- Standardized expressed oil (standardized to 0.6% thymoquinone): 4.5 g (5 mL) BID orally; 1 mL TID topically for arthritis

- Capsule or tablet of seed-expressed oil (*not a distilled essential oil*): 1 g/day

Optimal metabolic dose appears to be around 2 g/day

SAFETY AND PRECAUTION

The USFDA classifies "black cumin (black caraway), *Nigella sativa* L." as Generally Recognized as Safe (GRAS) for use as a spice, natural seasoning, or flavoring. Black seed is also permitted by the FDA as a component of dietary supplement products, with appropriate FDA notification and following of Good Manufacturing Practices.

Side Effects

Topical use may cause contact dermatitis.

Case Reports

A 2013 case report of a diabetic developing acute renal failure associated with (but not necessarily caused by) black seed.

Toxicity

High doses may be hepatotoxic. In mice, 21 g/kg induced hepatotoxicity. Oral LD50 of thymoquinone is 800–870 mg/kg in rats and mice (100–150 times higher than therapeutic level).

Pregnancy and Lactation

Insufficient human safety data.

Drug Interactions

- CYP: Inhibits CYP2D6, CYP2C19, CYP2C9, and CYP3A4
- Pgp: Increases P-glycoprotein activity

REFERENCES

Akhondian J, Parsa A, Rakhshande H. The effect of Nigella sativa L. (black cumin seed) on intractable pediatric seizures. Med Sci Monit 2007;13(12):CR555–9.

Akhondian J, Kianifar H, Raoofziaee M, Moayedpour A, Toosi MB, Khajedaluee M. The effect of thymoquinone on intractable pediatric seizures (pilot study). Epilepsy Res 2011;93(1):39–43.

Al-Azzawi M, AboZaid M, Ibrahem R, Sakr M. Therapeutic effects of black seed oil supplementation on chronic obstructive pulmonary disease patients: A randomized controlled double blind clinical trial. Heliyon 2020;6(8), e04711.

Alsamarai AM, Abdulsatar M, Ahmed Alobaidi AH. Evaluation of topical black seed oil in the treatment of allergic rhinitis. Antiinflamm Antiallergy Agents Med Chem 2014;13(1):75–82.

Amin F, Islam N, Anila N, Gilani AH. Clinical efficacy of the co-administration of turmeric and black seeds (Kalongi) in metabolic syndrome—a double blind randomized controlled trial—TAK-MetS trial. Complement Ther Med 2015;23(2):165–74.

Ansari ZM, Nasiruddin M, Khan RA, Haque SF. Protective role of *Nigella sativa* in diabetic nephropathy: a randomized clinical trial. Saudi J Kidney Dis Transpl 2017;28(1):9–14.

Badar A, Kaatabi H, Bamosa A, et al. Effect of Nigella sativa supplementation over a one-year period on lipid levels, BP and heart rate in type-2 diabetic patients receiving oral hypoglycemic agents: nonrandomized clinical trial. Ann Saudi Med 2017;37(1):56–63.

Bamosa A, Kaatabi H, Badar A, et al. Nigella sativa: a potential natural protective agent against cardiac dysfunction in patients with type 2 diabetes mellitus. J Family Community Med 2015;22(2):88–95.

Barakat EM, El Wakeel LM, Hagag RS. Effects of Nigella sativa on outcome of hepatitis C in Egypt. World J Gastroenterol 2013;19(16):2529–36.

Bin Sayeed MS, Asaduzzaman M, Morshed H, Hossain MM, Kadir MF, Rahman MR. The effect of Nigella sativa Linn. seed on memory, attention and cognition in healthy human volunteers. J Ethnopharmacol 2013;148(3):780–6.

Bin Sayeed MS, Shams T, Fahim Hossain S, et al. Nigella sativa L. seeds modulate mood, anxiety and cognition in healthy adolescent males. J Ethnopharmacol 2014;152(1):156–62.

Boskabady MH, Farhadi J. The possible prophylactic effect of Nigella sativa seed aqueous extract on respiratory symptoms and pulmonary function tests on chemical war victims: a randomized, double-blind, placebo-controlled trial. J Altern Complement Med 2008;14(9):1137–44.

Boskabady MH, Javan H, Sajady M, Rakhshandeh H. The possible prophylactic effect of Nigella sativa seed extract in asthmatic patients. Fundam Clin Pharmacol 2007;21(5):559–66.

Boskabady MH, Mohsenpoor N, Takaloo L. Anti-asthmatic effect of Nigella sativa in airways of asthmatic patients. Phytomedicine 2010;17(10):707–13.

Daryabeygi-Khotbehsara R, Golzarand M, Ghaffari MP, Djafarian K. Nigella sativa improves glucose homeostasis and serum lipids in type 2 diabetes: a systematic review and meta-analysis. Complement Ther Med 2017;35:6–13.

Dehkordi FR, Kamkhah AF. Antihypertensive effect of Nigella sativa seed extract in patients with mild HTN. Fundam Clin Pharmacol 2008;22(4):447–52.

Fallah Huseini H, Amini M, Mohtashami R, et al. BP lowering effect of Nigella sativa L. seed oil in healthy volunteers: a randomized, double-blind, placebo-controlled clinical trial. Phytother Res 2013 Dec;27(12):1849–53.

Farhangi MA, Dehghan P, Tajmiri S, Abbasi MM. The effects of Nigella sativa on thyroid function, serum vascular endothelial growth factor (VEGF)—1, Nesfatin-1 and anthropometric features in patients with Hashimoto's thyroiditis: a randomized controlled trial. BMC Complement Altern Med 2016;16(1):471.

Farhangi MA, Dehghan P, Tajmiri S. Powdered black cumin seed strongly improves serum lipids, atherogenic index of plasma and modulates anthropometric features in patients with Hashimoto's thyroiditis. Lipids Health Dis 2018;17(1):59.

Farzaneh E, Nia FR, Mehrtash M, Mirmoeini FS, Jalilvand M. The effects of 8-week Nigella sativa supplementation and aerobic training on lipid profile and VO2 max in sedentary overweight females. Int J Prev Med 2014;5(2):210–6.

Gheita TA, Kenawy SA. Effectiveness of Nigella sativa oil in the management of rheumatoid arthritis patients: a placebo controlled study. Phytother Res 2012;26(8):1246–8.

Ghorbani A, Zarvandi M, Rakhshandeh H. A randomized controlled trial of a herbal compound for improving metabolic parameters in diabetic patients with uncontrolled dyslipidemia. Endocr Metab Immune Disord Drug Targets 2019;6.

Ghorbanibirgani A, Khalili A, Rokhafrooz D. Comparing Nigella sativa oil and fish oil in treatment of Vitiligo. Iran Red Crescent Med J 2014;16(6), e4515.

Hadi V, Kheirouri S, Alizadeh M, Khabbazi A, Hosseini H. Effects of Nigella sativa oil extract on inflammatory cytokine response and oxidative stress status in patients with rheumatoid arthritis: a randomized, double-blind, placebo-controlled clinical trial. Avicenna J Phytomed 2016;6(1):34–43.

Hagag AA, AbdElaal AM, Elfaragy MS, Hassan SM, Elzamarany EA. Therapeutic value of black seed oil in methotrexate hepatotoxicity in Egyptian children with acute lymphoblastic leukemia. Infect Disord Drug Targets 2015;15(1):64–71.

Hallajzadeh J, Milajerdi A, Mobini M, et al. Effects of Nigella sativa on glycemic control, lipid profiles, and biomarkers of inflammatory and oxidative stress: a systematic review and meta-analysis of randomized controlled clinical trials. Phytother Res 2020;34(10):2586–608.

Hashem-Dabaghian F, Agah S, Taghavi-Shirazi M, Ghobadi A. Combination of *Nigella sativa* and honey in eradication of gastric *Helicobacter pylori* infection. Iran Red Crescent Med J 2016;18(11), e23771.

He T, Xiaohong X. The influence of Nigella sativa for asthma control: a meta-analysis. Am J Emerg Med 2020;38(3):589–93.

Huseini HF, Kianbakht S, Mirshamsi MH, Zarch AB. Effectiveness of topical Nigella sativa seed oil in the treatment of cyclic mastalgia: a randomized, triple-blind, active, and placebo-controlled clinical trial. Planta Med 2016;82(4):285–8.

Hussain M, Tunio AG, Akhtar L, Shaikh GS. Effects of nigella sativa on various parameters in patients of non-alcoholic fatty liver disease. J Ayub Med Coll Abbottabad 2017;29(3):403–7.

Ibrahim RM, Hamdan NS, Ismail M, et al. Protective effects of Nigella sativa on metabolic syndrome in menopausal women. Adv Pharm Bull 2014;4(1):29–33.

Işik H, Cevikbaş A, Gürer US, et al. Potential adjuvant effects of Nigella sativa seeds to improve specific immunotherapy in allergic rhinitis patients. Med Princ Pract 2010;19(3):206–11.

Kaatabi H, Bamosa AO, Lebda FM, Al Elq AH, Al-Sultan AI. Favorable impact of Nigella sativa seeds on lipid profile in type 2 diabetic patients. J Family Community Med 2012;19(3):155–61.

Kaatabi H, Bamosa AO, Badar A, et al. Nigella sativa improves glycemic control and ameliorates oxidative stress in patients with type 2 diabetes mellitus: placebo-controlled participant blinded clinical trial. PLoS One 2015;10(2), e0113486.

Kalus U, Pruss A, Bystron J, et al. Effect of Nigella sativa (black seed) on subjective feeling in patients with allergic diseases. Phytother Res 2003;17(10):1209–14.

Kapil H, Suresh DK, Bathla SC, Arora KS. Assessment of clinical efficacy of locally delivered 0.2% Thymoquinone gel in the treatment of periodontitis. Saudi Dent J 2018;30(4):348–54.

Kargozar R, Azizi H, Salari R. A review of effective herbal medicines in controlling menopausal symptoms. Electron Phys 2017;9(11):5826–33.

Kavandi H, Hajialilo M, Khabbazi A. Efficacy of *Nigella sativa* seeds oil in patients with Behcet's disease: a double-blind randomized controlled trial. Avicenna J Phytomed 2018;8(6):498–503.

Kheirouri S, Hadi V, Alizadeh M. Immunomodulatory effect of Nigella sativa oil on T lymphocytes in patients with rheumatoid arthritis. Immunol Invest 2016;45(4):271–83.

Kolahdooz M, Nasri S, Modarres SZ, Kianbakht S, Huseini HF. Effects of Nigella sativa L. seed oil on abnormal semen quality in infertile men: a randomized, double-blind, placebo-controlled clinical trial. Phytomedicine 2014;21(6):901–5.

Kooshki A, Forouzan R, Rakhshani MH, Mohammadi M. Effect of topical application of Nigella sativa oil and oral acetaminophen on pain in elderly with knee osteoarthritis: a crossover clinical trial. Electron Phys 2016;8(11):3193–7.

Koshak AE, Koshak EA. *Nigella sativa* L as a potential phytotherapy for coronavirus disease 2019: a mini review of in silico studies. Curr Ther Res Clin Exp 2020;93:100602.

Koshak A, Koshak E, Heinrich M. Medicinal benefits of *Nigella sativa* in bronchial asthma: a literature review. Saudi Pharm J 2017a;25(8):1130–6.

Koshak A, Wei L, Koshak E, et al. Nigella sativa supplementation improves asthma control and biomarkers: a randomized, double-blind, placebo-controlled trial. Phytother Res 2017b;31(3):403–9.

Latiff LA, Parhizkar S, Dollah MA, Hassan ST. Alternative supplement for enhancement of reproductive health and metabolic profile among perimenopausal women: a novel role of Nigella sativa. Iran J Basic Med Sci 2014;17(12):980–5.

Mahdavi R, Namazi N, Alizadeh M, Farajnia S. Effects of Nigella sativa oil with a low-calorie diet on cardiometabolic risk factors in obese women: a randomized controlled clinical trial. Food Funct 2015;6(6):2041–8.

Mahdavi R, Namazi N, Alizadeh M, Farajnia S. Nigella sativa oil with a calorie-restricted diet can improve biomarkers of systemic inflammation in obese women: a randomized double-blind, placebo-controlled clinical trial. J Clin Lipidol 2016;10(5):1203–11.

Mansoor K, Qadan F, Hinum A, et al. An open prospective pilot study of a herbal combination "relief" as a supportive dietetic measure during alcohol withdrawal. Neuro Endocrinol Lett 2018;39(1):1–8.

Mohtashami A, Entezari MH. Effects of *Nigella sativa* supplementation on blood parameters and anthropometric indices in adults: a systematic review on clinical trials. J Res Med Sci 2016;21:3.

Mohtashami R, Huseini HF, Heydari M, et al. Efficacy and safety of honey-based formulation of Nigella sativa seed oil in functional dyspepsia: a double blind randomized controlled clinical trial. J Ethnopharmacol 2015;175:147–52.

Molaie M, Darvishi B, Jafari Azar Z, Shirazi M, Amin G, Afshar S. Effects of a combination of Nigella sativa and Vitex agnus-castus with citalopram on healthy menopausal women with hot flushes: results from a subpopulation analysis. Gynecol Endocrinol 2019;35(1):58–61.

Mousa HFM, Abd-El-Fatah NK, Darwish OA, Shehata SF, Fadel SH. Effect of Nigella sativa seed administration on prevention of febrile neutropenia during chemotherapy among children with brain tumors. Childs Nerv Syst 2017;33(5):793–800.

Mousavi SM, Sheikhi A, Varkaneh HK, Zarezadeh M, Rahmani J, Milajerdi A. Effect of Nigella sativa supplementation on obesity indices: a systematic review and meta-analysis of randomized controlled trials. Complement Ther Med 2018;38:48–57.

Namazi N, Mahdavi R, Alizadeh M, Farajnia S. Oxidative stress responses to Nigella sativa oil concurrent with a low-calorie diet in obese women: a randomized, double-blind controlled clinical trial. Phytother Res 2015;29(11):1722–8.

Namazi N, Larijani B, Ayati MH, Abdollahi M. The effects of Nigella sativa L. on obesity: a systematic review and meta-analysis. J Ethnopharmacol 2018;219:173–81.

Nikakhlagh S, Rahim F, Aryani FH, Syahpoush A, Brougerdnya MG, Saki N. Herbal treatment of allergic rhinitis: the use of Nigella sativa. Am J Otolaryngol 2011;32(5):402–7.

Oysu C, Tosun A, Yilmaz HB, Sahin-Yilmaz A, Korkmaz D, Karaaslan A. Topical Nigella sativa for nasal symptoms in elderly. Auris Nasus Larynx 2014;41(3):269–72.

Pipalia PR, Annigeri RG, Mehta R. Clinicobiochemical evaluation of turmeric with black pepper and nigella sativa in management of oral submucous fibrosis-a double-blind, randomized preliminary study. Oral Surg Oral Med Oral Pathol Oral Radiol 2016;122(6):705–12.

Rafati S, Niakan M, Naseri M. Anti-microbial effect of Nigella sativa seed extract against staphylococcal skin Infection. Med J Islam Repub Iran 2014;28:42.

Rafati M, Ghasemi A, Saeedi M, et al. Nigella sativa L. for prevention of acute radiation dermatitis in breast cancer: a randomized, double-blind, placebo-controlled, clinical trial. Complement Ther Med 2019;47:102205.

Rezaeian A, Amoushahi KS. Effect of *Nigella sativa* nasal spray on the treatment of chronic rhinosinusitis without a nasal polyp. Allergy Rhinol (Providence) 2018;9. 2152656718800059.

Rizka A, Setiati S, Lydia A, Dewiasty E. Effect of Nigella sativa Seed Extract for HTN in elderly: a double-blind, randomized controlled trial. Acta Med Indones 2017;49(4):307–13.

Sabzghabaee AM, Dianatkhah M, Sarrafzadegan N, Asgary S, Ghannadi A. Clinical evaluation of Nigella sativa seeds for the treatment of hyperlipidemia: a randomized, placebo controlled clinical trial. Med Arch 2012;66(3):198–200.

Sahebkar A, Beccuti G, Simental-Mendía LE, Nobili V, Bo S. Nigella sativa (black seed) effects on plasma lipid concentrations in humans: a systematic review and meta-analysis of randomized placebo-controlled trials. Pharmacol Res 2016;106:37–50.

Salem EM, Yar T, Bamosa AO, et al. Comparative study of Nigella sativa and triple therapy in eradication of Helicobacter pylori in patients with non-ulcer dyspepsia. Saudi J Gastroenterol 2010;16(3):207–14.

Salem AM, Bamosa AO, Qutub HO, et al. Effect of Nigella sativa supplementation on lung function and inflammatory mediatorsin partly controlled asthma: a randomized controlled trial. Ann Saudi Med 2017;37(1):64–71.

Salimzadeh A, Ghourchian A, Choopani R, Hajimehdipoor H, Kamalinejad M, Abolhasani M. Effect of an orally formulated processed black cumin, from Iranian traditional medicine pharmacopoeia, in relieving symptoms of knee osteoarthritis: a prospective, randomized, double-blind and placebo-controlled clinical trial. Int J Rheum Dis 2017;20(6):691–701.

Shawki M, El Wakeel L, Shatla R, El-Saeed G, Ibrahim S, Badary O. The clinical outcome of adjuvant therapy with black seed oil on intractable paediatric seizures: a pilot study. Epileptic Disord 2013;15(3):295–301.

Soleymani S, Zargaran A, Farzaei M, et al. The effect of a hydrogel made byNigellasativa L. on acne vulgaris: a randomized double-blindclinicaltrial. Phytother Res 2020;34(11):3052–62.

Tavakkoli A, Mahdian V, Razavi BM, Hosseinzadeh H. Review on clinical trials of black seed (Nigella sativa) and its active constituent, thymoquinone. J Pharmacopuncture 2017;20(3):179–93.

Tuna HI, Babadag B, Ozkaraman A, Balci AG. Investigation of the effect of black cumin oil on pain in osteoarthritis geriatric individuals. Complement Ther Clin Pract 2018;31:290–4.

Yousefi M, Barikbin B, Kamalinejad M, et al. Comparison of therapeutic effect of topical Nigella with betamethasone and eucerin in hand eczema. J Eur Acad Dermatol Venereol 2013;27(12):1498–504.

Zarvandi M, Rakhshandeh H, Abazari M, Shafiee-Nick R, Ghorbani A. Safety and efficacy of a polyherbal formulation for the management of dyslipidemia and hyperglycemia in patients with advanced-stage of type-2 diabetes. Biomed Pharmacother 2017;89:69–75.

32

BURDOCK (*ARCTIUM LAPPA*)
Roots and Seeds

GENERAL OVERVIEW

Burdock has a long history of use in China, both as a food (stir-fried root) and as a medicine. It comes to mind for patients with skin conditions, dyspepsia, gastroparesis, liver disease, or akinetic gallbladder disease. As popular as this plant is globally, the evidence is relatively sparse. There are a few studies using the "fruit," which is the burr-like seed pod (possibly the inspiration for Velcro). Overall, burdock appears to be quite safe based on research and its long history of culinary and medicinal use. Burdock root is part of the Essiac tea and Hoxsey formulations that are commonly employed integratively in cancer treatment, but evidence for this application is also lacking.

Clinical research indicates that burdock, alone or in combination formulas, may be beneficial for diverticulitis prophylaxis, diabetic nephropathy, photoaging, acne, and inflammation.

IN VITRO AND ANIMAL RESEARCH

Burdock has cholagogic, choleretic, immunostimulant, and anti-inflammatory effects. It promotes hepatic detoxification enzymatic activity and is hepatoprotective through antioxidant activity. Burdock has been shown to improve hepatic function and protect the liver in mice after exposure to CCL4 or acetaminophen overdose (Lin et al., 2000). The bitter principles in burdock root promote gastric motility and digestion. A study in rats demonstrated improved gastric ulcer healing with burdock root, likely through restoration of SOD activity, prevention of GSH depletion, and reduction of gastric acidity (da Silva et al., 2013).

The root contains antidiabetic compounds. The antidiabetic effect was studied in streptozotocin-induced diabetic mice. The results showed that oral administration of burdock significantly decreased blood glucose and increased insulin levels in diabetic rats compared with the control group. In addition, TC, TG and LDL-C were all lower in the burdock group, whereas HDL-C was higher. The burdock group also had significantly decreased BUN and creatinine, and MDA levels in kidney and liver were reduced (Lu et al., 2012). No hypoglycemic effect of burdock root extract was observed in normal rats. Another rat study found that daily supplementation with burdock root 500–1000 mg/kg for 4 weeks led to a reduction in body weight. In this study, lipid synthesis was suppressed by downregulating or inhibiting various enzymes involved in lipid metabolism (Kuo et al., 2012).

The burdock constituent arctigenin has demonstrated ability to prevent renal fibrosis in rats through anti-inflammatory and antioxidant mechanisms. It was shown to reduce TGF-β1 and its receptor. It was shown to be comparable to losartan in renal protection (Li et al., 2017). Arctigenin has also demonstrated protective effects against scopolamine-induced memory impairment in mice with AD and against alcohol-induced neurotoxicity (Huang et al., 2014). This constituent has also been reported to exert antitumor activity by attenuating the tolerance of cancer cells to glucose deprivation (Gu et al., 2012).

In vitro studies using an extract from burdock fruit/seeds (high in the constituent arctiin) showed a stimulation of collagen synthesis and a decrease in interleukin-6 and TNF-α concentrations in canine dermal fibroblasts. In vitro studies on human dermal fibroblasts and monocyte-derived dendritic cells supplemented with pure arctiin showed a stimulation of collagen synthesis and a decrease in IL-6 and TNF-α concentration, respectively, relative to untreated control cells (Knott et al., 2008).

The lignans in burdock have been shown to promote longevity in roundworms. A study in mice demonstrated that burdock root supplementation elevated endurance and grip strength in a dose-dependent manner. It also significantly decreased lactate, ammonia, and CK levels after physical challenge and created few subchronic toxic effects (Chen et al., 2017). Burdock has been shown in mice to be synergistic with oseltamivir against influenza A (Hayashi et al., 2010). The polysaccharides in burdock have demonstrated antitussive properties in cats. Some constituents in burdock root have strong anticancer properties, particularly for pancreatic cancer cell lines.

HUMAN RESEARCH

Inflammatory Bowel Disorders: Acute Diverticulitis

A 22–30-month RCT in patients with chronic diverticular bleeding ($n = 91$) or acute diverticulitis ($n = 70$) compared a decoction of burdock root 1.5 g TID with a control group for a duration of treatment based on the respective diagnosis. Burdock showed significant preventive effects on recurrence of acute diverticulitis (recurrences in 10.6% and 31.8% with burdock and control, respectively). Recurrence-free duration was 59 months and 45 months with burdock and control, respectively ($P = 0.012$). There were no significant preventive effects on the chronic diverticular bleeding recurrence. The authors concluded that daily intake of burdock tea could be an effective strategy for prevention of acute diverticulitis recurrence (Mizuki et al., 2019).

Renal Disorders: Diabetic Nephropathy

A 3-month study in patients ($n = 54$) with diabetic nephropathy investigated a mixture of burdock *fruit* plus astragalus root compared with losartan. Symptoms, urinary protein, and albumin as well as lipid metabolism significantly improved after treatment with the burdock combination ($P < 0.05$), but in the control group improvement occurred only with respect to urinary albumin levels ($P < 0.05$) (Wang and Chen, 2004).

Musculoskeletal Disorders: Osteoarthritis

A 42-day RCT in patients ($n = 36$) with knee OA investigated acetaminophen 500 mg BID plus glucosamine 500 mg QD along with boiled water TID compared with the same drugs along with burdock root decoction 2 g/150 mL boiled water TID for effects on inflammation and oxidation. Levels of IL-6, hs-CRP, and MDA were decreased with burdock ($P = 0.002$; $P = 0.003$, and $P < 0.001$, respectively). Levels of TAC and SOD were increased with burdock ($P < 0.001$ and $P = 0.009$, respectively). The authors concluded that burdock root tea improved inflammatory status and oxidative stress in patients with knee OA (Maghsoumi-Norouzabad et al., 2016).

Dermatological Disorders

A 12-week RCT compared burdock *fruit* extract with a control vehicle for effects on aging skin. Compared with control vehicle, the procollagen and hyaluronan synthesis and the hyaluronan synthase-2 gene expression were all increased with burdock. Reduction of wrinkle volume in the crow's feet area was reduced to a significantly greater degree with burdock fruit than with control vehicle after 4 weeks (Knott et al., 2008).

A 6-month observational study in acne patients ($n = 34$) looked at homeopathic preparations of burdock starting with 6c potency and increasing to 1M (extremely dilute/potent). Objective assessment was change in acne lesion counts supplemented with Global Acne Grading System and Acne-Specific Quality of Life questionnaire (Acne-QoL). Improvement in lesion counts, grading system and questionnaire occurred ($P < 0.01$) (Miglani and Manchanda, 2014).

Oncologic Disorders

A Phase I clinical trial of an arctigenin-rich burdock fruit extract (GBS-01) was performed in patients ($n = 15$) with advanced pancreatic cancer refractory to gemcitabine. The extract was given orally at escalating doses from 1 to 4 g burdock fruit extract QD. None of the patients at any of the three dose levels showed any sign of dose-limiting toxicity by day 28. The main adverse events were mild increases in serum GGT, glucose, and increased T. bili. Of the 15 patients, one showed confirmed partial response and four patients had stable disease. The median progression-free and overall survival of the patients were 1.1 and 5.7 months, respectively. The authors concluded that the recommended dose of GBS-01 was 4 g/day of burdock fruit extract resulting in favorable clinical responses (Ikeda et al., 2016).

ACTIVE CONSTITUENTS

Root

- Carbohydrates
  - Oligosaccharides: inulin (up to 50%, immunostimulating via macrophage phagocytosis, anti-inflammatory, prebiotic, hypoglycemic)
  - Organic acids: acetic, proprionic, butyric, isovaleric
- Lipids
  - Fatty acids: lauric, myristic, stearic, palmitic
  - Polyacetylenes (immunomodulatory, anti-inflammatory): sulfur containing (antibacterial)
- Phenolic compounds
  - Phenolic acids: polyphenolic acid
  - Lignans: arctigenin, matairesinol, isolappaol A, lappaol C, lappaol F (inhibit the pro-inflammatory factors, nitric oxide, TNF-a, and IL-6, upregulate JNK-1) (Lappaol F and arctigenin have anticancer effects: cell cycle arrest, inhibition of proliferation, induction of apoptosis, and other mechanisms; antiviral, antiretroviral)
  - Flavonoids
    - Tannin: phlobaphone
- Terpenes
  - Sesquiterpene lactones: arctiopicrin
- Bitter compounds (stimulate gastric motility and digestive enzymes)

Fruit (Fructus Arctii)

- Phenolic compounds
  - Lignans: arctiin, arctigenin, neoarctin, matairesinol (antiviral, antiretroviral, anti-inflammatory, antiplatelet, anti-cancer), lappaol (antineoplastic)
- Steroids
  - Phytosterols: daucosterol

BURDOCK COMMONLY USED PREPARATIONS AND DOSAGE (FOR ADULTS UNLESS OTHERWISE SPECIFIED)

The following are examples of some available formulations and ranges of dosing for commercial herbal products. See Part III Introduction "How to prescribe medicinal herbs" for further guidance on herbal advising and prescribing.

Dried Root

- Decoction: 1 tsp per cup TID
- Fluid extract (1:1, 25%): 2–6 mL TID
- Tincture of dried root (1:5, 40%): 1–3 mL TID
- Powdered root extract: 1200 mg (1/2 tsp) QD
- Capsule or tablet of powdered root: 0.5–2 g BID-TID

Can be taken long-term in recommended doses

Fruit/Seed

- Extract: apply topically for wrinkles
- Extract: combined with astragalus for hyperglycemia, lipids, albuminuria

SAFETY AND PRECAUTION

Side Effects

May cause contact dermatitis or systemic allergic response in patients with inulin allergy. May cause diuretic effects.

Case Reports

Only one case of serious allergy to burdock is known. A 53-year-old Japanese man was diagnosed to be in anaphylactic shock after eating boiled burdock root.

Toxicity

Treatment of mice at 250 mg/kg for 8 weeks demonstrated no adverse histological effects on organs.

Pregnancy and Lactation

Avoid in pregnancy as may cause uterine smooth muscle contractions.

Drug Interactions

No reported interactions with drugs or herbs. However, it increases gut motility so may alter absorption of other herbs or pharmaceuticals given concurrently.

Increase in hepatic detoxification may increase metabolism of certain drugs. May augment effects of hypoglycemic agents and diuretics.

REFERENCES

Chen W, Hsu Y, Lee M, et al. Effect of burdock extract on physical performance and physiological fatigue in mice. J Vet Med Sci 2017 Oct;79(10):1698–706.

da Silva LM, Allemand A, Mendes DA, et al. Ethanolic extract of roots from Arctium lappa L. accelerates the healing of acetic acid-induced gastric ulcer in rats: Involvement of the antioxidant system. Food Chem Toxicol 2013;51:179–87.

Gu Y, Qi C, Sun X, Ma X, Zhang H, Hu L, Yuah J, Yu Q. Arctigenin preferentially induces tumor cell death under glucose deprivation by inhibiting cellular energy metabolism. Biochem Pharmacol 2012 Aug 15;84(4):468–76.

Hayashi K, Narutaki K, Nagaoka Y, Hayashi T, Uesato S. Therapeutic Effect of Arctiin and Arctigenin in Immunocompetent and Immunocompromised Mice Infected with Influenza A Virus. Biological & pharmaceutical bulletin. 2010;33:1199–205.

Huang K, Li LA, Meng YG, You YQ, Fu XY, Song L. Arctigenin promotes apoptosis in ovarian cancer cells via the iNOS/NO/STAT3/survivin signalling. Basic Clin Pharmacol Toxicol 2014;115(6):507–11.

Ikeda M, Sato A, Mochizuki N, et al. Phase I trial of GBS-01 for advanced pancreatic cancer refractory to gemcitabine. Cancer Sci 2016;107(12):1818–24.

Knott A, Reuschlein K, Mielke H, et al. Natural Arctium lappa fruit extract improves the clinical signs of aging skin. J Cosmet Dermatol 2008;7(4):281–9.

Kuo D, Hung M, Hung C, et al. Body weight management effect of burdock (*Arctium lappa* L.) root is associated with the activation of AMP-activated protein kinase in human HepG2 cells. Food Chem 2012;134(3):1320–6.

Li A, Zhang X, Shu M, et al. Arctigenin suppresses renal interstitial fibrosis in a rat model of obstructive nephropathy. Phytomedicine 2017;30:28–41.

Lin SC, Chung TC, Lin CC, Ueng TH, Lin YH, Lin SY, Wang LY. Hepatoprotective effects of Arctium lappa on carbon tetrachloride- and acetaminophen-induced liver damage. Am J Chin Med 2000;28(2):163–73.

Lu LC, Zhou W, Li ZH, et al. Effects of arctiin on streptozotocin-induced diabetic retinopathy in Sprague-Dawley rats. Planta Med 2012;78(12):1317–23.

Maghsoumi-Norouzabad L, Alipoor B, Abed R, Sadat BE, Mesgari-Abbasi M, Jafarabadi MA. Effects of Arctium lappa L. (Burdock) root tea on inflammatory status and oxidative stress in patients with knee osteoarthritis. Int J Rheum Dis 2016;19(3):255–61.

Miglani A, Manchanda RK. Observational study of Arctium lappa in the treatment of acne vulgaris. Homeopathy 2014;103(3):203–7.

Mizuki A, Tatemichi M, Nakazawa A, Tsukada N, Nagata H, Kinoshita Y. Effects of Burdock tea on recurrence of colonic diverticulitis and diverticular bleeding: an open-labelled randomized clinical trial. Sci Rep 2019;9:6793.

Wang HY, Chen YP. Clinical observation on treatment of diabetic nephropathy with compound fructus arctii mixture. Zhongguo Zhong Xi Yi Jie He Za Zhi 2004;24(7):589–92.

33 BUTTERBUR (*PETASITES HYBRIDUS*)
Leaf, Rhizome, Root

GENERAL OVERVIEW

This well-studied and efficacious herb requires attentive caution due to its pyrrolizidine alkaloid (PA) content, which is mostly in its roots, with lesser amounts in its leaves. PAs are known to cause hepatic veno-occlusive disease. Fortunately, most commercial preparations of butterbur extract guarantee zero to negligible amounts of PAs. Butterbur has a strongly evidence-based application for treatment of migraines, and has potential additional usefulness for allergic rhinitis, asthma, bladder spasms, and prevention of gastric ulcers. There has been enough good quality research demonstrating efficacy for migraines that the American Academy of Neurology and the American Headache Society have endorsed the use of butterbur root extract for prophylactic use in migraine headaches. As a rule, while the root may be beneficial for migraine prophylaxis, the leaf appears to have efficacy for allergic disorders.

Clinical research indicates that butterbur, alone or in combination formulas, may be beneficial for allergic rhinitis, asthma, overactive bladder, migraine headache prophylaxis, anxiety, and somatoform disorder.

IN VITRO AND ANIMAL RESEARCH

Butterbur has antispasmodic, anti-inflammatory, and antihistamine properties.

Pretreatment with bakkenolide B, a constituent of butterbur, significantly reduced microglial production of IL-1β, IL-6, IL-12, and TNF-α and increased AMPK phosphorylation in microglia, indicating it is an AMPK/Nrf2 pathway activator for suppressing abnormal neuroinflammation in neurodegenerative diseases. Activation of TRPA1 channels by a different constituent, isopetasin, has been shown to cause excitation of neuropeptide-containing nociceptors, followed by marked heterologous neuronal desensitization. Such attenuation in pain and neurogenic inflammation may account for the antimigraine action of butterbur. In cultured vascular smooth muscle cells S-petasin demonstrated a direct Ca2 + antagonism of L-type voltage-dependent calcium channels in vascular smooth muscle. Petasin inhibits the proliferation of colon cancer SW-620 cells via inactivating the Akt/mTOR pathway.

In a mouse model butterbur demonstrated suppressive properties for the pathogenesis of airway inflammation and is proposed as a potential agent for the treatment of asthma. Intravenous S-petasin in anesthetized rats produced a dose-dependent hypotensive effect. In animal models of gastrointestinal ulcers alcoholic extracts of butterbur were shown to block the ethanol-induced gastric damage and reduce small intestinal ulcerations induced in rats by indomethacin. Butterbur leaves have demonstrated neuroprotective activity against Aβ plaque-induced neurotoxicity.

HUMAN RESEARCH

Allergic Disorders: Allergic Rhinitis

For allergic rhinitis, butterbur leaf appears to have similar efficacy to antihistamines but with less sedation (fexofenadine in one trial and cetirizine in a second trial), but evidence is conflicting. Much of the research has used the butterbur formulation Ze 339, a 17.8–40 mg CO_2 extract standardized to 8 mg petasins.

A 2007 systematic review assessed the evidence for efficacy of butterbur in allergic rhinitis. The researchers selected 16 studies that met inclusion criteria, involving 10 different herbal products. Six RCTs suggested that butterbur was superior to placebo or similarly effective when compared with non-sedating antihistamines for intermittent allergic rhinitis. Two RCTs studied an Indian herbal combination, Aller-7, in patients with allergic rhinitis and reported positive results. The authors concluded that evidence suggested that butterbur may be an effective herbal treatment for intermittent allergic rhinitis (Guo et al., 2007).

A 2-week RCT in patients ($n = 330$) with allergic rhinitis compared butterbur extract (Ze 339) 8 mg TID with fexofenadine 180 mg QD and with placebo. Both butterbur and fexofenadine were significantly superior to placebo ($P < 0.001$) in improving daytime symptoms of allergic rhinitis and there were no differences between the two groups ($P = 0.37$). Physician global assessment, responder rates, and evening/night symptoms were better with both butterbur and fexofenadine than with placebo ($P < 0.001$). The authors concluded that this butterbur formulation and fexofenadine were similarly efficacious compared with placebo for allergic rhinitis (Schapowal, 2005).

A crossover RCT in patients ($n = 16$) with perennial allergic rhinitis and house dust mite sensitization compared butterbur extract 50 mg BID with fexofenadine 180 mg QD and with placebo QD or BID. Peak nasal inspiratory flow rates (PNIF) were measured. The maximum % fall in PNIF from baseline after a nasal adenosine monophosphate (AMP) challenge was 34%, 39%, and 46% with butterbur, fexofenadine, and placebo, respectively ($P < 0.05$) The area under the 60-min time–response curve (%-min) was 1052, 1194, and 1734 with butterbur, fexofenadine, and placebo, respectively ($P < 0.05$). Total nasal symptom score was 1.8, 1.8, and 2.8 with butterbur, fexofenadine, and placebo, respectively ($P < 0.05$). There were no significant differences between butterbur and fexofenadine for any outcomes. The authors concluded that butterbur and fexofenadine were equally effective in attenuating the nasal response to AMP and improving nasal symptoms (Lee et al., 2004).

A 2-week RCT in patients ($n = 186$) with allergic rhinitis compared butterbur (Ze 339) at high (TID) and low doses (BID) doses with placebo. Improvement in symptoms from baseline was significantly superior in both butterbur groups, relative to placebo, and a significant dose relationship was observed between the two butterbur doses. The clinicians' assessment of efficacy and the overall responder rates were significantly superior with butterbur than with placebo. Adverse events were similar across all three groups. The authors concluded that the effects of this formulation of butterbur were evident to patients and physicians (Schapowal, 2004).

A 2-week RCT in patients ($n = 125$) with allergic rhinitis compared butterbur (Ze 339) QID with cetirizine QHS. Improvements in SF-36 scores were similar between the two treatment groups for all items tested hierarchically. Butterbur and cetirizine were also similarly effective in global improvement scores on the clinical global impression scale (median score of 3.0 in both groups). Both treatments were well tolerated. In the cetirizine group, 8 out of 12 subjects reported adverse events associated with drowsiness and fatigue. The authors concluded that butterbur should be considered for treating allergic rhinitis when the sedative effects of antihistamines are not tolerated (Schapowal, 2002).

A serial allergen RCT in patients with respiratory allergies ($n = 8$) and volunteers without atopy ($n = 10$) compared butterbur (Ze 339) with acrivastine (a short-acting antihistamine) and with placebo for response to skin prick tests with different stimuli such as codeine, histamine, and methacholine. Wheal-and-flare reactions were assessed 90 min after a double dose of Ze 339, acrivastine, or placebo. An interval of at least 3 days was left between the skin tests. Butterbur did not inhibit skin test reactivity for any of the test solutions, but acrivastine did. The authors concluded that there was no skin test antihistamine effect of the butterbur formulation and that the mechanism by which butterbur is effective in the treatment of seasonal allergic rhinitis still needs to be elucidated (Gex-Collet et al., 2006).

A 1-week study in patients with allergic rhinitis investigated the effects butterbur (Ze 339) two tablets TID. Butterbur significantly improved daytime and nighttime nasal symptoms. Nasal flow increased from

403 to 844 cm^3/s. Inflammatory mediators in nasal fluids and serum declined significantly: histamine decreased from 154 to 53 pg/mL; LTB4 decreased from 313 to 181 pg/mL; and cysteinyl-LT decreased from 137 to 70 pg/mL. The authors concluded that Ze 339 may be effective in treating allergic rhinitis by decreasing levels of nasal inflammatory mediators (Thomet et al., 2002).

Pulmonary Disorders: Asthma

A 4-month non-randomized open trial in subjects ($n = 64$ adults, 16 children) with asthma looked at efficacy and tolerability of butterbur extract (Petadolex) in conjunction with routine asthma medication. The number, duration, and severity of asthma attacks decreased, while peak flow, FEV1, and all measured symptoms improved during therapy. More than 40% of patients using asthma medications at baseline reduced intake of these medications by the end of the study. The author concluded that this extract of butterbur was safe and effective in the treatment of asthma (Danesch, 2004).

Bladder Dysfunction: Overactive Bladder

An 8-week open-label clinical trial in women ($n = 24$) with overactive bladder investigated efficacy of butterbur extract Urovex. After 3 weeks, 17 women reported a significant reduction in the frequency of urination. Before they began taking butterbur, voiding intervals were 30 to 90 min, while 3 weeks later the intervals were 90 to 150 min (Bauer and Danesch, 1995).

Neurological Disorders: Migraine headache

Much of the research on butterbur for migraines utilized the formulation Petadolex, a proprietary root extract standardized to a minimum of 15% petasins and essentially free of PAs (content < 0.088 ppm).

A 2020 systematic review to assess herbal treatments for acute and prophylactic treatment of migraine headaches found 19 trials that met inclusion criteria, including studies of feverfew, butterbur, curcumin, menthol/peppermint oil, coriander, citron, Damask rose, chamomile, and lavender. Overall, there was positive, albeit limited evidence for butterbur, and mixed findings for feverfew. There were positive, preliminary findings for curcumin, citron, and coriander as a prophylactic treatment for migraine, and the

use of menthol and chamomile as an acute treatment. High risk for bias was noted in many of the studies. The authors concluded that several herbal medicines, via their multifactorial physiological influences, may enhance the treatment of migraine and that further high-quality research was warranted (Lopresti et al., 2020).

A 2006 systematic review to assess the efficacy of butterbur for prophylaxis of migraine headache selected studies that contained Petadolex 100–150 mg/day for 12–16 weeks. Two studies met inclusion criteria and were rated as being of high quality. One trial ($n = 60$) showed a significant reduction in migraine attacks with 100 mg Petadolex compared with placebo. The other trial ($n = 233$) reported a statistically significant reduction in frequency of migraine attacks with the 150 mg dose but not the 100 mg dose of Petadolex. The authors concluded that there was moderate evidence in support of the effectiveness for 3–4 months of daily prophylactic treatment with the butterbur root extract Petadolex 150 mg/day in the prophylaxis of migraine (Agosti et al., 2006).

A 3-month RCT in patients ($n = 60$) with migraine headache compared butterbur (Petadolex) 25 mg two capsules BID with placebo. The mean attack frequency per month decreased from 3.4 at baseline to 1.8 ($P = 0.0024$) and from 2.9 to 2.6 (N.S.) with butterbur and placebo, respectively. The responder rate (improvement of migraine frequency $\geq 50\%$) was 45% and 15% with butterbur and placebo, respectively. Butterbur was well tolerated. The authors concluded that butterbur may be effective in the prophylaxis of migraine (Diener et al., 2004).

A 12-week RCT in patients ($n = 60$) with migraines compared butterbur extract (Petadolex) 25 mg two capsules BID with placebo. The frequency of migraine attacks decreased by a maximum of 60% over baseline with butterbur, being a greater reduction than with placebo ($P < 0.05$). No adverse events were reported. The authors concluded that migraine patients may benefit from prophylactic treatment with Petadolex (Grossman and Schmidramsl, 2001).

A 4-month RCT in patients ($n = 245$) with migraine compared butterbur 75 mg BID or 50 mg BID with placebo BID. Migraine attack frequency was reduced by 48%, 36%, and 26% with butterbur 75 mg, butterbur 50 mg, and placebo, respectively (difference from placebo was $P= 0.0012$ and $P=0.127$ for the higher and lower doses of butterbur, respectively). The proportion of patients with $\geq 50\%$ reduction in attack frequency after 4 months was 68% with butterbur 75 mg and 49% with placebo ($P<0.05$). Results were also significant with 75 mg at 1, 2, and 3 months based on this endpoint. The most frequently reported adverse reactions possibly related to treatment were mild gastrointestinal events, predominantly burping. The authors concluded that butterbur 75 mg BID but not 50 mg BID was significantly more effective than placebo at reducing migraine headache frequency (Lipton et al., 2004).

An extended follow-up RCT in children ($n = 58$) with migraine compared butterbur root extract (Petadolex) with music therapy and with placebo for 12 weeks, all in addition to treatment as usual. Data analysis of subjects completing the respective study phase showed that during the 8-week post-treatment period, only music therapy was superior to placebo ($P = 0.005$), whereas in the 6-month follow-up period both music therapy and butterbur root extract were superior to placebo ($P = 0.018$ and $P = 0.044$, respectively). All groups showed a substantial reduction of attack frequency compared with baseline. The authors concluded that butterbur extract and music therapy might be superior to placebo in prophylaxis of pediatric migraine (Oelkers-Ax et al., 2008).

A 4-month open-label study in children and adolescents ($n = 108$) with migraine headaches assessed effects of butterbur 50–150 mg/day (based on age). A reduction by at least 50% in frequency of migraine attacks occurred in 77% of all patients. Overall, attack frequency was reduced by 63%. Slight-to-substantial improvement was reported by 91% of patients. Both doctors and patients reported improved well-being in about 90% of cases. Side effects occurred in 7.4% and included mostly eructation. No serious adverse events occurred. The authors concluded that butterbur root extract showed potential as an effective and well-tolerated migraine prophylaxis for children and teenagers (Pothmann and Danesh, 2005).

Psychiatric Disorders: Anxiety

A 3.5-year retrospective case-control study of hospitalized psychiatric patients ($n = 3252$) evaluated an herbal extract combination of passionflower, valerian, lemon balm, and butterbur (Ze 185) compared with no additional herbal therapy to investigate whether the herbal combination would change the prescription pattern of benzodiazepines. Data showed that both treatment modalities had a comparable clinical effectiveness but there were significantly fewer prescriptions of benzodiazepines with the herbal combination ($P=0.006$). The authors recommended that a RCT be performed (Keck et al., 2020).

An acutely dosed RCT in healthy men ($n=72$) investigated pre-dosing for 4 days with Ze 185, a fixed combination of valerian, passionflower, lemon balm, and butterbur, compared with pre-dosing with placebo and with a no-treatment control for effects on biological and affective responses to a standardized psychosocial stress paradigm. The stress paradigm induced significant and large cortisol and self-reported anxiety responses. Groups did not differ significantly in their salivary cortisol response to stress, but participants in the herbal group showed significantly attenuated responses in self-reported anxiety compared with placebo ($P=0.03$) and with no treatment ($P=0.05$). The authors suggested that the herbal combination reduced the self-reported anxiety response to stress without affecting the assumingly adaptive biological stress responses (Meier et al., 2018).

Psychiatric Disorders: Somatoform Disorder

A 2-week RCT in patients ($n = 182$) with somatoform disorders investigated Ze185, a four-herb combination containing valerian, passionflower, lemon balm, and butterbur compared with a three-herb combination without the butterbur and with placebo. The combination containing butterbur was significantly superior to the combination without butterbur, which was superior to placebo for changes in VAS-Anxiety scale, Beck Depression Inventory, and Clinical Global Impression. Nine non-serious adverse events were documented, but the distribution did not differ significantly between the treatment groups. The authors concluded that the herbal preparation Ze185 was an efficacious and safe short-term treatment in patients with somatoform disorders (Melzer et al., 2009).

ACTIVE CONSTITUENTS

Leaf, Rhizome, Root

- Phenolic compounds
  - Flavonoids (likely COX2 and PGE2 inhibition): tannins
- Terpenes
  - Sesquiterpenes (vascular and visceral smooth muscle spasmolytic, anti-inflammatory, antihistamine, leukotriene inhibition, calcium channel blockade, prostaglandin effects): petasin, exopetasin, isopetasin
- Alkaloids (potentially hepatotoxic): pyrrolizidine alkaloids
- Aromatic compounds: petasin, exopetasin, isopetasin

BUTTERBUR COMMONLY USED PREPARATIONS AND DOSAGE (FOR ADULTS UNLESS OTHERWISE SPECIFIED)

The following are examples of some available formulations and ranges of dosing for commercial herbal products. See Part III Introduction "How to prescribe medicinal herbs" for further guidance on herbal advising and prescribing.

Allergic Diseases—Leaf

- PA-free butterbur extract: 50–100 mg BID
- Butterbur leaf (PA-free) capsule or tablet of standardized CO_2 extract (standardized to 8 mg petasins): 17.8–40 mg BID to TID

Migraine Headaches—Root

- Butterbur root (PA-free) capsule or tablet of standardized extract (standardized to 1.25–7.5 mg petasin or isopetasin or 15% sesquiterpenes): 25–100 mg BID

For migraine headaches take daily for 6 months then slowly taper to lowest effective dose.

SAFETY AND PRECAUTION

Do not use products that have not guaranteed removal of pyrrolizidine alkaloids.

Side Effects

May cause belching, headache, itchy eyes, diarrhea, dyspnea, fatigue, and drowsiness. Petasin inhibits production in rat testicular cells, but is yet to be tested in humans. Allergic reactions may occur in people who are sensitive to plants such as ragweed, chrysanthemums, marigolds, and daisies.

Pregnancy and Lactation

Insufficient human safety data.

Drug Interactions

- CYP: None known as long as PA-free. Levels of PAs can be increased by drugs that induce CYP3A4.

REFERENCES

Agosti R, Duke RK, Chrubasik JE, Chrubasik S. Effectiveness of petasites hybridus preparations in the prophylaxis of migraine: a systematic review. Phytomedicine 2006;13(9-10):743–6.

Bauer HW, Danesch U. Therapeutische Aspekte in der Urologie mit Petadolex (Therapeutic aspects in the urology with Petadolex) Presse Symposium München 10/18/95, 1995.

Danesch U. *Petasites hybridus* (Butterbur root) extract in the treatment of asthma—an open trial. Altern Med Rev 2004;9(1):54–62.

Diener HC, Rahlfs VW, Danesch U. The first placebo-controlled trial of a special butterbur root extract for the prevention of migraine: reanalysis of efficacy criteria. Eur Neurol 2004;51:89–97.

Gex-Collet C, Imhof L, Brattstrom A, et al. The butterbur extract petasin has no effect on skin test reactivity induced by different stimuli: a randomized, double-blind crossover study using histamine, codeine, methacholine, and aeroallergen solutions. J Investig Allergol Clin Immunol 2006;16:156–61.

Grossman W, Schmidramsl H. An extract of Petasites hybridus is effective in the prophylaxis of migraine. Altern Med Rev 2001;6(3):303–10.

Guo R, Pittler MH, Ernst E. Herbal medicines for the treatment of allergic rhinitis: a systematic review. Ann Allergy Asthma Immunol 2007;99(6):483–95.

Keck ME, Nicolussi S, Spura K, Blohm C, Zahner C, Drewe J. Effect of the fixed combination of valerian, lemon balm, passionflower, and butterbur extracts (Ze 185) on the prescription pattern of benzodiazepines in hospitalized psychiatric patients-A retrospective case-control investigation. Phytother Res 2020;34(6):1436–45.

Lee DK, Gray RD, Robb FM, et al. A placebo-controlled evaluation of butterbur and fexofenadine on objective and subjective outcomes in perennial allergic rhinitis. Clin Exp Allergy 2004;34:646–9.

Lipton RB, Gobel H, Einhaupl KM, Wilks K, Mauskop A. *Petasites hybridus* root (butterbur) is an effective preventive treatment for migraine. Neurology 2004;63:2240–4.

Lopresti A, Smith S, Drummond P. Herbal treatments for migraine: A systematic review of randomised-controlled studies. Phytother Res 2020;34(10):2493–517.

Meier S, Haschke M, Zahner C, et al. Effects of a fixed herbal drug combination (Ze 185) to an experimental acute stress setting in healthy men—an explorative randomized placebo-controlled double-blind study. Phytomedicine 2018;39:85–92.

Melzer J, Schrader E, Brattström A, et al. Fixed herbal drug combination with and without butterbur (Ze 185) for the treatment of patients with somatoform disorders: randomized, placebo-controlled pharmaco-clinical trial. Phytother Res 2009;23:1303–8.

Oelkers-Ax R, Leins A, Parzer P, et al. Butterbur root extract and music therapy in the prevention of childhood migraine: an explorative study. Eur J Pain 2008;12(3):301–13.

Pothmann R, Danesh U. Migraine prevention in children and adolescents: Results of an open trial with a special butterbur root extract. Headache 2005;45:1–8.

Schapowal A. Petasites Study Group. "Randomised controlled trial of butterbur and cetirizine for treating seasonal allergic rhinitis". BMJ 2002;324(7330):144–6.

Schapowal A. Butterbur Ze339 for the treatment of intermittent allergic rhinitis: dose-dependent efficacy in a prospective, randomized, double-blind, placebo-controlled study. Arch Otolaryngol Head Neck Surg 2004;130(12):1381–6.

Schapowal A. A Study Group. "Treating intermittent allergic rhinitis: a prospective, randomized, placebo and antihistamine-controlled study of Butterbur extract Ze 339". Phytother Res 2005;19(6):530–7.

Thomet OA, Schapowal A, Heinisch IV, Wiesmann UN, Simon HU. Anti-inflammatory activity of an extract of Petasites hybridus in allergic rhinitis. Int Immunopharmacol 2002;2(7):997–1006.

34

CALENDULA (*CALENDULA OFFICINALIS*)
Flower

GENERAL OVERVIEW

Calendula is the quintessential wound healer and skin calmer. Its other common name is marigold, not to be confused with the common flowering plants that are bought at the local garden center. The healing benefits of calendula are due to a combination of soothing, tissue growth promoting, and antimicrobial properties. This herb is most commonly used as a topical application.

Clinical research indicates that calendula, alone or in combination formulas, may be beneficial for gingivitis, radiation mucositis, vaginal candidiasis, episiotomy healing, chronic prostatitis, diaper dermatitis, leg ulcers (venous and neuropathic), and radiation dermatitis.

IN VITRO AND ANIMAL RESEARCH

Calendula has been shown to have antiinflammatory, cytotoxic, antitumor, antimicrobial (antifungal, antibacterial, antiparasitic, anti-HIV) properties and to promote wound healing. It has a photoprotective effect thought to be associated with improved collagen synthesis in the subepidermal connective tissue. It inhibits gingival collagen degradation and MMP-2 activity. Fish studies have demonstrated protective properties to liver, kidney, and heart likely through antioxidant and antiinflammatory activity. Laboratory research has demonstrated that calendula may play a role in healing mucosal ulcers including lesions of the GI tract.

HUMAN RESEARCH

Oral and Dental Disorders

A 6-month RCT of patients ($n=240$) with gingivitis and bleeding gums compared a dilute tincture of calendula rinse BID with distilled water rinse. Calendula rinse showed a statistically significant reduction in plaque index, gingival index, sulcus bleeding index, and oral hygiene index, whereas the control group showed no reduction in scores after 3 months. At the third month scaling was performed and subsequently there was a statistically significant reduction in the scores of all parameters when the third month scores were compared with the sixth month scores in both groups ($P < 0.05$), but the test group showed a significantly greater reduction in PI, GI, SBI, and OHI-S scores compared with those of the control group (Khairnar et al., 2013).

A 14-day RCT of patients ($n=60$) with gingivitis compared the effects of a polyherbal mouthwash (containing calendula, rosemary, and ginger) with chlorhexidine and with placebo 5 g of each BID. Scores for modified gingival index, gingival bleeding index, and modified Quigley-Hein plaque index showed significant improvement from baseline for both the polyherbal and chlorhexidine mouthwash groups with no change in the placebo group. There was no significant difference in response between the polyherbal and chlorhexidine groups (Mahyari et al., 2016).

A 6-week RCT in patients ($n=40$) with head and neck cancers undergoing radiotherapy compared 2% calendula extract oral gel with placebo. Calendula mouthwash significantly decreased the scores on the oral mucositis assessment compared with placebo at week 2 (5.5 vs 6.8; $P=0.019$), week 3 (8.25 vs 10.95; $P<0.0001$) and week 6 (11.4 vs 13.35; $P=0.031$). The authors concluded that calendula could be effective in decreasing the intensity of radiotherapy-induced oral mucositis during treatment. They surmised that antioxidant capacity may be partly responsible for the effect (Babaee et al., 2013).

Women's Genitourinary Disorders: Vaginitis and Episiotomy

A 35-day RCT of women ($n=150$) with vaginal candidiasis compared calendula cream with clotrimazole 5 g QHS for seven nights. Follow-up testing at 15 and 35 days showed that the frequency of testing negative for candidiasis in the calendula group was significantly lower at 15 days (49% vs 74%, OR: 0.32) but higher at 35 days (77% vs 34%, OR: 3.1). The frequency of most signs and symptoms were almost equal in the two groups at the first follow-up but were significantly lower in the calendula group at the second follow-up. Sexual function had almost equally significant improvement in both groups. The authors concluded that calendula vaginal cream appeared to have been effective in the treatment of vaginal candidiasis and to have a delayed but greater long-term effect compared with clotrimazole (Saffari et al., 2017).

A 5-day RCT of primiparous women ($n=111$) who had undergone episiotomy compared calendula ointment with aloe ointment every 8 h, respectively, and with usual care (control) for rates of healing. The REEDA scale (redness, edema, ecchymosis, discharge, and approximation) showed a statistically significant difference between the control group and the treatment groups in favor of treatment groups ($P<0.001$). There was no significant difference in healing between calendula and aloe ointments (Eghdampour et al., 2013).

Men's Genitourinary Disorders: Chronic Prostatitis

A 3-month Phase II clinical trial in patients ($n=60$) with chronic prostatitis/chronic pelvic pain syndrome type III (CP/CPPSIII) compared rectal suppositories of curcumin 350 mg plus calendula 80 mg QD with placebo suppositories. The curcumin group had a significant improvement in NIH-Chronic Prostatitis Symptoms Index (from 20.5 to 15; $P<0.01$), IIEF-5 (from 18.5 to

22; $P<0.01$), Premature Ejaculation Diagnostic Tool (from 11 to 5.5; $P<0.01$), peak flow (from 14 to 16.8; $P<0.01$), and VAS (from 7.5 to 1.0; $P<0.01$), with all changes being significantly different from the placebo group. The authors concluded that there was clinical efficacy with curcumin and calendula suppositories in patients with CP/CPPSIII (Morgia et al., 2017).

Dermatological Disorders: Contact Dermatitis and Diaper Dermatitis

A 5-day study of experimentally induced contact dermatitis (ICD) in healthy adults compared cream preparations containing seven different types of calendula and rosemary. When the test products were applied at the same time as the irritating stimulus for ICD, a statistically significant protective effect of all cream preparations was observed through visual and quantified methods, but this benefit was not statistically significant and was not observed when the test creams were applied following the irritating stimulus (Fuchs et al., 2005).

A 10-day study of infants ($n=66$) with diaper dermatitis compared aloe cream with calendula ointment applied topically TID. Improvement in the severity of the diaper dermatitis was observed in both groups ($P<0.001$). The calendula group had significantly fewer rash sites compared with the aloe group ($P=0.001$). No adverse effect was reported from either of the medications. The authors concluded that topical aloe and, in particular, calendula could serve as safe and effective treatment for diaper dermatitis in infants (Panahi et al., 2012).

A 7-day RCT in infants ($n=73$) with nonsevere, noninfected diaper dermatitis compared 1.5% calendula ointment with 1.5% olive ointment. Measurements at days 0, 3, 5, and 7 revealed no significant difference between the olive oil and calendula groups in terms of severity of diaper dermatitis. No adverse effect was reported from either of the medications in this study. The authors concluded that olive ointment provided the same benefits as calendula ointment and could be used as an alternative in the healing of diaper dermatitis (Sharifi-Heris et al., 2018).

Dermatological Disorders: Wound Healing

A 2019 systematic review of the use of calendula for wound healing found 14 studies (seven animal and seven clinical) that met inclusion criteria. One human trial and five animal studies on acute wound healing showed faster resolution of the inflammation phase with increased production of granulation tissue in the test groups treated with calendula. Chronic wound healing studies were varied. Two RCTs on venous ulcers demonstrated decreased ulcer surface area compared with controls. A RCT on diabetic leg ulcer healing demonstrated no improvement with calendula. Burn healing also showed mixed results, and an RCT in patients suffering from partial-to-full thickness burns demonstrated no benefit from topical application of calendula extract compared with controls. For prevention of acute post radiation dermatitis, one study showed improvements compared with trolamine, while another found no improvement compared with aqua gel cream. The authors concluded that there was some evidence for the beneficial effects of calendula extract for wound healing, consistent with its role in traditional medicine, and that there was need for further research (Givol et al., 2019).

A 2008 systematic review was conducted on the efficacy of calendula for wound healing. Although six trials were identified, only one was of good quality. The review of the studies indicated that there was only weak evidence to support the topical administration of calendula in acute and chronic wounds (Leach, 2008).

A 30-week RCT in patients ($n=57$) with venous leg ulcers compared topical calendula extract with a control group. The proportion of the treatment patients achieving complete epithelialization was 72% and 32% in the treatment and control groups, respectively. Healing velocity per week was increased by 7.4% and 1.7% in calendula and control patients, respectively. No adverse events were observed. The authors concluded that calendula extract was an effective treatment for venous leg ulcers (Buzzi et al., 2016a).

A 3-week RCT in patients ($n=34$) with leg ulcers compared calendula ointment with saline dressings applied BID. By the third week, the total surface of the ulcers was decreased by 42% with calendula and 15% with saline dressings. Complete epithelialization occurred in 33% of patients using calendula and 31% using saline. The authors concluded that a statistically significant acceleration of wound healing was demonstrated with calendula ($P<0.05$) (Duran et al., 2005).

A 30-week pilot study in patients ($n=41$) with stable neuropathic ulcers of >3 months' duration assessed the effect of daily calendula extract spray plus saline-moistened, sterile, nonadherent gauze and bandages and foot offloading with adequate protective footwear. Complete wound closure after 11, 20, and 30 weeks of treatment occurred in 54%, 68%, and 78% of patients, respectively. Mean healing time was 15 weeks. After 30 weeks of treatment, the number of colonized wounds decreased from 29 at baseline to 5, and the number of odorous wounds decreased from 19 to 1. Ulcer bed planimetry data showed a significant reduction in the amount of exudate, fibrin slough, and necrotic tissue ($P=0.001$). No adverse events were observed during treatment (Buzzi et al., 2016b).

A 30-day RCT in patients ($n=32$) with diabetic foot ulcers compared low-level laser therapy (LLLT) plus calendula oil with LLLT alone for effects on ulcer healing. Analog pain scale showed reduced pain in both groups ($P<0.01$). Lesion area reduction with LLLT plus calendula and LLLT alone showed a significant difference in favor of calendula ($P=0.0032$ and $P=0.0428$, respectively) (Carvalho et al., 2016).

Dermatological Disorders: Radiation Dermatitis

An irradiation-linked RCT in patients ($n=51$) undergoing radiotherapy for head and neck cancer compared calendula oil with essential fatty acids applied BID during radiation therapy for prevention of radiation dermatitis. A higher incidence of Grade 1 and 2 radiodermatitis occurred in the EFA group compared with calendula ($P=0.00402$ and $P=0.0120$, respectively). The authors concluded that calendula showed better therapeutic response than essential fatty acids in the prevention and treatment of radiodermatitis (Schneider et al., 2015).

A Phase III RCT in patients ($n=254$) who were to receive postoperative radiation therapy for breast cancer compared calendula with trolamine applied to the irradiated fields after each session. The occurrence of acute dermatitis of Grade 2 or higher was significantly lower with calendula than with trolamine lower (41% vs 63%; $P<0.001$). Patients receiving calendula had less frequent interruption of radiotherapy and significantly reduced radiation-induced pain. The authors concluded that calendula was highly effective for the prevention of acute dermatitis of Grade 2 or higher and should be proposed for patients undergoing postoperative irradiation for breast cancer (Pommier et al., 2004).

ACTIVE CONSTITUENTS

- Carbohydrates
  - Polysaccharides (immune stimulating, demulcent): mucilage
- Lipids
  - Fatty acids: calendic acid
- Phenolic compounds
  - Flavonoids (antioxidant, antiinflammatory, antiviral): patulitrin, patuletin
- Terpenes
  - Triterpenoids (antiinflammatory, antiviral, antiretroviral, trichomonacidal, antitumor): faradiol-3-O-palmitate, faradiol-3-O-myristate, faradiol-3-O-laurate, arnidiol-3-O-palmitate, arnidiol-3-O-myristate, arnidiol-3-O-laurate, calenduladiol-3-O-palmitate, and calenduladiol-3-O-myristate
  - Triterpenoid saponins (decrease tissue swelling, increase capillary perfusion, antimutagenic, cytotoxic, antiviral, hypoglycemiant, gastroprotective): oleanolic acid (chemoprotective, hepatoprotective), ursolic acid (anti-HIV, anti-EBV, antiviral, AChEI, procollagen, proceremide, antitumor), calendasaponins A–D
  - Tetraterpenes/Carotenoids (stimulate granulation tissue): auroxanthin, lutein, β-carotene, flavoxanthin

CALENDULA COMMONLY USED PREPARATIONS AND DOSAGE (FOR ADULTS UNLESS OTHERWISE SPECIFIED)

The following are examples of some available formulations and ranges of dosing for commercial herbal products. See Part III Introduction "How to prescribe medicinal herbs" for further guidance on herbal advising and prescribing.

Dried Flower

- Oral infusion (tea): 1 tsp. per cup TID.
- Tincture (1:5, 60%–90%): 0.7–4 mL TID-QID.
- Topical preparations: creams, gels, ointments, oils, poultices, and suppositories applied TID.

Antifungal effects of tincture are only found using 90% ETOH for extraction.

SAFETY AND PRECAUTION

Side Effects

Side effects are rare. Calendula is known to cause allergic reactions including skin rash in patients with allergies to ragweed.

Toxicity

Oral administration of a single acute dose (2000 mg/kg) of calendula to rats resulted in no mortalities or signs of toxicity; subchronic doses (50, 250, and 1000 mg/kg/day) affected hemoglobin, erythrocytes, leukocytes, and blood clotting time. For blood chemistry parameters, ALT, AST, and ALP were affected. Histopathological examination of tissues showed slight abnormalities in hepatic parenchyma that were consistent with biochemical variations observed. Ethanolic extracts up to 1.0 g/kg did not induce any hematological alterations in mice and rats.

Pregnancy and Lactation

Insufficient human safety data.

Drug Interactions

No known drug or herb interactions.

REFERENCES

Babaee N, Moslemi D, Khalilpour M, et al. Antioxidant capacity of *Calendula officinalis* flowers extract and prevention of radiation induced oropharyngeal mucositis in patients with head and neck cancers: a randomized controlled clinical study. Daru 2013 Mar 7;21(1):18.

Buzzi M, de Freitas F, de Barros Winter M. Therapeutic effectiveness of a Calendula officinalis extract in venous leg ulcer healing. J Wound Care 2016a Dec 2;25(12):732–9.

Buzzi M, de Freitas F, Winter M. A prospective, descriptive study to assess the clinical benefits of using Calendula officinalis hydroglycolic extract for the topical treatment of diabetic foot ulcers. Ostomy Wound Manage 2016b Mar;62(3):8–24.

Carvalho AF, Feitosa MC, Coelho NP, et al. Low-level laser therapy and Calendula officinalis in repairing diabetic foot ulcers. Rev Esc Enferm USP 2016 Jul-Aug;50(4):628–34.

Duran V, Matic M, Jovanović M, et al. Results of the clinical examination of an ointment with marigold (Calendula officinalis) extract in the treatment of venous leg ulcers. Int J Tissue React 2005;27(3):101–6.

Eghdampour F, Jahdie F, Kheyrkhah M, Taghizadeh M, Naghizadeh S, Hagani H. The impact of Aloe and Calendula on perineal healing after episiotomy in Primiparous women: a randomized clinical trial. J Caring Sci 2013 Nov 30;2(4):279–86.

Fuchs SM, Schliemann-Willers S, Fischer TW, Elsner P. Protective effects of different marigold (Calendula officinalis L.) and rosemary cream preparations against sodium-lauryl-sulfate-induced irritant contact dermatitis. Skin Pharmacol Physiol 2005 Jul-Aug;18(4):195–200.

Givol O, Kornhaber R, Visentin D, Cleary M, Haik J, Harats M. A systematic review ofCalendulaofficinalis extract for wound healing. Wound Repair Regen 2019 Sep;27(5):548–61.

Khairnar MS, Pawar B, Marawar PP, Mani A. Evaluation of Calendula officinalis as an anti-plaque and anti-gingivitis agent. J Indian Soc Periodontol 2013 Nov;17(6):741–7.

Leach MJ. Calendula officinalis and wound healing: a systematic review. Wounds 2008 Aug;20(8):236–43.

Mahyari S, Mahyari B, Emami SA, et al. Evaluation of the efficacy of a polyherbal mouthwash containing Zingiber officinale, Rosmarinus officinalis and Calendula officinalis extracts in patients with gingivitis: a randomized double-blind placebo-controlled trial. Complement Ther Clin Pract 2016 Feb;22:93–8.

Morgia G, Russo GI, Urzì D, et al. A phase II, randomized, single-blinded, placebo-controlled clinical trial on the efficacy of Curcumina and Calendula suppositories for the treatment of patients with chronic prostatitis/chronic pelvic pain syndrome type III. Arch Ital Urol Androl 2017 Jun 30;89(2):110–3.

Panahi Y, Sharif MR, Sharif A, et al. A randomized comparative trial on the therapeutic efficacy of topical aloe and Calendula officinalis on diaper dermatitis in children. ScientificWorldJournal 2012;2012:810234.

Pommier P, Gomez F, Sunyach MP, et al. Phase III randomized trial of Calendula officinalis compared with trolamine for the prevention of acute dermatitis during irradiation for breast cancer. J Clin Oncol 2004;22(8):1447–53.

Saffari E, Mohammad-Alizadeh-Charandabi S, Adibpour M, Mirghafourvand M, Javadzadeh Y. Comparing the effects of Calendula officinalis and clotrimazole on vaginal Candidiasis: a randomized controlled trial. Women Health 2017 Nov-Dec;57(10):1145–60.

Schneider F, Danski MT, Vayego SA. Usage of Calendula officinalis in the prevention and treatment of radiodermatitis: a randomized double-blind controlled clinical trial. Rev Esc Enferm USP 2015 Apr;49(2):221–8.

Sharifi-Heris Z, Farahani L, Haghani H, Abdoli-Oskouee S, Hasanpoor-Azghady S. Comparison the effects of topical application of olive and calendula ointments on Children's diaper dermatitis: a triple-blind randomized clinical trial. Dermatol Ther 2018 Nov;31(6):e12731.

35

CHAMOMILE, GERMAN (*MATRICARIA RECUTITA/CHAMOMILLA*) AND CHAMOMILE, ROMAN (*CHAMAEMELUM NOBILE*)
Flower

GENERAL OVERVIEW

When Peter Rabbit arrived home psychologically traumatized by his encounter with Mr. McGregor, his mother gave him a tablespoonful of chamomile tea and sent him to bed. She knew what she was doing. Chamomile is known for its safe calming effects on the central nervous system, skin, and GI tract. Although there are two commonly used forms of chamomile as noted above, the more popular and better studied of the two is German chamomile. Regardless, both species share most properties. The chamomile blossom is packed with all the goodness of this plant. The flowers are used as a tea, a tincture, a cream, or an essential oil.

Clinical research indicates that chamomile, alone or in combination formulas, may be beneficial for gingivitis, hyperlipidemia, diabetes, functional dyspepsia, infantile colic, diarrhea, ulcerative colitis, menopause, carpal tunnel syndrome, wounds, anxiety, depression, short-term insomnia, attention-deficit/hyperactivity disorder, and cancer-related mucositis.

IN VITRO AND ANIMAL RESEARCH

In vitro studies show that chamomile extracts have antiinflammatory effects via COX2 and LOX inhibition and reduction of IL-1β and TNF-α. Chamomile inhibits histamine release from mast cells and has antihyperglycemic and intestinal antispasmodic activity. In an in vitro study of several anxiolytic plants, German chamomile was shown to inhibit glutamic acid decarboxylase activity, contributing to its anxiolytic effect. It is antibacterial (staph, group B strep, pneumococcus,

Helicobacter pylori, mycobacterium), antifungal (*Candida albicans*, trichophytons), and antiviral (*Herpes simplex*, poliovirus). Chamomile has demonstrated anticancer properties. The apigenin constituent, in particular, has been shown to selectively induce apoptosis of several cancer cell lines.

Animal studies have shown that German chamomile reduces inflammation, speeds wound healing, reduces muscle spasms, and serves as a mild sedative to help with sleep. At lower doses in animal research it reduced anxious behavior, while at higher doses it induced sleep. A chamomile mouthwash was found to reduce 5-fluorouracil-induced mucositis in hamsters. In another study, a chamomile extract was shown to provide gastroprotection against ethanol-induced ulceration by increasing GSH levels. Methanol extracts of chamomile have also demonstrated neuroprotective activity by decreasing lipid peroxidation and by increasing SOD, catalase, GSH, and total thiol levels.

HUMAN RESEARCH

Oral and Dental Disorders

An RCT in patients with gingival bleeding compared mouth rinses containing pomegranate and chamomile with a chlorhexidine 0.12% mouthwash. Efficacy for gingival bleeding with the herbal rinses was similar to that of chlorhexidine 0.12% (Batista et al., 2014).

A study in patients ($n=80$) in the ICU on ventilators compared three different mouthwashes (10% chamomile, 10% *Salvadora persica*, or 0.2% chlorhexidine gluconate) with placebo (saline mouthwash) for the oral colonization with *Staphylococcus aureus* and *Streptococcus pneumoniae*. Decreased rates of bacterial colonies after intervention in all four groups were significant ($P < 0.001$). The mouth wash with chlorhexidine ($P < 0.001$), *S. persica* ($P = 0.008$), and chamomile ($P = 0.01$) had a significant antibacterial effect on *S. aureus* and *S. pneumoniae* (Darvishi Khezri et al., 2013).

Ear, Nose, and Throat Disorders: Chronic Rhinosinusitis

A 3-week RCT in patients ($n = 74$) with chronic rhinosinusitis compared chamomile extract nasal drops with placebo drops instilled following saline irrigation TID. The adjusted mean QOL scores with chamomile and placebo drops were 34.3 and 45.9, respectively ($P = 0.001$). Endoscopic nasal examination at the end of the third week in the chamomile and placebo groups, respectively, revealed very mild inflammation/discharge in 24% and 46% and Grade 1 polyposis in 21.6% and 48% ($P < 0.05$). The authors concluded that chamomile extract was effective at further reducing clinical symptoms and improving QOL in patients with chronic rhinosinusitis (Nemati et al., 2020).

Cardiometabolic Disorders: Hyperlipidemia and Diabetes

An 8-week single-blind RCT in adults ($n = 64$) with T2DM investigated chamomile tea (3 g/150 mL hot water) TID immediately after meals compared with a control group (a water regimen for the same intervention period). Chamomile tea significantly decreased A1C ($P = 0.03$), serum insulin levels ($P < 0.001$), IR ($P < 0.001$), TC ($P = 0.001$), TG ($P < 0.001$), and LDL-C ($P = 0.05$) compared with the control group. No significant changes were shown in serum HDL cholesterol levels in both groups. The authors concluded that chamomile tea had some beneficial effects on glycemic control and serum lipids in T2DM patients (Rafraf et al., 2015).

Gastrointestinal Disorders: Functional Dyspepsia and Infantile Colic

A 2018 systematic review on dietary interventions for infantile colic selected 15 RCTs ($n = 1121$) for inclusion. Although the studies were small and at high risk of bias, the authors identified benefit from an extract of fennel, chamomile, and lemon balm in one study.

Average crying time for the herbal combination and placebo was 76.9 and 169.9 min/day, respectively, at the end of the 1-week study (Gordon et al., 2018).

A 4-week RCT in patients ($n = 60$) with functional dyspepsia compared Iberogast in two different formulations (chamomile, peppermint, caraway, licorice, lemon balm, angelica, celandine, and milk thistle with or without bitter candy tuft) with placebo for effects on gastrointestinal symptoms. The herbal preparations showed a clinically significant improvement in Gastrointestinal Symptom score compared with placebo after 2 and 4 weeks of treatment ($P < 0.001$). No statistically significant difference could be observed between the efficacy of two different herbal preparations ($P > 0.05$), but a solid improvement of GI symptoms could be achieved earlier with the herbal preparation containing bitter candy tuft ($P = 0.023$). The authors concluded that Iberogast and its modified formulation improved dyspeptic symptoms better than placebo and that bitter candy tuft had an additive effect (Madisch et al., 2001).

A 12-week partial crossover RCT in patients ($n = 120$) with functional dyspepsia compared STW 5-II (containing extracts from licorice, bitter candy tuft, chamomile, peppermint, caraway, and lemon balm) with placebo. Each patient received the treatment for three consecutive 4-week treatment blocks. The first two treatment blocks were fixed. For the third treatment period, medication was based upon the investigator's judgment of symptom improvement during the preceding treatment period. In patients without adequate control of symptoms, the treatment was switched, or if symptoms were controlled, the treatment was continued. During the first 4 weeks, the gastrointestinal symptom score decreased significantly in subjects on active treatment compared with placebo ($P < 0.001$). During the second 4-week period symptoms further improved in subjects who continued on active treatment or those who were switched to active treatment, while those switched to placebo deteriorated. After 8 weeks there was complete relief of symptoms in 43% and 3% of subjects on active treatment and placebo, respectively ($P < 0.001$). The authors concluded that this polyherbal preparation improved dyspeptic symptoms better than placebo (Madisch et al., 2004).

A 1-week RCT in breastfed infants ($n = 93$) with colic compared a polyherbal standardized extract combination (chamomile, lemon balm, and fennel) with placebo BID. The daily average crying time with the herbal formula decreased from 201 to 77 min/day. With placebo the crying time decreased from 199 to 169 min/day (*P* < 0.005). Crying time reduction was observed in 85% of subjects using the herbal formula and 49% of subjects given placebo (*P* < 0.005). No side effects were reported. The authors concluded that colic in breastfed infants improves within 1 week of treatment with this polyherbal formula (Savino et al., 2005).

A 1-week RCT in healthy term 2- to 8-week-old infants (*n* = 68) who had colic compared a polyherbal tea (German chamomile, vervain, licorice, fennel, and lemon balm) with a placebo tea (glucose, flavoring) up to 150 mL/dose up to TID. Parents reported that the tea eliminated colic in 57% of the infants, whereas placebo was helpful in 26% (*P* < 0.01). No adverse effects were noted in either group (Weizman et al., 1993).

A 28-day RCT in infants (*n* = 176) with colic investigated Colimil Plus (a mixture of chamomile, lemon balm, and tyndallized (sterilized) *Lactobacillus acidophilus* HA122) compared with *Lactobacillus reuteri* DSM 17938 and with simethicone for the treatment of infantile colic. Mean daily crying time at day 28 was significantly less with Colimil Plus (− 44 min; *P* < 0.001) and *Lactobacillus reuteri* (− 35 min; *P* < 0.001) when compared with simethicone. The mean difference between the former two groups was not statistically significant (*P* = 0.205). At day 28, 95% of the Colimil Plus group responded to treatment vs 86% of the *Lactobacillus reuteri* group and 68% of the simethicone group (*P* < 0.001). The authors concluded that the combination product and the *L. reuteri* product were significantly more effective than simethicone in infantile colic (Martinelli et al., 2017).

Gastrointestinal Disorders: Diarrhea and Ulcerative Colitis

A 3-day RCT in children (*n* = 79) with diarrhea compared a combination of apple pectin and chamomile with placebo. At the end of 3 days of treatment, the diarrhea had ended in 33 of 39 children with pectin-chamomile and in 23 of 40 children with placebo (*P* < 0.05). Pectin-chamomile reduced the duration of diarrhea by at least 5 h (*P* < 0.05) (de la Motte et al., 1997).

A 12-month RCT in patients (*n* = 96) with ulcerative colitis (UC) investigated the herbal combination of myrrh, chamomile, and coffee charcoal compared with mesalamine for UC disease activity. Mean clinical colitis activity index demonstrated no significant difference between the two treatment groups in the intention-to-treat (*P* = 0.121) or per-protocol (*P* = 0.251) analysis. Relapse rates in total were 53% and 45% in the herbal and mesalamine groups, respectively (*P* = 0.54). Safety profile and tolerability were good, and no significant differences were shown in relapse-free time, endoscopy, and fecal biomarkers (Langhorst et al., 2014).

Women's Genitourinary Disorders: Menopause

A 12-week RCT in postmenopausal women (*n* = 55) with hot flushes and refusing hormonal therapy compared Climex (a combination of dong quai and chamomile) five tablets daily between meals with placebo. Climex was significantly better than placebo for decreasing the number and intensity of hot flushes over baseline (90%–96% vs 15%–25%; *P* < 0.001). With the herbal combination there was a 68% reduction in daytime hot flushes and a 74% reduction in nighttime hot flushes after the first month. There was also a marked alleviation of sleep disturbances and fatigue. The authors concluded that Climex seemed to be effective for menopausal symptoms without apparent major adverse effects (Kupfersztain et al., 2003).

A 12-week RCT in menopausal women (*n* = 96) with dyspareunia and sexual dissatisfaction compared 5% chamomile vaginal gel with CEE vaginal cream and with placebo. By 12 weeks, mean sexual satisfaction scores were significantly better with both chamomile and estrogen compared with placebo (*P* < 0.001). Reductions in dyspareunia were also greater in the two intervention groups compared with placebo. The 95% CI for dyspareunia scores were 0.68–1.04 for chamomile, 0.63–0.98 for estrogen, and 1.8–2.1 for placebo (*P* < 0.001). The authors concluded that chamomile vaginal gel could reduce dyspareunia and increase sexual satisfaction in postmenopausal women (Bosak et al., 2020).

Musculoskeletal Disorders: Carpal Tunnel Syndrome

A 4-week pilot RCT in patients (*n* = 26) with severe carpal tunnel syndrome compared night splint plus topical chamomile oil BID with night splint plus placebo oil BID. Significant improvements in symptomatic and functional status were observed with chamomile compared with placebo ($P=0.019$ and $P=0.016$, respectively). However, electrodiagnostic parameters showed no significant changes between the two groups (Hashempur et al., 2015).

Dermatological Disorders: Wounds

A 28-day randomized trial in patients ($n=72$) with peristomal skin lesions compared chamomile solution compresses BID with 1% hydrocortisone ointment application QD. Lesions healed significantly faster with chamomile than with hydrocortisone (mean time to healing 8.9 and 14.5 days, respectively; $P=0.001$). Pain and itching also resolved faster with chamomile than with hydrocortisone (Charousaei et al., 2011).

A small RCT in patients ($n=14$) undergoing dermabrasion for tattoos compared chamomile extract with placebo for effects on healing. Wound weeping decreased and epithelialization increased with chamomile significantly better than with placebo (Glowania et al., 1987).

Psychiatric Disorders: Anxiety and Depression

A 2019 systematic review and meta-analysis to study the efficacy and safety of chamomile for the treatment of state anxiety, generalized anxiety disorder (GAD), sleep quality, and insomnia found 12 RCTs for inclusion. Based on the HAM-A scales, there were significant improvements in GAD after treatment for 2 weeks (MD $= -1.43$; $P=0.007$) and 4 weeks (MD $= -1.79$, $P=0.0097$). Meta-analysis of three RCTs did not show any difference in cases of anxiety (SMD $= -0.15$, $P=0.4214$). One RCT on insomnia found no significant change in insomnia severity index ($P>0.05$). However, an insomnia meta-analysis showed significant improvement in sleep quality after chamomile administration (SMD $= -0.73$, $P<0.005$). Mild adverse events were reported by three RCTs. The authors concluded that chamomile appeared to be efficacious and safe for sleep quality and GAD (Hieu et al., 2019).

A 2018 systematic review to identify single-herb medicines that may warrant further study for treatment of anxiety and depression in cancer patients found 100 studies involving 38 botanicals that met inclusion criteria. Among herbs most studied (≥ 6 RCTs each),

lavender, passionflower, and saffron produced benefits comparable to standard anxiolytics and antidepressants. Black cohosh, chamomile, and chasteberry were also promising. Overall, 45% of studies reported positive findings with fewer adverse effects compared with conventional medications. The authors concluded that saffron, black cohosh, chamomile, chasteberry, lavender, and passionflower appeared useful in mitigating anxiety or depression with favorable risk-benefit profiles compared with standard treatments, and these botanicals may benefit cancer patients by minimizing medication load and accompanying side effects (Yeung et al., 2018).

A 2013 systematic review looking at plants that had both preclinical and clinical evidence for antianxiety effects found 21 plants with human clinical trial evidence. Support for efficacy identified several herbs with efficacy for anxiety spectrum disorders including kava, lemon balm, chamomile, ginkgo, skullcap, milk thistle, passionflower, ashwagandha, rhodiola, echinacea, *Galphimia glauca*, *Centella asiatica*, and *Echium amoenum*. Acute anxiolytic activity was found for passionflower, sage, gotu kola, lemon balm, and bergamot. The review also specifically found that bacopa showed anxiolytic effects in people with cognitive decline (Sarris et al., 2013).

A 2010 review to evaluate effectiveness of herbal medicines for GAD found that kava had an unequivocal anxiolytic effect. Isolated studies with valerian, ginkgo, chamomile, passionflower, and *Galphimia glauca* showed a potential use for anxious diseases. Ginkgo and chamomile showed an effect size (Cohen's $d=0.47\text{-}0.87$) greater than or equal to benzodiazepines, buspirone and antidepressants (Cohen's $d=0.17\text{--}0.38$) (Faustino et al., 2010).

An 8-week RCT in patients ($n=57$) with mild-to-moderate GAD compared chamomile capsules (220 mg, standardized to 1.2% apigenin) with placebo, adjusted up to five capsules daily. There was a clinically meaningful and statistically significant reduction in HAM-A scores with chamomile over placebo ($P=0.047$) (Amsterdam et al., 2009).

The preceding trial was later analyzed for possible improvement in depression as well as anxiety in those subjects who also met criteria for depression. Chamomile was associated with a greater reduction for all participants in total HAM-D scores and HAM-D core mood item scores ($P < 0.05$ for both) as well as a clinically meaningful but nonsignificant trend for a greater reduction in total HAM-D scores and HAM-D core mood item scores in participants with current comorbid depression ($P = 0.6$). The authors concluded that chamomile may provide clinically meaningful antidepressant activity that occurs in addition to its previously observed anxiolytic activity (Amsterdam et al., 2012).

A two-phase RCT in patients ($n = 179$) with a primary diagnosis of moderate-to-severe GAD looked at the long-term antianxiety efficacy of chamomile. In Phase I, eligible participants received 12 weeks of open-label therapy with chamomile extract 500 mg TID. During Phase II, treatment responders ($n = 93$) were randomized to continuation of chamomile therapy or placebo for 26 weeks. Relapse occurred during Phase II in 15% with chamomile and 25.5% with placebo. Mean time to relapse was 11 weeks with chamomile and 6.3 weeks with placebo. Hazard of relapse was nonsignificantly lower for chamomile (HR = 0.52; $P = 0.16$). During follow-up, chamomile participants maintained significantly lower GAD symptoms than placebo ($P = 0.0032$), with significant reductions in BW ($P = 0.046$) and mean arterial BP ($P = 0.0063$). Both treatments had similar low adverse event rates. The authors concluded that long-term chamomile was safe and significantly reduced moderate-to-severe GAD symptoms but did not significantly reduce rate of relapse (Mao et al., 2016).

Further analysis of the preceding trial entailed categorizing patients into two groups: GAD without comorbid depression ($n = 100$) and GAD with comorbid depression ($n = 79$). The authors observed similar anxiolytic effects over time in both diagnostic subgroups. However, there was a greater reduction in HAM-D core symptom scores ($P < 0.023$), and a trend level reduction in HAM-D total scores ($P < 0.14$) and in BDI total scores ($P < 0.060$) in subjects with comorbid depression. The authors concluded that chamomile may produce clinically meaningful antidepressant effects in addition to its anxiolytic activity in subjects with GAD and comorbid depression (Amsterdam et al., 2020).

An 8-week open-label study in patients ($n = 79$) with moderate-to-severe GAD investigated the efficacy of chamomile 1500 mg/day. HAM-A, BAI, and Psychological General Well Being Index all showed statistically significant and clinically meaningful re-

ductions. Significant improvement over time was also observed on the GAD-7 rating. Adverse events were minor. The authors concluded that chamomile produced reductions in GAD symptoms over 8 weeks at a rate comparable to those observed during conventional anxiolytic drug therapy and with fewer adverse events (Keefe et al., 2016).

An open-label study of subjects ($n = 45$) with GAD looked at the effect of chamomile on salivary cortisol 3 days pretreatment and 3 days posttreatment. Samples were collected at 8 am, 12 pm, 4 pm, and 8 pm and correlated with GAD symptoms. Subjects who experienced more symptomatic improvement experienced significant increases in their morning salivary cortisol ($P < 0.001$) and a greater decrease in cortisol from morning to the rest of the day ($P < 0.001$) (Keefe et al., 2018).

An 8-week open-label trial looked at the impact of expectancies regarding treatment efficacy on the efficacy and side effects with chamomile. Primary outcome was patient-reported GAD-7 scores, with clinical response and treatment-emergent side effects as secondary outcomes. Expectancies were used to predict symptomatic and side effect outcomes. Higher efficacy expectancies at baseline predicted greater change on the GAD-7 ($P = 0.011$). Patients with higher side effect expectancies reported more side effects ($P = 0.038$) (Keefe et al., 2017).

Psychiatric Disorders: Insomnia

Overall, studies are not very impressive, but chamomile may be most beneficial for short-term insomnia and in the elderly.

A 2015 systematic review on the effects of a variety of herbs for insomnia found 14 RCTs ($n = 1602$) that met the inclusion criteria. Four singular herbs were identified in studies, one being chamomile. There was no statistically significant difference between any herbal medicine and placebo, or any herbal medicine and active control (pharmaceutical), for any of the 13 measures of clinical efficacy. As for safety, a similar or smaller number of adverse events per person were reported with chamomile when compared with placebo (Leach and Page, 2015).

A 6-week-day single-blinded RCT in elderly nursing home patients ($n = 60$) with baseline poor sleep compared 28 days of chamomile extract capsules

200 mg BID with placebo for effect on insomnia. Sleep quality based on the Pittsburgh Sleep Quality Index was significantly better with chamomile than with placebo following the intervention ($P < 0.05$). The authors concluded that chamomile extract could improve sleep quality among elderly people and could be used as a safe modality for promoting sleep in this group (Adib-Hajbaghery and Mousavi, 2017).

A 4-week open-label study in elderly patients ($n = 77$) in nursing homes investigated chamomile 400 mg BID after lunch and dinner compared with a control group for sleeping quality as measured by the Pittsburgh Sleep Quality Index questionnaire. Before intervention, the mean score of sleep quality between groups were similar. After 4 weeks of intervention, the Pittsburgh Sleep Quality Index questionnaire score was < 5 in 52% and 21% of the chamomile and control groups, respectively, and was 11–26 in 10% and 30% of the chamomile and control groups, respectively ($P < 0.001$). The authors concluded that chamomile extract had sedative properties and improved sleep in nursing home patients (Abdullahzadeh et al., 2017).

A 28-day RCT pilot trial in adults ($n = 34$) with *DSM-IV* primary insomnia compared chamomile 270 mg/day with placebo for effects on sleep. Although chamomile did produce a modest nonsignificant improvement in daytime functioning, there were no significant differences between groups in changes in sleep diary measures, including total sleep time, sleep efficiency, sleep latency, wake after sleep onset, sleep quality, and number of awakenings. Sleep latency, night-time awakenings, and Fatigue Severity Scale had moderate Cohen's *d* effect sizes in favor of chamomile. However, placebo performed better for total sleep time. There were no differences in adverse events reported by the chamomile group compared with placebo (Zick et al., 2011).

A 2-week RCT in postpartum women ($n = 80$) with poor sleep quality (Postpartum Sleep Quality Scale score ≥ 16) compared chamomile tea with usual care. Compared with the control group, the experimental group demonstrated significantly lower scores of physical-symptoms-related sleep inefficiency ($P = 0.015$) and the symptoms of depression ($P = 0.020$). However, the scores for all three instruments were similar for both groups at 4-week post-test, suggesting

that the positive effects of chamomile tea were limited to the immediate term (Chang and Chen, 2016).

Psychiatric Disorders: Attention-Deficit/Hyperactivity Disorder

Since chamomile has been shown to have SNRI activity, a small open-label trial of 14- to 16-year-old male patients ($n = 3$) diagnosed with ADHD were rated at baseline and while taking chamomile. Patients' mean scores improved for Conners' hyperactivity, inattention, and immaturity factors (Niederhofer, 2009).

Oncologic Disorders: Mucositis

A single-blinded nonrandomized controlled trial in patients ($n = 105$) undergoing radiotherapy due to head and neck cancer compared gargling with solutions of chamomile, honey, or water (control) on radiation side effects. Severe stomatitis occurred in 0%, 5.7%, and 17.6% of patients with honey, chamomile, and water, respectively. On the 14th day, stomatitis rates were 0%, 0%, and 17.6% with honey, chamomile, and water, respectively ($P < 0.001$) (Bahramnezhad et al., 2015).

A 22-day RCT in patients ($n = 38$) undergoing mucositis-inducing chemotherapy compared ice cubes with water to ice cubes with chamomile. Oral mucositis developed in 30% and 50% of the chamomile and control groups, respectively. Mouth pain score was higher in the control group on all evaluations ($P = 0.02$ for day 8; $P = 0.09$ for day 15, and $P = 0.14$ for day 22). Patients in the chamomile group never developed mucositis with Grade 2 or higher. On day 8, ulceration was present in 0% and 16% of the chamomile and control groups, respectively ($P = 0.10$) (Dos Reis et al., 2016).

A Phase II RCT in patients ($n = 40$) undergoing hematopoietic stem cell transplantation compared mouthwashes at different strengths of chamomile fluid extract (0.5%, 1%, or 2%) to standard care alone (control group). The 1% chamomile liquid reduced incidence, intensity, and duration of oral mucositis compared with the control group. No moderate or severe adverse effects were identified (Braga et al., 2015).

A 30-day RCT in children (n = 40) undergoing treatment for ALL compared daily chamomile syrup 2.5 mL with placebo for effects on neutropenia. An increasing trend of the ANC was observed with chamomile syrup while a decreasing trend occurred with placebo ($P = 0.019$). No serious AEs were reported. The authors concluded that chamomile syrup given adjunctively may improve immunity in children with leukemia by minimizing chemotherapy-induced neutropenia (Daneshfard et al., 2020).

ACTIVE CONSTITUENTS

- Carbohydrates
  - Polysaccharides (immunostimulating)
- Phenolic compounds
  - Coumarins: umbelliferone (antiinflammatory, venotonic, lymphatotonic, possibly anticoagulant, antispasmodic, antigenotoxic, hepatoprotective, antifungal), herniarin (antispasmodic, antigenotoxic, antimicrobial in presence of UV light)
  - Flavonoids: apigenin (antiinflammatory, antioxidant, antihistamine, hypotensive, antiserotonin release, GABA agonism, antispasmodic, antibacterial, chemopreventive, antineoplastic, ERB), luteolin (antiinflammatory, antispasmodic, antibacterial, hepatoprotective, antiestrogenic, antiproliferative), quercetin (antiinflammatory, antioxidant, hypotensive, antidiabetic, antispasmodic, neuroprotective, XO inhibition, antibacterial, anticancer), isohamnetin (antimicrobial); chamaemeloside (Roman chamomile—hypoglycemic)
- Terpenes
  - Sesquiterpenes: alpha bisabolol, alpha bisabololoxide A–C, chamazulene (see *Aromatic compounds*)
  - Sesquiterpene lactones: matricin (antiinflammatory)
- Aromatic compounds: alpha bisabolol (antimicrobial, antiinflammatory, antiulcer, antispasmodic), alpha bisabololoxide A-C (antiinflammatory, augments 5-fluorouracil in leukemic cells), chamazulene (only present after distillation: increases cortisol release, reduces histamine, antiinflammatory, hepatoregenerative, antifungal, antineoplastic), matricin (antiinflammatory), nobilin (antineoplastic), cis-spiroethers (antispasmodic), α-pinene, anthemic acid, *n*-butyl angelate and isoamyl angelate (Roman chamomile)

CHAMOMILE COMMONLY USED PREPARATIONS AND DOSAGE (FOR ADULTS UNLESS OTHERWISE SPECIFIED)

The following are examples of some available formulations and ranges of dosing for commercial herbal products. See Part III Introduction "How to prescribe medicinal herbs" for further guidance on herbal advising and prescribing.

Dried Flower

- Oral infusion (tea): 2–3 tsp. per cup TID-QID between meals or swished and gargled prn.
- Fluid extract (1:1, 45%) 1–4 mL TID.
- Tincture (1:5, 45%): 3–5 mL TID; 5–10 mL hs for insomnia.
- Powdered flower extract: 400–800 mg (1/6–1/3 tsp) QD-TID.
- Capsule or tablet of powdered flower extract: 250–700 mg BID with meals.
- Capsule or tablet of standardized extract (standardized to 3 mg/serving apigenin): one capsule QD-BID.
- Essential oil: add to essential oil diffuser or use 5–10 drops in steaming hot water for inhalation, or in full tub of bath water for skin irritation.
- Cream: 3%–10% chamomile applied TID for inflammatory skin disorders.

Chamomile tea (infusion) has been used for centuries in children as well as adults. As a general precaution, children under 5 years should be limited to no more than 4 oz of chamomile tea per day. For colicky infants 1–2 oz per day has been used.

SAFETY AND PRECAUTION

Side Effects

Although German chamomile is considered generally safe, atopic individuals and those allergic to ragweed or the Compositae family may develop allergic symptoms or worsening asthma. This may occur in less than 2% of patients. May cause excess sedation.

Case Report

Fatal anaphylaxis when chamomile enema was administered to allergic patient during labor. Several other reports exist on anaphylaxis related to chamomile exposure.

Pregnancy and Lactation

There have been two cases reported of premature constriction of ductus arteriosus following regular maternal consumption of chamomile tea. One case was at 20 weeks and the other case was at 35 weeks. So, although chamomile tea is generally thought of as being safe, regular consumption should be avoided. Galactagogue effects have been reported as well.

Disease Interactions

Chamomile has phytoestrogenic properties so should be avoided in women with estrogen-sensitive cancers.

Drug Interactions

- CYP: Inhibits CYP1A2, CYP2C9, CYP2D6, and CYP3A4.
- Possible interactions with anticoagulants, sedating medication, and anticonvulsants.
- May augment effects of antihypertensives, hypoglycemiants.
- May increase levels of cyclosporine.

REFERENCES

Abdullahzadeh M, Matourypour P, Ali NS. Investigation effect of oral chamomilla on sleep quality in elderly people in Isfahan: a randomized control trial. J Educ Health Promot 2017;6:53.

Adib-Hajbaghery M, Mousavi S. The effects of chamomile extract on sleep quality among elderly people: aclinical trial. Complement Ther Med 2017 Dec;35:109–14.

Amsterdam JD, Li Y, Soeller I, et al. A randomized, double-blind, placebo-controlled trial of oralMatricaria recutita (chamomile) extract therapy for generalized anxiety disorder. J Clin Psychopharmacol 2009 Aug;29(4):378–82.

Amsterdam JD, Shults J, Soeller I, et al. Chamomile (Matricaria recutita) may provide antidepressant activity in anxious, depressed humans: an exploratory study. Altern Ther Health Med 2012 Sep-Oct;18(5):44–9.

Amsterdam JD, Qing SL, Xie SX, Mao JJ. Putative antidepressant effect of chamomile (Matricaria chamomilla L.) oral extract in subjects with comorbid generalized anxiety disorder and depression. J Altern Complement Med 2020 Sep;26(9):813–9.

Bahramnezhad F, Dehghan Nayeri N, Bassampour SS, Khajeh M, Asgari P. Honey and radiation-induced stomatitis in patients with head and neck cancer. Iran Red Crescent Med J 2015 Oct 22;17(10):e19256.

Batista AL, Lins RD, de Souza CR, do Nascimento Barbosa D, Moura Belém N, Alves Celestino FJ. Clinical efficacy analysis of the mouth rinsing with pomegranate and chamomile plant extracts in the gingival bleeding reduction. Complement Ther Clin Pract 2014 Feb;20(1):93–8.

Bosak Z, Iravani M, Moghimipour E, Haghighizadeh M, Jelodarian P, Khazdair M. Evaluation of the influence ofchamomilevaginal gel on dyspareunia and sexual satisfaction in postmenopausal women: a randomized, double-blind, controlledclinicaltrial. Avicenna J Phytomed Sep-Oct 2020;10(5):481–91.

Braga FT, Santos AC, Bueno PC, et al. Use of Chamomilla recutita in the prevention and treatment of oral mucositis in patients undergoing hematopoietic stem cell transplantation: a randomized, controlled, phase II clinical trial. Cancer Nurs 2015 Jul-Aug;38(4):322–9.

Chang SM, Chen CH. Effects of an intervention with drinking chamomile tea on sleep quality and depression in sleep disturbed postnatal women: a randomized controlled trial. J Adv Nurs 2016 Feb;72(2):306–15.

Charousaei F, Dabirian A, Mojab F. Using chamomile solution or a 1% topical hydrocortisone ointment in the management of peristomal skin lesions in colostomy patients: results of a controlled clinical study. Ostomy Wound Manage 2011 May;57(5):28–36.

Daneshfard B, Shahriari S, Heiran A, Nimrouzi M, Yarmohammadi H. Effect of chamomile on chemotherapy-induced neutropenia in pediatric leukemia patients: a randomized triple-blind placebo-controlled clinical trial. Avicenna J Phytomed Jan-Feb 2020;10(1):58–69.

Darvishi Khezri H, Haidari Gorji MA, Morad A, Gorji H. Comparison of the antibacterial effects of matrica & Persica™ and chlorhexidine gluconate mouthwashes in mechanically ventilated ICU patients: a double blind randomized clinical trial. Rev Chilena Infectol 2013 Aug;30(4):361–73.

de la Motte S, Böse-O'Reilly S, Heinisch M, Harrison F. Double-blind comparison of an apple pectin-chamomile extract preparation with placebo in children with diarrhea. Arzneimittelforschung 1997 Nov;47(11):1247–9.

Dos Reis PE, Ciol MA, de Melo NS, Figueiredo PT, Leite AF, Manzi NM. Chamomile infusion cryotherapy to prevent oral mucositis induced by chemotherapy: a pilot study. Support Care Cancer 2016 Oct;24(10):4393–8.

Faustino TT, Almeida RB, Andreatini R. Medicinal plants for the treatment of generalized anxiety disorder: a review of controlled clinical studies. Braz J Psychiatry 2010 Dec;32(4):429–36.

Glowania HJ, Raulin C, Swoboda M. Effect of chamomile on wound healing—a clinical double-blind study. Z Hautkr 1987 Sep 1;62(17):1262. 1267–71.

Gordon M, Biagioli E, Sorrenti M, et al. Dietary modifications for infantile colic. Cochrane Database Syst Rev 2018 Oct 10;10, CD011029.

Hashempur MH, Lari ZN, Ghoreishi PS, et al. A pilot randomized double-blind placebo-controlled trial on topical chamomile (Matricaria chamomilla L.) oil for severe carpal tunnel syndrome. Complement Ther Clin Pract 2015 Nov;21(4):223–8.

Hieu T, Dibas M, Dila K, et al. Therapeutic efficacy and safety ofchamomilefor state anxiety, generalized anxiety disorder, insomnia, and sleep quality: a systematic review and meta-analysis of randomizedtrialsand quasi-randomizedtrials. Phytother Res 2019 Jun;33(6):1604–15.

Keefe JR, Mao JJ, Soeller I, Li QS, Amsterdam JD. Short-term open-labelchamomile (Matricaria chamomilla L.) therapy of moderate to severe generalized anxiety disorder. Phytomedicine 2016 Dec 15;23(14):1699–705.

Keefe JR, Amsterdam J, Li QS, Soeller I, DeRubeis R, Mao JJ. Specific expectancies are associated with symptomatic outcomes and side effect burden in a trial of chamomile extract for generalized anxiety disorder. J Psychiatr Res 2017 Jan;84:90–7.

Keefe JR, Guo W, Li QS, Amsterdam JD, Mao JJ. An exploratory study of salivary cortisol changes duringchamomileextract therapy of moderate to severe generalizedanxietydisorder. J Psychiatr Res 2018 Jan;96:189–95.

Kupfersztain C, Rotem C, Fagot R, Kaplan B. The immediate effect of natural plant extract, Angelica sinensis and Matricaria chamomilla (Climex) for the treatment of hot flushes during menopause. A preliminary report. Clin Exp Obstet Gynecol 2003;30(4):203–6.

Langhorst J, Frede A, Knott M, et al. Distinct kinetics in the frequency of peripheral CD4+ T cells in patients with ulcerative colitis experiencing a flare during treatment with mesalazine or with a herbal preparation of myrrh, chamomile, and coffee charcoal. PLoS One 2014 Aug 21;9(8):e104257.

Leach MJ, Page AT. Herbal medicine for insomnia: a systematic review and meta-analysis. Sleep Med Rev 2015 Dec;24:1–12.

Madisch A, Melderis H, Mayr G, Sassin I, Hotz J. A plant extract and its modified preparation in functional dyspepsia. Results of a double-blind placebo controlled comparative study. Z Gastroenterol 2001 Jul;39(7):511–7.

Madisch A, Holtmann G, Mayr G, VInson B, Hotz J. Treatment of functional dyspepsia with a herbal preparation. A double-blind, randomized, placebo-controlled, multicenter trial. Digestion 2004;69(1):45–52.

Mao JJ, Xie SX, Keefe JR, Soeller I, Li QS, Amsterdam JD. Long-termchamomile (Matricaria chamomilla L.) treatment for generalized anxiety disorder: a randomized clinical trial. Phytomedicine 2016 Dec 15;23(14):1735–42.

Martinelli M, Ummarino D, Giugliano FP, et al. Efficacy of a standardized extract of Matricariae chamomilla L., Melissa officinalis L. and tyndallized Lactobacillus acidophilus (HA122) in infantile colic: an open randomized controlled trial. Neurogastroenterol Motil 2017 Dec;29(12).

Nemati S, Yousefbeyk F, Ebrahimi S, FaghihHabibi A, Shakiba M, Ramezani H. Effects ofchamomileextract nasal drop on chronic rhinosinusitis treatment: a randomized double-blind study. Am J Otolaryngol 2020 Sep 28;42(1):102743.

Niederhofer H. Observational study: Matricaria chamomilla may improve some symptoms of attention-deficit hyperactivity disorder. Phytomedicine Apr 2009;16(4):284–6.

Rafraf M, Zemestani M, Asghari-Jafarabadi M. Effectiveness of chamomile tea on glycemic control and serum lipid profile in patients with type 2 diabetes. J Endocrinol Invest 2015 Feb;38(2):163–70.

Sarris J, McIntyre E, Camfield DA. Plant-based medicines for anxiety disorders, part 2: a review of clinical studies with supporting preclinical evidence. CNS Drugs 2013 Apr;27(4):301–19.

Savino F, Cresi F, Castagno E, Silvestro L, Oggero R. A randomized double-blind placebo-controlled trial of a standardized extract of *Matricaria recutita, Foeniculum vulgare* and *Melissa officinalis* (ColiMil) in the treatment of breastfed colicky infants. Phytother Res 2005;19(4):335–40.

Weizman Z, Alkrinawi S, Goldfarb D. Efficacy of herbal tea preparation in infantile colic. J Pediatr 1993;122(650):652.

Yeung KS, Hernandez M, Mao JJ, Haviland I, Gubili J. Herbal medicine for depression and anxiety: a systematic review with assessment of potential psycho-oncologic relevance. Phytother Res 2018 May;32(5):865–91.

Zick SM, Wright BD, Sen A, Arnedt JT. Preliminary examination of the efficacy and safety of a standardized chamomile extract for chronic primary insomnia: a randomized placebo-controlled pilot study. BMC Complement Altern Med 2011 Sep 22;11:78.

36

CHASTEBERRY/CHASTE TREE/VITEX (*VITEX AGNUS CASTUS*)
Fruit

GENERAL OVERVIEW

This herb's common name is misleading. While the berry of the chaste tree was indeed used by monks in the Middle Ages to promote chastity, modern application of this herb promotes, among other things, female fertility. Chasteberry has a potential role in stressed out young women who are having difficulty getting pregnant, likely because stress raises prolactin, and chasteberry reduces prolactin through dopamine agonist activity. Chasteberry may actually increase or decrease prolactin depending on the baseline prolactin level and the dosage used. One might consider chasteberry to be "woman's best friend" due to its beneficial effects for premenstrual syndrome and perimenopause in addition to its benefits for infertility. It can be used continuously, and the longer it is used the better the results, at least up to 6 months.

Clinical research indicates that chasteberry, alone or in combination formulas, may be beneficial for cyclical mastalgia, premenstrual syndrome, premenstrual dysphoric disorder, female infertility, perimenopause, menopause, hyperprolactinemia, bone healing, anxiety, depression, and insomnia.

IN VITRO AND ANIMAL RESEARCH

Chasteberry has opioidergic, dopaminergic, hepatoprotective, antiinflammatory, and antiproliferative properties in vitro. Much of the clinical efficacy of chasteberry stems from the agonist activity on dopamine-2 receptors. This activity comes from several different constituents. Activation of dopamine receptors may play a role not only directly with respect to mood, but also indirectly via reduction in prolactin

and the resultant improved ovarian follicle and corpus luteum development. It also has constituents that activate opioid receptors. The antiinflammatory effects are mostly attributed to casticin, which suppresses LOX and reduces T-cell activation better than prednisolone.

The effect of chasteberry on estrogen is complex. In vivo studies measuring serum levels of estrogen in female rats noted increased estrogen levels by 24.3% (vs 115.5% with estradiol). Yet it had no estrogenic impact on the uterus or bones. Chasteberry extract appears to have affinity for the β-subunit of the estrogen receptor exclusively. Although most animal research shows that chasteberry binds exclusively to the β-subunit, other research has indicated a reduction in the activity of the α-subunit of the estrogen receptor, so chasteberry may well serve as a SERM and the net effect may be antiestrogenic. To complicate matters further, chasteberry appears to have some aromatase activity, raising estrogen levels in menopausal mice presumably from androgenic precursors.

With respect to antiinflammatory and analgesic activity, research has been performed using hydroethanolic extracts and essential oils of chasteberry in mouse models of inflammation. The results showed that the oil was as effective as morphine and diclofenac in reducing pain and inflammation, respectively.

HUMAN RESEARCH

Breast Disorders: Mastalgia

A 3-month RCT in women ($n=114$) younger than 40 years with cyclical mastalgia compared chasteberry with flurbiprofen. VAS scores decreased from 7.1 to 3.1

and from 7.1 to 3.5 with chasteberry and flurbiprofen, respectively ($P = 0.25$). Significant improvement or full recovery occurred in 64.7% and 60.3% of patients with chasteberry and flurbiprofen, respectively ($P = 0.95$). The authors concluded that chasteberry and flurbiprofen significantly reduced cyclical mastalgia symptoms and had no superiority over each other (Dinç and Coşkun, 2014).

A three-cycle RCT in women with cyclical mastalgia compared chasteberry solution 30 drops (roughly 1 mL) BID with placebo. With chasteberry, the mean decrease in pain intensity on VAS was 21.4, 33.7, and 34.3 mm at 1, 2, and 3 months, respectively. With placebo the mean decrease in pain intensity was 10.6, 20.3, and 25.7 at 1, 2, and 3 months, respectively. The difference between chasteberry and placebo was significant at all three intervals ($P = 0.018$; $P = 0.006$; $P = 0.064$, respectively). There was no difference in the frequency of adverse events between groups. The authors concluded that chasteberry appeared to be effective and well tolerated in the treatment of cyclical mastalgia (Halaska et al., 1999).

Premenstrual Syndrome and Premenstrual Dysphoric Disorder

A 2019 meta-analysis was performed on RCTs evaluating the efficacy of chasteberry in PMS. Out of the 21 clinical trials, three studies ($n = 520$) met inclusion criteria, and these studies compared the efficacy of special extracts Ze 440 and BNO 1095 with placebo for the treatment of PMS. Women taking chasteberry were 2.57 times more likely to experience a remission in their symptoms compared with those taking the placebo. The authors concluded that, although several clinical trials had been carried out with chasteberry, most of the studies could not be used as evidence for efficacy due to incomplete reporting, especially concerning the description of the medication that was used (Csupor et al., 2019).

A 2017 systematic review to evaluate the efficacy of chasteberry for PMS and PMDD found eight RCTs that met inclusion criteria. Although the studies had wide variability in treatment forms and measurement outcomes, all trials were positive for chasteberry in the treatment of PMS or PMDD, and chasteberry was well tolerated. The authors concluded that the RCTs using chasteberry for treatment of PMS and PMDD suggested that chasteberry was a safe and efficacious alternative (Cerqueira et al., 2017).

A 2016 systematic review to evaluate the efficacy of chasteberry for treatment of PMS, dysmenorrhea, and infertility found 43 trials that met inclusion criteria. Chasteberry was shown to contribute to the treatment of PMS, dysmenorrhea, and infertility. The authors concluded that the dopaminergic compounds in the plant were beneficial for premenstrual mastodynia and other PMS symptoms (Rafieian-Kopaei, 2017).

A 2014 systematic review was performed to evaluate the effects of acupuncture and herbal medicine for PMS and PMDD. The search found eight studies in acupuncture and 11 studies in herbal medicine that met inclusion criteria. In herbal medicine, studies on chasteberry, St. John's wort, ginkgo, *Xiao yao san*, and *Elsholtzia splendens*, as well as all acupuncture studies gave significantly improved results regarding PMS and PMDD. Acupuncture and herbal medicine treatments showed a 50% or greater reduction of symptoms compared with baseline. The authors concluded that limited evidence supported the efficacy of alternative medicinal interventions such as acupuncture and herbal medicine in controlling PMS and PMDD (Jang et al., 2014).

A 2013 systematic review of RCTs investigating women's health assessed the evidence for the efficacy and safety of chasteberry. Twelve RCTs met inclusion criteria: eight studied PMS, two studied PMDD, and two studied latent hyperprolactinemia. For PMS, seven of eight trials found chasteberry to be superior to placebo, pyridoxine, and magnesium oxide. In PMDD, one study reported chasteberry to be equivalent to fluoxetine, while in the other fluoxetine outperformed chasteberry. In latent hyperprolactinemia, one trial reported it to be superior to placebo for reducing TRH-stimulated prolactin secretion, normalizing a shortened luteal phase, and increasing midluteal progesterone and estradiol levels. The second study found chasteberry to be comparable to bromocriptine for reducing serum prolactin levels and ameliorating cyclical mastalgia. Adverse events with chasteberry were mild and generally infrequent (van Die et al., 2013).

A 2011 systematic review evaluating the effects of herbal medicine for PMS found 17 RCTs that met inclusion criteria and selected 10 of them for analysis, four of which ($n = 500$) studied chasteberry. Chasteberry was reported to consistently ameliorate PMS better than placebo. Single trials also supported the use of either ginkgo or saffron. Evening primrose oil and St. John's wort did not differ from placebo. None of the herbs was associated with major health risks, although the small number of tested patients did not allow definitive conclusions on safety (Dante and Facchinetti, 2011).

A three-cycle RCT in women ($n = 217$) with moderate-to-severe PMS compared chasteberry 40 mg/day with placebo for total PMS diary scores (PMSD) and premenstrual tension syndrome scores (PMTS). From baseline to the third cycle, with chasteberry vs placebo, the total PMSD score decreased from 29.2 to 6.4 vs from 28.1 to 12.6. The decrease was significant for both groups ($P < .0001$). The difference in magnitude of decrease between groups was also significant ($P < 0.0001$). With chasteberry vs placebo, the total scores for PMTS decreased from 26.2 to 9.9 vs from 27.1 to 14.6, with the decrease in each group being significant and the difference in decrease also being significant in favor of chasteberry ($P < 0.01$ for both). No serious adverse events occurred in either group. The authors concluded that chasteberry was a safe, well-tolerated, and effective drug for treatment of moderate-to-severe PMS (He et al., 2009).

A three-cycle RCT in women ($n = 170$) with PMS compared chasteberry 20 mg (Ze 440) QD with placebo for efficacy and tolerability. Improvements in the self-assessment of irritability, mood alteration, anger, headache, breast fullness, and bloating were greater with chasteberry than with placebo ($P < 0.001$). Changes in each of the three clinical global impressions were significantly better with chasteberry than with placebo ($P < 0.001$). Responder rates (as defined by a 50% reduction in symptoms) were 52% and 24% for chasteberry and placebo, respectively. Mild adverse events were reported in less than 10% of women in each group. The authors concluded that chasteberry was an effective and well tolerated treatment for PMS symptoms (Berger et al., 2000).

A 3-month RCT in younger women ($n = 162$) with PMS compared daily chasteberry 8, 20, or 30 mg with placebo. Improvement in individual and total symptom score in the 20 mg group was significantly higher than in the placebo and 8 mg treatment groups. The

higher dose of 30 mg did not provide an additional decrease in symptom severity compared with the 20 mg treatment. Each of the treatments was well tolerated. The author concluded that chasteberry 20 mg QD was the optimal dosing for PMS (Schellenberg et al., 2012).

A three-cycle RCT in women ($n = 67$) with moderate-to-severe PMS compared a special chasteberry extract (BNO 1095) with placebo. By the third cycle, the premenstrual syndrome diary sum score decreased from 29.4 to 4.3 and from 28.78 to 11.8 with chasteberry and placebo, respectively. All four-symptom factor scores were significantly reduced by the third treatment cycle. There were significant differences in the PMSD sum score, score of negative affect, and water retention between the two groups at cycle 3 ($P < 0.05$). The authors concluded that chasteberry was effective in treating moderate-to-severe PMS, especially the symptoms of negative affect and fluid retention (Ma et al., 2010).

A six-cycle RCT in women ($n = 128$) with PMS compared chasteberry extract 40 drops (roughly 1.5 mL) daily with placebo starting 6 days before menses. Improvement in symptoms was significantly greater with chasteberry than with placebo ($P < 0.0001$). The authors concluded that chasteberry could be considered an effective and well-tolerated treatment for relief of mild and moderate symptoms of PMS (Zamani et al., 2012).

A 2-month rater-blinded RCT in patients ($n = 41$) with PMDD compared chasteberry with fluoxetine for efficacy. Response was noted to occur in 68.4% and 57.9% of patients with fluoxetine and chasteberry, respectively. The difference in response between groups was not statistically significant. The authors concluded that this preliminary study suggested that patients with PMDD respond well to treatment with both fluoxetine and chasteberry. However, fluoxetine was more effective for psychological symptoms, while chasteberry diminished physical symptoms (Atmaca et al., 2003).

A three-cycle open-label study in patients ($n = 1634$) with PMS investigated the efficacy and tolerance of a chasteberry extract. After three menstrual cycles, 93% of patients reported a decrease in the number of symptoms or even cessation of PMS complaints. The improvement was seen with all PMS complexes (depression, anxiety, craving, and hyperhydration). The treatment was rated as "good" or "very good" by 85% of physicians.

Status after treatment was rated as "very much better" or "much better" by 81% of patients, and tolerance of chasteberry was rated as "good" or "very good" by 94% of patients. The authors concluded that the risk/benefit ratio of the tested chasteberry extract was very good, with significant efficacy for all aspects of the multifaceted clinical picture of PMS (Loch et al., 2000).

An open-label trial in younger women ($n = 69$) with PMS investigated the effects chasteberry 20 mg QD for three cycles on 10 common PMS symptoms. After the first menstrual cycle, a statistically significant decrease in total VAS score was observed ($P < 0.001$), and the score continued to diminish for the following two cycles. Each of the 10 symptom scores decreased significantly in this manner. In addition, the responder rate increased in a time-dependent manner reaching 91% by the third menstrual cycle. Eight patients exhibited nonserious adverse events. The authors concluded that chasteberry improved PMS symptoms with no substantial adverse events (Momoeda et al., 2014).

A 16-week RCT in perimenopausal women ($n = 14$) studied a combination of chasteberry plus St. John's wort given BID compared with placebo for effects on PMS symptoms. PMS scores were measured on the Abrahams Menstrual Symptoms Questionnaire, comprising the subclusters of PMS-A (anxiety), PMS-D (depression), PMS-H (hyperhydration), and PMS-C (cravings). The herbal combination resulted in a greater reduction than placebo in total PMS-like scores ($P = 0.02$), the PMS-D cluster ($P = 0.006$), the PMS-C clusters ($P = 0.027$), the anxiety cluster ($P = 0.003$), and the hyperhydration cluster ($P = 0.002$). Results of trend analyses showed significant beneficial effects across the five phases for total PMS and all subscales with the herb but not with placebo. The authors concluded that chasteberry plus St. John's wort had potential clinical application in PMS-like symptoms in perimenopausal women (van Die et al., 2009).

Abnormal Bleeding Secondary to Intrauterine Device

A 4-month RCT in women ($n = 84$) with IUD-induced menstrual bleeding compared chasteberry TID with mefenamic acid TID given during menses. Both chasteberry and mefenamic acid decreased bleeding. Prior to the fourth month, the improvement in bleeding scores was statistically different between groups in favor of mefenamic acid. However, by the fourth month, bleeding had decreased 52% and 47.6% with mefenamic acid and chasteberry, respectively, a nonsignificant difference. The authors concluded that mefenamic acid and chasteberry were both effective for IUD induced bleeding; however, mefenamic acid had earlier efficacy (Yavarikia et al., 2013).

Ovarian Disorders: Female Infertility

A 3-month RCT in women ($n = 52$) with luteal phase defects due to latent hyperprolactinemia compared chasteberry 20 mg/day with placebo. Blood for hormonal analysis was taken at days 5–8 and day 20 of the menstrual cycle before and after 3 months of therapy. Latent hyperprolactinemia was analyzed by monitoring the prolactin release 15 and 30 min after i.v. injection of 200 mcg of TRH. After 3 months of chasteberry, prolactin release was reduced, shortened luteal phases were normalized, and deficits in the luteal progesterone synthesis were eliminated. Estradiol levels increased during the luteal phase in these patients. There was no change with placebo. Two women in the chasteberry group became pregnant during the study period. The authors concluded that chasteberry may be effective for treating luteal phase defects due to latent hyperprolactinemia (Milewicz et al., 1993).

A 3-month RCT in women ($n = 93$) with infertility compared FertilityBlend for Women (chasteberry, green tea, L-arginine, vitamins, and minerals), with placebo for effects on progesterone levels, basal body temperatures, menstrual cycle length, pregnancy rate, and side effects. After 3 months, the herbal group demonstrated a trend toward increased mean midluteal progesterone, especially among women with basal progesterone < 9 ng/mL, where the increase was highly significant. The average number of days with luteal phase basal temperatures greater than 98°F increased significantly with the herbal product, and both short and long cycles (< 27 days or > 32 days pretreatment) were normalized. The placebo group did not show any significant changes in these parameters. After 3 months, 26% vs 10% of women became pregnant with the herb vs placebo ($P = 0.01$). After 6 months 32% of the women in the herbal group had conceived. No significant side effects were noted (Westphal et al., 2006).

A 3-month RCT in women ($n = 96$) with infertility from amenorrhea, luteal insufficiency, or idiopathic infertility investigated Mastodynon, a homeopathic remedy containing chasteberry and other ingredients, 30 drops BID compared with placebo. Pregnancy or spontaneous menstruation and pregnancy in women with amenorrhea, or improved concentrations of luteal hormones in women with luteal insufficiency or idiopathic infertility, was achieved in 57.6% and 36% of women with the homeopathic product and placebo, respectively ($P=0.069$). Pregnancy occurred in seven women with amenorrhea and four women with luteal insufficiency, more than twice the frequency of the placebo group. No significant hormonal changes were found. The authors concluded that in women with infertility due to secondary amenorrhea or luteal insufficiency, treatment with Mastodynon could be recommended over a period of 3–6 months (Gerhard et al., 1998).

Ovarian Disorders: Perimenopause and Menopause

A 2017 review of clinical trials on herbal efficacy in menopausal symptoms used the search terms menopause, climacteric, hot flushes, flashes, herb, and phytoestrogens. The authors found that chasteberry, passionflower, sage, lemon balm, valerian, black cohosh, fenugreek, black seed, fennel, evening primrose, ginkgo, alfalfa, St. John's wort, Asian ginseng, anise, licorice, red clover, and wild soybean were effective in the treatment of acute menopausal syndrome with different mechanisms. The authors concluded that medicinal plants could play a role in the treatment of acute menopausal syndrome and that further studies were warranted (Kargozar et al., 2017).

A 2016 systematic review of Iranian herbal medicines for menopausal hot flushes found 19 RCTs that met inclusion criteria. Overall, studies showed that chasteberry, licorice, anise, soy, black cohosh, red clover, evening primrose, flaxseed, sage, passionflower, avocado plus soybean oil, St. John's wort, and valerian could alleviate hot flushes. The authors concluded that several herbal medicines were effective in relieving hot flushes and could be an alternative for women experiencing hot flushes (Ghazanfarpour et al., 2016).

An 8-week RCT in healthy menopausal women ($n=46$) with hot flushes studies a combination of black seed and chasteberry plus citalopram QD compared with placebo plus citalopram for control of hot flushes. The herbal combination demonstrated superiority over placebo for three MENQOL domain scores including vasomotor ($P<0.001$), physical ($P=0.036$), and psychosocial ($P<0.001$). There were no significant differences between groups for sexual function ($P=0.231$). The authors concluded that the addition of a combination of black seed and chasteberry to citalopram may improve menopausal symptoms (Molaie et al., 2019).

A 3-month open-label study in women with either mild or moderate-severe menopausal symptoms investigated the effect of a combination product containing chasteberry, black cohosh, hyaluronic acid, zinc, and ginger (ElleN) one tablet daily. Results showed a significant reduction in the Kupperman Index in both groups. The treatment was particularly effective against hot flushes associated with night insomnia and anxiety. The product was well tolerated and did not cause any side effects. The authors concluded that this combination product was able to reduce moderate-severe menopause symptoms (Cappelli et al., 2015).

A 3-month RCT in premenopausal and postmenopausal women ($n=50$) compared Phyto-Female Complex (black cohosh, dong quai, milk thistle, red clover, American ginseng, and chasteberry) with placebo BID for effect on menopausal symptoms. The women receiving Phyto-Female Complex showed a significantly superior mean reduction in menopausal symptoms compared with the placebo group. Improvements in menopausal symptoms increased over time. In the treatment group there was a 73% decrease in hot flushes and a 69% reduction of night sweats, as well as a decrease in hot flush intensity and a significant improvement in sleep quality, by 3 months. Hot flushes ceased completely in 47% and 19% of women with the herbal product and placebo, respectively. There were no changes in findings on vaginal ultrasonography or levels of relevant hormones (estradiol, FSH), liver enzymes, or TSH in either group. The authors concluded that Phyto-Female Complex was safe and effective for the relief of hot flushes and sleep disturbances in pre- and postmenopausal women, when used for at least 3 months (Rotem and Kaplan, 2007).

Prolactin in Men

A 14-day RCT in healthy male subjects ($n=20$) compared chasteberry extract (BP1095E1) 120, 240, and 480 mg/day with placebo for tolerance and prolactin secretion. A significantly greater-than-placebo increase in the 24-h prolactin secretion occurred with 120 mg of chasteberry, and there was a slight reduction in prolactin compared with placebo with the 480 mg dose. After TRH stimulation on day 14, the 1-h AUC of prolactin was significantly increased with chasteberry 120 mg and was significantly decreased with 480 mg compared with placebo. The authors concluded that the effects of chasteberry are dependent on the dose administered and the initial level of prolactin concentration. There were no significant adverse effects, changes in BP or heart rate, blood count, Quick's test (coagulation), clinical chemistry, testosterone, FSH, or LH (Merz et al., 1996).

Musculoskeletal Disorders: Bone Metabolism

An 8-week RCT in younger women ($n = 64$) with long bone fractures investigated chasteberry extract 4 mg plus magnesium oxide 250 mg compared with chasteberry or magnesium plus placebo or placebo plus placebo. The level of ALP in the chasteberry + placebo group increased from 188.33 to 240.40 ($P = 0.05$). Administration of chasteberry + Mg did not increase ALP activity. However, treatment with chasteberry + Mg significantly enhanced the osteocalcin level. Chasteberry + placebo produced an increase in the serum concentration of VEGF from 269.04 to 640.03 ($P < 0.05$) (*VEGF plays an important role in bone formation*). Callus formation in the chasteberry + Mg group was higher than the other groups, but the differences between the four groups were not significant ($P = 0.39$). The authors concluded that chasteberry plus magnesium may promote fracture healing, but that further research was warranted (Eftekhari et al., 2014).

Psychiatric Disorders: Anxiety and Depression

A 2018 systematic review to identify single-herb medicines that may warrant further study for treatment of anxiety and depression in cancer patients found 100 studies involving 38 botanicals that met inclusion criteria. Among herbs most studied (≥ 6 randomized controlled trials each), lavender, passionflower, and saffron produced benefits comparable to standard anxiolytics and antidepressants. Chasteberry, black cohosh, and chamomile were also considered promising. Overall, 45% of studies reported positive findings with fewer adverse effects compared with conventional medications. The authors concluded that saffron, black cohosh, chamomile, chasteberry, lavender, and passionflower appeared useful in mitigating anxiety or depression with favorable risk-benefit profiles compared with standard treatments, and these botanicals may benefit cancer patients by minimizing medication load and accompanying side effects (Yeung et al., 2018).

Psychiatric Disorders: Insomnia

A 14-day RCT in healthy young males ($n = 20$) compared chasteberry 120–480 mg/day with placebo for effects on circadian rhythm. A significant dose-dependent increase in the AUC for melatonin secretion was found ($P < 0.05$). The pattern of circadian rhythm of melatonin secretion did not change with chasteberry or placebo. The authors suggested that chasteberry may be beneficial for sleep disturbances (Dericks-Tan et al., 2003).

ACTIVE CONSTITUENTS

- Lipids
  - Essential fatty acids: oleic acid, linolenic acid, palmitic acid, stearic acid
- Phenolic compounds
  - Flavonoids (antiandrogenic, antibacterial): casticin (dopaminergic, opioid through the activation of mu- and delta-opioid receptor subtypes), orientin, isovitexin (hepatoprotective, anticarcinogenic, apoptotic, antistaphylococcal), vitexin, (antioxidant, antiinflammatory, hepatoprotective, estrogen-β agonism, antihyperalgesic, antiarthritis, neuroprotective, antidepressant, dopaminergic, serotonergic, anticancer), apigenin (antiinflammatory, antioxidant, antihistamine, hypotensive, antiserotonin release, GABA agonism, antispasmodic, antibacterial, chemopreventive, antineoplastic, ERB), penduletin, quercetagetin
- Terpenes
  - Monoterpenoids: cineole (antispasmodic, carminative, and antiseptic, antimicrobia)
    - Iridoid glycosides (antibacterial, indirect effects on hormones): agnuside, aucubin
  - Diterpenoids: rotundifuran, B-110, B-115, clerodanediols, vitexilactone, vitetrifolin D

- Steroids: viticosterone E
- Aromatic compounds (antifungal, antibacterial, insect-repellent): bornyl acetate, limonene (antineoplastic, detoxifying), pinene, cineole (antispasmodic, carminative and antiseptic, antimicrobial), sabinene

CHASTEBERRY/CHASTE TREE/VITEX COMMONLY USED PREPARATIONS AND DOSAGE (FOR ADULTS UNLESS OTHERWISE SPECIFIED)

The following are examples of some available formulations and ranges of dosing for commercial herbal products. See Part III Introduction "How to prescribe medicinal herbs" for further guidance on herbal advising and prescribing.

Dried Berries (Fruit/Seeds)

- Oral infusion (tea): 1 tsp per cup TID
- Fluid extract (1:1): 0.5–1 mL QAM
- Tincture (1:4, 60–75%): 2–4 mL QD
- Powdered berry extract: 800 mg (1/3 tsp) QD
- Capsule or tablet of powdered berry extract: 400–800 mg QD-TID
- Capsule or tablet of standardized extract (standardized to 0.5% agnusides): 225–300 mg BID*

Dosing for chasteberry is confusing. The German Commission E recommends 30–40 mg/day of whole berry or 175 mg/day of a standardized extract. This reflects studies that have shown that extracts of the whole berry are more efficacious than individual constituents. Although doses as low as 20 mg/day have been shown to be beneficial for women's issues, reputable manufacturers offer preparations containing higher doses. Studies in men were performed with higher doses.

Duration of therapy: minimum of 4 months; may be taken up to 18 months

SAFETY AND PRECAUTION

Side Effects

Mild side effects occur in < 2% and include gastrointestinal upset, urticaria, fatigue, headache, dry mouth, tachycardia, nausea, and agitation. Chasteberry has been reported to worsen preexisting acne.

Case Reports

A woman had a pituitary microadenoma tumor that was falsely masked by consumption of chasteberry.

A 31-year-old woman with a pituitary adenoma reached 80% of baseline levels after treatment with chasteberry but experienced no reduction in symptoms.

Toxicity

The LD_{50} of the ethanolic extract of chasteberry in female rats appears to be 12.5 g/kg. The European Medicines Agency cites indications of liver damage associated with 26 weeks of continued usage of unspecified doses of chasteberry but lists no citations to support this claim.

Pregnancy and Lactation

Insufficient human safety data. Chasteberry is not recommended for use during pregnancy or lactation, although it has a long successful history of use in Europe for lactation.

A 2008 systematic review evaluated evidence on the use, safety, and pharmacology of chasteberry, focusing on issues pertaining to pregnancy and lactation. The authors found that in pregnancy there was poor evidence based on theoretical and expert opinion and in vitro studies that chasteberry may have estrogenic and progestogenic activity, uterine stimulant activity, emmenagogue activity and miscarriage prevention. In lactation, theoretical and expert opinion conflicted as to whether chasteberry increased or decreased lactation. The authors concluded that health care providers should be aware of the uncertainties surrounding the safety of this herb in pregnancy and lactation, given the common use of this herb by potentially childbearing women (Dugoua et al., 2008)

Disease Interactions

Caution in patients with hormone-sensitive cancers due to possible hormonal effects.

Drug Interactions

- CYP: Inhibits CYP2C19 and CYP3A4
- Caution with dopamine agonists such as anti-Parkinson drugs due to theoretical interaction
- Caution with dopamine antagonists such as antipyschotics due to theoretical interaction

- May reduce efficacy of HRT due to SERM activity
- May reduce efficacy of oral contraceptives

A 2005 systematic review was performed to evaluate human safety data of chasteberry. Data from clinical trials, postmarketing surveillance studies, surveys, spontaneous reporting schemes, manufacturers, and herbalist organizations indicate that the adverse events following chasteberry treatment were mild and reversible. The most frequent adverse events were nausea, headache, gastrointestinal disturbances, menstrual disorders, acne, pruritus, and erythematous rash. No drug interactions were reported. The authors noted that use of chasteberry should be avoided during pregnancy or lactation and that theoretically it might also interfere with dopaminergic antagonists. The data available seemed to indicate that chasteberry is a safe herbal medicine (Daniele et al., 2005)

REFERENCES

Atmaca M, Kumru S, Tezcan E. Fluoxetine vs Vitex agnus castus extract in the treatment of premenstrual dysphoric disorder. Hum Psychopharmacol 2003 Apr;18(3):191–5.

Berger D, Schaffner W, Schrader E, et al. Efficacy of Vitex agnus castus L. extract Ze 440 in patients with pre-menstrual syndrome (PMS). Arch Gynecol Obstet 2000;264:150–3.

Cappelli V, Morgante G, Di Sabatino A, Massaro MG, De Leo V. Evaluation of the efficacy of a new nutraceutical product in the treatment of postmenopausal symptoms. Minerva Ginecol 2015 Dec;67(6):515–21.

Cerqueira R, Frey B, Leclerc E, Brietzke E. Vitex agnus castus for premenstrual syndrome and premenstrual dysphoric disorder: a systematic review. Arch Womens Ment Health 2017 Dec;20(6):713–9.

Csupor D, Lantos T, Hegyi P, et al. Vitex agnus-castus in premenstrual syndrome: a meta-analysis of double-blind randomised controlled trials. Complement Ther Med 2019 Dec;47:102190.

Daniele C, Thompson Coon J, Pittler MH, et al. Vitex agnus castus: a systematic review of adverse events. Drug Saf 2005;28(4):319–32.

Dante G, Facchinetti F. Herbal treatments for alleviating premenstrual symptoms: a systematic review. J Psychosom Obstet Gynaecol 2011 Mar;32(1):42–51.

Dericks-Tan JS, Schwinn P, Hildt C. Dose-dependent stimulation of melatonin secretion after administration of Agnus castus. Exp Clin Endocrinol Diabetes 2003 Feb;111(1):44-6.

Dinç T, Coşkun F. Comparison of fructus agni casti and flurbiprofen in the treatment of cyclic mastalgia in premenopausal women. Ulus Cerrahi Derg 2014 Mar 1;30(1):34–8.

Dugoua JJ, et al. Safety and efficacy of chastetree (Vitex agnus-castus) during pregnancy and lactation. Can J Clin Pharmacol 2008 Winter;15(1):e74-9.

Eftekhari MH, Rostami ZH, Emami MJ, Tabatabaee HR. Effects of "vitex agnus castus" extract and magnesium supplementation, alone and in combination, on osteogenic and angiogenic factors and fracture healing in women with long bone fracture. J Res Med Sci 2014 Jan;19(1):1–7.

Gerhard II, Patek A, Monga B, Blank A, Gorkow C. Mastodynon(R) bei weiblicher Sterilität. Forsch Komplementmed 1998;5(6):272–8.

Ghazanfarpour M, Sadeghi R, Abdolahian S, Latifnejad RR. The efficacy of Iranian herbal medicines in alleviating hot flashes: a systematic review. Int J Reprod Biomed (Yazd) 2016 Mr;14(3):155–66.

Halaska M, Beles P, Gorkow C, Sieder C. Treatment of cyclical mastalgia with a solution containing a Vitex agnus castus extract: results of a placebo-controlled double-blind study. Breast 1999;8:175–81.

He Z, Chen R, Zhou Y, et al. Treatment for premenstrual syndrome with Vitex agnus castus: a prospective, randomized, multicenter placebo-controlled study in China. Maturitas 2009 May 20;63(1):99–103.

Jang SH, Kim DI, Choi MS. Effects and treatment methods of acupuncture and herbal medicine for premenstrual syndrome/premenstrual dysphoric disorder: systematic review. BMC Complement Altern Med 2014 Jan 10;14:11.

Kargozar R, Azizi H, Salari R. A review of effective herbal medicines in controlling menopausal symptoms. Electron Physician 2017 Nov;9(11):5826–33.

Loch EG, Selle H, Boblitz N. Treatment of premenstrual syndrome with a phytopharmaceutical formulation containing Vitex agnus castus. J Womens Health Gend Based Med 2000 Apr;9(3):315-20.

Ma L, Lin S, Chen R, Wang X. Treatment of moderate to severe premenstrual syndrome with Vitex agnus castus (BNO 1095) in Chinese women. Gynecol Endocrinol 2010 Aug;26(8):612–6.

Merz PG, Gorkow C, Schrödter A, et al. The effects of a special Agnus castus extract (BP1095E1) on prolactin secretion in healthy male subjects. Exp Clin Endocrinol Diabetes 1996;104(6):447–53.

Milewicz A, Gejdel E, Sworen H, et al. Vitex agnus castus extract in the treatment of luteal phase defects due to latent hyperprolactinemia. Results of a randomized placebo-controlled double-blind study. Arzneimittelforschung 1993 Jul;43(7):752–6.

Molaie M, Darvishi B, Jafari Azar Z, Shirazi M, Amin G, Afshar S. Effects of a combination of Nigella sativa and Vitex agnus-castus with citalopram on healthy menopausal women with hot flushes: results from a subpopulation analysis. Gynecol Endocrinol 2019 Jan;35(1):58–61.

Momoeda M, Sasaki H, Tagashira E, Ogishima M, Takano Y, Ochiai K. Efficacy and safety of Vitex agnus-castus extract for treatment of premenstrual syndrome in Japanese patients: a prospective, open-label study. Adv Ther 2014 Mar;31(3):362–73.

Rafieian-Kopaei M, Movahedi M. Systematic review of premenstrual, postmenstrual and infertility disorders of Vitex Agnus Castus. Electron Physician 2017 Jan 25;9(1):3685–9.

Rotem C, Kaplan B. Phyto-Female Complex for the relief of hot flushes, night sweats and quality of sleep: randomized, controlled, double-blind pilot study. Gynecol Endocrinol 2007 Feb;23(2):117–22.

Schellenberg R, Zimmermann C, Drewe J, Hoexter G, Zahner C. Dose-dependent efficacy of the Vitex agnus castus extract Ze 440 in patients suffering from premenstrual syndrome. Phytomedicine 2012 Nov 15;19(14):1325–31.

van Die MD, Bone KM, Burger HG, Reece JE, Teede HJ. Effects of a combination of Hypericum perforatum and Vitex agnus-castus on PMS-like symptoms in late-perimenopausal women: findings from a subpopulation analysis. J Altern Complement Med 2009 Sep;15(9):1045–8.

van Die MD, Burger HG, Teede HJ, Bone KM. Vitex agnus-castus extracts for female reproductive disorders: a systematic review of clinical trials. Planta Med 2013 May;79(7):562–75.

Westphal LM, Polan ML, Trant AS. Double-blind, placebo-controlled study of Fertilityblend: a nutritional supplement for improving fertility in women. Clin Exp Obstet Gynecol 2006;33(4):205–8.

Yavarikia P, Shahnazi M, Hadavand Mirzaie S, Javadzadeh Y, Lutfi R. Comparing the effect of mefenamic Acid and vitex agnus on intrauterine device induced bleeding. J Caring Sci 2013 Aug 31;2(3):245–54.

Yeung KS, Hernandez M, Mao JJ, Haviland I, Gubili J. Herbal medicine for depression and anxiety: a systematic review with assessment of potential psycho-oncologic relevance. Phytother Res 2018 May;32(5):865–91.

Zamani M, Neghab N, Torabian S. Therapeutic effect of Vitex agnus castus in patients with premenstrual syndrome. Acta Med Iran 2012;50(2):101–6.

37

COLEUS (*COLEUS FORSKOHLII*)
Root

GENERAL OVERVIEW

One of the prized Ayurvedic herbs, coleus is a cardiovascular, respiratory, and metabolic herb. Coleus is traditionally used in Ayurvedic medicine to treat skin rashes, asthma, bronchitis, insomnia, epilepsy, and angina pectoris. There are several patents for coleus formulations that promote antispasmodic effects on respiratory smooth muscle, relief of coughs, treatment of asthma and allergies, prevention of hair loss, deceleration of aging, and promotion of weight loss. Forskolin, the most active constituent in coleus, has been extensively studied in preclinical research.

Clinical research indicates that coleus, alone or in combination formulas, may be beneficial for glaucoma, asthma, congestive heart failure, obesity, subarachnoid hemorrhage, and psoriasis.

IN VITRO AND ANIMAL RESEARCH

Organic extracts of coleus have demonstrated antiinflammatory, antimicrobial, antioxidant, cytotoxic, hypotensive, spasmolytic, hepatoprotective, antifeedant (preventing infestation), and antitumor properties. Coleus activates adenylyl cyclase with resultant inhibition of platelet activation and degranulation, inhibition of mast cell degranulation and histamine release, increased force of contraction of heart muscle, relaxation of arteries and other smooth muscles, increased insulin secretion, increased thyroid function, increased lipolysis, and decreased ocular aqueous flow. Consequently, it is a fat-reducing, hypotensive, bronchodilating, inflammation modulating, positive inotropic, lipolytic, thyroid hormone stimulating, mood elevating, and platelet aggregation inhibiting herb.

The main active constituent of coleus, forskolin is a direct, rapid, and reversible activator of adenylyl cyclase, which results in marked increases in the level of intracellular cAMP in a variety of mammalian tissues. Unfortunately, forskolin is poorly water-soluble, but a derivative has been created (colforsin daropate) that is more water-soluble and therefore more amenable to therapeutic applications. Forskolin has positive inotropic effects on the heart, increases heart rate, and lowers blood pressure. Forskolin inhibits the vascular contractility of rat aortas in a concentration-dependent manner and has relaxant effects on rat tail arteries.

Studies with human myocardial tissue have shown synergism with isoproterenol. Forskolin has a stronger effect on coronary arteries than on pacemaker cells and ventricular muscle, possibly due to the presence of different adenylyl cyclase subtypes. Forskolin possesses direct vasodilator activity in the cerebrum, myocardium, and kidneys. It potently inhibits platelet aggregation through several mechanisms. Forskolin has been shown to inhibit platelet aggregation induced by melanoma cells and to inhibit the hepatic metastasis of colon cancer.

Coleus has demonstrated induction of lipolysis in rat adipose tissue and promotion of subcutaneous fat decomposition. Forskolin reduces BW and obesity in rats and reduces alcohol consumption and alcohol-induced neuronal cell death. Animal studies have also demonstrated antiinflammatory, antidepressant, and antiseizure effects as well preventive effects against neurodegenerative disorders. Forskolin increases the motility of sperm cells in vitro in a dose-dependent manner.

Topically applied 1% forskolin suspension reduces intraocular pressure in animals and healthy human subjects and increases iris-ciliary blood flow. Forskolin has been shown in vitro and in animal research to relax airway smooth muscle and inhibit histamine release. It also reduces the expression of inflammatory mediators in airway smooth muscle cells in asthmatics and reduces airway smooth muscle cell mitogenesis and growth. Preclinical studies have shown that forskolin stimulates the release of insulin and glucagon and increases serum glucose and free fatty acid levels. The constituent also stimulates gastric acid, pepsinogen, and exocrine pancreatic secretion and has demonstrated antidiarrheal effects on par with loperamide.

Animal studies have also shown that forskolin relaxes detrusor muscles, inhibits uterine contractions, stimulates renal renin release, increases glomerular filtration and sodium excretion, and causes bladder epithelial cells to eject uropathogenic *E. coli*. Dermally applied, forskolin has been shown to induce melatonin production in cultured hamster pineal glands. It increases pigments in hair follicles and stimulates the growth of hair follicular keratinocytes, protecting keratinocytes against UVA radiation. It induces tanning with or without sunlight.

Antitumor effects of forskolin include inhibiting lung tumor colonization and metastasis, inhibiting human gastric adenocarcinoma cell growth, and inhibiting growth and promoting apoptosis in myeloid and lymphoid cells. It causes a partial reversal of doxorubicin resistance in multidrug resistant murine sarcoma cells and increases the cytotoxicity of doxorubicin in human ovarian cancer cells in vitro.

HUMAN RESEARCH

Ophthalmological Disorders: Glaucoma

A 30-day open-label, case-controlled study of patients ($n = 97$) with uncontrolled glaucoma investigated the efficacy of an oral supplement containing rutin and forskolin BID in addition to their usual drug treatment compared with drug treatment alone. The supplemental treatment group showed a further 10% decrease ($P < 0.01$) of their intraocular pressure (IOP), starting from 1 week after introduction of the oral supplement and lasting until the last evaluation before surgery 30 days later. The decrease was 15% ($P < 0.01$) in those subjects with IOP ≥ 21 mmHg at baseline. IOP values in the control group remained stable from the beginning to the end of the observation period, regardless of their baseline values (Vetrugno et al., 2012).

A study in young healthy adults ($n = 20$) assessed the effects of 50 μL of 1% forskolin instilled in one eye compared with the vehicle alone in the other eye, each applied twice at five-minute intervals. The maximum IOP fall of 2.4 mmHg after 1 h was not significant for forskolin. Two instillations of forskolin reduced the aqueous flow rate to 87% of the control, while the iris permeability factor was increased to 114% ($P < 0.005$). Pretreatment with topical 0.25% timolol in both eyes 1 h prior to drug administration did not significantly alter the forskolin effects (Seto et al., 1986).

Pulmonary Disorders: Asthma

An RCT in healthy subjects ($n = 36$) investigated IV infusion of colforsin daropate (water-soluble derivative of forskolin) 0.5 mcg/kg/min compared with saline 7.5 mL/h (control) in thiamylal-fentanyl-induced bronchoconstriction under anesthesia. Prior to administration of fentanyl, both groups had comparable rates of airway flow and compliance. In the control group, mean and expiratory airway resistance increased significantly, and dynamic lung compliance decreased significantly compared with the baseline. In the colforsin daropate group, there were no changes in airway resistance and lung compliance (Wajima et al., 2002).

A 120-min four-period crossover RCT of patients ($n = 16$) with asthma compared inhaled fenoterol dry powder capsules (0.4 mg) with fenoterol metered dose inhaler (0.4 mg) and with inhaled colforsin (forskolin) dry powder capsules (10 mg). All active drugs caused a significant increase in specific airway conductance ($P < 0.05$). Fenoterol MDI, fenoterol dry powder capsules, and colforsin dry powder capsules produced a mean flow increase from baseline of (0.51, 0.49, and 0.30 $s^{-1} \times kPa^{-1}$), respectively. Finger tremor amplitude increased with fenoterol metered dose inhaler, fenoterol dry powder, and colforsin dry powder by 63%, 16%, and 13%, respectively. A decrease in plasma potassium occurred with both fenoterol formulations (Bauer et al., 1993).

A 6-month single-blinded study in patients ($n = 40$) with mild persistent or moderate persistent asthma compared forskolin capsules given orally QD with sodium cromoglycate inhalations TID in preventing asthma attacks. The percentage of patients who had asthma attacks during the treatment period was 40% with forskolin and 85% with cromoglycate. FEV1 values were similar between the two groups (Gonzalez-Sanchez et al., 2006).

Cardiovascular Disorders: Hypertension and Congestive Heart Failure

A study of patients ($n = 15$) with dilated cardiomyopathy (DCM) compared dobutamine with forskolin on cardiac parameters. The patients received dobutamine 10 mcg/kg/min i.v. or forskolin 3 mcg/kg/min i.v.. There was no change in contractility with forskolin, but contractility increased by 25% with dobutamine. The preload decline (LVEDP) was 27% with forskolin and 19% with dobutamine. LV function improved 9% with forskolin and 34% with dobutamine. The authors concluded that forskolin infusion improved LV function to a lesser degree than dobutamine. It did so primarily by reduction of cardiac preload in DCM hearts without raising metabolic costs produced by dobutamine (Kramer et al., 1987).

An intraindividual comparison study in patients ($n = 12$) with stage III (NYHA) congestive cardiomyopathy compared intravenous forskolin with dobutamine and with sodium nitroprusside. Forskolin dose-dependently reduced cardiac pre- and afterload values, and led to a reduction in systolic, diastolic, and mean pulmonary artery pressure as well as pulmonary wedge pressure by greater than 50% concomitant with an increase in cardiac output and a slight increase in heart rate. Cardiac stroke volume and stroke volume index were increased by approximately 70%. The cardiovascular effects of dobutamine and nitroprusside were less pronounced unless the drugs were combined. The authors concluded that forskolin, with its receptor-independent mechanism of action, may be advantageous for the treatment of severe heart failure, especially in patients with catecholamine-insensitive heart failure (Baumann et al., 1990).

An Ayurvedic study of coleus looked at the effect of two different preparations in elderly patients ($n = 49$) with HTN. Analysis of the results showed that the treatment with both preparations was found to be beneficial. Overall, 75%–76% of the patients were "mildly improved" with respect to blood pressure (Jagtap et al., 2011).

Cardiometabolic Disorders: Metabolic Syndrome and Obesity

A 12-week RCT in overweight and obese subjects ($n = 30$) compared coleus extract 250 mg BID with placebo for effects on metabolic markers. All participants were advised to follow a hypocaloric diet throughout the study. By 12 weeks the coleus group showed a favorable improvement in insulin levels and insulin resistance compared with the placebo group ($P = 0.001$ and $P = 0.01$, respectively). Compared with baseline, significant reductions to waist and hip circumferences occurred with both coleus and placebo ($P = 0.02$ and $P = 0.01$, respectively). HDL-C increased in both groups ($P = 0.01$ for both). The authors concluded that coleus extract in conjunction with a hypocaloric diet may be useful in the management of metabolic risk factors (Loftus et al., 2015).

A 12-week RCT in overweight men ($n = 30$) compared 250 mg of coleus extract standardized to 10% forskolin BID with placebo. Forskolin was shown to significantly decrease body fat percentage and fat mass as determined by DXA compared with placebo ($P < 0.05$). There was also a positive difference in bone mass for forskolin administration ($P < 0.05$) and a trend toward a significant increase in lean body mass ($P = 0.097$). Serum-free testosterone levels were significantly increased in the forskolin group ($P \leq 0.05$). The authors concluded that forskolin favorably altered body composition while concurrently increasing bone mass and serum-free testosterone levels in overweight and obese men, indicating that forskolin was a possible therapeutic agent for the management and treatment of obesity (Godard et al., 2005).

A 12-week RCT in overweight individuals ($n = 30$) compared coleus extract 250 mg BID with placebo, each in conjunction with a low-calorie diet. Significant reductions in waist and hip circumference ($P = 0.02$ and $P = 0.01$, for coleus and placebo, respectively) and increases in HDL-C ($P = 0.01$ for both) were recorded in both groups after 12 weeks. The coleus group showed a favorable improvement in insulin concentration and insulin resistance compared with the placebo group

($P = 0.001$ and $P = 0.01$, respectively). The authors concluded that coleus in conjunction with a hypocaloric diet may be useful in the management of metabolic risk factors (Loftus et al., 2015).

A 12-week RCT in female patients ($n = 23$) on a weight-loss diet studied a coleus extract standardized to 10% forskolin 250 mg BID compared with placebo. No significant differences were observed in caloric or macronutrient intake. Coleus resulted in a decrease in body mass by 0.7 kg ($P = 0.10$) with no significant differences in fat mass. Subjects in the coleus group tended to report less fatigue ($P = 0.07$), hunger ($P = 0.02$), and fullness ($P = 0.04$). No clinically significant interactions were seen in metabolic markers, blood lipids, muscle and liver enzymes, electrolytes, red cells, white cells, insulin, TSH, T3, and T4, heart rate, blood pressure, or weekly reports of side effects. The authors concluded that coleus did not appear to promote weight loss but may help mitigate weight gain with no clinically significant side effects in overweight females (Henderson et al., 2005).

An 8-week open-label study in healthy overweight women ($n = 6$) investigated the effects of coleus extract standardized to 10% forskolin 250 mg BID AC in conjunction with previously established daily exercise and eating habits. Mean weight loss was 4.3 lbs. and 9.2 lbs. at 4 and 8 weeks, respectively, significantly different from baseline ($P < 0.05$). Body fat decreased from 34% to 30% to 26% at 0, 4, and 8 weeks, respectively ($P < 0.05$). Lean body mass increased from 67% to 70% to 74% at 0, 4, and 8 weeks, respectively ($P < 0.05$). SBP decreased from 114 to 110 to 104 mmHg at 0, 4, and 8 weeks, respectively. DBP decreased slightly and nonsignificantly. Pulse rate increased slightly and nonsignificantly (Badmaev et al., 2001).

Neurological Disorders: Subarachnoid Hemorrhage

A consecutive series of patients ($n = 29$) with cerebral vasospasm following subarachnoid hemorrhage received intra-arterial colforsin daropate (a water-soluble forskolin derivative). Treatment was performed in 53 procedures in 29 patients. Angiographic improvement was observed following all procedures (100%), and clinical improvement was observed following 36 of 42 procedures (86%) in symptomatic cases. Cerebral circulation time improved significantly. At the 3-month follow-up, 19 patients (66%) showed good recovery or moderate disability on the Glasgow Outcome Scale. Major adverse effects were headache and increased heart rate (Suzuki et al., 2010).

Dermatological Disorders: Psoriasis

Psoriasis may also be helped by forskolin. Psoriasis typically has a decreased ratio of cAMP to cGMP in the skin. This imbalance results in the increased rate of cell division that occurs with psoriasis. Although clinical evidence for this use is sparse, there are four case reports of improvement in psoriasis with forskolin (Ammon and Müller, 1985).

ACTIVE CONSTITUENTS

(constituents vary depending on region grown)

Entire Plant

- Phenolic compounds
  - Phenylpropanoids (antioxidant, antimutagenic, antitumor, antimicrobial): caffeic acid, rosmarinic acid (antimicrobial, antiinflammatory, antioxidant, antiallergic)
  - Flavonoids: luteolin (antiinflammatory, antispasmodic, antibacterial, hepatoprotective, antiestrogenic, antiproliferative), apigenin (antiinflammatory, antioxidant, antihistamine, hypotensive, antiserotonin release, GABA agonism, antispasmodic, antibacterial, chemopreventive, antineoplastic, ERB), acacetin, scutellarein, acacetin
- Terpenes
  - Terpenoids: forskolins G-J (adenylyl cyclase activation, bronchodilating, systemic and ocular antihypertensive, inotropic, chronotropic, antidepressant, erectogenic, antihistamine, antiinflammatory, thyrotropic, antiplatelet, antimetastatic), coleonol (adenylyl cyclase activation, antihypertensive, vascular and GI antispasmodic), colenol (stiumulates insulin and glucagon release, net hyperglycemic), betulic acid, arjunic acid, coleon U 11-acetate, 16-acetoxycoleon U11-acetate, xanthanthusins F-K, 13-epi-sclareol (antineoplastic for breast and uterus), forskoditerpenoids A & B (tracheal antispasmodic), 12-hydroxy-8,13E-labdadien-15-oic acid, coleolic acid,

coleonic acid; abietanes—royleanones, spirocoleons, quinone methides, acylhydroquinones, 6,7-seco-abietanoids, aromatic abietanoids, phenolic abietanoids, coleoside, coleoside B, colforsin daropate

- Steroids
  - Phytosterols: beta-sitosterol, sigmasterol
- Colexanthone
- Aromatic compounds

COLEUS COMMONLY USED PREPARATIONS AND DOSAGE (FOR ADULTS UNLESS OTHERWISE SPECIFIED)

The following are examples of some available formulations and ranges of dosing for commercial herbal products. See Part III Introduction "How to prescribe medicinal herbs" for further guidance on herbal advising and prescribing.

Leaf

- Capsule or tablet of standardized extract (standardized to 10%–18% forskolin): 50–250 mg BID.
  It is unclear whether oral dosing is effective for asthma since studies used aerosolized powder.
  It is unclear if oral dosing is effective for glaucoma since studies used eye drops. It is unclear if oral dosing is of any benefit for congestive cardiomyopathy since studies used intravenous forskolin.

SAFETY AND PRECAUTION

Side Effects

Coleus may increase gastric acid secretion, therefore it should be used with caution in patients with peptic ulcer disease (PUD). It also may aggravate hypotension or bleeding disorders and enlarge renal cysts.

Toxicity

In cats, the LD^{50} appears to be 68 mg/kg bodyweight forskolin.

Pregnancy and Lactation

Insufficient human safety data.

Disease Interactions

Avoid in active PUD due to increased gastric acid secretion.

Drug Interactions

- CYP: Induces CYP3A.
- May augment effects of hypoglycemic agents.
- Potential for interactions with anticoagulants, hypotensives, digoxin.

REFERENCES

Ammon HP, Müller AB. Forskolin: from an Ayurvedic remedy to a modern agent. Planta Med 1985 Dec;6:473–7.

Badmaev V, Majeed M, Conte A, Parker JE. Diterpene forskolin: a possible new compound for reduction of BW by increasing lean body mass. Townsend Lett 2001;2001(June);115.

Bauer K, Dietersdorfer F, Sertl K, et al. Pharmacodynamic effects of inhaled dry powder formulations of fenoterol and colforsin in asthma. Clin Pharmacol Ther 1993;53:76–83. 24.

Baumann G, et al. Cardiovascular effects of forskolin (HL 362) in patients with idiopathic congestive cardiomyopathy—a comparative study with dobutamine and sodium nitroprusside. J Cardiovasc Pharmacol 1990;16(1):93–100.

Godard MP, Johnson BA, Richmond SR. Body composition and hormonal adaptations associated with forskolin consumption in overweight and obese men. Obes Res 2005;13(8):1335–43.

Gonzalez-Sanchez R, et al. Forskolin vs sodium cromoglycate for prevention of asthma attacks: a single-blinded clinical trial. J Int Med Res 2006;34(2):200–7.

Henderson S, Magu B, Rasmussen C, et al. Effects of Coleus forskohlii supplementation on body composition and hematological profiles in mildly overweight women. J Intl Soc Sports Nutr 2005;2(2):54–62.

Jagtap M, Chandola HM, Ravishankar B. Clinical efficacy of *Coleus forskohlii (Willd.) Briq. (Makandi)* in HTN of geriatric population. Ayu 2011 Jan-Mar;32(1):59–65.

Kramer W, Thormann J, Kindler M, Schlepper M. Effects of forskolin on left ventricular function in dilated cardiomyopathy. Arzneimittelforschung 1987;37:364–7.

Loftus HL, Astell KJ, Mathai ML, Su XQ. *Coleus forskohlii* extract supplementation in conjunction with a hypocaloric diet reduces the risk factors of metabolic syndrome in overweight and obese subjects: a randomized controlled trial. Nutrients 2015 Nov;7(11):9508–22.

Seto C, Eguchi S, Araie M, et al. Acute effects of topical forskolin on aqueous humor dynamics in man. Jpn J Ophthalmol 1986;30:238–44.

Suzuki S, Ito O, Sayama T, Goto K. Intra-arterial colforsin daropate for the treatment of cerebral vasospasm after aneurysmal subarachnoid hemorrhage. Neuroradiology 2010 Sep;52(9):837–45.

Vetrugno M, et al. Oral administration of forskolin and rutin contributes to intraocular pressure control in primary open angle glaucoma patients under maximum tolerated medical therapy. J Ocul Pharmacol Ther 2012 Oct;28(5):536–41.

Wajima Z, et al. Intravenous colforsin daropate, a water-soluble forskolin derivative, prevents thiamylal-fentanyl-induced bronchoconstriction in humans. Crit Care Med 2002;30(4):820–6.

38 CRANBERRY (*VACCINIUM MACROCARPON*)
Fruit

GENERAL OVERVIEW

Cranberry is familiar to and widely applied by the medical community and lay community alike for urinary tract health. It has been extensively researched for its effects on the urinary tract with fairly positive, albeit conflicting, evidence for preventing recurrent urinary tract infections. Cranberry has also shown some positive benefits for urinary tract issues unique to men. The efficacy of cranberry on urinary tract infections has been shown to be due primarily to its ability to inhibit the adhesion of *Escherichia coli* to genitourinary epithelium.

Clinical research indicates that cranberry, alone or in combination formulas, may be beneficial for gingivitis, dental plaque, dyslipidemia, diabetes, *Helicobacter pylori*, intestinal dysbiosis, urinary tract infection prophylaxis, benign prostatic hyperplasia, rheumatoid arthritis, and prostate cancer.

IN VITRO AND ANIMAL RESEARCH

In vitro studies have shown that cranberry juice extracts and constituents exhibit antimicrobial, antiinflammatory, antioxidant, and antiadherence properties. Cranberry has shown inhibition of cyclooxygenases and the proinflammatory cytokine and chemokine responses induced by lipopolysaccharides in vitro.

The antiinfection effects of cranberry have been explored in a great deal of in vitro and animal research. Cranberry and other berry fruits have been reported to show direct antimicrobial effects against human pathogens, including *Salmonella* and *Staphylococcus aureus*. Whole berries or whole berry extracts may be more effective as antimicrobials than purified polyphenol extracts. Cranberry juice has been shown to inhibit adhesion of *Streptococcus pneumoniae* to human bronchial (Calu-3) cells and to directly inhibit growth of *S. pneumoniae*. Inhibition of oral acid production, attachment, and biofilm formation by *S. mutans* has been demonstrated with cranberry components. Cranberry has also been shown to regulate aggressive human periodontitis fibroblast inflammatory responses via NFK-b and MMP-3 inhibition. Additional research has demonstrated cranberry's ability to reduce *S. mutans* as well as *Porphyromonas gingivalis* counts in saliva due to the antiadhesion activity of proanthocyanidin.

Cranberry extracts standardized to 36 mg of proanthocyanidins were shown to increase antiadhesion activity ex vivo for uropathogenic P-fimbriated *E. coli* in human urine. Another study demonstrated the ability of cranberry to inhibit *E. coli* adhesion to vaginal and bladder epithelial cells. In vitro examinations of bacterial adherence to urinary epithelial cells have shown that preincubation of *Proteus*, *Pseudomonas*, and *E. coli* with cranberry resulted in decreased bacterial adhesion to epithelial cells. Cranberry juice also inhibits the adhesion of *H. pylori* to human gastric mucosa. The Type-A linkages of the proanthocyanidins in cranberry have been shown to provide the antiadhesion effect. High molecular weight materials from cranberry have been shown to dose-dependently inhibit influenza virus A and B from hemagglutinating red blood cells and to reduce the viruses' infectivity in vitro.

Cranberry extracts and proanthocyanidins have demonstrated antiproliferative effects against prostate, liver, lung, neuroblastoma, breast, ovarian, gastric, colon, esophageal, and oral cancer cells in vitro. Additional cranberry anticancer mechanisms that have been demonstrated include decreasing cyclins, cyclin-dependent kinase expression, MMP activity, VEGFR expression, and proliferating cell nuclear antigen expression. Cranberry also induces apoptosis, ROS, and microRNA modifications within cancer cells. In neuroblastoma cells it has demonstrated a positive effect on cyclophosphamide retention with synergistic cytotoxic benefits.

HUMAN RESEARCH

Oral and Dental Disorders

An 8-week RCT in participants ($n = 50$) with gingivitis compared a daily 750 mL dose of cranberry beverage with water. Gingival and plaque indices improved significantly with cranberry. *S. mutans* colonies were also reduced significantly compared with control. The authors concluded that the consumption of cranberry beverage improved gingival and *plaque indices* without posing a risk of caries, and that cranberry beverage could be recommended as a safe adjunct for non-surgical plaque treatment in patients with gingivitis (Woźniewicz et al., 2018).

A 14-day RCT in young adults ($n = 50$), compared 10 mL of chlorhexidine mouthwash with 10 mL of cranberry mouthwash BID for effects on plaque. Plaque samples were cultured on day 1 and day 14. The number of *S. mutans* colony forming units showed a 69% reduction with chlorhexidine and a 68% reduction with cranberry (N.S.). The authors concluded that cranberry mouthwash was equally effective as chlorhexidine mouthwash with beneficial local and systemic effects and could therefore be used effectively as an alternative to chlorhexidine mouthwash (Khairnar et al., 2015).

Cardiometabolic Disorders: Dyslipidemia and Diabetes

A 2019 systematic review of RCTs that looked at effects of blueberries and cranberries in T2DM found seven RCTs ($n = 270$) that met inclusion criteria. Daily cranberry juice (240 mL) consumption for 12 weeks and blueberry extract or powder supplementation (9.1 and 9.8 mg of anthocyanins, respectively) for 8–12 weeks showed a beneficial effect on glucose control in T2DM subjects. The authors concluded that there was a promising use of these berries in T2DM management (Rocha et al., 2018).

An 8-week RCT in middle-aged adults ($n = 56$) compared 240 mL BID of low-calorie cranberry juice with a matched placebo beverage for impact on cardiometabolic risk factors. Fasting serum TGs were lower after consuming the cranberry juice. Patients with a higher baseline TG showed larger treatment effects (1.15 mmoL/L vs 1.25 mmol/L, respectively; $P = 0.027$). Serum CRP was lower with cranberry that with placebo ($P = 0.0054$). DBP was lower with cranberry than with placebo (69.2 mmHg vs 71.6 mmHg, respectively; $P = 0.048$). FBG was lower with cranberry than placebo (5.32 mmoL/L vs 5.42 mmol/L, respectively; $P = 0.03$). HOMA-IR improved over baseline for cranberry ($P = 0.035$). The authors concluded that low-calorie cranberry juice could improve several cardiometabolic risk factors (Novotny et al., 2015).

An 8-week study of middle-aged men and women with abdominal obesity ($n = 78$) compared daily consumption of 450 mL of a cranberry beverage with placebo. Compared with placebo the cranberry drink lowered endothelin 1, NO, and the reduced/oxidized glutathione ratio ($P < 0.05$). IFN-γ was elevated over baseline with a single dose of cranberry drink ($P < 0.05$). At 8 weeks fasting CRP and serum insulin were lower than baseline ($P < 0.05$) and HDL cholesterol was increased compared with placebo ($P < 0.05$). The authors concluded that an acute dose of cranberry juice improved antioxidant status, while 8 weeks of daily consumption reduced cardiovascular disease risk factors by improving glucoregulation, downregulating inflammatory biomarkers, and increasing HDL cholesterol (Chew et al., 2018).

A 6-week study in insulin-resistant overweight or obese human subjects ($n = 41$) compared a beverage containing 333 mg of strawberry-cranberry polyphenols (SCP) daily with a flavor-matched beverage for controls. Insulin sensitivity increased in the intervention group compared with the control group ($P = 0.03$), and there was a lower first-phase insulin secretion response ($P = 0.002$). No differences were detected between the two groups for lipids and markers of inflammation and oxidative stress (Paquette et al., 2017).

A crossover RCT in obese participants ($n = 25$) with T2DM compared a high-fat breakfast alone with high-fat breakfast plus dried cranberries for postprandial effects. The study revealed that postprandial increases in glucose, IL-18 and MDA were significantly lower ($P < 0.05$), while total serum nitrite was higher in the cranberry group. No significant differences were noted in insulin, insulin resistance, lipid profiles, blood pressure, CRP, or IL-6 between the cranberry and control groups. The authors concluded that adding whole cranberries to a high-fat meal may improve postprandial blood glucose management and warranted further investigation (Schell et al., 2017).

Gastrointestinal Disorders: Peptic Ulcer Disease and *H. pylori* Infection

An 8-week RCT in patients ($n = 522$) with *H. pylori* evaluated dose-response effects of proanthocyanidin-standardized cranberry juice, cranberry powder, or their placebos on suppression of *H. pylori* at 2 and 8 weeks by ^{13}C-urea breath testing and eradication at 45 days postintervention. At week 2, *H. pylori*-negative rates in placebo, low-proanthocyanidin, medium-proanthocyanidin, and high-proanthocyanidin cranberry juice groups (23 mg, 44 mg, and 88 mg of proanthocyanidin per 240 mL serving, respectively) were 13.2%, 7.6%, 1.5%, and 13.8%, respectively. At week 8, in the same four groups, *H. pylori* negative rates were 7.3%, 7.6%, 4.5%, and 20%, respectively ($P < 0.05$). Encapsulated cranberry powder doses were not significantly effective at either time point. Cranberry juice and powder were well tolerated. The authors concluded that the percentage of *H. pylori*-negative participants increased from 2 to 8 weeks in subjects who consumed 88 mg proanthocyanidin/day and may help potentiate suppression of *H. pylori* infection (Li et al., 2020).

An 8-week RCT in *H. pylori*-positive patients ($n = 200$) with PUD were randomized to standard triple therapy or triple therapy plus cranberry capsules 500 mg BID for the 14-day duration of treatment. ^{13}C-urea breath testing showed that eradication of *H. pylori* was increased from 74% to 89% with the addition of cranberry ($P = 0.042$). The authors concluded that the addition of cranberry to triple therapy for *H. pylori* produced a higher rate of eradication than the standard regimen alone (Seyyedmajidi et al., 2016).

Gastrointestinal Disorders: Gut Dysbiosis

A 10-day crossover RCT in volunteers ($n = 11$) investigated the effects of an animal-based diet (which has been shown to adversely affect gut microbes) plus 30 g/day of placebo powder compared with the same animal-based diet plus 30 g/day of cranberry powder for 5 days to determine the effect of cranberry on gut microbes. Compared with the postintervention phase of control diet, the cranberry diet modified nine taxonomic clades, including a decrease in the abundance of Firmicutes and an increase in Bacteroidetes (reversing the effect of the animal-based diet) and improved bile acid composition and short-chain fatty acid composition. The authors concluded that cranberries attenuated the adverse impact of the animal-based diet on microbiota composition, bile acids, and short-chain fatty acids (Rodríguez-Morató et al., 2018).

A 2-week study in healthy adults ($n = 10$) investigated the effect of 42 g/day of sweetened dried cranberry ingestion on urinary proteome and fecal microbiome. The fecal assessment showed a beneficial shift in the Firmicutes:Bacteroidetes ratio as well as increases in commensal bacteria and decreases in or the absence of bacteria associated with negative health effects (Bekiares et al., 2018).

Nephrological and Urological Disorders: Overactive Bladder

A 24-week RCT in women ($n = 98$) with OAB compared dried cranberry powder 500 mg QD with placebo. The cranberry group showed a significant reduction compared with placebo in daily micturitions (-1.91, 16.4%, $P = 0.0406$), urgency episodes (-2.81, 57.3%, $P = 0.0069$), and Patient Perception of Bladder Condition scores (-0.66, 39.7%, $P = 0.0258$) at 24 weeks of follow-up. Mean volume per micturition, nocturia and the remaining survey outcomes did not differ significantly between the groups ($P > 0.05$). The authors concluded that further studies were warranted (Cho et al., 2021).

Nephrological and Urological Disorders: Urinary Tract Infection Prophylaxis

In a 2017 systematic review and meta-analysis of women with history of UTI, seven RCTs ($n = 1498$) were included and indicated that cranberry reduced the risk of UTI by 26% (PRR = 0.74; $I^2 = 54\%$). The authors concluded that cranberry may be effective in preventing UTI recurrence in generally healthy women; however, larger high-quality studies are needed to confirm these findings (Fu et al., 2017).

A 2013 systematic review with meta-analysis that was focused on dose, frequency, and form of cranberry as well as patient characteristics for prevention of UTIs found 13 trials ($n = 1616$) that met inclusion criteria. Excluding the trial with low baseline UTI rates, cranberry products were effective in preventing recurrent UTI (RR 0.62), especially in women with recurrent UTIs (RR = 0.53), women in general (RR = 0.49), children (RR = 0.33), cranberry juice drinkers (RR = 0.47), and people using cranberry-containing products more than twice daily (RR = 0.58). The authors concluded that cranberry-containing products were associated with protective effect against UTIs (Wang et al., 2012).

A 2012 Cochrane review looking at clinical trials on cranberry for preventing UTIs found 24 studies ($n = 4473$) that met inclusion criteria. Thirteen studies (2380 participants) investigated only cranberry juice or concentrate; 9 studies (1032 participants) investigated only cranberry tablets or capsules; 1 study compared cranberry juice and tablets; and 1 study compared cranberry capsules and tablets. Data included in the meta-analyses showed that, compared with placebo, water, or no treatment, cranberry products did not significantly reduce the occurrence of symptomatic UTI overall (RR = 0.86) or for any the subgroups: women with recurrent UTIs (RR = 0.74); older people (RR = 0.75); pregnant women (RR = 1.04); children with recurrent UTI (RR = 0.48); cancer patients (RR = 1.15); or people with neurogenic bladder or spinal injury (RR = 0.95). The effectiveness of cranberry was not significantly different from antibiotics for women (RR = 1.31) and children (RR = 0.69). The authors concluded that cranberry juice was less effective than previously indicated and that cranberry products were not significantly different from antibiotics for preventing UTIs in three small studies (Jepson et al., 2012).

A 60-day RCT in patients ($n = 36$) with recurrent UTIs investigated standard therapy plus a daily dose of a cranberry extract standardized to 36 mg of anthocyanidins (Anthocran) compared with standard therapy alone. The mean number of UTIs observed in the supplemented group vs control group was 0.31 vs 2.3 respectively ($P = 0.0001$). Rate of symptom-free status was 63% with cranberry product vs 23% in the control group ($P < 0.05$). The authors concluded that this standardized supplement had compelling evidence for efficacy as prophylaxis against recurrent UTIs (Ledda et al., 2017).

A 12-month RCT in premenopausal women ($n = 221$) with recurrent UTIs compared trimethoprim-sulfamethoxazole (TMP-SMX), 480 mg QD with cranberry capsules, 500 mg BID. The mean number of patients with at least one symptomatic UTI was greater in the cranberry group than in the TMP-SMX group (4.0 and 1.8, respectively; $P = 0.02$), and the proportion of patients with at least one symptomatic UTI was greater in the cranberry group than in the TMP-SMX group (78.2% and 71.1%, respectively). Median time to the first symptomatic UTI was 4 months for the cranberry and 8 months for the TMP-SMX group. TMP-SMX resistance after 1 month was present in 23.7% of fecal and 28.1% of asymptomatic urine *E. coli* isolates with cranberry and in 86.3% of fecal and 90.5% of asymptomatic urine *E. coli* isolates with TMP-SMX. There were also increased resistance rates for trimethoprim, amoxicillin, and ciprofloxacin in these *E. coli* isolates after 1 month in the TMP-SMX group. After discontinuation of TMP-SMX, resistance reached baseline levels after 3 months. Antibiotic resistance did not increase in the cranberry group. Cranberries and TMP-SMX were equally well tolerated. The authors concluded that in premenopausal women with recurrent UTIs, TMP-SMX, 480 mg QD, was more effective than cranberry capsules, 500 mg BID, in preventing recurrent UTIs, at the expense of emerging, transient antibiotic resistance (Beerepoot et al., 2011).

A 12-month RCT in older women ($n = 928$) residing in nursing homes compared cranberry capsules with placebo BID. In participants with high UTI risk at baseline the incidence of clinically defined UTI was lower with cranberry capsules than with placebo (62.8 vs 84.8 per 100 person-years at risk; $P = 0.04$). No difference in UTI incidence between cranberry and placebo was found in participants with low UTI risk. The authors concluded that in long-term care facility residents with high UTI risk at baseline, cranberry capsules reduced the incidence of clinically defined UTI, although it did not reduce the incidence of bacteriuria. No difference in incidence of UTI was found in residents with low UTI risk (Caljouw et al., 2014).

An RCT in patients ($n=62$) with double J catheters compared routine prophylactic therapy with prophylactic therapy plus cranberry 120 mg/day. Bacteriuria rates were 13% in the cranberry treated group vs 39% in controls ($P=0.04$). The authors concluded that cranberry had an adjuvant effect in the prevention of UTI in patients with JJ catheters (Barnoiu et al., 2015).

A 6-month open-label study in subjects ($n=34$) with long-term indwelling catheters and recurrent symptomatic catheter-associated UTIs investigated the impact of a cranberry supplement standardized to 36 mg proanthocyanidin QD. Cranberry was associated with a reduction in the number of symptomatic catheter-associated UTIs in all patients, and resistance to antibiotics was reduced by 28%. Colony counts were reduced by 59%. No subjects had adverse events while taking cranberry (Thomas et al., 2017).

A 4-month RCT in patients ($n=60$) who underwent ileal conduit diversion between 2013 and 2014 investigated cranberry capsule administration compared with training about UTIs and with no intervention. There were fewer UTIs with cranberry than with training about UTIs or control groups ($P<0.05$). The authors concluded that the use of cranberry capsules was effective in the prevention of UTIs in patients undergoing urostomy (Temiz and Cavdar, 2018).

A 6-week RCT in women ($n=160$) who were undergoing gynecologic surgery requiring urinary catheterization compared cranberry (equivalent to two 8-oz servings of cranberry juice per day for 6 weeks) with matching placebo, each given for 6 weeks after surgery, for impact on UTI rate. The UTI rate was lower in the cranberry group. Incidence of UTI was 19% and 38% in cranberry and placebo groups, respectively ($P=0.008$). Adverse events were similar between groups (Foxman et al., 2015).

Cranberry has been investigated for efficacy in children with urological diseases. A 1-year RCT in infants and children ($n=85$ younger than 1 year; $n=107$ older than 1 year of age) with recurrent UTIs compared cranberry with trimethoprim. The cumulative UTI rate was 46% and 17% in cranberry and trimethoprim groups, respectively, in children younger than 1 year of age, but the rate was 26% for both groups older than 1 year of age. The authors concluded that cranberry was safe and effective in the prophylaxis of recurrent UTI in infants and children,

with similar efficacy to trimethoprim in children older than 1 year (Fernández-Puentes et al., 2015).

Men's Genitourinary Disorders: Benign Prostatic Hyperplasia and Chronic Bacterial Prostatitis

In a 2-month pilot study, older men ($n=43$) with BPH, LUTS, and risk for recurrent UTIs were given either standard management or a standardized cranberry extract. After 2 months the UTI episodes decreased from 3.2 to 0.8 in the cranberry-treated group ($P=0.0001$) with no significant changes in the control group (Ledda et al., 2016).

A 6-month RCT in men ($n=124$) older than 45 years with LUTS and an IPSS score ≥ 8 compared cranberry powder 250 or 500 mg with placebo on LUTS and uroflowmetry. By 6 months both cranberry groups had reductions in IPSS scores (-3.1 for 250 mg and -4.1 for 500 mg; $P=0.05$ and <0.001, respectively). Placebo group had a 1.5 reduction in IPSS. The 500-mg cranberry group also had a significant improvement in Q_{max}, Q_{avg}, and PVR ($P<0.05$). The authors concluded that cranberry powder showed a clinically relevant, dose-dependent, and significant reduction in LUTS in men older than 45 years (Vidlar et al., 2016).

A 36-week RCT in patients ($n=120$) with chronic bacterial prostatitis and recurrent infections due to *E. coli* and *E. faecalis* evaluated treatment with 24 weeks of daily Bifiprost (a combination of cranberry, goji, and probiotics) plus saw palmetto 320 mg compared with 24 weeks of saw palmetto 320 mg alone, each group having received appropriate antibiotic treatment with subsequently negative cultures. At 24 and 36 weeks, the patients in the Bifiprost group experienced a significantly larger reduction in episodes of prostatitis than the patients in the saw palmetto alone group. There was also a significant difference in the mean NIH-CPSI scores between the two groups at 24 and 36 weeks. At 12 weeks of treatment, the mean NIH-CPSI score was reduced in both groups compared with baselines, but no significant differences were seen between groups; nor was there a difference in reduction of episodes of prostatitis between groups at this time point. The authors concluded that combining Bifiprost and saw palmetto 320 mg improved the prevention of episodes of CBP due to Enterobacteriaceae and ameliorated prostatitis-related symptoms after 6 months of therapy, with continued benefit extending 3 months beyond the end of therapy (Chiancone et al., 2019).

Autoimmune Disorders: Rheumatoid Arthritis

A 90-day prospective RCT on women diagnosed with RA ($n = 41$) compared low-calorie cranberry juice 500 mL/day with usual management for disease activity. Compared with baseline, the cranberry group showed a decrease in the Disease Activity Score 28 ($P = 0.048$) and anti-CCP ($P = 0.034$) after 90 days of treatment, but changes in inflammatory biomarkers were not found. The authors concluded that cranberry juice decreased disease activity and may have beneficial effects for RA patients (Thimóteo et al., 2018).

Oncologic Disorders: Prostate Cancer

A 30-day RCT of men ($n = 64$) with prostate cancer compared cranberry fruit powder 1500 mg/day with placebo given for 30 days prior to prostatectomy for effect on PSA. On the day of surgery, blood tests showed a 22% decrease in serum PSA. The authors noted that whole cranberry contains constituents may regulate the expression of androgen-responsive genes (Student et al., 2016).

Cranberry may prevent UTIs in men with prostate cancer. An irradiation-based RCT in men ($n = 41$) with prostate cancer undergoing irradiation compared cranberry extract standardized to 72 mg of proanthocyanidins QD with placebo during pelvic irradiation and for 2 weeks afterward. The incidence of cystitis was 65% with cranberry vs 90% with placebo ($P = 0.058$). Severe cystitis occurred in 30% with cranberry and 45% with placebo ($P = 0.30$). Overall, the incidence of pain/burning was significantly lower in the cranberry cohort ($P = 0.045$) (Hamilton et al., 2015).

A 7-week RCT in patients ($n = 924$) with prostate carcinoma treated by radiotherapy investigated standardized cranberry extract compared with no treatment, each given concurrently with irradiation. Lower urinary tract infections were detected in 11% vs 25% of those receiving cranberry vs control ($P = 0.0001$). The treatment also resulted in a 50% reduction in the use of antiinflammatory drugs and antibiotics. The treatment was very well tolerated and there were no serious side effects. The authors concluded that enteric-coated, standardized cranberry extract could be used as a prophylactic to reduce the incidence of UTIs and decrease antibiotic therapy in patients receiving pelvic irradiation for prostate cancer (Bonetta et al., 2017).

ACTIVE CONSTITUENTS

- Carbohydrates
  - Disaccharides: galabiose (antibacterial adherence)
  - Organic acids: benzoic acid, citric acid, malic acid, quinic acid
- Phenolic compounds
  - Phenolic acids: 3- and 5-caffeoylquinic acid (antibacterial)
  - Phenylpropanoid derivatives (antioxidant, antimutagenic, antitumor, antimicrobial): substituted cinnamic acids
  - Stilbenes
  - Flavonoids: anthocyanins (antioxidant, antineoplastic), flavonols (antibacterial, antineoplastic), flavonol glycosides (antineoplastic), proanthocyanidins (antibacterial adherence, antioxidant, antineoplastic), gallotannins, ellagitannins
    - ☐ Glycosides: myricetin-3-galactoside, quercetin-3-galactoside, prunin (antibacterial adherence), phlorizin (antibacterial adherence)
- Terpenes
  - Terpenoids: ursolic acid and its esters (anti-HIV, anti-EBV, antiviral, androgenic, AChEI, procollagen, proceremide, antitumor), coumaroyl iridoid glycosides (antineoplastic)

CRANBERRY COMMONLY USED PREPARATIONS AND DOSAGE (FOR ADULTS UNLESS OTHERWISE SPECIFIED)

The following are examples of some available formulations and ranges of dosing for commercial herbal products. See Part III Introduction "How to prescribe medicinal herbs" for further guidance on herbal advising and prescribing.

Berry

- Juice (unsweetened, high-quality): 300–500 mL QD-BID.
- Tincture (1:4, 50%): 3–5 mL TID.

- Encapsulated cranberry powder: 850–1000 mg QD-BID
- Cranberry powdered extract: 400–500 mg (1/4 tsp) QD-TID.
- Concentrated (50:1) extract: 500 mg equivalent to 25 g of fresh cranberries QD-BID.
- Capsule or tablet of standardized extract (standardized to total dose of 72 mg proanthocyanidins) QD.

SAFETY AND PRECAUTION

Side Effects

Ingesting large amounts of cranberry juice (three cups daily) has been associated with gastrointestinal upset including nausea, vomiting, and diarrhea.

Case Report

An elderly man who consumed only cranberry juice for 2 weeks while on warfarin suffered from a fatal internal hemorrhage.

Toxicity

According to one report, supplementation with an unspecified number of cranberry tablets for 7 days increased the urinary excretion of oxalate by 43%, suggesting that long-term use of cranberry supplements might increase the risk of urolithiasis.

Pregnancy and Lactation

No known contraindications at usual doses.

Drug Interactions

- CYP: Cranberry inhibits enteric CYP3A and CYP2C9 in vitro but not in humans. Studies in healthy humans and in vitro have found that cranberry juice does not significantly inhibit CYP1A2.
- UGT: Modulates UGT enzymes in vitro.
- Warfarin: Several cases of increased INR and two cases of internal bleeding in patients on warfarin. Although consumption of cranberry juice in large quantities (1–2 L daily or supplements for > 3–4 weeks) may alter warfarin effects, monitoring intake rather than total avoidance of cranberry juice by warfarin users may be warranted.

Although it is thought that cranberry interacts with warfarin through effects on the CYP2C9 enzyme, a clinical study showed no interaction between cranberry and flurbiprofen, which is also metabolized by CYP2C. Studies in healthy volunteers, patients taking warfarin, and laboratory animals indicate that moderate consumption of cranberry (up to 250 mL for up to 10 days) does not affect the anticoagulation effects of warfarin or INR.

- Tacrolimus: Concurrent use with cranberry extracts resulted in subtherapeutic serum levels of tacrolimus in a renal transplant patient. The levels returned to desired range following cessation of cranberry.
- Cyclosporin: An RCT showed that 240 mL of cranberry juice had no clinically significant effect on the disposition of a 200-mg dose of cyclosporin.

REFERENCES

Barnoiu OS, Sequeira-García Del Moral J, Sanchez-Martínez N, Díaz-Molina P, Flores-Sirvent L, Baena-González V. American cranberry (proanthocyanidin 120 mg): its value for the prevention of urinary tracts infections after ureteral catheter placement. Actas Urol Esp 2015 Mar;39(2):112–7.

Beerepoot MA, ter Riet G, Nys S, et al. Cranberries vs antibiotics to prevent urinary tract infections: a randomized double-blind non-inferiority trial in premenopausal women. Arch Int Med Jul 25 2011;171(14):1270–8.

Bekiares N, Krueger CG, Meudt JJ, Shanmuganayagam D, Reed JD. Effect of sweetened dried cranberry consumption on urinary proteome and fecal microbiome in healthy human subjects. OMICS 2018 Feb;22(2):145–53.

Bonetta A, Roviello G, Generali D, et al. Enteric-coated and highly standardized cranberry extract reduces antibiotic and nonsteroidal anti-inflammatory drug use for urinary tract infections during radiotherapy for prostate carcinoma. Res Rep Urol 2017 Apr 26;9:65–9.

Caljouw MA, van den Hout WB, Putter H, et al. Effectiveness of cranberry capsules to prevent urinary tract infections in vulnerable older persons: a double-blind randomized placebo-controlled trial in long-term care facilities. J Am Geriatr Soc Jan 2014;62(1):103–10.

Chew B, Mathison B, Kimble L, et al. Chronic consumption of a low calorie, high polyphenol cranberry beverage attenuates inflammation and improves glucoregulation and HDL cholesterol in healthy overweight humans: a randomized controlled trial. Eur J Nutr 2019 Apr;58(3):1223–35.

Chiancone F, Carrino M, Meccariello C, Pucci L, Fedelini M, Fedelini P. The use of a combination of *Vaccinium Macracarpon*, *Lycium barbarum* L. and probiotics (bifiprost) for the prevention of chronic bacterial prostatitis: a double-blind randomized study. Urol Int 2019;103(4):423–6.

Cho A, Eidelberg A, Butler DJ, et al. Efficacy of daily intake of dried cranberry500 mg in women with overactive bladder: a randomized, double-blind, placebo controlled study. J Urol 2021 Feb;205(2):507-513.

Fernández-Puentes V, Uberos J, Rodríguez-Belmonte R, Nogueras-Ocaña M, Blanca-Jover E, Narbona-López E. Efficacy and safety profile of cranberry in infants and children with recurrent urinary tract infection. Ann Pediatr (Barc) 2015 Jun;82(6):397–403.

Foxman B, Cronenwett AE, Spino C, Berger MB, Morgan DM. Cranberry juice capsules and urinary tract infection after surgery: results of a randomized trial. Am J Obstet Gynecol 2015 Aug;213(2). 194.e1–8.

Fu Z, Liska D, Talan D, Chung M. Cranberry reduces the risk of urinary tract infection recurrence in otherwise healthy women: a systematic review and meta-analysis. J Nutr 2017 Dec;147(12):2282–8.

Hamilton K, Bennett NC, Purdie G, et al. Standardized cranberry capsules for radiation cystitis in prostate cancer patients in New Zealand: a randomized double blinded, placebo controlled pilot study. Support Care Cancer Jan 2015;23(1):95–102.

Jepson RG, Williams G, Craig JC. Cranberries for preventing urinary tract infections. Cochrane Database Syst Rev 2012;10, CD001321.

Khairnar MR, Karibasappa GN, Dodamani AS, Vishwakarma P, Naik RG, Deshmukh MA. Comparative assessment of cranberry and chlorhexidine mouthwash on streptococcal colonization among dental students: a randomized parallel clinical trial. Contemp Clin Dent 2015 Jan-Mar;6(1):35–42.

Ledda A, Belcaro G, Dugall M, et al. Supplementation with high titer cranberry extract (Anthocran®) for the prevention of recurrent urinary tract infections in elderly men suffering from moderate prostatic hyperplasia: a pilot study. Eur Rev Med Pharmacol Sci 2016 Dec;20(24):5205–9.

Ledda A, Belcaro G, Dugall M, et al. Highly standardized cranberry extract supplementation (Anthocran®) as prophylaxis in young healthy subjects with recurrent urinary tract infections. Eur Rev Med Pharmacol Sci 2017 Jan;21(2):389–93.

Li Z, Ma J, Guo Y, et al. Suppression of helicobacter pylori infection by dailycranberryintake: a double-blind, randomized, placebo-controlled trial. J Gastroenterol Hepatol 2020 Aug;11.

Novotny JA, Baer DJ, Khoo C, Gebauer SK, Charron CS. Cranberry juice consumption lowers markers of cardiometabolic risk, including BP and circulating C-reactive protein, triglyceride, and glucose concentrations in adults. J Nutr 2015 Jun;145(6):1185–93.

Paquette M, Medina Larqué AS, Weisnagel SJ, et al. Strawberry and cranberry polyphenols improve insulin sensitivity in insulin-resistant, non-diabetic adults: a parallel, double-blind, controlled and randomised clinical trial. Br J Nutr 2017 Feb;117(4):519–31.

Rocha DMUP, Caldas APS, da Silva BP, Hermsdorff HHM, Alfenas RCG. Effects of blueberry and cranberry consumption on type 2 diabetes glycemic control: a systematic review. Crit Rev Food Sci Nutr 2018 Jan;18:1–13.

Rodríguez-Morató J, Matthan NR, Liu J, de la Torre R, Chen CO. Cranberries attenuate animal-based diet-induced changes in microbiota composition and functionality: a randomized crossover controlled feeding trial. J Nutr Biochem 2018 Dec;62:76–86.

Schell J, Betts NM, Foster M, Scofield RH, Basu A. Cranberries improve postprandial glucose excursions in type 2 diabetes. Food Funct 2017 Sep 20;8(9):3083–90.

Seyyedmajidi M, Ahmadi A, Hajiebrahimi S, et al. Addition of cranberry to proton pump inhibitor-based triple therapy for Helicobacter pylorieradication. J Res Pharm Pract 2016 Oct-Dec;5(4):248–51.

Student V, Vidlar A, Bouchal J, et al. Cranberry intervention in patients with prostate cancer prior to radical prostatectomy. Clinical, pathological and laboratory findings. Biomed Pap Med Fac Univ Palacky Olomouc Czech Repub 2016 Dec;160(4):559–65.

Temiz Z, Cavdar I. The effects of training and the use of cranberry capsule in preventing urinary tract infections after urostomy. Complement Ther Clin Pract 2018 May;31:111–7.

Thimóteo NSB, Iryioda TMV, Alfieri DF, et al. Cranberry juice decreases disease activity in women with rheumatoid arthritis. Nutrition 2018 Oct 10;60:112–7.

Thomas D, Rutman M, Cooper K, Abrams A, Finkelstein J, Chughtai B. Does cranberry have a role in catheter-associated urinary tract infections? Can Urol Assoc J 2017 Nov;11(11):E421–4.

Vidlar A, Student Jr V, Vostalova J, et al. Cranberry fruit powder (Flowens™) improves lower urinary tract symptoms in men: a double-blind, randomized, placebo-controlled study. World J Urol 2016 Mar;34(3):419–24.

Wang CH, Fang CC, Chen NC, et al. Cranberry-containing products for prevention of urinary tract infections in susceptible populations: a systematic review and meta-analysis of randomized controlled trials. Arch Intern Med Jul 9 2012;172(13):988–96.

Woźniewicz M, Nowaczyk PM, Kurhańska-Flisykowska A, et al. Consumption of cranberry functional beverage reduces gingival index and plaque index in patients with gingivitis. Nutr Res 2018 Oct;58:36–45.

39

DANDELION (*TARAXACUM OFFICINALE*)
Leaf and Root

GENERAL OVERVIEW

A resilient plant that invades proudly groomed lawns and sends folks to the local nursery for herbicidal lawn chemicals, dandelion has been used traditionally for the treatment of numerous disorders including gastric, renal, and hepatic ailments, diabetes, and cancer. It is considered a detoxifier and an antioxidant. Dandelion has beneficial constituents in its leaves, roots, and fruit (seed pods). Although human data are practically nonexistent, vast traditional use lends this plant some credibility as a powerhouse of healing. The European Scientific Cooperative on Phytotherapy (ESCOP) recommends using dandelion root to improve liver function and bile production, for indigestion, and for lack of appetite. The German Commission E has approved its use for loss of appetite, dyspepsia, and diuresis. Because toxicity has not been reported, consumption of dandelion is qualified under the Generally Recognized as Safe (GRAS) seal by the USFDA.

Although quite limited, clinical research indicates that dandelion, alone or in combination formulas, may be beneficial for hypertension, diabetes, dyspepsia, irritable bowel syndrome, and ovarian androgen excess.

IN VITRO AND ANIMAL RESEARCH

The leaf has diuretic, choleretic, and anti-inflammatory properties. The bitters in the leaves not only stimulate digestive secretions and gastric motility but also have laxative properties. The potassium-sparing diuretic effect is on level with pharmaceuticals. Dandelion has also been shown to have lipid-lowering and antioxidant activities.

The root has choleretic, cholagogic, tonic, anti-rheumatic, digestive-stimulant, alterative and depurative properties. It is detoxifying via promotion of biliary drainage. It is also hepatoprotective in cases of fatty liver.

In vitro research has demonstrated that the crude extract of dandelion leaf decreases growth of certain strains of breast cancer cells and blocks invasion of breast cancer and prostate cancer cells. Other research has shown that the aqueous extract of dandelion root induces programmed cell death in > 95% of colon cancer cells, regardless of their p53 status, by 48 hours of treatment. Other research has shown anticancer properties against melanoma and leukemia cell lines.

An in vitro and in vivo study in mice to measure the inhibition of pancreatic lipase compared dandelion leaf ethanolic extract with orlistat. Dandelion and orlistat inhibited porcine pancreatic lipase activity by 86.3% and 95.7%. A single oral dose of dandelion significantly inhibited increases in plasma triglyceride levels at 90 and 180 min and reduced the AUC of the TG response curve ($P < 0.05$). The authors concluded that dandelion inhibited pancreatic lipase (Zhang et al., 2008).

Mice on a high-fat diet were fed dandelion leaf extract to determine the effect on hepatic steatosis. The high-fat diet supplemented by dandelion dramatically reduced hepatic lipid accumulation compared with a high-fat diet alone. Dandelion supplementation also dramatically suppressed TG, TC, insulin, fasting glucose, and HOMA-IR induced by the high-fat diet. Further, it increased activation of AMPK in liver and muscle, suppressed lipid accumulation in the liver, and reduced insulin resistance and lipids via the AMPK pathway. The authors concluded that dandelion leaf extract may have promise for prevention and treatment of obesity related NAFLD (Davaatseren et al., 2013).

Various fractions of a 70% ethanolic extract of dandelion were administered to mice to determine gastric emptying. The percentage of gastric emptying was 48.8% (vehicle control), 75.3% (cisapride positive control), 68% (ethanolic extract of dandelion), 53% (ethyl acetate fraction), 54% (aqueous fraction), and 86% (butanol fraction). The butanol fraction had been shown to increase spontaneous contractions of the gastric fundus and antrum and decrease the spontaneous motility of the pyloric sphincter in vitro, an activity that was blocked by atropine. The authors concluded that the butanol fraction of dandelion ethanolic extract held promise as a prokinetic agent (Jin et al., 2011).

Dandelion leaf extract at a dose of 500 mg/kg was orally administered to rats once per day for 30 days consecutively, followed by 10 mg/kg sodium dichromate intraperitoneal injection for 10 days. Sodium dichromate caused acute liver damage, necrosis of hepatocytes, and DNA fragmentation. Animals that were pretreated with dandelion showed hepatoprotection, revealed by a significant reduction of oxidative damage for all tested markers (Hfaiedh et al., 2016).

A study in rats was undertaken to investigate the protective activity of dandelion fruit extract against sodium nitroprusside-induced decreased cellular viability and increased lipid peroxidation in the cortex, hippocampus, and striatum of rats in vitro. Slices of cortex, hippocampus, and striatum were treated with 50 μM sodium nitroprusside and dandelion fruit ethanolic extract (1–20 μg/mL) to determine cellular viability. The extract protected against decreases in cellular viability and increases in lipid peroxidation in the cortex, hippocampus, and striatum. The extract had scavenger activity against DPPH and NO at low concentrations and was able to protect against H_2O_2 and Fe^2+ induced deoxyribose oxidation. The authors concluded that dandelion fruit extract had antioxidant activity and protected brain slices against sodium nitroprusside-induced cellular death (Colle et al., 2012a,b).

Mice subjected to swimming, tail suspension, and open field tests were given dandelion leaf and root water extract to assess behavioral changes and adrenal axis hormone changes. Chronic treatment (14 days) at the doses of 50, 100, and 200 mg/kg significantly de-

creased the immobility time in both swimming (92.6, 85.1, and 77.4 s, respectively) and tail suspension (84.8, 72.1, and 56.9 s, respectively). Acute treatment (1 day) at a dose of 200 mg/kg also markedly decreased the immobility time in swimming (81.7 s) and tail suspension (73.2 s). There was no change with the open field test. Chronic treatment with 200 mg/kg attenuated an increase in CRH (from 5.8 ng/mL to 3.9 ng/mL). Chronic treatment with 200 mg/kg and 50 mg/kg attenuated the rise in corticosterone from 37.3 ng/mL to 19.8 ng/mL and 29.9 ng/mL, respectively. The authors concluded that dandelion water extract had antidepressant effects in models of behavioral despair and suggested that the mechanism involved the neuroendocrine system (Li et al., 2014).

Mice were treated with 2.5, 5, and 10 mg/kg of taraxasterol, a pentacyclic-triterpene constituent of dandelion, prior to a lethal dose of a lipopolysaccharide challenge. Taraxasterol significantly improved mouse survival and attenuated tissue injury of the lungs. The constituent also reduced TNF-α, IFN-γ, IL-1β, IL-6, NO, and PGE_2 levels in sera from mice with endotoxic shock. The authors concluded that taraxasterol had a protective effect on murine endotoxic shock induced by lipopolysaccharide through modulating inflammatory cytokine and mediator secretion (Zhang et al., 2014).

HUMAN RESEARCH

Cardiovascular Disorders: Hypertension

A 2-day open-label pilot trial in volunteers ($n = 17$) investigated the effects of dandelion leaf ethanolic extract 8 mL TID for one day on urinary output. Urinary frequency increased significantly after the first dose in all subjects ($P < 0.05$). There was also a significant ($P < 0.001$) increase in the excretion ratio (urination volume/fluid intake) in the 5-h period after the second dose of extract. The third dose did not change any of the measured parameters. The authors concluded that dandelion showed promise as a diuretic (Clare et al., 2009).

Cardiometabolic Disorders: Diabetes

A 12-week unblinded prospective study in patients ($n = 119$) with T2DM investigated the efficacy of a combination of dandelion plus stinging nettle, cinnamon, tarragon, and Morus alba as add-on therapy for glycemic and lipid response. At 12 weeks, A1C decreased from 9.0% to 7.1% (22% reduction; $P < 0.0001$), mean blood glucose decreased from 211 mg/dL to 133 mg/dL (37% reduction; $P < 0.0001$), mean TC decreased to 185 mg/dL (13% reduction; $P < 0.01$) and mean serum TG decreased to 160 mg/dL (40% reduction; $P < 0.001$). Of the 13 patients requiring insulin, five were able to get off insulin and five reduced their daily insulin requirements by at least 30%. No response was noted in 12% of patients. Clinical observations included improvements in vasculopathy, including reversal of established retinopathic changes in two patients. No major adverse effects were observed, with minor abdominal symptoms reported in 16 patients (16%). The authors concluded that this herbal combination reduced A1C, glucose, and lipids with good tolerability (Chatterji and Fogel, 2018).

Gastrointestinal Disorders: Dyspepsia and Irritable Bowel Syndrome

A 60-day open-label study in patients ($n = 311$) with functional dyspepsia investigated the effect of the combination product Cynarepa (dandelion, rosemary, artichoke leaf, and turmeric) on a 10-point scale. The herbal formula resulted in steadily increasing improvement in functional dyspepsia symptoms. A 50% reduction in the total scores of all symptoms was recorded in 38% of patients at 30 days and in 79% at 60 days. At 60 days, TC, LDL-C, and TG levels had decreased by 6%–8% over baseline values ($P < 0.001$); AST, ALT, and GGT concentrations had diminished by 13–20 U/l ($P < 0.01$) in patients with relatively elevated baseline values (Sannia, 2010).

An open-label trial in patients ($n = 24$) with chronic non-specific colitis assessed the effect of an herbal combination that included dandelion. The spontaneous and palpable pains along the large intestine disappeared in 95.83% of patients by the 15th day and those with constipation had normalization of bowel movements (Chakŭrski et al., 1981).

Women's Genitourinary Disorders
Androgen Excess

A pilot RCT in healthy premenopausal women ($n = 40$) investigated the hormonal effects of a combination botanical supplement (dandelion, schisandra, turmeric, rosemary, milk thistle, and artichoke leaf) compared with dietary changes (three servings/d crucifers or dark leafy greens, 30 g/day fiber, 1–2 L/day of water,

and limiting caffeine and alcohol consumption to one serving per week) and with placebo. During the early follicular phase, compared with placebo, the polyherbal product decreased DHEA (-13.2%; $P = 0.02$), DHEA-S (-14.6%; $P = 0.07$), androstenedione (-8.6%; $P = 0.05$), and estrone-sulfate (-12.0%; $P = 0.08$). When comparing dietary changes with placebo, no statistically significant differences were observed. There were no substantial effects on estrone-sulfate, total estradiol, free estradiol, testosterone, SHBG, insulin, IGF-I, or leptin. The authors concluded that early-follicular phase androgens were decreased with the polyherbal product (Greenlee et al., 2007).

ACTIVE CONSTITUENTS

Leaf and Root

- Carbohydrates: polysaccharides
- Amino acid derivatives
  - Peptides: taraxicum officinale antimicrobial peptides (ToAMPs 1-4)
- Phenolic compounds
  - Phenolic acids
  - Coumarins: aesculin (venotonic, lymphatotonic)
  - Flavonoids: isovitexin (hepatoprotective, anticarcinogenic, apoptotic, anti-staphylococcal)
- Terpenes
  - Terpenoids (bitter principles—promote gastric and digestive enzyme secretions, gastric motility, biliary drainage, anti-inflammatory, diuretic): taraxasterol, eudesmanolide, germacranolide types
    - ☐ Tetraterpenoids/Carotenoids (stimulate granulation tissue): lutein, β-carotene, lutein epoxide
- Steroids
  - Phytosterols: sitosterin, stigmasterin, phytosterin
- Potassium
- Vitamin A

Unique to Root

- Carbohydrates
  - Oligosaccharides (prebiotic): inulin (immunostimulating via macrophage phagocytosis, anti-inflammatory, prebiotic, hypoglycemic), kestose, mystose, and fructofuranosylnystose

- Phenolic compounds:
  - Flavonoids: hesperidin

Unique to Leaf

- Phenolic compounds
  - Phenylpropanoids (antioxidant, antimutagenic, antitumor, antimicrobial, anti-hylauronidase activity, immunomodulatory, anti-HIV, apoptotic): chicoric acid, chlorogenic acid, caffeic acid
  - Flavonoids: luteolin (anti-inflammatory, antispasmodic, antibacterial, hepatoprotective, anti-estrogenic, antiproliferative), vitexin (antioxidant, anti-inflammatory, hepatoprotective, estrogen-β agonism, anti-hyperalgesic, anti-arthritis, neuroprotective, antidepressant, dopaminergic, serotonergic, anti-cancer)
    - Anthocyanins (antioxidant, anti-inflammatory, antineoplastic)
- Terpenes
  - Sesquiterpenes lactones: eudesmanolides (diuretic, anti-inflammatory, increase gastric acid), taraxacin (bitter principle), lactucin, lactupiricin)

DANDELION COMMONLY USED PREPARATIONS AND DOSAGE (FOR ADULTS UNLESS OTHERWISE SPECIFIED)

The following are examples of some available formulations and ranges of dosing for commercial herbal products. See Part III Introduction "How to prescribe medicinal herbs" for further guidance on herbal advising and prescribing.

Leaf

- Infusion of dried leaf: 1–2 tsp per cup TID
- Succus (pressed sap from fresh plant): 5–10 mL BID
- Tincture (1:5, 25%–40%): 3–10 mL TID
- Encapsulated freeze-dried leaf: 180–250 mg QD-TID

Organically grown fresh spring leaves can be eaten raw in salads.

Root

- Decoction: 2–3 tsp per cup TID
- Tincture (1:5, 60%): 3–8 mL TID
- Powdered root extract (4:1): 1 g (1/3 tsp) BID
- Capsule or tablet of powdered root extract: 1–2 g QD-BID

SAFETY AND PRECAUTION

Side Effects

Contact dermatitis is a possible side effect. Avoid dandelion if ragweed or other flower allergies (Compositae allergies) exist. Some people with latex allergies are allergic to the milky latex in the leaves. Children are more likely to have allergic reactions to dandelion. The roots contain inulin and thus should be avoided in individuals with inulin allergy. Overconsumption of tea (10 + cups per day) may cause hyperoxaluria.

Case Reports

Contact dermatitis; TEN due to contact with leaves; hypoglycemia in diabetic woman on insulin after 2 weeks of dandelion greens in salad.

Toxicity

Higher than normal doses in rats produced testicular damage.

Pregnancy and Lactation

Dandelion leaf tea has commonly been used, but no formal studies of safety have been performed.

Disease Interactions

Avoid with common duct stones and use with caution with all forms of cholelithiasis due to risk of obstructing the common bile duct. Caution with GERD, PUD, or gastritis due to increase in acid production.

Drug Interactions

- CYP: Inhibits CYP1A2 and CYP3A4
- UGT: Induces UGT
- May augment effects of hypoglycemic agents
- Avoid with other diuretics and lithium
- Caution with antihypertensives and anticoagulants
- May reduce absorption of fluoroquinolones

REFERENCES

Chakŭrski I, Matev M, Koĭchev A, Angelova I, Stefanov G. Treatment of chronic colitis with an herbal combination of Taraxacum officinale, Hipericum perforatum, Melissa officinalis, Calendula officinalis and Foeniculum vulgare. Vutr Boles 1981;20(6):51–4.

Chatterji S, Fogel D. Study of the effect of the herbal composition SR2004 on hemoglobin A1C, fasting blood glucose, and lipids in patients with type 2 diabetes mellitus. Integr Med Res 2018;7(3):248–56.

Clare BA, Conroy RS, Spelman K. The diuretic effect in human subjects of an extract of *Taraxacum officinale* folium over a single day. J Altern Complement Med 2009;15(8):929–34.

Colle D, Arantes LP, Gubert P, da Luz SC, Athayde ML, Teixeira Rocha JB, Soares FA. Antioxidant properties of Taraxacum officinale leaf extract are involved in the protective effect against hepatoxicity induced by acetaminophen in mice. J Med Food 2012 Jun;15(6):549-56.

Colle D, Arantes LP, Rauber R, et al. Antioxidant properties of Taraxacum officinale fruit extract are involved in the protective effect against cellular death induced by sodium nitroprusside in brain of rats. Pharm Biol 2012b;50(7):883–91.

Davaatseren M, et al. Taraxacum official (dandelion) leaf extract alleviates high-fat diet-induced nonalcoholic fatty liver. Food Chem Toxicol 2013;58:30–6.

Greenlee H, Atkinson C, Stanczyk FZ, Lampe JW. A pilot and feasibility study on the effects of naturopathic botanical and dietary interventions on sex steroid hormone metabolism in premenopausal women. Cancer Epidemiol Biomarkers Prev 2007;16(8):1601–9.

Hfaiedh M, Brahmi D, Zourgui L. Hepatoprotective effect of Taraxacum officinale leaf extract on sodium dichromate-induced liver injury in rats. Environ Toxicol 2016;31(3):339–49.

Jin YR, et al. The effect of Taraxacum officinale on gastric emptying and smooth muscle motility in Rodents. Neurogastroenterol Motil 2011.

Li YC, et al. Antidepressant effects of the water extract from Taraxacum officinale leaves and roots in mice. Pharm Biol 2014.

Sannia A. Phytotherapy with a mixture of dry extracts with hepatoprotective effects containing artichoke leaves in the management of functional dyspepsia symptoms. Minerva Gastroenterol Dietol 2010;56(2):93–9.

Zhang J, et al. Pancreatic lipase inhibitory activity of taraxacum officinale in vitro and *in vivo*. Nutr Res Pract 2008.

Zhang X, Xiong H, Li H, Cheng Y. Protective effect of taraxasterol against LPS-induced endotoxic shock by modulating inflammatory responses in mice. Immunopharmacol Immunotoxicol 2014;36(1):11–6.

40

DONG QUAI (*ANGELICA SINENSIS*)
Root

GENERAL OVERVIEW

Dong quai is used extensively in traditional Chinese medicine (TCM) multi-herbal prescriptions for replenishing blood and treating abnormal menstruation and other women's diseases. It has been used in the treatment of cardiovascular disease, cerebrovascular disease, gynecologic disease, nervous system disease, and nephrotic syndrome. It is considered an adaptogen for women's issues and is known for its hematopoietic, antioxidant, and immunoregulatory activities. Dong quai has been part of a well-researched and effective TCM formula for menopause and menstrual cramps. It appears to require the synergism of other plants for optimal effects.

Clinical research indicates that dong quai, alone or in combination formulas, may be beneficial for pulmonary hypertension due to chronic obstructive pulmonary disease, coronary artery disease, portal hypertension, chronic abdominal pain, ulcerative colitis, perimenopause, menopause, stroke recovery, anemia of kidney disease, and tamoxifen-induced endometrial cancer.

IN VITRO AND ANIMAL RESEARCH

Dong quai has anticoagulant and antiplatelet activities and contains coumarins but to a lesser degree than other *Angelica* species. It also has immune-stimulant and hematopoietic activities attributed to its polysaccharides and B vitamin content. It contains chemicals with antispasmodic as well as uterotonic activities that appear to work synergistically to alleviate dysmenor-

rhea. Three of dong quai's chemical constituents have properties that may be beneficial for bone and joint health via anti-inflammation, chondrocyte maintenance, glycosaminoglycan synthesis, osteoblast proliferation, and hyaluronic acid deposition. The herb has also shown neuroprotective, antitumor, pro-apoptotic, and anti-metastatic properties.

Animal studies have shown that dong quai, when combined with astragalus, prevents renal fibrosis on par with enalapril. It has also been shown to have quinidine-like activity in the heart, correcting experimental atrial fibrillation and improving coronary arterial flow. When combined with *Ligusticum* it inhibits ROS and promotes endothelial NOS expression and has been shown to be cardioprotective after induction of myocardial injury. Other animal studies have shown dong quai polysaccharides to protect from the toxicities of cyclophosphamide, doxorubicin, and radiation.

Imperatorin, a chemical constituent of dong quai, was investigated in rat model of HTN in a 10-week trial. Mean BP was significantly reduced by treatment with imperatorin at 6.25, 12.5, and 25 mg/kg/day. Renal catalase and xanthine oxidase activities, glutathione levels, NO, and NOS levels were significantly increased with imperatorin. Plasma endothelin, renal angiotensin II, MDA levels, and 24-h urinary excretion of 8-iso-PGF2α were decreased with imperatorin (Cao et al., 2013).

A 4-week study looking at the anti-osteoporosis effects of dong quai in ovariectomized rats compared 17β-estradiol 10 mcg/kg i.p. once daily to dong quai extract 30, 100, and 300 mg/kg p.o. once daily and to no treatment. The BMD of rats treated with the extract at a dose of 300 mg/kg was significantly higher than that of the control, reaching the BMD of the estradiol group. Serum ALP, collagen type I C-telopeptide, and osteocalcin were significantly decreased in the extract group. The body and uterus weight and serum estradiol concentration were not affected, and no treatment-related toxicity was observed during extract administration in rats (Lim and Kim, 2014).

Two main constituents of dong quai, sodium ferulate and a polysaccharidic fraction, have been shown in animal research to have benefit for osteoarthritis. Sodium ferulate has marked anti-inflammatory and antiapoptotic properties by inhibiting TNF-TNFR signal transduction. The polysaccharidic fraction promotes proteoglycan biosynthesis in cartilage matrix by stimulating the activity of UGT, which synthesizes the chondroitin sulfate chains of aggrecan (Magdalou et al., 2015).

The dong quai constituent ligustilide has demonstrated neuroprotection in the brain of aging mice. Maze testing showed that ligustilide administration markedly improved behavioral performance of d-galactose treated mice. This action could be partly due to reduction of the level of MDA as well as an increase in the activity of Na+-K+-ATPase (Li et al., 2015). The polysaccharides in dong quai have been shown to protect PC12 neuronal cells from H2O2-induced cytotoxicity and reduce apoptosis and intracellular ROS levels. In a rat model of local cerebral ischemia, dong quai polysaccharides were shown to enhance antioxidant activity in cerebral cortical neurons, increase the number of microvessels, and improve blood flow after ischemia (Lei et al., 2014).

Dong quai has been reported to promote hair growth. A group of mice treated with dong quai showed noticeable hair regrowth, restoring the lengths of hair shafts and size of hair follicles. SBD-4, a patented root aqueous extract of dong quai, has been shown to increase the strength of healed wounds in older rats. In zebrafish and in human skin DNA microarray research, there appears to be skin repair and regeneration. When combined with several types of wound dressings, SBD-4 increased type I collagen production in human dermal fibroblasts, and when formulated in nanosilver hydrocolloid dressing, it was found effective in wound healing in four patients with chronic nonhealing ulcers (Zhao et al., 2012).

A 6-week mouse study compared dong quai at different strengths to vehicle in exercised mice to assess effects on ergogenic and anti-fatigue functions. Dong quai treatments significantly increased endurance swimming time and blood glucose level, and decreased serum lactate, ammonia, and CK levels. Liver and muscle glycogen contents were higher with dong quai than with vehicle (Yeh and Chung, 2014).

Dong quai displays potency in suppressing the growth of malignant brain tumor cells via cell cycle arrest and apoptosis. Dong quai upregulates expression of cyclin kinase inhibitors, including p16, to decrease the phosphorylation of Rb proteins, resulting in arrest at the G0–G1 phase. The expression of the p53 protein is increased by dong quai, likely underlying the increase in apoptosis. Dong quai not only suppresses the growth of human malignant brain tumors but also significantly prolongs survival. It also has anti-angiogenic activity. Dong quai extracts cultured for 24 h with mouse glioblastoma cells significantly inhibited the proliferative activity of the cells by 30%–50% as well as the expression of cathepsin B and VEGF. In vivo in mice, the growth of the tumor was inhibited by 30% at 20 mg/kg ($P < 0.05$) and by 60% at 60 mg/kg ($P < 0.05$). The extracts also significantly inhibited neovascular formation in the tumors (Lee et al., 2006).

Dong quai has been shown to not have estrogenic activity in menopausal women. However, in vitro studies have shown that the water extract of dong quai stimulates the growth of MCF-7 cells, possibly due to weak estrogen-agonistic activity, and augments the BT-20 cell proliferation independently of the estrogen receptor-mediated pathway. It is generally thought best to avoid this herb in the presence of estrogen-sensitive cancers.

HUMAN RESEARCH

The human evidence for dong quai in isolation is sparse and may under-represent the potential uses for this herb. In most of the research, treatment with dong quai entailed use of formulas that also contain 3–10 additional herbs, as is typical of TCM therapy. Therefore, efficacy cannot be ascribed to dong quai in isolation. However, preclinical evidence allows for some extrapolation as to the activities that dong quai contributes to such polyherbal formulas. An additional caveat for human evidence is that when used alone in trials, it is often administered intravenously.

Pulmonary Disorders: Chronic Obstructive Pulmonary Disease With Pulmonary Hypertension

A 10-day study in patients ($n = 60$) with COPD complicated by pulmonary HTN investigated daily injections of 25% dong quai compared with D5W. The levels of mean pulmonary arterial pressure, pulmonary vascular resistance, blood endothelin-1, AT-II, and end-diastolic flow were reduced by 18%, 27%, 20%, 36%, and 38%, respectively, with dong quai. PaO_2 was increased with dong quai ($P < 0.05$). The control group showed only insignificant differences in the parameters studied. The authors concluded that dong quai injection could improve pulmonary hemodynamics and increase PaO_2 in patients with COPD and pulmonary HTN (Xu and Li, 2000).

A study in patients ($n = 40$) with COPD and pulmonary HTN investigated 25% dong quai injections 250 mL QD compared with nifedipine 10 mg po TID, with dong quai plus nifedipine, and with placebo. Mean pulmonary arterial pressure was decreased and cardiac output and PaO_2 were increased significantly ($P < 0.05$; $P < 0.01$, respectively) in the combination group. In the nifedipine alone group, the PaO_2 decreased, and this appeared to be corrected with addition of dong quai (Xu et al., 1992).

Cardiovascular Disorders: Coronary Artery Disease

A 1-year RCT in patients ($n = 426$) with ACS and mild-to-moderate renal insufficiency (eGFR 30–89 mL/min) evaluated the effect of Western medicine alone (control group) compared with Western medicine plus six months of a TCM-based formula of Chuanxiong capsules (dong quai and *Ligusticum chuanxioing*) plus Xinyu capsules (American ginseng). After 1 year, the composite of cardiac death, nonfatal recurrent myocardial infarction, and ischemia-driven revascularization occurred in 16 patients in the control group and in 6 patients in the treatment group (ARR = 0.046;

RR = 0.38; $P = 0.040$). The composite of stroke, congestive heart failure, and readmission for ACS occurred in 15 patients in the control group and five cases in the combined therapy group (ARR = 0.041; RR = 0.34; $P = 0.033$). The eGFRs in the treatment and control groups were 75.1 mL/min and 72.03 mL/min, respectively ($P < 0.05$). The eGFR in the TCM group was significantly higher after the intervention than the baseline of 72.27 ($P < 0.05$). The authors concluded that Chinese herbal medicines plus Western medicine standard therapy improved cardiac and renal clinical outcomes in patients with ACS and mild-to-moderate renal insufficiency more than Western medicine alone (Zhang et al., 2020).

A study in patients with coronary artery disease compared injections of a combination of ginseng, astragalus, and dong quai with placebo (D10W) for effects on disease symptoms. With the polyherbal formula the frequency and severity of angina episodes were reduced by 90%, and the ischemic ST-T changes on ECG improved in 56% of cases. The tolerance to treadmill exercise was increased from 348 to 503 M. Left ventricular function improved (PEP/LVET ratio decreased from 0.45 to 0.36). Blood viscosity and erythrocyte electrophoretic time decreased. Platelet aggregation and platelet adhesion were inhibited by 27% and 59%, respectively. Thromboxane B2 levels decreased from 260 to 139 pg/mL. Plasma 6-keto-PGF1 alpha level increased from 33.45 to 57.5 pg/mL. The differences were all statistically significant ($P < 0.05$-0.01) compared with placebo (Liao et al., 1989).

Gastrointestinal Disorders: Portal Hypertension

An open-label study assessed the acute and chronic effect of dong quai on serum gastrin levels in patients with cirrhosis. The results showed that after intravenous infusion of dong quai, serum gastrin levels from the inferior vena cava, hepatic, and peripheral veins were significantly decreased. After long-term administration of the agent, the levels fell nearly to that of control subjects. The authors suggested that the effect of reducing serum gastrin levels by dong quai may improve portal hemodynamics and be beneficial for portal hypertensive mucosal lesions in cirrhosis (Huang et al., 1996).

Gastrointestinal Disorders: Chronic Abdominal Pain

A study in patients ($n = 207$) with chronic abdominal pain compared dong quai with atropine and with placebo for efficacy. The efficacy rate of abdominal pain in the three groups were 93.3%, 97.1%, and 0% with dong quai, atropine, and placebo, respectively. The difference between dong quai and atropine was not statistically significant ($P > 0.05$), and the difference between dong quai and placebo was significant ($P < 0.01$). The authors attributed the beneficial effect of dong quai to the blocking of muscarinic, alpha and H1 receptors, an analgesic effect, and an antiseptic effect (Sun and Wang, 1992).

Gastrointestinal Disorders: Ulcerative Colitis

A 3-week study in patients with active UC ($n = 39$), UC in remission ($n = 25$) and healthy volunteers ($n = 30$) compared routine treatment alone with routine treatment plus dong quai injection for impact on microcirculation. At baseline, the platelet counts, 1-min platelet aggregation rate, and levels of alpha granule membrane protein, thromboxane B2, and von Willebrand factor-related antigen in active UC were significantly higher than those in remissive UC, which were higher than normal controls ($P < 0.05$–0.01). These parameters were significantly improved after treatment in dong quai group ($P < 0.05$–0.01), whereas they all changed minimally in routine therapy group ($P > 0.05$). The authors concluded that dong quai can inhibit platelet activation, relieve vascular endothelial injury, and improve microcirculation in UC (Dong et al., 2004).

Women's Genitourinary Disorders: Perimenopause and Menopause

A 2003 systematic review to assess the efficacy of herbal medicinal products for treatment of menopausal symptoms selected 18 RCTs that met inclusion criteria. One study concerned dong quai, the others being black cohosh, red clover, kava, evening primrose oil, ginseng, and combination products. The authors concluded that there was no convincing evidence for any herbal medical product in the treatment of menopausal symptoms. However, the evidence for black cohosh was promising, albeit limited by the poor methodology of the trials. The studies involving red clover suggested it may be of benefit for more severe menopausal symptoms. There was some evidence for the use of kava, but safety concerns were raised. The evidence was inconclusive for the other herbal medicinal products reviewed (Huntley and Ernst, 2003).

A 12-week RCT in postmenopausal women ($n = 55$) with hot flushes and refusing hormonal therapy compared Climex (combination of dong quai and chamomile) five tablets daily between meals with placebo. There was a significant difference between Climex and placebo in the decrease in number and intensity of hot flushes from baseline to completion of treatment (90%-96% and 15%-25%, respectively; $P < 0.001$). With the herbal combination there was a 68% reduction in daytime hot flushes and a 74% reduction in nighttime hot flushes after the first month. There was also a marked alleviation of sleep disturbances and fatigue. The authors concluded that Climex seemed to be effective for menopausal symptoms without apparent major adverse effects (Kupfersztain et al., 2003).

A 3-month RCT in women ($n = 50$) who were pre- and postmenopausal compared Phyto-Female Complex (standardized extracts of dong quai, black cohosh, milk thistle, red clover, American ginseng, and chasteberry) with placebo for effects on menopausal symptoms. The women receiving Phyto-Female Complex reported a significantly greater mean reduction in menopausal symptoms than the placebo group. By 3 months there was a 73% decrease in hot flushes and a 69% reduction of night sweats, a decrease in hot flush intensity and a significant improvement in sleep quality. Hot flushes ceased completely in 47% of women in the study group compared with only 19% in the placebo group. There were no changes in findings on vaginal ultrasonography or levels of relevant hormones (estradiol, FSH), liver enzymes or TSH in either group. The authors concluded that this formulation was safe and effective for relief of hot flushes and sleep disturbances in pre- and post-menopausal women (Rotem and Kaplan, 2007).

A 6-month RCT in women ($n = 50$) with symptomatic menopause compared a combination of dong quai and astragalus with placebo. There was a significant reduction in the number of mild hot flushes per month with herbal treatment (from 18.9 to 8.6 at 6 months; $P < 0.01$) but not with placebo (from 26 to 12.4; $P = 0.062$). For moderate flushes, there was a significant reduction with placebo vs herbal treatment (from 18.9 to 11.1; $P < 0.05$, vs from 10.5 to 6.0; $P = 0.107$, respectively). There was no significant change in either treatment or placebo groups in the reporting of severe hot flushes. Episodes of night sweats decreased significantly in the placebo but not in the treatment group. In the vasomotor domain of the Menopause Specific Quality of Life, there was a significant reduction in scoring in the placebo but not in the treatment group. The authors concluded that there was no overall significant difference between dong quai plus astragalus and placebo for the treatment of menopausal vasomotor symptoms (Haines et al., 2008).

A 24-week RCT in postmenopausal women ($n = 71$) with FSH levels $> 30\,\mathrm{mIU/mL}$ and hot flushes compared dong quai with placebo for effects on endometrial and vaginal cells as well as symptoms. There were no significant differences between groups in endometrial thickness, vaginal maturation index, number of vasomotor flushes, or Kupperman Index. The authors concluded that when used alone, dong quai does not produce estrogen-like responses in tissue and did not relieve menopausal symptoms (Hirata et al., 1997).

Neurological Disorders: Stroke

A 25-day study in patients ($n = 1404$) with acute cerebral infarction investigated dong quai injection compared with sage and with low molecular dextran injections for effect on infarct volume and neurofunction deficits. The total effective rate was 78.7%, 63.6%, and 59.3% for dong quai, sage, and dextran, respectively. Dong quai was more effective than the other two groups ($P < 0.05$). The improvement of neurofunction deficit scores and Barthel scores were better with dong quai than with sage or dextran on the 25th day ($P < 0.01$), and the decrease in volume of infarct with dong quai was greater than that with dextran ($P < 0.01$). The authors concluded that dong quai injection had a therapeutic effect in treating acute cerebral infarction (Liu et al., 2004).

Hematologic Disorders: Anemia of Chronic Kidney Disease

A case report of a patient with chronic renal failure and anemia of chronic disease unresponsive to human erythropoietin (as occurs with 4% of patients in this group) indicated that after the patient self-initiated regular consumption of dong quai, there was significant improvement in hematopoiesis despite the patient having decreased the human erythropoietin dosing (Bradley et al., 1999).

Oncologic Disorders: Tamoxifen-Induced Endometrial Cancer

An epidemiologic study of patients newly diagnosed with invasive breast cancer who received tamoxifen treatment from January 1, 1998, to December 31, 2008 were investigated for usage of Chinese herbal products containing dong quai. Almost 50% of study subjects had used dong quai. Among 31,938 tamoxifen-treated breast cancer survivors, 157 cases of subsequent endometrial cancer were identified. The hazard ratio for development of endometrial cancer among breast cancer survivors aged 20–79 years who had taken dong quai after tamoxifen treatment was 0.61 relative to patients who had never taken dong quai. This effect was stronger in younger women (Wu et al., 2014).

ACTIVE CONSTITUENTS

- Carbohydrates
  - Polysaccharides (promote proteoglycan synthesis, neuroprotective, pro-circulatory): high molecular weight polysaccharide (immunostimulating, hematopoietic).
- Phenolic compounds
  - Phenylpropanoids (antioxidant, antimutagenic, antitumor, antimicrobial): ferulic acid (antiplatelet, anti-TNF)
  - Coumarins (low levels) (venotonic, lymphatotonic): angelol, angelicone, oxypeucedanin, osthole (antiproliferative, anti-inflammatory, hepatoprotective, neuroprotective, antiosteoporotic, anticonvulsant, antiplatelet, antiallergic, anticancer), and 7-desmethylsuberosin
  - Furaoncoumarins: psoralen, bergapten (anti-inflammatory, neuroprotective, dermatoprotective, photosensitizing, anticancer), imperatorin (antioxidant, antihypertensive)
- Steroids
  - Phytosterols: beta-sitosterol
- Aromatic compounds: asligustilide, butylidenephthalide (anti-cancer), and butylphthalide (antispasmodic), n-butylidenephthalide, ligustilide (neuro-protective), n-butylphthalide, senkyunolide A
- Vitamins A, B12, E, C, folinic acid, biotin

DONG QUAI COMMONLY USED PREPARATIONS AND DOSAGE (FOR ADULTS UNLESS OTHERWISE SPECIFIED)

The following are examples of some available formulations and ranges of dosing for commercial herbal products. See Part III Introduction "How to prescribe medicinal herbs" for further guidance on herbal advising and prescribing.

Root

- Decoction or infusion of dried root: 1 tsp per cup TID
- Tincture (1:5, 60%): 1–2 mL up to TID
- Powdered root: 1000 mg QD-TID
- Capsule or tablet of powdered root: 0.5–1 g QD-TID
- Essential oil: diffusion and other aromatherapy methods as directed by a certified aromatherapist

SAFETY AND PRECAUTION

Side Effects

Occasional photosensitivity (especially essential oil), bloating, anorexia, diarrhea, gynecomastia, and HTN

Case Reports

Several case reports of excessively prolonged INR when taken concurrently with warfarin.

Pregnant and Lactation

Potential hormonal effects. Avoid.

Disease Interactions

Patients with hormone-sensitive cancers should avoid dong quai due to possible estrogenic effects and to proliferative effects on breast cancer cells in vitro.

Drug Interactions

- CYP: Induces CYP3A4
- Possible synergism with lamivudine-zidovudine (in rabbits)
- General consensus is that it may potentiate anticoagulants. However, research suggests otherwise (see below)
- May exacerbate anemia with lisinopril

An RCT in healthy volunteers ($n = 25$) assessed the anticoagulant effects of three herbs (turmeric, Asian ginseng, and dong quai) compared with aspirin alone or aspirin plus the herbal product in 3-week phases with 2-week washouts. PT/APTT, platelet function by light transmission aggregometry, and thrombin generation assay by calibrated automated thrombogram were measured at baseline and after each phase. Inhibition of arachidonic-acid induced platelet aggregation occurred in 5/24 turmeric subjects, 2/24 dong quai subjects, and 1/23 ginseng subjects. Beyond that, there was no clinically relevant impact on platelet and coagulation function. Combination of these herbal products with aspirin respectively did not further aggravate platelet inhibition caused by aspirin. None of the herbs impaired PT/APTT or thrombin generation. There was no significant bleeding manifestation. The authors concluded that there was good evidence for lack of bleeding risks with turmeric, dong quai, and Asian ginseng either alone or in combination with aspirin (Fung et al., 2017).

REFERENCES

Bradley RR, Cunniff PJ, Pereira BJ, Jaber BL. Hematopoietic effect of Radix angelicae sinensis in a hemodialysis patient. Am J Kidney Dis 1999;34(2):349–54.

Cao YJ, He X, Wang N, He LC. Effects of imperatorin, the active component from Radix Angelicae (Baizhi), on the BP and oxidative stress in 2K,1C hypertensive rats. Phytomedicine 2013;20(12):1048–54.

Dong WG, Liu SP, Zhu HH, Luo HS, Yu JP. Abnormal function of platelets and role of angelica sinensis in patients with ulcerative colitis. World J Gastroenterol 2004;10(4):606–9.

Fung FY, Wong WH, Ang SK, et al. A randomized, double-blind, placebo-controlled study on the anti-haemostatic effects of Curcuma longa, Angelica sinensis and Panax ginseng. Phytomedicine 2017;32:88–96.

Haines CJ, Lam PM, Chung TK, et al. A randomized, double-blind, placebo-controlled study of the effect of a Chinese herbal medicine preparation (Dang Gui Buxue Tang) on menopausal symptoms in Hong Kong Chinese women. Climacteric 2008;11(3):244–51.

Hirata JD, Swiersz LM, Zell B, Small R, Ettinger B. Does dong quai have estrogenic effects in postmenopausal women? A double-blind, placebo-controlled trial. Fertil Steril 1997;68(6):981–6.

Huang Z, Guo B, Liang K. Effects of Radix angelicae sinensis on systemic and portal hemodynamics in cirrhotics with portal HTN. Zhonghua Nei Ke Za Zhi 1996;35(1):15–8.

Huntley AL, Ernst E. A systematic review of herbal medicinal products for the treatment of menopausal symptoms. Menopause 2003;10(5):465–76.

Kupfersztain C, Rotem C, Fagot R, Kaplan B. The immediate effect of natural plant extract, Angelica sinensis and Matricaria chamomilla (Climex) for the treatment of hot flushes during menopause. A preliminary report. Clin Exp Obstet Gynecol 2003;30(4):203–6.

Lee WH, Jin JS, Tsai WC, et al. Biological inhibitory effects of the Chinese herb danggui on brain astrocytoma. Pathobiology 2006;73(3):141–8.

Lei T, Li H, Fang Z, et al. Polysaccharides from Angelica sinensis alleviate neuronal cell injury caused by oxidative stress. Neural Regen Res 2014;9(3):260–267.

Li JJ, Zhu Q, Lu YP, et al. Ligustilide prevents cognitive impairment and attenuates neurotoxicity in D-galactose induced aging mice brain. Brain Res 2015;1595:19–28.

Liao JZ, Chen JJ, Wu ZM, et al. Clinical and experimental studies of coronary heart disease treated with yi-qi huo-xue injection. J Tradit Chin Med 1989;9(3):193–8.

Lim DW, Kim YT. Anti-osteoporotic effects of Angelica sinensis (Oliv.) Diels extract on ovariectomized rats and its oral toxicity in rats. Nutrients 2014;6(10):4362–72.

Liu YM, Zhang JJ, Jiang J. Observation on clinical effect of Angelica injection in treating acute cerebral infarction. Zhongguo Zhong Xi Yi Jie He Za Zhi 2004;24(3):205–8.

Magdalou J, Chen LB, Wang H, et al. Angelica sinensis and osteoarthritis: a natural therapeutic link? Biomed Mater Eng 2015;25(1 Suppl):179–86.

Rotem C, Kaplan B. Phyto-Female Complex for the relief of hot flushes, night sweats and quality of sleep: randomized, controlled, double-blind pilot study. Gynecol Endocrinol 2007;23(2):117–22.

Sun SW, Wang JF. Efficacy of danggui funing pill in treating 162 cases of abdominal pain. Zhongguo Zhong Xi Yi Jie He Za Zhi 1992;12(9):531–2. 517.

Wu CT, Lai JN, Tsai YT. The prescription pattern of Chinese herbal products that contain dang-qui and risk of endometrial cancer among tamoxifen-treated female breast cancer survivors in Taiwan: a population-based study. PLoS One 2014;9(12), e113887.

Xu J, Li G. Observation on short-term effects of Angelica injection on chronic obstructive pulmonary disease patients with pulmonary HTN. Zhongguo Zhong Xi Yi Jie He Za Zhi 2000;20(3):187–9.

Xu JY, Li BX, Cheng SY. Short-term effects of Angelica sinensis and nifedipine on chronic obstructive pulmonary disease in patients with pulmonary HTN. Zhongguo Zhong Xi Yi Jie He Za Zhi 1992;12(12). 716-8, 707.

Yeh TS, Huang CC, Chuang HL, Hsu MC. Angelica sinensis improves exercise performance and protects against physical fatigue in trained mice. Molecules 2014;19(4):3926–39.

Zhang DW, Wang SL, Wang PL, et al. The efficacy of Chinese herbal medicines on acute coronary syndrome with renal insufficiency after percutaneous coronary intervention. J Ethnopharmacol 2020;248:112354.

Zhao H, Deneau J, Che GO, et al. Angelica sinensis isolate SBD.4: composition, gene expression profiling, mechanism of action and effect on wounds, in rats and humans. Eur J Dermatol 2012;22(1):58–67.

41

ECHINACEA (*ECHINACEA PURPUREA, ECHINACEA ANGUSTIFOLIA*)
Leaf, Flower, Stem, Root

GENERAL OVERVIEW

Echinacea is one of the better known and widely used—and misused—herbs. Many patients rightfully reach for this at the first sign of a cold or other viral illness. There is good evidence that early intake of the aerial parts (leaves and flowers) will shorten the duration of the illness, including influenza, by a couple of days. The two species of echinacea that are used medicinally, *E. purpurea* and *E. angustifolia*, are fairly equivalent in their applications and efficacy.

Clinical research indicates that echinacea, alone or in combination formulas, may be beneficial for autoimmune uveitis, gingival recession, osteoarthritis, anxiety, eczema, athletic performance, inflammation, upper respiratory infection, intubation-induced microbial colonization, and influenza.

IN VITRO AND ANIMAL RESEARCH

Echinacea is more aptly described as an immunomodulator. It is both immunostimulatory and anti-inflammatory. Immune-modulating effects of a standardized echinacea root extract include upregulation of IL-2 and IL-8 and downregulation of the proinflammatory cytokines TNF-α and IL-6. It has been shown to stimulate NK cells and may increase interferon. Echinacea has been shown to directly stimulate WBC production and phagocytic activity and to increase antibody-dependent cellular cytotoxicity via TNF-α.

In vitro, echinacea has demonstrated direct antiviral activity against enveloped viruses such as coronavirus, yellow fever virus, herpes simplex virus, and parainfluenza virus. It appears to irreversibly alter the viral envelope and spike proteins. It also has been shown to prevent binding and cell entry of pathogenic influenza (H5N1, H7N7, and H1N1) in vitro. Echinaforce, a whole plant extract from *E. purpurea* has demonstrated in vitro activity against human coronavirus (HCoV) 229E, MERS-CoV, SARS-CoV-1, and SARS-CoV-2 in vitro. (Signer) In animal research, echinacea has demonstrated anxiolytic effects and increased resistance to *Listeria monocytogenes* and *Candida albicans*.

In vitro studies have shown echinacea's major constituent, chicoric acid, inhibits proliferation of human colon cancer cells in a dose- and time-dependent manner. It decreases telomerase activity and induces apoptosis in colon cancer cells. In leukemic mice it has been shown to have a suppressive effect on leukemic cells via IFN-γ activity.

HUMAN RESEARCH

Echinacea research is fraught with contradictions. This may be due to the part of the plant used (root or aerial parts), dosage, species (purpurea, angustifolia, or other), soil, climate, etc. Even the bacterial content in the plant has been found to make a difference in immune response. However, there are enough positive studies and anecdotal reports with this herb to convey some confidence in its potential applications.

Ophthalmological Disorders: Uveitis

A 9-month controlled trial in patients ($n=51$) with low-grade, steroid-dependent, autoimmune uveitis assessed the effect of echinacea on disease activity.

Thirty-two patients (21 with anterior uveitis and 11 with intermediate uveitis) received echinacea 150 mg BID as add-on therapy to topical dexamethasone and oral prednisone taper and were compared with 20 patients (10 with anterior uveitis and 9 with intermediate uveitis) who were treated with the conventional steroid therapy alone. At 9 months 19/21 patients with anterior uveitis and 9/11 with intermediate uveitis treated with echinacea had resolution of uveitis and stable or improved visual acuity. Steroid-off time was 209 and 146 days with anterior uveitis and intermediate uveitis, respectively. No adverse effects were noted with echinacea. Patients who did not receive echinacea required a longer treatment period with steroids with a steroid-off time of 121 and 87 days. The study authors concluded that systemic echinacea appeared to be safe and effective in the control of low-grade autoimmune idiopathic uveitis (Neri et al., 2006).

Oral and Dental Disorders: Gingival Recession and Plaque

In an 8-week open-label case series of patients ($n = 18$) with gingival recession > 1 mm, following routine intervention (scaling and root planing), patients received two 3-day courses of a polyherbal patch (containing elderberry, echinacea, and *Gotu kola)* concurrent with a botanical rinse (of the same herbal combination as the patch) administered twice daily throughout the treatment period. At the end of the treatment period, mean gingival recession decreased from 4.2 mm to 3.3 mm; Miller classification of marginal tissue recession improved from 1.9 to 1.0; Gingival Index scores decreased from 1.4 to 0.17; and Plaque Index scores decreased from 1.3 to 0.8. Gingival thickness increased from 0.7 mm to 1.2 mm. No adverse effects were reported with either the patch or rinse treatments. The authors concluded that the combined botanical patch-rinse treatment may be effective as adjuvant treatment to standard conservative care for gingival recession (Levine et al., 2013).

Women's and Men's Genitourinary Disorders: Genital Condylomas

A 12-month RCT in patients ($n = 125$) post-laser treatment for genital condylomas evaluated HPVADL18 (dry extracts of 200 mg *E. purpurea* roots plus *E. angustifolia)* given for 4 months compared with no additional treatment (control) for relapse incidence. The relapse incidence differed statistically between the two studied groups and progressively decreased during the 12 months after treatment in both groups. This effect was more pronounced in patients older than 25 years. By 6 months, 87.5% and 60.7% of treatment and control groups, respectively, tested negative for HPV ($P < 0.001$); for patients with more extensive disease, 80% and 16.7% of the treatment and control groups, respectively, tested negative. By 12 months, 95.3% and 72.1% of patients in the treatment and control groups, respectively, tested negative for HPV ($P < 0.0001$); for patients with more extensive disease, 100% and 16.7% of patients in the treatment and control groups, respectively, tested negative for HPV ($P < 0.05$). The authors concluded that echinacea promoted the immune process necessary to reduce relapse of genital condylomatosis (De Rosa et al., 2019).

Musculoskeletal Disorders: Osteoarthritis

A 30-day pilot study in patients ($n = 15$) with chronic OA-related knee pain not responding to NSAIDs assessed the effect of ginger 25 mg plus echinacea 5 mg. After supplementation, a significant improvement of 12.27 points was observed for Lysholm scale score ($P < 0.05$) and there was a change of -0.52 cm in knee circumference ($P < 0.01$) (Rondanelli et al., 2017).

Psychiatric Disorders: Anxiety

A 2013 systematic review looking at plants that had both pre-clinical and clinical evidence for anti-anxiety effects found 21 plants with human clinical trial evidence. Support for efficacy identified several herbs with efficacy for anxiety spectrum disorders including kava, lemon balm, chamomile, ginkgo, skullcap, milk thistle, passionflower, ashwagandha, rhodiola, echinacea, *Galphimia glauca, Centella asiatica,* and *Echium amooenum.* Acute anxiolytic activity was found for passionflower, sage, gotu kola, lemon balm, and bergamot. The review also specifically found that bacopa showed anxiolytic effects in people with cognitive decline (Sarris et al., 2013).

A 4-week RCT in patients scoring greater than 45 points on the state or trait subscale of the State Trait Anxiety Inventory compared echinacea root standardized extract 40 mg BID for 7 days with placebo to assess effects on anxiety. State anxiety scores decreased by approximately 11 points and 3 points by the end of the 7-day treatment period with echinacea and placebo, respectively ($P < 0.01$). The effect persisted over the following 3 weeks. The preparation performed better than placebo in patients with high baseline anxiety, but the changes were less robust. Neither BDI nor PSS scores were affected by the treatments. Adverse effects were only observed in the placebo group. The authors concluded that particular echinacea preparations had significant beneficial effects on anxiety (Haller et al., 2020).

A 3-week open label trial in healthy adults with anxiety assessed the effect of echinacea extract 20 or 40 mg/day for 7 days. The 40-mg dosage resulted in decreased State and Trait Anxiety scores within 3 days and remained stable for the duration of the study including the 2 weeks that followed treatment. The lower dose did not affect anxiety significantly (Haller et al., 2013).

Dermatological Disorders: Eczema

A 3-month side to side comparison RCT in patients ($n = 60$) with atopic eczema compared a topical echinacea preparation with a commonly used polyherbal eczema preparation (Imlan Creme) applied BID-TID. Both creams reduced the SCORAD score significantly compared with baseline at 1 month ($P < 0.001$ and $P < 0.001$, respectively) and at 2 months ($P < 0.001$ and $P = 0.008$, respectively). By 3 months, the echinacea product showed a significant improvement in local SCORAD over baseline ($P = 0.013$) and over the polyherbal formula ($P = 0.047$). The mean local SCORAD AUC was significantly lower with the echinacea cream compared with the reference product (654.0 vs 708.5; $P = 0.021$). Echinacea also resulted in significantly higher levels of overall epidermal lipids, ceramide EOS (omega-acylceramide, essential for skin barrier), and cholesterol at day 15 compared with baseline. The authors concluded that the echinacea topical product showed great potential in alleviating symptoms of atopic eczema by anti-inflammatory actions and by restoring the epidermal lipid barrier (Oláh et al., 2017).

Disorders of Vitality: Athletic Performance

A 28-day RCT in young men ($n = 24$) compared high doses of echinacea 2000 mg QID with placebo for effects on EPO and VO2$_{max}$. Echinacea and placebo, respectively, increased EPO at 7 days (15.7 IU/L and 10 IU/L), 14 days (18.8 IU/L and 11 IU/L), and 21 days

(16 IU/L and 9.2 IU/L). VO2$_{max}$ and running economy also improved significantly with echinacea (Whitehead et al., 2012).

Autoimmune Disorders: Uveitis (see *Ophthalmological Disorders* Above)

Inflammation

A 1-month open-label study in healthy subjects ($n = 10$) investigated the anti-inflammatory effects of a 10-mL dose of syrup containing 100 mg of echinacea extract (corresponding to 4.7 mg of echinacoside and 8 mg of a high molecular weight-20,000 Da—polysaccharide). The resulting blood samples showed a decreased expression and plasma levels of IL-6, TNF-α, and IL-8, and increased expression of IL-10. The authors concluded that echinacea had a role in the control of cytokine expression (Dapas et al., 2014).

Infectious Disease: Upper Respiratory Infections

A 2020 systematic review and meta-analysis was performed to assess the evidence for safety and efficacy of echinacea in preventing and treating URIs. The investigators found that echinacea showed benefit for prevention (RR = 0.78) of URI. For treatment of URI echinacea produced a mean difference in average duration of −0.45 days. For safety, the investigators found the RR of 1.09. The authors noted clinical heterogeneity and concluded that echinacea might have a preventive effect on the incidence of URIs, but the effect might not be clinically meaningful. They concluded there was no evince for an effect on the duration of URIs, and that echinacea was safe, at least in the short term (Sholto and Cunningham, 2019).

A 2018 systematic review of RCTs looking at herbal therapy for respiratory tract infections in children and adolescents found 11 RCTs ($n = 2180$) that met inclusion criteria. The review found that the four trials involving echinacea had conflicting evidence and therefore no concrete conclusion on effects of echinacea could be drawn. However, umckaloabo was found through meta-analysis to have evidence for efficacy (RR = 2.56; $P < 0.01$) and safety (adverse events RR = 1.06; $P = 0.9$) compared with placebo (six trials) (Anheyer et al., 2018).

A 2015 systematic review looking at the use of echinacea for recurrent respiratory tract infections identified six clinical studies ($n=2458$) for meta-analysis. Use of echinacea extracts was associated with reduced risk of recurrent respiratory infections (RR=0.649; $P<0.0001$). Ethanolic extracts from echinacea appeared to provide superior effects over pressed juices, and increased dosing during acute episodes further enhanced these effects. Three of the studies found that in individuals with higher susceptibility, stress, or a state of immunological weakness, echinacea halved the risk of recurrent respiratory infections (RR=0.5; $P<0.0001$). Similar preventive effects were observed with virologically confirmed recurrent infections (RR=0.420; $P=0.005$). Complications including pneumonia, otitis media/externa, and tonsillitis/pharyngitis were also less frequent with echinacea treatment (RR=0.503; $P<0.0001$). The authors concluded that echinacea potently lowers the risk of recurrent respiratory infections and complications and that immunomodulatory, antiviral, and anti-inflammatory effects might contribute to the observed benefits, which appeared strongest in susceptible individuals (Schapowal et al., 2015).

A 2015 Cochrane review of herbs effective in treating cough found 34 RCTs ($n=7083$) with eight studies of echinacea that met inclusion criteria. Most studies had a low risk of bias. The meta-analysis revealed strong evidence for andrographis (SMD=−1.00; $P<0.001$) and an ivy-primrose-thyme combination (RR=1.40; $P<0.001$) in treating cough; moderate evidence for umckaloabo (RR=4.60; $P<0.001$); and limited evidence for echinacea (SMD=−0.68; $P=0.04$). The authors concluded that andrographis, ivy-primrose-thyme, and umckaloabo were significantly superior to placebo in alleviating the frequency and severity of cough symptoms (Wagner et al., 2015).

A 4-month RCT ($n=755$) comparing placebo with an echinacea (*purpurea*) extract containing 95% leaves and 5% roots demonstrated efficacy and safety in preventing cold symptoms (672 and 852 total cold days with echinacea and placebo, respectively). A total of 293 adverse events occurred with echinacea and 306 with placebo. The authors concluded that compliant prophylactic intake of echinacea over a 4-month period appeared to provide a positive risk-to-benefit ratio (Jawad et al., 2012).

A 10-day three-arm RCT in children ($n=130$) with URIs investigated the efficacy of andrographis plus eleuthero compared with echinacea and with standard treatment. The andrographis-eleuthero treatment was found to be significantly more effective than echinacea when started at an early stage of uncomplicated common colds, and the symptoms were less severe in this group. Amount of nasal discharge and nasal congestion showed the greatest impact. Recovery time was also faster with andrographis-eleuthero over echinacea and placebo (Spasov et al., 2004).

A 5-day RCT in patients ($n=177$) with URI compared an herbal combination Kan Jang (which includes eleuthero, echinacea, justiciar, and moench) 30 mL/day with placebo and to bromhexine 24 mg/30 mL/day for URI efficacy. Both Kang Jang and bromohexine relieved cough more effectively than placebo with faster improvement by day 3 in the Kan Jang group. The authors concluded that this herbal combination exerted significant antitussive effects in URI and that the study further supported the therapeutic use of Kan Jang in upper respiratory tract infections (Barth et al., 2015).

Infectious Disease: Intubation-Induced Colonization

A clinical trial of patients ($n=70$) aged 18–65 years undergoing oral tracheal intubation compared echinacea with chlorhexidine for oral microbial colonization. The microbial flora significantly decreased after the intervention in both groups, more so with echinacea ($P<0.0001$ and $P<0.001$ with echinacea and chlorhexidine, respectively). After 4 days, the oral microbial flora count was lower with echinacea than with chlorhexidine ($P<0.001$) (Safarabadi et al., 2017).

Infectious Disease: Influenza

An RCT of patients ($n=473$) with early influenza symptoms (<48 h) compared 10 days of an echinacea preparation Echinaforce Hotdrink with 5 days of oseltamivir followed by 5 days of placebo. Recovery from illness after 5 days was 50% and 49% with the echinacea beverage and oseltamivir, respectively. Recovery at 10 days was 90% and 85%, respectively. Virologically confirmed influenza was similar between groups. Incidence of complications and adverse events were lower with the echinacea product compared with oseltamivir ($P=0.076$). The authors concluded that Echinaforce Hotdrink was as effective as oseltamivir in the early treatment of clinically diagnosed and virologically confirmed influenza virus infections with a reduced risk of complications and adverse events (Rauš et al., 2015).

ACTIVE CONSTITUENTS

Aerial Parts and Root

- Carbohydrates
  - Oligosaccharides: inulin (immuno-stimulating via macrophage phagocytosis, anti-inflammatory, prebiotic, hypoglycemic)
- Lipids
  - Alkamides (antibacterial, antifungal, anti-inflammatory; bind to human cannabinoid receptors 1&2 and inhibit TNF-α): isobutylamides, methylbutylamides
  - Polyacetylenes (immunomodulatory, anti-inflammatory, antibacterial, antifungal)
- Amino acid derivatives: glycoproteins
- Phenolic compounds
  - Phenylpropanoids (antioxidant, antimutagenic, antitumor, antimicrobial): caffeic acid (active against staph aureus), echinacoside (antioxidant, hepatoprotective, neuroprotective, antimicrobial), isochlorogenic acid, chlorogenic acid, chicoric acid (anti-hylauronidase activity, immunomodulatory, anti-HIV, apoptotic)
  - Flavonoids (anti-inflammatory)
- Alkaloids: pyrrolizidine saturated type
- Aromatic compounds

Alkamides, polyacetylenes, caffeic acid derivatives, and polysaccharides may work together to increase the production and activity of lymphocytes and macrophages.

ECHINACEA COMMONLY USED PREPARATIONS AND DOSAGE (FOR ADULTS UNLESS OTHERWISE SPECIFIED)

The following are examples of some available formulations and ranges of dosing for commercial herbal products. See Part III Introduction "How to prescribe medicinal herbs" for further guidance on herbal advising and prescribing.

Echinacea angustifolia and/or *purpurea*: Aerial Parts With or Without Root

- Decoction of root: 1–2 tsp per cup TID
- Fluid extract (1:1, 45%): 1 mL every 2 h on first day then TID thereafter
- Tincture of root (1:5, 45%–75%): 2–5 mL TID
- Tincture of aerial parts (1:5, 75%): 5 mL TID
- Powdered root extract: 0.5–1 g TID
- Capsule or tablet of powdered aerial part extract: 400–1200 mg 3–6 times per day
- Capsule or tablet of standardized extract (standardized to 3%–4% echinacoside): 300 to 600 mg TID

SAFETY AND PRECAUTION

Side Effects

Echinacea is generally well tolerated. It may lead to infrequent headache, dizziness, constipation, nausea, and throat irritation in high doses. It may cause allergic reactions in people allergic to the Compositae family of plants.

Case Reports

A few case reports of allergic reactions including anaphylaxis.

Pregnancy and Lactation

In a matched control study in women inadvertently exposed to echinacea during pregnancy, 112 of whom were exposed in the first trimester, there was no increased risk for major malformations. While this information is reassuring, no further evidence is available on this subject, so best to avoid.

Disease Interactions

Autoimmune disease: Theoretically anything that stimulates the immune system should be contraindicated in autoimmune disorders, but both the immune system and the actions of echinacea are complex. One study of patients with autoimmune uveitis showed that those taking echinacea had a faster response to treatment. However, the long-term safety of echinacea in the presence of autoimmune disease has not been studied so therapeutic use should be undertaken with caution.

HIV: May theoretically promote spread of virus due to potential to effects on TNF-α, IL-1, and IL-6.

Drug Interactions

- CYP: Inhibits CYP3A4 and CYP2C8
- Pgp: Inhibits P-glycoprotein activity
- Theoretical or research-proven interactions occur with immuno-suppressive drugs, chemotherapy, corticosteroids, anticoagulants, hepatotoxic drugs, and oseltamivir. Has also reduced metabolic products of prodrugs such as tamoxifen and oseltamivir

REFERENCES

Anheyer D, Cramer H, Lauche R, Saha FJ, Dobos G. Herbal medicine in children with respiratory tract infection: systematic review and meta-analysis. Acad Pediatr 2018;18(1):8–19.

Barth A, Hovhannisyan A, Jamalyan K, Narimanyan M. Antitussive effect of a fixed combination of justicia adhatoda, echinacea purpurea and eleutherococcus senticosus extracts in patients with acute upper respiratory tract infection: a comparative, randomized, double-blind, placebo-controlled study. Phytomedicine 2015;22(13):1195–200.

Dapas B, Dall'Acqua S, Bulla R, et al. Immunomodulation mediated by a herbal syrup containing a standardized Echinacea root extract: a pilot study in healthy human subjects on cytokine gene expression. Phytomedicine 2014;21(11):1406–10.

De Rosa N, Giampaolino P, Lavitola G, et al. Effect of immunomodulatory supplements based on Echinacea angustifolia and Echinacea purpurea on the posttreatment relapse incidence of genital condylomatosis: A Prospective Randomized Study. Biomed Res Int 2019;2019:3548396.

Haller J, Freund TF, Pelczer KG, Füredi J, Krecsak L, Zámbori J. The anxiolytic potential and psychotropic side effects of an echinacea preparation in laboratory animals and healthy volunteers. Phytother Res 2013;27(1):54–61.

Haller J, Krecsak L, Zámbori J. Double-blind placebo controlled trial of the anxiolytic effects of a standardized Echinacea extract. Phytother Res 2020;34(3):660–8.

Jawad M, Schoop R, Suter A, Klein P, Eccles R. Safety and efficacy profile of Echinacea purpurea to prevent common cold episodes: a randomized, double-blind, placebo-controlled trial. Evid Based Complement Alternat Med 2012;841315.

Levine WZ, Samuels N, Bar Sheshet ME, Grbic JT. A novel treatment of gingival recession using a botanical topical gingival patch and mouthrinse. J Contemp Dent Pract 2013;14(5):948–53.

Neri PG, Stagni E, Filippello M, et al. Oral Echinacea purpurea extract in low-grade, steroid-dependent, autoimmune idiopathic uveitis: a pilot study. J Ocul Pharmacol Ther 2006;22(6):431–6.

Oláh A, Szabó-Papp J, Soeberdt M, et al. Echinacea purpurea-derived alkylamides exhibit potent anti-inflammatory effects and alleviate clinical symptoms of atopic eczema. J Dermatol Sci 2017;88(1):67–77.

Rauš K, Pleschka S, Klein P, Schoop R, Fisher P. Effect of an echinacea-based hot drink vs oseltamivir in influenza treatment: a randomized, double-blind, double-dummy, multicenter, noninferiority clinical trial. Curr Ther Res Clin Exp 2015;77:66–72.

Rondanelli M, Riva A, Morazzoni P, et al. The effect and safety of highly standardized Ginger (Zingiber officinale) and Echinacea (Echinacea angustifolia) extract supplementation on inflammation and chronic pain in NSAIDs poor responders. A pilot study in subjects with knee arthrosis. Nat Prod Res 2017;31(11):1309–13.

Safarabadi M, Ghaznavi-Rad E, Pakniyat A, Rezaie K, Jadidi A. Comparing the effect of echinacea and chlorhexidine mouthwash on the microbial flora of intubated patients admitted to the intensive care unit. Iran J Nurs Midwifery Res 2017;22(6):481–5.

Sarris J, McIntyre E, Camfield DA. Plant-based medicines for anxiety disorders, part 2: a review of clinical studies with supporting preclinical evidence. CNS Drugs 2013;27(4):301–19.

Schapowal A, Klein P, Johnston SL. Echinacea reduces the risk of recurrent respiratory tract infections and complications: a meta-analysis of randomized controlled trials. Adv Ther 2015;32(3):187–200.

Sholto D, Cunningham R. Echinacea for the prevention and treatment of upper respiratory tract infections: a systematic review and meta-analysis. Complement Ther Med 2019;44:18–26.

Spasov AA, Ostrovskij OV, Chernikov MV, Wikman G. Comparative controlled study of Andrographis paniculata fixed combination, Kan Jang and an Echinacea preparation as adjuvant, in the treatment of uncomplicated respiratory disease in children. Phytother Res 2004;18(1):47–53.

Wagner L, Cramer H, Klose P, et al. Herbal medicine for cough: a systematic review and meta-analysis. Forsch Komplementmed 2015;22(6):359–68.

Whitehead MT, Martin TD, Scheett TP, et al. Running economy and maximal oxygen consumption after 4 weeks of oral Echinacea supplementation. J Strength Cond Res 2012;26(7):1928–33.

42

ELDERBERRY/ELDER BERRY AND FLOWER (*SAMBUCUS NIGRA*)
Fruit and Flower

GENERAL OVERVIEW

When it comes to influenza, elderberry should quickly come to mind. Elderberry is the namesake ingredient in the commonly available OTC syrup Sambucol. The elder flower, as well as the berry, contains the active constituents. Elderberry has Level B evidence for influenza.

Clinical research indicates that elderberry and elder flower, alone or in combination formulas, may be beneficial for gingival recession, hyperlipidemia, dyslipidemia, metabolic syndrome, obesity, chronic constipation, upper respiratory infection, influenza, and HIV. It has been assigned Level C evidence for several of these indications.

IN VITRO AND ANIMAL RESEARCH

Both the berries and flowers of the elder bush have antiviral, antibacterial, immune-modulating, antiinflammatory, antioxidant, and glucose-lowering properties. They also have demonstrated efficacy against herpes simplex virus (HSV).

Research has shown a cardiovascular protective benefit from elderberry due to antioxidant effects. Human aortic endothelial cells incorporate elderberry anthocyanins into both the membrane and cytosol, resulting in significantly enhanced resistance to ROS. Preliminary studies have also shown that elderberry may cause a reduction in TC, LDL-C, and TG. Unfortunately, HDL-C was also lowered. In mice, elderberry appeared to positively influence HDL dysfunction associated with chronic inflammation by impacting hepatic gene expression. The elder flower has

demonstrated antidiabetic properties that occur via activation of PPAR-γ, increased insulin secretion, and stimulation of insulin-dependent glucose uptake.

Elderberry extracts have immune-modulating activity via increased production of TNF-α, IL-1β, and IL 8–10, consequently activating and mobilizing phagocytes. Elderberries contain several anthocyanin flavonoids known to possess significant antioxidant properties (hint: when you see dark purples and reds in foods, they probably contain anthocyanin flavonoids with antioxidant properties).

Elder chemical constituents have been shown in the lab to neutralize the activity of the hemagglutinin spikes found on the surface of several viruses, blocking host cell recognition and entry. The flavonoids and proanthocyanidins in elder flowers and berries were shown to block HIV1 infection and may have additive effects with existing HIV drugs such as enfuvirtide. Elder also has antibacterial properties. One study demonstrated antimicrobial activity against both Gram-positive bacteria of *Streptococcus pyogenes* groups C and G and the Gram-negative bacterium *Branhamella catarrhalis* in liquid cultures. Numerous in vitro studies using Sambucol syrup (containing 3.8 g elderberry extract per 10 mL) have shown it neutralizes and reduces infectivity of influenza A and B viruses, HIV strains, and HSV-1.

HUMAN RESEARCH

Oral and Dental Disorders

In an 8-week open-label case series of patients ($n=18$) with gingival recession >1 mm, following routine intervention (scaling and root planing), patients received two 3-day courses of a polyherbal patch (containing elderberry, echinacea, and *Gotu kola)* concurrent with a botanical rinse containing the same three herbs administered twice daily throughout the treatment period. At the end of the treatment period, mean gingival recession decreased from 4.2 to 3.3 mm; Miller classification of marginal tissue recession improved from 1.9 to 1.0; Gingival Index scores decreased from 1.4 to 0.17; and Plaque Index scores decreased from 1.3 to 0.8. Gingival thickness increased from 0.7 to 1.2 mm. No adverse effects were reported with either the patch or the rinse treatments. The authors concluded that the combined botanical patch-rinse treatment may be effective as adjuvant treatment to standard conservative care for gingival recession (Levine et al., 2013).

Cardiometabolic Disorders: Hyperlipidemia, Dyslipidemia, Metabolic Syndrome, and Obesity

Human studies on lipid effects of elderberry are mixed. Two studies have shown a lowering of TC with no effect on other serum lipid levels. A 2-year RCT of a polyherbal product containing elder berries, calendula, and *Viola tricolor* demonstrated a reduction in carotid IMT progression (Kirichenko et al., 2016).

A 5-week crossover RCT in healthy subjects ($n=40$) aged 50–70 years studied daily consumption of a control beverage compared with a berry beverage containing 150 g blueberries, 50 g blackcurrant, 50 g elderberry, 50 g lingonberries, 50 g strawberry, and 100 g tomatoes. The berry intervention reduced TC and LDL-C compared with baseline (both $P<0.05$) and compared with the control beverage ($P<0.005$ and $P<0.01$, respectively). The control beverage increased glucose concentrations ($P<0.01$) and tended to increase insulin concentrations ($P=0.064$) from baseline, and increased insulin concentrations in comparison with the berry beverage ($P<0.05$). Subjects performed better in the working memory test after the berry beverage compared with after the control beverage ($P<0.05$). The authors concluded that the improvements in cardiometabolic risk markers and cognitive performance after the berry beverage indicated a preventive potential of berries with respect to T2DM, cardiovascular disease, and associated cognitive decline, possibly due to the polyphenols and dietary fiber (Nilsson et al., 2017).

An open-label study in participants ($n=80$) desiring to lose weight administered elderberry juice enriched with flower extract plus tablets containing berry powder and flower extract plus an asparagus powder tablet. After the diet, the mean weight, blood pressure, physical and emotional well-being, and QOL had significantly improved (Chrubasik et al., 2008).

Gastrointestinal Disorders: Constipation

A crossover RCT in patients ($n=20$) with chronic constipation compared a polyherbal product containing elderberry, fennel, *Pimpinella anisum*, and *Cassia angustifolia* with placebo for 5 days with a 9-day washout between crossovers. Mean colonic transit time was 15.7 h vs 42.3 h with the herbal product vs placebo, respectively ($P<0.001$). The number of evacuations per day increased during the use of the active tea, and significant differences were observed as of the second day of treatment ($P<0.001$). Patient perception of bowel function was improved ($P<0.01$), but quality of life did not show significant differences among the study periods. There was a small reduction in serum potassium levels during the active treatment. The authors concluded that the polyherbal compound had laxative efficacy and was a safe alternative option for chronic constipation (Picon et al., 2010).

Infectious Disease: Upper Respiratory Infection and Influenza

A 2019 meta-analysis of elderberry benefits ($n=180$) found that elderberry substantially reduced upper respiratory symptoms with a large mean size effect. The authors concluded that the findings presented an alternative to antibiotic misuse for upper respiratory symptoms due to viral infections as well as a potentially safer alternative to prescription drugs for upper respiratory infections (URIs) and influenza (Hawkins et al., 2019).

Two clinical studies showed that Sambucol syrup (containing 3.8 g elderberry extract per 10 mL) shortened the symptomatic phase of influenza by about 50% when given within the first 48 h of symptom onset. A four-dose pilot RCT ($n=64$) with early influenza-like symptoms compared a proprietary elderberry extract lozenge 175 mg BID with placebo. The extract treated group showed significant improvement in most of the symptoms by 24 h after the onset of the treatment, whereas the placebo group showed no improvement or an increase in severity of the symptoms at the same time point. By 48 h, symptoms were resolved in 28% and improved in 60% with elderberry compared with 0% and 16% with placebo. No adverse effects were observed in either group. The author concluded that the proprietary elderberry extract was safe and highly effective in treating flu-like symptoms (Kong, 2009).

Another RCT in patients ($n = 60$) suffering from influenza-like symptoms for ≤ 48 h compared 15 mL of elderberry syrup with placebo syrup QID for 5 days. Symptoms were relieved on average 4 days earlier and use of rescue medication was significantly less in those receiving elderberry extract compared with placebo. The authors concluded that elderberry extract seemed to offer an efficient, safe, and cost-effective treatment for influenza (Zakay-Rones et al., 2004).

An RCT of overseas airline travelers ($n = 312$) compared standardized elderberry extract 300 mg with placebo (each given BID starting ten days before travel, then TID during travel and for 5 days after arrival) for prevention of viral illness. The incidence of URIs following the travel episodes were insignificantly greater with placebo than with elderberry (17 vs 12; $P = 0.4$). The placebo group had a significantly longer total duration of cold episodes (117 days vs 57 days; $P = 0.02$) and the average symptom score over these days was also significantly higher (583 vs 247; $P = 0.05$). The authors concluded that prophylactic use of elderberry extract may produce a significant reduction of cold duration and severity in air travelers (Tiralongo et al., 2016).

A 15-day RCT in patients ($n = 380$) with up to 3 days of symptoms of rhinosinusitis (major symptom score 12–15) compared BNO 1016 (gentian root, primula flower, sorrel herb, elder flower, and verbena herb in a ratio of 3:3:3:3:1) with placebo TID. Treatment resulted in clinically relevant differences in mean major symptom scores over placebo ($P = 0.0008$), providing symptom relief 2 days earlier than placebo. NNT was 8 for the polyherbal product. Responder rates at days 10 and 14 and percentage of patients without signs of acute viral rhinosinusitis on ultrasound were superior with the herbal combination. The herb was well tolerated (Jund et al., 2012).

Infectious Disease: HIV

In a case report, a female, taking no HIV drugs used Sambucol syrup (containing 3.8 g elderberry extract per 10 mL), with olive leaf extract (which has reverse transcriptase activity) demonstrated a viral load decrease from 17,000 to 4000 (Konlee, 1998).

ACTIVE CONSTITUENTS

Flower and Berry

- Carbohydrates
  - Polysaccharides: mucilage (immune stimulating, demulcent)
- Amino acid derivatives: *Sambucus nigra* agglutinin III (antiviral, ribosome inactivating, antiproliferative) plastocyanin, *N*-phenylpropenoyl-L-amino acid amides
  - Cyanogenic glycosides: sambunigrin
- Phenolic compounds
  - Flavonoids: quercetin (antiinflammatory, antioxidant, hypotensive, antidiabetic, antispasmodic, neuroprotective, XO inhibition, antibacterial, anticancer), rutin (antioxidant, antiinflammatory, antidiabetic, nephroprotective, antiosteoporotic, antispasmodic, neuroprotective, antianxiety), hyperoside (antioxidant, antiinflammatory, antiproliferative, apoptotic, hepatoprotective, nephroprotective, antiosteoporotic)
    - Anthocyanins: cyanidin-3-glucoside and cyanidin-3-sambubioside (antioxidant, antiviral)
    - Tannins
- Terpenes: triterpenes
- Steroids: phytosterols
- Aromatic compounds

ELDER BERRY/FLOWER COMMONLY USED PREPARATIONS AND DOSAGE (FOR ADULTS UNLESS OTHERWISE SPECIFIED)

The following are examples of some available formulations and ranges of dosing for commercial herbal products. See Part III Introduction "How to prescribe medicinal herbs" for further guidance on herbal advising and prescribing.

Flower

- Infusion: 2 tsp. (dried or fresh) per cup TID.
- Dried: 2–4 g TID.

- Tincture of fresh flower (1:2, 25%): 2–4 mL TID.
- Tincture of dried flower (1:5, 40%): 2–4 mL TID.

Berry

- Decoction: 1–2 tsp. per cup, 1/2 cup TID.
- Juice concentrate (5:1 or 10:1): 250–500 mg BID-TID.
- Tincture (1:4, 40%): 1 mL BID-QID
- Capsule or tablet of powdered berry extract: 500 mg BID-TID for 3–4 days for influenza or continuously for cardiovascular prevention.
- Capsule or tablet of standardized extract (standardized to anthocyanins): 1500 mg per day for antioxidant benefits.
- Concentrated berry syrup (30:1): 176 mg/10 mL; 10 mL QID.
- Sambucol® original syrup contains 3.8 g black elderberry per 10 mL serving; recommended 10 mL QD to QID depending on intended use.

SAFETY AND PRECAUTION

Side Effects

Raw or unripe elderberries contain cyanogenic glycosides and must be selected properly and cooked sufficiently to avoid risk of cyanide toxicity (vomiting and diarrhea). Elderberry leaves and stems also contain cyanogenic glycosides and should not be ingested. Some patients may have allergy to elder fruit or flower.

Pregnancy and Lactation

No adverse events have been reported. Insufficient human safety data.

Disease Interactions

Caution with autoimmune disorders.

Drug Interactions

- Potential interactions with antidiabetic drugs, immunosuppressive drugs.
- May increase effects of diuretics and laxatives.

REFERENCES

Chrubasik C, Maier T, Dawid C, et al. An observational study and quantification of the actives in a supplement with *Sambucus nigra* and *Asparagus officinalis* used for weight reduction. Phytother Res 2008 Jul;22(7):913–8.

Hawkins J, Baker C, Cherry L, Dunne E. Black elderberry (Sambucus nigra) supplementation effectively treats upper respiratory symptoms: a meta-analysis of randomized, controlled clinical trials. Complement Ther Med 2019 Feb;42:361–5.

Jund R, Mondigler M, Steindl H, et al. Clinical efficacy of a dry extract of five herbal drugs in acute viral rhinosinusitis. Rhinology 2012 Dec;50(4):417–26.

Kirichenko TV, Sobenin IA, Nikolic D, Rizzo M, Orekhov AN. Anticytokine therapy for prevention of atherosclerosis. Phytomedicine 2016 Oct 15;23(11):1198–210.

Kong F. Pilot clinical study on a proprietary elderberry extract: efficacy in addressing influenza symptoms. Online J Pharmacol Pharmacokinet 2009;5:32–43.

Konlee M. A new triple combination therapy. Posit Health News 1998 Fall;(17):12–4.

Levine WZ, Samuels N, Bar Sheshet ME, Grbic JT. A novel treatment of gingival recession using a botanical topical gingival patch and mouthrinse. J Contemp Dent Pract 2013 Sep 1;14(5):948–53.

Nilsson A, Salo I, Plaza M, Björck I. Effects of a mixed berry beverage on cognitive functions and cardiometabolic risk markers; A randomized crossover study in healthy older adults. PLoS One 2017 Nov 15;12(11), e0188173.

Picon PD, Picon RV, Costa AF, et al. Randomized clinical trial of a phytotherapic compound containing Pimpinella anisum, Foeniculum vulgare, Sambucus nigra, and Cassia augustifolia for chronic constipation. BMC Complement Altern Med 2010;10:17.

Tiralongo E, Wee S, Lea R. Elderberry supplementation reduces cold duration and symptoms in air-travellers: a randomized, double-blind placebo-controlled clinical trial. Nutrients 2016 Apr;8(4):182.

Zakay-Rones Z, Thom E, Wollan T, et al. Randomized study of the efficacy and safety of oral elderberry extract in the treatment of influenza A and B virus infections. J Int Med Res Mar-Apr 2004;32(2):132–40.

43

ELEUTHERO/SIBERIAN GINSENG (*ELEUTHEROCOCCUS SENTICOSUS/ ACANTHOPANAX SENTICOSUS*)
Root

GENERAL OVERVIEW

Eleuthero, as its other name "Siberian ginseng" implies, is another adaptogenic herb. It has a history of use in folk and traditional Chinese medicine. Originating from Northern Asia, it has been used traditionally as an adaptogen, performance enhancer, and immunostimulant.

Clinical research indicates that eleuthero, alone or in combination formulas, may be beneficial for allergic rhinitis, peripheral edema, hyperlipidemia, dyslipidemia, male infertility, osteoporosis, stroke recovery, depression, bipolar disorder, cognitive performance, hangover, athletic performance, immune function, familial Mediterranean fever, upper respiratory infection, pneumonia, dysentery, and chemotherapy-suppressed immune function.

IN VITRO AND ANIMAL RESEARCH

In vitro studies of eleuthero have found constituents that bind to estrogen, progestin, mineralocorticoid, and glucocorticoid receptors. Eleutheroside E and syringaresinol-di-O-beta-D glucoside have antifatigue effects. Eleuthero has also been shown to suppress LPS-iNOS expression with a resultant reduction in NF-kB expression in macrophages and ROS production. Eleuthero root has been shown to inhibit replication of RNA viruses such as human rhinovirus, RSV, and influenza A, but not DNA viruses such as adenovirus or HSV. Eleutheroside E has demonstrated protective effects against Aβ-induced atrophies of axons and dendrites in rat cultured cortical neurons. Another key constituent of eleuthero, isofraxidin, inhibits cell

invasion and the expression of MMP-7 by human hepatoma cell lines HuH-7 and Hep G-2, possibly through the inhibition of ERK1/2 phosphorylation.

A study in rats showed eleuthero may be of therapeutic benefit in prevention of bone resorption in steroid-induced osteoporosis. Animal experiments have provided evidence that eleuthero can decrease sleep latency, increase sleep duration, reduce blood glucose levels, and inhibit leukemia cells.

HUMAN RESEARCH

Allergic Disorders: Allergic Rhinitis

In an ex vivo study of healthy patients ($n = 12$) nasal mucosal cells were incubated with tissue culture medium, skullcap with or without eleuthero, and/or vitamin C, and stimulated with anti-IgE for 30 min and 6 h to imitate the allergic early and late phases. Additionally, *Staphylococcus aureus* superantigen B stimulation for 6 h was used to imitate T-cell activation. The combination of skullcap and eleuthero had a more potent suppressive effect on the release of PGD2, histamine, and IL-5 than did skullcap alone. The combination also resulted in a significant inhibition of the *S. aureus* superantigen B-induced cytokines comparable with or superior to fluticasone propionate. Vitamin C increased ciliary beat frequency but had no antiinflammatory effects. The authors concluded that the combination of skullcap and eleuthero may be able to significantly block allergic early- and late-phase mediators and substantially suppress the release of proinflammatory Th1-, Th2-, and Th-17-derived cytokines (Zhang et al., 2012).

Cardiovascular Disorders: Leg Edema

An acutely dosed crossover RCT in healthy female volunteers ($n=50$) compared eleuthero with control and found that eleuthero significantly attenuated leg edema at 2 and 4 h after ingestion. The authors surmised that eleutheroside E was responsible for the reduction in edema by inducing phosphorylation of the endothelial-specific receptor Tie2, which stabilizes lymphatic endothelial cells. The authors concluded that the study demonstrated that eleuthero exerted its potent antiedema activity mainly by promoting lymphatic function (Fukada et al., 2016).

Cardiometabolic Disorders: Hyperlipidemia and Dyslipidemia

A 6-month RCT in postmenopausal women ($n=40$) compared eleuthero plus calcium with calcium alone for effects on serum lipid profiles, biomarkers of oxidative stress, and lymphocyte DNA damage. The treatment group had significant decreases from baseline in LDL-C (127 and 110.3 for baseline and treatment, respectively; $P<0.001$) and the LDL/HDL ratio (2.4 and 2.1 for baseline and treatment, respectively; $P<0.001$). Serum MDA concentrations decreased by 12.6% and 2.2% in the eleuthero and control groups, respectively, after 6 months (neither group achieved statistical significance). Protein-carbonyl levels (indicative of oxidative stress) and lymphocyte DNA damage decreased significantly in eleuthero and control groups ($P<0.001$ and $P<0.05$, respectively) after 6 months of supplementation. The authors concluded that supplementation with eleuthero may have beneficial effects against oxidative stress and may improve serum lipid profiles without subsequent side effects (Lee et al., 2008).

Men's Genitourinary Disorders: Male Infertility

An ex vivo study of semen samples from asthenospermic men ($n=12$) compared applications of eleuthero 10 g/L with theophylline 3 mmol/L and with caffeine 7 mmol/L for effects on sperm hardiness. The eleuthero application significantly increased sperm motility, the percentage of progressive motile sperm, straight line velocity, and curvilinear velocity compared with theophylline and caffeine ($P<0.05$) (Wu et al., 2009).

A Phase I clinical study in healthy males compared the effects of high doses of a combination of andrographis plus eleuthero (Kan jang) with high doses of Asian ginseng and with valerian on semen quality. The results of the study revealed a positive trend toward the number of spermatozoids, percentage of normokinetic forms, and fertility indexes with the andrographis-eleuthero combination. There was also a decrease in percentage of dyskinetic spermatozoids. There were no significant negative effects of the herbal combination on male semen quality and fertility. Asian ginseng also showed no significant negative effects on the fertility parameters, and there was a clear decrease in the percentage of dyskinetic forms of spermatozoids. Subjects receiving valerian showed a temporary increase in the percentage of normokinetic spermatozoids and a decrease in dyskinetic forms, but these changes had no effect on fertility indices. The authors concluded that the andrographis-eleuthero combination, Asian ginseng, and valerian were safe with respect to effects on human male sterility when administered at dose levels corresponding to approximately three times the human daily dose (Mkrtchyan et al., 2005).

Musculoskeletal Disorders: Osteoporosis

A 6-month RCT in postmenopausal women ($n=81$) younger than 65 years with osteopenia or osteoporosis investigated calcium 500 mg/day with or without eleuthero 3 g/day. The group receiving eleuthero showed a significant increase in serum osteocalcin levels and a reduction in MMP-10 levels (both indicating improved bone metabolism) compared with the control group ($P=0.041$). No significant changes in bone mineral density were observed by dual-energy X-ray absorptiometry (DXA). The eleuthero extract was generally well tolerated, and no differences were observed between the two groups in terms of adverse events. The authors concluded that eleuthero may have beneficial effects on bone remodeling in postmenopausal women and that it had no significant adverse events (Hwang et al., 2009).

Neurological Disorders: Stroke

A 2009 Cochrane review looked at the efficacy of eleuthero for acute ischemic stroke. Thirteen trials ($n=962$) were included. The outcome measure in all included trials was the improvement of neurological deficit after treatment. Eleuthero was associated with a significant increase in the number of participants whose neurological impairment improved (RR = 1.22). Two trials reported adverse events; five trials reported no adverse events. The authors noted there was a high risk of bias in all trials (Li et al., 2009).

Psychiatric Disorders: Depression and Bipolar Mood Disorder

A 2014 systematic review of an herbal combination product Shuganjieyu (St. John's wort and eleuthero) for treatment of depressive disorder identified seven RCTs (n = 595) for inclusion. Shuganjieyu capsule was superior to placebo in terms of response rate (RR = 2.42; P = 0.0001), remission rate (RR = 4.29; P = 0.004), the mean change from baseline in the HAM-D17 scores (MD = −4.17; P < 0.00001), and mean change from baseline in the Chinese medicine syndrome score scale (MD = −6.00; P < 0.00001). When added to venlafaxine, Shuganjieyu produced a higher response rate (RR = 1.56; P < 0.00001) and greater mean change from baseline in HAM-D17 and Chinese medicine syndrome score scale (MD = −0.74; P = 0.0002) than venlafaxine alone. The authors concluded that Shuganjieyu was superior to placebo for depressive disorder in terms of overall treatment of effectiveness and safety, and that both response rate and remission rate in patients treated with the combination of Shuganjieyu plus venlafaxine were significantly greater than in those treated with venlafaxine alone (Zhang et al., 2014).

A 6-week RCT in adolescents (n = 76) with bipolar mood disorder investigated eleuthero plus lithium compared with fluoxetine plus lithium for treatment response. After 6 weeks of treatment, the response rate and remission rate with eleuthero (67.6% and 71.8%, respectively) and fluoxetine (51.4% and 48.7%, respectively) were similar. Three patients in the fluoxetine group switched to mania compared with no patients in the eleuthero group. Adverse events for eleuthero and fluoxetine, respectively, were 5.4% and 10.3% for nausea; 2.7% and 0% for rash; 2.7% and 0% for diarrhea; 0% and 7.7% for anxiety; 0% and 7.7% for insomnia; 0% and 2.6% for constipation; and 0% and 2.6% for tinnitus. The authors concluded that there was no significant difference between lithium plus eleuthero and lithium plus fluoxetine in treatment of adolescents with bipolar disorder (Weng et al., 2007).

Psychiatric Disorders: Attention and Cognitive Performance

A pilot RCT in stressed-out adults (n = 40) compared the effects of a single dose of ADAPT-232 (a standardized combination of rhodiola, schisandra, and eleuthero) with placebo on cognitive attention, speed, and accuracy while performing stressful cognitive tasks. The results showed a significant difference (P < 0.05) in attention, speed, and accuracy between the two treatment groups with superiority in the herbal treatment group. No serious side effects were reported, although a few minor adverse events such as sleepiness and cold extremities were observed in both study groups (Aslanyan et al., 2010).

Disorders of Vitality: Hangovers, Stamina, and Athletic Performance

A 2017 systematic review to evaluate herbs for hangover benefit selected six studies for analysis. Of the interventions, the use of polysaccharide-rich extract of eleuthero, Korean red ginseng antihangover drink, Korean pear juice, KSS formula (pith of citrus tangerine, tanaka, ginger root, and brown sugar), and After-Effect (borage oil, fish oil, vitamins B1, B6, and C, magnesium, milk thistle, and prickly pear) were associated with a significant improvement of hangover symptoms, particularly tiredness, nausea/vomiting, and stomachache (P < 0.05) (Jayawardena et al., 2017).

An 8-week crossover RCT in recreationally trained males (n = 9) compared eleuthero 800 mg/day with placebo for effects on endurance capacity, cardiovascular functions, and metabolism. The results showed the VO2$_{peak}$ of the subjects increased 12% (P < 0.05), endurance time improved 23% (P < 0.05), and the highest heart rate increased 4% (P < 0.05) with eleuthero compared with placebo. The authors concluded that 8 weeks of eleuthero supplementation enhanced endurance capacity, elevated cardiovascular functions, and altered metabolism in favor of sparing glycogen in recreationally trained males (Kuo et al., 2010).

A 6-week RCT in athletes compared effects of eleuthero root extract 4 g/day with Asian ginseng root extract 2 g/day and with placebo on competitive club-level endurance. There were no significant changes from pre- to posttests on CD-4, CD-8, NK cells, and B lymphocytes in any of the groups. There were also no significant changes in testosterone, cortisol, or testosterone/cortisol in the ginseng group. However, in the eleuthero group, testosterone/cortisol decreased by 29% ($P=0.03$), mostly attributed to a trend toward increased cortisol. The authors concluded that eleuthero increased rather than decreased hormonal indices of stress, which may be consistent with animal research suggesting a threshold of stress below which eleuthero increases the stress response and above which eleuthero decreases the stress response (Gaffney et al., 2001).

A crossover RCT in healthy adults compared a polysaccharide-rich eleuthero extract with placebo before and after consuming 1.75 g/kg of pure alcohol. Blood alcohol showed little difference between groups. The Acute Hangover Scale (tired, headache, dizziness, stomachache, and nausea) was significantly improved the following morning in the eleuthero group. Glucose and CRP were significantly altered by alcohol in the placebo group, but these changes were significantly attenuated by eleuthero. The authors concluded that eleuthero may have potential to reduce the severity of the alcohol hangover by inhibiting the alcohol-induced hypoglycemia and inflammatory response (Bang et al., 2015).

A crossover RCT in healthy nonsmoking adult men ($n=20$) compared an herbal combination (eleuthero, goji berry, *Viscum album*, and *Inonotus obliquus*) with placebo in the hangover effect from drinking a bottle of Soju, which is a commercially available liquor (19% alcohol in 360 mL). Alcohol levels were significantly lower and antioxidant levels were significantly higher in the herbal group than in the control group at 2 h after drinking Soju ($P<0.05$, respectively), and acetaldehyde levels tended to be insignificantly lower in the herbal group. The author concluded that this herbal combination reduced oxidative stress and hangover by mitigating plasma alcohol concentrations and elevating antioxidant activity in healthy male adults (Hong, 2016).

An 8-week RCT in elderly patients ($n=20$) with HTN and taking digitoxin compared eleuthero 300 mg/day with placebo for effects on health-related quality of life. After 4 weeks of therapy, higher scores in social functioning scales were observed in the eleuthero group ($P=0.02$), but these differences did not persist to the 8-week time point. There were no differences in blood pressure. No adverse events were noted. Subjects given eleuthero were more likely to believe they had received active therapy than subjects given placebo (70% vs 20%; $P<0.05$). The authors concluded that eleuthero safely improved some aspects of mental health and social functioning in patients with HTN and CHF after 4 weeks of therapy, although these differences were attenuated with continued use (Cicero et al., 2004).

Immune Function

A 4-week RCT in healthy volunteers ($n=36$) compared eleuthero tincture 10 mL TID for 4 weeks with a placebo tincture for impact on the immune response. The eleuthero group demonstrated an increase in the absolute number of immunocompetent cells based on flow cytometry, with an especially pronounced effect on T lymphocytes, predominantly of the helper/inducer type, but also on cytotoxic and NK cells. In addition, a general enhancement of the activation state of T lymphocytes was observed. No side effects were observed during the trial or in 6 months of follow-up (Bohn et al., 1987).

Inflammation: Familial Mediterranean Fever

A 1-month Phase II RCT of young patients ($n=24$) with familial Mediterranean fever compared ImmunoGuard (a standardized fixed combination of eleuthero, andrographis, schisandra, and licorice extracts) four tablets TID with placebo. The patient's self-evaluation was based on symptoms of abdominal pain, chest pain, temperature, arthritis, myalgia, and erysipelas-like erythema. All three features (duration, frequency, and severity of attacks) showed significant improvement in the ImmunoGuard group compared with placebo. In both clinical assessment and self-evaluation, the severity of attacks was found to show the most significant improvement in the herbal group. The authors concluded that both the clinical and laboratory results of the clinical study suggested that ImmunoGuard was a safe and efficacious herbal drug for the management of patients with FMF (Amaryan et al., 2003).

Infectious Disease: Upper Respiratory Infections

A 2004 systematic review assessing the efficacy of andrographis alone or in combination with eleuthero for the symptomatic treatment of uncomplicated URIs selected four studies ($n=433$) that met inclusion criteria. The authors found that andrographis in fixed combination with eleuthero was more effective than placebo (MD = 2.13 points; $P = 0.0002$) on the symptom severity score. The authors concluded that evidence suggested andrographis alone or in combination with eleuthero may be more effective than placebo for uncomplicated acute URI (Poolsup et al., 2004).

A 5-day RCT in patients ($n = 185$) with acute URIs compared eleuthero plus andrographis (Kan Jang) with placebo. The eleuthero-andrographis group had a highly significant improvement in URI and sinusitis symptoms. Greatest improvements occurred for headache, nasal and throat symptoms, and general malaise. Temperature was moderately reduced with the herbal combination. The authors concluded that this eleuthero-andrographis combination had a positive effect in the treatment of acute URI and that it also relieved inflammatory symptoms of sinusitis. The product was well tolerated (Gabrielian et al., 2002).

A 5-day RCT in patients ($n = 177$) with URIs compared an herbal combination of eleuthero, echinacea, justiciar, and moench 30 mL/day with placebo and with bromhexine 24 mg/30 mL/day for URI efficacy. Both the herbal product and bromhexine relieved cough more effectively than placebo with faster improvement by day 3 in the herbal group. The authors concluded that this herbal combination exerted significant antitussive effects in URI and that the study further supported the therapeutic use of the herbal combination in URIs (Barth et al., 2015).

A 10-day three-arm RCT in children ($n = 130$) with URIs assessed the efficacy of eleuthero plus andrographis compared with echinacea and with standard treatment alone. The eleuthero-andrographis treatment was found to be significantly more effective than echinacea, when started at an early stage of uncomplicated common colds, and the symptoms were less severe in this group. The amount of nasal discharge and nasal congestion showed the greatest impact. Recovery time was also faster with eleuthero-andrographis compared with echinacea and with placebo. The herbal combination was well tolerated, and no side effects or adverse reactions were reported (Spasov et al., 2004).

Infectious Disease: Pneumonia

A 10- to 15-day RCT in patients ($n = 60$) with pneumonia investigated the efficacy of ADAPT-232 (a standardized combination of eleuthero, schisandra, and rhodiola) BID plus the standard treatment of cefazolin, bromhexine, and theophylline compared with standard treatment plus placebo. The mean duration of treatment with antibiotics required to bring about recovery from the acute phase of the disease was 2 days shorter with the herbal product compared with placebo. Patients in the herbal group scored higher in QOL domains at the beginning of the rehabilitation period, and significantly higher on the fifth day after clinical convalescence, than did the placebo group. The authors concluded that adjuvant therapy with ADAPT-232 had a positive effect on the recovery of patients with pneumonia (Narimanian et al., 2005).

Infectious Disease: Dysentery

An RCT in children ($n = 100$) ages 1–14 years with dysentery compared eleuthero plus erythromycin with erythromycin alone. The dysentery process was similar between groups. The eleuthero group showed an earlier recovery than the erythromycin alone group. The authors concluded that use of eleuthero in combination with erythromycin for the treatment of children with dysentery was recommended (Vereshchagin, 1978).

Oncologic Disorders: Ovarian Cancer

A 4-week RCT in stage III–IV ovarian cancer patients ($n = 28$) compared the immunological effects of AdMax (eleuthero, rhodiola, schisandra, and *Rhaponticum carthamoides*) 270 mg/day with a control group for 4 weeks. Patients were treated with a dose of cisplatin 75 mg/m^2 and cyclophosphamide 600 mg/m^2, and labs were followed up at 4 weeks. In patients who took AdMax following the chemotherapy, the mean numbers of CD3, CD4, CD5, and CD8 cells were increased compared with those who did not take the herbal combination. Also, the mean amounts of IgG and IgM were also increased in the herbal group compared with control. The authors concluded that the combination of extracts from adaptogenic plants may boost the suppressed immunity in ovarian cancer patients who are undergoing chemotherapy (Kormosh et al., 2006).

ACTIVE CONSTITUENTS

Root

- Carbohydrates
  - Polysaccharides (immunostimulant)

- Lipids
  - Waxes (emollient, moisturizing): eleutheroside D (antifatigue), eleutheroside E or acanthoside D (protective effects against Aβ, antifatigue)
- Phenolic compounds
  - Phenylpropanoids (antioxidant, antimutagenic, antitumor, antimicrobial): eleutheroside B (syringin), chlorogenic acid
  - Coumarins: isofraxidin (inhibits cell invasion and the expression of MMP-7 by human hepatoma cell lines)
  - Lignans: sesamin
  - Flavonoids: quercetin (antiinflammatory, antioxidant, hypotensive, antidiabetic, antispasmodic, neuroprotective, XO inhibition, antibacterial, anticancer)
- Terpenes:
  - Triterpenoids: copteroside B, silphioside F, tauroside, mesembryanthemoidigenic acid
  - Triterpenoid saponins: eleutheroside A, ciwujianosides A1–4, B, C1–4, D1–3, E, sessiloside, hederasaponin B, chiisanoside, gypsogenin

ELEUTHERO/SIBERIAN GINSENG COMMONLY USED PREPARATIONS AND DOSAGE

Dried Root

- Decoction: 5 g per cup 2–5 times per day.
- Tincture (1:5, 50%): 1–4 mL up to TID.
- Powdered root: 500 mg (1/5 tsp) up to QID.
- Capsule or tablet of powdered root: 1–2 g per day.
- Capsule or tablet of powdered root extract: 250 mg up to TID.
- Capsule or tablet of standardized root extract (standardized to 1% eleutheroside B and E): 100–250 mg BID.

For adaptogenic uses, eleuthero is often taken for 6-8 weeks followed by a 2-week break.

SAFETY AND PRECAUTION

Side Effects

Hypertensive effects have been reported. Most ADRs noted in clinical studies were mild. Possible allergic reactions have been reported.

Case Reports

Subarachnoid hemorrhage was reported in a 53-year-old woman following use of an herbal supplement containing red clover, dong quai, and eleuthero for perimenopausal hot flashes. Symptoms resolved after supplement discontinuation.

Toxicity

The acute LD_{50} in mice for eleuthero appears to be greater than 25 g/kg of the dry root. In an acute and subchronic study in mice, doses up to 4000 mg/kg/day were associated with no adverse effect levels.

Pregnancy and Lactation

Insufficient human safety data. Animal data are reassuring despite concerns raised about fetal toxicity in vitro.

Disease Interactions

Avoid in the perioperative period.
Use with caution in patients with bipolar disorder or anxiety.
Avoid in patients with estrogen sensitive cancer.

Drug Interactions

- CYP: Induces CYP3A4. Eleutherosides B and E from eleuthero may inhibit CYP2C9 and CYP2E1.
- Digoxin: In a case report, Siberian ginseng elevated serum digoxin levels. May falsely elevate serum digoxin assays.

REFERENCES

Amaryan G, Astvatsatryan V, Gabrielyan E, Panossian A, Panosyan V, Wikman G. Double-blind, placebo-controlled, randomized, pilot clinical trial of ImmunoGuard—a standardized fixed combination of Andrographis paniculata Nees, with Eleutherococcus senticosus maxim, Schizandra chinensis bail. and Glycyrrhiza glabra L. extracts in patients with familial Mediterranean fever. Phytomedicine 2003 May;10(4):271–85.

Aslanyan G, Amroyan E, Gabrielyan E, Nylander M, Wikman G, Panossian A. Double-blind, placebo-controlled, randomised study of single dose effects of ADAPT-232 on cognitive functions. Phytomedicine 2010 Jun;17(7):494–9.

Bang JS, Chung YH, Chung SJ, et al. Clinical effect of a polysaccharide-rich extract of Acanthopanax senticosus on alcohol hangover. Pharmazie 2015 Apr;70(4):269–73.

Barth A, Hovhannisyan A, Jamalyan K, Narimanyan M. Antitussive effect of a fixed combination of Justicia adhatoda, Echinacea purpurea and Eleutherococcus senticosus extracts in patients with acute upper respiratory tract infection: a comparative, randomized, double-blind, placebo-controlled study. Phytomedicine 2015 Dec 1;22(13):1195–200.

Bohn B, Nebe CT, Birr C. Flow-cytometric studies with Eleutherococcus senticosus extract as an immunomodulatory agent. Arzneimittelforschung 1987 Oct;37(10):1193–6.

Cicero AF, Derosa G, Brillante R, Bernardi R, Nascetti S, Gaddi A. Effects of Siberian ginseng (*Eleutherococcus senticosus* maxim.) on elderly quality of life: a randomized clinical trial. Arch Gerontol Geriatr Suppl 2004;(9):69–73.

Fukada K, Kajiya-Sawane M, Matsumoto Y, Hasegawa T, Fukaya Y, Kajiya K. Antiedema effects of Siberian ginseng in humans and its molecular mechanism of lymphatic vascular function in vitro. Nutr Res 2016 Jul;36(7):689–95.

Gabrielian ES, Shukarian AK, Goukasova GI, et al. A double blind, placebo-controlled study of Andrographis paniculata fixed combination Kan Jang in the treatment of acute upper respiratory tract infections including sinusitis. Phytomedicine 2002 Oct;9(7):589–97.

Gaffney BT, Hügel HM, Rich PA. The effects of Eleutherococcus senticosus and Panax ginseng on steroidal hormone indices of stress and lymphocyte subset numbers in endurance athletes. Life Sci 2001 Dec 14;70(4):431–42.

Hong YH. Effects of the herb mixture, DTS20, on oxidative stress and plasma alcoholic metabolites after alcohol consumption in healthy young men. Integr Med Res 2016 Dec;5(4):309–16.

Hwang Y-C, Jeong I-K, Ahn KJ, Chung HY. The effects of *Acanthopanax senticosus* extract on bone turnover and bone mineral density in Korean postmenopausal women. J Bone Miner Metab September 2009;27(5):584–90.

Jayawardena R, Thejani T, Ranasinghe P, Fernando D, Verster JC. Interventions for treatment and/or prevention of alcohol hangover: systematic review. Hum Psychopharmacol 2017 Sep;32(5).

Kormosh N, Laktionov K, Antoshechkina M. Effect of a combination of extract from several plants on cell-mediated and humoral immunity of patients with advanced ovarian cancer. Phytother Res 2006 May;20(5):424–5.

Kuo J, Chen KW, Cheng IS, Tsai PH, Lu YJ, Lee NY. The effect of eight weeks of supplementation withEleutherococcus senticosuson endurance capacity and metabolism in human. Chin J Physiol 2010 Apr 30;53(2):105–11.

Lee YJ, Chung HY, Kwak HK, Yoon S. The effects of A. senticosus supplementation on serum lipid profiles, biomarkers of oxidative stress, and lymphocyte DNA damage in postmenopausal women. Biochem Biophys Res Commun 2008;375(1):44–8.

Li W, Liu M, Feng S, et al. Acanthopanax for acute ischaemic stroke. Cochrane Database Syst Rev 2009 Jul 8;3, CD007032.

Mkrtchyan A, Panosyan V, Panossian A, Wikman G, Wagner H. A phase I clinical study of Andrographis paniculata fixed combination Kan Jang versus ginseng and valerian on the semen quality of healthy male subjects. Phytomedicine 2005 Jun;12(6–7):403–9.

Narimanian M, Badalyan M, Panosyan V, et al. Impact of Chisan® (ADAPT-232) on the quality-of life and its efficacy as an adjuvant in the treatment of acute non-specific pneumonia. Phytomedicine 2005;12:723–9.

Poolsup N, Suthisisang C, Prathanturarug S, Asawamekin A, Chanchareon U. Andrographis paniculata in the symptomatic treatment of uncomplicated upper respiratory tract infection: systematic review of randomized controlled trials. J Clin Pharm Ther 2004 Feb;29(1):37–45.

Spasov AA, Ostrovskij OV, Chernikov MV, Wikman G. Comparative controlled study of Andrographis paniculata fixed combination, Kan Jang and an Echinacea preparation as adjuvant, in the treatment of uncomplicated respiratory disease in children. Phytother Res 2004 Jan;18(1):47–53.

Vereshchagin IA. Treatment of dysentery in children with a combination of monomycin and Eleutherococcus. Antibiotiki 1978 Jul;23(7):633–6.

Weng S, Tang J, Wang G, Wang X, Wang H. Comparison of the addition of Siberian ginseng (Acanthopanax senticosus) Vs fluoxetine to Lithium for the treatment of bipolar disorder in adolescents: a randomized, double-blind trial. Curr Ther Res Clin Exp 2007 Jul;68(4):280–90.

Wu W, Liu JH, Yin CP, Zhang CH. A comparative study of the effects of Acanthopanacis senticosi injection, theophylline and caffeine on human sperm mobility in vitro. Zhonghua Nan Ke Xue 2009 Mar;15(3):278–81.

Zhang N, Van Crombruggen K, Holtappels G, Bachert C. A herbal composition of Scutellaria baicalensis and Eleutherococcus senticosus shows potent anti-inflammatory effects in an ex vivo human mucosal tissue model. Evid Based Complement Alternat Med 2012;673145.

Zhang X, Kang D, Zhang L, Peng L. Shuganjieyu capsule for major depressive disorder (MDD) in adults: a systematic review. Aging Ment Health 2014;18(8):941–53.

44 FENNEL (*FOENICULUM VULGARE*)
Seed, Leaf, Root

GENERAL OVERVIEW

Fennel has been used traditionally for its gastrointestinal benefits. The seed is the source of the active constituents, which can be extracted and applied as an essential oil. The whole seed is commonly used as a tea for infantile colic, indigestion, dysmenorrhea, and lactation promotion. Preclinical evidence also indicates that fennel has potential applications for glaucoma and menopausal symptoms.

Clinical research indicates that fennel, alone or in combination formulas, may be beneficial for endothelial dysfunction, infantile colic, irritable bowel syndrome, constipation, primary dysmenorrhea, menopause, sexual dysfunction, and hirsutism.

IN VITRO AND ANIMAL RESEARCH

Fennel has demonstrated antispasmodic, diuretic, antiinflammatory, analgesic, secretomotor, secretolytic, galactagogue, emmenagogue, and antioxidant effects.

Fennel seed essential oil has been shown to stimulate both pancreatic α-cells and insulin secretion. It has also been shown to increase gastric acid secretion and GI motility and have antispasmodic effects at higher doses. It reduces GI and bladder smooth muscle contractions induced by acetylcholine. This latter effect appears to be related to calcium channel mechanisms. The effects of fennel essential oil on isolated rat uterus showed a reduction in frequency of contractions induced by PGE2 but not contractions induced by oxytocin.

In evaluating the oculohypotensive activity of fennel, ophthalmic applications of aqueous extract of fennel produced a 17.5%, 21%, and 22% reduction of intraocular pressure (IOP) in normotensive rabbits at 0.3%, 0.6%, and 1.2% concentrations, respectively. Thereafter, a steroid-induced model of glaucoma in rabbits given the 0.6% dose produced a maximum mean IOP lowering of 32%. The results were noted to be similar to timolol (Agarwal et al., 2007).

Rat stomachs were assessed for acid secretion in response to contact with a variety of different spices including fennel. Fennel was shown to increase acid secretion at a rate only second to red pepper (greater than cardamom, black pepper, cumin, or coriander). Contrary to red pepper, this effect was not blocked by atropine in the fennel group, suggesting the acid secretion with fennel is not due to cholinergic mechanisms. In the presence of ASA-induced mucosal injury, fennel did not increase acid secretion. Thus, despite a basic increase in acid secretion, fennel appears to have built-in gastroprotective effects (Vasudevan et al., 2000). In an ulcer-induction model in rats, fennel was shown to significantly ($P < 0.001$) reduce ethanol-induced gastric damage attributed in part to reduction in lipid peroxidation and an increase in antioxidant activity (Birdane et al., 2007).

An acetone extract of fennel seeds in male rats produced a decreased total protein concentration in testes and vas deferens and an increased total protein in seminal vesicles and prostate glands, with a decrease in acid phosphatase. In female rats this same extract caused increased vaginal cornification and ovulation, increased mammary gland weight, and increased weight of estrogen-sensitive tissues at higher doses, suggesting estrogenic activity (Malini et al., 1985). Research on goats has demonstrated an increase in milk production attributed to the estrogenic activity.

An alcoholic extract of fennel was shown to ameliorate the amnesic effect of scopolamine and aging in mice suggesting an AChE inhibition. Nitrates and nitrates from fennel seeds have been shown to promote NO in red blood cells ex vivo. A study to evaluate anxiolytic potential of fennel seeds in mice compared fennel seed in 2% of diet or in 4% of diet against controls. Anxious behavior was decreased in both fennel groups compared with the control group.

In vitro research on anethole, one of the main constituents of fennel seed, has demonstrated anti-inflammatory and anticarcinogenic effects by modulating TNF-induced cellular responses. It has been shown to suppress the NF-κB-dependent gene expression induced by TNF. Anethole has been shown to inhibit platelet aggregation induced by arachidonic acid, collagen, ADP, and U46619. It also inhibited thrombin-induced clot retraction. The antithrombotic dose appeared to be free of the prohemorrhagic side effect that is seen with ASA. Anethole has also demonstrated NO-independent vasorelaxant properties in rat aorta.

Estragole, another active constituent, is a procarcinogen but appears to have minimal actual carcinogenic risk due to inactivation by hepatic enzymes. Nevertheless, studies in rats have demonstrated a high rate of development of hepatomas at high doses. However, in a CCl4 model of hepatotoxicity in rats, fennel resulted in decreased liver enzymes, indicating hepatoprotective properties of fennel seed as a whole.

HUMAN RESEARCH

Cardiovascular Disorders: Endothelial Dysfunction

An unblinded study in healthy volunteers ($n=5$) assessed the effect of chewing 1 g of fennel seeds for 1 min. The salivary nitric oxide concentrations increased slightly more than twofold (Swaminathan et al., 2012).

Gastrointestinal Disorders: Infantile Colic

A 2018 systematic review on dietary interventions for infantile colic selected 15 RCTs ($n=1121$) for inclusion. Although the studies were small and at high risk of bias, the authors identified benefit from an extract of fennel, chamomile, and lemon balm in one study. Average crying times for the herbal combination and

placebo were 76.9 and 169.9 min/day, respectively, at the end of the 1-week study (Gordon et al., 2018).

A 2011 systematic review on complementary medicines for infantile colic found 15 RCTs that met inclusion criteria. The authors noted that there were some encouraging results for fennel extract, mixed herbal tea, and sugar solutions, although all trials had major limitations (Perry et al., 2011).

A 1-week RCT in infants ($n=125$) with colic compared fennel seed oil (one to four teaspoons of a water emulsion with 0.1% fennel seed oil, up to QID) with placebo. There was a complete resolution of colic in 65% of fennel infants, compared with 24% of placebo infants ($P<0.01$). There was a significant improvement of colic with fennel compared with placebo (ARR=41%, NNT=2). Side effects were not reported for infants in either group during the trial. The authors concluded that fennel seed oil emulsion was superior to placebo in decreasing intensity of infantile colic (Alexandrovich et al., 2003).

A 1-week RCT in breastfed infants ($n=93$) with colic compared a polyherbal standardized extract combination (chamomile, lemon balm and fennel) with placebo BID. The daily average crying time with the herbal formula decreased from 201 to 77 min/day. With placebo the crying time decreased from 199 to 169 min/day ($P<0.005$). Crying time reduction was observed in 85% of subjects given the herbal formula and 49% of subjects given placebo ($P<0.005$). No side effects were reported. The authors concluded that colic in breastfed infants improves within 1 week of treatment with this polyherbal formula (Savino et al., 2005).

A 1-week RCT in healthy term 2- to 8-week-old infants ($n=68$) who had colic compared a polyherbal tea (German chamomile, vervain, licorice, fennel, and lemon balm) with a placebo tea (glucose) up to 150 mL/dose up to TID. Parents reported that the tea eliminated the colic in 57% of the infants, whereas placebo was helpful in 26% ($P<0.01$). No adverse effects were noted in either group (Weizman et al., 1993).

Gastrointestinal Disorders: Irritable Bowel Syndrome and Constipation

A 30-day RCT in patients ($n=121$) with mild-to-moderate symptoms of IBS compared a combination of curcumin plus fennel essential oil with placebo two capsules BID. A significant decrease in the mean relative IBS-Symptom Severity Score (IBS-SSS) was observed after 30 days with curcumin-fennel vs placebo (50% vs 26%; $P < 0.001$). This result matched the reduction of abdominal pain and all the other symptoms of the IBS-SSS. The percentage of symptom-free patients with curcumin-fennel vs placebo was 26% vs 7%; $P = 0.005$). All domains of IBS-QOL improved consistently. The authors concluded that the curcumin-fennel combination significantly improved symptoms and quality of life in IBS patients over 30 days (Portincasa et al., 2016).

A 2-week open-label pilot study in treatment-resistant IBS patients ($n = 5$) assessed the effect of fennel seeds chewed after meals (four sugar-coated seeds per meal for 1 week then gradually increased to 8–12 seeds). After 2 weeks of therapy, there was marked improvement with less abdominal cramps, less dependence on Imodium and analgesics and less clinic visits. The subjects indicated that they had more control of their social life. The authors concluded that fennel seeds should be considered as a useful adjunctive therapeutic modality in refractory cases of IBS (Amjad and Jafary, 2000).

A 5-day crossover RCT in patients ($n = 20$) with chronic constipation compared 3 g/day of an herbal tea containing a combination of fennel, anise, elderberry, and senna with placebo tea. Mean colonic transit time as assessed by X-ray was 15.7 h with active treatment and 42.3 h with placebo ($P < 0.001$). The number of evacuations per day increased during use of the active tea and patient perception of bowel function was improved ($P < 0.01$), but quality of life did not show significant differences among the study periods. There were no significant differences in adverse effects except for a small reduction in serum potassium levels during the active treatment (Picon et al., 2010).

Women's Genitourinary Disorders: Primary Dysmenorrhea

A 2-month RCT in adolescent females ($n = 110$) with primary dysmenorrhea compared fennel with mefenamic acid for pain relief. Pain was either diminished or eliminated in 80% of the fennel group and 73% of the mefenamic acid group. Inactivity was no longer necessary in 80% of the fennel group and 62% of the mefenamic group. The difference between groups was not statistically significant (Modaress Nejad and Asadipour, 2006).

A three-cycle sequential RCT of women ($n = 30$) with moderate-to-severe primary dysmenorrhea compared mefenamic acid 250 mg QID on the second cycle with 2% fennel fruit 25 drops (roughly 1 mL) every 4 h in the third cycle, each given at onset of menses. Both drugs effectively relieved menstrual pain compared with the control cycle ($P < 0.001$). The mean onset of action was 67.5 min for mefenamic acid and 75 min for fennel ($P = 0.57$). Mefenamic acid had a more potent effect than fennel on the second and third menstrual days ($P < 0.05$), however, the difference on the other days was not significant. Five cases (16.6%) withdrew from the study due to fennel's odor and one case (3.11%) reported a mild increase in the amount of her menstrual flow with fennel. The authors concluded that fennel could be used as a safe and effective herbal drug for primary dysmenorrhea but may have a lower potency than mefenamic acid (Namavar Jahromi et al., 2003).

Women's Genitourinary Disorders: Oligomenorrhea

A 6-month RCT in patients ($n = 61$) with oligomenorrhea evaluated fennel tea plus dry cupping compared with metformin for effect on menses. Menstrual cycle length after 3 months with fennel plus cupping and with metformin was 32.59 and 40.66 days, respectively. After 6 months, the intermenstrual length with fennel plus cupping and with metformin was 30.7 and 43.1 days. Mean pain severity decreased significantly with fennel. The authors concluded that fennel seed infusion plus dry cupping was a safe and effective therapeutic intervention in the management of oligomenorrhea (Mokaberinejad et al., 2019).

Women's Genitourinary Disorders: Perimenopause and Menopause

A 2019 systematic review to look at the effectiveness of phytoestrogens on vaginal health and dyspareunia in peri- and postmenopausal women found 2 systematic reviews and 11 RCTs that met inclusion criteria. Comparison of fennel 5% vaginal cream and placebo gel showed significant differences in superficial cells ($P < 0.01$), parabasal cells ($P < 0.01$), and intermediate cells ($P < 0.01$), whereas no difference was found between oral fennel and placebo with respect to these parameters. Isoflavones increased the maturation value and attenuated vaginal atrophy. Topical iso-flavones had beneficial effects on vaginal atrophy. Similar efficacy was found between *Pueraria mirifica* and conjugated estrogen cream on dryness ($P=0.277$), soreness ($P=0.124$), irritation ($P=0.469$), discharge ($P=0.225$), and dyspareunia ($P=0.089$). The conjugated estrogen cream was more effective than *Pueraria mirifica* ($P<0.005$) for maturation index improvement. Administration of 80 mg red clover oil had a significant effect on superficial ($P<0.005$), intermediate ($P<0.005$), and parabasal cells and vaginal dryness ($P<0.005$) compared with placebo. Flaxseed had a trivial effect on maturation value. Genistein had an effect on the genital score with severity of dyspareunia decreasing by 27%. The authors concluded that phytoestrogens had various effects based on administration route and type of vaginal atrophy (Dizavandi et al., 2019).

A 2017 review of clinical trials on herbal efficacy in menopausal symptoms used search terms menopause, climacteric, hot flushes, flashes, herb, and phytoestrogens. The authors found that passionflower, sage, lemon balm, valerian, black cohosh, fenugreek, black seed, chasteberry, fennel, evening primrose, ginkgo, alfalfa, St. John's wort, Asian ginseng, anise, licorice, red clover, and wild soybean were effective in the treatment of acute menopausal syndrome with different mechanisms. The authors concluded that medicinal plants could play a role in the treatment of acute menopausal syndrome and that further studies were warranted (Kargozar et al., 2017).

A 10-week RCT in postmenopausal women ($n=90$) compared fennel 100 mg BID with placebo for 8 weeks. The fennel group showed a significant decrease in the mean Menopausal Rating Scale score with significant differences between the mean score at baseline and those at 4, 8, and 10 weeks after onset of treatment ($P<0.001$), whereas there were no significant differences in the placebo group. The differences between fennel and placebo were also significant ($P<0.001$). The authors concluded that fennel was an effective and safe treatment to reduce menopausal symptoms in postmenopausal women without serious side effects (Rahimikian et al., 2017).

An 8-week RCT in postmenopausal women ($n=60$) with vaginal atrophy compared 5% fennel vaginal cream with placebo 5 g/day. The number of superficial cells increased significantly with fennel compared with placebo (76 vs 12; $P<0.001$). The number of intermediate

and parabasal cells decreased significantly with fennel compared with placebo ($P<0.001$) and the vaginal pH decreased significantly with fennel compared with placebo (100% vs 7.4% of subjects; $P<0.001$). All women in the fennel group had a vaginal maturation index of 65–100 at 8 weeks, whereas 41% of the women in the control group had a maturation vaginal index of 50–64 ($P<0.001$). The authors concluded that fennel was an effective means to manage the symptoms of vaginal atrophy in postmenopausal women and without side effects (Yaralizadeh et al., 2016).

Women's Genitourinary Disorders: Female Sexual Dysfunction

A 2018 systematic review to evaluate the effectiveness of phytoestrogens on sexual disorders and severity of dyspareunia in women found that the phytoestrogens isolated from fennel, French maritime pine bark, maca, and fenugreek significantly improved sexual function, whereas the phytoestrogens isolated from Korean red ginseng, flaxseed, red clover, and soy did not lead to significant effects on sexual function (Najafi and Ghazanfarpour, 2018).

An 8-week RCT in postmenopausal women ($n=60$) with sexual dysfunction compared fennel vaginal cream with placebo 5 g QHS. All areas of sexual function including arousal, lubrication, orgasm, sexual satisfaction, and pain improved in both fennel and placebo groups after 8 weeks; however, the differences with the fennel group were more evident ($P<0.05$). The total Female Sexual Function Index score was 8.2 and 8 before the intervention and 33.8 and 19 after the intervention with fennel and placebo, respectively ($P<0.001$). The authors concluded that fennel vaginal cream was an effective means of improving sexual activity in postmenopausal women and that the use of this product in women who have sexual dysfunction and contraindications for hormone therapy was recommended (Abedi et al., 2018).

Dermatological Disorders: Hirsutism

A 24-week RCT in women ($n=44$) with mild-to-moderate idiopathic hirsutism compared 3% fennel gel with placebo gel applied topically. The thickness of hairs was reduced from 98 to 76 μm with fennel ($P<0.001$). Isolated itching or itching with irritation occurred in a total of eight patients, six of which were using fennel. The authors concluded that fennel gel 3% was effective in decreasing hair thickness in women with idiopathic mild to moderate hirsutism (Akha et al., 2014).

A 24-week RCT in women ($n = 38$) with hirsutism compared a 1% or 2% fennel cream with 0% (placebo) cream applied topically. The mean values of hair diameter reduction were 7.8%, 18.3%, and −0.5% for patients receiving 1%, 2%, and 0% creams, respectively. The hair thickness was reduced from 90 to 75 μm in the active treatment group and increased slightly in the control group after 24 weeks ($P < 0.001$). The authors concluded that the efficacy of treatment with the cream containing 2% fennel was better than the cream containing 1% fennel and these two were more potent than placebo (Javidnia et al., 2003).

ACTIVE CONSTITUENTS

- Phenolic compounds
  - Phenylpropanoids (antioxidant, antimutagenic, antitumor, antimicrobial): anethole, estragole
- Terpenes:
  - Monoterpenes: limonene (antineoplastic, detoxifying)
  - Tetraterpenes: β-carotene
- Aromatic compounds (hypoglycemic): anethole (dopaminergic, antineoplastic, antiinflammatory, antispasmodic), fenchone, estragole, alpha-pinene, beta-pinene, alpha-phellandrene, β-phellandrene, alpha-terpineol, beta-myrcene, camphene, p-cymene, safrole, limonene (antineoplastic, detoxifying)
- Vitamin C

FENNEL COMMONLY USED PREPARATIONS AND DOSAGE (FOR ADULTS UNLESS OTHERWISE SPECIFIED)

The following are examples of some available formulations and ranges of dosing for commercial herbal products. See Part III Introduction "How to prescribe medicinal herbs" for further guidance on herbal advising and prescribing.

Seed

- Whole seeds: 4–8 seeds chewed with meals (for IBS).
- Oral infusion (tea): 1/2–1 tsp. of ground seeds per cup TID pc.

- Tincture (1:5,40%): 1-2 mL TID.
- Powdered seed: 1 g (1/2) tsp. QD-BID.
- Capsule or tablet of powdered seed: 480 mg TID.
- Essential oil: should be administered under guidance of certified aromatherapist due to risks for toxicity.

SAFETY AND PRECAUTION

Side Effects

Rare allergic reactions may occur, as fennel is cross-reactive with allergies to the celery family of plants and to peaches. May cause premature gynecomastia in children with regular prolonged use. May lower seizure threshold. May be confused with giant fennel (*Ferula communis*), which has coumarin properties and bleeding risk.

Case Reports

A 12-month-old girl showed premature thelarche after being given 2–3 teaspoons of fennel tea daily for 6 months.

A woman with well-controlled epilepsy developed a generalized tonic-clonic seizure after ingesting cakes containing an unknown quantity of fennel essential oil.

Four cases of acute methemoglobinemia have been reported after young children ate homemade fennel purée.

Toxicity

Acute (24-h, 500, 1000, or 3000 mg/kg) and chronic (90-day, 100 mg/kg) oral toxicity studies of ethanolic extracts of fennel aerial parts in mice found no mortality. The treated male mice gained significant weight during chronic treatment while a loss or no significant change in weight was noticed in the female mice treated with the same extracts. There were no spermatotoxic effects.

Risk for toxicity is greater with the essential oil. Fennel essential oil (0.37, 0.75, and 1.5 mg/kg) was administered to mature male mice for 35 days and was shown to adversely affect cellular DNA and RNA as well as sperm count and morphology. Estragole has carcinogenic potential at oral intake of 0.23% by weight of rat diet for 1 year, inducing hepatoma in 56% of rats.

Pregnancy and Lactation

May be toxic to fetal cells. Avoid during pregnancy. Although fennel tea has traditionally been used to promote lactation, there are case reports of adverse newborn effects when the mother consumed large quantities of fennel tea when combined with anise (both herbs contain anethole). Some sources recommend limiting fennel tea consumption during lactation to 2 weeks.

Disease Interactions

Avoid in patients with estrogen-dependent cancers due to potential estrogenic activity.
Caution with seizure disorder as may reduce seizure threshold.

Drug Interactions

- Reduces efficacy of fluroquinolones.
- Caution with antiplatelet drugs due to platelet inhibition effects.

REFERENCES

Abedi P, Najafian M, Yaralizadeh M, Namjoyan F. Effect of fennel vaginal cream on sexual function in postmenopausal women: a double blind randomized controlled trial. J Med Life 2018 Jan-Mar;11(1):24–8.

Agarwal R, Sunder S, Gupta S, Srivastava S. Oculohypotensive effects of *Foeniculum vulgare* in experimental models of glaucoma. Indian J Physiol Pharmacol November 2007;52(1):77–83.

Akha O, Rabiei K, Kashi Z, et al. The effect of fennel (Foeniculum vulgare) gel 3% in decreasing hair thickness in idiopathic mild to moderate hirsutism, a randomized placebo controlled clinical trial. Caspian J Intern Med 2014 Winter;5(1):26–9.

Alexandrovich I, Rakovitskaya O, Kolmo E, Sidorova T, Shushunov S. The effect of fennel (Foeniculum vulgare) seed oil emulsion in infantile colic: a randomized, placebo-controlled study. Altern Ther Health Med 2003 Jul-Aug;9(4):58–61.

Amjad H, Jafary HA. Foeniculum vulgare therapy in irritable bowel syndrome. Am J Gastroenterol 2000;95:2491.

Birdane F, Cemek M, Birdane Y, Gülçin I, Büyükokuroğlu M. Beneficial effects of *Foeniculum vulgare* on ethanol-induced acute gastric mucosal injury in rats. World J Gastroenterol 2007 Jan 28;13(4):607–11.

Dizavandi FR, Ghazanfarpour M, Roozbeh N, Kargarfard L, Khadivzadeh T, Dashti S. An overview of the phytoestrogen effect on vaginal health and dyspareunia in peri- and post-menopausal women. Post Reprod Health 2019 Mar;25(1):11–20.

Gordon M, Biagioli E, Sorrenti M, et al. Dietary modifications for infantile colic. Cochrane Database Syst Rev 2018 Oct 10;10, CD011029.

Javidnia K, Dastgheib L, Mohammadi Samani S, Nasiri A. Antihirsutism activity of fennel (fruits of Foeniculum vulgare)

extract. A double-blind placebo-controlled study. Phytomedicine 2003;10(6–7):455–8.

Kargozar R, Azizi H, Salari R. A review of effective herbal medicines in controlling menopausal symptoms. Electron Physician 2017 Nov;9(11):5826–33.

Malini T, Vanithakumari G, Megala N, Anusya S, Devi K, Elango V. Effect of Foeniculum vulgare mill. Seed extract on the genital organs of male and female rats. Indian J Physiol Pharmacol 1985 Jan-Mar;29(1):21–6.

Modaress Nejad V, Asadipour M. Comparison of the effectiveness of fennel and mefenamic acid on pain intensity in dysmenorrhoea. East Mediterr Health J 2006 May-Jul;12(3–4):423–7.

Mokaberinejad R, Rampisheh Z, Aliasl J, Akhtari E. The comparison of fennel infusion plus dry cupping versus metformin in management of oligomenorrhoea in patients with polycystic ovary syndrome: a randomised clinical trial. J Obstet Gynaecol 2019 Jul;39(5):652–8.

Najafi NM, Ghazanfarpour M. Effect of phytoestrogens on sexual function in menopausal women: a systematic review and meta-analysis. Climacteric 2018 Oct;21(5):437–45.

Namavar Jahromi B, Tartifizadeh A, Khabnadideh S. Comparison of fennel and mefenamic acid for the treatment of primary dysmenorrhea. Int J Gynaecol Obstet 2003 Feb;80(2):153–7.

Perry R, Hunt K, Ernst E. Nutritional supplements and other complementary medicines for infantile colic: a systematic review. Pediatrics 2011 Apr;127(4):720-33.

Picon PD, Picon RV, Costa AF, et al. Randomized clinical trial of a phytotherapic compound containing Pimpinella anisum, Foeniculum vulgare, Sambucus nigra, and Cassia augustifolia for chronic constipation. BMC Complement Altern Med 2010 Apr 30;10:17.

Portincasa P, Bonfrate L, Scribano ML, et al. Curcumin and fennel essential oil improve symptoms and quality of life in patients with irritable bowel syndrome. J Gastrointestin Liver Dis 2016 Jun;25(2):151–7.

Rahimikian F, Rahimi R, Golzareh P, Bekhradi R, Mehran A. Effect of Foeniculum vulgare mill. (fennel) on menopausal symptoms in postmenopausal women: a randomized, triple-blind, placebo-controlled trial. Menopause 2017 Sep;24(9):1017–21.

Savino F, Cresi F, Castagno E, Silvestro L, Oggero R. A randomized double-blind placebo-controlled trial of a standardized extract of Matricariae recutita, Foeniculum vulgare and Melissa officinalis (ColiMil®) in the treatment of breastfed colicky infants. Phytother Res 2005 Apr;19(4):335–40.

Swaminathan A, Sridhara SR, Sinha S, et al. Nitrites derived from Foeniculum vulgare (fennel) seeds promotes vascular functions. J Food Sci 2012 Dec;77(12):H273–9.

Vasudevan K, Vembar S, Veeraraghavan K, Haranath PS. Influence of intragastric perfusion of aqueous spice extracts on acid secretion in anesthetized albino rats. Indian J Gastroenterol. 2000 Apr-Jun;19(2):53-6. PMID: 10812814.

Weizman Z, Alkrinawi S, Goldfarb D. Efficacy of herbal tea preparation in infantile colic. J Pediatr 1993;122(650):652.

Yaralizadeh M, Abedi P, Najar S, Namjoyan F, Saki A. Effect of Foeniculum vulgare (fennel) vaginal cream on vaginal atrophy in postmenopausal women: a double-blind randomized placebo-controlled trial. Maturitas 2016 Feb;84:75–80.

45

FENUGREEK (*TRIGONELLA FOENUM-GRAECUM*)
Seed

GENERAL OVERVIEW

Fenugreek seeds have traditionally been used as a cooking spice in India and carry a Generally Recognized as Safe (GRAS) designation by the USFDA. The seed extract is used for imitation maple flavoring. Because it is high in steroidal saponins, fenugreek is used in the commercial production of steroids. It has been used in Ayurvedic medicine as a demulcent, laxative, galactagogue, antiinflammatory, and vulnerary herb. It is used in modern herbalism for diabetes, boils, cellulitis, and tuberculosis. It is also used to enhance male libido, manage dysmenorrhea, induce labor, and promote lactation.

Clinical research indicates that fenugreek, alone or in combination formulas, may be beneficial for hyperlipidemia, diabetes, obesity, lactation, dysmenorrhea, polycystic ovary syndrome, menopause, female and male sexual dysfunction, Parkinson's disease, and athletic performance.

IN VITRO AND ANIMAL RESEARCH

In vitro and animal studies indicate that fenugreek has hypocholesterolemic, hypolipidemic, hypoglycemic, antioxidant, antiplatelet, antimicrobial, and hepatoprotective effects. There is animal evidence for benefit with peripheral neuropathy.

Studies have demonstrated the ability of fenugreek to significantly reduce serum cholesterol in dogs and rats. In both cholesterol and blood sugar testing, the defatted portion, but not the lipid extract, of the seed demonstrated cholesterol-reducing activity. The method of

action is unknown but may be due to saponins, alkaloids, or the galactomannan fiber content of the seed. The saponins present in fenugreek are transformed in the GI tract to sapogenins. Sapogenins increase biliary cholesterol secretion. Based on an in vitro study, fenugreek may also increase intraluminal binding of cholesterol, which results in increased fecal excretion of bile acids and neutral sterols. The high pectin content may explain the triglyceride-lowering effect of fenugreek. Pectin also absorbs bile acid salts resulting in an increase in hepatic cholesterol conversion to bile salts which are excreted along with the fiber and saponins present in fenugreek. In vitro evidence in diabetic human erythrocytes showed that polyphenolic acids from fenugreek seeds exhibited a concentration-dependent inhibition of lipid peroxidation.

Fenugreek has been shown to have several mechanisms for lowering blood sugar. Fenugreek seed extract dose-dependently increases glucose transport rates by increasing GLUT4 translocation across the plasma membrane. The seed powder increases pyruvate kinase and reduces PEP carboxykinase thereby reducing hepatic and renal gluconeogenesis. The soluble dietary fiber fraction blunts an increase in serum glucose, improves glucose uptake, and increases hepatic glycogen. The seed extract alters the reduction in hepatic glucokinase and hexokinase activity that is commonly increased in diabetes mellitus. An in vitro study indicated that fenugreek seed extract phosphorylates several proteins, including the insulin receptor, insulin receptor substrate 1, and the p85 subunit of phosphoinositide 3-kinases, in both adipocytes and human hepatoma cells, suggesting that some of fenugreek's effects may be due to activation of the insulin-signaling pathway in adipocytes and liver cells. The powdered leaves of fenugreek have demonstrated an effect similar to glyburide in rats and mice. In diabetic dogs, fenugreek seeds reduced blood glucose, plasma glucagon, and somatostatin levels as well as carbohydrate-induced hyperglycemia. Some animal studies have shown that fenugreek seeds delay gastric emptying due to the pectin content, slowing carbohydrate absorption.

The alkaloid trigonelline in fenugreek has hypoglycemic, hypolipidemic, neuroprotective, antimigraine, sedative, memory-improving, antibacterial, antiviral, and antitumor activities. It has been shown to reduce diabetic auditory neuropathy and platelet aggregation. The amino acid 4-hyroxyisoleucine in fenugreek seeds increases glucose-induced insulin release in vitro in human and rat pancreatic islet cells. When administered to type 2 diabetic rats, this amino acid increased peripheral glucose utilization and decreased hepatic glucose production, thereby improving insulin resistance. Chronic ingestion of 4-hydroxyisoleucine significantly reduced insulinemia.

Antiinflammatory and diuretic activities of fenugreek have been demonstrated in animals. Fenugreek and its constituent trigonelline have been shown to be renoprotective in diabetic rats through antioxidant mechanisms and to prevent calcium oxalate urolithiasis.

A study in mice who were treated with neuropathic doses of pyridoxine showed that fenugreek reversed neuropathic changes. In a rat study, fenugreek extract showed analgesic activity that may be similar to NSAIDs via the spinal 5-HT system or purinergic receptors. It has also been shown to raise hemoglobin, glutathione, and plasma antioxidant levels. It raises T4 and reduces T3 in rats. The fenugreek constituent protodioscin has been demonstrated to trigger release of nitric oxide in the corpus cavernosum and to produce increases in testosterone, DHT, and DHEA in animal studies. An extract of fenugreek leaf repels some insects.

Research has indicated that fenugreek has chemopreventive properties against certain cancers and reduces the toxicity associated with some antineoplastic drugs. Fenugreek has been shown to act as an estrogen receptor modulator and stimulate breast cancer cells in vitro. However, in MCF-7 estrogen receptor-positive breast cancer cells, fenugreek extract induced cell cycle arrest as well as apoptosis. The steroidal saponin dioscin has been shown to suppress cell viability of ovarian cancer cells through several pathways. In rats, dietary fenugreek seeds have been shown to inhibit colon carcinogenesis. Diosgenin suppressed total colonic aberrant crypt foci formation likely through inhibition of bcl-2 and induction of caspase-3 protein expression, thereby inducing apoptosis and inhibiting cell growth. Diosgenin has also been shown to inhibit NF-κB-regulated gene expression. Another constituent in fenugreek, protodioscin, has been shown to strongly inhibit growth and promote apoptosis of HL-60 cells through fragmentation of DNA.

HUMAN RESEARCH

Cardiometabolic Disorders: Hyperlipidemia

A 2020 systematic review to evaluate the effects of fenugreek on cardiovascular risk factors found 12 studies that met inclusion criteria. The reviewers found that fenugreek seed could reduce FBS greater than placebo (WMD: -12.94 mg/dL, I^2: 85%, $P = 0.0001$); reduce A1C greater than placebo (WMD: -0.58%, I^2:0%, $P = 0.61$); reduce TC greater than placebo (WMD: -9.13 mg/dL, I^2:0, $P = 0.48$); and reduce LDL-C greater than placebo (WMD: -11.11 mg/dL, I^2:1.41%, $P = 0.36$). No significant changes were observed in other cardiometabolic parameters. The authors concluded that fenugreek seed as an adjuvant therapy may reduce serum levels of FBS, LDL-C and A1C. They cautioned that there was high heterogeneity in glycemic status and that further studies were warranted (Khodamoradi et al., 2020).

A 2010 systematic review looking at herbal medicine (including traditional Chinese medicine formulations) for hyperlipidemia identified 53 RCTs that met criteria. There were significant decreases in TC and LDL-C after treatment with fenugreek as well as milk thistle, licorice, yarrow, guggul, Daming capsule, chunghyul-dan, garlic powder, black tea, green tea, soy drink enriched with plant sterols, *Satureja khuzestanica*, *Monascus purpureus*, Went rice, C. Koch, Ningzhi capsule, cherry, composite salvia dropping pill (CSDP), shanzha xiaozhi capsule, Ba-wei-wan (hachimijiogan), rhubarb stalk, *Rheum ribes*, and primrose oil. Data were conflicting for red yeast rice, garlic and guggul.

No significant adverse effects or increased mortality were observed. The authors concluded that 22 natural products were found effective in the treatment of hyperlipidemia and that further research was warranted (Hasani-Ranjbar et al., 2010).

A 24-week open-label study in patients with T2DM ($n=60$) assessed the lipid effects of powdered fenugreek seed 12.5 g BID in soup prior to lunch and dinner. TC decreased by 14% (from 241 to 207 mg/dL) and TG decreased by 18% (from 207 to 172 mg/dL). HDL-C increased insignificantly (Sharma et al., 1996).

An open-label study in hypercholesterolemic adults ($n=20$) looked at the effect of consumption of germinated fenugreek seed powder at 12.5 and 18.0 g on the blood lipid profiles. The findings revealed that consumption of 18.0 g of the germinated seed resulted in a significant reduction in TC and LDL-C levels with no significant changes in other lipid parameters (Sowmya and Rajyalakshmi, 1999).

An open-label study investigated 100 g of defatted fenugreek powder (basically the fiber portion) added to unleavened bread compared with unleavened bread alone. Fenugreek in the experimental diet significantly reduced TC and LDL-C by 25%, VLDL-C by 32%, and TG by 38% (Prasanna, 2000).

A 12-week RCT in diabetic patients ($n=50$) with dyslipidemia despite statin therapy investigated a combination of aloe, black seed, fenugreek, garlic, milk thistle, and psyllium (one sachet BID) plus conventional therapy compared with conventional therapy alone. Each sachet contained 300 mg of aloe leaf gel, 1.8 g of black seed, 300 mg of garlic, 2.5 g of fenugreek seed, 1 g of psyllium seed, and 500 mg of milk thistle seed. The levels of serum TG, TC, LDL-C, and A1C, but not FBS, showed a significant in-group improvement in the intervention group. Renal and hepatic transaminases were unchanged with the herbal compound. The authors concluded that this herbal compound was a safe and effective adjunctive treatment in lowering serum lipids in diabetic patients with uncontrolled dyslipidemia (Ghorbani et al., 2019).

A 40-day Phase I open-label clinical trial in diabetic patients ($n=30$) with uncontrolled hyperglycemia and dyslipidemia despite standard therapy compared a polyherbal formulation containing garlic, aloe, black seed, psyllium, fenugreek, and milk thistle one sachet BID in addition to their usual medications. The herbal formula significantly decreased fasting blood glucose from 162 to 146 mg/dL and A1C from 8.4% to 7.7%. LDL-C decreased significantly from 138 to 108 mg/dL, and TG decreased from 203 to 166 mg/dL. There were no changes in liver function, kidney function, or hematologic parameters. The authors concluded that the formulation was safe and effective in lowering blood glucose and serum lipids in patients with advanced-stage T2DM. After consumption of the herbal combination, two patients complained of mild nausea, and two patients reported diarrhea (Zarvandi et al., 2017).

Cardiometabolic Disorders: Prediabetes, Diabetes, and Obesity

A 2020 systematic review to evaluate the effects of fenugreek on cardiovascular risk factors found 12 studies that met inclusion criteria. The reviewers found that fenugreek seed could reduce FBS greater than placebo (WMD: -12.94 mg/dL, I^2: 85%, $P=0.0001$); reduce A1C greater than placebo (WMD: -0.58%, I^2:0%, $P=0.61$); reduce TC greater than placebo (WMD: -9.13 mg/dL, I^2:0, $P=0.48$); and reduce LDL-C greater than placebo (WMD: -11.11 mg/dL, I^2:1.41%, $P=0.36$). No significant changes were observed in other cardiometabolic parameters. The authors concluded that fenugreek seed as an adjuvant therapy may reduce serum levels of FBS, LDL-C, and A1C. They cautioned that there was high heterogeneity in glycemic status and that further studies were warranted (Khodamoradi et al., 2020).

A 2014 systematic review on the long-term effect of fenugreek on glycemia found 10 trials that met inclusion criteria. Fenugreek significantly changed fasting blood glucose by -0.96 mmol/L ($I^2=80\%$); 2-h postload glucose by -2.19 mmol/L ($I^2=71\%$;); and A1C by -0.85% ($I^2=0\%$) compared with control interventions. Significant effects on fasting and 2 h glucose were only found for studies that administered medium or high doses of fenugreek in diabetics. The authors concluded that fenugreek has supportive evidence for glycemic control in diabetics (Neelakantan et al., 2014).

A 2011 systematic review and meta-analysis regarding herbs for glycemic control in diabetics identified nine RCTs ($n=487$) that met inclusion criteria. Milk thistle, fenugreek, and sweet potato significantly improved glycemia, while cinnamon did not. The pooled mean differences in A1C were (-1.92%;

$P=0.008$; -1.13%; $P=0.03$; and -0.3% $P=0.02$) for milk thistle, fenugreek, and sweet potato, respectively. The authors concluded that supplementation with milk thistle, fenugreek, and/or *Ipomoea batatas* may improve glycemic control in T2DM (Suksomboon et al., 2011).

A 2009 review was undertaken to evaluate CAM interventions for glycemic control in T2DM. Their main findings were that gymnema reduced A1C levels in two small open-label trials. In addition, they found that chromium reduced A1C and FBS in a large meta-analysis, cinnamon improved FBS but had unknown effects on A1C, and bitter melon had no effect in two small trials. Green tea and fenugreek each reduced FBS levels in 1 of 3 small trials. Vanadium reduced FBS in small, uncontrolled trials. The authors concluded that chromium, and possibly gymnema, appeared to improve glycemic control (Nahas and Moher, 2009).

A 3-year RCT in patients ($n=140$) with pre-diabetes compared diet and lifestyle alone with diet and lifestyle plus fenugreek powder 5 g in water BID AC to assess progression to T2DM. At the end of the study, the cumulative incidence rate of diabetes was significantly less with fenugreek compared with control (22.97% vs 54.55%; $P<0.01$). Those in the fenugreek group had significantly lower fasting and postprandial blood glucose concentrations compared with baseline, ($P<0.05$ and $P<0.01$, respectively), whereas these values did not significantly change in the control group. Glucose levels normalized in 34.6% of the fenugreek group vs 18.3% of the control group by the end of the study. Also, LDL-C significantly decreased from baseline in the fenugreek group ($P<0.05$) but not in the control group. No significant differences were observed in the other lipids (TC, TG, and HDL-C), BMI, or BP in either group. The estimated odds ratio indicated a 4.2 greater chance of developing T2DM in the control group compared with the fenugreek group. The authors concluded that dietary supplementation of fenugreek 10 g/day in prediabetic subjects was associated with lower conversion to diabetes possibly due to its decreased insulin resistance (Gaddam et al., 2015).

A 2-month RCT in patients ($n=25$) with newly diagnosed T2DM compared fenugreek seed extract 1 g/day with placebo. FBS changed from a baseline average of 148 mg/dL to 119 mg/dL ($P<0.05$) with fenugreek and from 137 mg/dL to 113 mg/dL (N.S.) with placebo. Two-hour PPG decreased from 211 mg/dL to 181 mg/dL with fenugreek and increased from 219 mg/dL to 242 mg/dL with placebo, the difference not being significant. However, the area under the curve (AUC) of blood glucose decreased from 27,597 to 2327 with fenugreek ($P<0.01$), while it increased from 25,411 to 27,842 with placebo (N.S.). The AUC for insulin was decreased from 5630 to 2492 with fenugreek ($P<0.01$) vs from 5928 to 4177 with placebo (N.S.). Insulin sensitivity increased from 57 to 113 vs from 67 to 92 with fenugreek vs placebo, respectively ($P<0.05$). TG decreased and HDL-C increased significantly with fenugreek compared with placebo ($P<0.05$). Fenugreek was associated with transient dyspepsia and abdominal distension in 20% of patients. The authors concluded that adjunct use of fenugreek seeds improved glycemic control and decreased insulin resistance in mild T2DM, with a favorable effect on TGs (Gupta et al., 2001).

A 90-day RCT in subjects ($n=154$) with T2DM compared fenugreek seed powder 500 mg BID with placebo. Decreases in FBS occurred in 83% and 62% of the fenugreek and placebo groups, respectively. Postprandial glucose decreased in 89% and 72% of the fenugreek and placebo groups, respectively. A1C levels decreased significantly in both groups. A significant increase in fasting and postprandial C-peptide levels occurred in both groups with no significant difference between groups. Reduction in antidiabetic medications was able to take place in 49% and 18% of the fenugreek and placebo groups. The authors concluded that fenugreek seed powder was safe and effective in improving symptoms of T2DM (Verma et al., 2016).

A RCT in nonobese male and female subjects ($n=18$) studied a fenugreek extract that contained 90% total fiber and 78.9% soluble fiber (galactomannan), 4 or 8 g of powder in a beverage compared with a control beverage for satiety. The AUC for satiety was significantly higher for the 8 g fenugreek extract, when compared with the 4 g dose and the control ($P=0.008$ and $P=0.002$, respectively). The hunger AUC was significantly lower for the 8 g fenugreek extract compared with the 4 g fenugreek extract and the control ($P=0.010$ and $P=0.031$, respectively) with no significant differences between the 4 g dose and control groups. The AUC for postprandial insulin and peak insulin were significantly higher after the 8 g fenugreek extract compared with the low-dose fenugreek or control ($P = 0.01$ and $P = 0.07$, respectively). Unfortunately, palatability ratings for 8 g of fenugreek were significantly lower than control (Matthern et al., 2009).

Women's Disorders: Lactation

A 4-week RCT in mother/infant duos ($n = 78$) with breast milk insufficiency compared an herbal tea (containing 7.5 g fenugreek seed powder plus 3 g black tea powder) with a control tea (containing 3 g black tea powder) given TID between meals. After 4 weeks, weight, head circumference, number of wet diapers, frequency of defecation, and number of breastfeeding times increased significantly over baseline in the fenugreek group ($P < 0.001$ for all) compared with the control group. Growth in height difference between the two groups was not significant (Ghasemi et al., 2015).

Women's Genitourinary Disorders: Dysmenorrhea

A 2-month RCT in college students ($n = 101$) with dysmenorrhea compared fenugreek seeds 900 mg TID with placebo on days 1–3 of the menstrual cycle. After 2 months, pain severity decreased from 6.4 to 3.25 in the treatment group and from 6.1 to 5.9 in the placebo group. After each cycle, pain severity in the fenugreek group was significantly less than in the placebo group ($P < 0.001$), and duration of pain was significantly decreased in the treatment group ($P = 0.01$) (Younesy et al., 2014).

Women's Genitourinary Disorders: Polycystic Ovary Syndrome

A 3-month open-label study of patients with PCOS ($n = 50$) investigated the effect of an extract of fenugreek seed standardized to 40% furostanolic saponins, 1 g/day. Significant increases in LH (from 10.3 IU/L to 13.9 IU/L) and FSH (from 5.3 IU/L to 8.3 IU/L) and significant reductions in right but not left ovary volumes (from 14 cm to 10 cm) occurred. Regular menses resumed in 71% of patients. Reduction in cyst size occurred in 46% of patients, and 36% had no cysts at the end of the study. Liver and kidney function remained unchanged. Pregnancy occurred in 12% of patients during the study. Overall, 94% of patients saw im-

provements in some aspect of their PCOS. There was no effect on blood glucose (Swaroop et al., 2015).

Women's Genitourinary Disorders: Menopause

A 2017 review of clinical trials on herbal efficacy in menopausal symptoms used search terms menopause, climacteric, hot flushes, flashes, herb, and phytoestrogens. The authors found that passionflower, sage, lemon balm, valerian, black cohosh, fenugreek, black seed, chasteberry, fennel, evening primrose, ginkgo, alfalfa, St. John's wort, Asian ginseng, anise, licorice, red clover, and wild soybean were effective in the treatment of acute menopausal syndrome with different mechanisms. The authors concluded that medicinal plants could play a role in the treatment of acute menopausal syndrome and that further studies were warranted (Kargozar et al., 2017).

A 12-week RCT in women ($n = 88$) with moderate to severe symptoms of early menopause studied fenugreek seed husk extract (rich in protodioscin, trigonelline, and 4-hydroxyisoleucine) 1 g/day compared with placebo. The fenugreek group had a significant improvement in climacteric scale total score compared with baseline ($P < 0.001$) and with placebo ($P < 0.001$). Psychological, vasomotor, physical, and libido scores were all improved in the treatment group compared with placebo ($P < 0.001$ for all). Insomnia decreased by 75%, mood swings decreased by 68%, irritability decreased by 65%, night sweats decreased by 57%, headaches decreased by 54%, and hot flushes decreased by 48%. Approximately 32% of the fenugreek group reported no hot flushes at study end. Quality of life improved significantly in 73% of the treatment group while a similar increase was not observed for the placebo group. Plasma estradiol increased 120% and 5% in the treatment group and placebo group, respectively. Patients receiving fenugreek who had hypercholesterolemia at baseline had significant decreases in TC, LDL, and TG levels ($P < 0.05$ for all). There were no significant changes in anthropometric measures, although there was a trend toward improvement in BW ($P < 0.06$) and hip circumference ($P < 0.08$). No adverse events were reported (Shamshad Begum et al., 2016).

A 12-week RCT in menopausal women ($n = 115$) compared fenugreek dehusked seed extract 600 mg/day with placebo. There was a significant reduction in menopausal symptoms in the active group compared with the placebo group as assessed by total Menopause-Specific Quality of Life questionnaire ($P < 0.001$). There were significant improvements in the vasomotor ($P < 0.001$), psychosocial ($P < 0.001$), physical ($P < 0.001$), and sexual symptom ($P < 0.001$) domains. There were also significantly less daytime hot flushes and night sweats with fenugreek ($P < 0.001$). The average estradiol levels were similar in both groups after treatment. The authors concluded that this formulation of fenugreek may reduce menopausal symptoms in healthy women (Steels et al., 2017).

A 12-week RCT in postmenopausal women ($n = 60$) studied the vaginal effects of fenugreek 5% vaginal cream 0.5 g twice weekly compared with CEE vaginal cream 0.5 g containing 0.3 mg of conjugated estrogens given twice weekly. After the 12-week intervention, the mean score for atrophic vaginitis signs with fenugreek was 3.1, a significant difference from baseline, but with CEE outperforming fenugreek ($P = 0.001$). The vaginal maturation index was less than 49% in 86.7% and 46.7% of the participants in the fenugreek and estrogen groups, respectively. This was a significant difference in favor of the control group ($P = 0.001$). The authors concluded that fenugreek extract could be effective in treating signs of atrophic vaginitis but was not as effective as low-dose conjugated estrogen cream (Safary et al., 2020).

Women's Genitourinary Disorders: Female Sexual Dysfunction

A 2018 systematic review to evaluate the effectiveness of phytoestrogens on sexual disorders and severity of dyspareunia in women found that the phytoestrogens isolated from fennel, French maritime pine bark, maca and fenugreek significantly improved sexual function whereas the phytoestrogens isolated from Korean red ginseng, flaxseed, red clover, and soy did not lead to significant effects on sexual function (Najafi and Ghazanfarpour, 2018).

A 2-month exploratory, prospective, noncontrolled, observational study in postmenopausal women ($n = 29$) with sexual dysfunction as defined by a Female Sexual Function Index (FSFI) score < 25.83 assessed the effects of Libicare®, a polyherbal oral food supplement containing fenugreek, tribulus, ginkgo, and *Temera diffusa*, two tablets daily. FSFI mean score showed a significant increase from 20.15 at baseline to 25.03 after treatment ($P = 0.0011$). The FSFI score was increased in 86% of the subjects. All FSFI domains, except dyspareunia, showed significant increases. The highest increase was observed in the desire domain ($P = 0.0004$). A significant increase in testosterone level occurred in roughly half of the subjects, from 0.41 to 0.50 pg/mL. A significant decrease in SHBG level occurred in 95% of subjects from 85 to 73 nmol/L ($P = 0.0001$). The authors concluded that this polyherbal formula provided a significant improvement in sexual function and related hormone levels (Palacios et al., 2019).

Men's Genitourinary Disorders: Male Sexual Dysfunction

A 12-week RCT in healthy older males ($n = 120$) compared standardized fenugreek seed extract 600 mg (standardized to 50% saponin glycosides) QD with placebo for effects on androgen deficiency and sexual function. Compared with placebo, the fenugreek seed extract significantly improved the Aging Male Questionnaire score. The DSIF-SR score increased from 66.2 to 76.3 with fenugreek ($P < 0.01$) and decreased from 57.8 to 57.0 with placebo. Sexual arousal scores increased from 12.9 to 16.8 with fenugreek ($P < 0.001$) and from 10.8 to 11 with placebo. Sexual drive/relationship increased from 11.1 to 12.8 with fenugreek ($P < 0.01$) and from 10.4 to 10.6 with placebo. Total testosterone increased from 12.3 to 13.8 nmol/L with fenugreek ($P = 0.001$) and from 13.2 to 13.5 nmol/L with placebo. The fenugreek seed extract was well tolerated, with no serious adverse effects reported. The authors concluded that fenugreek was a safe and effective treatment for reducing symptoms of possible androgen deficiency, improving sexual function, and increasing serum testosterone in healthy middle-aged and older men (Rao et al., 2016).

A 6-week RCT of healthy males ($n = 60$) interested in raising their libido compared 600 mg/day of fenugreek extract powder containing magnesium, zinc, and pyridoxine with a placebo of 50 mg rice bran. Scores on a sexual functioning scale (DISF-SR) at 3 and 6 weeks increased from 67 to 75 and 82, respectively, in the fenugreek group, while the scores decreased in the placebo group. Improved libido as well as improved general energy were reported in 81% of the fenugreek group. Serum prolactin and testosterone levels remained within normal reference ranges (Steels et al., 2011).

Neurological Disorders: Parkinson's Disease

In a 6-month RCT in patients ($n = 50$) with PD compared an extract of fenugreek seed standardized to trigonelline and hydroxyleucine 300 mg BID with placebo. The treatment group showed no significant differences for total Unified Parkinson's Disease Rating Scale (UPDRS) total scores. However, the total UPDRS scores showed a slower rise of 0.098% with fenugreek as opposed to a steep rise of 13.36% with placebo. Clinically important differences of 5.3 for total UPDRS scores and of 4.8 for scores of the motor subsection of UPDRS were found with fenugreek. Hoehn and Yahr stage was lowered in 21.7% of patients with fenugreek vs 5.3% of patients with placebo. The authors concluded that the standardized extract of fenugreek could be a useful adjuvant treatment with ʟ-dopa in management of patients with PD (Nathan et al., 2014).

Disorders of Vitality: Athletic Performance

An 8-week RCT in male participants ($n = 138$) compared Testofen, an extract of fenugreek, 600 or 300 mg/day with placebo for changes in muscular strength and endurance, body composition, functional threshold power, and sex hormones in response to an exercise program. All groups improved their maximal leg press from baseline to 8 weeks; however, both Testofen-treated groups improved more than placebo ($P < 0.05$). The 600 mg group showed decreases in body mass and body fat (-1.2 kg and −1.4%, respectively) and increases in lean mass (1.8%) and testosterone concentration from baseline to 8 weeks. The authors concluded that Testofen could be an effective ergogenic aid for individuals wanting to rapidly improve their exercise performance capabilities and body composition above and beyond that of calisthenic exercise alone (Rao et al., 2020).

A study in trained male cyclists compared effects of a dextrose beverage alone (control) and a dextrose beverage with the addition of 4-hydroxyisoleucine isolated from fenugreek seeds. There was a significant 63% increase in muscle glycogen concentration from immediately post exercise to 4h after exercise with the addition of the fenugreek isolate compared with the control group. The authors concluded that when 4-hydroxyisoleucine was added to a high oral dose of dextrose, rates of postexercise glycogen resynthesis were enhanced above dextrose alone (Ruby et al., 2005).

ACTIVE CONSTITUENTS

Seeds

- Carbohydrates
  - Polysaccharides: mucilaginous fiber, galactomannan
  - Organic acids: 2-oxoglutarate
- Lipids: fatty acids
- Amino acid derivatives:
  - Amino acids: 4-hydroxyisoleucine (hypoglycemic, muscle glycogenic)
- Phenolic compounds
  - Phenolic acids (antioxidant): protocatechuic acid, quinic acid, gallic acid
  - Coumarins (venotonic, lymphatotonic)
  - Flavonoids
    - C-glycoside flavones (antioxidant): luteolin-7-O-glycoside, apigenin-7-O-glycoside
- Terpenes
  - Triterpenoid saponins: yamogenin
- Steroids
  - Steroidal saponins (antilipemic): fenusides, diosgenin (antineoplastic)
    - Trigoneosides: trigofaenoside A, glycoside D,
    - Glycosides of diosgenin: protodioscin (aphrodisiac, antineoplastic)
- Alkaloids: trigonelline aka trigonellic acid (hypoglycemic, hypolipidemic, hypotensive, neuroprotective, antimigraine, sedative, memory-improving, antipyretic, antibacterial, antiviral, antitumor)
- Aromatic compounds: neryl acetate, camphor, β-pinene, β-caryophyllene, 2,5-dimethylpyrazine, geranial

FENUGREEK COMMONLY USED PREPARATIONS AND DOSAGE (FOR ADULTS UNLESS OTHERWISE SPECIFIED)

The following are examples of some available formulations and ranges of dosing for commercial herbal products. See Part III Introduction "How to prescribe medicinal herbs" for further guidance on herbal advising and prescribing.

Seeds

- Seeds: 3–30 g with each meal (eaten, made into flour, baked into bread, brewed into tea, pressed into oil. Due to bitter taste, debitterized seeds preferred if available).
- Infusion: 5–7.5 g of powdered seeds in hot water TID (for breastmilk production).
- Tincture (1:2.5, 75%): 280 mg (0.7 mL) up to five times per day.
- Powdered seed: 1 g (1/2 tsp) up to TID.
- Capsule or tablet of powdered seed: 2 g QD-TID (for lactation, menopause, PCOS, dysmenorrhea).
- Capsule or tablet of standardized extract (standardized to 50% fenusides): 350–600 mg per day (for male libido and menopause).

SAFETY AND PRECAUTION

Side Effects

No adverse reactions to fenugreek have been found when taken in culinary quantities. May cause body secretions to smell like maple syrup due to the metabolite sotolon.

Allergic reactions including rhinorrhea, wheezing, numbness of head, facial angioedema, and fainting were reported following inhalation and external application of fenugreek seed powder.

Toxicity

In mice an oral dose of 3 g/kg bodyweight of ethanol-extract of fenugreek failed to show adverse effects. Potential for hypoglycemia and bleeding.

Pregnancy and Lactation

One study showed teratogenic potential at large doses in rats, so avoid during pregnancy. Considered safe with breastfeeding when standard dosages are employed.

Disease Interactions

Fenugreek acts as an estrogen receptor modulator and was shown to stimulate breast cancer cells in vitro. May raise testosterone. Avoid with hormone-sensitive cancers.

Drug Interactions

- May potentiate the effects of warfarin.
- May interfere with cytotoxic effects of cyclophosphamide.
- Alters bioavailability of theophylline in animals.
- May augment effects of hypoglycemic agents.

REFERENCES

Gaddam A, Galla C, Thummisetti S, Marikanty RK, Palanisamy UD, Rao PV. Role of fenugreek in the prevention of type 2 diabetes mellitus in prediabetes. J Diabetes Metab Disord October 2, 2015;14:74.

Ghasemi V, Kheirkhah M, Vahedi M. The effect of herbal tea containing fenugreek seed on the signs of breast milk sufficiency in Iranian girl infants. Iran Red Crescent Med J August 15, 2015;17(8):e21848.

Ghorbani A, Zarvandi M, Rakhshandeh H. A randomized controlled trial of a herbal compound for improving metabolic parameters in diabetic patients with uncontrolled dyslipidemia. Endocr Metab Immune Disord Drug Targets 2019 Feb;6.

Gupta A, Gupta R, Lal B. Effect of Trigonella foenum-graecum (fenugreek) seeds on glycaemic control and insulin resistance in type 2 diabetes mellitus: a double blind placebo controlled study. J Assoc Physicians India 2001 Nov;49:1057–61.

Hasani-Ranjbar S, Nayebi N, Moradi L, Mehri A, Larijani B, Abdollahi M. The efficacy and safety of herbal medicines used in the treatment of hyperlipidemia; a systematic review. Curr Pharm Des 2010;16(26):2935–47.

Kargozar R, Azizi H, Salari R. A review of effective herbal medicines in controlling menopausal symptoms. Electron Physician 2017 Nov;9(11):5826–33.

Khodamoradi K, Khosropanah MH, Ayati Z, et al. The effects of fenugreek on cardiometabolic risk factors in adults: a systematic review and meta-analysis. Complement Ther Med 2020 Aug;52:102416.

Matthern JR, Raatz SK, Thomas W, Slavin JL. Effect of fenugreek fiber on satiety, blood glucose and insulin response and energy intake in obese subjects. Phytother Res Nov 2009;23(11):1543–8.

Nahas R, Moher M. Complementary and alternative medicine for the treatment of type 2 diabetes. Can Fam Physician 2009 Jun;55(6):591–6.

Najafi NM, Ghazanfarpour M. Effect of phytoestrogens on sexual function in menopausal women: a systematic review and meta-analysis. Climacteric 2018 Oct;21(5):437–45.

Nathan J, Panjwani S, Mohan V, Joshi V, Thakurdesai PA. Efficacy and safety of standardized extract of Trigonella foenum-graecum L seeds as an adjuvant to L-Dopa in the management of patients with Parkinson's disease. Phytother Res 2014 Feb;28(2):172–8.

Neelakantan N, Narayanan M, de Souza RJ, van Dam RM. Effect of fenugreek (Trigonella foenum-graecum L.) intake on glycemia: a meta-analysis of clinical trials. Nutr J 2014 Jan 18;13:7.

Palacios S, Soler E, Ramírez M, Lilue M, Khorsandi D, Losa F. Effect of a multi-ingredient-based food supplement on sexual function in women with low sexual desire. BMC Womens Health 2019 Apr 30;19(1):58.

Prasanna M. Hypolipidemic effect of fenugreek: a clinical study. Indian J Pharm 2000;32:34–6.

Rao A, Steels E, Inder WJ, Abraham S, Vitetta L. Testofen, a specialised Trigonella foenum-graecum seed extract reduces age-related symptoms of androgen decrease, increases testosterone levels and improves sexual function in healthy aging males in a double-blind randomised clinical study. Aging Male 2016 Jun;19(2):134–42.

Rao A, Mallard A, Grant R. Testofen * (Fenugreek extract) increases strength and muscle mass compared to placebo in response to calisthenics. A randomised control trial. Trans Sports Med 2020 March. https://doi.org/10.1002/tsm2.153.

Ruby BC, Gaskill SE, Slivka D, Harger SG. The addition of fenugreek extract (Trigonella foenum-graecum) to glucose feeding increases muscle glycogen resynthesis after exercise. Amino Acids 2005 Feb;28(1):71–6.

Safary M, Hakimi S, Mobaraki-Asl N, Amiri P, Tvassoli H, Delazar A. Comparison of the effects of fenugreek vaginal cream and ultra low- dose estrogen on atrophic vaginitis. Curr Drug Deliv 2020;17(9):815–22.

Shamshad Begum S, Jayalakshmi HK, Vidyavathi HG, et al. A novel extract of fenugreek husk (FenuSMART™) alleviates postmenopausal symptoms and helps to establish the hormonal balance: a randomized, double-blind, placebo-controlled study. Phytother Res 2016 Nov;30(11):1775–84.

Sharma RD, Sarkar A, Hazra DK, et al. Hypolipidaemic effect of fenugreek seeds: a chronic study in non-insulin dependent diabetic patients. Phytother Res 1996;10:332–4.

Sowmya P, Rajyalakshmi P. Hypocholesterolemic effect of germinated fenugreek seeds in human subjects. Plant Food Hum Nutr Dec 1999;53:359–65.

Steels E, Rao A, Vitetta L. Physiological aspects of male libido enhanced by standardized Trigonella foenum-graecum extract and mineral formulation. Phytother Res 2011 Sep;25(9):1294–300.

Steels E, Steele ML, Harold M, Coulson S. Efficacy of a proprietary Trigonella foenum-graecum L. De-husked seed extract in reducing menopausal symptoms in otherwise healthy women: a double-blind, randomized, placebo-controlled study. Phytother Res 2017 Sep;31(9):1316–22.

Suksomboon N, Poolsup N, Boonkaew S, Suthisisang CC. Meta-analysis of the effect of herbal supplement on glycemic control in type 2 diabetes. J Ethnopharmacol 2011 Oct 11;137(3):1328–33.

Swaroop A, Jaipuriar AS, Gupta SK, et al. Efficacy of a novel fenugreek seed extract (Trigonella foenum-graecum, Furocyst™) in polycystic ovary syndrome (PCOS). Int J Med Sci October 3, 2015;12(10):825–31.

Verma N, Usman K, Patel N, Jain A, Dhakre S, Swaroop A, Bagchi M, Kumar P, Preuss HG, Bagchi D. A multicenter clinical study to determine the efficacy of a novel fenugreek seed (Trigonella foenum-graecum) extract (Fenfuro™) in patients with type 2 diabetes. Food Nutr Res. 2016 Oct 11;60:32382. https://doi.org/10.3402/fnr.v60.32382.

Younesy S, Amiraliakbari S, Esmaeili S, Alavimajd H, Nouraei S. Effects of fenugreek seed on the severity and systemic symptoms of dysmenorrhea. J Reprod Infertil January 2014;15(1):41–8.

Zarvandi M, Rakhshandeh H, Abazari M, Shafiee-Nick R, Ghorbani A. Safety and efficacy of a polyherbal formulation for the management of dyslipidemia and hyperglycemia in patients with advanced-stage of type-2 diabetes. Biomed Pharmacother 2017 May;89:69–75.

46

FRANKINCENSE/BOSWELLIA (*BOSWELLIA SERRATA/SACRA/ CARTERII*)
Bark Resin

GENERAL OVERVIEW

Frankincense, the aromatic resin of Christian nativity fame, probably deserved its high regard by the three wise men. At the very least it may have helped Mary recover from childbirth. The resin has been used in the Middle East for more than 6000 years, mostly in religious rites. The source of the medicine is the gum oleoresin found on the underside of the tree's bark. There are five main species of *Boswellia* from which frankincense is derived. The best known are *B. serrata* (Indian Frankincense), *B. carterii*, and *B. sacra*. The former is particularly antiinflammatory and analgesic and has been the subject of the preponderance of research on frankincense. Frankincense has modern herbal application for the long list of diseases that are fundamentally inflammatory.

Clinical research indicates that frankincense, alone or in combination formulas, may be beneficial for gingivitis, asthma, diabetes, irritable bowel syndrome, collagenous colitis, Crohn's disease, urinary tract infection, stress urinary incontinence, breast density, mastalgia, menorrhagia, osteoarthritis (OA), memory impairment, psoriasis, eczema, photoaging, rheumatoid arthritis (RA), chemotherapy-induced peripheral neuropathy, and radiation-induced brain edema.

IN VITRO AND ANIMAL RESEARCH

The main mode of action of frankincense is through blocking various inflammatory pathways. Studies have demonstrated NSAID-level antiinflammatory properties without NSAID adverse gastric effects or depletion of joint glycosaminoglycans. Its major component, boswellic acid, has been shown to be a potent inhibitor of 5-LOX production. It inhibits production of 5-HETE and LTB4, both of which are responsible for bronchoconstriction, chemotaxis, and increased vascular permeability. Frankincense also inhibits COX-1 and blocks human leukocyte elastase, which may play a role in emphysema and cystic fibrosis. Animal studies have shown a defatted alcoholic extract of frankincense decreased PMN infiltration and migration, decreased antibody synthesis, and strongly inhibited the complement pathway. In vitro studies show gum resin extracts of frankincense have an antiplatelet effect by inhibiting clotting factors Xa and XIa. Two boswellic acid components have been shown to alter multidrug-resistant proteins. The essential oil of frankincense has antimicrobial activity.

Frankincense shows in vitro and animal research benefit for various cancers. It inhibits NF-κB and TNF-α production and has cytotoxic properties via induction of p21 expression through a p53-independent pathway. Frankincense is a potent inhibitor of angiogenesis and invasiveness. Studies have been positive with pancreatic, colorectal, prostate, breast, cervical, myeloma, leukemia, and glioma cell lines. One of the boswellic acid components, acetyl-11-keto-beta-boswellic acid (AKBA), was found to inhibit human prostate tumor growth via inhibition of angiogenesis induced by VEGFR2 signaling pathways.

351

HUMAN RESEARCH

General Benefits

Most of the clinical trials on frankincense have used *B. serrata* or the chief constituent boswellic acid. Also, many of the trials included additional herbs or supplements such as turmeric, which is thought to work synergistically with frankincense. A 2008 systematic review of general frankincense evidence found seven trials that met inclusion criteria. The author concluded that frankincense extracts were clinically effective for asthma, RA, Crohn's disease, OA, and collagenous colitis with no serious safety issues (Ernst, 2008).

Oral and Dental Disorders

An RCT in patients ($n = 75$) with moderate plaque-induced gingivitis compared applications of frankincense extract 100 mg with frankincense powder 200 mg and with placebo. Scaling and root planing (SRP) in association with frankincense application (either extract or powder) led to a decrease in inflammatory indices in comparison with the groups without SRP plus drug therapy ($P < 0.001$). No significant differences were observed between powder and extract therapies ($P > 0.05$) or between patients that received either additional SRP and treatment alone ($P = 0.169$) (Khosravi Samani et al., 2011).

Pulmonary Disorders: Asthma

A 4-week RCT in asthmatic subjects ($n = 32$) investigated ICS plus LABAs compared with ICS plus LABAs plus a lecithin-based frankincense delivery system (Casperome) 500 mg orally QD. Subjects receiving the addition of the frankincense formulation showed a decrease in the number of inhalations needed compared with patients who did not receive the herbal therapy. The treatment was well tolerated and only mild-to-moderate adverse events were noted (Ferrara et al., 2015).

A 6-week RCT in patients ($n = 80$) with asthma compared frankincense extract 300 mg orally TID with placebo. Parameters including dyspnea, rhonchi, number of attacks, FEV1, FVC and PEFR, eosinophilic count, and ESR improved in 70% and 27% of frankincense and placebo groups, respectively. The authors concluded that the findings indicated a definite role for gum resin of frankincense in the treatment of bronchial asthma (Gupta et al., 1998).

A 21-day RCT in patients ($n = 54$) with chronic asthma compared frankincense with licorice and with prednisolone for improvement of pulmonary function. FEV1 was increased from 62% to 81% and from 61% to 72.4% with licorice and frankincense, respectively. FVC increased from 1.08 to 3.6, from 0.72 to 2.63, and from 1.05 to 2.25 with licorice, frankincense, and prednisolone, respectively. Symptomatic improvement was greater with licorice than with frankincense. The authors concluded that licorice was superior to frankincense for chronic asthma (Al-Jawad et al., 2012).

Cardiometabolic Disorders: Diabetes and Metabolic Syndrome

A 3-month RCT in patients ($n = 60$) with T2DM studied an herbal blend containing milk thistle, nettle, and frankincense compared with placebo for glycemic control. The mean FBS, A1C, and TG with the herbal combination were significantly less than with placebo after 3 months of the intervention. The authors concluded that there was a potential antihyperglycemic and TG-lowering effect of the herbal formulation, while it did not have any significant lowering effect on cholesterol or BP (Khalili et al., 2017).

Bowel Disorders: Irritable Bowel Syndrome and Inflammatory Bowel Disease

A 2017 Cochrane review of treatments for collagenous colitis included 12 RCTs for analysis. The authors concluded that there was low-quality evidence that budesonide may be an effective therapy for active and inactive collagenous colitis but that due to small sample sizes and low study quality there was uncertainty about the benefits and harms of therapy with Pepto-Bismol, frankincense extract, mesalamine with or without cholestyramine, prednisolone, and probiotics. The small study ($n = 30$) involving frankincense showed that diarrhea resolved in 44% of those taking 400 mg TID for 8 weeks (vs 27% of those taking placebo) (Kafil et al., 2017).

A 6-month RCT in patients ($n = 69$) with mild IBS compared standard management (diet and PRN anticholinergics) with a frankincense lecithin-based delivery form (Casperome) 250 mg/day. At 3- and 6-month follow-up the frankincense group showed lower mean score values for almost all self-assessed IBS symptoms. A significantly lower need for rescue medications and consultations or medical evaluation/admissions was found in the frankincense group. The incidence of adverse events, mainly dry mouth, was minimal albeit significantly higher in the standard-management group. The authors concluded that the frankincense lecithin-based delivery form in the study appeared to be effective and safe in improving signs and symptoms in IBS subjects (Riva et al., 2019).

A 4-week RCT in subjects ($n=71$) with IBS investigated hyoscine butylbromide PRN compared with papaverine 10 mg plus belladonna 10 mg PRN and with a frankincense lecithin-based delivery form (Casperome) 250 mg/day, for 4 weeks. In all groups, the abdominal pain, altered bowel movements, meteorism, and cramps improved during the observational period. Only in the Casperome-supplemented group did the number of subjects with any IBS symptoms significantly decrease, from 58% to 12.5%. The number of subjects who needed medical attention significantly decreased to 4.1% with Caspersome. In addition, frankincense supplementation was correlated with a lower incidence of dry mouth (Belcaro et al., 2017).

A 6-week RCT in patients ($n=30$) with grade II to III ulcerative colitis compared frankincense gum resin 350 mg TID with sulfasalazine 1 g TID. In the frankincense and sulfasalazine groups remission rates were 82% and 75%, respectively. There were similar changes between groups in stool properties; histopathology and electron microscopy of rectal biopsies; and blood parameters including Hgb, serum iron, calcium, phosphorus, proteins, total leukocytes, and eosinophils (Gupta et al., 1997).

A head-to-head comparison trial in patients ($n=102$) with Crohn's disease compared a resin extract of frankincense (H15) with mesalamine. The mean scores on the Crohn's Disease Activity Index decreased between enrolment and end of therapy by 90 and 53 points with frankincense and mesalamine, respectively. The difference was not statistically significant. The authors concluded that the frankincense extract was not inferior to mesalamine for Crohn's disease (Gerhardt et al., 2001).

Nephrological and Urological Disorders: Urinary Tract Infection and Stress Urinary Incontinence

A 3-month RCT in adult females ($n=93$) with uncomplicated UTI compared an herbal combination containing L-methionine, hibiscus, and frankincense BID

for 7 days with short-term antibiotic treatment according to international guidelines. Both groups showed a statistically significant improvement in quality-of-life scores compared with baseline assessment at 30 days and 3 months ($P<0.001$). At 3 months, a statistically significant difference in QOL was reported between the two groups (99.1 vs 98.1 with phytotherapy vs antibiotics, respectively; $P<0.003$). A transition from UTI to asymptomatic bacteriuria was observed in 26% patients in the herbal group, while no patients in the antibiotic group demonstrated bacteriuria ($P=0.007$). The authors concluded that this phytotherapeutic combination was able to improve patients' quality of life, reducing symptoms in acute setting and preventing the recurrences, but that asymptomatic bacteriuria was greater with phytotherapy than with antibiotics (Cai et al., 2018).

An 8-week RCT in patients ($n=60$) with stress urinary incontinence compared a combination of frankincense and *Cyperus scariosus* 2 g BID plus pelvic floor exercises with placebo plus pelvic floor exercises. The improvement in the herb and placebo groups as measured by the 1-h pad test was 60% and 37%, respectively ($P=0.035$). The improvement from baseline was also significant ($P<0.001$) in both groups. No adverse effects were noted. The authors concluded that the herbal treatment was more effective than pelvic floor exercises alone for treatment of stress urinary incontinence (SUI) (Arkalgud Rangaswamy et al., 2014).

Women's Disorders: Breast Density and Mastalgia

A 6-month RCT in women ($n=76$) with symptomatic fibrocystic breast disease compared a combination product containing boswellic acid, betaine, and myo-inositol (myo-inositol has already been proven to modulate some factors involved in the genesis of breast diseases, such as fibrosis and metabolic and endocrine causes) with placebo. After 6 months of treatment, statistically significant differences between the two groups were recorded for pain relief (56% vs 17%) and breast density reduction (60% vs 9%). Furthermore, benign breast mass dimension showed a reduction in the experimental group (40% vs 16%). The authors concluded that the combination of boswellic acid, betaine, and myo-inositol was effective in the treatment of breast pain and radiologically and histologically confirmed benign breast mass and in the reduction of breast density without any side effects (Pasta et al., 2016b).

A 6-month RCT study in patients 30 years old and younger ($n = 64$) with breast fibroadenoma investigated the combination of frankincense, betaine, myo-inositol, B vitamins, and N-acetylcysteine compared with B vitamins and N-acetylcysteine alone. A significant clinical improvement was observed with the frankincense formula. Fibroadenoma median volume reduction averaged 18% in the experimental group and 6% in the placebo group, and 39% of patients receiving the frankincense formula showed a reduction of fibroadenoma volume compared with 18% of patients receiving placebo ($P = 0.005$) (Pasta et al., 2016a).

Women's Genitourinary Disorders: Menorrhagia

A 2-month RCT in patients ($n = 102$) with heavy menstrual bleeding studied the effects of ibuprofen 200 mg plus either frankincense 300 mg, ginger 300 mg, or placebo each given TID for 7 days starting with onset of menses. Duration of menstrual bleeding was decreased with frankincense (-1.77 days; $P = 0.003$) and ginger (-1.8 days; $P = 0.001$), but not with placebo (-0.52 days; $P = 0.42$). The amount of bleeding was decreased in all ($P < 0.05$), with no difference among the study groups. QOL was improved more in the frankincense (-25.7; $P < 0.001$) and ginger (-29.2; $P < 0.001$) groups compared with the placebo group (-15.07, $P < 0.001$) with between-group differences being significant ($P = 0.02$). The authors concluded that ginger and frankincense seemed to be effective complementary treatments for heavy menstrual bleeding (Eshaghian et al., 2019).

Musculoskeletal Disorders: Osteoarthritis and Musculoskeletal Pain

A 2018 systematic review looked at trials comparing curcuminoids (from turmeric) or frankincense formulations with placebo or NSAIDs for OA. The authors included 11 RCTs ($n = 1009$) and found that both curcuminoid and frankincense formulations were statistically significantly more effective than placebo for pain relief and functional improvement. There were no significant differences between curcuminoids or frankincense and placebo in safety outcomes. Curcuminoids

showed no statistically significant differences in efficacy outcomes compared with NSAIDs; patients receiving curcuminoids were significantly less likely to experience gastrointestinal adverse events. No RCTs compared frankincense against approved NSAIDs (Bannuru et al., 2018).

A 2018 systematic review to investigate the efficacy and safety of dietary supplements for patients with OA found 69 studies that met inclusion criteria. Of the 20 supplements investigated, seven (collagen hydrolysate, passion fruit peel extract, turmeric, curcumin, frankincense, pycnogenol, and L-carnitine) demonstrated large and clinically important effects for pain reduction and improved function at short term (effect size > 0.80). Another six supplements (undenatured type II collagen, avocado soybean unsaponifiables, MSM, diacerein, glucosamine, and chondroitin) revealed statistically significant improvements in pain and function but were of unclear clinical importance. Only green-lipped mussel extract and undenatured type II collagen had clinically important effects on pain and function at medium term. For long-term pain reduction, there were no supplements identified with clinically important effects. Chondroitin demonstrated statistically significant but not clinically important structural benefits. There were no differences between supplements and placebo for safety outcomes, except for diacerein. The authors concluded that supplements provided moderate and clinically meaningful treatment effects on pain and function in patients with hand, hip, or knee OA at short term, although the quality of evidence was very low (Liu et al., 2018).

A 2014 Cochrane review of herbal therapies for osteoarthritis selected 49 RCTs ($n = 5980$) for review. Due to differing interventions, meta-analyses were restricted to frankincense alone and avocado soybean unsaponifiables (two-herb combination products). Five studies of three different extracts from frankincense were included. High-quality evidence from two studies (85 participants) indicated that 90 days of treatment with 100 mg of enriched frankincense extract improved symptoms better than placebo. Frankincense reduced pain by a mean of 17 points with NNT = 2. WOMAC scores were improved by eight points with frankincense, NNT = 4. Moderate-quality evidence indicated that adverse events were probably reduced with enriched frankincense (18/48 events vs 30/48 events with placebo, RR = 0.60). The authors concluded that several medicinal plant products, including extracts of *B. serrata*, showed trends of benefits that warranted further investigation because the risk of adverse events appears to be low (Cameron and Chrubasik, 2014).

A 6-month open-label study in patients (*n* = 66) with knee OA compared boswellia extract 333 mg TID with valdecoxib 10 mg QD. Pain, stiffness, and difficulty in performing daily activities showed statistically significant improvement with 2 months of treatment with frankincense. This benefit lasted until 1 month after stopping the intervention. With valdecoxib the statistically significant improvement in all parameters was reported after 1 month of therapy, but the effect persisted only as long as drug therapy continued. Three patients with frankincense and two with valdecoxib group complained of gastric acidity. One patient with frankincense complained of diarrhea and abdominal cramps. The authors concluded that frankincense showed a slower onset of action, but the effect persisted even after stopping therapy while the action of valdecoxib became evident faster but waned rapidly after stopping the treatment (Sontakke et al., 2007).

A 90-day RCT in patients with OA (*n* = 75) compared two different doses of a standardized extract of frankincense with placebo. With the lower dose (100 mg/day) there was a 40% improvement in WOMAC pain scores after 90 days. In the 250 mg/day group there was a 52% improvement in WOMAC pain score and a 62% decrease in WOMAC stiffness score as well as a 46% reduction in synovial fluid MMP-3 concentration at day 90. The MMP-3 level in the placebo group remained nearly unchanged throughout the study. Improvement in pain scores and physical ability scores started to occur at 7 days after the start of treatment, and improvement continued throughout the 90 days of treatment. The authors concluded that the standardized extract of frankincense reduced pain and improved physical functioning significantly in OA patients and was safe for human consumption. They postulated that the herb exerted its beneficial effects by controlling inflammatory responses through a reduction in proinflammatory modulators, and that it may improve joint health by reducing the enzymatic degradation of cartilage in OA patients (Sengupta et al., 2008).

A 16-week crossover RCT in patients (*n* = 30) with OA of the knee compared frankincense extract with placebo. After the first 8 weeks of treatment, washout was given and then the groups were crossed over to receive the opposite intervention for 8 weeks. All patients receiving frankincense reported decreased knee pain, increased knee flexion, increased walking distance, and decreased frequency of swelling with the findings having statistical significance over placebo response. Radiologically there was no change. Frankincense was well tolerated by the subjects except for minor GI effects (Kimmatkar et al., 2003).

A 4-week RCT in patients (*n* = 56) with symptomatic knee arthrosis investigated Phytoproflex (an extract containing boswellic acid 90%, curcumin 20%, and valeric acid 0.8%) plus standard management compared with standard management alone. The Karnofsky Scale at 4 weeks was improved in both groups: from 74 to 89 ($P < 0.05$) with the herbal supplement and from 75 to 79 ($P < 0.05$) with standard management. The effects in the supplement group were significantly higher than those in the control group ($P < 0.05$). The WOMAC Score was decreased significantly more in the supplement group for pain, stiffness, and physical functions ($P < 0.05$). Social/emotional functions also improved better with Phytoproflex ($P < 0.05$). Both groups improved their walking distance at 4 weeks with a higher improvement in the supplement group ($P < 0.05$). The need for other drugs or tests during the registry period was reduced more with Phytoproflex ($P < 0.05$). The author concluded that Phytoproflex could be safely used as an effective, supplementary management in most OA patients (Belcaro et al., 2018).

A 2-week trial in patients (*n* = 23) with painful "stress" arthritis of the hand compared standard management with standard management plus supplementation with a standardized phytosomal preparation of frankincense (FlexiQule), 150 mg TID. After 2 weeks, the ESR was normal in the supplement group and mildly elevated in controls ($P < 0.05\%$). The decrease in hyperthermic areas was faster and greater with frankincense ($P < 0.05$), and the decrease in pain was significantly faster. Functional scores were also better with the supplement ($P < 0.05$). Adjunct pharmaceutical use did not occur in the frankincense group, while in the control group three subjects eventually used NSAIDs to control pain and stiffness and one used a corticosteroid (Belcaro et al., 2015).

A 4-week RCT in young healthy rugby players ($n = 52$) with acute knee pain and inflammation compared standard management alone with standard management plus a frankincense lecithin-based delivery system (Casperome). A significant beneficial effect of frankincense vs standard management alone was observed for all the parameters evaluated: local pain on effort, pain-free walking distance, minimal joint effusion, structural damage and intramuscular hematomas, thermal imaging of the anterior knee, VAS for pain, need for concomitant drugs and medical attention, and measurement of inflammatory biomarkers. The authors concluded that Casperome supplementation may be an effective and safe integrated approach for the treatment of osteo-muscular pain and inflammation (Franceschi et al., 2016).

A 6-month RCT in patients ($n = 122$) with full-thickness supraspinatus tendon tear treated by arthroscopy compared a combination of frankincense plus turmeric with placebo. Treatment was initiated 3 weeks prior to arthroscopy and continued for 2 months. The herbal group demonstrated significantly lower overall pain scores in at 1 week ($P = 0.0477$), and lower but not significantly different scores at 2 weeks ($P = 0.0988$); at subsequent time points, differences were not significant ($P > 0.05$). The authors concluded that the combination product, added to standard analgesics, alleviated short and partially mid-term pain, while long-term pain was unchanged. The authors surmised that this limitation could probably be addressed by a dosage increase over the first 4 weeks and by extending treatment by one or 2 months (Merolla et al., 2015).

A 12-week RCT in patients ($n = 201$) with OA studied the effects of a combination of curcuminoids and frankincense (350 mg and 150 mg, respectively) TID compared with curcuminoids alone (333 mg) TID and with placebo TID. Favorable effects of both preparations compared with placebo were observed by the end of the 12 weeks. A significant effect of the combination product compared with placebo was observed both in physical performance tests and the WOMAC joint pain index, while superior efficacy of curcuminoid alone vs placebo was observed only in physical performance tests. The treatments were well tolerated. The authors concluded that curcumin complex or its combination with boswellic acid reduced pain-related symptoms in patients with OA, and that curcumin in combination with boswellic acid was more effective (Haroyan et al., 2018).

A 12-week RCT in patients ($n = 30$) with knee OA compared turmeric 350 mg plus frankincense 150 mg BID with celecoxib for safety and efficacy. In the herbal group 86% and 21% of the subjects were in the moderate/severe category at baseline and at 12 weeks, respectively. In the celecoxib group, 79% and 50% of patients were in the moderate/severe category at baseline and 12 weeks, respectively. Statistically significant improvements in the proportion of individuals scoring a walking distance of > 1000 m were observed within the two groups over a period of 12 weeks. In the herbal group, 93% of subjects could walk > 1000 m compared with 86% in the celecoxib group following treatment, with the difference between groups being nonsignificant. Joint-line tenderness decreased more with the herbal product than with the drug. Crepitus and tenderness decreased significantly and equally in both groups. The treatment was well tolerated and did not produce any adverse effect in patients (Kizhakkedath, 2013).

A 6-month RCT in subjects ($n = 54$) with moderate knee OA compared standard management alone with standard management plus Movardol, a supplement containing glucosamine, ginger, and frankincense, TID for 1 week then BID. Significant improvements in the functional outcomes and pain-free walking distance were observed after 1, 3, and 6 months in OA patients taking the supplement. All the signs and symptoms of disease assessed by WOMAC tended to regress over a 6-month period in the supplemented group, and inflammatory markers and plasma content of ROS decreased over 6 months in this group as well. The supplement appeared to be safe and well tolerated (Bolognesi et al., 2016).

A clinical trial in patients ($n = 60$) ages 40–70 years with OA investigated three weekly intraarticular injections of hyaluronic acid 1.6% compared with oral supplementation of Syalox 300 Plus (a combination of hyaluronic acid 300 mg + *B. serrata* extract 100 mg) one Table tablet QD for 20 days and afterward Syalox 150 (hyaluronic acid 150 mg) one Table QD for an additional 20 days. The American Knee Society Score of the patients in both groups was significantly increased by the treatment, and VAS score was significantly reduced. Better results were reported in younger patients who received the injections and older subjects who took the oral supplement. The authors concluded that HA injection and oral administration may have beneficial therapeutic effects on patients with early OA. Different outcomes in younger and older subjects suggested administration of a combined therapy first with local infiltrations and then with the oral combination (Ricci et al., 2017).

A pilot study in patients ($n = 13$) who had experienced baseline persistent musculoskeletal pain for at least 4 months (mean duration 5 years) in ≥ 1 body parts without relief from traditional treatments investigated the efficacy of a polyherbal combination including stinging nettle, frankincense, horsetail, garlic, celery, and thiamine (350 mg BID for 14 days). The average VAS pain subscale score was 58 at baseline and 23 at 14 days ($P < 0.05$). The average VAS subscale score for functional mobility was 57 at baseline and 29 at follow-up ($P < 0.05$). No adverse effects were reported. The authors concluded that the complex of five herbs, plus vitamin B1, should be considered as a valuable alternative treatment in the management of chronic musculoskeletal pain (Hedaya, 2017).

A 32-week RCT in patients ($n = 90$) with OA compared an Ayurvedic combination containing ashwagandha, frankincense, ginger, and turmeric with placebo. The mean reduction in pain VAS for herb vs placebo was 2.7 vs 1.3 at week 16 and 2.8 vs 1.8 at week 32 ($P < 0.05$). The improvement in the WOMAC scores at week 16 and week 32 were also significantly superior ($P < 0.01$) with the combination herbal product. Both the groups reported mild adverse events without any significant difference between groups (Chopra et al., 2004).

Neurological Disorders: Stroke

A 1-month RCT in patients ($n = 80$) within 72 h of onset of ischemic stroke, with NIH Stroke Scale (NIHSS) scores of 4–20, assessed the 1-month impact of boswellic acids on NIHSS score and inflammation markers compared with placebo. According to NIHSS evaluation, the boswellic acid group demonstrated a significant recovery in neurological function during the 1-month follow-up, compared with the placebo. The levels of the plasma inflammatory markers TNF-α, IL-1β, IL-6, IL-8, and PGE2 were significantly decreased in boswellic acid group 7 days

after the intervention. The authors concluded, based on this preliminary trial, that boswellic acids could improve clinical outcome in the early phases of stroke along with promising changes in plasma inflammatory factors (Baram et al., 2019).

Neurological Disorders: Cognitive Impairment

A 1-month RCT in 70-year-old adults ($n = 70$) with memory impairment investigated a combination of lemon balm plus frankincense tablets compared with placebo for effects on memory scales. Comparison of the two groups showed that the total scores of the Wechsler Memory Scale-Revised and the subscales, including immediate auditory, immediate memory, immediate visual, and working memory, were increased after consumption of the combination herbal product ($P < 0.0001$). The authors concluded that the frankincense plus lemon balm tablet in older adults could be beneficial for improvement of memory (Taghizadeh et al., 2018).

Dermatological Disorders: Psoriasis, Eczema, and Photoaging

An RCT in patients with psoriasis or erythematous eczema compared Bosexil (a lecithin-frankincense formulation) with bilberry seed oil and with placebo. In patients with psoriasis, both scales and erythema improved with both frankincense and bilberry seed oil treatment compared with placebo. The frankincense formulation improved scales (70% of cases) and erythema (50% of cases) without any case of worsening. In patients with eczema, frankincense, bilberry, and placebo improved itch by 60%, 66.7%, and 10%, respectively; erythema improved by 60%, 78%, and 10%, respectively. The authors concluded that this frankincense formulation could be promising for the treatment of psoriasis and erythematous eczema (Togni et al., 2014).

A 2-month randomized split-faced trial in women ($n = 15$) with photoaging investigated a base cream containing 0.5% boswellic acids compared with the base cream alone applied BID for 30 days. At baseline, at the end of the treatment, and after a 2-month follow-up, clinical findings as assessed with the Dover classification scale for photoaging and by biophysical and echographic measurements showed a significant improvement of tactile roughness and fine lines in the side of the face treated with boswellic acid. There was an improvement of elasticity, a decrease of sebum excretion, and a change of echographic parameters suggesting a reshaping of dermal tissue. The treatment was well tolerated without adverse effects. The authors concluded that the topical application of boswellic acids may represent a suitable treatment option for selected features of skin photoaging (Pedretti et al., 2010).

Autoimmune Disorders

See *Bowel Disorders: Irritable Bowel Syndrome and Inflammatory Bowel Disease.*

Oncologic Disorders: Chemotherapy-Induced Peripheral Neuropathy and Radiation-Induced Brain Edema

A prospective study in patients ($n=25$) with chemotherapy-induced peripheral neuropathy administered a dietary supplement with α-lipoic (CIPN) acid, frankincense, MSM and bromelain (Opera) at onset of neuropathic symptoms for 12 weeks. Analysis of VAS data showed reduction in pain perceived by patients. According to the neuropathy scales used, both pain and sensory and motor neuropathic impairments decreased after 12 weeks of treatments. Treatment with the supplement was well tolerated. The authors concluded that OPERA was able to improve CIPN symptoms with no significant toxicity or interaction (Desideri et al., 2017).

A study in patients ($n=44$) with primary or secondary malignant brain tumors compared radiotherapy plus frankincense 4200 mg/day with radiotherapy plus placebo. Compared with baseline there was a >75% reduction of cerebral edema in 60% of patients treated with frankincense and 26% of patients given placebo ($P=0.023$). Aside from minor GI discomfort there were no ADRs with frankincense. The authors concluded that frankincense significantly reduced cerebral edema measured by MRI and could potentially be steroid sparing for patients receiving brain irradiation (Kirste et al., 2011).

A 34-week RCT in patients ($n=20$) with glioblastoma multiforme treated with surgery, radiotherapy, and chemotherapy with temozolomide assessed the effects of an innovative phytosomal delivery form of boswellic acids extract (Monoselect AKBA) 4500 mg/day for a maximum of 34 weeks. Patients tended to have reduced or stable edema, the percentage of which increased over the observation period. Two patients were able to undergo a more complete surgical resection due to the reductions in their brain edema. Several patients were able to reduce their steroid dose or were dexamethasone free during the study. Patients' QOL and psychological state were stable throughout the study. The authors concluded that this form of boswellic acid extract, through antiinflammatory properties, might exert a beneficial effect in reducing radiochemotherapy-induced cerebral edema, allowing for a reduction in steroid use and improving resectability (Di Pierro et al., 2019).

ACTIVE CONSTITUENTS

Gum-Resin Found Under Bark

- Carbohydrates:
  - Polysaccharides: gums (analgesic, sedative, demulcent)
- Terpenes:
  - Terpenoids (13% monoterpenes, 1% sesquiterpenes, 42.5% diterpenes, triterpenes): boswellic acid (noncompetitive inhibitor of 5-lipoxygenase, antiinflammatory, antineoplastic, antilipemic, antistaphylococcal,), α-boswellic acid, β-boswellic acid, 3-acetyl-β-boswellic acid, acetyl-11-keto-β-boswellic acid aka AKBA (most active for ulcerative colitis, antiinflammatory, antineoplastic), boswellic acid acetate (antineoplastic), lupeolic acid, acetyl-lupeolic acid, incensole acetate, α and β-Amyrin (antiinflammatory, antiviral, antineoplastic, antilipemic, antioxidant, immunostimulant, antibone loss, apoptotic)
- Aromatic compounds: alpha-thujene, pinene, dipentene, phellandrene, sclarene, *p*-cymene

FRANKINCENSE COMMONLY USED PREPARATIONS AND DOSAGE (FOR ADULTS UNLESS OTHERWISE SPECIFIED)

The following are examples of some available formulations and ranges of dosing for commercial herbal products. See Part III Introduction "How to prescribe medicinal herbs" for further guidance on herbal advising and prescribing.

Gum-Resin

- Powdered resin standardized extract (standardized to >65% boswellic acids): 500 mg (1/5 tsp) QD-BID.
- Capsule or tablet of standardized extract of gum resin (standardized to 37.6%–65% boswellic acids): 300–500 mg QD-TID.

Brand name products that have higher concentrations of AKBA are dosed lower, in the range of 100–250 mg QAM.

For ulcerative colitis, the dose used in the study was 550 mg TID standardized to AKBA content.

SAFETY AND PRECAUTION

Side Effects

Rare side effects including diarrhea, skin rash, and nausea may occur. Allergic contact dermatitis may occur with topical cream. Ingestion of straight resin may result in bezoar.

Toxicity

Boswellia serrata was found safe at a daily dose of 500 mg/kg in rats. Rats given 1000 mg/kg did not gain weight as rapidly as rats on 100 and 500 mg/kg doses. Higher doses may be linked to upregulation of metabolic activity due to guggulsterone content of the herb.

Pregnancy and Lactation

Acetyl-11-keto-β-boswellic acid (AKBA) from *B. serrata* induced pericardial edema, yolk-sac edema, abnormal melanin, spinal curvature, hatching inhibition, and shortened body length in zebrafish embryos. Avoid.

Drug Interactions

- Pgp: Inhibits Pgp.
- Modulates activity of OATP1B3 (anion transporter).
- Modulates activity of MRP2 (multidrug resistant protein).
- Theoretical potential for interacting with anticoagulants due to platelet-inhibiting properties.

REFERENCES

Al-Jawad F, Al-Razzuqi R, Hashim H, Al-Bayati N. Glycyrrhiza glabra vs Boswellia carterii in chronic bronchial asthma: a comparative study of efficacy. Ind J Allergy Asthma Immunol January–June 2012;26(1):6–8.

Arkalgud Rangaswamy P, Sultana A, Rahman K, Nagapattinam S. Efficacy of Boswellia serrata L. and Cyperus scariosus L. plus pelvic floor muscle training in stress incontinence in women of reproductive age. Complement Ther Clin Pract 2014 Nov;20(4):230–6.

Bannuru RR, Osani MC, Al-Eid F, Wang C. Efficacy of curcumin and Boswellia for knee osteoarthritis: systematic review and meta-analysis. Semin Arthritis Rheum 2018 Dec;48(3):416–29.

Baram SM, Karima S, Shateri S, et al. Functional improvement and immune-inflammatory cytokines profile of ischaemic stroke patients after treatment with boswellic acids: a randomized, double-blind, placebo-controlled, pilot trial. Inflammopharmacology 2019 Dec;27(6):1101–12.

Belcaro G, Feragalli B, Cornelli U, Dugall M. Hand 'stress' arthritis in young subjects: effects of Flexique (pharma-standard Boswellia extract). A preliminary case report. Minerva Gastroenterol Dietol 2015 Oct;22.

Belcaro G, Gizzi G, Pellegrini L, et al. Supplementation with a lecithin-based delivery form of Boswellia serrata extract (Casperome®) controls symptoms of mild irritable bowel syndrome. Eur Rev Med Pharmacol Sci 2017 May;21(9):2249–54.

Belcaro G, Dugall M, Luzzi R, et al. Phytoproflex®: supplementary management of osteoarthrosis: a supplement registry. Minerva Med 2018 Apr;109(2):88–94.

Bolognesi G, Belcaro G, Feragalli B, et al. Movardol® (N-acetylglucosamine, Boswellia serrata, ginger) supplementation in the management of knee osteoarthritis: preliminary results from a 6-month registry study. Eur Rev Med Pharmacol Sci 2016 Dec;20(24):5198–204.

Cai T, Cocci A, Tiscione D, et al. L-Methionine associated with Hibiscus sabdariffa and Boswellia serrata extracts are not inferior to antibiotic treatment for symptoms relief in patients affected by recurrent uncomplicated urinary tract infections: focus on antibiotic-sparing approach. Arch Ital Urol Androl 2018 Jun 30;90(2):97–100.

Cameron M, Chrubasik S. Oral herbal therapies for treating osteoarthritis. Cochrane Database Syst Rev 2014 May 22;5, CD002947.

Chopra A, Lavin P, Patwardhan B, Chitre D. A 32-week randomized, placebo-controlled clinical evaluation of RA-11, an Ayurvedic drug, on osteoarthritis of the knees. J Clin Rheumatol 2004 Oct;10(5):236–45.

Desideri I, Francolini G, Becherini C, et al. Use of an alpha lipoic, methylsulfonylmethane and bromelain dietary supplement (Opera) for chemotherapy-induced peripheral neuropathy management, a prospective study. Med Oncol 2017 Mar;34(3):46.

Di Pierro F, Simonetti G, Petruzzi A, et al. A novel lecithin-based delivery form of Boswellic acids as complementary treatment of radiochemotherapy-induced cerebral edema in patients with glioblastoma multiforme: a longitudinal pilot experience. J Neurosurg Sci 2019 Jun;63(3):286–91.

Ernst E. Frankincense: systematic review. BMJ 2008 Dec 17;337:a2813.

Eshaghian R, Mazaheri M, Ghanadian M, Rouholamin S, Feizi A, Babaeian M. The effect of frankincense (Boswellia serrata, oleoresin) and ginger (Zingiber officinale, rhizoma) on heavy menstrual bleeding: a randomized, placebo-controlled, clinical trial. Complement Ther Med 2019 Feb;42–7.

Ferrara T, De Vincentiis G, Di Pierro F. Functional study on Boswellia phytosome as complementary intervention in asthmatic patients. Eur Rev Med Pharmacol Sci 2015 Oct;19(19):3757–62.

Franceschi F, Togni S, Belcaro G, et al. A novel lecithin-based delivery form of Boswellic acids (Casperome®) for the management of osteo-muscular pain: a registry study in young rugby players. Eur Rev Med Pharmacol Sci 2016 Oct;20(19):4156–61.

Gerhardt H, Seifert F, Buvari P, Vogelsang H, Repges R. Therapy of active Crohn disease with Boswellia serrata extract H 15. Z Gastroenterol 2001 Jan;39(1):11–7.

Gupta I, Parihar A, Malhotra P, et al. Effects of Boswellia serrata gum resin in patients with ulcerative colitis. Eur J Med Res 1997 Jan;2(1):37–43.

Gupta I, Gupta V, Parihar A, et al. Effects of Boswellia serrata gum resin in patients with bronchial asthma: results of a double-blind, placebo-controlled, 6-week clinical study. Eur J Med Res 1998 Nov 17;3(11):511–4.

Haroyan A, Mukuchyan V, Mkrtchyan N, et al. Efficacy and safety of curcumin and its combination with boswellic acid in osteoarthritis: a comparative, randomized, double-blind, placebo-controlled study. BMC Complement Altern Med 2018 Jan 9;18(1):7.

Hedaya R. Five herbs plus thiamine reduce pain and improve functional mobility in patients with pain: a pilot study. Altern Ther Health Med 2017 Jan;23(1):14–9.

Kafil TS, Nguyen TM, Patton PH, MacDonald JK, Chande N, McDonald J. Cochrane: treatments for collagenous colitis, https://www.cochrane.org/CD003575/IBD_treatments-collagenous-colitis; 11 November 2017.

Khalili N, Fereydoonzadeh R, Mohtashami R, Mehrzadi S, Heydari M, Huseini HF. Silymarin, Olibanum, and Nettle. A mixed herbal formulation in the treatment of type ii diabetes: a randomized, double-blind, placebo-controlled, clinical trial. J Evid Based Complement Altern Med 2017 Oct;22(4):603–8.

Khosravi Samani M, Mahmoodian H, Moghadamnia A, Poorsattar Bejeh Mir A, Chitsazan M. The effect of Frankincense in the treatment of moderate plaque-induced gingivitis: a double blinded randomized clinical trial. Daru 2011;19(4):288–94.

Kimmatkar N, Thawani V, Hingorani L, Khiyani R. Efficacy and tolerability of Boswellia serrata extract in treatment of osteoarthritis of knee—a randomized double blind placebo controlled trial. Phytomedicine 2003 Jan;10(1):3–7.

Kirste S, Treier M, Wehrle SJ, et al. Boswellia serrata acts on cerebral edema in patients irradiated for brain tumors: a prospective, randomized, placebo-controlled, double-blind pilot trial. Cancer 2011;117:3788–95.

Kizhakkedath R. Clinical evaluation of a formulation containing Curcuma longa and Boswellia serrata extracts in the management of knee osteoarthritis. Mol Med Rep 2013 Nov;8(5):1542–8.

Liu X, Machado GC, Eyles JP, Ravi V, Hunter DJ. Dietary supplements for treating osteoarthritis: a systematic review and meta-analysis. Br J Sports Med 2018 Feb;52(3):167–75.

Merolla G, Dellabiancia F, Ingardia A, Paladini P, Porcellini G. Co-analgesic therapy for arthroscopic supraspinatus tendon repair pain using a dietary supplement containing Boswellia serrata and Curcuma longa: a prospective randomized placebo-controlled study. Musculoskelet Surg 2015 Sep;99(Suppl 1):S43–52.

Pasta V, Dinicola S, Giuliani A, et al. A randomized trial of Boswellia in association with betaine and myo-inositol in the management of breast fibroadenomas. Eur Rev Med Pharmacol Sci 2016a My;20(9):1860–5.

Pasta V, Dinicola S, Giuliani A, et al. A randomized pilot study of inositol in association with betaine and Boswellia in the management of mastalgia and benign breast lump in premenopausal women. Breast Cancer (Auckl) 2016b Apr 20;10:37–43.

Pedretti A, Capezzera R, Zane C, Facchinetti E, Calzavara-Pinton P. Effects of topical boswellic acid on photo and age-damaged skin: clinical, biophysical, and echographic evaluations in a double-blind, randomized, split-face study. Planta Med 2010 Apr;76(6):555–60.

Ricci M, Micheloni GM, Berti M, et al. Clinical comparison of oral administration and viscosupplementation of hyaluronic acid (HA) in early knee osteoarthritis. Musculoskelet Surg 2017 Apr;101(1):45–9.

Riva A, Giacomelli L, Togni S, et al. Oral administration of a lecithin-based delivery form of boswellic acids (Casperome®) for the prevention of symptoms of irritable bowel syndrome: a randomized clinical study. Minerva Gastroenterol Dietol 2019 Mar;65(1):30–5.

Sengupta K, Alluri KV, Satish AR, et al. A double blind, randomized, placebo-controlled study of the efficacy and safety of 5-Loxin® for treatment of osteoarthritis of the knee. Arthritis Res Ther 2008;10(4):R85.

Sontakke S, Thawani V, Pimpalkhute S, Kabra P, Babhulkar S, Hingorani L. Open, randomized, controlled clinical trial of Boswellia serrata extract compared with valdecoxib in osteoarthritis of the knee. Indian J Pharmacol Feb 2007;39(1):27–9.

Taghizadeh M, Maghaminejad F, Aghajani M, Rahmani M, Mahboubi M. The effect of tablet containing Boswellia serrata and Melisa officinalis extract on older adults' memory: a randomized controlled trial. Arch Gerontol Geriatr 2018 Mar-Apr;75:146–50.

Togni S, Maramaldi G, Di Pierro F, Biondi M. A cosmeceutical formulation based on boswellic acids for the treatment of erythematous eczema and psoriasis. Clin Cosmet Investig Dermatol 2014 Nov 11;7:321–7.

47

GINGER (*ZINGIBER OFFICINALE*)
Root

GENERAL OVERVIEW

Ginger is recognized by conventional medical practitioners for its anti-nausea and anti-inflammatory effects. It improves digestion by stimulating salivary flow, gastric motility, gastric acid production, bile flow, and gall bladder kinesis, so may be beneficial for a host of functional gastrointestinal complaints. Ginger has been shown to have several gastrointestinal benefits in clinical trials.

Clinical research indicates that ginger, alone or in combination formulas, may be beneficial for gingivitis, coronary artery disease, hyperlipidemia, nausea and vomiting of pregnancy, motion sickness, post-operative nausea, chemotherapy-induced nausea, gastroparesis, dysmenorrhea, menorrhagia, menopause, male infertility, osteoarthritis, muscle pain, migraine headache, and colorectal cancer prevention.

IN VITRO AND ANIMAL RESEARCH

In vitro research has shown that ginger or its chemical constituents have antiplatelet, antioxidant, and anti-inflammatory activity. The antioxidant activity in one study was equal to that of ascorbic acid. The anti-inflammatory activity is due to COX-1, COX-2, PGI-2, 5-LOX, and thromboxane inhibition. Although ginger extracts inhibit platelet aggregation and thromboxane synthesis, several studies using ginger orally did not find any significant anticoagulant effects in vivo.

The constituents 6-gingerol and 6-shogaol have antipyretic, analgesic, anti-inflammatory, antitussive, and hypotensive effects as demonstrated in animal models. Research with rats has shown a reduction in BP

and heart rate from ginger. The gingerols and shogaol found in the fresh root increase uptake of calcium by the myocardium increasing contractility. In mice and rats ginger has been shown to improve insulin sensitivity and to lower serum glucose, cholesterol, and triglycerides. Raw ginger reversed diabetic proteinuria and promoted weight loss in diabetic rats.

The GI effects of ginger are complex with mixed results likely due to different preparations (dried, fresh, alcohol extract, etc.). Ginger's main active constituents have been shown to increase bile acid and digestive enzyme activity. Ginger appears to increase gastric tone and motility due to anticholinergic and antiserotonergic activity. Conversely, ginger has been shown to inhibit gastric contraction in other studies. Four animal studies have demonstrated the antiemetic activity of ginger extracts and the shogaols and gingerols in ginger. 6-shogaol has the greatest potency for inhibiting the 5-HT response that leads to nausea. The anti-ulcer activity of ginger has also been demonstrated in animal models.

High doses of ginger have been shown to raise sperm count in rats. There is also evidence of neural protection against insult from Aβ. Antibacterial, antifungal, and anti-helminthic activity has been demonstrated. Specific activity has been demonstrated against *Helicobacter pylori*, *Staphylococcus aureus*, *Pseudomonas aeruginosa*, *Salmonella typhimurium*, *Escherichia coli*, *Micrococcus luteus*, and *Candida albicans*. Fresh ginger has antiviral activity through stimulation of IFN-β antiviral activity.

Anticancer activities that have been demonstrated with ginger include induction of apoptosis of gastric cancer cells and inhibition of cell-cycle progression by gingerol. Ginger also inhibits VEGF and IL-I in ovarian cancer cells. Shogaol inhibits tumor growth by damaging microtubules and inducing mitotic arrest. In rodent models, ginger has demonstrated antitumor activity and increased immunologic function. Pretreatment of mice with a ginger rhizome reduced the severity of radiation sickness, GI syndrome, bone marrow suppression and overall mortality, likely through antioxidant effects.

HUMAN RESEARCH

General Overview

A 2020 systematic review to provide a comprehensive assessment of the clinical effects of ginger in all reported areas found 109 studies for inclusion. There was consistent support for the improvement of nausea and vomiting in pregnancy, inflammation, metabolic syndrome, digestive function, and colorectal cancer's markers. Other proposed benefits for ginger found conflicting studies. Only 39.4% of the clinical trials were of a high quality of evidence. The researchers concluded that further studies with adequate designs were warranted to validate the reported clinical functions of ginger (Anh et al., 2020).

Oral and Dental Disorders

A 14-day RCT of patients ($n=60$) with gingivitis compared the effects of a polyherbal mouthwash (containing calendula, rosemary, and ginger) with chlorhexidine and with placebo 5 g of each BID. Scores for modified gingival index, gingival bleeding index, and modified Quigley-Hein plaque index showed significant improvement from baseline for both the polyherbal and chlorhexidine mouthwash groups with no change in the placebo group. There was no significant difference in response between the polyherbal and chlorhexidine groups (Mahyari et al., 2016).

Cardiometabolic Disorders: Hyperlipidemia and Coronary Artery Disease

A 45-day RCT in patients ($n=85$) attending a cardiac clinic compared ginger 1 g TID with placebo with respect to effects on lipids. The ginger group showed a significant reduction in TG, TC, LDL-C, and VLDL-C compared with baseline levels ($P<0.05$). All lipid changes except for VLDL were significantly greater with ginger than with placebo ($P<0.05$) (Alizadeh-Navaei et al., 2008).

An open-label study in healthy adult volunteers ($n=30$) investigated the effect of ginger 5 g on fibrinolytic activity when that activity had been reduced by dietary fat. Administration of 50 g of fat decreased fibrinolytic activity from a baseline of 64 to 52 units ($P<0.001$) and adding ginger to the fat increased fibrinolytic activity from baseline ($P<0.001$) (Verma and Bordia, 2001).

Cardiometabolic Disorders: Diabetes

A 2019 systematic review to compare the effects of dietary ginger on the baseline and follow-up levels of FBS and A1C in T2DM found eight studies ($n=454$) that met inclusion criteria. The results showed significant improvements in A1C with ginger consumption (WMD: 0.46, $P=0.02$), but no significant difference between baseline and follow-up values for FBS in patients who consumed ginger (WMD = 1.38, $P=0.16$). Patients in the placebo or control groups had no significant changes with either FBS or A1C. The authors concluded that dietary ginger might have an impact on glucose control over a longer period of time in patients with T2DM (Huang et al., 2019).

A 90-day RCT in adult patients ($n=103$) with T2DM whose A1Cs on antidiabetic drugs were between 6% and 10% evaluated ginger 600 mg BID with breakfast and lunch compared with placebo for glycemic and lipid effects. With ginger the FBG decreased from 203.6 mg/dL to 174 mg/dL ($P<0.001$), and with placebo FBG decreased from 185.2 mg/dL to 175.9 mg/dL ($P=0.041$). With ginger the A1C decreased from 8.4% to 8.14% ($P=0.144$), and with placebo A1C decreased from 8.36% to 8.29% ($P=0.36$). The authors concluded that ginger could help in the treatment of T2DM (Carvalho et al., 2020).

Gastrointestinal Disorders: Nausea, Vomiting, and Gastroparesis

(See also Oncology: Chemotherapy-Induced Nausea and Vomiting)

A 2009 systematic review looking at therapies for post-operative nausea and vomiting selected 21 studies ($n=2286$) that met inclusion criteria. The authors concluded there was some limited evidence to support providing ginger in doses between 1 g and 1.5 g to prevent or reduce the level of nausea but not vomiting postoperatively and to reduce the need for rescue medication. Other modalities found to be effective included acupressure or capsaicin application to certain acupoints, and inhalation of isopropyl alcohol (Hewitt and Watts, 2009).

A 2006 systematic review of the effects of a fixed dose of ginger on 24-h postoperative nausea and vomiting found five RCTs ($n = 363$) that met inclusion criteria for meta-analysis. The summary RR of ginger for postoperative nausea and vomiting and postoperative vomiting were 0.69 and 0.61, respectively. Only one side effect, abdominal discomfort, was reported. The authors concluded that a fixed dose at least 1 g of ginger is more effective than placebo for the prevention of postoperative nausea and vomiting (Chaiyakunapruk et al., 2006).

A 2005 systematic review looking at the evidence for safety and efficacy of ginger therapy for nausea and vomiting during pregnancy selected six RCTs ($n = 675$) plus a prospective observational study that met inclusion criteria. Four of the six RCTs ($n = 246$) showed superiority of ginger over placebo; the other two RCTs ($n = 429$) indicated that ginger was as effective as the reference drug (vitamin B6) in relieving the severity of nausea and vomiting episodes. The observational study and RCTs (including follow-up periods) showed the absence of significant side effects or adverse effects on pregnancy outcomes. There were no spontaneous or case reports of adverse events during ginger treatment in pregnancy. The authors concluded that ginger may be an effective treatment for nausea and vomiting in pregnancy. However, they cautioned that more observational studies, with a larger sample size, are needed to confirm the encouraging preliminary data on ginger safety (Borrelli et al., 2005).

A 2000 systematic review of evidence of ginger for nausea and vomiting of various causes identified six studies for review. Three on postoperative nausea and vomiting were identified and two of these suggested that ginger was superior to placebo and equally effective as metoclopramide. The pooled ARR for the incidence of postoperative nausea, however, indicated a non-significant difference between the ginger and placebo groups for ginger 1 g taken before surgery (ARR = 0.052). The remaining three studies found

favorable evidence for seasickness, morning sickness and chemotherapy-induced nausea, respectively (Ernst and Pittler, 2000).

A 4-day RCT in pregnant women ($n = 126$) with nausea and vomiting compared ginger 650 mg with pyridoxine 25 mg TID. Both ginger and pyridoxine significantly reduced nausea and vomiting scores from 8.7 to 5.4 and from 8.3 to 5.7, respectively ($P < 0.05$). The mean score change after treatment was greater with ginger than with pyridoxine (3.3 vs 2.6; $P < 0.05$). The authors concluded that both ginger and pyridoxine were effective for treatment of nausea and vomiting in pregnancy, and that ginger was more effective than the vitamin. Side effects from ginger were reported to be minor (Chittumma et al., 2007).

A 4-day RCT in pregnant women ($n = 70$) with nausea compared ginger 1 g/day with pyridoxine 40 mg/day for four days. Compared with baseline, the decrease in the VAS of post-therapy nausea in the ginger group was significantly greater than that for the pyridoxine group ($P = 0.024$). In the ginger group, 29/35 women reported an improvement in nausea symptoms, compared with 23/34 women in the pyridoxine group ($P = 0.52$) (Ensiyeh and Sakineh, 2009).

A 7-day RCT in pregnant women ($n = 170$) with nausea and vomiting compared ginger 500 mg BID with dimenhydrinate 50 mg TID. There was no significant difference in the VAS for nausea scores between groups. Vomiting episodes were greater with ginger on the first and second days of the treatment but no difference in vomiting episodes was noted during the days 3–7 of treatment. Drowsiness occurred in 6% of ginger group and 78% of dimenhydrinate group ($P < 0.01$). The authors concluded that ginger was as effective as dimenhydrinate in the treatment of nausea and vomiting during pregnancy and had fewer side effects (Pongrojpaw et al., 2007).

A 4-day RCT in women ($n = 120$) in the first trimester of pregnancy compared ginger extract 125 mg QID for 4 days with placebo. The nausea experience score was significantly less for the ginger extract group relative to the placebo group after the first day and all subsequent days of treatment. Retching was also reduced by ginger extract although to a lesser extent. No significant effect was observed for vomiting. Follow-up of the pregnancies revealed normal ranges of birthweight, gestational age, Apgar scores, and frequencies of congenital abnormalities compared with the general population. The authors concluded that ginger could be considered as a useful treatment option for women suffering from morning sickness (Willetts et al., 2003).

A 4-day single-blinded study in pregnant women ($n = 67$) with nausea and vomiting compared ginger 250 mg QID with placebo. The ginger group demonstrated a greater rate of improvement than the placebo group (85% vs 56%; $P < 0.01$) and a reduction in vomiting episodes (50% vs 9%; $P < 0.05$). The authors concluded that ginger was an effective herbal remedy for decreasing nausea and vomiting during pregnancy (Ozgoli et al., 2009b).

A study in volunteers ($n = 13$) with a history of motion sickness assessed the efficacy of pretreating spinning activity with ginger 1 g and 2 g. Both ginger groups demonstrated a reduction in nausea, tachygastria, and plasma vasopressin. Ginger also prolonged the latency before nausea onset and shortened the recovery time following the spinning activity (Lien et al., 2003).

A single-day RCT in patients ($n = 120$) patients who underwent major gynecologic surgery compared ginger 1 g taken 1 h before the procedure with placebo given 1 h prior to procedure. The ginger group experienced significantly less nausea than the placebo group (48% vs 67%) with the greatest differences occurring at 2 h and 6 h post-op (Nanthakomon and Pongrojpaw, 2006).

A single-day RCT in patients ($n = 120$) undergoing gynecological laparoscopy studied ginger 2 g compared with droperidol 1.24 mg, with combined ginger plus droperidol at same doses, and with placebo. There were no significant differences in the incidence of postoperative nausea, which was 32%, 20%, 22%, and 33%, and vomiting, which was 35%, 15%, 25%, and 25% in the four groups, respectively. The authors concluded that ginger powder 2 g, droperidol 1.25 mg, or both were ineffective in reducing the incidence of postoperative nausea and vomiting after gynecological laparoscopy (Visalyaputra et al., 1998).

Another surgically related RCT in post-operative laparoscopy patients ($n = 60$) compared ginger 500 mg TID with placebo TID for post-operative nausea and vomiting. Median nausea and vomiting at 2 h post-op were similar between groups. At 6 h post-op, the median VAS for nausea was significantly lower in the ginger group (0.55 vs 2.80; $P = 0.015$). At 6 h, 23.3% of the ginger group and 47% of the placebo group had an episode of vomiting ($P = 0.058$). The authors concluded that ginger showed efficacy for prevention of nausea and borderline significance for prevention vomiting after gynecological laparoscopy at 6 h post-op (Apariman et al., 2006).

An open-label controlled study in healthy young male volunteers ($n = 14$) examined the effect of ginger dried powder 1 g in water on LES and esophageal peristalsis compared with water alone. The study showed that after the ginger consumption, the LES resting pressures remained unchanged, but the percent relaxation with swallowing was significantly increased throughout the 180 min. In addition, the velocity of contraction waves was decreased throughout the study period. The authors proposed an anti-flatulent effect through increased gastric gas expulsion capacity (Lohsiriwat et al., 2010).

A single-day RCT in healthy volunteers ($n = 24$) compared ginger 1200 mg with placebo for effects on gastric emptying. In the ginger group, the antral area decreased more rapidly ($P < 0.001$) and the gastric half-emptying time was less than with placebo (13 vs 27 min; $P < 0.01$). The frequency of antral contractions was greater with ginger ($P < 0.005$). Fundus dimensions did not differ, and there was no significant difference in any GI symptoms. The authors concluded that ginger accelerated gastric emptying and stimulated antral contractions in healthy volunteers, with potential benefit for patients symptomatic of gastroparesis (Wu et al., 2008).

A placebo-controlled study in healthy humans ($n = 22$) compared ginger 2 g with placebo for effect on gastric motility during hyperglycemic clamping and with the addition of misoprostol 400 μg (to produce a prostaglandin effect). After placebo, hyperglycemia reduced normal peristaltic activity from 94% to 10%, and the dominant frequencies increased from 3 to 4 cpm. Tachygastria increased from 2% to 29% ($P < 0.05$). These hyperglycemia effects on normal gastric activity, dominant frequencies, and tachygastria were significantly reduced by ginger ($P < 0.05$). However, ginger did not correct the abnormalities produced by misoprostol compared with placebo suggesting that ginger prevents the hyperglycemic slow-wave dysrhythmias, but not those produced by prostaglandin. The authors concluded that ginger likely acted to blunt production of prostaglandins rather than inhibiting their action (Gonlachanvit et al., 2003).

Gastrointestinal Disorders: Ulcerative Colitis

A 12-week RCT in patients ($n=46$) with mild-to-moderate UC compared encapsulated ginger powder 2000 mg/day with placebo. After 6 and 12 weeks, MDA was reduced significantly ($P=0.003$ and $P<0.001$, respectively). There was no significant effect on TAC. At 12 weeks, the scores of severity of disease activity were significantly improved with ginger compared with placebo ($P=0.017$), and ginger was associated with an increased QOL ($P=0.039$). The authors concluded that ginger could improve treatment of patients with UC and that further studies were warranted (Nikkhah-Bodaghi et al., 2019).

Women's Genitourinary Disorders: Dysmenorrhea and Menorrhagia

A 2015 systematic review on the use of ginger for primary dysmenorrhea identified seven studies that met selection criteria. Four of the RCTs compared the therapeutic efficacy of ginger with a placebo during the first 3–4 days of the menstrual cycle and were included in the meta-analysis. The meta-analysis of these data showed a significant effect of ginger in reducing pain VAS in subjects having primary dysmenorrhea ($RR=-1.85$; $P=0.0003$). The authors concluded that there was suggestive evidence for the effectiveness of 750–2000 mg ginger powder during the first 3–4 days of menstrual cycle for primary dysmenorrhea (Daily et al., 2015).

A 3-day RCT in female college students ($n=150$) with primary dysmenorrhea compared ginger 250 mg with mefenamic acid 250 mg and with ibuprofen 400 mg, each given at onset of menses. The severity of dysmenorrhea decreased in all groups and no differences were found between the groups in severity of dysmenorrhea, pain relief, or satisfaction with the treatment ($P>0.05$). No severe side effects occurred. The authors concluded that ginger was as effective as mefenamic acid and ibuprofen in relieving pain in women with primary dysmenorrhea (Ozgoli et al., 2009a).

A 2-month RCT in patients ($n=102$) with heavy menstrual bleeding compared ibuprofen 200 mg plus either frankincense 300 mg, ginger 300 mg, or placebo TID for 7 days starting with onset of menses. Duration of menstrual bleeding was decreased with frankincense (-1.77 days; $P=0.003$) and ginger (-1.8 days; $P=0.001$), but not with placebo (-0.52 days; $P=0.42$). The amount of bleeding was decreased in all ($P<0.05$), with no difference among the study groups. QOL was improved more with frankincense (-25.7; $P<0.001$) and ginger (-29.2; $P<0.001$) than with placebo (-15.07, $P<0.001$), and between-group differences were significant ($P=0.02$). The authors concluded that ginger and frankincense seemed to be effective complementary treatments for heavy menstrual bleeding (Eshaghian et al., 2019).

Women's Genitourinary Disorders: Perimenopause and Menopause

A 3-month open-label study in women with either mild or moderate-severe menopausal symptoms investigated the effect of ElleN, a combination product containing chasteberry, black cohosh, hyaluronic acid, zinc, and ginger, one tablet daily. Results showed a significant reduction in the Kupperman Index for both the mildly and moderately-severe symptomatic groups. The treatment was particularly effective against hot flushes associated with night insomnia and anxiety. The product was well tolerated and did not cause any side effects. The authors concluded that this combination product was able to reduce mildly and moderately-severe menopause symptoms (Cappelli et al., 2015).

Men's Genitourinary Disorders: Male Infertility

A one-year open-label longitudinal study in younger men ($n=75$) with infertility looked at the effects of ginger supplementation. By the end of the year of treatment there was an increase in sperm count by up to 16%, sperm motility by up to 47%, and sperm viability and morphology by up to 40% ($P<0.01$, respectively). Ejaculate volume increased by up to 36%. MDA was reduced significantly from baseline ($P<0.01$), and GSH was increased significantly from baseline ($P<0.01$). FSH, LH, and testosterone levels were also increased significantly. The authors concluded that ginger caused a significant reduction in serum MDA and a significant increase in serum GSH, LH, FSH, and testosterone (Mares and Najam, 2012).

Musculoskeletal Disorders: Osteoarthritis and Muscle Pain

A 72-week crossover RCT in patients ($n = 29$) with knee OA compared ginger 250 mg QID with placebo TID with crossover at 3 months. By the end of 24 weeks of crossover treatments there was a significant difference between the VAS of pain and disability of the two groups ($P < 0.001$). This difference was not apparent at the end of the first 12 weeks. This suggests a cumulative benefit with ginger in knee OA, the response of which may distort findings of shorter studies (Wigler et al., 2003).

A 6-month RCT in subjects ($n = 54$) with moderate knee OA compared standard management alone with standard management plus Movardol, a supplement containing glucosamine, ginger, and frankincense, TID for 1 week then BID. Significant improvements in the functional outcomes and pain-free walking distance were observed after 1, 3, and 6 months in OA patients taking the supplement. All the signs and symptoms of disease assessed by WOMAC tended to regress over a 6-month period in the supplemented group, and inflammatory markers and plasma content of ROS decreased over 6 months in this group as well. The supplement appeared to be safe and well tolerated (Bolognesi et al., 2016).

A 32-week RCT in patients ($n = 90$) with OA compared an Ayurvedic combination containing ashwagandha, frankincense, ginger, and turmeric with placebo. The mean reduction in pain VAS for the herbal combination vs placebo was 2.7 vs 1.3 at week 16 and 2.8 vs 1.8 at week 32 ($P < 0.05$). The improvements in the WOMAC scores at week 16 and week 32 were also significantly superior ($P < 0.01$) with the combination herbal product. Both of the groups reported mild adverse events without any significant difference between groups (Chopra et al., 2004).

A 30-day pilot study in patients ($n = 15$) with chronic OA-related knee pain not responding to NSAIDs assessed the effect of a standardized supplement of ginger 25 mg plus echinacea 5 mg. After supplementation, a significant improvement of 12.27 points was observed for Lysholm scale score ($P < 0.05$) and there was

a change of -0.52 cm in knee circumference ($P < 0.01$) (Rondanelli et al., 2017).

Two 11-day RCTs in volunteers ($n = 34$ and 40, respectively) compared ginger 2 g (raw or heated, respectively) with placebo for muscle pain related to exercise (18 eccentric actions of the elbow flexors to induce pain and inflammation). Raw and heat-treated ginger resulted in similar pain reductions 24 h after eccentric exercise compared with placebo (25%, $P = 0.041$; 23%, $P = 0.049$, respectively). The authors concluded that daily consumption of raw and heat-treated ginger resulted in moderate-to-large reductions in muscle pain following exercise-induced muscle injury, and that this study further demonstrated ginger's effectiveness as a pain reliever (Black et al., 2010).

Neurological Disorders: Migraine Headache

A 1-month RCT in patients ($n = 100$) with migraines without aura compared ginger with sumatriptan administered abortively. Two hours after using either drug, mean headache severity decreased significantly, producing a 4.7-unit reduction in pain VAS with sumatriptan and a 4.6-unit reduction with ginger ($P < 0.001$, respectively). Efficacy of ginger powder and sumatriptan was similar. Clinical adverse effects of ginger powder were less than sumatriptan. Patients' satisfaction and willingness to continue did not differ. The authors concluded that the effectiveness of ginger powder in the treatment of common migraine attacks was statistically comparable to sumatriptan with less side effects (Maghbooli et al., 2014).

An acutely dosed RCT in patients ($n = 60$) who sought medical care in the ER for an acute migraine compared ginger 400 mg with placebo, each in addition to ketoprofen 100 mg IV. Patients treated with ginger showed significantly better clinical response after 1 h ($P = 0.04$), 1.5 h ($P = 0.01$), and 2 h ($P = 0.04$). Ginger treatment promoted reduction in pain and improvement in functional status at all times assessed. The authors concluded that the addition of ginger to NSAIDs may contribute to the treatment of migraine attack (Martins et al., 2019).

Inflammation

A 2020 systematic review and meta-analysis to investigate the efficacy of ginger on circulating levels of CRP, hs-CRP, TNF-α, soluble ICAM, and IL-6 concentrations found 16 RCTs ($n = 1010$) that met inclusion criteria for meta-analysis. Ginger was associated with a significant reduction of circulating CRP (SMD: -5.11, $I^2 = 98.1\%$), hs-CRP (SMD: -0.88, $I^2 = 90.8\%$), and TNF-α levels (SMD: -0.85, $I^2 = 89.4\%$). The reviewers did not find a significant impact of ginger on IL-6 or soluble ICAM levels. The authors concluded that ginger produced a significant impact in lowering circulating CRP, hs-CRP and TNF-α level, and larger trials were warranted (Morvaridzadeh et al., 2020).

A 2020 systematic review and meta-analysis to investigate the effects of ginger on inflammation and oxidative stress found 25 studies that met inclusion criteria for meta-analysis. Pooled results indicated a statistically significant effect of ginger compared with controls on serum CRP, TNF-α, IL-6, TAC, and MDA levels. The effects of ginger on serum PGE2 were marginally significant. The authors concluded that ginger had a significant effect on serum inflammatory and oxidative stress markers (Jalali et al., 2020).

Autoimmune Disorders: Rheumatoid Arthritis

(See also Gastrointestinal Disorders: Ulcerative Colitis)

A 12-week RCT in patients ($n = 70$) with RA compared ginger 1500 mg/day with placebo for impacts on the expression of immunity and inflammation intermediate genes. The study followed disease activity scores and gene expression of NF-κB, PPAR-γ, FoxP3, T-bet, GATA-3, and RORγt as immunity and inflammation intermediate factors. After 12 weeks of ginger, FoxP3 gene expression increased significantly over baseline and compared with placebo ($P = 0.01$). T-bet and RORγt gene expression decreased significantly with ginger compared with placebo ($P < 0.05$). PPAR-γ gene expression increased significantly from baseline with ginger ($P = 0.047$), but the difference was not significant from placebo ($P = 0.12$). With ginger, the reduction in disease activity score was significant compared with baseline and with placebo. The authors concluded that that ginger could improve RA by decreasing disease manifestations via increasing FoxP3 genes expression and by decreasing RORγt and T-bet genes expression (Aryaeian et al., 2019).

Oncologic Disorders: Colorectal Cancer Prevention

A 28-day pilot RCT in volunteers ($n = 20$) at increased risk for colorectal cancer compared ginger 2 g QD with placebo. Colorectal biopsies were performed pre- and post-treatment to evaluate numerous indexes of proliferation, apoptosis, and differentiation. In the ginger group, relative to placebo, BAX expression decreased 15.6% ($P = 0.78$) in the whole crypts with even more difference in the higher risk proliferation zone of the crypts ($P = 0.67$). In addition, hTERT (telomerase) expression in the whole crypts decreased by 41.2% ($P = 0.05$); and MIB-1 (a cellular proliferation protein gene) expression decreased in the whole crypts 16.9% ($P = 0.39$). The authors concluded that ginger may reduce proliferation in the normal-appearing colorectal epithelium and increase apoptosis and differentiation relative to proliferation, especially in the differentiation zone of the crypts, in people at increased risk for colorectal cancer (Citronberg et al., 2013).

A 28-day RCT in healthy volunteers ($n = 30$) compared ginger 2 g/day with placebo for effects on colonic eicosanoids as assessed through sigmoidoscopic biopsies. There were no significant differences in mean percent change between baseline and day 28 for any of the eicosanoids, when normalized to protein. With ginger compared with placebo there was a significant decrease in mean percent change in PGE2 ($P = 0.05$) and 5-HETE ($P = 0.04$), and a trend toward significant decreases in 12-HETE ($P = 0.09$) and 15-HETE ($P = 0.06$) normalized to free arachidonic acid. There was no difference between the groups in terms of total adverse events ($P = 0.55$) The authors concluded that ginger had the potential to decrease eicosanoid levels, perhaps by inhibiting their synthesis from arachidonic acid. Ginger also seemed to be tolerable and safe (Zick et al., 2011).

A 28-day RCT study in participants ($n = 50$) with normal ($n = 30$) or elevated ($n = 20$) risk for colon cancer compared ginger 2 g/day with placebo for 28 days for effect on COX activity. Colon biopsies were performed pre- and post-treatment. After ginger consumption, participants at increased risk for CRC had a 24% reduced colonic COX-1 protein level compared with a 19% reduction with placebo ($P = 0.03$). This difference did not occur in the participants at normal risk for CRC. The authors concluded that ginger significantly lowered COX-1 protein expression in participants at increased risk for CRC but not in those at normal risk for CRC (Jiang et al., 2005).

Oncologic Disorders: Chemotherapy-Induced Nausea and Vomiting

A 2019 systematic review to evaluate the effects of ginger on the incidence, duration, and severity of chemotherapy-induced nausea and vomiting (CINV) found 18 studies that met inclusion criteria. The likelihood of acute vomiting ($n = 301$) was reduced by 60% with ginger $\leq 1\,g/day$ for > 3 days, compared with control groups (OR = 0.4, $I^2 = 20\%$; $P = 0.01$). The likelihood of fatigue ($n = 219$) was reduced by 80% with ginger of any dose for < 3 days (OR = 0.2, $I^2 = 0\%$, $P = 0.03$). No statistically significant association was found between ginger and likelihood of overall or delayed vomiting, likelihood or severity of nausea, or other outcomes related to chemotherapy-induced nausea and vomiting. The authors concluded that ginger might benefit CINV as well as fatigue. Further research was recommended (Crichton et al., 2019).

A 2019 systematic review undertaking a comprehensive overview of the current evidence regarding the effectiveness of ginger for controlling CINV in breast cancer patients found nine studies that met inclusion criteria. Two studies had examined the effect of ginger on the frequency of nausea, five studies on the frequency of vomiting, seven studies on the severity of nausea, and three studies on severity of vomiting. The investigators concluded that the research suggested that ginger may reduce nausea in the acute phase of chemotherapy in patients with breast cancer and that more research was warranted (Saneei Totmaj et al., 2019).

A chemotherapy based RCT in women ($n = 100$) with advanced breast cancer on standard chemotherapy compared ginger 500 mg TID plus a standard antiemetic regimen (granisetron plus dexamethasone) with the standard antiemetic regimen alone for 4 days from the initiation of chemotherapy. A significantly lower prevalence of nausea was observed in the ginger group during 6 to 24 h post-chemotherapy. No other significant additional benefit from ginger was observed for prevalence or severity of nausea, vomiting, and retching in any of the assessed periods. The authors concluded that the addition of ginger 1.5 g/day to standard antiemetic therapy in patients with advanced breast cancer effectively reduced the prevalence of nausea 6 to 24 h post-chemotherapy without any additional advantage for ginger in reducing prevalence or severity of acute or delayed CINV (Panahi et al., 2012).

A chemotherapy based RCT in bone sarcoma patients ($n = 57$) compared ginger root powdered capsules with placebo as anti-emetic add-on therapy during 60 chemotherapy cycles of cisplatin plus doxorubicin. Acute moderate to severe nausea and vomiting were observed in 93% and 77%, respectively, of cycles in the control group vs 56% and 33%, respectively, of cycles in experimental group (between-group difference $P = 0.003$ and 0.002, respectively). Delayed (4–6 days post chemo) moderate to severe nausea and vomiting were observed in 73% and 47%, respectively, of cycles in the control group compared with 26% and 15%, respectively, of cycles in the experimental group (between-group difference $P < 0.001$ and $P = 0.022$, respectively). The authors concluded that ginger root powder was effective at reducing severity of acute and delayed CINV as additional therapy to ondansetron and dexamethasone in patients receiving high emetogenic chemotherapy (Pillai et al., 2011).

A multicenter RCT in cancer patients ($n = 744$) compared ginger 0.5 g, 1 g, or 1.5 g (1–2 capsules of 250 mg BID) with placebo in addition to standard anti-emetic therapy. All doses of ginger significantly reduced acute nausea severity compared with placebo on day 1 of chemotherapy ($P = 0.003$). The largest reduction in nausea intensity occurred with 0.5 g and 1.0 g of ginger ($P = 0.017$ and $P = 0.036$, respectively). The authors concluded that ginger supplementation at a daily dose of 0.5 g–1.0 g significantly reduced the severity of acute chemotherapy-induced nausea in adult cancer patients (Ryan et al., 2012).

ACTIVE CONSTITUENTS

Root

- Amino acid derivatives
  - Enzymes: zingibain (a proteolytic enzyme)
- Phenolic compounds
  - Phenylpropanoids: gingerols 6, 8, 10 (fresh ginger - anti-nausea, anti-5HT3 receptor, antiplatelet, antioxidant, anti-inflammatory, an-

drogenic, antineoplastic via apoptosis, VEGF inhibition and cell-cycle inhibition), paradols, zingerone, shogoals 6 & 10 (dried ginger, antitussive, antinociceptive), (10)-dehydrogingerdione, (6)- and (10)-gingerdione, vallinoids, galanals A and B

- Polyphenol: gingerenone A (anti-obesity, anti-inflammatory, anti-staphylococcal)
- Terpenes
  - Sesquiterpenes: zingiberene (carminative), bisabolenes
  - Diterpenoids: galanal A & B (apoptosis inducers, immune modulators), galanolactone (acetone extracts -competitive inhibitor at serotonin 5-HT3 receptors)
- Aromatic compounds (antilipid, vasodilating, antispasmodic, antioxidant): zingiberene, bisabolene

GINGER COMMONLY USED PREPARATIONS AND DOSAGE (FOR ADULTS UNLESS OTHERWISE SPECIFIED)

The following are examples of some available formulations and ranges of dosing for commercial herbal products. See Part III Introduction "How to prescribe medicinal herbs" for further guidance on herbal advising and prescribing.

Root

- Infusion of grated fresh root: 1 tsp. per cup TID prn nausea
- Fluid extract (1:1, 40%): 0.25–1 mL TID
- Tincture (1:5, 40%–90%): 1.5–3 mL TID
- Fresh root grated: 5 g per day
- Powdered root extract: 500 mg (1/5 tsp) QD-BID
- Capsule or tablet of powdered root extract: 550 mg QD-BID

Can be candied, applied as compress, or incorporated into cough syrup.

For motion sickness 500 mg dried root or powdered root extract before and every 2 h during travel.

For boosting testosterone, the dose would likely need to be in the 10–15 g range. However, safety at these high doses has not been fully evaluated.

For nausea of pregnancy a ginger infusion made from fresh grated root up to 1 g daily prn.

Use half the adult dose if younger than 6 years.

Use of dried ginger is less likely to affect platelets and bleeding risk, although overall risk for bleeding has been shown to be low.

SAFETY AND PRECAUTION

Side Effects

High doses may cause heartburn. Topically may cause contact dermatitis. May increase bleeding in patients with bleeding disorders. May increase abdominal pain in patients with gallstones due to cholagogic effect.

Toxicity

Rats given up to 2000 mg/kg for 35 days showed no significant adverse changes in blood chemistry or organ weight except a decrease in testicle size likely due to the androgenic activity of high doses. Lower dosages (500 mg/kg) have been tested for up to 13 weeks in rats of both genders with no side effects noted.

Pregnancy and Lactation

An extract given to pregnant rats resulted in no deaths or treatment-related adverse effects. However, in another similar study, embryonic loss in the treatment group was double that of the control group. Because ginger contains some compounds that cause chromosomal mutation in vitro, there is theoretical concern about the safety of using ginger during pregnancy.

A comparison study compared pregnancy outcomes in women ($n = 187$) who were either taking ginger in the first trimester of pregnancy or who were exposed to nonteratogenic drugs (comparison group) that were not antiemetic medications. There were no statistical differences in the outcomes between the ginger group and the comparison group with the exception of more infants weighing less than 2500 g in the comparison group (12 vs 3; $P < .001$). The authors concluded that ginger did not appear to increase the rates of major malformations above the baseline rate of 1% to 3% and that it had a mild effect in the treatment of NVP (Portnoi et al., 2003).

A more recent (2013) and larger ($n = 1020$) population-based cohort study in Norway found that the use of ginger during pregnancy was not associated with an increased risk of congenital malformations, still birth/perinatal birth, low birth weight, or preterm birth (Heitmann et al., 2013). Given this clinical research and a long history of heavy culinary use in some cultures it is reasonable to conclude that prudent use of ginger for morning sickness is safe in amounts up to 1 g per day on a PRN basis for short-term use. High doses (15 g/day) could possibly exert and androgenic effect.

Disease Interactions

■ Anticoagulation: May increase bleeding in patients with bleeding disorders.
■ Gallbladder disease: May increase abdominal pain in patients with gallstones due to cholagogic effect.
■ Surgery: Although a systematic review failed to show increased risk for bleeding, it is best to avoid due to theoretical platelet effects and fibrinolytic effects (but see studies below).

A systematic review assessing the effect of ginger on platelet function found seven trials that met inclusion criteria. Effects of ginger on platelet function were equivocal, with lower doses (1–4 g/day) having no effect on platelet function whereas studies using 5–10 g/day showed inhibition. Given that the antinausea effect of ginger occurs at 1 g/day the authors concluded that it was possible that the safety window between efficacy and adverse platelet events was wide enough to support the use of ginger in patients undergoing chemotherapy (Marx et al., 2015).

A 1-day RCT in healthy male volunteers ($n=8$) compared ginger 2 g with placebo with respect to platelet function at 3 h and 24 h post ingestion. There were no differences between ginger and placebo in bleeding time, platelet count, thromboelastography, and whole blood platelet aggregometry. It was concluded that the effect of ginger on thromboxane synthetase activity is dose dependent, or only occurs with fresh ginger, and that up to 2 g of dried ginger is unlikely to cause platelet dysfunction when used therapeutically (Lumb, 1994).

In another placebo-controlled study in subjects with CAD, ginger 4 g/day for 3 months did not affect ADP- and epinephrine-induced platelet aggregation, fibrinolytic activity, and fibrinogen level. However, a single dose of 10 g powdered ginger administered to these CAD patients produced a significant reduction in platelet aggregation with no effect on blood lipids and blood sugar (Bordia et al., 1997).

Drug Interactions

■ May increase absorption of drugs due to increased gastric motility.
■ May reduce blood concentrations of cyclosporine.
■ May reduce absorption of fat-soluble vitamins and iron.
■ May increase risk of bleeding in patients on anticoagulants (but see studies above).
■ May augment effects of hypoglycemic agents.

The synergistic effect of ginger and nifedipine on antiplatelet aggregation in human subjects was studied in Taiwan. The study demonstrated that both aspirin and ginger could potentiate the antiplatelet aggregation effect of nifedipine, suggesting that ginger and nifedipine have a synergistic effect on antiplatelet aggregation (Young et al., 2006).

An open label, three-way crossover randomized study in healthy male subjects ($n=12$), investigated the effects of ginkgo and ginger on warfarin. The subjects received a single 25 mg dose of warfarin either alone or after 7 days pretreatment plus 7 days posttreatment with recommended doses of ginkgo or ginger. INR and platelet aggregation were not affected by administration of ginkgo or ginger alone. Ginkgo and ginger at the recommended doses did not significantly affect clotting status or the pharmacokinetics or pharmacodynamics of warfarin (Jiang et al., 2013).

REFERENCES

Alizadeh-Navaei R, Roozbeh F, Saravi M, Pouramir M, Jalali F, Moghadamnia AA. Investigation of the effect of ginger on the lipid levels. A double blind controlled clinical trial. Saudi Med J 2008;29(9):1280–4.

Anh NH, Kim SJ, Long NP, et al. Ginger on human health: a comprehensive systematic review of 109 randomized controlled trials. Nutrients 2020;12(1):157.

Apariman S, Ratchanon S, Wiriyasirivej B. Effectiveness of ginger for prevention of nausea and vomiting after gynecological laparoscopy. J Med Assoc Thai 2006;89(12):2003–9.

Aryaeian N, Shahram F, Mahmoudi M, et al. The effect of ginger supplementation on some immunity and inflammation intermediate genes expression in patients with active rheumatoid arthritis. Gene 2019;698:179–85.

Black CD, Herring MP, Hurley DJ, O'Connor PJ. Ginger (*Zingiber officinale*) reduces muscle pain caused by eccentric exercise. J Pain 2010;11(9):894–903.

Bolognesi G, Belcaro G, Feragalli B, et al. Movardol® (N-acetylglucosamine, *Boswellia serrata*, ginger) supplementation in the management of knee osteoarthritis: preliminary results from a 6-month registry study. Eur Rev Med Pharmacol Sci 2016;20(24):5198–204.

Bordia A, Verma SK, Srivastava KC. Effect of ginger (*Zingiber officinale* Rosc.) and fenugreek (*Trigonella foenumgraecum* L.) on blood lipids, blood sugar and platelet aggregation in patients with coronary artery disease. Prostaglandins Leukot Essent Fatty Acids 1997;56(5):379–84.

Borrelli F, Capasso R, Aviello G, Pittler MH, Izzo AA. Effectiveness and safety of ginger in the treatment of pregnancy-induced nausea and vomiting. Obstet Gynecol 2005;105(4):849–56.

Cappelli V, Morgante G, Di Sabatino A, Massaro MG, De Leo V. Evaluation of the efficacy of a new nutraceutical product in the treatment of postmenopausal symptoms. Minerva Ginecol 2015;67(6):515–21.

Carvalho GCN, Lira-Neto JCG, Araújo MFM, Freitas RWJF, Zanetti ML, Damasceno MMC. Effectiveness of ginger in reducing metabolic levels in people with diabetes: a randomized trial. Rev Lat Am Enfermagem 2020;28:e3369.

Chaiyakunapruk N, Kitikannakorn N, Nathisuwan S, Leeprakobboon K, Leelasettagool C. The efficacy of ginger for the prevention of postoperative nausea and vomiting: a meta-analysis. Am J Obstet Gynecol 2006;194(1):95–9.

Chittumma P, Kaewkiattikun K, Wiriyasiriwach B. Comparison of the effectiveness of ginger and vitamin B6 for treatment of nausea and vomiting in early pregnancy: a randomized double-blind controlled trial. J Med Assoc Thai 2007;90(1):15–20.

Chopra A, Lavin P, Patwardhan B, Chitre D. A 32-week randomized, placebo-controlled clinical evaluation of RA-11, an Ayurvedic drug, on osteoarthritis of the knees. J Clin Rheumatol 2004;10(5):236–45.

Citronberg J, Bostick R, Ahearn T, et al. Effects of ginger supplementation on cell-cycle biomarkers in the normal-appearing colonic mucosa of patients at increased risk for colorectal cancer: results from a pilot, randomized, and controlled trial. Cancer Prev Res 2013;6(4):271–81.

Crichton M, Marshall S, Marx W, McCarthy AL, Isenring E. Efficacy of ginger (*Zingiber officinale*) in ameliorating chemotherapy-induced nausea and vomiting and chemotherapy-related outcomes: a systematic review update and meta-analysis. J Acad Nutr Diet 2019;119(12):2055–68.

Daily JW, Zhang X, da Kim S, Park S. Efficacy of ginger for alleviating the symptoms of primary dysmenorrhea: a systematic review and meta-analysis of randomized clinical trials. Pain Med 2015;16(12):2243–55.

Ensiyeh J, Sakineh MA. Comparing ginger and vitamin B6 for the treatment of nausea and vomiting in pregnancy: a randomised controlled trial. Midwifery 2009;25(6):649–53.

Ernst E, Pittler MH. Efficacy of ginger for nausea and vomiting: a systematic review of randomized clinical trials. Br J Anaesth 2000;84(3):367–71.

Eshaghian R, Mazaheri M, Ghanadian M, Rouholamin S, Feizi A, Babaeian M. The effect of frankincense (*Boswellia serrata*, oleo-resin) and ginger (*Zingiber officinale*, rhizoma) on heavy menstrual bleeding: a randomized, placebo-controlled, clinical trial. Complement Ther Med 2019;42–7.

Gonlachanvit S, Chen YH, Hasler WL, Sun WM, Owyang C. Ginger reduces hyperglycemia-evoked gastric dysrhythmias in healthy humans: possible role of endogenous prostaglandins. J Pharmacol Exp Ther 2003;307(3):1098–103.

Heitmann K, Nordeng H, Holst L. Safety of ginger use in pregnancy: results from a large population-based cohort study. Eur J Clin Pharmacol 2013;69(2):269–77.

Hewitt V, Watts R. The effectiveness of non-invasive complementary therapies in reducing postoperative nausea and vomiting following abdominal laparoscopic surgery in women: a systematic review. JBI Libr Syst Rev 2009;7(19):850–907.

Huang FY, Deng T, Meng LX, Ma XL. Dietary ginger as a traditional therapy for blood sugar control in patients with type 2 diabetes mellitus: a systematic review and meta-analysis. Medicine (Baltimore) 2019;98(13):e15054.

Jalali M, Mahmoodi M, Moosavian SP, et al. The effects of ginger supplementation on markers of inflammatory and oxidative stress: a systematic review and meta-analysis of clinical trials. Phytother Res 2020;34(8):1723–33.

Jiang X, Williams KM, Liauw WS, et al. Effect of ginkgo and ginger on the pharmacokinetics and pharmacodynamics of warfarin in healthy subjects. Br J Clin Pharmacol 2005;59(4):425–32.

Jiang Y, Turgeon DK, Wright BD, et al. Effect of ginger root on cyclooxygenase-1 and 15-hydroxyprostaglandin dehydrongenase expression in colonic mucosa of human at normal and increased risk of colorectal cancer. Eur J Cancer Prev 2013;22(5):455–60.

Lien HC, Sun WM, Chen YH, Kim H, Hasler W, Owyang C. Effects of ginger on motion sickness and gastric slow-wave dysrhythmias induced by circular vection. Am J Physiol Gastrointest Liver Physiol 2003;284(3):G481–9.

Lohsiriwat S, Rukkiat M, Chaikomin R, Leelakusolvong S. Effect of ginger on lower esophageal sphincter pressure. J Med Assoc Thai 2010;93(3):366–72.

Lumb AB. Effect of dried ginger on human platelet function. Thromb Haemost 1994;71(1):110–1.

Maghbooli M, Golipour F, Esfandabadi AM, Youse M. Comparison between the efficacy of ginger and sumatriptan in the ablative treatment of the common migraine. Phytother Res 2014;28(3):412–5.

Mahyari S, Mahyari B, Emami SA, et al. Evaluation of the efficacy of a polyherbal mouthwash containing *Zingiber officinale*, *Rosmarinus officinalis* and *Calendula officinalis* extracts in patients with gingivitis: a randomized double-blind placebo-controlled trial. Complement Ther Clin Pract 2016;22:93–8.

Mares WAA-K, Najam WS. The effect of Ginger on semen parameters and serum FSH, LH & testosterone of infertile men. Tikrit Med J 2012;18(2):322–9.

Martins LB, Rodrigues AMDS, Rodrigues DF, Dos Santos LC, Teixeira AL, Ferreira AVM. Double-blind placebo-controlled randomized clinical trial of ginger (*Zingiber officinale* Rosc.) addition in migraine acute treatment. Cephalalgia 2019;39(1):68–76.

Marx W, McKavanagh D, McCarthy A, et al. The effect of ginger (*Zingiber officinale*) on platelet aggregation: a systematic literature. Review. PLoS One 2015;10(10):e0141119.

Morvaridzadeh M, Fazelian S, Agah S, et al. Effect of ginger (*Zingiber officinale*) on inflammatory markers: a systematic review and meta-analysis of randomized controlled trials. Cytokine 2020;135:155224.

Nanthakomon T, Pongrojpaw D. The efficacy of ginger in prevention of postoperative nausea and vomiting after major gynecologic surgery. J Med Assoc Thai 2006;89(Suppl 4):S130–6.

Nikkhah-Bodaghi M, Maleki I, Agah S, Hekmatdoost A. *Zingiber officinale* and oxidative stress in patients with ulcerative colitis: a randomized, placebo-controlled, clinical trial. Complement Ther Med 2019;43:1–6.

Ozgoli G, Goli M, Moattar F. Comparison of effects of ginger, mefenamic acid, and ibuprofen on pain in women with primary dysmenorrhea. J Altern Complement Med 2009a;15(2):129–32.

Ozgoli G, Goli M, Simbar M. Effects of ginger capsules on pregnancy, nausea, and vomiting. J Altern Complement Med 2009b;15(3):243–6.

Panahi Y, Saadat A, Sahebkar A, Hashemian F, Taghikhani M, Abolhasani E. Effect of ginger on acute and delayed chemotherapy-induced nausea and vomiting: a pilot, randomized, open-label clinical trial. Integr Cancer Ther 2012;11(3):204–11.

Pillai AK, Sharma KK, Gupta YK, Bakhshi S. Anti-emetic effect of ginger powder vs placebo as an add-on therapy in children and young adults receiving high emetogenic chemotherapy. Pediatr Blood Cancer 2011;56(2):234–8.

Pongrojpaw D, Somprasit C, Chanthasenanont A. A randomized comparison of ginger and dimenhydrinate in the treatment of nausea and vomiting in pregnancy. J Med Assoc Thai 2007;90(9):1703–9.

Portnoi G, Chng LA, Karimi-Tabesh L, Koren G, Tan MP, Einarson A. Prospective comparative study of the safety and effectiveness of ginger for the treatment of nausea and vomiting in pregnancy. Am J Obstet Gynecol 2003;189(5):1374–7.

Rondanelli M, Riva A, Morazzoni P, et al. The effect and safety of highly standardized Ginger (*Zingiber officinale*) and Echinacea (*Echinacea angustifolia*) extract supplementation on inflammation and chronic pain in NSAIDs poor responders. A pilot study in subjects with knee arthrosis. Nat Prod Res 2017;31(11):1309–13.

Ryan JL, Heckler CE, Roscoe J, et al. Ginger (*Zingiber officinale*) reduces acute chemotherapy-induced nausea: a URCC CCOP study of 576 patients. Support Care Cancer 2012;20(7):1479–89.

Saneei Totmaj A, Emamat H, Jarrahi F, Zarrati M. The effect of ginger (*Zingiber officinale*) on chemotherapy-induced nausea and vomiting in breast cancer patients: a systematic literature review of randomized controlled trials. Phytother Res 2019;33(8):1957–65.

Verma SK, Bordia A. Ginger, fat and fibrinolysis. Indian J Med Sci 2001;55(2):83–6.

Visalyaputra S, Petchpaisit N, Somcharoen K, Choavaratana R. The efficacy of ginger root in the prevention of postoperative nausea and vomiting after outpatient gynaecological laparoscopy. Anaesthesia 1998;53(5):506–10.

Wigler I, Grotto I, Caspi D, Yaron M. The effects of Zintona EC (a ginger extract) on symptomatic gonarthritis. Osteoarthr Cartil 2003;11(11):783–9.

Willetts KE, Ekangaki A, Eden JA. Effect of a ginger extract on pregnancy-induced nausea: a randomised controlled trial. Aust N Z J Obstet Gynaecol 2003;43(2):139–44.

Wu KL, Rayner CK, Chuah SK, et al. Effects of ginger on gastric emptying and motility in healthy humans. Eur J Gastroenterol Hepatol 2008;20(5):436–40.

Young HY, Liao JC, Chang YS, Luo YL, Lu MC, Peng WH. Synergistic effect of ginger and nifedipine on human platelet aggregation: a study in hypertensive patients and normal volunteers. Am J Chin Med 2006;34(4):545–51.

Zick SM, Turgeon DK, Vareed SK, et al. Phase II study of the effects of ginger root extract on eicosanoids in colon mucosa in people at normal risk for colorectal cancer. Cancer Prev Res 2011;4(11):1929–37.

48 GINKGO (*GINKGO BILOBA*)
Leaf

GENERAL OVERVIEW

With more than 300 clinical trials under its belt today, ginkgo made its debut into mainstream medicine in the late 1990s. Like the pharmaceutical acetylcholinesterase inhibitors that it has been compared with, it has slipped out of the limelight of clinical medicine due to underwhelming benefit for treatment of dementia. For what it's worth, the World Federation of Societies of Biological Psychiatry guidelines list EGb 761 (a standardized extract of ginkgo) as having the same strength of evidence as AChEIs and NMDA antagonists. EGb 761 has Level B evidence for improving cognition, behavior, and activities of daily living in both Alzheimer's disease and vascular dementia. Given these findings and endorsements, it is reasonable to give it a try in appropriate older candidates with memory issues. It has other neuropsychiatric as well as vascular applications that are noteworthy albeit lesser known.

Clinical research indicates that ginkgo, alone or in combination formulas, may be beneficial for macular degeneration, glaucoma, periodontitis, tinnitus, vertigo, hyperlipidemia, dyslipidemia, diabetes, peripheral artery disease, chronic hepatitis, diabetic nephropathy, premenstrual syndrome, premenstrual dysphoric disorder, menopausal sexual dysfunction, acute mountain sickness, migraine headache, mild cognitive impairment, dementia, behavioral and psychological symptoms of dementia, postoperative delirium, anxiety, depression, attention-deficit/hyperactivity disorder, schizophrenia, tardive dyskinesia, and xeroderma.

IN VITRO AND ANIMAL RESEARCH

Ginkgo has been shown to have antioxidant and vasodilating properties via NO. Administration of *Ginkgo biloba* extract to diabetic rats with cataracts was shown to inhibit aldose reductase activity, stimulate GSH production, decrease MDA and advanced glycosylation end product levels, and delay the progression of lens opacification. Ginkgo promotes cerebral blood flow in animal models. It prevents decline in cholinergic receptor density in the rat hippocampus. It also reduces platelet aggregation and adhesion via PAF inhibition, lowers fibrinogen levels, and stabilizes RBC membranes. It lowers plasma viscosity. While ginkgo increases brain glucose and oxygen utilization, it also decreases hyperglycemic endothelial inflammation via inhibition of IL-6.

Some constituents in ginkgo have been shown to inhibit MAO-A and MAO-B. Ginkgo has also been shown to reverse the loss of serotonin receptors that occur with aging. Ginkgo has been shown in various studies in rodents to be neuroprotective, hepatoprotective, and cardioprotective against ischemia and toxic injury. It has also been shown to reduce cataract development in rats exposed to radiation, toxins, or elevated glucose.

Some ginkgo constituents inhibit proliferation and promote apoptosis and differentiation of gastric cancer cells. Additionally, ginkgo inhibits aromatase, which may be beneficial in breast cancer survivors.

HUMAN RESEARCH

Ophthalmological Disorders

A 2013 systematic review of efficacy of ginkgo for age-related macular degeneration identified two published trials ($n = 119$) that met inclusion criteria. Both trials lasted six months and both reported some positive effects of ginkgo on vision. The author concluded that the level of efficacy of ginkgo was insufficient to conclude that the herb prevented progression of age-related macular degeneration (AMD) (Evans, 2013).

A crossover RCT in patients ($n = 27$) with bilateral visual field damage resulting from normal tension glaucoma compared ginkgo with placebo by administering ginkgo 40 mg TID for 4 weeks, followed by a wash-out period of 8 weeks, then 4 weeks of placebo treatment. Other patients underwent the same regimen in reverse order. Following ginkgo treatment, improvement in visual field indices showed a decrease in mean deviation from 11.4 dB at baseline to 8.8 dB ($P = 0.0001$). Corrected pattern standard deviation at baseline vs after ginkgo was 10.9 dB vs 8.1 dB ($P = 0.0001$). No significant changes were found in intraocular pressure (IOP), blood pressure, or heart rate after placebo or ginkgo treatment. The authors concluded that ginkgo appeared to improve preexisting visual field damage in some patients with normal tension glaucoma (Quaranta et al., 2003).

A retrospective analysis of eye health parameters was carried out over 12–59 months by chart review of 332 subjects with normal tension glaucoma (209 men and 123 women) who were treated with anthocyanins ($n = 132$), *Ginkgo biloba* extract ($n = 103$), or no medication ($n = 97$). After a mean of 23 months of anthocyanin treatment, the mean best corrected visual acuity for all eyes improved from 0.16 to 0.11 logMAR units ($P = 0.008$), and visual field mean deviation improved from -6.44 to -5.34 ($P = 0.001$). With ginkgo treatment, visual field mean deviation improved from -5.25 to -4.31 ($P = 0.002$). The authors concluded that anthocyanins and ginkgo may be helpful in improving visual function in some individuals with normal tension glaucoma (Shim et al., 2012).

Oral and Dental Disorders

A 6-month RCT in patients ($n = 30$) with moderate-to-severe periodontitis compared efficacy of ginkgo gel with minocycline gel, each treatment given in addition to usual care. The detection rates of the most common periodontal pathogens decreased comparably in both groups 1 week after treatment. The plaque indexes and bleeding indexes were not significantly different between the experimental group and the control group after treatment ($P > 0.05$). The attachment loss decreased with time for both groups. The authors concluded that the inhibition effects of ginkgo and minocycline hydrochloride were comparable for major periodontal pathogens in the short term (Cheng et al., 2014).

Ear, Nose, and Throat Disorders: Tinnitus and Vertigo

A 2018 meta-analysis was conducted to evaluate the effects of a standardized ginkgo extract (EGb 761) 240 mg/day on tinnitus and dizziness associated with dementia. Five trials met inclusion criteria. Overall, the ginkgo extract was superior to placebo with decrease from baseline for tinnitus (WMD = -1.06; $P = 0.003$) and for dizziness (WMD = -0.77; $P = 0.03$). The authors concluded that there was support for the notion that EGb 761 was effective in alleviating concomitant neurosensory symptoms in patients with dementia (Spiegel et al., 2018).

A 12-week RCT in patients ($n = 197$) with subchronic or chronic tinnitus compared a ginkgo standardized extract (EGb 761) 120 mg BID with pentoxifylline 600 mg BID. For both treatment groups, significant improvements were observed in the Mini-Tinnitus Questionnaire, the 11-Point Box Scales for tinnitus loudness and annoyance, the Hospital Anxiety and Depression Scale anxiety score and the Sheehan Disability Scale. There was no relevant difference regarding tinnitus-related outcomes between the two treatment groups. Adverse events were documented for 20 and 36 events in ginkgo and pentoxifylline groups, respectively, with no serious adverse events. The authors concluded that EGb 761 and pentoxifylline were similarly effective in reducing the loudness and annoyance of tinnitus as well as overall suffering of the patients, and there were fewer adverse events with the ginkgo product (Procházková et al., 2018).

A prospective study in patients whose tinnitus did not improve after 6 weeks of treatment with betahistine 72 mg (36 of 84 patients) investigated the efficacy of ginkgo 120 mg plus hyperbaric oxygen. The tinnitus disappeared in 5%, was alleviated in 36%, and showed overall improvement in 42%. The average intensity of tinnitus before and after treatment was 41 dB and 38 dB, respectively ($P = 0.046$). The authors concluded that both betahistine and ginkgo plus hyperbaric oxygen produced statistically significant improvements, and they recommended hyperbaric oxygen therapy for the general public (Holy et al., 2016).

A 90-day RCT in adults ($n = 33$) with tinnitus compared ginkgo extract (EGb 761), digital hearing aids, and ginkgo plus hearing aids for beneficial effects. The researchers found a significant improvement in self-perception of tinnitus loudness and severity after 90 days of treatment in all three groups. Hearing aids were more effective in patients with a shorter tinnitus onset time and ginkgo was effective regardless of tinnitus duration. The authors concluded that ginkgo and/or hearing aids could improve tinnitus (Radunz et al., 2020).

A 12-week RCT in patients ($n = 160$) with vertigo compared a standardized extract of ginkgo (EGb761) 240 mg/day with betahistine 32 mg/day. Both treatment groups were comparable at baseline and improved in all outcome measures during treatment. There was no significant intergroup difference in changes in an 11-point numeric analogue scale, the Vertigo Symptom Scale-short form, the Clinical Global Impression Scales, and the Sheehan Disability Scale. Numerically, improvements in patients receiving ginkgo were slightly more pronounced on all scales. Clinical global impression was rated "very much improved" or "much improved" in 79% and 70% of patients treated with ginkgo and betahistine, respectively. Ginkgo showed better tolerability than betahistine. The authors concluded that ginkgo and betahistine were similarly effective in the treatment of vertigo, but EGb 761 was better tolerated (Sokolova et al., 2014).

A six-month RCT in patients ($n = 29$) with vestibular neuritis compared methylprednisolone plus ginkgo with ginkgo alone for 2 weeks along with vestibular exercises for both groups. Both groups showed statistically significant improvements in caloric weakness and video head impulse tests at one- and six-month follow-up evaluations compared with the initial examination; however, differences between groups were not significant. The rates of normaliza-

tion of canal paresis at 1 and 6 months were 50% and 64% in the ginkgo-alone group and 33% and 60% in the steroid-plus-ginkgo group, respectively, with no differences between the two groups. The rates of video head impulse test normalization at 1 and 6 months after treatment were 57% and 78% in the ginkgo-alone group and 53% and 87% in the steroid-plus-ginkgo group, respectively, with no differences between the two groups. There were no significant differences in the improvement of composite scores of sensory organization tests or dizziness handicap indexes between the two groups. The authors concluded that methylprednisolone had no additional benefit in patients with vestibular neuritis who underwent vestibular exercises and received ginkgo (Yoo et al., 2017).

Cardiometabolic Disorders: Hyperlipidemia and Dyslipidemia

A 2019 systematic review investigating the effects of a combination of Asian ginseng and ginkgo on physiological and psychological outcomes in humans identified eight studies meeting the criteria. All studies used the combination brand Gincosan. The most consistent results found were benefits to aspects of the circulatory/cardiovascular system in patient populations and "secondary memory" performance in patient and healthy populations. The authors concluded that this combination of ginseng and ginkgo could improve aspects of physiological and cognitive function in humans; however, evidence for synergy required further investigation (Reay et al., 2019).

A 2018 meta-analysis sought to investigate whether adjuvant treatment with ginkgo added to statins had incremental benefits in patients with dyslipidemia. Eight RCTs ($n = 664$) were included. Compared with statin therapy alone, the combination of statins and ginkgo achieved greater reductions in TG (MD $= -28$ mg/dL), TC (MD $= -23$ mg/dL), and LDL-C (MD $= -12$ mg/dL), and a greater increment in HDL-C (MD $= 10$ mg/d/L). Subgroup analyses showed that ginkgo plus simvastatin appeared to achieve a greater reduction in serum levels of TG, TC, and LDL-C than when combined with atorvastatin. The authors concluded that adjuvant treatment with ginkgo appeared to improve blood lipid parameters better than statin therapy alone (Fan et al., 2018).

Cardiometabolic Disorders: Diabetes

A 2020 systematic review and meta-analysis to assess the influence of ginkgo on cardiometabolic parameters in T2DM patients found seven studies ($n = 768$) for inclusion. The meta-analysis found a significant effect of ginkgo on A1C (WMD = 0.26, $P = 0.034$) and serum HDL-C (WMD = 1.99, $P = 0.030$). The authors concluded that ginkgo could significantly modulate A1C and HDL-C levels, but that more research was warranted (Tabrizi et al., 2020).

A 90-day RCT in patients ($n = 60$) with T2DM investigated the effect of augmenting metformin with ginkgo extract 120 mg compared with placebo augmentation. Augmentation with ginkgo significantly decreased A1C (from 8.6% at to 7.7%; $P < 0.001$), fasting serum glucose (from 194 mg/dL to 155 mg/dL; $P < 0.001$), and insulin (from 18.5 μU/mL to 13.4 μU/mL; $P = 0.006$). There were also decreases in BMI from 34 kg/m^2 to 31.6 kg/m^2 ($P < 0.001$), WC from 106 cm to 102.6 cm ($P < 0.001$), and visceral adiposity index from 192 to 159 ($P = 0.007$). Ginkgo extract did not negatively impact the liver, kidney, or hematopoietic functions. The authors concluded that ginkgo as an adjuvant was effective in improving metformin treatment outcomes in T2DM patients (Aziz et al., 2018).

Cardiovascular Disorders: Peripheral Artery Disease

A 2013 systematic review of the research on ginkgo for intermittent claudication identified 14 trials ($n = 739$) that met inclusion criteria. Following treatment with ginkgo the absolute claudication distance increased with an overall effect size of 3.57 kcal ($P = 0.06$), compared with placebo, translating to an increase of 64.5 m on a flat treadmill with an average speed of 3.2 km/h. The authors noted that publication bias leading to missing data or "negative" trials was likely to have inflated the effect size, and they concluded that there was no evidence that ginkgo had a clinically significant benefit for patients with peripheral artery disease (Nicolaï et al., 2013).

Gastrointestinal Disorders: Chronic Hepatitis

A 4-week RCT in patients ($n = 64$) with chronic hepatitis B investigated IV polyunsaturated phosphatidylcholine plus either a standardized extract of ginkgo (EGb 761) or placebo for effects on liver fibrosis and hepatic microcirculation. In the ginkgo group, there was a significant reduction of blood transforming growth factor β1, PAF, and endothelin-1 ($P < 0.05$), whereas this was not observed with placebo. In both groups, there were significant decreases in ALT, TBili, and PT ($P < 0.05$), and significant increases in albumin ($P < 0.05$). Liver biopsies showed that hepatic inflammation and fibrosis were reduced only with ginkgo. Electron microscopy showed red blood cell aggregates and microthrombosis disappeared or decreased in sinusoids, collagen deposits in sinusoidal lumen and the perisinusoidal space decreased, and sinusoidal capillarization improved. The authors concluded that this ginkgo extract could improve sinusoidal microcirculation, alleviate inflammation, and inhibit fibrosis through multiple mechanisms and was effective in the treatment of chronic liver diseases (Zhang et al., 2016).

Nephrological and Urological Disorders: Diabetic Nephropathy

A 2013 systematic review investigated the effectiveness and safety of a ginkgo for patients with early diabetic nephropathy. Sixteen RCTs met inclusion criteria. The review found that ginkgo decreased the urinary albumin excretion rate, FBS, serum creatinine, and BUN. The extract also improved hemorheology. No serious adverse effects were reported. The authors concluded that ginkgo had potential value in treating early diabetic nephropathy, especially with high baseline urinary albumin excretion. Better studies were recommended (Zhang et al., 2008).

Women's Genitourinary Disorders: Premenstrual Syndrome and Premenstrual Dysphoric Disorder

A 2014 systematic review was performed to evaluate the effects of acupuncture and herbal medicine for PMS and PMDD. The search found 8 studies in acupuncture and 11 studies in herbal medicine that met inclusion criteria. Herbal medicine studies on chasteberry, St. John's wort, ginkgo, *Xiao yao san*, and *Elsholtzia splendens* as well as all acupuncture modalities studied gave significantly improved results regarding PMS and PMDD. Acupuncture and herbal medicine treatments showed a 50% or better reduction of symptoms compared with baseline. The authors concluded that limited evidence supported the efficacy of alternative medicinal interventions such as acupuncture and herbal medicine in controlling PMS and PMDD (Jang et al., 2014).

A 2011 systematic review evaluating the effects of herbal medicine for PMS found 17 RCTs that met inclusion criteria and selected ten of them for analysis. Single trials supported the use of either ginkgo or saffron. Four trials (*n* = 500) indicated that chasteberry consistently ameliorated PMS better than placebo. Evening primrose oil and St. John's wort did not differ from placebo. None of the herbs was associated with major health risks, although the reduced number of tested patients did not allow definitive conclusions on safety (Dante and Facchinetti, 2011).

Women's Genitourinary Disorders: Perimenopause and Menopause

A 2017 review of clinical trials on herbal efficacy in menopausal symptoms used search terms menopause, climacteric, hot flushes, flashes, herb, and phytoestrogens. The authors found that ginkgo, passionflower, sage, lemon balm, valerian, black cohosh, fenugreek, black cumin, chasteberry, fennel, evening primrose, alfalfa, St. John's wort, Asian ginseng, anise, licorice, red clover, and wild soybean were effective in the treatment of acute menopausal syndrome with different mechanisms. The authors concluded that medicinal plants could play a role in the treatment of acute menopausal syndrome and that further studies were warranted (Kargozar et al., 2017).

A 2007 systematic review looking at herbs and supplements for menopausal mood disorders found one RCT of ginseng in postmenopausal women reporting improvements in mood and anxiety. Five of seven trials of St. John's wort showed benefit for mild-to-moderate depression. All three RCTs of ginkgo found no effect on depression. Kava significantly reduced anxiety in four of eight RCTs. Black cohosh significantly reduced depression and anxiety in all studies reviewed. The authors concluded that St. John's wort and black cohosh appeared to be the most useful in alleviating mood and anxiety changes during menopause, that ginseng may be effective, but required more research, and that kava held promise for decreasing anxiety in peri- and postmenopausal women. Ginkgo did not appear to be beneficial for menopausal depression (Geller and Studee, 2007).

Women's Genitourinary Disorders: Female Sexual Dysfunction

A 30-day RCT in healthy female volunteers (*n* = 80) with menopausal reduced sexual desire compared ginkgo 120–240 mg/day with placebo with respect to sexual function. Sexual desire as measured on the Sabbatsberg Sexual Rating Scale was significantly improved in the ginkgo group compared with the placebo group (*P* = 0.02). The authors concluded that ginkgo had a positive effect on the sexual desire of menopausal women (Pebdani et al., 2014).

A 12-week RCT in patients (*n* = 24) with sexual impairment due to antidepressants compared ginkgo 240 mg/day with placebo. HAM-A and HAM-D ratings and simple global assessments of alertness and memory were made at 0, 6 and 12 weeks. While there were some spectacular individual responses in both groups, there were no statistically significant differences, and no differences in side-effects (Wheatley, 2004).

A two-month RCT in patients (*n* = 37) with sexual dysfunction while on antidepressants compared ginkgo with placebo. While there was improvement in some aspects of sexual function compared with baseline in both groups, there was no statistically significant difference between ginkgo and placebo at 2, 4, and 8 weeks after medication (Kang et al., 2002).

A two-month exploratory, prospective, noncontrolled, observational study in postmenopausal women (*n* = 29) with sexual dysfunction as defined by a Female Sexual Function Index (FSFI) score < 25.83 assessed the effects of Libicare, a polyherbal product containing ginkgo, fenugreek, tribulus, and *Temera diffusa*, two tablets daily. FSFI mean score showed a significant increase from 20.15 at baseline to 25.03 after treatment (*P* = 0.0011). The FSFI score was increased in 86% of the subjects. All FSFI domains, except dyspareunia, showed significant increases. The highest increase was observed in the desire domain (*P* = 0.0004). A significant increase in testosterone level occurred in roughly half of the subjects, from 0.41 to 0.50 pg/mL. A significant decrease in SHBG level occurred in 95% of subjects from 85 to 73 nmoL/L (*P* = 0.0001). The authors concluded that this polyherbal formula provided a significant improvement in sexual function and related hormone levels (Palacios et al., 2019).

Neurological Disorders: Headache

A 2018 systematic review and meta-analysis evaluating the efficacy of ginkgo for acute mountain sickness selected seven study groups in six published articles ($n = 451$) that met all eligibility criteria. In the primary meta-analysis of all study groups, ginkgo showed a non-significant trend for acute mountain sickness prophylaxis, (RR = 0.68; $P = 0.08$) with substantial heterogeneity. The pooled risk difference showed a significant reduction in acute mountain sickness from 45% to 6% with ginkgo ($P = 0.011$) (Tsai et al., 2018).

An open trial in patients ($n = 25$) who had migraine with aura investigated the possible efficacy of a ginkgo constituent ginkgolide B in the treatment of acute aura. After recording symptoms in the first attack patients were instructed to take abortively two capsules of Migrasoll (a combination of phytosomal ginkgo terpenes 60 mg, coenzyme Q10 11 mg, and riboflavin 8.7 mg) at the onset of the second attack. Aura duration was reduced by Migrasoll intake from 33.6 min in the first (untreated) attack to 21.9 min during the second attack ($P < 0.001$). In general, there was a marked amelioration of the features of the aura in the treated attack. The pain phase disappeared in 18% of patients with the ginkgo product. No serious adverse events were reported (Allais et al., 2013).

Neurological Disorders: Stroke

A 2020 systematic review and meta-analysis to evaluate the effectiveness and safety of long-term use of ginkgo during convalescence from ischemic stroke found 15 RCTs ($n = 1829$) that met inclusion criteria. For acute ischemic stroke, adding ginkgo to conventional therapy led to higher Barthel index scores (MD = 5.72) and lower neurological function deficit scores (MD = -1.39). For convalescing patients, ginkgo was superior for reducing dependence (MD: 7.17) and neurological function deficit scores (MD: -1.15) compared with placebo or conventional therapy. The difference in vascular events (RR = 0.70), recurrence rate (RR: 0.57), and mortality (RR: 1.07) did not reach statistical significance. The authors concluded that ginkgo appeared to improve neurological function and dependence compared with conventional therapy at difference stages following ischemic stroke and appeared generally safe (Ji et al., 2020).

Neurological Disorders: Cognitive Impairment, Dementia, and Alzheimer's Disease

A 2019 meta-analysis investigated the therapeutic benefits and tolerability of a standardized ginkgo extract (EGb 761) 240 mg/day compared with donepezil, galantamine, rivastigmine, and memantine in mild-to-moderate AD patients. Ginkgo and memantine showed no therapeutic benefits in all study outcomes. For cognition, all AChEIs were significantly better than placebo. Galantamine was better than rivastigmine (oral and patch), ginkgo, and memantine. The global impression ratings were more improved with donepezil than with galantamine or with ginkgo (RR = 1.40 for both) (Thancharoen et al., 2019).

A 2017 overview of systematic reviews assessing the efficacy of ginkgo for dementia selected 12 systematic reviews that met eligibility criteria. The authors concluded that, overall, the available evidence suggested that ginkgo had potentially beneficial effects over placebo on cognitive performance, ADLs, and clinical global impression in the treatment of dementia at doses greater than 200 mg/day (usually 240 mg/day) administered for 22 weeks or longer, and that ginkgo appeared to be safe for human consumption (Yuan et al., 2017).

A 2016 overview of systematic reviews assessed the effects of non-pharmacological, pharmacological, and alternative therapies on ADL function in people with dementia. A total of 23 systematic reviews were included in the overview. Interventions that were reported to be effective in minimizing decline in ADL function were: exercise (SMD = 0.68), dyadic interventions for caregivers and care receivers (SMD = 0.37), donepezil 10 mg (SMD = 0.18), selegiline (SMD = 0.27), huperzine A (SMD = 1.48), and ginkgo (SMD = 0.36). Only donepezil was given a moderate grade of evidence. All others were graded as "low" or "very low." (Laver et al., 2016).

A 2016 overview of systematic reviews assessing ginkgo for prevention of cognitive decline and for intervention in mild cognitive impairment and dementia identified 10 systematic reviews that met selection criteria. Medication with ginkgo showed improvement in cognition, neuropsychiatric symptoms, and daily activities, and the effect was dose-dependent with efficacy convincingly demonstrated only when 240 mg/day was applied. Compared with placebo, overall adverse events and serious adverse events were at the same level as placebo, with less adverse events in favor of ginkgo in the subgroup of AD patients, and fewer incidences in vertigo, tinnitus, angina pectoris, and headache. The authors concluded that ginkgo was safe and effective for MCI and dementia, but that the question on efficacy to prevent cognitive decline was still open (Zhang et al., 2013).

A 2015 systematic review to assess new evidence on the clinical and adverse effects of a standardized ginkgo extract (EGb761) for cognitive impairment and dementia selected nine trials ($n = 2561$) that met inclusion criteria. In the meta-analysis, the changed scores for cognition were in favor of ginkgo compared with placebo (WMD $= -2.86$); the change in scores for ADLs were also in favor of ginkgo compared with placebo (SMD $= -0.36$); and Clinicians' Global Impression of Change scale showed a significant difference from placebo (OR: 1.88). In subgroup analysis of patients with neuropsychiatric symptoms, ginkgo improved cognitive function, ADLs, Clinician's Global Impression, and neuropsychiatric symptoms with statistical superiority over the whole group. In subgroup analysis of patients with AD, there was no statistical superiority for the main outcomes. Safety data revealed no important safety concerns. All the benefits identified were associated with EGb761 at a dose of 240 mg/day (Tan et al., 2015).

A 2015 systematic review assessing the efficacy of ginkgo (EGb 761) in dementia with behavioral and psychological symptoms (BPSD) identified four studies ($n = 1628$) that met inclusion criteria. Change from baseline in cognition, BPSD (including caregiver distress rating), ADLs, clinical global impression, and quality of life favored ginkgo ($P < 0.001$ for all comparisons). The authors concluded that the pooled analyses provided evidence of efficacy of EGb 761 at 240 mg/day in the treatment of out-patients suffering from AD or vascular or mixed dementia with BPSD (von Gunten et al., 2016).

A six-year multicenter RCT conducted between 2000 and 2008 in 3069 volunteers aged 75 years with normal cognition ($n = 2587$) or MCI ($n = 482$) compared ginkgo extract 120 mg BID with placebo for effects on cognitive decline. Dementia developed in 277 subjects in the ginkgo arm and 246 subjects

in the placebo arm. Overall dementia rate was 3.3 per 100 person-years with ginkgo and 2.9 per 100 person-years with placebo. The HR for ginkgo compared with placebo for all-cause dementia and for AD was 1.12 ($P = 0.21$) and 1.16 ($P = 0.11$), respectively, and the HR for progression to dementia in subjects with MCI was 1.13 ($P = 0.39$), indicating no effect. The authors concluded that ginkgo 120 mg BID was not effective in reducing overall incidence of dementia or AD in elderly individuals or those with MCI (DeKosky et al., 2008).

A 12-month RCT in patients ($n = 828$) with mild-to-moderate Alzheimer's dementia undergoing treatment with AChEIs investigated the drug combined with ginkgo compared with the drug alone. Significantly different changes in the MMSE scores over the 12-month follow-up were reported between patients on combined therapy compared with those taking only AChEIs. The changes in the ADAS-Cog scores between the two groups did not show statistically significant differences, although similar trends were noticed. The effects were only observed at 12 months and were not apparent at 6 months. There was no difference between groups in the ADL scores. The authors concluded that ginkgo could provide some added cognitive benefits in AD patients already under AChEI treatment (Canevelli et al., 2014).

A perioperative RCT in elderly patients ($n = 57$) with a history of post-operative delirium investigated ginkgo standardized extract (EGb761) 80 mg TID plus oxygen inhalation compared with oxygen inhalation alone. While there was no significant difference between the two groups in postoperative delirium onset time, the duration of postoperative delirium was 16 h and 35 h with and without ginkgo respectively ($P < 0.001$). The authors concluded that ginkgo could shorten the course of post-operative delirium in elderly patients (Xie et al., 2018).

A six-month RCT in patients ($n = 50$) with MCI and associated dual-task-related gait impairment compared ginkgo standardized extract (Symfona forte) 120 mg BID with placebo. After 6 months, dual-task-related cadence increased with ginkgo compared with placebo ($P = 0.019$). In addition, non-significant trends were found after the six-month treatment for dual-task-related gait velocity and stride time variability. The authors concluded that the self-reported unspecified improvements from ginkgo among MCI patients may be correlated with improvements in gait (Gschwind et al., 2017).

An RCT in patients ($n = 60$) with vertebral artery ischemia undergoing total hip replacement compared ginkgo 1 mg/kg with normal saline given after induction anesthesia. Although there were no significant differences in pO2 or a-vO2 difference during surgery between groups, the ginkgo group had higher jugular venous O2 and internal jugular venous oxygen saturation, and a lower rate a-v O2 (cerebral oxygen extraction) difference, and arteriovenous glucose and lactate content differences at the end of surgery and on post-op day 1 than those in the control group ($P < 0.05$). The authors concluded that ginkgo could improve cerebral oxygen supply, decrease cerebral oxygen extraction rate and consumption, and help maintain the balance between cerebral oxygen supply and consumption (Xu et al., 2015).

An acutely dosed RCT in volunteers ($n = 112$) compared ginkgo with rhodiola, with a combination of the two herbs, and with placebo for effects on a psychomotor vigilance task and short-term working memory accuracy. The herbal combination improved the psychomotor vigilance task performance and low-to-moderate working memory accuracy ($P < 0.01$), while there was no improvement with placebo ($P > 0.05$). The combined effect of rhodiola plus ginkgo led to a more significant effect on psychomotor vigilance task performance, all levels of short-term working memory accuracy, and critical fusion versus flicker ($P < 0.01$), with the improvement being greater than either herb used alone (Al-Kuraishy, 2015).

A four-week RCT in patients ($n = 66$) diagnosed with MCI compared a daily dose of Memo (a combination of lyophilized royal jelly 750 mg plus standardized extracts of ginkgo 120 mg and Asian ginseng 150 mg) with placebo for effects on MMSE scores. The mean change in MMSE score in the group treated with the combination product was significantly greater than in the control group (+2.07 vs +0.13, respectively; $P < 0.0001$). The authors concluded that this combination formula could be beneficial in treating age-related cognitive decline as well as in the early phases of pathologic cognitive impairments such as vascular dementia or AD (Yakoot et al., 2013).

Psychiatric Disorders: Anxiety and Depression

A 2013 systematic review looking at plants that had both pre-clinical and clinical evidence for anti-anxiety effects found 21 plants with human clinical trial evidence. Support for efficacy identified several herbs with efficacy for anxiety spectrum disorders including ginkgo, kava, lemon balm, chamomile, skullcap, milk thistle, passionflower, ashwagandha, rhodiola, echinacea, *Galphimia glauca*, *Centella asiatica*, and *Echium amooenum*. Acute anxiolytic activity was found for passionflower, sage, gotu kola, lemon balm, and bergamot. The review also specifically found that bacopa showed anxiolytic effects in people with cognitive decline (Sarris et al., 2013).

A 2010 review to evaluate effectiveness of herbal medicines for GAD found that kava had an unequivocal anxiolytic effect. Isolated studies with valerian, ginkgo, chamomile, passionflower, and *Galphimia glauca* showed a potential use for anxious diseases. Ginkgo and chamomile showed an effect size (Cohen's $d = 0.47–0.87$) similar to or greater than standard anxiolytics drugs (benzodiazepines, buspirone and antidepressants, $d = 0.17–0.38$) (Faustino et al., 2010).

A 12-week RCT in elderly patients ($n = 136$) with depression studied a standardized extract of ginkgo (EGb 761) plus citalopram compared with citalopram alone. The time of onset of efficacy was significantly shorter in the ginkgo augmentation group compared with citalopram alone (6.2 vs 14 days; $P < 0.05$). There were significant differences in HAM-D and HAM-A scores between groups ($P < 0.05$ for both). The ginkgo group showed an increase in correct numbers and classifications and a decrease in numbers of persistent errors on cognitive testing. S100B (a protein marker of brain injury; elevated levels indicate depression) was decreased in both groups with the change being greater in the ginkgo group. The authors concluded that EGb 761 was an adjunctive treatment that could effectively improve depressive symptoms and reduce expression of serum S100B (Dai et al., 2018).

Psychiatric Disorders: Attention-Deficit/Hyperactivity Disorder

A 2017 systematic review looking at natural products for ADHD in children selected nine RCTs ($n = 464$) that met inclusion criteria. Low evidence could be found for lemon balm, valerian, and passionflower. Limited evidence could be found for pine bark extract and ginkgo. The other herbal preparations showed no efficacy in the treatment of ADHD symptoms (Anheyer et al., 2017).

A six-week RCT in children and adolescents with ADHD investigated methylphenidate (20–30 mg/day) plus ginkgo (80–120 mg/day) compared with methylphenidate plus placebo. Greater reductions were observed with ginkgo for the ADHD-RS-IV parent rating inattention score (-7.7 vs -5.3; $P<0.001$) and total score (-13.1 vs -10.2; $P=0.001$) as well as teacher rating inattention score (-7.3 vs -6.0; $P=0.004$). Parent-rated response rate (defined as >27% improvement from baseline in ADHD-RS-IV) was higher with ginkgo compared with placebo (93% vs 58%; $P=0.002$). The authors concluded that ginkgo was an effective complementary treatment for ADHD (Shakibaei et al., 2015).

A 3–5-week open label clinical pilot study in children ($n=20$) with ADHD investigated the response to standardized ginkgo extract (EGb 761) up to 240 mg/ day. Following ginkgo administration, possible improvements in QOL, ADHD core symptoms and continuous performance tests were detected. Symptom improvement correlated with the brain electrical activity test amplitudes. The authors concluded that this study provided preliminary evidence to suggest that EGb 761 at a maximal dosage of 240 mg/day might be a clinically useful alternative treatment for children with ADHD (Uebel-von Sandersleben et al., 2014).

A four-week open-label study in children ($n=36$) diagnosed with ADHD assessed the effects of adding a combination product containing American ginseng 200 mg and ginkgo 50 mg BID in addition to their usual medication. After 2 weeks of treatment, the proportion of the subjects exhibiting improvement ranged from 31% for the anxious-shy attribute to 67% for the psychosomatic attribute. After 4 weeks of treatment, the proportion of subjects exhibiting improvement ranged from 44% for the social problems attribute to 74% for the Conners' ADHD index and the *DSM-IV* hyperactive-impulsive attribute. The authors concluded that the combination of American ginseng plus ginkgo may improve symptoms of ADHD and that further research was warranted (Lyon et al., 2001).

Psychiatric Disorders: Schizophrenia

A 2016 meta-analysis of studies of ginkgo for tardive dyskinesia identified three RCTs ($n=299$) of antipsychotics plus ginkgo compared with antipsychotics plus placebo or antipsychotic therapy alone. Ginkgo 240 mg/day outperformed the control groups in reducing the severity of TD and clinical symptoms as measured by the Abnormal Involuntary Movement Scale (WMD $=-2.30$; $P<0.00001$) and the adverse drug reactions as assessed by the Treatment Emergent Symptom Scale ($n=142$, WMD $=-2.38$; $P=0.004$). The authors concluded that adjunctive ginkgo appeared to be an effective and safe option for improving TD in the treatment of schizophrenia patients (Zhang et al., 2016).

A 2015 systematic review assessing the efficacy and safety of ginkgo extract as an adjuvant therapy to antipsychotics in chronic schizophrenia treatment identified eight RCTs ($n=1033$) for analysis. The result showed that ginkgo had a significant difference in ameliorating total and negative symptoms of chronic schizophrenia as an adjuvant therapy to antipsychotics (Chen et al., 2015).

Dermatological Disorders: Xeroderma

A 28-day clinical trial compared a ginkgo topical formula with a mixture of tea and rooibos for effects on skin. The ginkgo preparation increased skin moisturization by 28% and smoothness by 4% and reduced roughness by 0.4% and wrinkles by 4.6%. The tea and rooibos formula reduced wrinkles by 10% but was inferior to ginkgo for skin moisturization ($P=0.05$) (Chuarienthong et al., 2010).

ACTIVE CONSTITUENTS

- Carbohydrates
  - Polysaccharides (affect the expression of c-myc, bcl-2, and c-fos genes, which can inhibit proliferation and induce apoptosis and differentiation of human gastric tumor cells)
  - Organic acids: hydroxykinurenic acid, kynurenic acid, protocatechic, acid vanillic acid, shikimic acid, ginkgols (antineoplastic), D-glucaric acid and ginkgolic acid (toxic—should be limited to 5 ppm)

- Phenolic compounds
  - Alkylphenols
  - Flavonoids: quercetin (anti-inflammatory, antioxidant, hypotensive, antidiabetic, antispasmodic, neuroprotective, XO inhibition, antibacterial, anti-cancer), kaempferol (anti-inflammatory, antidepressant, strengthens capillaries), isorhamnetin
    - Flavone glycosides (increase tissue oxygen and glucose utilization, antioxidant)
    - Proanthocyanidins
- Terpenes
  - Diterpene lactones: ginkgolides A, B, C, and others (anti-inflammatory bronchodilation, neuroprotective, endothelial relaxation, decrease cortisol response to ACTH) (ginkgolide B is potent PAF antagonist), bilobalide (chemopreventive, suppresses hypoxia-induced membrane breakdown in brain)

GINKGO COMMMONLY USED PREPARATIONS AND DOSAGE (FOR ADULTS UNLESS OTHERWISE SPECIFIED)

The following are examples of some available formulations and ranges of dosing for commercial herbal products. See Part III Introduction "How to prescribe medicinal herbs" for further guidance on herbal advising and prescribing.

Leaf

- Infusion (5-min) of dried leaf: 1 Tbsp per cup TID
- Tincture (1:5, 25%): 2–4 mL TID
- Powdered leaf extract: 175 mg (1/16 tsp) BID-TID
- Capsule or tablet of concentrated powdered leaf (10:1): 50–60 mg BID
- Capsule or tablet of standardized extract (*see note below*): 40–160 mg QD-BID; max 240 mg per day
- *May take 6 weeks to see effects; even up to 1 year in some studies. Some recommend a 6-week pause every 6 months.*
- *Best to use standardized extract to minimize the content of toxic ginkgolic acid. The most studied standardized extracts are EGb-761 (24% ginkgo flavone glycosides, 6% terpenoids), and LI 1370 (25% ginkgo flavone glycosides, 6% terpenoids).*

SAFETY AND PRECAUTION

Side Effects

Occasional nausea, vomiting, increased salivation, loss of appetite, headaches, dizziness, tinnitus, peripheral visual shimmering, hypersensitivity reactions have been reported. Side effects are rare with the standardized extract.

Case Reports

Reports of subdural hematomas and hyphema have been reported in association with ginkgo intake.

Toxicity

High doses (20 mg/kg) of five different bioflavonoids (amentoflavone, sciadopitysin, ginkgetin, isoginkgetin, and bilobetin) in ginkgo were noted to have hepatotoxic and nephrotoxic effects in rats. A 6-month human trial using 120 mg BID of a standardized extract in 47 elderly subjects did not reveal any adverse effects or hepatotoxicity.

Pregnancy and Lactation

Insufficient human safety data.

Disease Interactions

- Caution in patients with coagulation disorders, G6PD deficiency.
- Avoid in peri-operative period due to risk of bleeding.

Drug Interactions

- CYP: Inhibits CYP2B6 and CYP3A4 (but data are conflicting).
- Pgp: May interfere with drugs that are transported by P-glycoprotein.
- UGT: Can increase side effects of drugs metabolized by UGT enzymes.
- MATE1 substrates: Isorhamnetin, a compound present in ginkgo was shown to be a strong inhibitor of the human multidrug and toxic compounds extrusion transporter 1 (hMATE1), responsible for the excretion of various drugs in the kidney and liver.

- Although in vivo studies have failed to demonstrate increased bleeding with ginkgo, avoid with anticoagulants, ASA, NSAIDs. Caution with SSRIs and SNRIs.
- Avoid with MAO inhibitors.
- Avoid with older anti-psychotics or prochlorperazine as may further lower seizure threshold. May augment effects of hypoglycemic agents.
- May inhibit effects of efavirenz.
- May inhibit metabolism of amlodipine.

A 2005 systematic review to look at the risk of bleeding with ginkgo identified 12 case reports of bleeding in patients that were taking ginkgo, with the bleeding being attributed to ginkgo due to the known anti-platelet activities of the herb. However, the reviewers concluded that the suggestion of causality was far from compelling, as causality was rated no higher than "possible," and a search of five large databases identified relatively few case reports of bleeding associated with ginkgo use despite the widespread use of ginkgo worldwide. The authors also noted that the results of several controlled studies did not support the link between bleeding and ginkgo use. The authors recommended that more systematic research was warranted (Ernst et al., 2005).

An open label, three-way crossover randomized study in healthy male subjects ($n = 12$), investigated the effects of ginkgo and ginger on warfarin. The subjects received a single 25 mg dose of warfarin either alone or after 7 days pretreatment plus 7 days posttreatment with recommended doses of ginkgo or ginger. INR and platelet aggregation were not affected by administration of ginkgo or ginger alone. Ginkgo and ginger at the recommended doses did not significantly affect clotting status or the pharmacokinetics or pharmacodynamics of warfarin (Jiang et al., 2005).

REFERENCES

Al-Kuraishy HM. Central additive effect of *Ginkgo biloba* and *Rhodiola rosea* on psychomotor vigilance task and short-term working memory accuracy. J Intercult Ethnopharmacol 2015;5(1):7–13.

Allais G, D'Andrea G, Maggio M, Benedetto C. The efficacy of ginkgolide B in the acute treatment of migraine aura: an open preliminary trial. Neurol Sci 2013;34(Suppl 1):S161–3.

Anheyer D, Lauche R, Schumann D, Dobos G, Cramer H. Herbal medicines in children with attention deficit hyperactivity disorder (ADHD): a systematic review. Complement Ther Med 2017;30:14–23.

Aziz TA, Hussain SA, Mahwi TO, Ahmed ZA, Rahman HS, Rasedee A. The efficacy and safety of *Ginkgo biloba* extract as an adjuvant in type 2 diabetes mellitus patients ineffectively managed with metformin: a double-blind, randomized, placebo-controlled trial. Drug Des Devel Ther 2018;12:735–42.

Canevelli M, Adali N, Kelaiditi E, et al. Effects of Gingko biloba supplementation in Alzheimer's disease patients receiving cholinesterase inhibitors: data from the ICTUS study. Phytomedicine 2014;21(6):888–92.

Chen X, Hong Y, Zheng P. Efficacy and safety of extract of *Ginkgo biloba* as an adjunct therapy in chronic schizophrenia: a systematic review of randomized, double-blind, placebo-controlled studies with meta-analysis. Psychiatry Res 2015;228(1):121–7.

Cheng Q, Gao W, Cao B, Liu Y, Zeng Z, Wang Z. Comparison of the effects of *Ginkgo biloba* extract and minocycline hydrochlovide on periodontitis. Zhonghua Kou Qiang Yi Xue Za Zhi 2014;49(6):347–51.

Chuarienthong P, Lourith N, Leelapornpisid P. Clinical efficacy comparison of anti-wrinkle cosmetics containing herbal flavonoids. Int J Sci 2010;32(2):99–106.

Dai CX, Hu CC, Shang YS, Xie J. Role of *Ginkgo biloba* extract as an adjunctive treatment of elderly patients with depression and on the expression of serum S100B. Medicine (Baltimore) 2018;97(39):e12421.

Dante G, Facchinetti F. Herbal treatments for alleviating premenstrual symptoms: a systematic review. J Psychosom Obstet Gynaecol 2011;32(1):42–51.

DeKosky ST, Williamson JD, Fitzpatrick AL, et al. Ginkgo evaluation of memory study investigators. *Ginkgo biloba* for prevention of dementia: a randomized controlled trial. JAMA 2008;300(19):2253–62.

Ernst E, Canter PH, Coon JT. Does *Ginkgo biloba* increase the risk of bleeding? A systematic review of case reports. Perfusion 2005;18:52–6.

Evans JR. Ginkgo biloba extract for age-related macular degeneration. Cochrane Database Syst Rev 2013;1, CD001775.

Fan Y, Jin X, Man C, Gong D. Does adjuvant treatment with ginkgo biloba to statins have additional benefits in patients with dyslipidemia? Front Pharmacol 2018;9:659.

Faustino TT, Almeida RB, Andreatini R. Medicinal plants for the treatment of generalized anxiety disorder: a review of controlled clinical studies. Braz J Psychiatry 2010;32(4):429–36.

Geller SE, Studee L. Botanical and dietary supplements for mood and anxiety in menopausal women. Menopause 2007;14(3 Pt 1):541–9.

Gschwind YJ, Bridenbaugh SA, Reinhard S, Granacher U, Monsch AU, Kressig RW. Ginkgo biloba special extract LI 1370 improves dual-task walking in patients with MCI: a randomised, double-blind, placebo-controlled exploratory study. Aging Clin Exp Res 2017;29(4):609–19.

Holy R, Prazenica P, Stolarikova E, et al. Hyperbaric oxygen therapy in tinnitus with normal hearing in association with combined treatment. Undersea Hyperb Med 2016;43(3):201–5.

Jang SH, Kim DI, Choi MS. Effects and treatment methods of acupuncture and herbal medicine for premenstrual syndrome/premenstrual dysphoric disorder: systematic review. BMC Complement Altern Med 2014;14:11.

Ji H, Zhou X, Wei W, Wu W, Yao S. *Ginkgo biloba* extract as an adjunctive treatment for ischemic stroke: a systematic review and meta-analysis of randomized clinical trials. Medicine (Baltimore) 2020;99(2):e18568.

Jiang X, Williams KM, Liauw WS, et al. Effect of ginkgo and ginger on the pharmacokinetics and pharmacodynamics of warfarin in healthy subjects. Br J Clin Pharmacol 2005;59(4):425–32.

Kang BJ, Lee SJ, Kim MD, Cho MJ. A placebo-controlled, double-blind trial of Ginkgo biloba for antidepressant-induced sexual dysfunction. Hum Psychopharmacol 2002;17(6):279–84.

Kargozar R, Azizi H, Salari R. A review of effective herbal medicines in controlling menopausal symptoms. Electron Physician 2017;9(11):5826–33.

Laver K, Dyer S, Whitehead C, Clemson L, Crotty M. Interventions to delay functional decline in people with dementia: a systematic review of systematic reviews. BMJ Open 2016;6(4):e010767.

Lyon MR, Cline JC, Totosy de Zepetnek J, Shan JJ, Pang P, Benishin C. Effect of the herbal extract combination *Panax quinquefolium* and *Ginkgo biloba* on attention-deficit hyperactivity disorder: a pilot study. J Psychiatry Neurosci 2001;26(3):221–8.

Nicolaï SP, Kruidenier LM, Bendermacher BL, et al. Ginkgo biloba for intermittent claudication. Cochrane Database Syst Rev 2013;6, CD006888.

Palacios S, Soler E, Ramírez M, Lilue M, Khorsandi D, Losa F. Effect of a multi-ingredient-based food supplement on sexual function in women with low sexual desire. BMC Womens Health 2019;19(1):58.

Pebdani MA, Taavoni S, Seyedfatemi N, Haghani H. Triple-blind, placebo-controlled trial of *Ginkgo biloba* extract on sexual desire in postmenopausal women in Tehran. Iran J Nurs Midwifery Res 2014;19(3):262–5.

Procházková K, Šejna I, Skutil J, Hahn A. *Ginkgo biloba* extract EGb 761 vs pentoxifylline in chronic tinnitus: a randomized, double-blind clinical trial. Int J Clin Pharmacol 2018;40(5):1335–41.

Quaranta L, Bettelli S, Uva MG, Semeraro F, Turano R, Gandolfo E. Effect of *Ginkgo biloba* extract on preexisting visual field damage in normal tension glaucoma. Ophthalmology 2003;110:359–62.

Radunz CL, Okuyama CE, Branco-Barreiro FCA, Pereira RMS, Diniz SN. Clinical randomized trial study of hearing aids effectiveness in association with *Ginkgo biloba* extract (EGb 761) on tinnitus improvement. Braz J Otorhinolaryngol 2020;86(6):734–42.

Reay JL, van Schaik P, Wilson CJ. A systematic review of research investigating the physiological and psychological effects of combining *Ginkgo biloba* and *Panax ginseng* into a single treatment in humans: implications for research design and analysis. Brain Behav 2019;9(3):e01217.

Sarris J, McIntyre E, Camfield DA. Plant-based medicines for anxiety disorders, part 2: a review of clinical studies with supporting preclinical evidence. CNS Drugs 2013;27(4):301–19.

Shakibaei F, Radmanesh M, Salari E, Mahaki B. *Ginkgo biloba* in the treatment of attention-deficit/hyperactivity disorder in children and adolescents. A randomized, placebo-controlled, trial. Complement Ther Clin Pract 2015;21(2):61–7.

Shim SH, Kim JM, Choi CY, Kim CY, Park KH. Ginkgo biloba extract and bilberry anthocyanins improve visual function in patients with normal tension glaucoma. J Med Food 2012;15(9):818–23.

Sokolova L, Hoerr R, Mishchenko T. Treatment of vertigo: a randomized, double-blind trial comparing efficacy and safety of *Ginkgo biloba* extract EGb 761 and Betahistine. Int J Otolaryngol 2014;2014:682439.

Spiegel R, Kalla R, Mantokoudis G, et al. *Ginkgo biloba* extract EGb 761 alleviates neurosensory symptoms in patients with dementia: a meta-analysis of treatment effects on tinnitus and dizziness in randomized, placebo-controlled trials. Clin Interv Aging 2018;13:1121–7.

Tabrizi R, Nowrouzi-Sohrabi P, Hessami K, et al. Effects of *Ginkgo biloba* intake on cardiometabolic parameters in patients with type 2 diabetes mellitus: a systematic review and meta-analysis of clinical trials. Phytother Res 2020;35:246–55.

Tan MS, Yu JT, Tan CC, et al. Efficacy and adverse effects of ginkgo biloba for cognitive impairment and dementia: a systematic review and meta-analysis. J Alzheimers Dis 2015;43(2):589–603.

Thancharoen O, Limwattananon C, Waleekhachonloet O, Rattanachotphanit T, Limwattananon P, Limpawattana P. Ginkgo biloba extract (EGb761), cholinesterase inhibitors, and memantine for the treatment of mild-to-moderate Alzheimer's disease: a network meta-analysis. Drugs Aging 2019;36(5):435–52.

Tsai TY, Wang SH, Lee YK, Su YC. *Ginkgo biloba* extract for prevention of acute mountain sickness: a systematic review and meta-analysis of randomised controlled trials. BMJ Open 2018;8(8):e022005.

Uebel-von Sanderslebe H, Rothenberger A, Albrecht B, Rothenberger LG, Klement S, Bock N. Ginkgo biloba extract EGb 761® in children with ADHD. Z Kinder Jugendpsychiatr Psychother 2014;42(5):337–47.

von Gunten A, Schlaefke S, Überla K. Efficacy of *Ginkgo biloba* extract EGb 761 in dementia with behavioural and psychological symptoms: a systematic review. World J Biol Psychiatry 2016;17(8):622–33.

Wheatley D. Triple-blind, placebo-controlled trial of *Ginkgo biloba* in sexual dysfunction due to antidepressant drugs. Hum Psychopharmacol 2004;19(8):545–8.

Xie KJ, Zhang W, Yuan JB, Zhou J, Lian YY, Fang J. Therapeutic effect of *Ginkgo biloba* extract on postoperative delirium in aged patients. Zhonghua Yi Xue Za Zhi 2018;98(18):1430–3.

Xu L, Hu Z, Shen J, McQuillan PM. Effects of *Ginkgo biloba* extract on cerebral oxygen and glucose metabolism in elderly patients with pre-existing cerebral ischemia. Complement Ther Med 2015;23(2):220–5.

Yakoot M, Salem A, Helmy S. Effect of Memo®, a natural formula combination, on mini-mental state examination scores in patients with mild cognitive impairment. Clin Interv Aging 2013;8:975–81.

Yoo MH, Yang CJ, Kim SA, et al. Efficacy of steroid therapy based on symptomatic and functional improvement in patients with vestibular neuritis: a prospective randomized controlled trial. Eur Arch Otorhinolaryngol 2017;274(6):2443–51.

Yuan Q, Wang CW, Shi J, Lin ZX. Effects of *Ginkgo biloba* on dementia: an overview of systematic reviews. J Ethnopharmacol 2017;195:1–9.

Zhang CF, Zhang CQ, Zhu YH, Wang J, Xu HW, Ren WH. *Ginkgo biloba* extract EGb 761 alleviates hepatic fibrosis and sinusoidal microcirculation disturbance in patients with chronic hepatitis B. Gastroenterology Res 2008;1(1):20–8.

Zhang L, Mao W, Guo X, et al. *Ginkgo biloba* extract for patients with early diabetic nephropathy: a systematic review. Evid Based Complement Alternat Med 2013;2013, 689142.

Zhang HF, Huang LB, Zhong YB, et al. An overview of systematic reviews of *Ginkgo biloba* extracts for mild cognitive impairment and dementia. Front Aging Neurosci 2016;8:276.

49

GINSENGS: ASIAN/KOREAN/ CHINESE (*PANAX GINSENG*) AND AMERICAN *(PANAX QUINQUEFOLIUS)*
Root

GENERAL OVERVIEW

Known as adaptogens, the ginsengs are useful for patients who are "failing to thrive" and for those who want to improve their resilience. Several plants with adaptogenic properties have been casually or formally referred to as gingsengs, including eleuthero ("Siberian ginseng"), gynostemma ("southern ginseng"), and rhodiola (Nordic ginseng), but this chapter is focused on the two true ginsengs: American and Asian. They are being presented together for ease of reference and for proximal comparisons, perhaps to the dismay of anyone intimately familiar with these two adaptogens. Asian ginseng is also known as Korean ginseng (including Korean red ginseng or KRG). Asian and American ginseng do have differences that will hopefully be elucidated. Based on available clinical evidence, Asian ginseng would be the preferred ginseng for congestive heart failure, menopause, or erectile dysfunction while American ginseng would be preferred for diabetes, cognitive enhancement, and prevention or treatment of upper respiratory infections.

Usually when people say "ginseng" they are referring to *Panax ginseng* (Asian/Korean/Chinese ginseng), as this plant has been subjected to much more research than American ginseng. *Panax* is derived from the Latin root panacea, so you get the picture. It is reasonable to assume roughly similar actions for American ginseng, but the following information will provide notes on the differences in constituents and activity. For both plants, the active constituents come from the roots. However, the leaves of ginseng have also been shown to have some beneficial properties

such as immune enhancement. The ginsengs are best avoided in more "activated" patients or those with hypertension, although some studies have shown a reduction in BP from ginseng. Asian ginseng is thought to be particularly more activating than the American form.

Another nuance to point out about ginseng is that there are two distinct forms of *Panax ginseng*: red and white ginseng. The difference is the method of processing that results in different pigment compositions. White ginseng is produced by harvesting the root and drying it in the sun, while KRG is steamed after harvest and then dried. The content of ginsenoside compounds differs slightly between the red and white forms. Growing time also impacts ginsenoside content, with roots from plants older than five years being more potent and quite a bit more expensive than roots from one- or two-year-old plants.

Clinical research indicates that Asian ginseng, alone or in combination formulas, may be beneficial for dry eyes, hearing loss prophylaxis, hypertension, coronary artery disease, congestive heart failure, endothelial dysfunction, diabetes, obesity, menopause, erectile dysfunction, male infertility, cognitive impairment, dementia, Alzheimer's disease, cognitive performance, stress resilience, photoaging, alopecia areata, fatigue, hangover, stamina, athletic performance, vaccine response, immune function, HIV, cancer prophylaxis, cancer survival, and cancer quality of life.

Clinical research indicates that American ginseng, alone or in combination formulas, may be beneficial for hypertension, diabetes, menopause, cognitive performance, attention-deficit/hyperactivity disorder, schizophrenia, upper respiratory infection prophylaxis, and cancer-related fatigue.

IN VITRO AND ANIMAL RESEARCH

In vitro experiments reveal enhanced NK cell activity and increased immune cell phagocytosis after ginsenoside exposure. Ginseng has demonstrated anti-inflammatory effects through several mechanisms including inhibition of COX-2, iNOS, and NF-κB. Ginseng may improve nitric oxide synthesis in endothelium of the heart, lung, kidneys, and corpus cavernosum. Ginseng has been shown to have both angiogenesis-promoting and angiogenesis-inhibiting properties. This appears to be due to varying amounts of its constituents Rg1 (promotes angiogenesis) and Rb1 (inhibits angiogenesis). Asian and American ginseng appear to contain predominantly Rb1, which may therefore have a role in cancer prevention and management. Rb1 also improves the release of acetylcholine and enhances post-synaptic uptake of choline.

American ginseng and Korean red ginseng have been shown to stimulate insulin secretion in isolated rat pancreatic cells. Various other constituents of ginseng have been shown to have glucose-lowering capabilities through several mechanisms including calcium channels, beta-adrenoreceptors, intestinal absorption, glucose uptake, and hepatic mechanisms. Several different ginsenosides have been shown to activate AMPK pathways.

Ginseng saponins are thought to decrease serum prolactin, thereby increasing libido in cases of male impotence. Endurance studies in rodents have indicated that ginseng may lead to an increase in survival under physical and chemical stress and an alteration of the mechanism of fuel homeostasis during prolonged exercise. In tests of in vivo efficacy, ginseng was compared with ashwagandha in mice. For swimming endurance, swimming time on average was 163 min with placebo, 536 min with ginseng, and 474 min with ashwagandha. In the anabolic portion of the study, both treated groups gained more BW than placebo, more so with ashwagandha.

Another ginsenoside, Rh2, increases insulin levels and decreases plasma glucose levels in rats via muscarinic stimulation. Rg3 blocks the nuclear translocation of the protein ß-catenin in colon cancer cells thus reducing cancer potential. Differentiation of HL-60 (promyelocytic cells) was induced by ginsenosides Rh2 and Rh3. Rp1 reduces breast cancer cell proliferation by decreasing the stability of the IGF-1R protein in breast cancer cells.

HUMAN RESEARCH: ASIAN GINSENG

There are ample clinical trials on Asian ginseng currently. From 2002 to 2017, 134 ginseng clinical studies were registered, with many still ongoing. The Asian ginseng studies tend to be of higher quality than the rest of the herbal field. In fact, there is a journal specifically for reporting research on Asian ginseng. Roughly 95% of the trials employed randomized allocation to study arms, 80% were double-blind studies using placebo as one of the control groups, and 70% were published as completed trials. Most studies had small sample size (n < 100) and were not privately funded. Unfortunately, there is still a lot of heterogeneity with respect to ginseng species and variety, indications, dose, duration, and participant characteristics.

Ophthalmological Disorders

An 8-week RCT in patients ($n=49$) with glaucoma compared KRG (3 g/day) with placebo for effects on dry eyes secondary to glaucoma medication. After the 8-week intervention, ginseng supplementation significantly improved tear film stability and total Ocular Surface Disease Index score, compared with placebo ($P < 0.01$). The authors concluded that KRG supplementation may provide an additional treatment option for dry eyes in patients with glaucoma using antiglaucoma eye drops (Bae et al., 2015).

Ear, Nose, and Throat Disorders: Hearing Loss Prophylaxis

A 2018 meta-analysis investigated antioxidant supplementation on the auditory thresholds in patients of different age groups with sensorineural hearing loss. Ten publications were selected for further evaluation. When compared with *N*-acetylcysteine and ginseng groups, the increase in threshold at the 4 kHz frequency was significantly higher in the control group (1.9; $P < 0.0001$). At 6 kHz, the threshold increase was non-significantly higher in the control group (1.42; $P=0.28$). The authors concluded that ginseng was the antioxidant agent that showed the best effect in preventing auditory threshold worsening at the frequency of 4 kHz, but not 6 kHz, in patients with sensorineural hearing loss caused by exposure to high sound pressure levels (Souza et al., 2018).

Cardiovascular Disorders: Hypertension

A 2016 systematic review of ginseng for BP effects included nine RCTs for analysis. Two studies reported positive effects of KRG on acute reduction of both SBP and DBP (-6.5 and -5.2; $P=0.0002$ and $P=0.0001$, respectively). Two other trials failed to do so with American ginseng. Two studies showed positive long-term effects of KRG on reducing SBP and DBP compared with placebo (-2.92 and -3.19; $P=0.04$ and $P=0.008$, respectively) (Lee et al., 2017).

A 28-day RCT in healthy adults ($n=30$) compared Asian ginseng extract 200 mg/day with placebo for effects on BP and 12-lead ECGs at 50 min, 2 h, and 5 h following ingestion. Compared with placebo, ginseng increased the QTc interval by 0.015 s at 2 h on day 1 ($P=0.03$) and reduced DBP from 75 mmHg at baseline to 70 mmHg at the same time point ($P=0.02$). The observed effects were not believed to be clinically significant. No other statistically significant changes were found in electrocardiographic or hemodynamic variables on days 1 or 28. The authors concluded that Asian ginseng 200 mg/day increased the QTc interval and decreased DBP 2 h after ingestion in healthy adults on the first day of therapy (Caron et al., 2002).

A 12-week RCT in patients ($n=80$) with T2DM evaluated the hypotensive effects of a combination of ginsenoside Rg3-enriched KRG and American ginseng 2.25 g TID compared with placebo. A reduction in central systolic BP relative to placebo (-4.69 mmHg, $P=0.04$) was observed. This was characterized by a decrease in end-systolic pressure (-6.60 mmHg, $P=0.01$) and the AUC for systolic and diastolic BP (-132.80, $P=0.04$; -220.90, $P=0.02$, respectively). There was no significant change in reactive hyperemia index, pulse-wave velocity, or other related pulse wave components. The authors concluded that the combination of KRG and American ginseng may have utility for modest BP benefit in addition to its other benefits in T2DM (Jovanovski et al., 2020).

A single-dose RCT with crossover in young healthy volunteers compared consumption of 32 oz of an energy drink, a control drink with 800 mg of Panax ginseng, or matching placebo-control drink over 45 min with respect to cardiovascular safety. The energy drink produced a significant increase in QTc interval and SBP 2 h post energy drink consumption compared with placebo (3.4 ms vs -3.2 ms and 2 mmHg vs -2.7 mmHg; ($P=0.014$; $P=0.030$ respectively). The ginseng-control drink did not have a significant impact on ECG or BP parameters. The authors concluded that certain energy drinks consumed at a high volume significantly increase the QTc interval and SBP by >6 ms and 4 mmHg, respectively, but that *Panax ginseng* alone did not have a significant impact on ECG or BP parameters (Shah et al., 2016).

An RCT with crossover design in healthy subjects ($n=23$) compared vascular effects of 400 mg of Rg3 ginsenoside-enriched KRG with 400 mg of wheat bran as control on two separate visits separated by a seven-day washout period. At 3 h after the intervention, the ginseng group showed significant reductions in the augmentation index (a measure of arterial stiffness; -4.3; $P=0.03$), central and brachial mean arterial pressure (-4.8 mmHg and -4.4 mmHg, respectively; $P=0.01$ for both), central SBP and DBP (-5.0 mmHg and -3.9 mmHg, respectively; $P=0.01$ for both), and brachial SBP and DBP (-4.4 mmHg and -3.6 mmHg, respectively; $P=0.048$ and $P=0.01$, respectively) compared with control. The authors concluded that Rg3 ginsenoside-enriched KRG acutely lowered central and peripheral arterial pressures in healthy adults (Jovanovski et al., 2014a).

Cardiovascular Disorders: Coronary Artery Disease and Congestive Heart Failure

A 2011 systematic review looking at the TCM formula Shen-Mai (also called Shengmai, a formula containing schisandra, Asian ginseng, and *Liriope spicata*) as a complementary treatment for heart failure in China selected six RCTs ($n=440$) that met inclusion criteria. Compared with usual treatment alone, Shengmai plus usual treatment in five trials indicated an improvement in NYHA classification (RR=0.37). Other possible benefits included improved EF, CO, stroke volume, exercise test, and ratio of peak early-to-late diastolic filling velocity. Only one RCT with 40 patients compared

Shengmai with placebo, and improvements were seen in stroke volume, health, cardiac indexes, and myocardial contractility. The authors concluded that Shen-Mai alone or in addition to usual treatment could be beneficial for heart failure compared with placebo or with usual treatment alone (Zheng et al., 2011).

An RCT in patients ($n = 45$) with class IV CHF studied the hemodynamic effects of digoxin 0.25 mg/day alone compared with KRG 0.4 g/day alone and with KRG plus digoxin. Improvement of hemodynamic and biochemical indexes (improving from Class IV to Class III HF) occurred in 87% of patients with digoxin or ginseng alone and in 93% with combined treatment. The improvement in HR and MAP was greater with KRG and the combination than with digoxin alone. The improvement in cardiac index was greatest in the combination group ($P < 0.05$). Stroke volume index improvement was greatest with combined treatment followed by ginseng alone followed by digoxin alone. The authors concluded that KRG and digoxin had synergism for the treatment of CHF, and KRG was an effective and safe adjuvant without any side effects (Ding et al., 1995).

A 1-week RCT in patients ($n = 240$) with CHF and CAD compared Shenmai injection (a combination of KRG plus *Ophiopogon japonicus*) 100 mL/day with placebo in addition to standard medicines for the treatment of CHF. During treatment, the NYHA functional classification gradually improved in both groups, but the Shenmai group demonstrated a significantly greater improvement compared with the placebo group ($P = 0.001$). Six-minute walking distance, SF-36 score, and TCM syndrome score with Shenmai were also superior to placebo. Shenmai was well tolerated with no apparent safety concerns. The authors concluded that integrative treatment with standard medicine plus Shenmai injection could further improve NYHA functional classification for patients with CHF and CAD (Xian et al., 2016).

A study in patients with CAD compared injections of a combination of ginseng, astragalus, and dong quai with placebo (D10W) for effects on disease symptoms. With the polyherbal formula the frequency and severity of angina episodes were reduced by 90%, and the ischemic ST-T changes on ECG improved in 56% of cases. The tolerance to treadmill exercise was increased from 348 to 503 m. The PEP/LVET ratio

decreased from 0.45 to 0.36, indicative of improved left ventricular function. Blood viscosity and erythrocyte electrophoretic time decreased. Platelet aggregation and platelet adhesion were inhibited by 27% and 59% respectively. Thromboxane B2 levels decreased from 260 to 139 pg/mL. Plasma 6-keto-PGF1α level increased from 33.45 to 57.5 pg/mL. The differences were all statistically significant ($P < 0.05$-0.01) compared with placebo (Liao et al., 1989).

A 14-day RCT in patients ($n = 40$) with CHF investigated the effects of standard heart failure therapy plus Shenfu decoction granules (a combination of Asian ginseng and *Aconitum carmichaeli* Debx) compared with standard therapy alone (control group). Minnesota Living with Heart Failure Questionnaire scores were improved by 35 and 24 points in the herb and control groups, respectively ($P < 0.01$). Both physical and emotional scores were significantly higher in the herbal group than in the control group (21 vs 17 and 5 vs 1, respectively; $P < 0.05$ for both). Circulating ALT was significantly decreased by herbal treatment (-13.3 IU/L vs -0.6 IU/L; $P < 0.01$). The grading of cardiac function increased by 1.6 and 1.1, and LVEF increased by 18% and 8% in the herbal and control groups, respectively ($P < 0.05$ for both). The level of TNF-α declined from 65 to 58 in the herbal group ($P < 0.05$), while declining insignificantly in the control group from 61 to 58 ($P > 0.05$). The authors concluded that compared with standard heart failure treatment, Shenfu decoction as adjuvant therapy significantly improved QOL and hepatic injury in CHF patients (Wei et al., 2015).

Cardiovascular Disorders: Endothelial Dysfunction

An acutely dosed RCT in healthy subjects ($n = 16$) compared the vascular effects of four separate doses of a 3-g extract of KRG with bioequivalent doses of ginseng ginsenosides or polysaccharides and with placebo. KRG significantly improved flow-mediated vasodilatation by 2.6% at 180 min compared with the control group change of 0.8% ($P = 0.003$). The ginsenoside extract, but not the polysaccharide fraction, produced a comparable response (1.7% and 0.10%, respectively). BP remained unchanged for all treatments ($P = 0.45$). The authors concluded that KRG acutely improved endothelial function in healthy individuals, attributable to its ginsenoside containing fraction (Jovanovski et al., 2014b).

A 12-week RCT in female patients ($n = 80$) with cold hypersensitivity in the extremities compared KRG powder capsules 3 g BID for 8 weeks with placebo. The ginseng group had significantly higher skin temperature of the hands and feet, lower VAS scores, higher recovered temperature of the right fifth finger, and less parasympathetic activity than the placebo group at 8 weeks. No significant differences were noted in distal-dorsal difference of the hands and Short Form Health Survey-36 scores. The authors concluded that peripheral vasodilation by KRG may alleviate cold hypersensitivity in the hands and feet (Park et al., 2014a).

Cardiometabolic Disorders: Dyslipidemia and Hyperlipidemia

A 2020 systematic review and meta-analysis to evaluate the efficacy of ginseng on plasma lipids found 27 studies ($n = 1245$) that met inclusion criteria. The meta-analysis revealed that, overall, ginseng did not significantly change TC, TG, LDL-C, or HDL-C. However, high-dose ginseng did produce significant reductions in TC, LDL-C, and TG, with sustained impact in long-term interventions. The authors concluded that further research was warranted (Ziaei et al., 2020).

Cardiometabolic Disorders: Diabetes and Obesity

A 2014 systematic review looking at Asian ginseng and diabetes included 16 trials for analysis. Ginseng significantly reduced fasting blood glucose compared with control (MD = -0.31 mmol/L, $P = 0.03$). Although there was no significant effect on fasting plasma insulin or HOMA-IR, parallel trials (but not crossover trials) did show significant reductions in A1C (MD = 0.22%, $P = 0.01$) (Shishtar et al., 2014).

A 12-week RCT in patients ($n = 72$) with impaired fasting glucose compared ginseng berry extract with placebo for effects on glucose metabolism. The ginseng berry extract decreased serum concentrations of fasting glucose by 3.7% ($P = 0.035$), 60-min post-glucose load glucose by 10.7% ($P = 0.006$), and the AUC for glucose by 7.7% ($P = 0.024$) only in those with a fasting glucose level of 110 mg/dL or higher, while the placebo group did not exhibit a statistically significant

decrease. Safety profiles were not different between the two groups (Choi et al., 2018).

An 8-week RCT in patients ($n = 36$) with T2DM compared Asian ginseng (100 or 200 mg) with placebo. Ginseng produced improved mood, improved psycho-physical performance, and reduced FBG and BW. The 200-mg dose of ginseng improved A1C, type III collagen and physical activity. The AUC for 2-h BG was reduced from 27 to 22.6 ($P < 0.001$) in the eight ginseng-treated patients who had normalized BG. Placebo reduced BW and altered the serum lipid profile but did not alter FBS. The authors concluded that ginseng may be a useful adjunct in the treatment of T2DM (Sotaniemi et al., 1995).

An 8-week RCT in subjects ($n = 23$) with FBG between 5.6 mM and 6.9 mM compared hydrolyzed Asian ginseng extract 960 mg/day with placebo for effects on blood glucose. FBG and postprandial glucose were significantly decreased in the ginseng group compared with the placebo group ($P = 0.017$ and $P = 0.01$, respectively). No clinically significant changes in any safety parameter were observed. The authors concluded that hydrolyzed ginseng was a potent anti-diabetic agent that did not produce noticeable adverse effects (Park et al., 2014b).

A 12-week crossover RCT in patients ($n = 19$) with well-controlled T2DM compared KRG 2 g/meal TID with placebo in addition their usual anti-diabetic therapy. There was no change in the A1C, and participants remained well controlled (A1C = 6.5%) throughout. Ginseng treatment reduced the 75 g OGTT glucose indices by 8%–11% and fasting and OGTT plasma insulin indices by 33%–38%. Ginseng also increased fasting and OGTT insulin sensitivity indexes by 33%, compared with placebo ($P < 0.05$). Safety and compliance outcomes remained unchanged. The authors concluded that although clinical efficacy based on A1C was not demonstrated, 12 weeks of KRG treatment safely maintained good glycemic control and improved postprandial glucose and insulin beyond usual therapy in people with well-controlled T2DM (Vuksan et al., 2008).

An acutely dosed study in healthy subjects ($n = 13$) compared 10 different treatments: 3 g of either whole root KRG, 30% KRG ethanolic extract, 50% KRG ethanolic extract, 70% KRG ethanolic extract, or American ginseng ethanolic extracts of similar strengths, and compared with two cornstarch placebos. Treatments were given 40 min prior to a 50 g OGTT. There was no difference in attenuation of PPG among the tested ginseng preparations. However, increased insulin sensitivity was demonstrated with the 30% extract of KRG and the 50% extract of American ginseng compared with placebo ($P < 0.05$). The authors concluded that the insulin-sensitizing effects of KRG 30% extract and American ginseng 50% extract suggest that other root parts, including other ginsenosides not typically measured, may influence postprandial glucose and insulin parameters (De Souza et al., 2015).

An 8-week open-label study in obese middle-aged Korean women ($n = 10$) assessed the effects of Asian ginseng extract on body composition parameters, metabolic biomarkers, and gut microbiota. Significant changes were observed in BW and BMI. Significant differences of baseline gut microbiota were observed between the subjects who did and those who did not lose weight with ginseng. The authors concluded that ginseng exerted a weight loss effect and slight effects on gut microbiota, and that its anti-obesity effects differed depending on the composition of gut microbiota prior to ginseng intake (Song et al., 2014).

Women's Genitourinary Disorders: Menopause and Female Sexual Function

A 2018 systematic review to evaluate the effectiveness of phytoestrogens on sexual disorders and severity of dyspareunia in women found that the phytoestrogens isolated from maca as well as French maritime pine bark, fennel, and fenugreek significantly improved sexual function, whereas the phytoestrogens isolated from KRG, flaxseed, red clover, and soy did not lead to significant effects on sexual function (Najafi and Ghazanfarpour, 2018).

A 2017 review of clinical trials on herbal efficacy in menopausal symptoms used search terms menopause, climacteric, hot flushes, flashes, herb, and phytoestrogens. The authors found that Asian ginseng, passionflower, sage, lemon balm, valerian, black cohosh, fenugreek, black cumin, chasteberry, fennel, evening primrose, ginkgo, alfalfa, St. John's wort, anise, licorice, red clover, and wild soybean were effective in the treatment of acute menopausal syndrome with different mechanisms. The authors concluded that medicinal plants could play a role in the treatment of acute menopausal syndrome and that further studies were warranted (Kargozar et al., 2017).

A 2016 systematic review looking at the effects of KRG on menopausal symptoms included 10 RCTs for evaluation. One RCT did not show a significant difference in hot flush frequency between KRG and placebo. The second RCT reported positive effects of KRG on menopausal symptoms. The third RCT found beneficial effects of ginseng on depression, well-being, and general health. Four RCTs failed to show significant differences in various hormones except for DHEA between KRG and placebo controls. Two other RCTs showed no effects of ginseng on endometrial thickness in menopausal women. The authors concluded that there was positive evidence of ginseng for sexual function and KRG for sexual arousal and total hot flushes score in menopausal women (Lee et al., 2016a).

A 2013 systematic review of studies looking at the effects of ginseng for menopausal women identified four RCTs for inclusion. Results were favorable for KRG on symptoms of sexual arousal, global health, or menopausal symptoms, but one study failed to find a difference in hot flush frequency. The authors concluded that the overall evidence for use of ginseng in menopause was limited due to low number of trials and low sample size (Kim et al., 2013b).

A 2007 systematic review looking at herbs and supplements for menopausal mood disorders found one RCT of ginseng in postmenopausal women reporting improvements in mood and anxiety. Five of seven trials of St. John's wort showed benefit for mild-to-moderate depression. All three RCTs of ginkgo found no effect on depression. Kava significantly reduced anxiety in four of eight RCTs. Black cohosh significantly reduced depression and anxiety in all studies reviewed. The authors concluded that St. John's wort and black cohosh appeared to be the most useful in alleviating mood and anxiety changes during menopause, that ginseng may be effective but required more research, and that Kava held promise for decreasing anxiety in peri- and postmenopausal women (Geller and Studee, 2007).

A 2003 systematic review to assess the efficacy of herbal medicinal products for treatment of menopausal symptoms selected 18 RCTs that met inclusion criteria. One study concerned dong quai, the others being black cohosh, red clover, kava, evening primrose oil, ginseng, and combination products.

The authors concluded that there was no convincing evidence for any herbal medical product in the treatment of menopausal symptoms. However, the evidence for black cohosh was promising, albeit limited by the poor methodology of the trials. The studies involving red clover suggested it may be of benefit for more severe menopausal symptoms. There was some evidence for the use of kava, but safety concerns meant this herbal product was not a therapeutic option at the time of the study. The evidence was inconclusive for the other herbal medicinal products reviewed (Huntley and Ernst, 2003).

A 4-week RCT in postmenopausal women ($n = 62$) with sexual dysfunction compared Asian ginseng 500 mg BID with placebo for impact on sexual function. After the intervention, the mean total score of Female Sexual Function Index was significantly higher with ginseng than with placebo (AMD = 6.32, $P < 0.001$). The mean total score of quality of life and menopausal symptoms were significantly lower with ginseng than with placebo (AMD = -20.79, $P < 0.001$; and AMD = -8.25, $P < 0.001$, respectively). The authors concluded that ginseng improved sexual function and quality of life and mitigated symptoms in menopausal women (Ghorbani et al., 2019).

Men's Genitourinary Disorders: Male Sexual Dysfunction

A 2018 systematic review to evaluate the efficacy of herbal medicines in erectile dysfunction (ED) identified 24 RCTs ($n = 2080$) for inclusion. Among these, five investigated ginseng ($n = 399$), three investigated saffron ($n = 397$), and two investigated tribulus ($n = 202$). Twelve studies investigated combinations of herbs and/or supplements. Ginseng significantly improved erectile function (IIEF-5 score: 140 with ginseng, 96 with placebo; SMD = 0.43; $P < 0.01$). *P. pinaster* and maca showed very preliminary positive results, and saffron and tribulus produced mixed results. Adverse events were recorded in 19 of 24 trials, with no significant differences between placebo and verum in placebo-controlled studies. The authors concluded that there was encouraging evidence to suggest that ginseng may be an effective herbal treatment for ED (Borrelli et al., 2018).

A 12-week RCT in patients ($n = 60$) with mild-to-moderate ED compared KRG 1 g TID with placebo.

The IIEF-5 score after the treatment was significantly higher in the ginseng group compared with baseline (from 16.4 to 21.0; $P < 0.0001$), while there was no difference before and after the treatment in the placebo group (from 17.0 to 17.7; $P > 0.05$). With ginseng, 67% of patients reported improved erection, with significant improvement in the global efficacy question ($P < 0.01$); in the placebo group there was no significance. Rigidity, penetration, and maintenance were significantly greater with ginseng than with placebo ($P < 0.01$). There was a significant improvement in total IIEF-5 score for the ginseng group compared with placebo ($P < 0.001$). The levels of serum testosterone, prolactin, and cholesterol after the treatment were not significantly different between the ginseng and placebo groups ($P > 0.05$). The authors concluded that KRG could be an effective alternative to invasive approaches for treating male ED (de Andrade et al., 2007).

An acutely dosed RCT in patients ($n = 90$) with ED compared KRG with trazodone and with placebo for effects on erectile function. The ginseng group showed changes in early detumescence and erectile parameters such as penile rigidity and girth, libido, and patient satisfactions that were significantly greater than those in the trazodone and placebo groups ($P < 0.05$). The overall therapeutic efficacies on ED were 60% for the ginseng group and 30% for the placebo and trazodone-treated groups ($P < 0.05$). The authors concluded that KRG was shown to have superior effects compared with placebo or trazodone for ED (Choi et al., 1995).

Men's Genitourinary Disorders: Male Infertility

An open-label case-controlled study investigated the effects Asian ginseng in men with idiopathic oligo-asthenospermia or varicocele-related oligo-asthenospermia and age-matched volunteers ($n = 66$). Use of ginseng extract showed an increase in spermatozoa number/ml and progressive oscillating motility; an increase in plasma total and free testosterone, DHT, FSH, and LH levels; and a decrease in prolactin. Based on these findings, the authors hypothesized that ginsenosides may have an effect at different levels of the hypothalamic-pituitary-testis axis (Salvati et al., 1996).

A 12-week RCT in male infertility patients ($n = 80$) with varicocele compared non-varicocelectomy plus placebo with varicocelectomy plus placebo, with non-varicocelectomy plus KRG 1.5 g/day, and with vari-cocelectomy plus KRG 1.5 g/day. All groups entailing an intervention (varicocelectomy and/or KRG) showed significant improvements in sperm concentrations, motility, morphology, and viability at the end of the study. The authors concluded that KRG may be a useful agent for the treatment of male infertility (Park et al., 2016).

A Phase I clinical toxicity study in healthy males evaluated the effects of high doses of Asian ginseng compared with a combination of andrographis plus eleuthero (Kan jang) and with high doses of valerian for possible adverse effects on semen quality. Asian ginseng showed no significant negative effects on the fertility parameters, and there was a clear decrease in the percentage of dyskinetic forms of spermatozoids. There was a positive trend toward the number of spermatozoids, percentage of normokinetic forms, and fertility indexes with the andrographis combination. There was also a decrease in percentage of dyskinetic spermatozoids. There were no significant negative effects of the herbal combination on male semen quality and fertility. Subjects receiving valerian showed a temporary increase in the percentage of normokinetic spermatozoids and a decrease in dyskinetic forms, but these changes had no effect on fertility indices. The authors concluded that Asian ginseng, the combination of andrographis plus eleuthero, and valerian were safe with respect to effects on human male sterility when administered at dose levels corresponding to approximately three times the human daily dose (Mkrtchyan et al., 2005).

Neurological Disorders: Cognitive Impairment and Dementia

A 2019 systematic review investigating the effects of a combination of Asian ginseng and ginkgo treatments on physiological and psychological outcomes in humans identified eight studies meeting the criteria. All studies used the combination brand Gincosan. The most consistent results found were benefits to aspects of the circulatory/cardiovascular system in patients with disease and "secondary memory" performance in patient and healthy populations. The authors concluded that this combination of ginseng and ginkgo could improve aspects of physiological and cognitive function in humans; however, evidence for synergy required further investigation (Reay et al., 2005).

A 2016 systematic review and meta-analysis on ginseng for AD found four RCTs ($n = 259$) to review. They found that the effectiveness of combined treatment (adding ginseng to conventional treatment) was inconsistent (Wang et al., 2016).

A 2013 systematic review searched to capture clinical studies into the neurocognitive effects of modafinil, ginseng, and bacopa. The highest effect sizes (Cohen's d) for cognitive outcomes were 0.77 with modafinil (visuospatial memory accuracy), 0.86 with ginseng (simple reaction time), and 0.95 with bacopa (delayed word recall). These data indicated that neurocognitive enhancement from well-characterized nutraceuticals can produce cognition-enhancing effects of similar magnitude to those from pharmaceutical interventions (Neale et al., 2013).

A 4-week RCT in patients ($n = 66$) diagnosed with MCI compared a daily dose of Memo, a combination of lyophilized royal jelly 750 mg plus standardized extracts of ginkgo 120 mg and Asian ginseng 150 mg, with placebo for effects on MMSE scores. The mean change in MMSE scores in the group treated with the combination product was significantly greater than in the control group ($+2.07$ vs $+0.13$, respectively; $P < 0.0001$). The authors concluded that this combination formula could be beneficial in treating age-related cognitive decline as well as the early phases of pathologic cognitive impairments such as vascular dementia or AD (Yakoot et al., 2013).

A 12-week open-label RCT in patients ($n = 61$) with AD compared low-dose and high-dose KRG (4.5 g/day and 9 g/day) with a control group. The patients in the high-dose ginseng group showed significant improvement on the ADAS and Clinical Dementia Rating scales after 12 weeks compared with those in the control group ($P = 0.032$ and $P = 0.006$, respectively). The ginseng treatment groups showed improvement from baseline MMSE scores when compared with the control group (1.42 vs -0.48), but this improvement was not statistically significant. The authors concluded that KRG showed good efficacy for the treatment of AD (He et al., 2018).

In a 2-year follow-up to this study the dose of KRG was maintained at 4.5 g/day or 9 g/day. At 24 weeks, the MMSE score reached maximal improvement and remained without significant decline at the 48th and 96th weeks. ADAS-cog showed similar findings. The authors concluded that the research indicated feasible efficacy of ginseng in long-term follow-up of AD (Heo et al., 2011).

Psychiatric Disorders: General Cognitive Performance and Stress Resilience

A 1-month RCT in healthy volunteers ($n = 65$) compared Asian ginseng 500 mg/day with placebo for effects on serum MDA levels when subjected to daily psychomotor stress (performance task and visual working memory accuracy testing). The participants in the control group showed significant increases in MDA serum levels ($P = 0.0004$), which were related to a significant increase in the perceived stress scale ($P < 0.0001$), while ginseng led to a significant reduction in MDA serum levels ($P < 0.01$), with a smaller but still significant increase in perceived stress scale ($P = 0.02$). The authors concluded that Asian ginseng produced a significant reduction in oxidative stress and augmented eustress levels in healthy volunteers after 1 month of therapy (Al-Kuraishy and Al-Gareeb, 2017).

An acutely dosed RCT in healthy young subjects ($n = 28$) investigated the cognitive and mood effects of single doses of guarana extract 75 mg, Asian ginseng 200 mg, and their combination (75 mg + 200 mg) compared with placebo. In comparison with placebo, all the treatments resulted in improved task performance throughout the day. Both ginseng and the ginseng-guarana combination enhanced the speed of attention task and memory task performance. With guarana alone, attention tasks were improved, but accuracy was decreased (Kennedy et al., 2004).

Dermatological Disorders: Photoaging and Alopecia

A 12-week left-right comparative RCT in subjects ($n = 23$) compared a topical application of an enzyme-modified ginseng extract with placebo for preventive effects on eye-wrinkle formation. The ginseng group significantly reduced the global photodamage score compared with placebo. Total roughness and smoothness depth were significantly decreased with use of ginseng. The subjects reported post-study that ginseng was more potent than placebo in softening and moisturizing the skin. The authors concluded that enzyme-modified ginseng was a promising anti-aging candidate that could be used as an ingredient in natural functional food and cosmetic products (Hwang et al., 2015).

A 12-week clinical study in patients ($n = 50$) with alopecia areata studied the hair growth efficacy and safety of KRG plus intralesional corticosteroids compared with intralesional corticosteroids alone. At 12 weeks the average hair number in the combination group increased from 44/cm² at baseline to 101/cm² and the average hair thickness increased from 0.062 mm to 0.085 mm. In the intralesional injection alone group, the hair density increased from 40/cm² to 91/cm² and average hair thickness increased from 0.058 mm to 0.078 mm. The difference between groups was not statistically significant for either parameter. However, when global photographs were reviewed in a blinded manner by an expert panel of three dermatologists at the end of the trial using a four-point scale, the average score of the ginseng add-on group was 3.6 and that of the other group was 3.1 ($P < 0.05$). The authors concluded that treatment with KRG could result in improved hair regrowth for patients with alopecia areata (Oh and Son, 2012).

Disorders of Vitality: Fatigue and Hangover

A 2018 systematic review evaluating the safety and efficacy of Asian ginseng and American ginseng for fatigue selected 10 studies for analysis. The authors found that there was a low risk of adverse events associated with the use of ginseng and modest evidence for its efficacy for fatigue (Arring et al., 2018).

A 2017 systematic review to evaluate herbs for hangover benefit selected six studies for analysis. Of the interventions, the use of KRG, polysaccharide-rich extract of eleuthero, anti-hangover drink, Korean pear juice, KSS formula (pith of citrus tangerine, tanaka, ginger root, and brown sugar) and After-Effect (borage oil, fish oil, vitamins B1, B6, and C, magnesium, milk thistle, and prickly pear) were associated with a significant improvement of hangover symptoms, particularly tiredness, nausea, vomiting, and stomachache ($P < 0.05$) (Jayawardena et al., 2017).

A 2016 systematic review and meta-analysis looking at efficacy of ginseng supplements for fatigue reduction and physical performance enhancement selected 12 RCTs ($n = 630$) for the final analysis. The authors found in four RCTs a statistically significant efficacy of ginseng supplements for fatigue reduction

(SMD = 0.34). However, in eight RCTs, ginseng was not associated with physical performance enhancement (SMD = −0.01). The authors concluded that larger RCTs were required to confirm the efficacy of ginseng supplements on fatigue reduction (Bach et al., 2016).

A 2016 systematic review evaluating the effect of KRG supplementation on exercise performance and fatigue recovery selected 14 studies for analysis. The authors found that aerobic and anaerobic capacity demonstrated no overall improvement and that the antioxidant function as measured by levels of SOD and MDA showed mixed results (Lee et al., 2016b).

A 4-week RCT in patients ($n = 90$) with idiopathic chronic fatigue compared Asian ginseng extract 1 g/day or 2 g/day with placebo. After 4 weeks, the mental numeric self-rating score with 1 g of ginseng decreased from 20.4 to 15.1; the 2-g ginseng dose was associated with a decrease from 20.7 to 13.8. With placebo the change was from 20.9 to 18.8 (ginseng vs placebo; $P < 0.01$). Ginseng decreased the total numeric self-rating score insignificantly compared with placebo ($P > 0.05$). The higher dose of ginseng reduced the VAS score from 7.3 to 4.4 compared with the placebo reduction from 7.1 to 5.8 ($P < 0.01$). Oxidation measures were decreased, and antioxidant measures were increased by ginseng compared with placebo. The authors postulated that the anti-fatigue effects of ginseng were mediated through antioxidant mechanisms (Kim et al., 2013a).

A 12-week RCT in patients ($n = 38$) with fibromyalgia compared Asian ginseng 100 mg/day with amitriptyline 25 mg/day and with placebo. For the ginseng group, ratings on the VAS revealed a reduction from baseline in pain ($P < 0.0001$) and improvements in fatigue ($P < 0.0001$), sleep ($P < 0.001$), tender points, and quality of life. However, there were no significant differences between groups with respect to anxiety. Improvements occurred in the ginseng group compared with baseline ($P < 0.0001$), but amitriptyline resulted in significantly greater improvements ($P < 0.05$) (Braz et al., 2013).

Disorders of Vitality: Stamina and Athletic Performance

A three-cycle trial in healthy subjects ($n = 19$) compared a high-dose (960 mg) or low-dose (160 mg) enzyme-fermented ginseng supplement with pla-

cebo for effects on hormonal and inflammatory responses to physical stress. Participants completed three 14-day treatment cycles with different doses (high: 960 mg; low: 160 mg; placebo: 0 mg), each cycle being followed by intense physical exercise. Based on serial blood testing for HPA axis and antioxidant activity, ginseng supplementation was found to produce a stress-inducible dose-dependent reduction in circulating cortisol and an increase in antioxidant activity. The authors concluded that 24 h after intense exercise, a high-dose ginseng significantly reduced muscle damage and HPA responses to physical stress in humans, possibly due to increased antioxidant expression. Additionally, this group of subjects rated perceived exertion after each set of exercises as well as muscle pain/soreness. Psychomotor performance and peak power were measured. Both high- and low-dose ginseng significantly reduced change in muscle soreness at 24 h post exercise. Analysis of peak power demonstrated the presence of responders ($n = 13$) and non-responders ($n = 6$). Responders showed a significant effect of the high-dose ginseng for maintenance of neuromuscular function. The authors proposed that the appearance of responders and non-responders could explain the mixed literature base on the ergogenic properties of ginseng (Caldwell et al., 2018).

A 12-week RCT in sedentary individuals ($n = 117$) compared low-dose ginsenoside (100 mg/day) and high-dose ginsenoside (500 mg/day) with placebo for enhancement of aerobic capacity during a supervised aerobic and resistance exercise training course. After exercise training, the VO2$_{max}$ increased from 28.6 to 33.7 and from 30.4 to 32.8 with the high-dose ginsenoside and placebo, respectively ($P = 0.029$). Aerobic threshold increased from 19.3 to 20.9 mL/kg/min in the high-dose group, whereas it did not change with placebo ($P = 0.038$). There was no difference in VO2$_{max}$ between the low-dose ginsenoside and placebo groups and there were no differences in muscular strength during exercise training among the three groups. The authors concluded that high-dose ginsenoside supplementation augmented the improvement of aerobic capacity associated with exercise training (Lee et al., 2018).

An acutely dosed RCT in untrained men ($n = 12$) compared exercise plus ginseng with exercise plus placebo for effects on intensive exercise-induced changes in muscle epigenetics. Skeletal muscle biopsies were performed before and after the intervention to measure the methylation of H3K-36 histone protein. There was a significant increase in histone H3-k36 protein methylation following intensive exercise in the placebo group, but this did not occur in the ginseng group. The authors concluded that the methylation caused by intense physical exercise (and by extension other forms of physical stress) could be reduced by ginseng extract (Naghavi Moghadam et al., 2019).

Immune Function

A 12-week RCT in volunteer patients ($n = 227$) compared standardized ginseng extract 100 mg QD with placebo for immune response to influenza vaccination at week 4. The ginseng group experienced fewer episodes of influenza or common cold between 4 and 12 weeks than did the placebo group (15 and 42 cases, respectively; $P < 0.001$). Antibody titers by week 8 rose to an average of 272 units and 171 units with ginseng and placebo, respectively ($P < 0.0001$). Natural killer activity levels were nearly twice as high in the ginseng group compared with the placebo group ($P < 0.0001$). Ginseng appeared to be safe and well tolerated (Scaglione et al., 1996).

A 14-week RCT in healthy volunteers ($n = 72$) compared an acidic polysaccharide from Asian ginseng (Y-75) 6 g/day with placebo for effects on immune enhancement. The polysaccharide significantly increased NK cell cytotoxic activity from baseline by 35.2% at 8 weeks and 40.2% at 14 weeks. The phagocytic activity of peripheral blood cells and serum level of TNF-α were increased by 25.2% and 38.2%, respectively, at 8 weeks, and by 39.4% and 44.5%, respectively, at 14 weeks. The changes from baseline were statistically significant. Differences in the efficacy with the polysaccharide compared with placebo were also significant. The authors concluded that Y-75 was shown to be a safe and potentially effective natural alternative for enhancing immune function (Cho et al., 2001, 2014, 2017).

Immune Disorders: Inflammation

A 2020 meta-analysis to assess effects of ginseng supplementation on CRP/hs-CRP levels found nine studies that met inclusion criteria. Meta-analysis found a non-significant decrease in CRP with ginseng (WMD = −0.1, $P = 0.27$) and significant het-

erogeneity in the studies. Subgroup analysis showed that ginseng could significantly reduce CRP levels by 0.51 ($P < 0.001$, $I^2 = 0.0\%$) in patients with baseline CRP > 3 mg/dL. The authors concluded that ginseng could decrease CRP/hsCRP levels in patients with baseline elevated levels (Saboori et al., 2019).

Infectious Disease: HIV

A 20-year study in HIV patients ($n = 1751$) looked at the effects of KRG on the HIV nef gene (gross deletions in the nef gene are associated with long-term nonprogression of infected patients). The study was divided into three phases: baseline, KRG alone, and KRG plus HAART. The proportion of defective nef genes was significantly greater with ginseng (15.6%) than with baseline (5.7%), control (5.6%), ginseng plus HAART (7.8%), and HAART (6.6%) ($P < 0.01$). Small in-frame deletions or insertions were significantly more frequent in the ginseng group compared with controls ($P < 0.01$). Significantly fewer instances of genetic defects were detected in samples taken during the ginseng plus HAART phase (7.8%; $P < 0.01$). The authors concluded that KRG treatment might induce genetic defects in the nef gene (Cho et al., 2001, 2014, 2017).

Oncologic Disorders: General Cancer Prophylaxis

A paired case-control retrospective study of cancer patients ($n = 905 + 905$) investigated the effect of ginseng consumption on the risk of cancer. Of the 905 cases, 62% had a history of ginseng intake compared with 75% of controls ($P < 0.01$), with the odds ratio of cancer for ginseng intake of 0.56. ORs for cancer were 0.37 with fresh ginseng extract, 0.57 with white ginseng extract, 0.30 with white ginseng powder, and 0.20 with red ginseng. Overall, the risk decreased as the frequency and duration of ginseng intake increased. When analyzed for cancer type, the odds ratios were 0.47 for cancer of the lip, oral cavity, and pharynx; 0.20 for esophageal cancer; 0.36 for stomach cancer; 0.42 for colorectal cancer; 0.48 for liver cancer; 0.22 for pancreatic cancer; 0.18 for laryngeal cancer; 0.55 for lung cancer; and 0.15 for ovarian cancer. In cancers of the female breast, uterine cervix, urinary bladder, and thyroid gland, however, there was no reduction with ginseng intake, which might explain why men showed a stronger benefit (Yun and Choi, 1998).

Oncologic Disorders: Lung Cancer

A 2018 meta-analysis looked at the safety and efficacy of injections of Aidi (a combination extract including *Mylabris phalerata*, astragalus root, Asian ginseng root, and eleuthero) in combination with platinum-based chemotherapy for stage IIIB/IV NSCLC. The authors selected 42 RCTs ($n=4081$) for inclusion. Compared with platinum-based chemotherapy alone, Aidi injection plus platinum-based chemotherapy increased relative benefit of disease control rate (RR = 1.13; $P<0.00001$), objective response rate (RR = 1.26; $P<0.00001$), improved 1-, 2-, 3-year survival rates (RR = 1.14, 1.31, 1.88; $P=0.03$, 0.02, 0.0005, respectively), and QOL (RR = 1.80; $P<0.00001$). The combination also reduced severe (grade 3 and 4) toxicities by 36% (RR = 0.64; $P<0.00001$). The authors concluded that addition of Aidi injection to platinum-based chemotherapy improved the clinical efficacy and alleviated the toxicity of chemotherapy in patients with stage IIIB/IV NSCLC (Wang et al., 2018).

A longitudinal RCT in patients ($n=414$) with stage III–IV NSCLC investigated the effects of chemotherapy plus ginseng enriched with ginsenoside Rg3 compared with chemotherapy plus placebo. The median overall survival was 12 months in the experimental group and 8.5 months in the control group ($P<0.05$). Reductions in Hgb and WBCs after the first and second cycles were milder the with ginseng ($P<0.05$). After two courses of treatment, the Karnofsky performance scale (measure of functional status, with lower score indicating impairment) was 80 in the ginseng group and 77 in the control group, while the TCM symptoms score was 2.5 in the experimental group and 2.9 in the control group ($P<0.05$). The authors concluded that a combination of TCM with Western medicine (chemotherapy) could prolong the survival of patients with advanced NSCLC and could improve patients' symptoms and reduce chemotherapy-induced myelosuppression (Zhang et al., 2018).

Oncologic Disorders: Breast Cancer and Ovarian Cancer

A 6-year study in patients ($n=1455$) with breast cancer studied the association of ginseng use with survival and quality of life (QOL). Approximately 27% of study participants were regular ginseng users before cancer diagnosis. Compared with patients who never used ginseng, regular users had a significantly reduced risk of total mortality (HR = 0.71) and disease-specific mortality or recurrence (HR = 0.70). Ginseng use after cancer diagnosis, particularly current use, was positively associated with QOL scores, with the strongest effect in the psychological and social well-being domains and this effect appeared to be cumulative (Cui et al., 2006).

A 3-month RCT in patients ($n=30$) with epithelial ovarian cancer compared KRG 3 g/day with placebo for toxicity, quality of life, and survival after adjuvant chemotherapy. Ginseng reduced micronuclei yield in comparison with placebo despite no difference of binucleated cell index. Although ginseng increased ALT and AST significantly, they were within the normal range. There were no differences in adverse events between placebo and ginseng groups. Ginseng was associated with improved emotional functioning and decreased symptoms of fatigue, nausea, vomiting, dyspnea, anxiety, and daytime somnolence. There were no differences in survival. The authors concluded that KRG may be safe and effective to reduce genotoxicity and improve HRQOL despite no benefit of survival (Kim et al., 2017).

Oncologic Disorders: Gastric and Colorectal Cancer

A 2014 systematic review to evaluate the clinical evidence for the addition of herbal medicines to FOLFOX 4 for advanced colorectal cancer selected 13 RCTs for analysis. Meta-analysis found the addition of herbal medicine improved tumor response rate (RR = 1.25), 1-year survival (RR = 1.51), and quality of life in terms of Karnofsky Performance Status gains (RR = 1.84) and alleviated grade 3 and 4 chemotherapy-related adverse effects including neutropenia (RR = 0.33), nausea and vomiting (RR = 0.34), and neurotoxicity (RR = 0.39), compared with FOLFOX4 alone. The most frequently studied herbs were astragalus, Asian ginseng, *Atractylodes macrocephala*, *Poria cocos*, *Coix lachrymajobi*, and *Sophora flavescens* (Chen et al., 2014).

A chemotherapy-connected RCT in colorectal cancer patients ($n=438$) undergoing mFOLFOX-6 therapy compared KRG with placebo for 16 weeks to assess impact on cancer-related fatigue. KRG up to 16 weeks improved fatigue over baseline compared with placebo. On the Brief Fatigue Inventory, "Mood" and "Walking ability" showed most notable improvements ($P=0.038$, $P=0.023$, respectively). In the per-protocol group, KRG led to improved fatigue compared with the placebo ($P = 0.019$), especially in "Fatigue right now," "Mood," "Relations with others," "Walking ability," and "Enjoyment of life" at 16 weeks ($P = 0.045$, $P = 0.006$, $P = 0.028$, $P = 0.003$, $P = 0.036$, respectively). Neutropenia was more frequent with KRG. However, the incidence of all adverse events was similar. The authors concluded that KRG could be safely and effectively combined with mFOLFOX-6 chemotherapy in colorectal cancer patients to reduce cancer-related fatigue (Kim et al., 2020).

A 9-day RCT in gastric cancer patients ($n = 58$) compared parenteral Shen-Mai (also called Shengmai, a TCM formula containing schisandra, ginseng, and *Liriope spicata*) therapy alone with enteral nutrition alone and with a combination of Shen-Mai and parenteral nutrition for impact on postoperative fatigue. Conditions of recovery, post-operative mood, and sleep quality were better, and the postoperative fatigue was reduced more significantly in the combined treatment group than in the other two groups ($P < 0.05$). Additionally, pre-albumin, CD3, CD4, and CD4/CD8 were significantly higher with combined treatment ($P < 0.05$). The authors concluded that combining Shen-Mai with enteral nutrition could improve mood, sleep, and postoperative fatigue through improving nutritional status and immune function, thus speeding up the recovery of patients (Dong et al., 2010).

Oncologic Disorders: Leukemia

A 2-year study to investigate the effects of ginseng on immune function in children ($n = 30$) following treatment for leukemia and solid cancers compared KRG extract 60 mg/kg/day with a control group. Although lymphocyte subpopulations (T cell, B cell, NK cell, T4, T8, and T4/T8 ratio) and serum immunoglobulin subclasses (IgG, IgA, and IgM) did not show significant differences between the study and the control groups, the cytokines of the ginseng group decreased more rapidly than that of the control group. The authors concluded that KRG might have a stabilizing effect on the inflammatory cytokines in children with cancer after chemotherapy (Lee et al., 2012).

Oncologic Disorders: Quality of Life During Treatment

A 2016 meta-analysis was conducted to assess the effectiveness of integrative management of chemotherapy-induced nausea and vomiting. The authors identified 27 RCTs ($n = 1843$), in which the traditional plant-based medicines plus oxaliplatin showed significantly reduced nausea and vomiting (RR = 0.65) with or without the addition of conventional anti-emetics. The six plants associated with significant reductions in nausea and vomiting were *Atractylodes macrocephala*, *Poria cocos*, *Coix lacryma-jobi*, Chinese licorice, astragalus, and Asian ginseng. Experimental studies of these six plants have reported possible mechanisms for this benefit: inhibitory effects on nausea and vomiting (or its animal equivalent), regulation of gastrointestinal motility, gastroprotective effects, and antioxidant actions (Chen et al., 2016).

A 4-week RCT in patients with cancer undergoing chemotherapy or radiotherapy compared Shen-Mai-San (also called Shengmai San, a TCM formula containing schisandra, ginseng, and *Liriope spicata*) with placebo for quality of life. Based on measurements using the European Organization for Research and Treatment of Cancer Quality of Life questionnaire (QOL-C30) Shen-Mai-San was found to be effective for treating cancer-related fatigue and had anti-fatigue activity. This supported the TCM approach to addressing Qi and Yin deficiency in the face of chemotherapy or radiotherapy for cancer (Lo et al., 2012).

HUMAN RESEARCH: AMERICAN GINSENG

Several of the following studies, particularly for diabetes and URIs, were undertaken by the same authors who were studying proprietary extracts of American ginseng standardized to a particular constituent.

Cardiovascular Disorders: Hypertension

A 12-week RCT in patients ($n = 64$) with well-controlled essential HTN and T2DM on conventional medication compared American ginseng 3 g daily with placebo, both in addition to usual care for vascular effects. Arterial stiffness, as measured by the augmentation index, was lowered by 5.3% in the ginseng group ($P = 0.04$). SBP was reduced by 12% with ginseng ($P < 0.001$). The authors concluded that the addition of American ginseng to conventional therapy in T2DM and HTN improved arterial stiffness and attenuated SBP (Mucalo, 2013).

A 12-week RCT in patients ($n = 80$) with T2DM evaluated the hypotensive effects of a combination of ginsenoside Rg3-enriched KRG and American ginseng 2.25 g TID compared with placebo. A reduction in central systolic BP relative to placebo (-4.69 mmHg, $P = 0.04$) was observed. This was characterized by a decrease in end-systolic pressure (-6.60 mmHg, $P = 0.01$) and AUC for systolic and diastolic BP (-132.80, $P = 0.04$; -220.90, $P = 0.02$, respectively). There was no significant change in reactive hyperemia index, pulse-wave velocity, or other related pulse wave components. The authors concluded that the combination of KRG and American ginseng may have utility for modest BP benefit in addition to its other benefits in T2DM (Jovanovski et al., 2020).

Cardiometabolic Disorders: Diabetes

A 4-week RCT in patients ($n = 84$) with CAD and impaired fasting glucose, impaired glucose tolerance, or T2DM compared a standardized extract of American ginseng plus usual care with a control group of Western medicine alone. FBG decreased in both groups ($P < 0.01$), showing a greater trend with American ginseng (26% vs 21%). There were no obvious changes in fasting insulin or insulin sensitivity ($P > 0.05$). HOMA-β value, a measure of β-cell function, increased markedly in the ginseng group after treatment from 3.48 to 4.19 ($P < 0.01$) with no change in the control group. TC and LDL-C decreased from baseline with ginseng ($P < 0.05$), with a difference between groups in TC ($P < 0.05$) after treatment (Zhang et al., 2007).

A 16-day crossover RCT in healthy nondiabetic adults ($n = 12$) compared the effect of American ginseng 1, 2, and 3 g daily with placebo on post-glucose load BG. Glycemia was lower over the last 45 min of the test after all three doses of ginseng than after placebo ($P < 0.05$). There were no significant differences between doses. The reductions in AUC for the three doses were 14.4%, 10.6%, and 9.1%, respectively. Glycemia in the last hour of the test and the AUC were significantly lower when ginseng was administered 40 min before the challenge than when it was administered 20, 10, or 0 min before the challenge ($P < 0.05$). The authors concluded that American ginseng reduced postprandial glycemia in subjects without diabetes, and that the reductions were time dependent but not dose dependent, requiring the dose

to be administered no later than 40 min before the challenge (Vuksan et al., 2001).

A crossover RCT in patients ($n = 24$) with T2DM compared American ginseng 1 g TID AC with placebo in addition to usual medications for additive hypoglycemic efficacy. The subjects were treated for 8 weeks, followed by a 4-week washout period, then crossed over to the opposite arm for 8 weeks. Compared with placebo American ginseng significantly reduced A1C (-0.29%; $P = 0.041$), FBG (-0.71 mmol/L; $P = 0.008$), SBP (-5.6 mmHg; $P < 0.001$), and mean percent end-difference of LDL-C and LDL-C/HDL (-12.3% and -13.9%, respectively). American ginseng also increased NOx ($+1.85$ μmol/L; $P < 0.03$). The authors concluded that American ginseng may be a safe and effective adjunct to conventional treatment for T2DM (Vuksan et al., 2019).

A time-dependent dosing RCT in healthy adults ($n = 10$) and adults with T2DM ($n = 9$) compared American ginseng 3 g with placebo given 40 or 0 min before a 25-g oral glucose challenge on four separate occasions. In the healthy subjects, no differences were found in postprandial glycemia between placebo and ginseng when administered at the same time as the glucose challenge, but when ginseng was taken 40 min before the glucose challenge, significant reductions were observed ($P < 0.05$). Reductions in the glycemic AUC were 18% in the latter group. In the subjects with T2DM, there were significant reductions in glycemia at both dosing times (40 min before or concurrently with the glucose load; $P < 0.05$). Reductions in the glycemic AUC were 19% in the pre-dosing diabetic group and 22% in the concurrent-dosing diabetic group. The authors concluded that in non-diabetic patients, American ginseng should be taken with meals to avoid potential for hypoglycemia (Vuksan et al., 2000a).

A variably dosed and timed RCT in patients ($n = 10$) with T2DM compared American ginseng 3, 6, or 9 g with placebo given at different intervals (120, 80, 40, or 0 min) prior to a 25-g oral glucose load. Analysis demonstrated that dosage, but not time of administration, significantly affected glucose ($P < 0.05$) and the AUC ($P = 0.037$). The AUC was reduced by 20%, 15%, and 16% with 3, 6 or 9 g, respectively, compared with placebo ($P < 0.05$). Compared with placebo, incremental glycemia was decreased at 30 min by 16%, 18%, and 18%, respectively. At 45 min glycemia was decreased by 12%, 14%, and 14%, respectively. At 120 min glycemia was decreased by 59%, 41%, and 45%, respectively. The authors concluded that American ginseng reduced PPG irrespective of dose and time of administration. No more than 3 g of American ginseng was required at any time in relation to the challenge to achieve reductions (Vuksan et al., 2000b).

A similar RCT, this time in nondiabetic individuals ($n = 10$), compared the same three doses (3, 6, or 9 g) of American ginseng with placebo given on 12 separate occasions at 120, 80, or 40 min prior to 25 g oral glucose. Compared with the placebo, 3-, 6-, and 9-g doses reduced postprandial incremental glucose at 30, 45, and 60 min ($P < 0.05$); 3 g and 9 g did so at 90 min as well. At 60 min, the 9-g dose reduced incremental postprandial glucose relative to the 3-g dose ($P < 0.05$). All doses reduced the incremental glucose AUC (3 g, 27%; 6 g, 29%; 9 g, 38%; $P < 0.05$ for all). The timing of the dosing of American ginseng did not influence the outcomes. The authors concluded that 3, 6, or 9 g of American ginseng taken 40, 80, or 120 min before a glucose challenge similarly affected glucose tolerance in nondiabetic individuals (Vuksan et al., 2000c).

A 12-week RCT in patients ($n = 74$) with T2DM compared an extract of American ginseng standardized to 10% ginsenosides 3 g/day with placebo to determine safety. Outcomes included measures of kidney function (urates and creatinine), liver function (AST and ALT), and hemostatic function (PT/INR). There was no change in any of the measures of safety between treatments from baseline. The number or severity of adverse events did not differ between American ginseng and placebo (Mucalo, 2014).

Women's Genitourinary Disorders: Menopause

A 3-month RCT in premenopausal and postmenopausal women ($n = 50$) compared Phyto-Female Complex (American ginseng, black cohosh, dong quai, milk thistle, red clover, and chasteberry) with placebo BID for effect on menopausal symptoms. The women receiving Phyto-Female Complex reported a significantly superior mean reduction in menopausal symptoms with the herbal complex than with placebo. The effect of treatment improvements in menopausal symptoms increased over time; by 3 months there was a 73% decrease in hot flushes, a 69% decrease in night sweats, and a decrease in hot flush intensity. There was

also a significant improvement in sleep quality. Hot flushes ceased completely in 47% and 19% of women with the herbal product and placebo, respectively. There were no changes in findings on vaginal ultrasonography or levels of estradiol, FSH, liver enzymes, or TSH in either group. The authors concluded that Phyto-Female Complex was safe and effective for the relief of hot flushes and sleep disturbances in pre- and postmenopausal women, at least for 3 months' use (Rotem and Kaplan, 2007).

Psychiatric Disorders: Attention-Deficit/ Hyperactivity Disorder and Cognitive Performance

An acutely dosed crossover RCT in healthy middle-aged volunteers ($n = 52$) compared American ginseng 200 mg with placebo for memory effects at 1, 3, and 6 h following treatment. Compared with placebo, American ginseng improved cognitive performance on the "Working Memory" factor at 3 h, particularly spatial working memory. There were no significant effects on mood or blood glucose levels (Ossoukhova et al., 2015).

An acutely dosed RCT in healthy young adults ($n = 32$) compared an extract of American ginseng standardized to 10.6% ginsenosides at three doses (100, 200, 400 mg) with placebo for cognitive and mood effects at 1, 3, and 6 h after treatment. There was a significant improvement of working memory performance with American ginseng. The Corsi block performance was improved by all doses at all testing times. There were differential effects of all doses on other working memory tasks across the testing day. Choice reaction time accuracy and calmness were significantly improved by 100 mg. There were no changes in blood glucose levels. The authors concluded that American ginseng provided robust working memory enhancement following administration, and that these effects were distinct from those of Asian ginseng, suggesting that psychopharmacological properties depend critically on ginsenoside profiles (Scholey et al., 2010).

A 4-week open-label study in children ($n = 36$) diagnosed with ADHD assessed the effects of adding BID dosing of a combination product containing American ginseng 200 mg and ginkgo 50 mg in addition to their usual medication. After 2 weeks of treatment, the proportion of the subjects exhibiting improvement ranged from 31% for the anxious-shy attribute to 67% for the psychosomatic attribute. After 4 weeks of treatment, the proportion of subjects exhibiting improvement ranged from 44% for the social problems attribute to 74% for the Conners' ADHD index and the *DSM-IV* hyperactive-impulsive attribute. The authors concluded that a combination of American ginseng plus ginkgo may improve symptoms of ADHD and that further research was warranted (Lyon et al., 2001).

Psychiatric Disorders: Schizophrenia

A 4-week RCT in patients ($n=64$) with schizophrenia compared an extract of American ginseng standardized to ginsenosides with placebo for effects on verbal working memory and visual working memory. Visual working memory was significantly improved in the treatment group, but not in the placebo group. Perhaps more importantly, extrapyramidal symptoms were significantly reduced after 4 weeks of treatment with the herb but not with placebo. The authors concluded that the standardized extract of American ginseng had potential as an adjunct therapy in schizophrenia, for improvement in working memory, and for reduction in medication-related side effects, and it had considerable potential to improve functional outcome (Chen et al., 2014).

Infectious Disease: Upper Respiratory Infection and Influenza

A 2011 systematic review of American ginseng for effect on URI included five trials ($n=747$). American ginseng preparations significantly reduced the total number of common colds by 25% compared with placebo. There was a tendency toward a lower incidence of having at least one URI in the ginseng group compared with the placebo group (five trials; RR=0.70). Compared with placebo, ginseng significantly shortened the duration of URIs by 6.2 days. The authors concluded that there was insufficient evidence to conclude that ginseng reduced the incidence or severity of common colds, but that American ginseng appeared to be effective in shortening the duration of colds or URIs in healthy adults when taken preventively for durations of 8–16 weeks (Seida et al., 2011).

A 4-month RCT in elderly community-dwelling adults ($n=43$) studied COLD-fX, an extract of American ginseng rich in poly-furanosyl-pyranosyl-saccharides, 200 mg BID compared with placebo in the

prevention of URIs. Subjects also received influenza vaccination 1 month into the trial. The frequency and duration of URIs during the first 2 months was similar between groups. In the final 2 months, 32% and 62% of subjects in the treatment and placebo groups, respectively, reported URIs. In addition, the duration of symptoms was shorter with American ginseng (5.6 days vs 12.6 days) (McElhaney et al., 2004).

A 4-month RCT in subjects ($n=323$) with a history of at least two colds in the previous year compared COLD-fX, a poly-furanosyl-pyranosyl-saccharide-rich extract of American ginseng, with placebo for effect on incidence of URIs. The mean number of colds per person was lower in the ginseng group than in the placebo group (0.68 vs 0.93). The proportion of subjects with two or more Jackson-verified colds during the 4-month period was significantly lower in the ginseng group (10% vs 23%) and the total symptom score was lower with ginseng (77 vs 112). The total number of days cold symptoms were reported was 10.8 and 16.5 days with ginseng and placebo, respectively. The authors concluded that the poly-furanosyl-pyranosyl-saccharide-rich extract of American ginseng reduced the mean number of colds and severity of symptoms (Predy et al., 2005).

A 6-month RCT in influenza-vaccinated community-dwelling adults ($n=783$) compared CVT-E002 (a proprietary extract of American ginseng) 400 mg or 800 mg with placebo for effect on URI incidence. The incidence of URIs was 5.5%, 5.2%, and 4.6% with placebo, 400 mg, and 800 mg, respectively ($P=0.89$). Jackson-confirmed URIs were significantly lower in the treated groups ($P<0.04$). The severity and duration of Jackson-confirmed URIs was also lower in the treatment groups. The authors concluded that this extract of American ginseng may prevent symptoms of URIs and could be safely used (McElhaney et al., 2006).

An 8-week and a 12-week RCT in institutionalized elderly patients ($n=196$) compared a standardized extract of American ginseng 200 mg BID with placebo for effect on acute respiratory illness due to either influenza or RSV during the 2000 and 2001 influenza seasons. Analysis revealed that the incidence of laboratory-confirmed influenza illness was greater with placebo than with the herb (7% vs 1%; OR: 7.73; $P=0.033$). Combined data for influenza and RSV illness were also greater with placebo than with the herb (9% vs 1%; OR: 10.5; $P=0.009$), for an overall 89%

relative risk reduction of acute respiratory illness with standardized American ginseng extract. The author concluded that the standardized extract of American ginseng was potentially effective for preventing acute respiratory illness due to influenza and RSV (McElhaney et al., 2011).

Oncologic Disorders: Cancer-Related Fatigue

An 8-week RCT in fatigued cancer survivors (*n* = 364) compared American ginseng 2 g/day with placebo for effect on fatigue. Changes from baseline in the general subscale of the Multidimensional Fatigue Symptom Inventory-Short Form were 14.4 and 20 in the ginseng arm and 8.2 and 10.3 in the placebo arm at 4 weeks and 8 weeks, respectively (*P* = 0.07 and *P* = 0.003, respectively). Greater benefit was reported in patients receiving active cancer treatment compared with those who had completed treatment. There were no discernible toxicities associated with the treatment. The authors concluded that American ginseng 2 g/day may be of benefit for cancer-related fatigue and that there were no discernible toxicities associated with the treatment (Barton et al., 2013).

ACTIVE CONSTITUENTS: ASIAN GINSENG

Root

- Carbohydrates
  - Oligosaccharides
  - Polysaccharides (immune stimulating, antineoplastic): β-glucans, ginsenan PA, ginseng acidic polysaccharide (inhibits *H. pylori* adhesion)
  - Organic acids: acetic acid
- Lipids
  - Fatty acids: linolenic acid
  - Polyacetylenes (antineoplastic, immunomodulatory, anti-inflammatory): ginsenoynes A-K, falcarinol, falcarintriol panaxydol, panaxytriol (anti-5HT-3A receptor), panaxynol
- Amino acid derivatives
  - Peptidoglycan: panaxans (hypotensive)
  - Amino acids: arginine
  - Amines
    □ Methylxanthines: caffeine, theophylline, theobromine

- Terpenes
  - Sesquiterpenes: B-elemene, panasinsanol A and B, and ginsenol
  - Triterpenes: oleanolic acid (chemoprotective, hepatoprotective), panaxadial, panaxans, panaxatriol
  - Steroidal saponins (corticosteroid-like action; antiallergic; bronchorelaxant; coronary vasodilating; hepatoprotective; GABA, NE, dopamine, glutamate, and serotonin reuptake inhibition; CNS depressant; neuroregenerative, analgesic; increase cellular and humoral immunity; hematopoietic; angiogenic; antineoplastic; some vasoconstrict and others vasodilate, some increase cardiac contractility and others decrease cardiac contractility; some are hemostatic and others are anticoagulant, some are CNS stimulant and others are CNS depressant): 40 distinct ginsenosides that vary in quantity between white and red ginseng, including ginsenosides F1, F2, F3, R0, Ra1, Ra2, Rb1 (anti-neovascular, anticonvulsant, analgesic, tranquilizing, hypotensive, anti-ulcer, vulnerary, anti-inflammatory), Rb2 (vulnerary), Rb3, Rc, Rd, Rd2, Re, Rf, Rg1 (immunostimulant), Rg2, Rg3, Rh1, Rh2, Rh3, Rs3, Rs4, Ia, Re, notoginsenoside-Fe, notoginsenoside R1 (fibrinolytic), ginpanaxosides. *Panax ginseng has much higher amounts of Rg1 than American ginseng, which has more Rb1. Rg1 and Rb1 are thought to have opposing pharmacological roles. Rg1 is thought to be a slight central nervous system stimulant, hypertensive, anti-fatigue agent, anabolic (stimulates DNA, protein, and lipid synthesis), and mental acuity and intellectual performance enhancer.*

ACTIVE CONSTITUENTS: AMERICAN GINSENG

Root

- Carbohydrates
  - Polysaccharides: poly-furanosyl-pyranosyl-saccharides
- Lipids
  - Polyacetylenes (immunomodulatory, anti-inflammatory): panaxynol, falcarindiol, panasydol, panaxytriol

- Amino acid derivatives
  - Protein: quinquerginsin
- Terpenes
  - Triterpenes
    - Steroidal saponins: ginsenosides Rb1 (higher amounts than in KRG, anti-neovascular, anti-convulsant, analgesic, tranquilizing, hypotensive, anti-ulcer, vulnerary, anti-inflammatory), Rb 2, Rc, Rd, Re, Ro, Rg1 (stimulates humoral and cell-mediated immunity, increases T helper cells, T lymphocytes, NK cells); Metabolite Compound K (antiproliferative), mRb1, mRb2, mRc, mRd, quinquenosides I-V, pseudoginsenoside F11

GINSENGS COMMONLY USED PREPARATIONS AND DOSAGE (FOR ADULTS UNLESS OTHERWISE SPECIFIED)

The following are examples of some available formulations and ranges of dosing for commercial herbal products. See Part III Introduction "How to prescribe medicinal herbs" for further guidance on herbal advising and prescribing.

Ginsengs are best taken earlier in day. For long-term maintenance, use lower dosage range and take in pulsed schedule (for example 2-3 weeks on and 1-2 weeks off.) German Commission E stated that Asian ginseng could be used up to 3 months, with repeated courses of treatment if needed. Conversely, it is generally recommended that American ginseng be taken for long periods of time for efficacy.

Asian/Korean/Chinese Ginseng Root

- Decoction of dried root: 1/2 tsp per cup TID
- Tincture of root (1:5, 60%): 1–3 mL TID
- Fluid extract (1:2 concentration) from crude root: 1–6 mL QD
- Powdered root extract: 1 g (1/3 tsp) QD-BID
- Capsule or tablet of powdered root extract: 500–1000 mg QD-TID
- Capsule or tablet of standardized root extract (standardized to 4%-7% ginsenosides): 250–525 mg QD-BID at breakfast and lunch

American Ginseng Root

- Decoction of dried root: 1–3 g per cup
- Tincture of root (1:5, 50%): 3–5 mL TID

- Powdered root extract: 1 g (1/3 tsp) QD-BID
- Capsule or tablet of powdered root extract: 1–3 g per day
- Capsule or tablet of standardized root extract (standardized to 5%–9% ginsenosides): 200–500 mg BID

In non-diabetics, American ginseng should be taken with meals rather than before meals to avoid postprandial hypoglycemia.

SAFETY AND PRECAUTION FOR THE GINSENGS

Side Effects

Variable and questionable reports of dry mouth, nosebleed, tachycardia, nausea, vomiting, diarrhea, insomnia, restlessness, and anxiety have been reported. Asian ginseng may increase BP in some individuals, so caution is advised. However, a 2014 meta-analysis of the effects of Asian ginseng on BP concluded, "No significant effect of ginseng on SBP, DBP and MAP was found. Stratified analysis, although not significant, appears to favor SBP improvement in diabetes, metabolic syndrome and obesity." American ginseng may cause hypoglycemia in non-diabetics if taken between meals.

Case Reports

Precipitation of mania, male gynecomastia, and oro-buco-lingual dyskinesia have been reported in isolated cases.

Large doses (3–9 g) of Asian ginseng have been associated with disturbance in accommodation and dizziness.

A 41-year-old man taking an herbal combination of tribulus, oat, and Asian ginseng was hospitalized with massive pulmonary embolism. The same combination was associated with three case reports of acute coronary syndrome.

Toxicity

No acute or chronic toxicity has been found with Asian ginseng, per the World Health Organization (WHO). A systematic review found a low incidence of harm with Asian ginseng. Dosage of 4.5 g for 12 weeks showed lack of toxicity.

Pregnancy and Lactation

Despite a long history of safe use in traditional Chinese medicine during pregnancy and lactation, there is insufficient human safety data. Althogh ginsenosides Rb1, Rg1 and Re have demonstrated embryotoxic and teratogenic effects in rodent whole embryo cultures, in vivo animal data are reassuring.

Disease Interactions

- Avoid in the perioperative period
- Use with caution in patients with bipolar disorder or anxiety
- Avoid in patients with estrogen sensitive cancer Caution in patients with hypertension

Drug Interactions

- CYP: Induces CYP3A4
- American ginseng decreases the anticoagulant effects of warfarin
- May augment effects of hypoglycemic agents
- Avoid with MAO inhibitors
- May increase risk of hepatotoxicity with imatinib
- May increase drug levels of raltegravir Caution with digoxin

An RCT in healthy volunteers ($n = 25$) assessed the anticoagulant effects of three herbs, turmeric, Asian ginseng, and dong quai, compared with aspirin alone or aspirin plus the herbal product in 3-week phases with 2-week washouts. PT/APTT, platelet function by light transmission aggregometry, and thrombin generation assay by calibrated automated thrombogram were measured at baseline and after each phase. Inhibition of arachidonic-acid induced platelet aggregation occurred in 5/24 turmeric subjects, 2/24 dong quai subjects, and 1/23 ginseng subjects. Beyond that, there was no clinically relevant impact on platelet and coagulation function. Combination of these herbal products with aspirin, respectively, did not further aggravate platelet inhibition caused by aspirin. None of the herbs impaired PT/APTT or thrombin generation. There was no significant bleeding manifestation. The authors concluded that there was good evidence for lack of bleeding risks with turmeric, dong quai, and Asian ginseng either alone or in combination with aspirin (Fung et al., 2017).

REFERENCES

Asian Ginseng

Al-Kuraishy HM, Al-Gareeb AI. Eustress and malondialdehyde (MDA): role of panax ginseng: randomized placebo controlled study. Iran J Psychiatry 2017;12(3):194–200.

Arring NM, Millstine D, Marks LA, Nail LM. Ginseng as a treatment for fatigue: a systematic review. J Altern Complement Med 2018;24(7):624–33.

Bach HV, Kim J, Myung S-K, Cho YA. Efficacy of ginseng supplements on fatigue and physical performance: a meta-analysis. J Korean Med Sci 2016;31(12):1879–86.

Bae HW, Kim JH, Kim S, et al. Effect of Korean Red Ginseng supplementation on dry eye syndrome in glaucoma patients—a randomized, double-blind, placebo-controlled study. J Ginseng Res 2015;39(1):7–13.

Borrelli F, Colalto C, Delfino DV, Iriti M, Izzo AA. Herbal dietary supplements for erectile dysfunction: a systematic review and meta-analysis. Drugs 2018;78(6):643–73.

Braz AS, Morais LC, Paula AP, Diniz MF, Almeida RN. Effects of Panax ginseng extract in patients with fibromyalgia: a 12-week, randomized, double-blind, placebo-controlled trial. Braz J Psychiatry 2013;35(1):21–8.

Caldwell LK, DuPont WH, Beeler MK, et al. The effects of a Asian ginseng, GINST15, on perceptual effort, psychomotor performance, and physical performance in men and women. J Sports Sci Med 2018;17(1):92–100.

Caron MF, Hotsko AL, Robertson S, Mandybur L, Kluger J, White CM. Electrocardiographic and hemodynamic effects of Panax ginseng. Ann Pharmacother 2002;36(5):758–63.

Chen M, May BH, Zhou IW, Xue CC, Zhang AL. FOLFOX 4 combined with herbal medicine for advanced colorectal cancer: a systematic review. Phytother Res 2014;28(7):976–91.

Chen MH, May BH, Zhou IW, Zhang AL, Xue CC. Integrative medicine for relief of nausea and vomiting in the treatment of colorectal cancer using oxaliplatin-based chemotherapy: a systematic review and meta-analysis. Phytother Res 2016;30(5):741–53.

Cho YK, et al. Long-term intake of Korean red ginseng in HIV-1-infected patients: development of resistance mutation to zidovudine is delayed. Int Immunopharmacol 2001;1:1295–305.

Cho YJ, Son HJ, Kim KS. A 14-week randomized, placebo-controlled, double-blind clinical trial to evaluate the efficacy and safety of ginseng polysaccharide (Y-75). J Transl Med 2014;12:283.

Cho YK, Kim JE, Woo JH. Genetic defects in the *nef* gene are associated with Korean Red Ginseng intake: monitoring of *nef* sequence polymorphisms over 20 years. J Ginseng Res 2017;41(2):144–50.

Choi HK, Seong DH, Rha KH. Clinical efficacy of Korean red ginseng for erectile dysfunction. Int J Impot Res 1995;7(3):181–6.

Choi HS, Kim S, Kim MJ, et al. Efficacy and safety of *Panax ginseng* berry extract on glycemic control: a 12-wk randomized, double-blind, and placebo-controlled clinical trial. J Ginseng Res 2018;42(1):90–7.

Cui Y, Shu XO, Gao YT, et al. Association of ginseng use with survival and quality of life among breast cancer patients. Am J Epidemiol 2006;163:645–53.

de Andrade E, de Mesquita AA, Claro Jde A, et al. Study of the efficacy of Korean red ginseng in the treatment of erectile dysfunction. Asian J Androl 2007;9(2):241–4.

De Souza LR, Jenkins AL, Jovanovski E, Rahelić D, Vuksan V. Ethanol extraction preparation of American ginseng (Panax quinquefolius L) and Korean red ginseng (Panax ginseng C.A. Meyer): differential effects on postprandial insulinemia in healthy individuals. J Ethnopharmacol 2015;159:55–61.

Ding DZ, Shen TK, Cui YZ. Effects of red ginseng on the congestive heart failure and its mechanism. Zhongguo Zhong Xi Yi Jie He Za Zhi 1995;15(6):325–7.

Dong QT, Zhang XD, Yu Z. Integrated Chinese and Western medical treatment on postoperative fatigue syndrome in patients with gastric cancer. Zhongguo Zhong Xi Yi Jie He Za Zhi 2010;30(10):1036–40.

Engelberg D, McCutcheon A, Wiseman S. A case of ginseng-induced mania. J Clin Psychopharmacol 2001;21:535–6.

Farzaei MH, Shahpiri Z, Bahramsoltani R, Nia MM, Najafi F, Rahimi R. Efficacy and tolerability of phytomedicines in multiple sclerosis patients: a review. CNS Drugs 2017;31(10):867–89.

Flanagan SD, DuPont WH, Caldwell LK, et al. The effects of a Asian ginseng, GINST15, on hypo-pituitary-adrenal and oxidative activity induced by intense work stress. J Med Food 2018;21(1):104–12.

Fung FY, Wong WH, Ang SK, et al. A randomized, double-blind, placebo-controlled study on the anti-haemostatic effects of Curcuma longa, Angelica sinensis and Panax ginseng. Phytomedicine 2017;32:88–96.

Geller SE, Studee L. Botanical and dietary supplements for mood and anxiety in menopausal women. Menopause 2007;14(3 Pt 1):541–9.

Ghorbani Z, Mirghafourvand M, Charandabi SM, Javadzadeh Y. The effect of ginseng on sexual dysfunction in menopausal women: a double-blind, randomized, controlled trial. Complement Ther Med 2019;45:57–64.

He BC, Gao JL, Luo X, et al. Ginsenoside Rg3 inhibits colorectal tumor growth through the down-regulation of Wnt/ß-catenin signaling. Int J Oncol 2011;38(2):437–45.

He Y, Yang J, Lv Y, et al. A review of ginseng clinical trials registered in the WHO International Clinical Trials Registry Platform. Biomed Res Int 2018;2018:1843142.

Heo JH, Lee ST, Chu K, et al. An open-label trial of Korean red ginseng as an adjuvant treatment for cognitive impairment in patients with Alzheimer's disease. Eur J Neurol 2008;15(8):865–8.

Heo JH, Lee ST, Chu K, Oh MJ, Park HJ, Shim JY. Improvement of cognitive deficit in Alzheimer's disease patients by long term treatment with Korean red ginseng. J Ginseng Res 2011;35(4):457–61.

Hong B, Ji YH, Hong JH, et al. A double-blind crossover study evaluating the efficacy of Korean red ginseng in patients with erectile dysfunction: a preliminary report. J Urol 2002;168:2070–3.

Huntley AL, Ernst E. A systematic review of herbal medicinal products for the treatment of menopausal symptoms. Menopause 2003;10(5):465–76.

Hwang E, Park SY, Jo H, et al. Efficacy and safety of enzyme-modified panax ginseng for anti-wrinkle therapy in healthy skin: A Single-Center, Randomized, Double-Blind, Placebo-Controlled Study. Rejuvenation Res 2015;18(5):449–57.

Jayawardena R, Thejani T, Ranasinghe P, Fernando D, Verster JC. Interventions for treatment and/or prevention of alcohol hangover: systematic review. Hum Psychopharmacol 2017;32(5).

Jovanovski E, Bateman EA, Bhardwaj J, et al. Effect of Rg3-enriched Korean red ginseng (Panax ginseng) on arterial stiffness and BP in healthy individuals: a randomized controlled trial. J Am Soc Hypertens 2014a;8(8):537–41.

Jovanovski E, Peeva V, Sievenpiper JL, et al. Modulation of endothelial function by Korean red ginseng (Panax ginseng C.A. Meyer) and its components in healthy individuals: a randomized controlled trial. Cardiovasc Ther 2014b;32(4):163–9.

Jovanovski E, Lea-Duvnjak-Smircic, Komishon A, et al. Vascular effects of combined enriched Korean Red ginseng (Panax Ginseng) and American ginseng (Panax quinquefolius) administration in individuals with hypertension and type 2 diabetes: A randomized controlled trial. Complement Ther Med 2020;49:102338.

Kang JH, Song KH, Woo JK, et al. Ginsenoside Rp1 from Panax ginseng exhibits anticancer activity by down-regulation of the IGF-1R/Akt pathway in breast cancer cells. Plant Foods Hum Nutr 2011;12.

Kargozar R, Azizi H, Salari R. A review of effective herbal medicines in controlling menopausal symptoms. Electron Phys 2017;9(11):5826–33.

Kennedy DO, Haskell CF, Wesnes KA, Scholey AB. Improved cognitive performance in human volunteers following administration of guarana (Paullinia cupana) extract: comparison and interaction with Panax ginseng. Pharmacol Biochem Behav 2004;79(3):401–11.

Kim HG, Cho JH, Yoo SR, et al. Antifatigue effects of Panax ginseng C.A. Meyer: a randomised, double-blind, placebo-controlled trial. PLoS One 2013a;8(4), e61271.

Kim M-S, Lim H-J, Yang HJ, Lee MS, Shin B-C, Ernst E. Ginseng for managing menopause symptoms: a systematic review of randomized clinical trials. J Ginseng Res 2013b;37(1):30–6.

Kim HS, Kim MK, Lee M, Kwon BS, Suh DH, Song YS. Effect of red ginseng on genotoxicity and health-related quality of life after adjuvant chemotherapy in patients with epithelial ovarian cancer: a randomized, double blind, placebo-controlled trial. Nutrients 2017;9(7). pii: E772.

Kim JW, Han SW, Cho JY, et al. Korean red ginseng for cancer-related fatigue in colorectal cancer patients with chemotherapy: a randomised phase III trial. Eur J Cancer 2020;130:51–62.

Lee Y, Jin Y, Lim W, et al. A ginsenoside-Rh1, a component of ginseng saponin, activates estrogen receptor in human breast carcinoma MCF-7 cells. J Steroid Biochem Mol Biol 2003;84(4):463–8.

Lee JM, Hah JO, Kim HS. The effect of red ginseng extract on inflammatory cytokines after chemotherapy in children. J Ginseng Res 2012;36(4):383–90.

Lee HW, Choi J, Lee Y, Kil KJ, Lee MS. Ginseng for managing menopausal woman's health: a systematic review of double-blind, randomized, placebo-controlled trials. Medicine (Baltimore) 2016a;95(38), e4914.

Lee NH, Jung HC, Lee S. Red ginseng as an ergogenic aid: a systematic review of clinical trials. J Exerc Nutrition Biochem 2016b;20(4):13–9.

Lee HW, Lim HJ, Jun JH, Choi J, Lee MS. Ginseng for treating HTN: a systematic review and meta-analysis of double blind, randomized, placebo-controlled trials. Curr Vasc Pharmacol 2017;15(6):549–56.

Lee ES, Yang YJ, Lee JH, Yoon YS. Effect of high-dose ginsenoside complex (UG0712) supplementation on physical performance of healthy adults during a 12-week supervised exercise program: A randomized placebo-controlled clinical trial. J Ginseng Res 2018;42(2):192–8.

Liao JZ, Chen JJ, Wu ZM, et al. Clinical and experimental studies of coronary heart disease treated with yi-qi huo-xue injection. J Tradit Chin Med 1989;9(3):193–8.

Lo LC, Chen CY, Chen ST, Chen HC, Lee TC, Chang CS. Therapeutic efficacy of traditional Chinese medicine, Shen-Mai San, in cancer patients undergoing chemotherapy or radiotherapy: study protocol for a randomized, double-blind, placebo-controlled trial. Trials 2012;13:232.

Ma SW, Benzie IF, Chu TT, et al. Effect of Panax ginseng supplementation on biomarkers of glucose tolerance, antioxidant status and oxidative stress in type 2 diabetic subjects: results of a placebo-controlled human intervention trial. Diabetes Obes Metab 2008;18.

Mkrtchyan A, Panosyan V, Panossian A, Wikman G, Wagner H. A phase I clinical study of Andrographis paniculata fixed combination Kan Jang versus ginseng and valerian on the semen quality of healthy male subjects. Phytomedicine 2005;12(6-7):403–9.

Naghavi Moghadam AA, Shiravand M, Rezapour S, Khoshdel A, Bazgir B, Mardani M. Effect of a session of intensive exercise withginsengsupplementation on histone H3 protein methylation of skeletal muscle of nonathlete men. Mol Genet Genomic Med 2019;7(5), e651.

Nah JJ, Hahn JH, Chung S, et al. Effect of ginsenosides, active components of ginseng, on capsaicin-induced pain-related behavior. Neuropharmacology 2000;39:2180–4.

Najafi NM, Ghazanfarpour M. Effect of phytoestrogens on sexual function in menopausal women: a systematic review and meta-analysis. Climacteric 2018;21(5):437–45.

Nakamura K, Goto Y, Sazuka T, Imamura Y, Komiya A, Ichikawa T. Koujin powder (red ginseng powder) with ninjin-youeito for fatigue due to targeted therapy for advanced renal cell carcinoma: a retrospective cohort study. Nihon Hinyokika Gakkai Zasshi 2017;108(4):194–9.

Neale C, Camfield D, Reay J, Stough C, Scholey A. Cognitive effects of 2 nutraceuticals Ginseng and Bacopa benchmarked against modafinil: a review and comparison of effect sizes. Br J Clin Pharmacol 2013;75(3):728–37.

Norelli LJ, Xu C. Manic psychosis associated with ginseng: a report of 2 cases and discussion of the literature. J Diet Suppl 2014;1.

Oh GN, Son SW. Efficacy of Korean red ginseng in the treatment of alopecia areata. J Ginseng Res 2012;36(4):391–5.

Park KS, Park KI, Kim JW, et al. Efficacy and safety of Korean red ginseng for cold hypersensitivity in the hands and feet: a randomized, double-blind, placebo-controlled trial. J Ethnopharmacol 2014a;158(Pt A):25–32.

Park SH, Oh MR, Choi EK, et al. An 8-wk, randomized, double-blind, placebo-controlled clinical trial for the antidiabetic effects of hydrolyzed ginseng extract. J Ginseng Res 2014b;38(4):239–43.

Park HJ, Choe S, Park NC. Effects of Korean red ginseng on semen parameters in male infertility patients: a randomized, placebo-controlled, double-blind clinical study. Chin J Integr Med 2016;22(7):490–5.

Reay JL, Kennedy DO, Scholey AB. Single doses of Panax ginseng (G115) reduce blood glucose levels and improve cognitive performance during sustained mental activity. J Psychopharmacol 2005;19:357–65.

Reay JL, van Schaik P, Wilson CJ. A systematic review of research investigating the physiological and psychological effects of combining Ginkgo biloba and Panax ginseng into a single treatment in humans: implications for research design and analysis. Brain Behav 2019;9(3), e01217.

Saboori S, Falahi E, Yousefi Rad E, Asbaghi O, Khosroshahi MZ. Effects of ginsengon C-reactive protein level: a systematic review and meta-analysis of clinical trials. Complement Ther Med 2019;45:98–103.

Scaglione F, Cattaneo G, Alessandria M, Cogo R. Efficacy and safety of the standardised Ginseng extract G115 for potentiating vaccination against the influenza syndrome and protection against the common cold [corrected]. Drugs Exp Clin Res 1996;22(2):65–72.

Shah SA, Occiano A, Nguyen TA, et al. Electrocardiographic and BP effects of energy drinks and Panax ginseng in healthy volunteers: a randomized clinical trial. Int J Cardiol 2016;218:318–23.

Shin HR, Kim JY, Yun TK, et al. The cancer-preventive potential of Panax ginseng: a review of human and experimental evidence. Cancer Causes Control 2000;11:565–76 [review].

Shishtar E, Sievenpiper JL, Djedovic V, et al. The effect of ginseng (The Genus *Panax*) on glycemic control: a systematic review and meta-analysis of randomized controlled clinical trials. PLoS One 2014;9(9), e107391.

Song MY, Kim BS, Kim H. Influence of Panax ginseng on obesity and gut microbiota in obese middle-aged Korean women. J Ginseng Res 2014;38(2):106–15.

Sotaniemi EA, Haapakoski E, Rautio A. Ginseng therapy in non-insulin-dependent diabetic patients. Diabetes Care 1995;18:1373–5.

Souza M, Costa K, Vitorino PA, Bueno NB, Menezes PL. Effect of antioxidant supplementation on the auditory threshold in sensorineural hearing loss: a meta-analysis. Braz J Otorhinolaryngol 2018;84(3):368–80.

Teves MA, Wright JE, Welch MJ, et al. Effects of ginseng on repeated bouts of exhaustive exercise. Med Sci Sports Exerc 1983;15:162.

Vuksan V, Sung MK, Sievenpiper JL, et al. Korean red ginseng (Panax ginseng) improves glucose and insulin regulation in well-controlled, type 2 diabetes: results of a randomized, double-blind, placebo-controlled study of efficacy and safety. Nutr Metab Cardiovasc Dis 2008;18(1):46–56.

Wang Y, Yang G, Gong J, et al. Ginseng for Alzheimer's disease: a systematic review and meta-analysis of randomized controlled trials. Curr Top Med Chem 2016;16(5):529–36.

Wang J, Li G, Yu L, Mo T, Wu Q, Zhou Z. Aidi injection plus platinum-based chemotherapy for stage IIIB/IV non-small cell lung cancer: a meta-analysis of 42 RCTs following the PRISMA guidelines. J Ethnopharmacol 2018;221:137–50.

Wei H, Wu H, Yu W, Yan X, Zhang X. Shenfu decoction as adjuvant therapy for improving quality of life and hepatic dysfunction in patients with symptomatic chronic heart failure. J Ethnopharmacol 2015;169:347–55.

Xian S, Yang Z, Lee J, et al. A randomized, double-blind, multicenter, placebo-controlled clinical study on the efficacy and safety of Shenmai injection in patients with chronic heart failure. J Ethnopharmacol 2016;186:136–42.

Yakoot M, Salem A, Helmy S. Effect of Memo*, a natural formula combination, on Mini-Mental State Examination scores in patients with mild cognitive impairment. Clin Interv Aging 2013;8:975–81.

Yan B, Liu Y, Shi A, et al. Investigation of the antifatigue effects of asian ginseng on professional athletes by gas chromatography-time-of-flight-mass spectrometry-based metabolomics. J AOAC Int 2018;101(3):701–7.

Yennurajalingam S, Tannir NM, Williams JL, et al. A double-blind, randomized, placebo-controlled trial of Panax ginseng for cancer-related fatigue in patients with advanced cancer. J Natl Compr Canc Netw 2017;15(9):1111–20.

Yun TK, Choi SY. Preventive effect of ginseng intake against various human cancers: a case-control study on 1987 pairs. Cancer Epidemiol Biomarkers Prev 1995;4:401–8.

Yun TK, Choi SY. Non-organ specific cancer prevention of ginseng: a prospective study in Korea. Int J Epidemiol 1998;27:359–64.

Zhang Y, Wang XQ, Liu H, Liu J, Hou W, Lin HS. A multicenter, large-sample, randomized clinical trial on improving the median survival time of advanced non-small cell lung cancer by combination of Ginseng Rg3 and chemotherapy. Zhonghua Zhong Liu Za Zhi 2018;40(4):295–9.

Zheng H, Chen Y, Chen J, Kwong J, Xiong W. Shengmai (a traditional Chinese herbal medicine) for heart failure. Cochrane Database Syst Rev 2011;2, CD005052.

Ziaei R, Ghavami A, Ghaedi E, Hadi A, Javadian P, Clark CCT. The efficacy of ginsengsupplementation on plasma lipid concentration in adults: a systematic review and meta-analysis. Complement Ther Med 2020;48:102239.

American Ginseng

Attele AS, Wu JA, Yuan CS. Ginseng pharmacology: multiple constituents and multiple actions. Biochem Pharmacol 1999;58:1685–93.

Barton DL, Liu H, Dakhil SR, et al. Wisconsin Ginseng (Panax quinquefolius) to improve cancer-related fatigue: a randomized, double-blind trial, N07C2. J Natl Cancer Inst 2013;105(16):1230–8.

Chen EY, Hui CL. HT1001, a proprietary North American ginseng extract, improves working memory in schizophrenia: a double-blind, placebo-controlled study. Phytother Res 2012;26(8):1166–72.

High KP, Case D, Hurd D, et al. A randomized, controlled trial of Panax quinquefolius extract (CVT-E002) to reduce respiratory infection in patients with chronic lymphocytic leukemia. J Support Oncol 2012;10(5):195–201.

Li XL, Wang CZ, Sun S, et al. American ginseng berry enhances chemopreventive effect of 5-FU on human colorectal cancer cells. Oncol Rep 2009;22(4):943–52.

Li B, Wang CZ, He TC, et al. Antioxidants potentiate American ginseng-induced killing of colorectal cancer cells. Cancer Letters 2010;289(1):62–70.

Li B, Zhao J, Wang CZ, et al. Ginsenoside Rh2 induces apoptosis and paraptosis-like cell death in colorectal cancer cells through activation of p53. Cancer Lett 2011;301(2):185–92.

Lyon MR, Cline JC, Totosy de Zepetnek J, Shan JJ, Pang P, Benishin C. Effect of the herbal extract combination Panax quinquefolium and Ginkgo biloba on attention-deficit hyperactivity disorder: a pilot study. J Psychiatry Neurosci 2001;26(3):221–8.

McElhaney JE, Gravenstein S, Cole SK, et al. A placebo-controlled trial of a proprietary extract of North American ginseng (CVT-E002) to prevent acute respiratory illness in institutionalized older adults. J Am Geriatr Soc 2004;52:13–9 [PubMed].

McElhaney JE, Goel V, Toane B, Hooten J, Shan JJ. Efficacy of COLD-fX in the prevention of respiratory symptoms in community-dwelling adults: a randomized, double-blinded, placebo-controlled trial. J Altern Complement Med 2006;12(2):153–7.

McElhaney JE, Simor AE, McNeil S, Predy GN. Efficacy and safety of CVT-E002, a proprietary extract of Panax quinquefolius in the prevention of respiratory infections in influenza-vaccinated community-dwelling adults: a multicenter, randomized, double-blind, and placebo-controlled trial. Influenza Res Treat 2011;2011:759051.

Mucalo I, Jovanovski E, Rahelić D, Božikov V, Romić Z, Vuksan V. Effect of American ginseng (Panax quinquefolius L.) on arterial stiffness in subjects with type-2 diabetes and concomitant HTN. J Ethnopharmacol 2013;150(1):148–53.

Mucalo I, Jovanovski E, Vuksan V, Božikov V, Romić Z, Rahelić D. American ginseng extract (Panax quinquefolius L.) is safe in long-term use in type 2 diabetic patients. Evid Based Complement Alternat Med 2014;2014:969168.

Ossoukhova A, Owen L, Savage K, et al. Improved working memory performance following administration of a single dose of American ginseng (Panax quinquefolius L.) to healthy middle-age adults. Hum Psychopharmacol 2015;30(2):108–22.

Predy GN, et al. Efficacy of an extract of North American ginseng containing poly-furanosyl-pyranosyl-saccharides for preventing upper respiratory tract infectons: a randomized controlled trial. CMAJ 2005;173(9):1043–8.

Rotem C, Kaplan B. Phyto-female complex for the relief of hot flushes, night sweats and quality of sleep: randomized, controlled, double-blind pilot study. Gynecol Endocrinol 2007;23(2):117–22.

Salvati G, Genovesi G, Marcellini L, et al. Effects of Panax Ginseng C.A. Meyer saponins on male fertility. Panminerva Med 1996;38(4):249–54.

Scholey A, Ossoukhova A, Owen L, et al. Effects of American ginseng (Panax quinquefolius) on neurocognitive function: an acute, randomised, double-blind, placebo-controlled, crossover study. Psychopharmacology (Berl) 2010;212(3):345–56.

Seida JK, Durec T, Kuhle S. North American (Panax quinquefolius) and Asian Ginseng (Panax ginseng) preparations for prevention of the common cold in healthy adults: a systematic review. Evid Based Complement Alternat Med 2011;282151.

Vuksan V, Sievenpiper JL, Koo VY, et al. American ginseng (Panax quinquefolius L) reduces postprandial glycemia in nondiabetic subjects and subjects with type 2 diabetes mellitus. Arch Intern Med 2000a;160(7):1009–13.

Vuksan V, Stavro MP, Sievenpiper JL, et al. Similar postprandial glycemic reductions with escalation of dose and administration time of American ginseng in type 2 diabetes. Diabetes Care 2000b;23(9):1221–6.

Vuksan V, Stavro MP, Sievenpiper JL, et al. American ginseng improves glycemia in individuals with normal glucose tolerance: effect of dose and time escalation. J Am Coll Nutr 2000c;19(6):738–44.

Vuksan V, Sievenpiper JL, Wong J, et al. American ginseng (Panax quinquefolius L.) attenuates postprandial glycemia in a time-dependent but not dose-dependent manner in healthy individuals. Am J Clin Nutr 2001;73(4):753–8.

Vuksan V, Xu ZZ, Jovanovski E, et al. Efficacy and safety of American ginseng (Panax quinquefolisu L.) extract on glycemic control and cardiovascular risk factors in individuals with type 2 diabetes: a double-blind, randomized, cross-over clinical trial. Eur J Nutr 2019;58(3):1237–45.

Yuan CS, et al. Brief Communication: American Ginseng reduces Warfarin's effect in healthy patients. Ann Intern Med 2004;141:23–7.

Zhang Y, Lu S, Liu YY. Effect of panax quinquefolius saponin on insulin sensitivity in patients of coronary heart disease with blood glucose abnormality. Zhongguo Zhong Xi Yi Jie He Za Zhi 2007;27(12):1066–9.

50

GOJI BERRY/WOLFBERRY (*LYCIUM BARBARUM*)
Fruit

GENERAL OVERVIEW

Goji berries are known for their potent antioxidant effects. However, their scope of potential benefits extends well beyond the subduing of free radicals. Goji has been used traditionally in Chinese medicine for dermatitis, myalgias, nose bleeds, and insomnia. Traditional Chinese medicine considers goji berries to have the ability to maintain eye health and tonify the liver, kidneys, and lungs via boosting and balancing yin and yang in the body.

Clinical research indicates that goji, alone or in combination formulas, may be beneficial for macular degeneration, dyslipidemia, metabolic syndrome, diabetes, vitality, hangover, immune function, and as an adjuvant to biological cancer therapy.

IN VITRO AND ANIMAL RESEARCH

In vitro and animal research have provided evidence for a wide array of potential benefits from goji berries (henceforth referred to simply as *goji*), particularly the polysaccharides. Goji has shown antioxidant, antiaging, antiinflammatory, antiviral, immunomodulating, retinal-protective, hepatoprotective, neuroprotective, antidiabetic, lipid-lowering, and anticancer properties. It is both radiosensitizing and photoprotective.

Goji polysaccharides have been shown to protect retinal ganglion cells in experimental models of glaucoma. Animal research has demonstrated that goji berries increase macular pigmentation, a surrogate marker for protection against macular degeneration.

Goji polysaccharides have shown hypoglycemic activity by increasing glucose metabolism, insulin secretion, and pancreatic β-cell proliferation and by reducing insulin resistance. Goji polysaccharide (LBP) has been shown to reduce insulin resistance in vitro through P13K/AKT signaling, which has been shown in vitro to induce phosphorylation of Nrf2, increase detoxification and antioxidant enzyme expression, reduce ROS levels, regulate phosphorylation levels of GSK3β and JNK, and reverse glycolytic and gluconeogenic gene expression via Nrf2. The polysaccharides have also demonstrated potential benefit in male reproduction by increasing the quality, quantity, and motility of sperm, improving sexual performance, and protecting the testis against toxic insults.

Several benefits of goji have been demonstrated in rat models for diabetes, stroke, and AD. The polysaccharides in goji have been shown to reduce the symptoms of mice with AD and to enhance neurogenesis in the hippocampus and subventricular zone, improving learning and memory abilities.

In vitro goji has been shown to inhibit growth of ER-positive breast cancer cells. The polysaccharides have been shown to inhibit the growth of leukemia HL-60 cells and increase expression of IL-2 and TNF-α. They also prevent cardiotoxicity from doxorubicin. In cervical cancer cells the polysaccharides have been shown to induce cell cycle arrest, increasing NO content, NOS, and iNOS activities, and inducing apoptosis through the mitochondrial pathway.

HUMAN RESEARCH

Ophthalmological Disorders

A 90-day RCT in elderly subjects ($n = 150$) compared goji milk containing 13.7 g/day of goji with placebo for effects on the macula. After 90 days, ophthalmic exams showed that the placebo group had hypopigmentation and soft drusen accumulation in the macula, whereas the goji group remained stable. Both plasma zeaxanthin level and antioxidant capacity increased significantly in the goji group, by 26% and 57%, respectively, but did not change in the placebo group. No adverse events were reported in either group. The authors concluded that daily dietary supplementation with goji berry increased plasma zeaxanthin and antioxidant levels and protected from hypopigmentation and soft drusen accumulation in the macula of elderly subjects. However, the mechanism of action was unclear, given the lack of relationship between change in plasma zeaxanthin and change in macular characteristics (Bucheli et al., 2011).

A 12-month RCT in patients ($n = 42$) with retinitis pigmentosa compared daily goji berry granules with placebo for effect on visual acuity (VA). At 12 months there were no deteriorations of either 90% or 10% contrast VA in the goji group compared with the placebo group ($P = 0.001$) and there was no thinning of the macular layer with goji, while thinning occurred with placebo ($P = 0.008$). No significant differences were found in the sensitivity of visual field or in any parameters of ffERG between the two groups. No significant adverse effects were reported in the treatment group. The authors concluded that goji berry supplementation provided a neuroprotective effect for the retina and could help delay or minimize cone degeneration in retinitis pigmentosa (Chan et al., 2007).

Cardiometabolic Disorders: Dyslipidemia, Metabolic Syndrome, and Diabetes

A 2018 systematic review of the effects of goji on cardiometabolic risk factors selected seven RCTs ($n = 548$) for review. In the meta-analysis, the pooled estimate showed that goji significantly reduced fasting glucose concentrations (-6.5 mg/dL) and marginally reduced concentrations of TC (-11.6 mg/dL; $P = 0.189$) and TG (-17.7 mg/dL; $P = 0.122$). No benefit was found in relation to bodyweight and blood pressure. The authors concluded that goji might have a favorable effect on glucose control (Guo et al., 2017).

An 8-week RCT in overweight subjects ($n = 53$) with hypercholesterolemia compared consumption of goji berry extract 13.5 g/day with placebo. After 8 weeks there was a slight but significant decrease in erythrocyte SOD activity and an increase in catalase activity, suggesting antioxidant activity. The authors concluded that goji intake had antioxidant and anti-inflammatory effects in overweight and hypercholesterolemic subjects by modulating mRNA expression (Lee et al., 2017).

A 3-month RCT in patients ($n = 67$) with T2DM compared goji polysaccharides 300 mg/day with placebo for metabolic effects. Serum glucose was found to be significantly decreased and the insulinogenic index increased with goji. The effect was more pronounced in the subjects who were not taking hypoglycemic medicine during the study. HDL-C levels were also increased in the goji group. The authors concluded that goji was a potential add-on treatment for T2DM (Cai et al., 2015).

A 14-day RCT in healthy subjects ($n = 29$) compared goji juice 120 mL/day with placebo for effects on metabolic rate, postprandial energy expenditure, waist circumference (WC), and other morphometric changes. The postprandial energy expenditure increased in the first 4 h postintake over baseline and was 10% higher in the goji group than in the placebo group at 1 h ($P < 0.05$). Goji was found to significantly decrease waist circumference from baseline by 5.5 cm compared with placebo (0.9 cm reduction; $P < 0.01$). The authors concluded that goji consumption increased metabolic rate and reduced WC, relative to placebo-treated subjects (Amagase and Nance, 2011).

A 45-day RCT in patients ($n = 50$) with metabolic syndrome evaluated goji berries 14 g/day plus a healthy diet compared with a healthy diet alone for metabolic effects. A significant reduction in transaminases as well as an improvement in lipid profile occurred in the goji group. WC also decreased significantly with the addition of goji compared with control. Increased glutathione and catalase levels and a reduction of lipid peroxidation also occurred in the goji group. The authors concluded that goji was an effective dietary supplement for the prevention of cardiovascular diseases in individuals with metabolic syndrome (de Souza Zanchet et al., 2017).

A 30-day RCT in healthy adults ($n = 50$) compared goji drink 120 mL/day with placebo for antioxidant effects. Antioxidant markers, consisting of serum levels of SOD, glutathione peroxidase, and MDA (indicative of lipid peroxidation) were examined pre- and post-intervention. In the goji group, SOD and glutathione peroxidase increased significantly by 8.4% and 9.9%, respectively. MDA levels were significantly decreased by 8.7%. The antioxidant markers improved insignificantly in the placebo group, and the difference between the improvements with goji and placebo was statistically significant. The authors concluded that goji increased antioxidant efficacies in humans by stimulating endogenous factors, and they suggested that continued use beyond 30 days might help prevent or reduce free radical-related conditions (Amagase et al., 2009a).

Disorders of Vitality: Vitality and Hangover

A 14-day RCT in healthy adults ($n = 34$) compared a goji beverage 120 mL/day (equivalent to 150 g of goji berries) with placebo on several health and well-being parameters. Between day 1 and day 14 the goji group demonstrated significant improvements in ratings for energy level, athletic performance, quality of sleep, ease of awakening, ability to focus on activities, mental acuity, calmness, and feelings of health, contentment, stress reduction, fatigue reduction, and happiness. In contrast, the placebo group showed only two significant changes: heartburn and happiness. The authors concluded that 14 days of goji increased subjective feelings of general well-being and improved neurologic/psychologic performance and gastrointestinal functions (Amagase and Nance, 2008).

A 30-day RCT in healthy adults ($n = 39$) compared goji juice with placebo for adrenal steroid response and fatigue after an exercise challenge. Relative to the placebo group, tiredness and overall health were significantly improved in the goji group. Cortisol, DHEA, and lactic acid levels were significantly increased by the exercise prior to supplementation with goji, but after 30 days of goji, increases in cortisol and DHEA levels were significantly attenuated. The authors concluded that goji attenuated the adrenal steroid response and reduced the feeling of tiredness after exercise (Amagase and Nance, 2012).

A crossover RCT in healthy nonsmoking adult men ($n = 20$) compared an herbal combination (including goji, eleuthero, *Viscum album*, and *Inonotus obliquus*) with placebo in hangover effect from drinking a bottle of Soju, which is a commercially available liquor (19% alcohol in 360 mL). Alcohol levels and antioxidant levels in the herbal group were significantly lower than in the control group at 2 h after the beverage consumption ($P < 0.05$, respectively), and acetaldehyde levels tended to be insignificantly lower in the herbal group. The author concluded that this herbal combination reduced oxidative stress and hangover by mitigating plasma alcohol concentrations and elevating antioxidant activity in healthy male adults (Hong, 2016).

Immune Function

A 3-month RCT in healthy elderly subjects ($n = 150$) compared a goji-milk beverage 13.7 g/day with placebo on the immune response to the influenza vaccination and general inflammatory and physical status. The subjects receiving goji milk had significantly higher postvaccination serum influenza-specific IgG levels and seroconversion rate, between days 30 and 90, compared with those receiving placebo. The herbal supplementation had no significant effect on delayed-type hypersensitivity response and inflammatory markers. No serious adverse reactions were reported during the trial. The authors concluded that long-term dietary supplementation with goji milk in elderly subjects enhanced their capacity to respond to antigenic challenges without overstimulating their immune system, supporting a contribution to reinforcing immune defense in this population (Vidal et al., 2012).

A 30-day RCT in healthy older adults ($n = 60$) studied a goji beverage 120 mL/day (equivalent to 150 g of fresh fruit) compared with placebo with respect to immune parameters. The goji group showed a statistically significant increase in the number of lymphocytes and levels of IL-2 and IgG compared with baseline and with the placebo group. The number of CD4, CD8, and NK cells and levels of IL-4 and IgA were not significantly altered. The placebo group showed no significant changes in any immune measures. In addition, the goji group showed a significant increase in general feelings of well-being, such as fatigue and sleep, and showed a tendency for increased short-term memory and focus between pre- and postintervention, while the placebo group showed no significant positive changes in these measures. The authors concluded that daily consumption of goji significantly increased several immunological responses and subjective feelings of general well-being without any adverse reactions (Amagase et al., 2009b).

Oncologic Disorders

An RCT in patients ($n = 79$) with advanced cancer compared treatment with goji polysaccharides plus LAK/IL-2 with LAK/IL-2 alone. The response rate of patients treated with LAK/IL-2 plus goji polysaccharides was 40.9%, while that of patients treated with LAK/IL-2 alone was 16.1% ($P < 0.05$). The objective regression of cancer was achieved in patients with malignant melanoma, renal cell carcinoma, colorectal carcinoma, lung cancer, nasopharyngeal carcinoma, and malignant hydrothorax. The mean remission in patients treated with LAK/IL-2 plus goji polysaccharides also lasted significantly longer. LAK/IL-2 plus goji polysaccharide treatment led to more marked increase in NK and LAK cell activity than LAK/IL-2 without goji. The authors concluded that goji could be used as an adjuvant in the biotherapy of cancer (Cao et al., 1994).

ACTIVE CONSTITUENTS

Berries

- Carbohydrates
  - Polysaccharides: *Lycium barbarum* polysaccharide (LBP) (antitumor, immune-enhancing, hypoglycemic, neuroprotective, radiosensitizing, hepatoprotective via NF-kB and MAPK, photoprotective)
  - Organic acids: Vitamin C (includes 2-O-β-D-glucopyranosyl-L-ascorbic acid)
- Lipids
  - Phospholipids: cerebroside
- Amino acid derivatives
  - Amino acids: betaine (gastric acidification)
- Phenolic compounds
  - Coumarins: scopoletin AKA chrysatropic acid (antiinflammatory, α-glucosidase inhibitor, AChE inhibitor, neuroprotective, antipsychotic, melanogenic, anticancer), escopoletin (anticancer), gelseminic acid, and scopoletol
- Terpenes
  - Tetraterpene/Carotenoids: zeaxanthin (antioxidant, macular pigment component) β-carotene, β-cryptoxanthin, mutatoxanthin

- Steroids
  - Phytosterols: β-sitosterol (reduces GI cholesterol absorption, inhibits 5-α-reductase), lanosterol, sigmasterol, cyclosterol, campesterol

GOJI BERRY COMMONLY USED PREPARATIONS AND DOSAGE (FOR ADULTS UNLESS OTHERWISE SPECIFIED)

The following are examples of some available formulations and ranges of dosing for commercial herbal products. See Part III Introduction "How to prescribe medicinal herbs" for further guidance on herbal advising and prescribing.

Berry

- Infusion of dried berries: 5–15 g per day.
- Whole dried berries: 15 g ingested daily.
- Goji juice: 120 mL daily.
- Goji juice powder: 8 g (one Tbsp) in smoothie QD.
- Capsule or tablet of powdered berry extract: 500–700 mg BID-QID.
- Capsule or tablet of standardized extract (standardized to 40% polysaccharides): 400–500 mg TID.

Best absorbed when formulated with hot milk.

A crossover comparison study in healthy volunteers ($n = 12$) looked at the bioavailability of zeaxanthin in goji berries from three different freeze-dried formulations: goji berries homogenized in hot nonfat milk, warm nonfat milk, or hot water. The triacylglycerol-rich lipoprotein zeaxanthin peaked at 6 h postingestion for all formulations. Mean area under the curve results were 9.73, 3.24, and 3.14 nmol × h/L for the hot milk, warm milk, and hot water formulations, respectively, indicating that zeaxanthin bioavailability from hot milk formulation is significantly greater ($P < 0.001$) (Benzie et al., 2006).

SAFETY AND PRECAUTION

Side Effects

Possible allergic reaction in sensitive individuals.

Case Reports

Systemic photosensitivity in 53-year-old man also taking cat's claw.

Anaphylactic reaction reported, cross-reactivity to tomato.

Pregnancy and Lactation

No data. Nutritional consumption of berries as part of diet (in moderation) likely safe.

Drug Interactions

- CYP: Induces CYP3A4.
- Possible increased INR with warfarin.

REFERENCES

Amagase H, Nance DM. A randomized, double-blind, placebo-controlled, clinical study of the general effects of a standardized Lycium barbarum (goji) juice, GoChi. J Altern Complement Med 2008 May;14(4):403–12.

Amagase H, Nance DM. Lycium barbarum increases caloric expenditure and decreases waist circumference in healthy overweight men and women: pilot study. J Am Coll Nutr 2011 Oct;30(5):304–9.

Amagase H, Nance DM. *Lycium barbarum* fruit (goji) attenuates the adrenal steroid response to an exercise challenge and the feeling of tiredness: a randomized, double-blind, placebo-controlled human clinical study. J Food Res 2012;1(2).

Amagase H, Sun B, Borek C. Lycium barbarum (goji) juice improves *in vivo* antioxidant biomarkers in serum of healthy adults. Nutr Res 2009a Jn;29(1):19–25.

Amagase H, Sun B, Nance DM. Immunomodulatory effects of a standardized Lycium barbarum fruit juice in Chinese older healthy human subjects. J Med Food 2009b Oct;12(5):1159–65.

Benzie IF, Chung WY, Wang J, Richelle M, Bucheli P. Enhanced bioavailability of zeaxanthin in a milk-based formulation of wolfberry (Gou qi Zi; Fructus barbarum L.). Br J Nutr 2006 Jul;96(1):154–60.

Bucheli P, Vidal K, Shen L, et al. Goji berry effects on macular characteristics and plasma antioxidant levels. Optom Vis Sci 2011 Feb;88(2):257–62.

Cai H, Liu F, Zuo P, et al. Practical application of antidiabetic efficacy of Lycium barbarum polysaccharide in patients with type 2 diabetes. Med Chem 2015;11(4):383–90.

Cao GW, Yang WG, Du P. Observation of the effects of LAK/IL-2 therapy combining with Lycium barbarum polysaccharides in the treatment of 75 cancer patients. Zhonghua Zhong Liu Za Zhi 1994 Nov;16(6):428–31.

Chan HC, Chang RC, Koon-Ching Ip A, et al. Neuroprotective effects of Lycium barbarum Lynn on protecting retinal ganglion cells in an ocular HTN model of glaucoma. Exp Neurol 2007;203(1):269–73.

de Souza Zanchet MZ, Nardi GM, Oliveira Souza Bratti L, Filippin-Monteiro FB, Locatelli C. *Lycium barbarum* reduces abdominal fat and improves lipid profile and antioxidant status in patients with metabolic syndrome. Oxid Med Cell Longev 2017;2017:9763210.

Guo XF, Li ZH, Cai H, Li D. The effects of Lycium barbarum L. (L. barbarum) on cardiometabolic risk factors: a meta-analysis of randomized controlled trials. Food Funct 2017 May 24;8(5):1741–8.

Hong YH. Effects of the herb mixture, DTS20, on oxidative stress and plasma alcoholic metabolites after alcohol consumption in healthy young men. Integr Med Res 2016 Dec;5(4):309–16.

Lee YJ, Ahn Y, Kwon O, et al. Dietary wolfberry extract modifies oxidative stress by controlling the expression of inflammatory mRNAs in overweight and hypercholesterolemic subjects: a randomized, double-blind, placebo-controlled trial. J Agric Food Chem 2017 Jan 18;65(2):309–16.

Vidal K, Bucheli P, Gao Q, et al. Immunomodulatory effects of dietary supplementation with a milk-based wolfberry formulation in healthy elderly: a randomized, double-blind, placebo-controlled trial. Rejuvenation Res 2012 Feb;15(1):89–97.

51

GYMNEMA/GURMAR (*GYMNEMA SYLVESTRE*)
Leaf

GENERAL OVERVIEW

As a natural therapy for hyperglycemia, gymnema occupies a unique position due to its evidence for use in type 1 diabetes as well as type 2 diabetes. The leaves have been used for more than 2000 years in India to treat "honey urine." Gymnema may act by enhancing insulin secretion through an increased number of pancreatic β-cells and through improved cell function. It also appears to reduce intestinal absorption of glucose, enhance tissue glucose uptake, and inhibit glycolysis. It has demonstrated other incretin-mimetic activity as well. Not only does it appear to lower blood glucose, but it has also been shown to reduce taste perception of sweetness and increase perception of bitterness (hence the Hindi name Gurmar or "sugar destroyer"), possibly leading to a decrease in consumption of simple carbohydrates. Evidence suggests that this effect varies among individuals.

There is also evidence suggesting possible efficacy of gymnema for dyslipidemia. Most of the studies have been of poor quality and were reported before the turn of the millennium. While the herb needs more high-quality evidence, it is a worthy blip on the clinician's radar.

Clinical research indicates that gymnema, alone or in combination formulas, may be beneficial for diabetes and weight gain.

IN VITRO AND ANIMAL RESEARCH

In vitro research has demonstrated that gymnema has antiinflammatory and antioxidant activity. In rats, gymnema reduced the level of lipid peroxidation by 32% in serum, 10% in the liver, and 9% in the kidney. The more acidic methanol extracts of gymnema demonstrate good activity toward a broad spectrum of pathogens including cariogenic bacteria, *Bacillus pumilus*, *B. subtilis*, *Pseudomona aeruginosa*, and *Staphylococcus aureus*.

Animal evidence indicates that gymnema may be useful for dyslipidemia and obesity. In a study on the effect of gymnema on lipids, rats in the control group that were fed a high-cholesterol diet showed increases in TC, TG, LDL-C, and VLDL-C and significant decreases in HDL-C, while the group administered gymnema at a dose of 200 mg/kg showed a significant reduction in the levels of all lipids with increases in HDL-C (Bishayee and Chatterjee, 1994). In a different study, rats given a hexane extract of gymnema leaves for 45 days showed a significant reduction in weight gain with improvements in TC, TG, LDL, and HDL levels (Shigematsu et al., 2001a).

Multiple animal studies have reported hypoglycemic effects associated with the ingestion of gymnema leaves. A study in streptozotocin-treated rats showed that gymnema caused regeneration of islet cells, promoted insulin secretion, and normalized blood glucose (Shanmugasundaram et al., 1990a). Other studies have demonstrated a reduction of glucose absorption from the intestine, improvement in uptake of glucose into cells, and prevention of adrenal hormones from stimulating hepatic gluconeogenesis. Another study in streptozotocin-treated mice showed that hepatic gluconeogenesis and ketogenesis returned to normal levels after the administration of an ethanolic leaf extract of gymnema. One active constituent, gymnemic acid IV, decreased blood glucose levels by 14%–60% within 6 h of administration compared with glibenclamide. It did not decrease BG in normal mice. Gymnemic acid IV also increased plasma insulin levels in that study (Sugihara et al., 2000).

Gymnema has also shown significant hepatoprotective effects against D-galactosamine-induced hepatotoxicity and wound healing properties in rats. A study on beryllium nitrate-treated rats showed that gymnema produced a slight increase in BW and protein, indicating protection against beryllium toxicity (Prakash et al., 1986).

Gymnema leaf water-soluble and petroleum ether extracts were found to be significantly effective in controlling inflammatory arthritis in rats. The tannins and saponins are mostly responsible for the antiinflammatory activity of the plant. In one rat study it was found that gymnema aqueous extract at a concentration of 300 mg/kg significantly decreased the paw edema volume by 48% within 4 h of administration, while phenylbutazone decreased the paw edema volume by 58% (Malik et al., 2008).

Gymnema has demonstrated some anticancer and immunostimulant activity. The saponin gymnemagenol has been shown to have direct inhibitory activity against *HeLa* cancer cell proliferation and was not toxic to the growth of normal cells under in vitro conditions. The aqueous leaf extract of gymnema showed robust immunostimulatory activity in human neutrophils in vitro.

HUMAN RESEARCH

Human evidence for gymnema is sparse and of poor quality, which is not to say the herb is not effective, but rather that more studies are desperately needed for this promising traditional herb.

Cardiometabolic Disorders: Diabetes

A 2009 review was undertaken to evaluate CAM interventions for glycemic control in T2DM. The main findings were that gymnema reduced A1C levels in two small open-label trials. In addition, researchers found that chromium reduced A1C and FBS in a large meta-analysis, cinnamon improved FBS but had unknown effects on A1C, and bitter melon had no effect in two small trials. Green tea and fenugreek each reduced FBS in one of three small trials. Vanadium reduced FBS in

small, uncontrolled trials. The authors concluded that chromium, and possibly gymnema, appeared to improve glycemic control (Nahas and Moher, 2009).

A 90-day open-label trial in patients ($n = 65$) with DM investigated the effect of gymnema extract (Beta Fast GXR) BID. After 90 days, the gymnema supplementation reduced mean daily preprandial plasma glucose concentrations by 11% (from 161 to 144 mg/dL), and the 2-h PPG was reduced by 13% (from 207 to 180 mg/dL). A1C was reduced from 8.8% to 8.2%. All measurements showed greater reductions in subjects whose baseline A1C was ≥ 9%. In addition, 11 patients (16%) had a decrease in prescription medicine intake. The authors concluded that gymnema supplementation in all patients with diabetes had a positive result, and in patients with the poorest control benefits were even greater (Joffe and Freed, 2001).

A 20-month open-label study in patients ($n = 22$) with T2DM and on conventional diabetic therapy investigated the effectiveness of GS4, an extract from the leaves of gymnema, 400 mg/day in addition to usual therapy compared with usual therapy alone (control). The average A1C decreased from 12% to 8.5%, and FBS decreased from 174 to 124 mg/dL with the addition of gymnema. TC and TG were reduced from 260 to 231 mg/dL and from 170 to 140 mg/dL, respectively, in the gymnema group ($P < 0.001$ for all). Insulin levels were increased. Five of the 22 subjects were able to discontinue their conventional drug and maintain their blood glucose homeostasis with the gymnema extract alone. The authors concluded that the β cells may be regenerated/repaired in T2DM patients on GS4 supplementation (Baskaran et al., 1990).

A 12-week RCT in patients ($n = 24$) with metabolic syndrome compared gymnema 300 mg BID with placebo. With gymnema there were significant decreases from baseline in body weight (from 81.3 to 77.9 kg, $P = 0.02$), BMI (from 31.2 to 30.4 kg/m^2, $P = 0.02$), and VLDL-C (from 0.45 to 0.35 mmol/dL, $P = 0.05$). The authors concluded that gymnema administration decreased BW, BMI, and VLDL levels in subjects with metabolic syndrome without changes in insulin secretion and insulin sensitivity (Zuñiga et al., 2017).

A 40-day RCT comparing three different herbs including gymnema was carried out on patients ($n = 32$) with T2DM. The groups were divided to receive capsules of gymnema 500 mg, *Citrullus colocynthis*, *Artemisia absinthium*, or placebo BID for 30 days. Glucose reductions for gymnema, *Citrullus*, and *Artemisia* were 37%, 35%, and 32%, respectively ($P < 0.05$ for all). The reductions reversed after discontinuation of the herbs. LDL-C reduction was 13%, 9% and 6% with gymnema, *Citrullus*, and *Artemisia*, respectively (N.S.). The authors concluded that powdered gymnema, *Citrulus colocynthis*, and *Artemisia absinthium* had good antidiabetic features, but no significant effect on lipid profiles in patients with T2DM (Li et al., 2015).

An 8-week polyherbal combination (gymnema, turmeric, *Salacia oblonga*, *Tinospora cordifolia*, *Emblica officinalis*, and *Moringa pterygosperma gaertn*) was given to patients ($n = 89$) newly diagnosed with T2DM and healthy age-matched volunteers ($n = 50$) at a total dose of 1000 mg/day. Significant improvements were seen in fasting and postprandial glucose, A1C, TC, HDL-C, LDL-C, and TG. There were no adverse effects on liver or kidney function. The authors concluded that short-term supplementation of this polyherbal combination attenuates hyperglycemia and acts as a hypolipidemic agent in patients with diabetes (Kurian et al., 2014).

A 30-month nonrandomized open-label trial in patients ($n = 64$) with T1DM studied insulin as usual ($n = 37$) compared with insulin plus gymnema water extract ($n = 27$) 200 mg BID for 6–30 months (insulin-only group was followed for 10–12 months). In the gymnema group, mean insulin requirements were reduced by 50%, accompanied by significant reductions in mean fasting blood glucose levels, from 232 to 152 mg/dL. A1C levels were also reduced. The insulin-only group exhibited no significant mean decreases in insulin requirements or BG levels. Subjective measures of well-being also improved with gymnema. The authors concluded that gymnema water extract appeared to enhance endogenous insulin, possibly by regeneration or revitalization of the residual β cells in insulin-dependent diabetes mellitus (Shanmugasundaram et al., 1990b).

An older (1983) 10-day open-label trial in healthy young adults ($n = 10$) and middle-aged uncomplicated and untreated diabetic adults ($n = 6$) assessed the glycemic effects of gymnema 2 g TID. Gymnema

significantly reduced FBS levels compared with baseline in both normal and diabetic subjects (from 80 to 69 mg/dL in normal subjects, $P < 0.05$); from 136 to 111 mg/dL in diabetic subjects, $P < 0.02$). The herb significantly reduced mean OGTT glucose levels from pretreatment levels in the diabetic group for both the 30 and 120-min measurements (from 220 to 181 mg/dL at 30 min, $P < 0.05$; from 153 to 121 mg/dL at 120 min, $P < 0.01$). In the nondiabetic subjects there were nonsignificant reductions in postglucose load values. The authors concluded that gymnema had definite hypoglycemic activity in both normal and diabetic subjects (Khare et al., 1983).

Cardiometabolic Disorders: Obesity

A study in fasted normal weight subjects assessed the effects of a gymnema extract on consumption of a load sweetened with sucrose (1.1 g/kg) or aspartame (0.011 g/kg), or no added sweetener. Sweetness perception of the load was reduced in half of the subjects and that group subsequently ate less total and sweet calories than those whose sweetness had not been decreased (Brala and Hagen, 1983).

ACTIVE CONSTITUENTS

Leaf

- Lipids
  - Alkanes: hentriacontane, pentatriacontane
- Amino acid derivatives
  - Polypeptides: gurmarin (reduces sweet perception under acidic conditions, likely via interference with Na+/K+ ATPase activity of taste receptors or from neural inhibition.
- Phenolic compounds
  - Phenylpropanoids (antioxidant, antimutagenic, antitumor, antimicrobial): hydroxycinnamic acids
  - Coumarins (venotonic, lymphatotonic): coumarols
  - Flavonoids: flavones
    - ☐ Tannins (antiinflammatory)
  - Quinones: anthraquinones
- Terpenes:
  - Triterpenoids: gymnemic acids I–VII, VIII–XVIII (hypoglycemic, reduced intestinal

glucose absorption, antiobesity, antisweet), gymnemagenin/gymnemic acid A (hypoglycemic), gymnemosides A–F, lupeol (antiarthritic), alternoside II (reduces sweet perception), β-amyrin related glycosides (hypoglycemic, hypolipidemic)

- Triterpenoid saponins: gymnema saponins III–V (antisweet), gymnemasins A–D, saponin I (antisweet), saponin glycosides (antiarthritic)
- Steroids:
  - Phytosterols: stigmasterol (antiinflammatory):
- Cyclic alcohols: D-quercitol, conduritol A (hypoglycemic)
- Phytin

GYMNEMA/GURMAR COMMONLY USED PREPARATIONS AND DOSAGE (FOR ADULTS UNLESS OTHERWISE SPECIFIED)

The following are examples of some available formulations and ranges of dosing for commercial herbal products. See Part III Introduction "How to prescribe medicinal herbs" for further guidance on herbal advising and prescribing.

Leaf

- Decoction: (ratio of herb to water not specified in study) 2 mL TID.
- Whole leaf powder (traditional use): 2–4 g per day.
- Powdered leaf extract: 500 mg (1/4 tsp) QD-BID.
- Capsule or tablet of powdered leaf extract: 500 mg TID.
- Capsule or tablet of standardized extract (standardized to 25% gymnemic acids): 125–450 mg QD-BID.
- Capsule or tablet of standardized (6:1) extract (standardized to gymnemic acids): 400 mg QD.

SAFETY AND PRECAUTION

Side Effects

Hypoglycemia is a potential side effect. Possible cross-reaction with allergies to milkweed family may occur.

Case Report

One case report of toxic hepatitis, possibly due to the use of gymnema.

Toxicity

There was no toxic effect over 52 weeks in rats treated with gymnema at doses equivalent to 500 mg/kg/day in humans.

Pregnancy/Lactation

Insufficient human safety data.

Drug Interactions

- CYP: Animal research found gymnema to be safe for CYP3A4-mediated inhibitory herb-drug interaction in rats.
- May augment effects of hypoglycemic agents.

REFERENCES

Baskaran K, Kizar Ahamath B, Radha Shanmugasundaram K, Shanmugasundaram ER. Antidiabetic effect of a leaf extract from Gymnema sylvestre in non-insulin-dependent diabetes mellitus patients. J Ethnopharmacol 1990 Oct;30(3):295–300.

Bishayee A, Chatterjee M. Hypolipidemic and antiatherosclerotic effects of oral *Gymnema sylvestre* R.Br. leaf extract in albino rats fed on a high fat diet. Phytother Res 1994;8:118–20.

Brala PM, Hagen RL. Effects of sweetness perception and caloric value of a preload on short term intake. Physiol Behav 1983 Jan;30(1):1–9.

Joffe DJ, Freed SH. Effect of extended release *Gymnema sylvestre* leaf extract (B Fast GXR) alone or in combination with oral hypoglycemics or insulin regimens for type 1 and type 2 diabetes. Diabetes in Control Newsletter 2001;76.

Khare AK, Tondon RN, Tewari JP. Hypoglycaemic activity of an indigenous drug (Gymnema sylvestre, 'Gurmar') in normal and diabetic persons. Indian J Physiol Pharmacol 1983 Jul-Sep;27(3):257–8.

Kurian GA, Manjusha V, Nair SS, Varghese T, Padikkala J. Short-term effect of G-400, polyherbal formulation in the management of hyperglycemia and hyperlipidemia conditions in patients with type 2 diabetes mellitus. Nutrition 2014 Oct;30(10):1158–64.

Li Y, Zheng M, Zhai X, et al. Effect of gymnema sylvestre, citrullus colocynthis and artemisia absinthium on blood glucose and lipid profile in diabetic human. Acta Pol Pharm 2015 Sep-Oct;72(5):981–5.

Malik J, Manvi F, Alagawadi K, Noolvi M. Evaluation of antiinflammatory activity of Gymnema sylvestre leaves extract in rats. Int J Green Pharmacy 2008 Apr-June; 2 (2):114-115.

Nahas R, Moher M. Complementary and alternative medicine for the treatment of type 2 diabetes. Can Fam Physician 2009 Jun;55(6):591–6.

Prakash AO, Mather S, Mather R. Effect of feeding *Gymnema sylvestre* leaves on blood glucose in beryllium nitrate treated rats. J Ethnopharmacol 1986;18:143–4.

Shanmugasundaram ER, Gopinath KL, Radha Shanmugasundaram K, Rajendran VM. Possible regeneration of the islets of Langerhans in streptozotocin diabetic rats given *Gymnema sylvestre* leaf extracts. J Ethnopharmacol 1990a;30:265–79.

Shanmugasundaram ER, Rajeswari G, Baskaran K, Rajesh Kumar BR, Radha Shanmugasundaram K, Kizar AB. Use of Gymnema sylvestre leaf extract in the control of blood glucose in insulin-dependent diabetes mellitus. J Ethnopharmacol 1990 Oct;30(3):281–94.

Shigematsu N, Asano R, Shimosaka M, Okazaki M. Effect of administration with the extract of *Gymnema sylvestre* R. Br leaves on lipid metabolism in rats. Biol Pharm Bull 2001a;24:713–7.

Sugihara Y, Nojima H, Matsuda H, et al. Antihyperglycemic effects of gymnemic acid IV, a compound derived from *Gymnema sylvestre* leaves in streptozotocin-diabetic mice. J Asian Nat Prod Res 2000;2:321–7.

Zuñiga LY, González-Ortiz M, Martínez-Abundis E. Effect of-Gymnemasylvestre administration on metabolic syndrome, insulin sensitivity, and insulin secretion. J Med Food 2017 Aug;20(8):750–4.

52

GYNOSTEMMA/JIAOGULAN (*GYNOSTEMMA PENTAPHYLLUM*)
Leaf

GENERAL OVERVIEW

Gynostemma, aka "Southern ginseng" has been widely used in China for diabetes, hyperlipidemia, cardiovascular disease, fatty liver disease, and obesity. It shares many properties with Asian ginseng due to its content of ginsenosides. It may be more antidiabetic than Asian ginseng due to the unique gypenosides in gynostemma. One of the advantages of gynostemma over other adaptogenic herbs is that the medicinal properties are in the leaves as well as the roots, so it is unnecessary to kill the plant to reap the rewards.

Clinical research indicates that gynostemma, alone or in combination formulas, may be beneficial for oxidation, diabetes, obesity, nonalcoholic fatty liver disease, cognitive performance, and cancer metastasis and relapse.

IN VITRO AND ANIMAL RESEARCH

In vitro research demonstrates that gynostemma has antiinflammatory, antioxidant, lipid regulatory, hypoglycemic, immune potentiating, neuroprotective, anxiolytic, antiproliferative, and antitumor activities. Polysaccharides from gynostemma have been shown to improved cellular immune response by increasing levels of TNF-α, IFN-γ, IL-10, and IL-12. Chemical constituents of gynostemma have demonstrated moderate cytotoxicity and antiproliferative properties against hepatic, colon, lung, stomach, glioblastoma, breast, melanoma, and prostate cancer cell lines. Anticancer activities of gynostemma that have been demonstrated in vitro include cell cycle arrest, induction of apopto-

sis, inhibition of invasion and metastasis, suppression of proliferation via inhibition of glycolysis, and enhancement of innate immune mechanisms.

Airway hyperresponsiveness and eosinophil infiltration were significantly reduced in mice given gynostemma extracts via decreased Th2 cytokines and increased IFN-γ. IV gynostemma given to guinea pigs demonstrated cardioprotective effects against vasospasm and arrhythmias. Gynostemma has been shown in animal studies to be a potent AMPK activator. One of the gypenosides, phanoside, has been shown in rodents to stimulate insulin secretion. It has been shown to reduce obesity in mice and to exert antihyperlipidemic effects by elevating the levels of phosphatidylcholine and decreasing the levels of trimethylamine N-oxide.

The gypenosides in gynostemma have been shown to protect gastrointestinal mucosa from the ulcerogenic effects of NSAIDs, *Helicobacter pylori*, alcohol, and stress. Animal studies have suggested a neuroprotective effect in PD. The gypenosides have been shown to attenuate white matter lesions induced by chronic hypoperfusion in rats. Gynostemma also appears to protect against scopolamine-induced learning impairment in mice. An endurance study in rats showed that the polysaccharide component of gynostemma could extend the exhaustive swimming time of rats, decrease the blood lactic acid and BUN, and increase hemoglobin, liver glycogen, and muscle glycogen concentrations.

Gypenosides have reduced tumor size, inhibited tumorigenesis, and promoted survival in mice with various cancers. They have also enhanced the anticancer effects of 5-fluorouracil in colorectal cancer cells and xenografts. The polysaccharides in gynostemma have been shown to reduce tumorigenesis and increase immune response in mice. A review of research on gynostemma and cancer concluded that gynostemma could have potential curative effects on cancer. Multiple mechanisms of action have been proposed including cell cycle arrest, apoptosis, inhibition of invasion and metastasis, inhibition of glycolysis, and immunomodulating activities (Li et al., 2016).

HUMAN RESEARCH

Cardiometabolic Disorders: Oxidation

A 1-month RCT in healthy patients ($n = 610$) aged 50–90 years compared gypenosides 20 mg/day with borax and with placebo. With gypenosides, the SOD levels in elderly subjects (70–90 years old) increased 283% and free radicals were reduced by 21%. In middle-aged (50–69 years old) subjects there was a 116% increase in SOD and a 16% decrease in free radicals. There were no changes in the placebo or borax groups (Liu et al., 1994).

Cardiometabolic Disorders: Diabetes and Obesity

A 12-week RCT in patients ($n = 24$) with newly diagnosed T2DM compared gynostemma powder tea 3 g in 60 mL water with green tea prepared similarly each given BID 30 min before breakfast and dinner. Patients were also instructed to follow a diabetic diet and to walk 30 min 3 days a week during the study period. Following treatment, FBG significantly declined compared with baseline in the gynostemma group ($P < 0.001$) but not in the green tea group. Posttreatment FBG levels were significantly lower with gynostemma compared with green tea ($P < 0.01$). A1C decreased compared with baseline levels in both groups, but the gynostemma group experienced a greater change than the green tea group ($P < 0.001$). The HOMA-IR results declined from baseline to a greater degree with gynostemma than with green tea ($P < 0.05$). The authors concluded that gynostemma resulted in a prompt improvement of glycemia and insulin sensitivity, providing a basis for a novel, effective, and safe approach for using gynostemma tea to treat T2DM patients (Huyen et al., 2010).

A 12-week RCT in patients ($n = 25$) newly diagnosed with T2DM investigated the antidiabetic effects and safety of gynostemma extract as add-on therapy to gliclazide 30 mg QD. After a 4-week run-in with the sulfonylurea alone, the patients were randomized to gliclazide plus gynostemma 3 g BID or gliclazide plus green tea. In addition, the patients followed a diabetic diet and were instructed to walk 30 min daily at least 5 days per week. As expected, after the gliclazide run-in, the FBG and A1C decreased significantly ($P < 0.001$ for both parameters). Increased C-peptide and insulin levels and improved lipid profiles were also reported. Following add-on treatment for 8 weeks, FBG was significantly decreased further by 2.9 and 0.9 mmol/L with gynostemma and green tea, respectively ($P < 0.001$). The A1C values decreased from 9% to 7% in the gynostemma extract group, and from 8.8% to 8.1% in the green tea group ($P = 0.001$). Therapy with gynostemma extract also significantly reduced the 30- and 120-min OGTT postload values ($P < 0.02$ for both). No major changes were seen in circulating insulin or C-peptide levels, or in HOMA-IR and HOMA-β. No significant changes in BW or the other secondary outcome parameters were noted, and no adverse effects were reported. The authors concluded that gynostemma extract in addition to a sulfonylurea offered an alternative to addition of other oral medication to treat type 2 diabetic patients (Huyen et al., 2012).

A 12-week RCT in healthy overweight and obese patients ($n = 80$) investigated the gynostemma constituent actiponin 450 mg QD compared with placebo for effects on fat mass. The actiponin group and placebo group had a 6% and 1% decrease, respectively, in total abdominal fat area. The treatment group also had an 11% decrease in visceral fat compared with a 3% decrease in the placebo group. The actiponin group also showed decreases in BW, body fat mass, percent body fat, and BMI. The authors concluded that actiponin was a potent antiobesity reagent that did not produce any significant adverse effects and that actiponin supplementation may be effective for treating obese individuals (Park et al., 2014).

Gastrointestinal: Nonalcoholic Fatty Liver Disease

A 4-month nonblinded study in patients ($n = 56$) with NAFLD investigated gynostemma tea TID plus the AHA diet compared with the AHA diet alone. Following 4 months of gynostemma, subjects showed significant decreases in BMI ($P < 0.001$), AST ($P = 0.015$), ALP ($P < 0.001$), insulin ($P = 0.017$), and HOMA-IR ($P = 0.028$). The decreases in these parameters were not statistically significant in the diet-only group, but the decreases were also not significantly different between the two groups. TG and uric acid were significantly decreased with gynostemma ($P = 0.089$ and $P = 0.006$, respectively), while these measures increased in the diet-only group. There were significant improvements in the fatty liver score with both gynostemma and diet-only ($P < 0.001$ and $P = 0.003$, respectively). The authors concluded that gynostemma was an effective adjunct to diet therapy for patients with NAFLD (Chou et al., 2006).

Psychiatric Disorders: Anxiety

An 8-week RCT in healthy adults ($n = 72$) who had perceived chronic stress and anxiety and had a score of 40–60 on the State-Trait Anxiety Inventory (STAI) compared gynostemma 200 mg BID with placebo. Study subjects were exposed to repetitive loads of mental stress by performing the serial subtraction tasks for 5 min every other day. After the 8-week intervention, the gynostemma group had lower scores on the Trait-STAI by 16.8% compared with placebo ($P = 0.041$). The total STAI score decreased by 17.8% with gynostemma, a greater improvement that with placebo ($P = 0.067$). There were no significant differences in the score changes for S-STAI, HAM-A, and BAI from baseline between the two groups. There were no associated AEs. The authors concluded that gynostemma reduced "anxiety proneness" in subjects under chronic psychological stress, and it could be used as a regimen to safely reduce stress and anxiety, but that more studies were needed (Choi et al., 2019).

Psychiatric Disorders: Cognitive Performance

A 2-month trial in healthy older patients ($n = 91$) investigated a panglycoside gynostemma extract, 60 mg TID for 2 months compared with a control group for antioxidant and cognitive effects. The gynostemma product resulted in increased erythrocyte SOD levels ($P < 0.01$), decreased lipid peroxidase levels ($P < 0.01$), and increased memory quotients ($P < 0.05$) compared with baseline, whereas these measures were unchanged

in the control group. The authors concluded that the panglycoside extract of gynostemma was beneficial to older patients and would promote their health (Hong et al., 2001).

Oncologic Disorders

An RCT of patients ($n = 59$) with advanced malignant tumors compared a gynostemma soup formula with a control group. Relapse and metastasis rates were 72% and 55%, respectively, in the control group and 12% and 8.5%, respectively, in the gynostemma group. The study also revealed improved T lymphocyte transformation, and acid α-naphthyl acetate esterase activity increased by 8.2% following gynostemma treatment (Wang and Zhao, 1993).

A 5-year observational study showed that the treatment of cancer patients with a gynostemma formula led to significant reductions in cancer relapse and metastasis rates, as well as reduced mortality and improved immune function (Wang et al., 1997).

Gynostemma has been reported to enhance NK cell activity in breast cancer patients (Yu and Wang, 1997). It has been shown to increase T lymphocyte transformation rate and decrease IgG and IgM levels in cancer patients, particularly lung cancer patients, after chemotherapy (Wang and Cao, 1989). It has been shown to have synergy with chemotherapy (Zhou and Bai, 2015).

ACTIVE CONSTITUENTS

- Carbohydrates
  - Polysaccharides (immunostimulant): GPP1a, GPP2b, GPP3a, PGSP, GPB1
  - Organic acids: allantoin
- Phenolic compounds
  - Phenylpropanoids (antioxidant, antimutagenic, antitumor, antimicrobial): caffeic acid
  - Flavonoids: quercetin (antiinflammatory, antioxidant, hypotensive, antidiabetic, antispasmodic, neuroprotective, XO inhibition, antibacterial, anticancer), rutin (antioxidant, antiinflammatory, antidiabetic, nephroprotective, antiosteoporotic, antispasmodic, neuroprotective, antianxiety), kaempferol (antiinflammatory, antidepressant, strengthens capillaries), vitexin (antioxidant,

antiinflammatory, hepatoprotective, estrogen-β agonism, antihyperalgesic, antiarthritis, neuroprotective, antidepressant, dopaminergic, serotonergic, anticancer), ombuoside, ombuin, isorhamnetin

- Terpenes
    - Triterpenoid saponins: gypenosides (actiponin, phanoside, damulens, and others: AMPK activation, PTP1B inhibition, cytotoxicity against hepatic adenocarcinoma cell lines, inducer of p53 tumor suppressor gene).
    - Tetraterpenes/Carotenoids (stimulate granulation tissue): *cis*-neoxanthin, violaxanthin, auoxanthin, luteoxanthin, lutein, α-carotene, and β-carotene
- Steroids:
    - Steroidal saponins: ginsenosides Rb1, Rb3, Rd, F2 (antineovascular, anticonvulsant, analgesic, tranquilizing, hypotensive, antiulcer, vulnerary, antiinflammatory, stimulates humoral and cell-mediated immunity, increases T helper cells, T lymphocytes, NK cells)
    - Phytosterols

GYNOSTEMMA/JIAOGULAN COMMONLY USED PREPARATIONS AND DOSAGE (FOR ADULTS UNLESS OTHERWISE SPECIFIED)

The following are examples of some available formulations and ranges of dosing for commercial herbal products. See Part III Introduction "How to prescribe medicinal herbs" for further guidance on herbal advising and prescribing.

Leaf

Infusion: 3–6 g of leaves per cup BID.

Powdered leaf extract: 500–750 mg (1/5–1/3 tsp) QD.

Capsule or tablet of powdered leaf extract: 100–450 mg BID.

Capsule or tablet of concentrated powdered (12:1) extract: 250 mg QD.

Capsule or tablet of standardized extract (standardized to 45% gypenosides): 500–820 mg QD.

Gypenosides: 100–500 mg per day.

Tea (infusion) is the most commonly used form of gynostemma.

SAFETY AND PRECAUTION

Side Effects

None reported. An 8-week safety study in humans taking 400 mg/day found no adverse effects or significant changes in several laboratory parameters.

Toxicity

High doses up to 750 mg/kg in rats (equivalent to 120 mg/kg/day of leaf as water extract in humans) showed no adverse effects.

Pregnancy and Lactation

Insufficient human data.

Drug Interactions

- CYP: Gypenosides might cause herb-drug interactions via inhibition of CYP2D6.
- Potential for reducing efficacy of immunosuppressive drugs.
- Caution with anticoagulants and antiplatelet drugs.
- May augment effects of hypoglycemic agents.

REFERENCES

Choi EK, Won YH, Kim SY, et al. Supplementation with extract of Gynostemmapentaphyllum leaves reduces anxiety in healthy subjects with chronic psychological stress: a randomized, double-blind, placebo-controlledclinicaltrial. Phytomedicine 2019 Jan;52:198–205.

Chou S, Chen K, Hwang J, et al. The add-on effects of Gynostemma pentaphyllum on NAFLD. Altern Ther 2006;12(3):34–9.

Hong Y, Yongxing M, Shuzhen X, Jiemin G. Approaching the antisenescence effect of pan glycoside extract of Gynostemma pentaphyllum (Thunb) Mak. Shanghai Med Pharm J 2001;11.

Huyen VT, Phan DV, Thang P, Hoa NK, Ostenson CG. Antidiabetic effect of Gynostemma pentaphyllum tea in randomly assigned type 2 diabetic patients. Horm Metab Res 2010 May;42(5):353–7.

Huyen VTT, Phan DV, Thang P, Ky PT, Hoa NK, Ostenson CG. Antidiabetic effects of add-on *Gynostemma pentaphyllum* extract therapy with sulfonylureas in type 2 diabetic patients. Evid Based Complement Alternat Med 2012;452313.

Li Y, Lin W, Huang J, Xie Y, Ma W. Anticancer effects of *Gynostemma pentaphyllum* (Thunb.) Makino (*Jiaogulan*). Chin Med 2016;11:43.

Liu S-X, Wang J-R. Experimental and clinical study on treatment of cancer with *Gynostemma pentaphyllum* Makin. Zhongguo Zhong Xi Yi Jie He Wai Ke Za Zhi 1996;110–1.

Liu J, et al. Effects of gypenosides-containing tonics on the serum SOD activity and MDA content in middle aged persons. J Guiyang Med Coll 1994;19(1):17.

Park SH, Huh TL, Kim SY, et al. Antiobesity effect of Gynostemma pentaphyllum extract (actiponin): a randomized, double-blind, placebo-controlled trial. Obesity (Silver Spring) 2014 Jan;22(1):63–71.

Wang J, Cao B. Immunological effects of jiaogulan granule in 19 cancer patients. Zhejiang Zhong Yi Za Zhi 1989;24:449.

Wang J-M, Wang J-R, Bi H-G, Fu G-X, Zhao J-B. Jiaogulan soup prevent recurrence of cancer metastasis on cancer patients after chemotherapy. Hebei Zhong Yi 1997;19:23–4.

Wang J-R, Zhao J-B. The effect of preventing recurrence of cancer metastasis on jiaogulan soup in clinical study. Zhejiang Zhong Yi Za Zhii 1993;28:529–30.

Yu S-Q, Wang J-R. Jiaogulan formula increase NK cell activity in breast cancer patients. Zhong Yi Yao Yan Jiu 1997;13:7–8.

Zhou K, Bai S. The quality of randomized parallel controlled study of chemotherapy in advanced gastric cancer and improve survival of yiqi jianpi qingre huoxue method. Shiyong Zhongyi Neike Zazhi 2015;29:42–4.

53

HAWTHORN (*CRATAEGUS OXYCANTHA*, *LAEVIGATA*, AND SEVERAL OTHER SPECIES)
Leaf, Flower, Fruit

GENERAL OVERVIEW

Hawthorn holds its activity in the flowers and leaves as well as the berries, a fortunate discovery for harvesters who have had to mindfully avoid the large thorns that surround the berries. Hawthorn is considered one of the best cardiovascular herbs, being both cardiotonic and antiarrhythmic. Hawthorn is also sedating, adaptogenic, antioxidant, vasodilating, diuretic, and hypotensive. It is used in modern herbalism for congestive heart failure, angina, hypertension, and orthostatic hypotension. It is also gastroprotective and supportive of cartilage and bone.

Clinical research indicates that hawthorn, alone or in combination formulas, may be beneficial for hypertension, coronary artery disease, congestive heart failure, orthostatic hypotension, nonalcoholic fatty liver disease.

IN VITRO AND ANIMAL RESEARCH

The oligomeric procyanidins in hawthorn have been shown to have antioxidant properties. The flavonoids that are found more in the leaves and flowers than in the berries are negative chronotropic, positive inotropic, positive dromotropic, negative bathmotropic, vasodilating, and antioxidant. The cardiac action of the flavonoids is thought to be via inhibition of cAMP phosphodiesterase.

Animal research has demonstrated improved coronary circulation and negative chronotropic and positive inotropic cardiac effects as well as ACE inhibition and mild diuresis. Antiarrhythmic effects have been demonstrated as well. Research in rats has shown a beneficial effect on lipids, in part through increased hepatic uptake and biliary elimination of LDL-C. Other animal research has demonstrated myocardial protection from ischemic damage and reperfusion injury as well as reduction in HTN-related hypertrophy. Hawthorn has been shown to improve endothelial functions such as NO synthesis and to delay endothelial senescence. The BP-lowering effect of hawthorn has been linked to NO-mediated vasodilation.

A 65-week controlled study in rats assessed the ability and mechanism of a standardized hawthorn extract WS 1442 to prevent age-related endothelial dysfunction. Aging was associated with decreased endothelium-dependent relaxation and induction of endothelium-dependent contractile responses to acetylcholine. Both age-related impairment of endothelium-dependent relaxations and induction of endothelium-dependent contractile responses were improved with hawthorn treatment and with COX inhibitors. The excessive vascular oxidative stress and an upregulation of COX-1 and COX-2 observed in the arteries of old rats were improved with hawthorn treatment (Idris-Khodja et al., 2012).

HUMAN RESEARCH

Almost all clinical studies of hawthorn, thus far, have been conducted with standardized hydroalcoholic extracts from leaves and flowers. A large volume of the research on hawthorn for CHF has been done with an extract WS 1442. This product is a dry extract from hawthorn leaves with flowers (4–6.6:1), extraction solvent of ethanol 45% (w/w), adjusted to 17.3%–20.1% of oligomeric procyanidins. Importantly, it has demonstrated benefit for both HFrEF and HFpEF. Given that studies with non-standardized hawthorn extracts do not give as impressive results as WS 1442, using the standardized formula would be a safer bet for CHF.

Cardiovascular Disorders: Hypertension

A 30-day RCT in patients with three or more cardiovascular risk factors (HTN, obesity, hyperlipidemia, smoking, sedentary, family history, DM) compared a dietary supplement containing beet root plus hawthorn (Neo40Daily) with placebo BID to assess impact on systemic nitric oxide levels. Patients taking the dietary supplement showed significant increases in both plasma nitrite ($P < 0.01$) and nitrate ($P < 0.0001$), indicating an increase in systemic NO availability. TGs decreased significantly in those with elevated baseline TGs in 72% of patients (from 232 to 168 mg/dL; $P = 0.02$). The authors concluded that the strategy of formulating a combination of natural products and botanicals chosen specifically for their NO activity showed promise in restoring NO homeostasis in human subjects at risk for cardiovascular disease (Zand et al., 2011).

A 10-week pilot RCT in patients ($n = 36$) with mild HTN compared magnesium 600 mg QD with hawthorn 500 mg QD, with magnesium plus hawthorn, and with placebo for effects on blood pressure. Systolic and diastolic BP declined in all treatment groups similarly. However, factorial contrast analysis in ANOVA showed a promising reduction ($P = 0.081$) in the resting diastolic BP at week 10 in the 19 subjects who were assigned to the hawthorn extract, compared with the other groups. Furthermore, a trend toward a reduction in anxiety ($P = 0.094$) was also observed in those taking hawthorn compared with the other groups. The authors recommended further study with higher doses of hawthorn (Walker et al., 2006).

A crossover RCT in prehypertensive or mildly hypertensive adults ($n = 21$) compared a hawthorn extract (standardized to 50 mg oligomeric procyanidin per 250 mg) with placebo to determine optimal dosing. Randomly sequenced doses of hawthorn extract (1000, 1500, and 2500 mg) and placebo were assigned to each participant. Doses were taken twice daily for 3.5 days followed by measurement of brachial artery flow-mediated dilation and a 4-day washout before proceeding to the next dosing period. There was no evidence of a dose-response effect for flow-mediated dilation or absolute change in brachial artery diameter and blood pressure. The authors concluded that they found no evidence of a dose-response effect of hawthorn extract and postulated that if hawthorn has a BP-lowering effect it is likely mediated via a nitric oxide-independent mechanism (Asher et al., 2012).

A 16-week RCT in diabetic patients ($n = 79$) with HTN compared hawthorn extract 1200 mg QD with placebo. The DBP decreased from 85.6 to 83.3 mmHg in the hawthorn group and increased from 84.5 to 85 mmHg in the placebo group ($P = 0.035$): There was no difference between groups in SBP reduction from baseline (3.6 and 0.8 mmHg for hawthorn and placebo groups, respectively; $P = 0.329$). No herb-drug interactions were found. The authors concluded that this study demonstrated a hypotensive effect of hawthorn in patients with diabetes taking medication (Walker et al., 2002).

A 4-month RCT in patients ($n = 92$) with mild HTN compared Iranian hawthorn (*Crataegus curvisepala*) extract TID with placebo. The hawthorn group had a decrease in both systolic and diastolic BP after 3 months ($P < 0.05$). The authors concluded that *Crataegus curvisepala* had a time-dependent antihypertensive effect (Asgary et al., 2004).

Cardiovascular Disorders: Coronary Artery Disease

A 12-week RCT in patients ($n = 80$) with stable angina compared hawthorn extract, aerobic exercise alone, aerobic exercise plus hawthorn, and no intervention (control) for effects on intercellular adhesion molecule (ICAM-1) and E-selectin levels. All experimental groups showed a reduction in serum levels of ICAM-1 and E-selectin ($P < 0.01$). Exercise plus hawthorn produced a significantly greater improvement in serum levels of ICAM-1 compared with hawthorn alone and with control, but not compared with exercise alone ($P = 0.021$; $P = 0.000$, and $P = 0.068$, respectively). Exercise plus hawthorn and hawthorn alone produced significantly greater changes in E-selectin compared with control, but exercise alone did not produce a significant difference from controls ($P = 0.021$; $P = 0.000$, and $P = 0.052$, respectively). The authors concluded that aerobic exercise in combination with hawthorn extract was an effective complementary strategy to significantly lower the risk of atherosclerosis and heart problems (Jalaly et al., 2015).

A 6-month RCT in diabetic subjects ($n = 49$) with coronary heart disease compared micronized flower and leaf of English hawthorn (*Crataegus laevigata*) 400 mg TID with placebo for effects on secondary targets. Neutrophil elastase (a source of inflammation) decreased in the hawthorn group from 35.8 to 33.2 ng/mL and increased in the placebo group from 31 to 36.7 ng/mL ($P < 0.0001$). Hawthorn added to statins decreased LDL-C from 105 mg/dL at baseline to 93 mg/dL at 6 months ($P = 0.03$), and non-HDL-C from 131 to 119.6 mg/dL ($P < 0.001$). Differences between groups did not reach statistical significance at 6 months. No changes were noted in CBC, CRP, and MDA. The authors concluded that *C. laevigata* decreased neutrophil elastase and showed a trend to lower LDL-C compared with placebo as add-on treatment for diabetic subjects with chronic CHD (Dalli et al., 2011).

Cardiovascular Disorders: Congestive Heart Failure

A 2018 review of WS 1442 found in nonclinical studies that the product had positive inotropic and antiarrhythmic properties and protected the myocardium from ischemic damage, reperfusion injury, and HTN-related hypertrophy, improved endothelial functions such as NO synthesis, and delayed endothelial senescence. Furthermore, RCTs in patients with heart failure have demonstrated that WS 1442 increased functional capacity, alleviated disabling symptoms, and improved HR-QOL. A favorable safety profile for the product has been demonstrated in clinical trials and postmarketing surveillance. The authors concluded that WS 1442 may help to close the therapeutic gap between systolic and diastolic heart failure for which evidence of efficacy for other cardioactive drugs was sparse (Holubarsch et al., 2018).

A 2017 systematic review of literature on nutraceuticals for congestive heart failure found reports on hawthorn, coenzyme Q10, ʟ-carnitine, ᴅ-ribose, carnosine, vitamin D, some probiotics, Omega-3 PUFAs, and beet nitrates. All these substances were associated with improvements in functional parameters such as EF, SV, and CO in patients with CHF, with minimal side effects. The benefits were shown to be greater with early heart failure. The proposed mechanisms included antioxidant, antiinflammatory, antiischemic, and antiaggregant effects. The authors concluded that supplementation with nutraceuticals may be a useful option for effective management of CHF, with the advantage of excellent clinical tolerance (Cicero and Colletti, 2017).

A 2008 systematic review to assess the use of hawthorn for CHF found 14 trials that met inclusion criteria. In most of the studies, hawthorn was used as an adjunct to conventional treatment. Ten trials ($n = 855$) in patients with NYHA II–III CHF underwent meta-analysis. Treatment with hawthorn was more beneficial than placebo for maximal workload improvement (WMD = 5.35 W; $P < 0.02$) and for exercise tolerance (WMD = 1.22 W × min). The pressure-heart rate product also showed a beneficial decrease with hawthorn treatment (WMD = − 19.22 mmHg/min). Symptoms such as shortness of breath and fatigue improved significantly with hawthorn treatment compared with placebo (WMD = − 5.47). Reported adverse events were infrequent, mild, and transient; they included nausea, dizziness, and cardiac and gastrointestinal complaints. The authors concluded that there was suggestive evidence of significant benefit in symptom control and physiologic outcomes from hawthorn as adjunctive treatment for chronic heart failure (Pittler et al., 2008).

A 2011 pooled analysis on hawthorn for CHF reviewed data from 10 studies ($n = 687$) comparing hawthorn with placebo. Treatment effects on physiologic outcome parameters and on symptoms were analyzed for their association with baseline severity and gender. LVEF improved from baseline with hawthorn regardless of baseline. The in maximal workload and increase in pressure-heart rate product at 50 W ergometric exercise improved with hawthorn to a degree proportional to baseline. Improvement of typical symptoms like reduced exercise tolerance, exertional dyspnea, weakness, fatigue, and palpitations improved more with hawthorn and more so in patients with more severe symptoms. There were no gender differences in response magnitude. The authors concluded that hawthorn exerted effects of physiologic outcomes and typical symptoms by baseline severity but not by gender (Eggeling et al., 2011).

A 24-month RCT in patients ($n = 2681$) with NYHA II–III CHF and LVEF ≤35% compared a standardized extract of hawthorn (WS 1442) with placebo for time to first cardiac event. Average time to first cardiac event was 620 days with hawthorn and 606 days with placebo (event rates: 27.9% and 28.9%, respectively; HR = 0.95; $P = 0.476$). There was an insignificant trend for cardiac mortality reduction with hawthorn (HR = 0.89; $P = 0.269$). In the subgroup with LVEF ≥25%, hawthorn reduced sudden cardiac death by 39.7% (HR 0.59; $P = 0.025$). Adverse events were comparable in both groups. The authors concluded that hawthorn had no significant effect on reducing cardiac events but was safe to use in patients on optimal medication for HFrEF and that it could potentially reduce incidence of sudden cardiac death in those with better ventricular function (Holubarsch et al., 2008).

A 16-week RCT in patients ($n = 209$) with NYHA III CHF compared two different strengths of hawthorn extract (WS 1442 900 or 1800 mg QD) with placebo for effect on exercise capacity. Maximal workload showed a statistically significant increase with the higher dose of hawthorn compared with the lower dose and with placebo. Typical heart failure symptoms as rated by the patients were reduced to a significantly greater extent with both doses of WS 1442 than with placebo. Both efficacy and tolerability were rated by both patients and investigators as best with the higher dose of hawthorn, and the incidence of adverse events was lowest in this higher dose group, particularly with respect to dizziness and vertigo. The authors concluded that there was a dose-dependent effect of WS 1442 on exercise capacity and clinical signs and symptoms in patients with heart failure (Tauchert et al., 1994).

A cohort study in patients ($n = 952$) with NYHA II CHF studied hawthorn extract (WS 1442) alone compared with hawthorn plus conventional therapy and with conventional therapy alone. In the first 2 years, the hawthorn groups had equal or greater improvement in symptoms compared with the conventional therapy group. After 2 years, fatigue, dyspnea on exertion, and palpitations were significantly less marked in the hawthorn groups than in the conventional therapy group ($P = 0.036$; $P = 0.020$, and $P = 0.048$, respectively). The authors concluded that there was clear benefit for patients with CHF treated with WS 1442. Hawthorn alone or in addition to pharmaceutical medication resulted in objective improvements at comparable costs (Habs, 2004).

A 24-week observational study in patients ($n = 1011$) with NYHA II CHF assessed the effects of a standardized extract of hawthorn (WS 1442) 450 mg BID. A significant improvement in clinical symptoms (reduced performance with ETT, fatigue, palpitations, and exercise dyspnea) was observed. Ankle edema and nocturia disappeared in 83% and 50%, respectively, of those patients who had the symptoms. There was a noted reduction in blood pressure, an increase in maximal exercise tolerance, an increase in ejection fraction and fractional shortening, and a reduction in the difference in the resting heart rate and pressure/heart rate product. Telemetric monitoring showed a reduction in arrhythmias. Maximal exercise showed a reduction in the number of patients showing ST depressions, arrhythmias, and ventricular extrasystoles. Almost two thirds of patients felt better or much better following the 24 weeks of treatment. More than three quarters of the participating physicians noted a "good" or "very good" efficacy, and 98.7% noted a "good" or "very good" tolerance. The authors concluded that high-dose hawthorn therapy is efficient and well-tolerated in patients with NYHA II CHF (Tauchert et al., 1999).

An 8-week RCT in patients ($n = 143$) with NYHA II CHF compared hawthorn extract 30 drops TID with placebo for effects on exercise tolerance. Both groups showed improvement in exercise tolerance. The hawthorn group had 8.3 W greater improvement over placebo ($P = 0.045$). The change in pressure-heart rate product at 50 W was insignificantly superior in the hawthorn group. The subjective assessment of cardiac symptoms and the patient and investigator overall assessment of efficacy were similar for the two groups. The authors concluded that, since dyspnea on exertion improved with hawthorn, NYHA II patients may expect an improvement in their heart failure condition under long term therapy with the standardized extract of hawthorn (Degenring et al., 2003).

A 2-month RCT in patients ($n = 132$) with NYHA II CHF compared hawthorn extract 300 mg TID with captopril 12.5 mg TID for beneficial effects on CHF. Ergometry, pressure-heart rate product, and score for five typical symptoms (fatigue, shortness of breath) were not significantly different between groups. Both showed a statistically significant increase ($P < 0.01$) in maximum tolerated exercise performance (from 83 to 97 W with hawthorn and from 83 to 99 W with captopril). Both treatments reduced pressure-heart rate product and reduced symptom severity of by 50% (Tauchert, 2002).

A 12-week RCT in patients ($n = 88$) with NYHA II CHF compared a standardized extract of fresh hawthorn berries (Rob 10) 25 drops TID with placebo. The hawthorn group showed an increase in exercise time of 38.9 s over placebo, and quality of life improved in favor of hawthorn. Total Minnesota Questionnaire scores decreased by 31% with hawthorn and by 18% with placebo. The Dyspnea-Fatigue Index increased 12% with hawthorn and 8% with placebo. Subjective dyspnea decreased by 11% with hawthorn and 4% with placebo. The authors concluded that this standardized extract of hawthorn showed efficacy and safety in patients with NYHA II CHF (Rietbrock et al., 2001).

A 12-week RCT in patients ($n = 40$) with NYHA II CHF compared a standardized hawthorn extract (WS 1442) TID with placebo. With hawthorn, the exercise tolerance increased by 66.3 W × min (10.8%) compared with a reduction of 105.3 W × min (-16.9%) with placebo ($P = 0.06$). The pressure-heart rate product decreased more with hawthorn than placebo (-26.8% and -2.7%, respectively). The hawthorn extract was safe and well tolerated. The authors concluded that WS 1442 was clinically effective in patients with NYHA II CHF (Zapfe Jun, 2001).

An 8-week RCT in patients ($n = 30$) with NYHA II CHF compared hawthorn extract WS 1442 BID with placebo. The hawthorn group showed a statistically significant advantage over placebo in terms of changes in pressure rate product (at a load of 50 W) and in the score of subjective improvement and heart rate. In both groups, both systolic and diastolic BP were mildly reduced. No adverse reactions occurred (Leuchtgens, 1993).

A 6-month RCT in patients ($n = 120$) with NYHA II–III CHF on conventional medical therapy compared addition of hawthorn 450 mg BID with placebo. There were no significant differences between groups in the change in 6 min walk distance ($P = 0.61$), or on measures of QOL, functional capacity, neurohor-

mones, oxidative stress, or inflammation. A modest difference in LVEF favored hawthorn ($P = 0.04$). There were significantly more adverse events reported in the hawthorn group ($P = 0.02$), although most were noncardiac (Zick et al., 2009).

An 8-week open-label trial in sedentary patients ($n = 140$) with NYHA II HFpEF assessed the effects of exercise training with or without a hawthorn extract (WS 1442) 450 mg BID. Skeletal O2 utilization increased, decreased, or undulated with increasing exercise intensity in individual patients and was not altered by training alone. The hawthorn extract improved the 2 km walking time over baseline to a greater degree than exercise alone (-12.7% and -8.4%, respectively; $P = 0.019$), and tended to improve symptoms and skeletal muscle O2 utilization. The authors concluded that both endurance training and hawthorn were safe and well tolerated in combination with standard drug treatment (Härtel et al., 2014).

An 8-week RCT in patients ($n = 212$) with NYHA II CHF investigated a **homeopathic** hawthorn preparation (Cralonin) compared with a combination of ACEI plus diuretics (control group) for effect on variables of CHF. Both treatment regimens improved scores on most variables studied, with the greatest effect on the pressure-heart rate product after exercise (average score reduction 15.4% in the Cralonin group and 16.0% in the control group). Stringent noninferiority of Cralonin was demonstrated on seven variables. Medium-stringent noninferiority was indicated by 13 variables. The hawthorn preparation did not meet noninferiority for SBP during exercise and DBP at rest, but the differences between treatments were not significant. Both treatments were well tolerated. The authors concluded that the hawthorn-based homeopathic preparation was noninferior to ACEI plus diuretic treatment on all parameters except for BP reduction (Schröder et al., 2003).

Cardiovascular Disorders: Orthostatic Hypotension

A 2019 systematic review and metaanalysis to evaluate the efficacy of Korodin, a fixed combination of hawthorn extract and camphor, for orthostatic hypotension found four RCTs ($n = 221$) that met inclusion criteria. The analysis determined that the fixed combination significantly increased systolic and diastolic BP compared with placebo ($P=0.017$ and $P=0.049$, respectively) and had a beneficial but not statistically significant effect on cognitive performance ($P=0.071$). The authors concluded that this fixed combination of hawthorn and camphor was an effective and presumably safe complementary therapy for the treatment of hypotension (Csupor et al., 2019).

An acutely dosed RCT in healthy volunteers ($n=54$) compared Korodin (a combination of camphor and hawthorn berry extract) 20 drops QID with placebo on four separate occasions for effects on BP and attention. Greater increases in BP occurred after the Korodin administrations in comparison with the placebo administrations. The performance in two parameters of the d2 Test of Attention was consistently superior after intake of Korodin. The herbal product was well tolerated (Erfurt et al., 2014).

A 2003 epidemiological retrospective cohort study in patients ($n=399$) with orthostatic hypotension looked at the efficacy of an herbal drug combination containing D-camphor and hawthorn compared with a control group (conventional drugs: etilefrine, oxilofrine, midodrine, norfenefrine, or dihydroergotamine). The adjusted odds ratio for improvement with the herbal combination was 5.6, and the adjusted mean increase in SBP was twofold compared with the control group. The authors concluded that the herbal combination was effective and safe in the treatment of orthostatic hypotension in medical practice for all age groups and was independent of initial blood pressures (Hempel et al., 2005).

Gastrointestinal Disorders: Nonalcoholic Fatty Liver Disease

A 2012 systematic review and metaanalysis of RCTs to evaluate the efficacy and safety of TCM in the treatment of NAFLD included 419 TCM studies ($n=25,661$) for metaanalysis. Compared with Western medicine for NAFLD, TCM had a better effect on the normalization of ALT and disappearance of radiological steatosis. TCM formulations had an average of 10 herbs. Hawthorn berry (321 times in 17,670 patients) was the most frequently used herb in the treatment of NAFLD. The authors concluded that TCM was of modest benefit in the treatment of NAFLD (Shi et al., 2012).

Psychiatric Disorders: Anxiety

A 3-month RCT in patients ($n=264$) with mild-to-moderate generalized anxiety compared a combination of hawthorn, California poppy, and magnesium BID with placebo for effects on anxiety. Total and somatic Hamilton scale scores and subjective patient-rated anxiety fell more with the hawthorn combination than with placebo during treatment. Clinical improvement, as measured by the mean difference between final and pretreatment scores for anxiety was -10.6 and -8.9 with hawthorn and placebo, respectively ($P=0.005$). For somatic scores, the improvement was -6.5 and -5.7 with hawthorn and placebo, respectively ($P=0.054$). Subjectively assessed anxiety score improvement was -38.5 and -29.2 with hawthorn and placebo, respectively ($P=0.005$). Adverse events, which were mainly mild or moderate digestive or psychopathological symptoms, occurred in 11.5% with hawthorn and 9.7% with placebo. The authors concluded that the fixed quantities of hawthorn, California poppy, and magnesium proved to be safe and more effective than placebo in treating mild-to-moderate anxiety disorders (Hanus et al., 2004).

A 28-day RCT in patients ($n=182$) with adjustment disorder with anxious mood investigated Euphytose, a polyherbal product containing hawthorn, passionflower, valerian, *Ballota*, *Cola*, and *Paullinia* (the combination being theoretically both calming and stimulating) compared with placebo, two tablets TID for effects on anxiety. Comparing the two groups, 42.9% and 25.3% of the herbal and placebo groups, respectively, had a HAM-A score of less than 10 by day 28 ($P=0.012$). The authors noted that from day 7 to day 28 there was a significant difference ($P=0.042$) between the groups, indicating that Euphytose was better than placebo in the treatment of adjustment disorder with anxious mood (Bourin et al., 1997).

ACTIVE CONSTITUENTS

Leaf and Flower

- Phenolic compounds
  - Phenylpropanoids (antioxidant, antimutagenic, antitumor, antimicrobial): caffeic acid, chlorogenic acid
  - Flavonoids/"crataemon" (antioxidant, antiarrhythmogenic, hypotensive, negative chronotropic, positive inotropic, antilipemic,

coronary and general vasodilating, anti-oxidant; improves integrity of blood vessels and capillaries): hyperoside (antioxidant, antiinflammatory, antiproliferative, apoptotic, hepatoprotective, nephroprotective, antiosteoporotic), vitexin 2'-0-rhamnoside, vitexin 4'-0-rhamnoside, acetyl-2-vutexin 2'-0-rhamnoside, quercetin (antiinflammatory, antioxidant, hypotensive, antidiabetic, antispasmodic, neuroprotective, XO inhibition, antibacterial, anticancer), isovitexin (hepatoprotective, anticarcinogenic, apoptotic, antistapyholcoccal)

  □ Oligomeric procyanidins: procyanidin B-2, epicatechin, catechin (antioxidant, improve coronary circulation, negative chronotropic and positive inotropic cardiac effects)
- Terpenes
  - Triterpenes: eleanolic acid, crataegolic acid, uvalol
  - Triterpenoid saponins: ursolic acid (anti-HIV, anti-EBV, antiviral, androgenic, AChEI, pro-collagen, pro-ceramide, antitumor)
- Alkaloids: phenethylamine, *O*-methoxyphenethylamine, tyramine (inotropic)

Fruit

- Phenolic compounds
  - Flavonoids: hyperoside (antioxidant, antiinflammatory, antiproliferative, apoptotic, hepatoprotective, nephroprotective, antiosteoporotic), quercetin (antiinflammatory, antioxidant, hypotensive, antidiabetic, antispasmodic, neuroprotective, XO inhibition, antibacterial, anticancer), rutin (antioxidant, antiinflammatory, antidiabetic, nephroprotective, antiosteoporotic, antispasmodic, neuroprotective, antianxiety), 2'-0-rhamnoside
    □ Oligomeric procyanidins
    □ Anthocyanidins (stabilize collagen in cartilage and bone)
- Terpenes
  - Triterpenoid saponins: ursolic acid (anti-HIV, anti-EBV, antiviral, androgenic, AChEI, pro-collagen, pro-ceramide, antitumor), oleanolic acid (chemoprotective, hepatoprotective), crataegolic acid

HAWTHORN COMMONLY USED PREPARATIONS AND DOSAGE (FOR ADULTS UNLESS OTHERWISE SPECIFIED)

The following are examples of some available formulations and ranges of dosing for commercial herbal products. See Part III Introduction "How to prescribe medicinal herbs" for further guidance on herbal advising and prescribing.

Dried Leaf and/or Flower

- Infusion or decoction: 2 tsp per cup TID.
- Fluid extract (1:1, 25%): 1–2 mL TID.
- Tincture (1:5, 45%): 1–2.5 mL BID-TID.
- Capsule or tablet of powdered berry: 1.08 g BID-TID.
- Capsule or tablet of powdered leaf, flower, and berry extract: 500 mg BID.
- Capsule or tablet of standardized extract (standardized to 1.8%–2.2% vitexin or 18.75% OPCs): 80–900 mg QD-BID.

One study in CHF indicated that 1800 mg per day of the standardized extract was optimal.

Takes at least 2 months for efficacy to become manifest and is safe taken long-term.

Fruit

- Fluid extract (1:1, 25%) 0.5–1 mL TID.
- Tincture of fruit (1:5, 45%) 1–2 mL TID.

SAFETY AND PRECAUTION

Side Effects

Nausea, sweating, fatigue, mild rash, headache, dizziness, palpitations, drowsiness, and agitation have been reported.

Toxicity

Overdose may produce hypotension and arrhythmias.

A combination of hawthorn, passionflower, and valerian was administered in high doses to rats, mice, and dogs, both acute and chronically for 180 days. Weight gain/loss, general physical conditions, water/food consumption, and anatomo-pathological examination of the organs were not adversely affected.

Pregnancy and Lactation

Insufficient human safety data.

Hawthorn did not have an adverse effect on embryonic development in pregnant rats receiving 56 times the human dose as a daily gavage, nor did it have adverse effects in vitro.

Disease Interactions

Increased risk for postoperative bleeding.

Drug Interactions

- CYP: Induces CYP3A4 by activating pregnane X receptor (PXR).
- UGT: Modulates UGT enzymes in vitro and can increase the side effects of drugs metabolized by them.
- Theoretically may interact with vasodilating medications and may affect drugs used for heart failure, HTN, angina, and arrhythmias. However, large studies in patients on multiple CHF medications failed to demonstrate any herb-drug interactions with hawthorn.

A crossover RCT with 7-day washout in healthy volunteers ($n = 20$) assessed EKG effects, especially QTc, of a single dose of hawthorn 160 mg compared with placebo at 1-, 2-, 4-, and 6-h post dose. No significant differences in 4- or 6-h QT_c interval were seen between hawthorn and placebo. Maximum postdose QT_c intervals in the hawthorn and placebo groups were similar (346 and 346, respectively; $P = 0.979$). No significant adverse events were seen. The authors concluded that a single dose of oral hawthorn had no effect on electrocardiographic parameters in healthy volunteers.

Trexler et al. (2018)

- Theoretical interaction with digoxin, as hawthorn contains alkaloids that are structurally similar to digoxin. This has not been studied, but as a general precaution avoid or use cautiously in patients on digoxin.

A study in healthy volunteers ($n = 8$) studied the pharmacokinetics of digoxin 0.25 mg QD for 10 days alone compared with digoxin plus hawthorn extract WS 1442 450 mg BID for 21 days. Following 3 weeks of concomitant therapy, hawthorn did not significantly alter the pharmacokinetic parameters for digoxin. This suggests that both hawthorn and digoxin, in the doses and dosage form studied, may be co-administered safely.

Tankanow et al. (2003)

REFERENCES

Asgary S, Naderi GH, Sadeghi M, Kelishadi R, Amiri M. Antihypertensive effect of Iranian *Crataegus curvisepala* Lind.: a randomized, double-blind study. Drugs Exp Clin Res 2004;30(5–6):221–5.

Asher GN, Viera AJ, Weaver MA, Dominik R, Caughey M, Hinderliter AL. Effect of hawthorn standardized extract on flow mediated dilation in prehypertensive and mildly hypertensive adults: a randomized, controlled crossover trial. BMC Complement Altern Med 2012;12:26.

Bourin M, Bougerol T, Guitton B, Broutin E. A combination of plant extracts in the treatment of outpatients with adjustment disorder with anxious mood: controlled study vs placebo. Fundam Clin Pharmacol 1997;11:127–32.

Cicero AFG, Colletti A. Nutraceuticals and dietary supplements to improve quality of life and outcomes in heart failure patients. Curr Pharm Des 2017;23(8):1265–72.

Csupor D, Viczián R, Lantos T, et al. The combination of hawthorn extract and camphor significantly increases blood pressure: a meta-analysis and systematic review. Phytomedicine 2019;152:984.

Dalli E, Colomer E, Tormos MC, et al. *Crataegus laevigata* decreases neutrophil elastase and has hypolipidemic effect: a randomized, double-blind, placebo-controlled trial. Phytomedicine 2011;18(8–9):769–75.

Degenring FH, Suter A, Weber M, Saller R. A randomised double blind placebo controlled clinical trial of a standardised extract of fresh Crataegus berries (Crataegisan) in the treatment of patients with congestive heart failure NYHA II. Phytomedicine 2003;10(5):363–9.

Eggeling T, Regitz-Zagrosek V, Zimmermann A, Burkart M. Baseline severity but not gender modulates quantified Crataegus extract effects in early heart failure—a pooled analysis of clinical trials. Phytomedicine 2011;18(14):1214–9.

Erfurt L, Schandry R, Rubenbauer S, Braun U. The effects of repeated administration of camphor-crataegus berry extract combination on BP and on attentional performance—a randomized, placebo-controlled, double-blind study. Phytomedicine 2014;21(11):1349–55.

Habs M. Prospective, comparative cohort studies and their contribution to the benefit assessments of therapeutic options: heart failure treatment with and without Hawthorn special extract WS 1442. Forsch Komplementarmed Klass Naturheilkd 2004;11(Suppl. 1):36–9.

Hanus M, Lafon J, Mathieu M. Double-blind, randomised, placebo-controlled study to evaluate the efficacy and safety of a fixed combination containing two plant extracts (*Crataegus oxyacantha* and

Eschscholtzia californica) and magnesium in mild-to-moderate anxiety disorders. Curr Med Res Opin 2004;20(1):63–71.

Härtel S, Kutzner C, Westphal E, et al. Effects of endurance exercise training and *Crataegus* extract WS* 1442 in patients with heart failure with preserved ejection fraction—a randomized controlled trial. Sports 2014;2(3):59–75.

Hempel B, Kroll M, Schneider B. Efficacy and safety of a herbal drug containing hawthorn berries and D-camphor in hypotension and orthostatic circulatory disorders/results of a retrospective epidemiologic cohort study. Arzneimittelforschung 2005;55(8):443–50.

Holubarsch CJ, Colucci WS, Meinertz T, Gaus W, Tendera M, Survival and Prognosis: Investigation of Crataegus Extract WS 1442 in CHF (SPICE) Trial Study Group. The efficacy and safety of Crataegus extract WS 1442 in patients with heart failure: the SPICE trial. Eur J Heart Fail 2008;10(12):1255–63.

Holubarsch C, Colucci WS, Eha J. Benefit-risk assessment of *Crataegus* extract WS 1442: an evidence-based review. Am J Cardiovasc Drugs 2018;18(1):25–36.

Idris-Khodja N, Auger C, Koch E, Schini-Kerth VB. Crataegus special extract WS(®)1442 prevents aging-related endothelial dysfunction. Phytomedicine 2012;19(8–9):699–706.

Jalaly L, Sharifi G, Faramarzi M, et al. Comparison of the effects of *Crataegus oxyacantha* extract, aerobic exercise and their combination on the serum levels of ICAM-1 and E-selectin in patients with stable angina pectoris. Daru 2015;23:54.

Leuchtgens H. Crataegus special extract WS 1442 in NYHA II heart failure. A placebo controlled randomized double-blind study. Fortschr Med 1993;111:352–4.

Pittler MH, Guo R, Ernst E. Hawthorn extract for treating chronic heart failure. Cochrane Database Syst Rev 2008;1:CD005312.

Rietbrock N, Hamel M, Hempel B, Mitrovic V, Schmidt T, Wolf GK. Actions of standardized extracts of Crataegus berries on exercise tolerance and quality of life in patients with congestive heart failure. Arzneimittelforschung 2001;51(10):793–8.

Schröder D, Weiser M, Klein P. Efficacy of a homeopathic Crataegus preparation compared with usual therapy for mild (NYHA II)

cardiac insufficiency: results of an observational cohort study. Eur J Heart Fail 2003;5(3):319–26.

Shi KQ, Fan YC, Liu WY, Li LF, Chen YP, Zheng MH. Traditional Chinese medicines benefit to NAFLD: a systematic review and meta-analysis. Mol Biol Rep 2012;39(10):9715–22.

Tankanow R, Tamer HR, Streetman DS, et al. Interaction study between digoxin and a preparation of hawthorn (*Crataegus oxyacantha*). J Clin Pharmacol 2003;43(6):637–42.

Tauchert M. Efficacy and safety of crataegus extract WS 1442 in comparison with placebo in patients with chronic stable New York Heart Association class-III heart failure. Am Heart J 2002;143(5):910–5.

Tauchert M, Ploch M, Hübner W-D. Effectiveness of hawthorn extract LI 132 compared with the ACE inhibitor Captopril: multicenter double-blind study with 132 patients NYHA stage II. Münch Med Wochenschr 1994;132(Suppl):S27–33.

Tauchert M, Gildor A, Lipinski J. High-dose Crataegus extract WS 1442 in the treatment of NYHA stage II heart failure. Herz 1999;24(7):586.

Trexler SE, Nguyen E, Gromek SM, Balunas MJ, Baker WL. Electrocardiographic effects of hawthorn (Crataegus oxyacantha) in healthy volunteers: a randomized controlled trial. Phytother Res 2018;32(8):1642–6.

Walker AF, Marakis G, Morris AP, Robinson PA. Promising hypotensive effect of hawthorn extract: a randomized double-blind pilot study of mild, essential HTN. Phytother Res 2002;16(1):48–54.

Walker AF, Marakis G, Simpson E, et al. Hypotensive effects of hawthorn for patients with diabetes taking prescription drugs: a randomized controlled trial. Br J Gen Pract 2006;56(527):437–43.

Zand J, Lanza F, Garg HK, Bryan NS. All-natural nitrite and nitrate containing dietary supplement promotes nitric oxide production and reduces triglycerides in humans. Nutr Res 2011;31(4):262–9.

Zapfe Jun G. Clinical efficacy of crataegus extract WS 1442 in congestive heart failure NYHA class II. Phytomedicine 2001;8(4):262–6.

Zick SM, Vautaw BM, Gillespie B, Aaronson KD. Hawthorn extract randomized blinded chronic heart failure (HERB CHF) trial. Eur J Heart Fail 2009;11(10):990–9.

54

HOLY BASIL/TULSI (*OCIMUM TENUIFLORUM/SANCTUM*)
Leaf

GENERAL OVERVIEW

Holy basil has broad applications in Ayurvedic medicine. It fits the definition of an adaptogen, and like gynostemma, it offers adaptogenic benefits through its leaves rather than its roots. The leaf of holy basil has been used traditionally for more than 3000 years for fever, mouth diseases, earache, hiccups, asthma, bronchitis, liver disease, gastric disorders, joint pains, neuralgia, headache, epilepsy, skin diseases, wounds, blood diseases, and parasitic infestations. The roots and stems of the plant have been used on mosquito and snake bites and for malaria. In more recent times holy basil has been used for diabetes, menstrual disorders, male hypogonadism, male infertility, cough, and malaria.

Clinical research indicates that holy basil, alone or in combination formulas, may be beneficial for gingivitis, dental plaque, hypertension, dyslipidemia, diabetes, obesity, anxiety, stress, cognitive performance, immune function, and viral encephalitis.

IN VITRO AND ANIMAL RESEARCH

In vitro and animal studies with holy basil leaf have demonstrated antioxidant, antiinflammatory, immunomodulatory, hepatoprotective, radioprotective, antimicrobial, anticonvulsant, antidiabetic, and anticancer effects. Holy basil has been shown to have a hepatic membrane stabilizing effect that prevents toxin-induced liver damage. The hepatoprotective effect appears to be synergistic when added to milk thistle. It has been shown to promote body elimination of cadmium. In vitro research has also demonstrated that holy basil has strong AChE inhibition. Maximum inhibition was found to be 83% at 320 μg/mL (Kandhan et al., 2018).

In a study in rats with experimentally induced diabetes, an aqueous extract of holy basil significantly decreased blood glucose, serum lipid profile, and serum levels of AST, ALT, ALP, LDH, CK-MB, creatinine, and BUN. Experimentally induced low insulin levels were increased by holy basil. Lipid peroxidation was reduced via increased activities of antioxidant enzymes in the liver, kidney, and cardiac tissue with preservation of these organs. The authors concluded that holy basil had antihyperglycemic, antihyperlipidemic, and free radical scavenging effects providing organ protection from diabetes, and that the phenolic compounds may be responsible for these activities (Suanarunsawat et al., 2014).

In mice, holy basil resulted in increased swimming survival time. When the constituents ocimarin and ocimumosides A and B were given to rats, an antistress effect was observed. Its antistress effectiveness was on par with imipramine, and this property has been shown to protect rats from stress-related cardiovascular changes (Sood et al., 2006). Animal studies have also demonstrated cardio-protection postischemia, improved wound healing, and gastro-protection against aspirin. Studies in mice have also shown reduced pain sensitivity with the analgesic action being exerted both centrally and peripherally and involving both the opioid and the serotonergic systems (Khanna and Bhatia, 2003).

Ursolic acid in holy basil appears to function as an androgenic analogue, reducing LH and secondarily spermatogenesis. A rabbit study showed holy basil 2 g per day reduced sperm count and reproductive potential (Sethi et al., 2010). This same constituent also potentiates apoptosis in cancer cells through a non-P53 pathway.

HUMAN RESEARCH

Oral and Dental Disorders

A 30-day RCT in medical students ($n = 108$) compared holy basil mouthwash with chlorhexidine mouthwash and with normal saline mouth rinse for effects on plaque and gingival scores. Holy basil was found to be equally as effective as chlorhexidine in reducing plaque and gingivitis, with a reduction in gingival bleeding and plaque indices in both groups at 15 and 30 days compared with the saline group. Holy basil produced no side effects. The authors concluded that holy basil mouth rinse decreased periodontal indices by reducing plaque accumulation, gingival inflammation, and bleeding and that it had no side effects compared with chlorhexidine (Gupta et al., 2014).

A 3-day RCT in children ($n = 40$) compared dental application of holy basil essential oil with that of triple antibiotic ointment for microbial effects. There was a statistically significant reduction in CFUs taken from root canals after using holy basil essential oil. However, triple antibiotic ointment resulted in a greater reduction in CFUs. The authors concluded that holy basil could be used in cases of long-standing infection owing to its antimicrobial efficacy and antiinflammatory potential as an intracanal medicament in primary teeth (Ahirwar et al., 2018).

Cardiometabolic Disorders: Dyslipidemia, Diabetes, and Obesity

A 2017 systematic review of holy basil with respect to general health conditions selected 24 studies that met inclusion criteria ($n = 1111$). The authors noted that studies of glycemic impact showed more dramatic reductions in fasting and postprandial glucose if carried out for 12–13 weeks rather than for just 3–4 weeks. A1C was significantly decreased when holy basil was added to hypoglycemic medication compared with the

drug alone. Uric acid levels, lipid profiles, and BMI also improved. The authors concluded that the literature suggested that holy basil was a safe herbal intervention that may assist in normalizing glucose, blood pressure, and lipid profiles, and dealing with psychological and immunological stress (Jamshidi and Cohen, 2017).

A 90-day RCT in patients ($n = 60$) with T2DM compared glibenclamide 5 mg/day alone with glibenclamide 5 mg/day plus holy basil 250 mg BID. In the glibenclamide-alone group FBS decreased from 174 to 114 mg/dL and PPG decreased from 247 to 152 mg/dL ($P < 0.05$ for both compared with baseline). With glibenclamide plus holy basil the FBS decreased from 171 to 103 mg/dL and the PPG decreased from 254 to 143 mg/dL ($P < 0.05$ for both compared with baseline). A1C decreased from 7.6% to 5.3% with glibenclamide alone and from 7.7% to 5% with glibenclamide plus holy basil. Hypoglycemic episodes were not different between groups. The authors concluded that holy basil could be used as adjuvant therapy in T2DM (Somasundaram et al., 2012).

A 4-week RCT in patients with T2DM ($n = 16$) compared 2.5 g of powdered holy basil leaves with placebo for effects on fasting and postprandial blood glucose and serum cholesterol levels. FBG fell from 135 mg/dL at baseline to 99 mg/dL at 4 weeks with holy basil ($P < 0.001$). When compared with placebo, postprandial blood glucose fell by 15.8 mg/dL, a 7.3% reduction ($P < 0.02$) (Agrawal et al., 1996).

An open label 45-day trial in patients ($n = 40$) with T2DM investigated the effects of holy basil 3 g/day. The FBS decreased significantly only in the male subjects from 388 mg/dL to 368 mg/dL ($P < 0.01$). The 2-h PPG decreased from 556 to 520 mg/dL in women and from 610 to 516 mg/dL in men ($P < 0.01$ for both). The study was too short to evaluate changes in A1C. The authors concluded that holy basil could be used as an adjunct to diet and medication in T2DM (Gandhi et al., 2016).

An 8-week open-label RCT in overweight and obese subjects ($n = 30$) compared holy basil 250 mg with a control group. Compared with no treatment, holy basil resulted in improvements in serum TG ($P = 0.019$), LDL-C ($P = 0.001$), HDL-C ($P = 0.001$), VLDL-C ($P = 0.019$), BMI ($P = 0.005$); insulin ($P = 0.021$), and insulin resistance ($P = 0.049$). There was no significant alteration of the liver enzymes. The authors concluded that holy basil had beneficial effects on various biochemical parameters in young overweight and obese individuals (Satapathy et al., 2017).

Psychiatric Disorders: Anxiety, Stress, and Cognitive Performance

A 60-day open-label study in patients ($n = 35$) with GAD assessed the efficacy of holy basil 500 mg BID on anxiety as measured on the Brief Psychiatric Rating Scale. Holy basil attenuated generalized anxiety ($P < 0.001$) as well as correlated stress and depression ($P < 0.001$). It also improved adaptability and attention ($P < 0.001$). The authors concluded that holy basil may be useful in the treatment of GAD (Bhattacharyya et al., 2008).

A 6-week RCT in volunteers ($n = 150$) compared a holy basil extract 1200 mg/day with placebo for effects on stress-related symptoms. After 6 weeks of intervention, scores of symptoms such as forgetfulness, sexual problems of recent origin, frequent feeling of exhaustion, and frequent sleep problems of recent origin as well as total symptom scores decreased significantly ($P \leq 0.05$) in the holy basil group compared with the placebo group. The overall improvement with holy basil was found to be 1.6 times or 39% greater than placebo in the control of general stress symptoms. No adverse events were reported during the study. The authors concluded that holy basil extract was effective and well tolerated by all of the generally stressed patients over the study period (Saxena et al., 2012).

A 30-day RCT in healthy volunteers ($n = 44$) compared holy basil extract 300 mg/day with placebo for effects on cognition and stress. After an initial improvement in both study groups for the first 15 days, the placebo group improvement plateaued, but the holy basil group experienced additional significant improvement in cognitive parameters. The parameters that improved included reaction times and error rates of cognitive tests. Holy basil showed a significant improvement in P300 latency (an indicator of memory impairment), while the improvements in salivary cortisol and State-Trait Anxiety Inventory were not significantly superior to placebo. The authors concluded that holy basil leaf extract had potential cognition-enhancing properties in humans (Sampath et al., 2015).

Immune Function

A 4-week RCT in healthy human subjects ($n = 24$) compared holy basil leaf extract 300 mg with placebo for impact on immune function. Compared with placebo, the herb produced an increase in IFN-γ ($P = 0.039$), IL-4 ($P = 0.001$), NK cell activity ($P = 0.017$), and T-helper cells ($P = 0.001$) in humans. Ex vivo the immune cells from patients treated with holy basil mounted a greater inflammatory response. The authors concluded that holy basil had immunomodulatory activity in healthy individuals (Mondal et al., 2011).

Infectious Disease: Viral Encephalitis

In an open-label trial, holy basil powder 2.5 g QID was compared with standard management during an outbreak of viral encephalitis in northern India in 1978. Survival with holy basil was 60% vs 0% with conventional management (Das et al., 1983).

ACTIVE CONSTITUENTS

- Carbohydrates: polysaccharides
- Lipids
  - Fatty acids: stearic, palmitic, oleic, linoleic, and linolenic acids
  - Glycoglycerolipids: ocimumosides A and B (antistress, antioxidant, nootropic)
- Phenolic compounds
  - Phenylpropanoids (antioxidant, antimutagenic, antitumor, antimicrobial): eugenol
  - Coumarins: ocimarin (antistress)
  - Flavonoids: apigenin (antiinflammatory, antioxidant, antihistamine, hypotensive, antiserotonin release, GABA agonism, antispasmodic, antibacterial, chemopreventive, antineoplastic, ERB), orientin, vicenin, cirsilineol, cirsimaritin, isothymusin, isothymonin
- Terpenes
  - Terpenoid saponins: ursolic acid (anti-HIV, anti-EBV, antiviral, androgenic, AChEI, procollagen, pro-ceremide, antitumor)
  - Tetraterpenes/Carotenoids (stimulate granulation tissue): lutein
- Aromatic compounds: eugenol (chief constituent), methyl eugenol, cinnamyl acetate, β-elemene, caryophyllene

HOLY BASIL COMMONLY USED PREPARATIONS AND DOSAGE (FOR ADULTS UNLESS OTHERWISE SPECIFIED)

The following are examples of some available formulations and ranges of dosing for commercial herbal products. See Part III Introduction "How to prescribe medicinal herbs" for further guidance on herbal advising and prescribing.

Leaf

- Infusion of dried herb: 1 tsp per cup BID.
- Powdered leaf: 250–500 mg (1/5–1/2 tsp) QD-BID.
- Capsule or tablet of powdered leaf: 600–800 mg QD-BID.
- Capsule or tablet of freeze-dried leaf: 200 mg TID.
- Capsule or tablet of powdered leaf extract: 250–500 mg QD to BID.
- Capsule or tablet of standardized extract (standardized to minimum 2% ursolic acid): 450–500 mg QD-BID.

SAFETY AND PRECAUTION

Side Effects

None reported. Theoretically may cause hypoglycemia. May reduce sperm count, motility, and speed and increase anomalies.

Toxicity

Ethanol extract showed no toxicity in high doses in rats acutely and subacutely. Oil extract with 70% eugenol content demonstrated toxicity at 42.5 mL/kg.

Pregnancy and Lactation

Insufficient human data.

Drug Interactions

- May increase hypoglycemia with antidiabetic drugs.
- May augment anticoagulant drugs.

REFERENCES

Agrawal P, Rai V, Singh RB. Randomized placebo-controlled, single blind trial of holy basil leaves in patients with noninsulin-dependent diabetes mellitus. Int J Clin Pharmacol Ther 1996;34(9):406–9.

Ahirwar P, Shashikiran ND, Sundarraj RK, Singhla S, Thakur RA, Maran S. A clinical trial comparing antimicrobial efficacy of "essential oil of *Ocimum sanctum*" with triple antibiotic paste as an intracanal medicament in primary molars. J Indian Soc Pedod Prev Dent 2018;36(2):191–7.

Bhattacharyya D, Sur TK, Jana U, Debnath PK. Controlled programmed trial of *Ocimum sanctum* leaf on generalized anxiety disorders. Nepal Med Coll J 2008;10(3):176–9.

Das S, Chandra A, Agarwal S, Singh N. *Ocimum sanctum* (tulsi) in the treatment of viral encephalitis. Antiseptic 1983;80:323–27.

Gandhi R, Chauhan B, Jadeja G. Effect of *Ocimum sanctum* (tulsi) powder on hyperglycemic patient. Indian J Appl Res 2016;6(5):62–64.

Gupta D, Bhaskar DJ, Gupta RK, et al. A randomized controlled clinical trial of *Ocimum sanctum* and chlorhexidine mouthwash on dental plaque and gingival inflammation. J Ayurveda Integr Med 2014;5(2):109–16.

Jamshidi N, Cohen MM. The clinical efficacy and safety of tulsi in humans: a systematic review of the literature. Evid Based Complement Alternat Med 2017;2017:9217567.

Kandhan T, et al. AChE activity of *Ocimum sanctum* leaf extract. J Adv Pharm Educ Res 2018:8(1):41–44.

Khanna N, Bhatia J. Antinociceptive action of *Ocimum sanctum* (tulsi) in mice: possible mechanisms involved. J Ethnopharmacol 2003;88(2–3):293–6.

Mondal S, Varma S, Bamola VD, et al. Double-blinded randomized controlled trial for immunomodulatory effects of tulsi (*Ocimum sanctum* Linn.) leaf extract on healthy volunteers. J Ethnopharmacol 2011;136(3):452–6.

Sampath S, Mahapatra SC, Padhi MM, Sharma R, Talwar A. Holy basil (*Ocimum sanctum* Linn.) leaf extract enhances specific cognitive parameters in healthy adult volunteers: a placebo-controlled study. Indian J Physiol Pharmacol 2015;59(1):69–77.

Satapathy S, Das N, Bandyopadhyay D, Mahapatra SC, Sahu DS, Meda M. Effect of tulsi (*Ocimum sanctum* Linn.) supplementation on metabolic parameters and liver enzymes in young overweight and obese subjects. Indian J Clin Biochem 2017;32(3):357–63.

Saxena RC, Singh R, Kumar P, et al. Efficacy of an extract of *Ocimum tenuiflorum* (OciBest) in the management of general stress: a double-blind, Placebo-Controlled Study. Evid Based Complement Alternat Med 2012;2012:894509.

Sethi J, et al. Effect of tulsi (*Ocimum sanctum* Linn.) on sperm count and reproductive hormones in male albino rabbits. Int J Ayurveda Res 2010 Oct;1(4):208-10.

Somasundaram G, Manimekalai K, Kartik JS, Pandiamunian J. Evaluation of the antidiabetic effect of *Ocimum sanctum* in type 2 diabetes patients. Int J Life Sci Pharma Res 2012;2(3):75–81.

Sood S, Narang D, Thomas MK, et al. Effect of *Ocimum sanctum* Linn. on cardiac changes in rats subjected to chronic restraint stress. J Ethnopharmacol 2006;108:423–7.

Suanarunsawat T, Ayutthaya WD, Thirawarapan S, Poungshompoo S. Anti-oxidative, antihyperglycemic and lipid-lowering effects of aqueous extracts of *Ocimum sanctum* L leaves in diabetic rats. Food Nutr Sci 2014;5:801–11.

55

HOPS/HOP (*HUMULUS LUPULUS*)
Strobiles

GENERAL OVERVIEW

More commonly known and highly regarded for the flavor it imparts to India pale ales, hops is a versatile medicinal herb. The active ingredients come from the strobiles, the female inflorescences of the plant. Hops may be useful for dyspepsia, insomnia, and a host of menopausal issues. Its constituents are chemopreventive, antitumor, antiangiogenic, antiinflammatory, and antidiabetic. Hops is often paired with valerian to promote sleep, a combination that has been well-supported by human studies. Hops may also reduce triglycerides, reduce arthritic pain, and prevent bone loss.

Clinical research indicates that hops, alone or in combination formulas, may be beneficial for endothelial dysfunction, metabolic syndrome, menopause, psychological stress, and insomnia.

IN VITRO AND ANIMAL RESEARCH

In vitro tests of hops have demonstrated antiproliferative, anticarcinogenic, antigenotoxic, and antiinflammatory effects. The xanthohumol prenyl-flavonoid in hops is more antioxidant than vitamin C or vitamin E. Hops has been associated with a decrease of plasma glucose, lipid levels, and weight of white adipose tissue in diabetic mice. Isohumulones, the bitter compounds derived from hops that are present in beer, were found to activate PPAR-α and -γ. Mice fed a high-fat diet that were treated with isohumulones showed reduced plasma glucose, TG, and free fatty acid levels by 65.3%,

62.6%, and 73.1%, respectively. Additionally, the mice experienced a decrease in size and an increase in apoptosis of their hypertrophic adipocytes.

The rho iso-α acids (RIAA) in hops have been shown to modulate insulin signaling in vitro. Iso-α acids are converted from α acids during brewing, leading to the flavor and bitterness of beer. Iso-α-acids have been shown to prevent diet-induced obesity in mice. RIAA have also been shown to inhibit LPS-stimulated PGE2 formation with more than 200-fold selectivity of COX-2 over COX-1. This occurs only when RIAA is added prior to, but not after, LPS stimulation, indicating that RIAA inhibits inducible but not constitutive COX-2. In gastric mucosa there has been little PGE2 inhibition, indicating that RIAA may have a lower potential for the gastrointestinal and cardiovascular toxicity observed with COX inhibitors. A combination of RIAA from hops and proanthocyanidins from *Acacia nilotica* was shown to modulate insulin signaling in vitro. In a separate study this combination was also shown to synergistically increase TG deposition and adiponectin secretion in adipocytes under hyperinsulinemic conditions and to reduce glucose and insulin in obese mice.

Matured hop bitter acids (MHBA) are produced when beer is stored for long periods of time. MHBA have been shown to reduce body fat in rodents at least in part by increasing thermogenesis in brown adipose tissue. MHBA have similar structures to iso-α acids but are less bitter and therefore more palatable. In an in vitro model, a mixture of tetrahydro-iso-α acids (THIAA) plus niacin was shown to inhibit several

TNF-α-induced cytokines in human aortic endothelial cells and in human monocytic cells and was significantly more efficacious than niacin alone.

The bitter compounds in hops have been used traditionally to improve appetite and digestion. Rats given hops orally demonstrated increased gastric secretion, presumably due to the bitter principles. This effect did not occur when the hops was administered via intra-gastric administration. One of the key prenyl-flavonoids in hops, xanthohumol demonstrated benefit in preventing liver fibrosis and toxin-induced hepatitis in murine and rat models. The mechanism appeared to be through inhibition of hepatic stellate cells, reduction in NF-κB, inhibition of lipid peroxidation, induction of NADPH-quinone oxidoreductase, and induction of Nrf2. Xanthohumol was also shown to inhibit hyaluronan export via binding of multidrug resistance-associated protein 5.

Xanthohumol has been shown to prevent loss of proteoglycan and collagen as well as MMP-dependent shedding of I-CAM in culture medium. These activities suggest a role in osteoarthritis prevention. Through similar mechanisms xanthohumol may have a role in preventing or partially reversing skin aging. Xanthohumol inhibits MMP-1, MMP-8, and elastase activity, and stimulates biosynthesis of fibrillar collagens, elastin, and fibrillins. Hops has demonstrated beneficial properties for preservation of bone mineral density. In vitro studies demonstrated that specific phytoestrogen compounds found in hops exert estrogen-like activities on bone metabolism affecting both ERα and ERβ. Xanthohumol has been shown in vitro and in murine models to inhibit osteoclastogenesis. In addition, hops is high in silica, a mineral that is critical to bone maintenance.

In a study in ovariectomized rats, hops reversed the induced rise in skin temperature suggesting a role for reduction in menopausal hot flushes. The estrogenic constituent in hops extract is thought to be 8-prenylnaringenin (8-PN), which has 10% of the binding activity of 17-β-estradiol. Research done in estrogen-sensitive human cells compared the estrogenic activity of different licorice species against that of hops. The estrogenic activity decreased in the order hops > G. uralensis > G. inflata > G. glabra. In 1998 8-PN was identified as the most potent phytoestrogen known so far. 8-PN is present in small quantities in most hops extracts, but hops extracts enriched with 8-PN have been developed particularly for menopausal symptoms. The presence of phytoestrogenic activity in hops raises some concern for women with breast cancer. However, laboratory research is conflicting. One in vitro study showed an increased proliferation of breast cancer cell lines and another study showed the opposite. In vivo animal studies indicate that the estrogenic effect is minimal if there is any at all. Some of the flavonoids from hops have been shown to inhibit aromatase activity and breast cancer cell proliferation and increase breast cancer cell apoptosis in vitro. Some laboratory research has shown that hops may reduce risk for colon and prostate cancer, extending the potential benefits of hops to men.

Lupulin, the yellow resin in the flower, is thought to be the source of sedating and calming chemicals in the plant. Some of the sleep-inducing activity may be through action on melatonin receptors. The β acids in hops extract affect the plateau of GABA currents in a dose-dependent manner. Hops' volatile oil, 2-methyl-3-buten-2-ol (dimethylvinyl carbinol), is also believed to contribute to the plant's sedative properties. This volatile oil increases in amount during storage and possibly after ingestion. To further understand the calming and sedating aspects of various herbs, an in vitro study of several anxiolytic plants was performed. While lemon balm exhibited the greatest inhibition of GABA-transaminase activity, gotu kola and valerian stimulated glutamic acid decarboxylase activity, and German chamomile and hops inhibited glutamic acid decarboxylase activity.

The α and β acids in hops have been shown to be effective against Gram-positive bacteria and *Mycobacterium tuberculosis*. An interesting historical note is that brewery workers in England in the late 19th century had a fourfold lower incidence and a 30% lower mortality rate from tuberculosis. Hops polyphenols have been shown to significantly reduce growth of *Streptococcus mutans* and reduce oral lactic acid production and water-soluble glucan, contributors to dental plaque and caries.

HUMAN RESEARCH

Oral and Dental Disorders

A 3-day RCT in healthy subjects ($n = 28$) compared hops polyphenols 7 and 20 mg with placebo, one tablet dissolved orally 7 times a day for effect on dental plaque formation. Initially, an in vitro portion of the study had demonstrated that 0.5% hops polyphenol significantly reduced the growth of *S. mutans* compared with the control ($P < 0.01$), and that after an 18-h incubation, the hops polyphenol at 0.1% and 0.5% significantly reduced lactic acid production ($P < 0.05$ and $P < 0.001$, respectively). At 0.01%, 0.1%, and 0.5% it also suppressed production of water-insoluble glucan, a major component of plaque ($P < 0.01$; $P < 0.001$, and $P < 0.001$, respectively). In the clinical part of the trial, the high-dosage group exhibited a reduction in the plaque scoring system compared with the control group (1.37 vs 2.41, respectively; $P < 0.05$) (Yaegaki et al., 2008).

A crossover RCT in healthy volunteers ($n = 29$) compared hops bract polyphenols 0.1% rinse with placebo rinse following plaque removal and a subsequent 3-day abstention from oral hygiene other than the mouth rinse. The mean amount of plaque with the hops rinse was significantly less than that after the placebo rinse ($P < 0.001$). The number of *S. mutans* in the plaque samples after the hops rinse was significantly lower than after the placebo rinse ($P < 0.05$) (Shinada et al., 2007).

Allergic Disorders

A 12-week RCT in subjects ($n = 39$) with Japanese cedar allergy compared oral hops water extract 100 mg with placebo for improvement of symptoms. The nasal symptom score was reduced to a significantly greater degree in the hops group than in the placebo group. Improvements were observed in nasal swelling, nasal color, amount of nasal discharge, and characteristics of nasal discharge in the hops group after 12 weeks of treatment. Nasal eosinophils were not significant in the hops group, as opposed to the placebo group. The authors concluded that an oral administration of hops water extract may be effective in alleviating the allergic symptoms related to Japanese cedar allergy (Segawa et al., 2007).

Cardiovascular Disorders: Endothelial Dysfunction

A crossover RCT in subjects ($n = 23$) including 12 smokers and 11 nonsmokers compared isomerized hops extract rich in isohumulones with placebo for effects on endothelial function in a high oxidative stress state. At baseline, the flow-mediated dilation (FMD) of the smokers was significantly lower than that of the

nonsmokers. The FMD increased significantly after 30 and 120 min of the hops extract in both smokers and nonsmokers. Hops protected the human aortic endothelial cells from hypoxia-induced cell death as assessed by cell viability and reduced the angiotensin II-induced intracellular ROS level. The authors concluded that ingestion of isomerized hops extract appeared to exert acute beneficial effects on the endothelial function in both the smokers and nonsmokers, and that in vitro experiments suggested that the effect may be through reducing intracellular oxidative stress (Tomita et al., 2017).

A pilot study in volunteers ($n = 11$) with dyslipidemia studied the effects of tetrahydro-iso-α acids (THIAA) 125 mg from hops plus niacin 500 given BID compared with placebo on endothelial-regulated FMD. There was a clinically relevant increase in FMD with THIAA compared with a trend toward an FMD decrease with placebo. The between-arm difference was statistically significant. THIAA plus niacin treatment also improved TC, LDL-C, and uric acid. No significant improvement in these parameters was observed with placebo. The hs-CRP was significantly increased only in the placebo arm. The authors concluded that a THIAA and niacin combination may provide benefits for endothelial function in those with dyslipidemia (Lamb et al., 2012).

Cardiometabolic Disorders: Dyslipidemia, Diabetes, Metabolic Syndrome, and Obesity

A 28-day study in obese patients ($n = 9$) assessed the effects of an isohumulone drug (KDT501) given in escalating doses up to 1000 mg BID. After KDT501 treatment, plasma TGs were reduced at 4 h during a lipid tolerance test. Plasma adiponectin and high-molecular-weight adiponectin increased significantly, and plasma TNF-α decreased significantly. There were no significant changes in OGTT results or insulin sensitivity measures. The drug was well tolerated. The authors concluded that administration of isohumulone reduced measures of systemic inflammation and improved postmeal plasma TG levels, which may be beneficial in participants with insulin resistance or metabolic syndrome (Kern et al., 2017).

A 12-week RCT in subjects ($n = 200$) who were overweight compared matured hops extract (high in matured hops bitter acids) with placebo. There was a significant negative correlation between the change in visceral fat area and daily steps taken in the hops group ($r = -0.208$; $P = 0.048$). There was no significant correlation in total fat area or subcutaneous fat area. The interaction effect between hops and physical activity was suggested to be synergistic ($P = 0.055$). The authors concluded that the matured hops extract when combined with light intensity exercise could induce a greater reduction in visceral fat area, which would be beneficial for obese or overweight individuals in reducing obesity and obesity-related diseases (Suzuki et al., 2018).

A 12-week RCT in patients ($n = 104$) with metabolic syndrome investigated rho-iso-α acid (RIAA) from hops 100 mg plus proanthocyanidins from *Acacia nilotica* 500 mg one or two tablets TID compared with placebo. Subjects taking three tablets daily of the combination product showed greater reductions than placebo in TGs, TG/HDL, fasting insulin, and HOMA-IR scores. The authors concluded that this hops-*Acacia* constituent combination favorably modulated the dysregulation of metabolic syndrome (Minich et al., 2010).

A 12-week RCT in patients ($n = 94$) with prediabetes compared 16, 32, or 48 mg of isohumulones daily with placebo. After 4 weeks, FBS was decreased in the 32- and 48-mg groups but did not change in the placebo group. A1C was also significantly decreased after 4 weeks in the 16-mg group and after 8 weeks in the 32- and 48-mg groups. BMI was significantly decreased, and the decrease in total fat area was greater in the 48-mg group compared with the placebo group. The authors concluded that isohumulones had beneficial effects in diabetes and obesity (Obara et al., 2009).

A 3-week RCT in men ($n = 30$) who were required to fast for 24 h once a week for 3 weeks evaluated the effects of 100 or 250 mg of a bitter hops extract (Amarasate) BID compared with placebo, each given twice per day at 16 and 20 h into the fast. From 18 to 24 h, both the 100- and 250-mg treatment groups exhibited a greater than 10% reduction in hunger ($P < .05$). The expected noontime increase in hunger present in the placebo group was absent with both doses of hops. The authors concluded that bitter compounds may regulate appetite independently of meal timing and may be useful in reducing hunger during intermittent fasting (Walker et al., 2019).

Women's Genitourinary Disorders: Menopause

A 12-week RCT in women ($n = 120$) in early menopause compared hops with placebo for menopausal symptoms. The mean Greene Climacteric Scale score was significantly lower with hops than with placebo (AMD $= -10.0$, -18.6, and -23.4) at the end of 4, 8, and 12 weeks, respectively. The number of hot flushes was significantly lower with hops than with placebo (-8.4, -17.1, and -23.8) at 4, 8, and 12 weeks, respectively. The authors concluded that hops effectively reduced early menopausal symptoms (Aghamiri et al., 2016).

A 16-week crossover RCT in menopausal women ($n = 36$) compared hops extract standardized to 8-prenylnaringenin 100 µg/day with placebo for 8 weeks each for relief of menopausal discomforts. Both the active treatment and placebo produced significant improvements over baseline on the Kupperman Index, Menopause Rating Scale, and VAS. Placebo improvements were slightly greater at 8 weeks. After 16 weeks only the active treatment that crossed over from placebo further reduced all outcome measures, and the time-specific estimates of treatment efficacy indicated significant reductions on the Kupperman Index ($P = 0.02$) and VAS ($P = 0.03$) and a marginally significant reduction on the Menopause Rating Scale ($P = 0.06$) after 16 weeks. Placebo after active treatment resulted in an increase for all outcome measures by 16 weeks. The authors concluded that results from the second treatment period suggest superiority of the standardized hops extract over placebo (Erkkola et al., 2010).

A 12-week RCT in menopausal women ($n = 67$) investigated a hops extract standardized to 8- prenylnaringenin 100 µg QD compared with the same extract at 250 µg QD and with placebo for effects on menopausal symptoms. All three groups showed a significant reduction of the Kupperman Index after both 6 and 12 weeks. A trend for a more rapid decrease of symptoms was noticed for both active groups compared with placebo. The hops extract at 100 µg of 8-PN was significantly superior to placebo after 6 weeks ($P = 0.023$) but not after 12 weeks ($P = 0.086$). Surprisingly, the higher dose was less active than the lower dose after both 6 and 12 weeks. The hot flush score reduction was significantly greater than placebo for both doses of hops after 6 weeks ($P < 0.01$). The authors concluded that daily intake of this standardized hop extract exerted favorable effects on vasomotor symptoms and other menopausal discomforts (Heyerick et al., 2006).

A 12-week open-label trial in postmenopausal women ($n = 100$) with urogenital atrophy investigated the effects of a gel containing hyaluronic acid, liposomes, and phytoestrogens from hops extract, plus vitamin E, 2.5 g daily for 1 week then twice weekly for 11 weeks. The results showed statistically significant reductions of vaginal dryness and all other symptoms and signs since the first week of treatment. No treatment-related adverse events were reported by the subjects and the treatment course showed a high level of acceptability by the subjects. The authors concluded that this combination gel, which included hops phytoestrogens could be considered an effective and safe alternative treatment of genital atrophy in postmenopausal women, especially when HRT was not recommended (Morali et al., 2006).

Musculoskeletal Disorders: Osteoporosis and Osteoarthritis

A 14-week RCT in postmenopausal women ($n = 51$) with metabolic syndrome investigated a modified Mediterranean-style low-glycemic-load diet and aerobic exercise plus placebo compared with the same diet and exercise protocol plus 200 mg hops rho iso-α acids, 100 mg berberine sulfate trihydrate, 500 IU vitamin D_3, and 500 µg vitamin K_1 BID for effects on bone metabolism. Compared with baseline, the intervention arm exhibited an approximate 25% mean decrease ($P < 0.001$) in serum osteocalcin, whereas the placebo arm exhibited a 21% increase ($P = 0.003$). Serum 25-OH D increased 23% ($P = 0.001$) in the intervention arm and decreased 12% ($P = 0.03$) in the placebo arm. The between-arm differences for osteocalcin and 25-hydroxyvitamin D were statistically significant. Serum IGF-I was statistically increased in both arms, but the between-arm differences were not statistically significant. Subanalysis showed that among those in the highest tertile of baseline IGF-I, the intervention arm exhibited a significant increase in amino-terminal propeptide of type I collagen, whereas the placebo arm showed a significant decrease. The authors concluded that treatment with rho iso-α acids, berberine, vitamin D_3, and vitamin K_1 produced a more favorable bone biomarker profile indicative of healthy bone metabolism in postmenopausal women with metabolic syndrome (Lamb et al., 2011).

An 8-week open-label observational trial in patients ($n = 54$) with OA, rheumatoid arthritis and fibromyalgia investigated the efficacy of Meta050, a proprietary standardized combination of reduced iso-α acids from hops, rosemary extract, and oleanolic acid, 440 mg TID X 4 weeks then 880 mg BID X 4 weeks. A statistically significant decrease in pain of 50% and 40%, respectively, was observed in arthritis subjects using the visual analog scale and the abridged arthritis impact measurement scale ($P < 0.0001$ and $P < 0.0001$, respectively). Fibromyalgia subject scores did not significantly improve. A decreasing trend of CRP was also observed in subjects with elevated baseline CRP. No serious side effects were observed. The authors concluded that this standardized combination of reduced iso-α acids at a dosage of 440 mg TID had a beneficial effect on pain in arthritis subjects (Lukaczer et al., 2005).

A 6-week open-label pilot study in patients ($n = 13$) with knee OA found that rho iso-α acids 500 mg BID produced a 54% reduction in WOMAC global scores ($P < 0.0010$). WOMAC subscales of pain, stiffness, and physical function assessment showed an average 45% reduction in scores. VAS scores for pain showed reduction as well ($P < 0.01$) (Hall et al., 2008).

Neurological Disorders: Cognitive Decline

A 12-week RCT in older adults ($n = 100$) with perceived cognitive decline compared matured hop bitter acids (MHBA) with placebo for cognitive effects. At 12 weeks, Symbol Digit Modalities Test (SDMT) score assessing divided attention was significantly higher ($P = 0.045$) and β-endorphin (a marker for stress) was significantly lower ($P = 0.043$) in the subjects receiving MHBA. Memory retrieval and the Ray Verbal Learning Test also significantly improved with MHBA in the subgroup with perceived subjective cognitive decline and without requirement for medical assistance. The authors concluded that MHBA intake improved cognitive function, attention, and mood in older adults (Fukuda et al., 2020b).

Psychiatric Disorders: Anxiety and Depression

An RCT in healthy volunteers ($n = 50$) compared a beverage containing β-eudesmol, an oxygenated sesquiterpene in immature hops, with placebo for effects on objective and subjective markers related to sympathetic nerve activity after the application of mental stress. The beverages were given 5 min before taking the Trier Social Stress Test as a mental stressor. Saliva 3-methoxy-4-hydroxyphenylglycol (MHPG), a major product of noradrenaline breakdown and a representative marker of sympathetic nerve activity, was significantly lower just after the mental stressor test in the β-eudesmol group compared with the placebo group. Saliva cortisol was not significantly different between the two groups (Ohara et al., 2018).

A 4-week by 4-week crossover RCT in patients ($n = 36$) with mild depression based on Depression Anxiety Stress Scale-21 compared hops with placebo for effect on mood. With hops compared with baseline, there were significantly decreased DASS-21 scores for anxiety (9.2 and 5.1 for baseline and hops, respectively), depression (11.9 and 9.2, respectively), and stress (19.1 and 11.6, respectively; $P < 0.05$ for all). These changes were significantly greater compared with those caused by the placebo (all $P < 0.05$). The authors concluded that in otherwise healthy young adults reporting at least mild depression, anxiety, and stress symptoms, daily supplementation with a hops dry extract could significantly improve all these symptoms over a 4-week period (Kyrou et al., 2017).

A crossover RCT in healthy volunteers ($n = 16$) investigated a multiherbal lozenge containing lavender, hops, lemon balm, and oat compared with a placebo lozenge with respect to EEG patterns. After baseline recording each subject sucked a lozenge and 2 h later a second one. Recording was performed immediately after finishing the lozenge and in hourly intervals thereafter. Increases in α-1, α-2, and β-1 electrical power occurred at the electrode positions Cz, P3, T3, and T5, and these increases were even more pronounced after a second application 2 h later. The authors concluded that this herbal lozenge could lead to improved coping with psychological and emotional stress (Dimpfel and Suter, 2008).

Psychiatric Disorders: Insomnia

A 2010 systematic review to evaluate the efficacy of valerian and hops in the treatment of primary insomnia found 12 studies that used valerian with or without hops. These studies were associated with improvements in some sleep parameters such as sleep latency and quality of sleep, but further studies were recommended by the authors (Salter and Brownie, 2010).

A 2-week RCT in patients ($n = 91$) with primary insomnia investigated NSF-3, an herbal combination containing valerian, hops, and passionflower, one tablet QHS compared with zolpidem 10 mg QHS. There was a significant improvement in total sleep time, sleep latency, number of nightly awakenings, and insomnia severity index scores in both groups. No statistically significant difference was observed between the groups. Epworth Sleepiness Scale scores did not change significantly over the study period. Mild adverse events were reported in 12 herbal subjects and 16 zolpidem subjects. The authors concluded that this combination of valerian, hops, and passionflower was a safe and effective short-term alternative to zolpidem for primary insomnia (Maroo et al., 2013).

A 28-day RCT in patients ($n = 184$) with mild insomnia investigated standardized extracts of valerian and hops for 28 days compared with placebo for 28 days and with diphenhydramine 50 mg for 2 weeks followed by placebo. Subjective sleep parameters improved modestly with the herbal combination and with diphenhydramine. The herbal combination produced slightly greater reductions of sleep latency than did placebo and diphenhydramine by 14 days and greater reductions than placebo by 28 days of treatment. Diphenhydramine produced significantly greater increases in sleep efficiency and a trend toward increased total sleep time relative to placebo during the first 14 days of treatment. There was no significant group difference on any of the sleep continuity variables measured by polysomnography, and no alteration in stages 3–4 sleep and REM sleep with any of the treatments. Patients in the herbal and diphenhydramine groups rated their insomnia severity lower relative to placebo at the end of 14 days of treatment. Quality of life was significantly more improved in the herbal group relative to the placebo group at the end of 28 days. There were no significant residual effects and no serious adverse events with either valerian-hops or diphenhydramine and no rebound insomnia following their discontinuation. The authors concluded that there was a modest hypnotic effect with the herbal combination and with diphenhydramine relative to placebo, and that there was an improved quality of life with the valerian-hops combination (Morin et al., 2005).

A single-dose study of patients ($n = 42$) who were characterized as poor sleepers investigated the acute effects of a valerian-hops combination fluid extract 2 mL in 50 mL water compared with a similar placebo given 15 min before EEG recording during the night. Time spent in sleep was significantly greater for the herbal group compared with the placebo group ($P < 0.01$). The difference with respect to time spent in deeper sleep was also significantly superior with the herbal treatment ($P < 0.01$). Sleep quality as derived from the sleep inventory SF-A subscore was also superior with the herbal combination ($P < 0.0001$). The authors concluded that valerian-hops fluid extract could be used successfully for sleep as a single administration (Dimpfel et al., 2004).

A clinical trial in patients with nonorganic insomnia studied a fixed extract combination of valerian 500 mg plus hops 120 mg compared with valerian 500 mg alone and with placebo for effect on sleep latency. Objective sleep parameters were registered by means of a transportable home recorder system. The fixed extract combination was significantly superior to placebo in reducing the sleep latency. The single valerian extract was not superior to placebo (Koetter et al., 2007).

A 3-week RCT in patients with sleep disorders compared a hops-valerian combination with a benzodiazepine for 2 weeks with an additional week of follow-up. Sleep quality, fitness, and quality of life were determined by psychometric tests, psychopathologic scales, and sleep-questionnaires at the beginning and end of therapy. The equivalence of both therapies according to sleep quality, fitness, and quality of life was proven by a Mann-Whitney-Statistic of 0.50. The patients' state of health improved during therapy while showing a deterioration after cessation with both preparations. Withdrawal symptoms were documented only with the benzodiazepine. Stomach complaints were reported equally in both groups (Schmitz and Jäckel, 1998).

An RCT in healthy volunteers ($n = 80$) assessed residual sedative effects of valerian-hops tablets compared with valerian syrup, with flunitrazepam, and with placebo. The subjective perception of sleep quality was improved in all three medication groups when compared with placebo. A very slight impairment of vigilance 1–2 h after taking the valerian was statistically significant as well as a retardation in the

processing of complex information for valerian plus hops. Objectively measurable impairment of performance on the morning after medication occurred only in the flunitrazepam group, a finding that was even more pronounced in the subjective questionnaires. Mild side effects were reported in 10% of the herbal and placebo groups and in 50% of the flunitrazepam group. The authors concluded that residual sedative effects observed in some earlier studies could not be confirmed for the recommended doses of the two herbal remedies but instead showed improved subjective reports of alertness, activity, and well-being. However, a slight impairment of performance during the first few hours after ingestion should be anticipated. The authors noted that impairment of vigilance on the morning after ingestion of benzodiazepines constituted a potential hazard and that plant remedies such as those examined in this study should be considered as viable alternatives (Gerhard et al., 1996).

A 20-day RCT in patients ($n = 120$) with sleep disturbances compared Vagonette (an herbal compound containing valerian, hops, and jujube) 2 QHS with placebo. The group receiving the herbal combination showed a faster onset of sleep and longer total sleep time with fewer nocturnal awakenings compared with the placebo group ($P < 0.001$). Daily symptom scores showed significant reductions in tension and irritability, difficulty in concentration, and fatigue intensity with the herbal product compared with placebo ($P < 0.001$). There were no reported adverse reactions with the herbal combination, and 98% of subjects judged the product as having from good to excellent safety and tolerability (Palmieri et al., 2017).

A 3-week controlled trial in volunteers ($n = 30$) assessed the effects of nonalcoholic beer on sleep quality. The first 7 days were used as the control, and during the following 14 days the students ingested nonalcoholic beer during dinner. Subjective Sleep Quality improved and sleep latency decreased during the beer-drinking portion of the study compared with the initial control week ($P < 0.05$). The overall rating Global Score of Quality of Sleep also improved significantly ($P < 0.05$) (Franco et al., 2014).

A 2-week pilot study in patients ($n = 30$) with mild-moderate nonorganic insomnia investigated Ze 91,019 (valerian 250 mg plus hops 60 mg) two tablets HS for effects of polysomnography. A polysomnographic re-examination after 2 weeks of treatment revealed declines in the sleep latency and wake time. Stage 1 sleep was reduced and slow wave sleep was increased. In addition, the patients reported being more refreshed in the morning. No adverse events were observed (Fussel et al., 2000).

Psychiatric Disorders: General Cognitive Performance

A 12-week RCT in healthy adults ($n = 60$) ages 45–64 years with self-awareness of cognitive decline compared matured hop bitter acids (MHBAs) 35 mg/day with placebo for cognitive and mood effects. The change in verbal fluency score at week 6 compared with baseline was significantly higher with MHBAs compared with placebo ($P = 0.034$). Stroop test score at week 12 was significantly lower with MHBAs-compared with placebo ($P = 0.019$). Subjective fatigue and anxiety at week 12 were significantly improved with MHBAs compared with placebo ($P = 0.008$ and .043, respectively). The authors concluded that hop-derived bitter acids might be beneficial for cognition and mood (Fukuda et al., 2020a).

Dermatological Disorders: Oily Skin and Body Odor

A 17-day split-face RCT in healthy volunteers ($n = 21$) with normal-to-oily skin compared a face cleanser with hops and willow bark plus disodium cocoyl glutamate (as a mild cleansing agent) with a standard face cleanser containing sodium laurel sulfate, each applied BID for 15 days, for effect on skin sebum production. The sebum level was determined using a Sebumeter and skin redness was measured using a Mexameter. The botanical face cleanser significantly reduced the sebum level ($P < 0.01$) in the test area that persisted through day 17. The control cleanser showed a statistically relevant degreasing effect on day 15, but after cessation of application the sebum level increased again by day 17. None of the cleansers caused skin irritation as determined by skin redness measurements. The authors concluded that the botanical skin cleanser had a continuous degreasing effect without reactive seborrhea after the treatment break (Weber et al., 2019).

An open-label study in volunteers ($n = 6$) assessed supercritical hops extract for antibacterial properties

and for antiodor properties when added to zinc ricinoleate prepared into a deodorant stick. The extract was submitted to a zone of inhibition test and an agar-dilution assay against *C. xerosis* and *S. epidermidis*. MIC values of 6.25 and 25 μg/mL against *Corynebacterium xerosis* and *S. aureus*, respectively, were obtained. In the clinical odor evaluation, the mean malodor score dropped from 6.28 to 1.80, 1.82, and 2.24 after 8, 12, and 24 h, respectively. The authors concluded that hops had good in vitro antibacterial properties and, in combination with zinc ricinoleate in an appropriate base, reduced odor (Dumas et al., 2009).

Oncologic Disorders: Cancer Prophylaxis

A randomized crossover trial in volunteers ($n = 22$) provided a beverage with 12 mg/day of the hops flavonoid xanthohumol to assess effects on DNA stability. A decrease of oxidatively damaged purines and protection against ROS-induced DNA damage was found after the consumption of the beverage; also, the excretion of 8-oxo-7,8-dihydro-2′-deoxyguanosine and 8-oxo-guanosine in urine was reduced. The authors concluded that low doses of xanthohumol protected humans against oxidative DNA damage (Gerhauser et al., 2002).

ACTIVE CONSTITUENTS

Strobiles

- Carbohydrates:
  - Organic acids (antiproliferative, antiinflammatory)
- Phenolic compounds:
  - Polyphenols
  - Prenyl-flavonoids (antiproliferative, antineoplastic, antiinflammatory): xanthohumol (antiangioigenic via inhibition of NF-kB and Akt pathway, antineoplastic); isoxanthohumol; 8-prenylaringen (8-PN) (most estrogenic; low quantities, requires certain intestinal bacteria to metabolize xanthohumol to 8-PN, antiinflammatory). Prenyl flavonoids from hops inhibit aromatase activity
  - Phloroglucinol derivatives (antibacterial, sedative): humulones (α acids), lupulones (β acids, estrogenic), 2-methyl-3-butenol, isohumulone,

isocohumulone (activate PPAR-α and -γ, reduce insulin resistance), humulon (antiin-flammatory), colupulone

- Aromatic compounds (sedative-hypnotic, antimicrobial): myrcene, α-humulene, β-acryophyllene, farnesene

HOPS COMMONLY USED PREPARATIONS AND DOSAGE (FOR ADULTS UNLESS OTHERWISE SPECIFIED)

The following are examples of some available formulations and ranges of dosing for commercial herbal products. See Part III Introduction "How to prescribe medicinal herbs" for further guidance on herbal advising and prescribing.

Dried Strobiles

- Infusion: 1–2 tsp per cup TID or HS prn insomnia.
- Fluid extract (1:1, 45%): 0.5–1 mL TID or HS prn insomnia.
- Tincture (1:5, 40%–75%): 1–4 mL BID or TID.
- Powdered strobile concentrated (5:1) extract: 520 mg (1/4 tsp) QD.
- Capsule or tablet of freeze-dried strobiles: 200 mg QD-TID.
- Capsule or tablet of powdered strobile extract: 340–620 mg QD.

SAFETY AND PRECAUTION

Side Effects

May cause drowsiness and contact dermatitis. High rates of hops allergies have been reported in hop farmers.

Case Reports

Postmenopausal bleeding has been reported in women taking hop-soy supplements.

Toxicity

No chromosomal abnormalities were observed with the 2000 mg/kg dose of a matured hops extract; no deaths or signs of toxicity were recorded in the acute and subchronic safety studies. The NOAEL was found to be over 3484 mg/kg BW/day (males) or 4022 mg/kg BW/day (females).

A 14-day clinical study assessed the safety of RIAA 900 mg/day. When compared with naproxen 1000 mg/day with respect to GI safety, RIAA produced no change while naproxen increased fecal calprotectin 200%. RIAA did not reduce prostacyclin or change the urinary prostacyclin/thromboxane B2 ratio, indicating there is no increase in platelet activation and aggregation.

Pregnancy and Lactation

Insufficient human safety data.

Disease Interactions

Based on lack of research and some evidence that hop has phytoestrogenic effects, patients with hormone-sensitive cancer should avoid hops extracts.

Drug Interactions

- CYP: Inhibits CYP3A11 and CYP2C9. Drugs that induce CYP1A2 may increase the estrogenic effect of hops extracts.
- May increase effects of sedative drugs.
- Some hops species may slow clearance of acetaminophen.

REFERENCES

Aghamiri V, Mirghafourvand M, Mohammad-Alizadeh-Charandabi S, Nazemiyeh H. The effect of hop (*Humulus lupulus* L.) on early menopausal symptoms and hot flushes: a randomized placebo-controlled trial. Complement Ther Clin Pract 2016;23:130–5.

Dimpfel W, Suter A. Sleep improving effects of a single dose administration of a valerian/hops fluid extract—a double blind, randomized, placebo-controlled sleep-EEG study in a parallel design using electrohypnograms. Eur J Med Res 2008;13(5):200–4.

Dimpfel W, Pischel I, Lehnfeld R. Effects of lozenge containing lavender oil, extracts from hops, lemon balm and oat on electrical brain activity of volunteers. Eur J Med Res 2004;9(9):423–31.

Dumas ER, Michaud AE, Bergeron C, Lafrance JL, Mortillo S, Gafner S. Deodorant effects of a supercritical hops extract: antibacterial activity against Corynebacterium xerosis and *Staphylococcus epidermidis* and efficacy testing of a hops/zinc ricinoleate stick in humans through the sensory evaluation of axillary deodorancy. J Cosmet Dermatol 2009;8(3):197–204.

Erkkola R, Vervarcke S, Vansteelandt S, Rompotti P, De Keukeleire D, Heyerick A. A randomized, double-blind, placebo-controlled, crossover pilot study on the use of a standardized hop extract to alleviate menopausal discomforts. Phytomedicine 2010;17(6):389–96.

Franco L, Bravo R, Galán C, Rodríguez AB, Barriga C, Cubero J. Effect of non-alcoholic beer on subjective sleep quality in a university stressed population. Acta Physiol Hung 2014;101(3):353–61.

Fukuda T, Obara K, Saito J, Umeda S, Ano Y. Effects of hop bitter acids, bitter components in beer, on cognition in healthy adults: a randomized controlled trial. J Agric Food Chem 2020a;68(1):206–12.

Fukuda T, Ohnuma T, Obara K, Kondo S, Arai H, Ano Y. Supplementation with matured hop bitter acids improves cognitive performance and mood state in healthy older adults with subjective cognitive decline. J Alzheimers Dis 2020b;76(1):387–98. https://doi.org/10.3233/JAD-200229.

Fussel A, Wolf A, Brattström A. Effect of a fixed valerian-hop extract combination (Ze 9109) on sleep polygraphy in patients with non-organic insomnia: a pilot study. Eur J Med Res 2000;5:385–90.

Gerhard U, Linnenbrink N, Georghiadou C, Hobi V. Vigilance-decreasing effects of 2 plant-derived sedatives. Praxis (Bern 1994) 1996;85(15):473–81.

Gerhauser C, Alt A, Heiss E, et al. Cancer chemopreventive activity of xanthohumol, a natural product derived from hop. Mol Cancer Ther 2002;1(11):959–69.

Hall AJ, Babish JG, Darland GK, et al. Safety, efficacy and anti-inflammatory activity of rho iso-α-acids from hops. Phytochemistry 2008;69(7):1534–47.

Heyerick A, Vervarcke S, Depypere H, Bracke M, De Keukeleire D. A first prospective, randomized, double-blind, placebo-controlled study on the use of a standardized hop extract to alleviate menopausal discomforts. Maturitas 2006;54(2):164–75.

Kern PA, Finlin BS, Ross D, et al. Effects of KDT501 on metabolic parameters in insulin-resistant prediabetic humans. J Endocr Soc 2017;1(6):650–9.

Koetter U, Schrader E, Käufeler R, Brattström A. A randomized, double blind, placebo-controlled, prospective clinical study to demonstrate clinical efficacy of a fixed valerian hops extract combination (Ze 91019) in patients suffering from non-organic sleep disorder. Phytother Res 2007;21(9):847–51.

Kyrou I, Christou A, Panagiotakos D, et al. Effects of a hops (Humulus lupulus L.) dry extract supplement on self-reported depression, anxiety and stress levels in apparently healthy young adults: a randomized, placebo-controlled, double-blind, crossover pilot study. Hormones (Athens) 2017;16(2):171–80.

Lamb JJ, Holick MF, Lerman RH, et al. Nutritional supplementation of hop rho iso-α acids, berberine, vitamin D_3, and vitamin K_1 produces a favorable bone biomarker profile supporting healthy bone metabolism in postmenopausal women with metabolic syndrome. Nutr Res 2011;31(5):347–55.

Lamb JJ, Konda VR, Desai A, Bland JS, Tripp ML. The effects of tetrahydro-iso-α acids and niacin on monocyte-endothelial cell interactions and flow-mediated vasodilation. Glob Adv Health Med 2012;1(4):84–91.

Lukaczer D, Darland G, Tripp M, et al. A pilot trial evaluating Meta050, a proprietary combination of reduced iso-α acids, rosemary extract and oleanolic acid in patients with arthritis and fibromyalgia. Phytother Res 2005;19(10):864–9.

Maroo N, Hazra A, Das T. Efficacy and safety of a polyherbal sedative-hypnotic formulation NSF-3 in primary insomnia in comparison with zolpidem: a randomized controlled trial. Indian J Pharmacol 2013;45(1):34–9. https://doi.org/10.4103/0253-7613.106432.

Minich DM, Lerman RH, Darland G, et al. Hop and acacia phytochemicals decreased lipotoxicity in 3T3-L1 adipocytes, db/db mice, and individuals with metabolic syndrome. J Nutr Metab 2010. pii:467316.

Morali G, Polatti F, Metelitsa EN, Mascarucci P, Magnani P, Marre GB. Open, non-controlled clinical studies to assess the efficacy and safety of a medical device in form of gel topically and intravaginally used in postmenopausal women with genital atrophy. Arzneimittelforschung 2006;56(3):230–8.

Morin CM, Koetter U, Bastien CH, Ware JC, Wooten V. Valerian-hops combination and diphenhydramine for treating insomnia: a randomized placebo-controlled clinical trial. Sleep 2005;28(11):1307–13.

Obara K, Mizutani M, Hitomi Y, Yajima H, Kondo K. Isohumulones, the bitter component of beer, improve hyperglycemia and decrease body fat in Japanese subjects with prediabetes. Clin Nutr 2009;28(3):278–84.

Ohara K, Misaizu A, Kaneko Y, et al. β-Eudesmol, an oxygenized sesquiterpene, reduces the increase in saliva 3-methoxy-4-hydroxyphenylglycol after the "trier social stress test" in healthy humans: a randomized, double-blind, placebo-controlled crossover study. Nutrients 2018;11(1). pii:E9.

Palmieri G, Contaldi P, Fogliame G. Evaluation of effectiveness and safety of a herbal compound in primary insomnia symptoms and sleep disturbances not related to medical or psychiatric causes. Nat Sci Sleep 2017;9:163–9.

Salter S, Brownie S. Treating primary insomnia—the efficacy of valerian and hops. Aust Fam Physician 2010;39(6):433–7.

Schmitz M, Jäckel M. Comparative study for assessing quality of life of patients with exogenous sleep disorders (temporary sleep onset and sleep interruption disorders) treated with a hops-valarian preparation and a benzodiazepine drug. Wien Med Wochenschr 1998;148(13):291–8.

Segawa S, Takata Y, Wakita Y, et al. Clinical effects of a hop water extract on Japanese cedar pollinosis during the pollen season: a double-blind, placebo-controlled trial. Biosci Biotechnol Biochem 2007;71(8):1955–62 [Epub 2007 Aug. 7].

Shinada K, Tagashira M, Watanabe H, et al. Hop bract polyphenols reduced three-day dental plaque regrowth. J Dent Res 2007;86(9):848–51.

Suzuki S, Yamazaki T, Takahashi C, Kaneko Y, Morimoto-Kobayashi Y, Katayama M. The relationship between the effect of matured hop extract and physical activity on reducing body fat: re-analysis of data from a randomized, double-blind, placebo-controlled parallel group study. Nutr J 2018;17(1):98.

Tomita J, Mochizuki S, Fujimoto S, et al. Acute improvement of endothelial functions after oral ingestion of isohumulones, bitter components of beer. Biochem Biophys Res Commun 2017;484(4):740–5.

Walker E, Lo K, Tham S, et al. New Zealand bitter hops extract reduces hunger during a 24 h water only fast. Nutrients 2019;11(11):2754.

Weber N, Schwabe K, Schempp CM, Wölfle U. Effect of a botanical cleansing lotion on skin sebum and erythema of the face: a randomized controlled blinded half-side comparison. J Cosmet Dermatol 2019;18(3):821–6.

Yaegaki K, Tanaka T, Sato T, et al. Hop polyphenols suppress production of water-insoluble glucan by Streptococcus mutans and dental plaque growth in vivo. J Clin Dent 2008;19(2):74–8.

56

HORSE CHESTNUT (*AESCULUS HIPPOCASTANUM*)
Seed

GENERAL OVERVIEW

Horse chestnut seed extract (HCSE) is a useful product with clinical evidence for chronic venous insufficiency (CVI). Conclusions from systematic reviews and meta-analyses state that horse chestnut extract is a safe and well-tolerated treatment for CVI. It has venotonic, vascular protective, antispasmodic, anti-edematous, anti-allergic, anti-inflammatory, astringent, vasodilator, bitter, and diuretic properties. It can be used both topically and systemically for capillary and venous-related soft tissue edema. In addition to benefits for chronic venous insufficiency, clinical trials indicate that HCSE or its constituent escin may be beneficial for hearing loss and varicocele-related infertility.

IN VITRO AND ANIMAL RESEARCH

In vitro studies have shown that HCSE induces contraction of isolated vein, which is thought to be mediated through 5-HT2A receptors. In addition, contraction forces generated by non-muscle cells such as fibroblasts have been demonstrated with horse chestnut. However, the venotonic efficacy of HCSE is believed to be due primarily to an inhibitory effect on the catalytic breakdown of capillary wall proteoglycans.

The chief constituent in HCSE is escin (aka aescin), which is a mixture of triterpenoid saponins. Escin has been shown to have anti-inflammatory, neuroprotective, and antitumor effects. It improves capillary stability and inhibits hyaluronidase. Escin stimulates release of PGF2α leading to an anti-exudative effect through downregulation of inflammatory genes and upregulation of GM-CSF. PGF2α inhibits catabolism of venous tissue mucopolysaccharides and improves venous contractility.

In animal research, HCSE has been shown to reduce the localized edema associated with inflammation and to reduce capillary permeability to water, thus decreasing exudation into intercellular spaces. B-escin has been shown in mouse models to dose-dependently inhibit the early phase of allergic reactions by blocking mast cell activation and degranulation. It also prevents extravasation of fluids into tissue in the skin and inhibits the late response after antigen challenge in a lung allergy model of ovalbumin-sensitized mice. Allergic airway inflammation was suppressed via reduction of leucocytes, eosinophils, IL-5, and IL-13 in the bronchoalveolar lavage fluid. In both early and late allergic phase models, the inhibitory effect of β-escin was comparable to that of dexamethasone.

Escin has demonstrated antitumor potential against leukemia and multiple myeloma. It appears to potentiate TNF-induced apoptosis and inhibit tumor cell invasion. Escin also suppresses NF-κB through inhibition κB kinase complex, thus down-regulating Bcl-2 (the cellular inhibitor of apoptosis protein-2), cyclin D1, COX-2, ICAM-1, MMP-9, and VEGF. B-escin has also been shown in vitro to inhibit human hepatocellular carcinoma SMMC-7721 cells when combined with fluorouracil. These two substances appear to have a synergistic effect on cell-cycle arrest, apoptosis, caspases, and Bcl-2 expression. B-escin appears to also have synergism with gemcitabine through effects on NF-kB.

451

HUMAN RESEARCH

One of the earlier herbal trials to hit mainstream medical media concerned HCSE and was published in The Lancet in 1996. It indicated beneficial effects of HCSE for patients with chronic venous insufficiency (Diehm et al., 1996).

Ear, Nose, and Throat Disorders: Hearing Loss

A 44-day RCT in patients ($n=34$) with various inner ear causes of hearing loss investigated a fixed combination of escin plus troxerutin (a flavonoid derived from rutin) compared with pentoxifylline. After treatment with the combination of escin and troxerutin, hearing threshold improved more than 10 dB in 23 of 34 subjects ($P < 0.05$). With pentoxifylline hearing also improved, although to a lesser degree. Both drugs were well tolerated; major adverse drug effects were not observed with either treatment (Siegers et al., 2008).

Cardiovascular Disorders: Chronic Venous Insufficiency

A 2015 review of the evidence for efficacy of horse chestnut from in vitro, in vivo, and clinical trials concluded that the results of studies had proven that HCSE not only significantly improved subjective symptoms in patients with CVI like calf spasm, leg pain, pruritus, and fatigue, but it also reduced leg volume and ankle and calf circumferences. The preparations containing HCSE had similar effectiveness as compression therapy and as a preparation with O-(β-hydroxyethyl)-rutosides (four studies on the latter). The review also concluded that HCSE had been proven to be safe and very well tolerated (Dudek-Makech and Studzinksa-Sroka, 2015).

A 2012 systematic review on the efficacy of oral HCSE for CVI found seven placebo-controlled trials that assessed leg pain, edema, and pruritis. Six trials reported significant reductions of leg pain and reductions of edema in the HCSE groups compared with the placebo groups, and the seventh study reported a statistically significant improvement compared with baseline. One trial suggested a WMD of 42.4 mm measured on a 100 mm VAS. Of the seven trials that measured leg volume, six ($n=502$) suggested a WMD of 32.1 mL in favor

of horse chestnut compared with placebo. One trial indicated that horse chestnut may be as effective as treatment with compression stockings. Adverse events were usually mild and infrequent. The authors concluded that HCSE was an efficacious and safe short-term treatment for CVI (Pittler and Ernst, 2012).

A 2006 review of four clinical trials in patients with CVI and one study in patients with varicose veins demonstrated the effectiveness of Aesculaforce (fresh HCSE as tincture, tablets 20 mg or 50 mg, or topical gel) through the objective measure of reduction in lower leg edema and the subjective alleviation of leg pain, heaviness, and itching. The authors concluded that this HCSE preparation offered a safe and well-tolerated alternative treatment for patients with mild-to-moderate venous insufficiency (Suter et al., 2006).

A 2002 systematic review included, for the first time, data from both RCTs and large-scale observational studies regarding outcomes as well as adverse events of HCSE for CVI. It included 13 RCTs of patients ($n=1051$) with CVI and three observational studies ($n=10,725$). Overall, the RCTs indicated that HCSE improved symptoms in patients with CVI, including a reduction in leg volume by 46.4 mL, a fourfold increase in the likelihood of improvement in leg pain, a 1.5-fold increased likelihood for improvement of edema and a 1.7-fold increase in likelihood for improvement of itching. There was insufficient evidence to demonstrate the herb's effect on leg fatigue/heaviness or calf cramps. Observational studies showed significant effectiveness regarding pain, edema, and leg fatigue/heaviness. No severe adverse events were reported, and HCSE did not significantly increase mild adverse events (Siebert et al., 2002).

The first systematic review of HCSE for efficacy with CVI occurred in 1998. This review found that the superiority of horse chestnut was suggested by all placebo-controlled studies. The use of horse chestnut was associated with a decrease of the lower-leg volume and a reduction in leg circumference at the calf and ankle. Symptoms such as leg pain, pruritus, and a feeling of fatigue and tenseness were reduced. Five comparative trials against the reference medication indicated that HCSE and O-(β-hydroxyethyl)-rutosides were equally effective. One trial suggested a therapeutic equivalence of HCSE and compression therapy. Adverse effects were usually mild and infrequent (Pittler and Ernst, 1998).

A 12-week RCT in patients ($n = 54$) with venous leg ulcers compared HCSE with placebo. The difference between groups in the number of healed leg ulcers and change in wound surface area, depth, volume, pain, and exudate was not statistically significant. However, horse chestnut did have a significant effect on the percentage of wound slough over time ($P = 0.045$) and on the number of dressing changes at week 12 ($P = 0.009$). The authors concluded that although the study did not support the claim of facilitating venous ulcer healing, the significant improvement in wound slough and visit frequency indicated it may be useful in management of venous leg ulcers. A cost-benefit analysis of HCSE therapy was conducted considering the cost of the herbal product, dressing materials, travel, staff salaries, and infrastructure for each patient. HCSE therapy combined with conventional therapy was found to be more cost-effective than conventional therapy alone with an average savings of 95 Australian dollars in organizational costs and 10 Australian dollars in dressing materials per patient (Leach et al., 2006a,b).

A 12-week RCT in patients ($n = 240$) with CVI compared HCSE standardized to 50 mg of escin BID with placebo. Lower leg volume of the more severely affected limb decreased on average by 43.8 mL with HCSE and 46.7 mL with compression therapy, while it increased by 9.8 mL with placebo. Significant edema reductions were achieved by HCSE ($P = 0.005$) and compression ($P = 0.002$) compared with placebo, and the two therapies were shown to be equivalent ($P = 0.001$). Both HCSE and compression therapy were well tolerated, and no serious treatment-related events were reported. The authors concluded that compression stocking therapy and HCSE therapy were alternative therapies for treating edema of CVI (Diehm et al., 1996).

An 8-week open-label study was carried out to assess the safety and tolerability of HCSE 50 mg BID in the treatment of CVI. In total, 91 adverse events were reported, of which only four were rated as probably related to the study drug. Patients judged the tolerability of the study medication at visits 2 and 3 to be "good" or "fairly good" (90% and 95%, respectively). Both the ankle and lower leg circumference decreased, with a difference in the median

value between baseline and 8 weeks for all symptoms being significant. The majority of patients rated efficacy to be "very good" or "good" (Dickson et al., 2004).

A 4-week open controlled study in patients ($n = 40$) with CVI compared French maritime pine bark extract 360 mg/day with HCSE 600 mg/day. The pine bark extract significantly reduced the circumference of the lower limbs and improved subjective symptoms. It also significantly decreased serum TC and LDL-C values but had no effect on HDL-C. HCSE only moderately but insignificantly reduced the circumference of the lower limbs and marginally improved symptoms and had no effect on lipid values (Koch, 2002).

An 18-week RCT in postmenopausal women ($n = 137$) with CVI investigated HCSE 600 mg/day for 12 weeks compared with oxerutins (O-(β-hydroxyethyl)-rutosides)1000 mg/day for 12 weeks and with oxerutins 1000 mg/day for 4 weeks then 500 mg/day for 8 weeks. Leg volume was reduced by 3004 mL-d, 5273 mL-d, and 3187 mL-d with HCSE, full dose oxerutins, and reduced dose oxerutins, respectively. Based on follow-up measurements at the 18th week, both compounds exhibited a substantial carry-over effect (Rehn et al., 1996).

Men's Genitourinary Disorders: Male Infertility

A 2-month RCT in patients ($n = 219$) with varicocele-associated infertility investigated escin 30 mg BID compared with surgery and with control. Sperm density improvement rates were 38.5%, 68.8%, and 57.5%, in the control, the surgery, and the escin groups, respectively. The improvements with surgery and escin were significantly better than with the control group ($P < 0.05$ for both). Sperm motility improvement rates were 46.2%, 77.1%, and 55.7% in the control, surgery, and escin groups, respectively. A significant difference was observed only between the surgery and the control groups ($P < 0.05$). In the escin group, severity of varicocele was correlated with a variation in response (response rates 41.7%, 64%, and 20.0%, for mild, moderate, and severe disease, respectively; $P < 0.05$). The authors concluded that escin was a safe and effective drug to improve sperm quality in patients with varicocele-associated infertility (Fang et al., 2010).

Dermatological Disorders: Wrinkles and Photoaging

A 9-week study in healthy female volunteers ($n=40$) assessed the efficacy of a gel containing HCSE 3% applied topically to the skin around the eye TID. After 6 and 9 weeks, significant decreases in the VAS wrinkle scores at the corners of the eye or in the lower eyelid skin were observed compared with controls. The authors concluded that that an extract of horse chestnuts can generate contraction forces in fibroblasts and is a potent anti-aging ingredient (Fujimura et al., 2006).

ACTIVE CONSTITUENTS

Seeds

- Lipids
  - Fatty acids: including linolenic acid, palmitic acid, and steric acid
- Phenolic compounds
  - Polyphenols: proanthocyanidin A2 (antioxidant)
    - Coumarins scopeletin glucoside, aesculetin (anticancer), fraxin (anti-inflammatory, antioxidant, vascular integrity, hepatoprotective), aesculin (venotonic, lymphatotonic). *Aesculin (a coumarin glycoside) found on the bark, leaves, and seeds needs to be removed from extracts as it is toxic.*
    - Flavonoids: quercitin, tamarixetin, rutin (antioxidant, anti-inflammatory, antidiabetic, nephroprotective, anti-osteoporotic, antispasmodic, neuroprotective, antianxiety), kaempferol (anti-inflammatory, antidepressant, strengthens capillaries)
    - Tannins
- Terpenes
  - Triterpenoid saponins
    - Escin/escins: β-escins and α-escins (Ia, Ib, IIa, IIb, IIIa, IIIb, IV, V, VI and isoescins Ia, Ib and V) (anti-inflammatory, venotonic)
- Steroids:
  - Phytosterols: stigmasterol, α-spinaserol, β-sitosterol (reduces GI cholesterol absorption, inhibits 5-α-reductase)

Bark

- Alkaloids: quinine (antiprotozoal, spasmolytic, anti-arthritic)

HORSE CHESTNUT COMMONLY USED PREPARATIONS AND DOSAGE (FOR ADULTS UNLESS OTHERWISE SPECIFIED)

The following are examples of some available formulations and ranges of dosing for commercial herbal products. See Part III Introduction "How to prescribe medicinal herbs" for further guidance on herbal advising and prescribing.

Seed

- Tincture (1:5, 40%): 1–4 mL TID; alternatively (1:2.6, 65%) 0. 5–0.7 mL TID
- Powdered extract: 300 mg (1/6 tsp) QD-BID.
- Capsule or tablet of standardized extract (standardized to 16%–20% escin): 200–300 mg BID (or 100–150 mg escin daily)
- Topical: 2%–3% escin applied TID-QID
- *Aesculin (coumarin glycoside) found on the seeds needs to be removed during preparation as it is toxic.*
- Not recommended for children.

SAFETY AND PRECAUTION

Side Effects

Generally, well tolerated at recommended doses and proper preparation (removal of aesculin). May cause nausea, headache, and itching.

Case Reports

Contact urticaria. Anaphylactic shock reported in two cases. Life-threatening rupture of renal angiomyolipoma. Anaphylaxis, toxic nephropathy, and renal failure have been reported after IV administration.

Toxicity

Avoid the use of raw horse chestnut seed, bark, flower, or leaves due to toxicity. Higher than recommended doses can cause hemolysis, acute renal failure, and nausea. The LD50 for a single dose of extract from horse chestnut seeds was 10.6 mg/g of BW for chicks and 10.7 mg/g of BW for hamsters. The LD50 for chicks given two consecutive daily doses of horse chestnut seed was 6.5 mg/g. α-escin has been found to be toxic for bone marrow cells of mice but only when administered at a high dose of 80% LD50.

Pregnancy and Lactation

Insufficient human safety data. Studies in pregnant humans have not revealed any adverse effects.

Disease Interactions

May worsen gastroparesis or GERD due to inhibition of gastric emptying.

Drug Interactions

- CYP: Escin was shown to both inhibit and induce CYP1A2, CYP2C9 and CYP3A4 enzymes
- Theoretically may interact with anticoagulants due to inhibition of platelet aggregation (but research points to aesculin as the risky component and this is removed from most available preparations)
- May interact with highly protein-bound drugs via interference with protein-binding.
- Enhances the efficacy of gemcitabine

REFERENCES

Dickson S, Gallagher J, McIntyre L, Suter A, Tan J. An open study to assess the safety and efficacy of Aesculus hippocastanum tablets (Aesculaforce 50 mg) in the treatment of chronic venous insufficiency. J Herb Pharmacother 2004;4(2):19–32.

Diehm C, Trampisch HJ, Lange S, Schmidt C. Comparison of leg compression stocking and oral horse-chestnut seed extract therapy in patients with chronic venous insufficiency. Lancet 1996;347(8997):292–4.

Dudek-Makech M, Studzinksa-Sroka E. Horse chestnut—efficacy and safety in chronic venous insufficiency: an overview. Rev Brasil Farmacog 2015;29(5).

Fang Y, Zhao L, Yan F, et al. Escin improves sperm quality in male patients with varicocele-associated infertility. Phytomedicine 2010;17(3-4):192–6.

Fujimura T, Tsukahara K, Moriwaki S, Hotta M, Kitahara T, Takema Y. A horse chestnut extract, which induces contraction forces in fibroblasts, is a potent anti-aging ingredient. J Cosmet Sci 2006;57(5):369–76.

Koch R. Comparative study of venostasin and pycnogenol in chronic venous insufficiency. Phytother Res 2002;16(Suppl 1):S1–5.

Leach MJ, Pincombe J, Foster G. Clinical efficacy of horsechestnut seed extract in the treatment of venous ulceration. J Wound Care 2006a;15:159–67.

Leach MJ, Pincombe J, Foster G. Using horsechestnut seed extract in the treatment of venous leg ulcers: a cost-benefit analysis. Ostomy Wound Manage 2006b;52(4). 68-70, 72-4, 76-8.

Pittler MH, Ernst E. Horse-chestnut seed extract for chronic venous insufficiency. A criteria-based systematic review. Arch Dermatol 1998;134:1356–60.

Pittler MH, Ernst E. Horse chestnut seed extract for chronic venous insufficiency. Cochrane Database Syst Rev 2006;1, CD003230. Review.

Pittler MH, Ernst E. Horse chestnut seed extract for chronic venous insufficiency. Cochrane Database Syst Rev 2012;11, CD003230.

Rehn D, Unkauf M, Klein P, et al. Comparative clinical efficacy and tolerability of oxerutins and horse chestnut extract in patients with chronic venous insufficiency. Arzneimittelforschung 1996;46:483–7.

Siebert U, Brach M, Sroczynski G, Berla K. Efficacy, routine effectiveness, and safety of horsechestnut seed extract in the treatment of chronic venous insufficiency. A meta-analysis of randomized controlled trials and large observational studies. Int Angiol 2002;21:305–15.

Siegers CP, Syed Ali S, Tegtmeier M. Escin and troxerutin as a successful combination for the treatment of inner ear disturbances. Phytomedicine 2008;15:160–3.

Suter A, Bommer S, Rechner J. Treatment of patients with venous insufficiency with fresh plant horse chestnut seed extract: a review of 5 clinical studies. Adv Ther 2006;23:179–90.

57

HORSETAIL (*EQUISETUM ARVENSE*)
Above-Ground Parts

GENERAL INFORMATION

Horsetail is high in silica so may be beneficial for bones, nail, hair, and connective tissue. It is used traditionally for benign prostatic hyperplasia (BPH), prostatitis, interstitial cystitis, and childhood enuresis. It is generally thought to be beneficial for healing mucosa in the genitourinary and respiratory systems. Horsetail is used as a tonic (maintenance of health) for connective tissue and bones and is therefore thought to be useful for prevention and treatment of osteoporosis and arthritis. It can be used as a mild diuretic. Horsetail may play a role in gout management through increased uric acid excretion.

Research on this herb is sparse; however, clinical research indicates that horsetail, alone or in combination formulas, may be beneficial for fluid retention, osteoporosis, wound-healing, and psoriatic nail disease.

Horsetail contains the enzyme thiaminase, so it needs to be taken for limited periods of time or intermittently along with thiamine supplementation. Thiaminase is neutralized by alcohol, temperature, and alkalinity, so tinctures, fluid extracts, or preparations of the herb subjected to 100°C temperatures during manufacturing are preferred for medicinal use.

IN VITRO AND ANIMAL RESEARCH

Horsetail's various constituents demonstrate immunostimulant, WBC stimulant, connective tissue tonic, anti-rheumatic, anti-inflammatory, astringent, anti-hemorrhagic, hemostatic, diuretic, and vulnerary properties. The silicates in horsetail stimulate leukocyte activity. Silica in its various forms has also been shown in animal and human research to promote growth of collagen in skin, hair, and nails, and to improve hair loss and skin changes related to aging. The flavonoids and saponins in horsetail have demonstrated a diuretic effect. The horsetail constituents petrosin, onitin, and luteolin have exhibited hepatoprotective activities on tacrine-induced cytotoxicity in human liver cells.

A study in rats investigated a bone supplement (calcium plus Vitamin D, L-lysine, L-proline, L-arginine, and L-ascorbic acid) compared with the same supplement plus horsetail and with raloxifene for effects on bone density. The bone supplement had already been shown to promote bone mineralization in ovariectomized rats. Both supplement groups produced beneficial changes in serum biomarkers, bone mineral content, and femur bone histology. There were significant changes in formation and resorption markers of bone as well as in cortical bone thickness and trabecular width in these groups. The supplements appeared to be as effective as raloxifene. The group with added horsetail also restored lipid profiles to near normal levels compared with ovariectomized group (Kotwal and Badole, 2016).

A study of anti-inflammatory and nociceptive effects of horsetail was performed in mice. Horsetail extract up to 100 mg/kg reduced the writhing induced by acetic acid up to 98% in a dose-dependent manner. The 50 mg/kg and 100 mg/kg doses reduced licking time by 80% and 95% of mice, respectively, in the first phase following formalin exposure, but only the higher dose reduced licking time (by 35%) in the second phase. The effect was not reversed by naloxone. The 50 mg/kg dose reduced the paw edema at 2 h (25%) and 4 h (30%) after carrageenan administration (Do Monte et al., 2004).

A combination of *Herniaria glabra*, *Agropyron repens*, horsetail, and elderberry was given in varying doses (30–500 mg/kg) to rats with experimental nephrolithiasis. Animals treated with 125 mg/kg of the formula had significantly lower calcium oxalate crystal deposit content compared with the control group. All doses significantly decreased the number of microcalcifications compared with the control group. The number of kidneys affected by subcapsular fibrosis was significantly higher in control group than in the herbal groups. Diuresis was significantly higher than control with 125 and 500 mg/kg of the formula (Crescenti et al., 2015).

The ethanolic extract of horsetail (50 and 100 mg/kg) was comparable to diazepam in reducing anxiety behaviors in mice without producing the sedating aspects of diazepam. (Singh et al., 2011) Chronic administration of horsetail extract at dose of 50 mg/kg intraperitoneally to mice improved both short- and long-term retention of inhibitory avoidance tasks and ameliorated the cognitive performance and working memory version of the Morris Water Maze. No toxicity manifestations were observed during treatment. The authors found evidence that the cognitive enhancement may be attributed at least in part to its antioxidant action (Guilherme dos Santos et al., 2005).

Studies in streptozotocin-treated rats showed that different doses (50–150 mg/kg) of methanolic extracts of horsetail reduced blood sugar significantly compared with control groups (Safiyeh et al., 2007). In another similar study using 50 and 150 mg/kg of horsetail methanolic extract for 5 weeks, concurrent histological studies of the pancreas showed comparable regeneration between the two horsetail extract groups (Soleimani). Streptozotocin-induced diabetic mice showed improved wound healing with horsetail ointment 5% and 10% ($P < 0.05$). By day 14, the horsetail group showed 99.7% and 99.9% wound closure ratios and higher dermal and epidermal regeneration, angiogenesis, and granulation tissue thickness ($P < 0.05$) (Ozay et al., 2013).

HUMAN RESEARCH

Nephrological and Urological Disorders: Fluid Retention

A crossover RCT in healthy male volunteers ($n = 36$) compared the diuretic effects of horsetail extract 900 mg/day × 4 days with HCTZ 25 mg/day and with placebo. Each crossover period was separated by 10-day washout periods. Horsetail produced a diuretic effect that was stronger than that of placebo and was equivalent to that of HCTZ without causing significant changes in the elimination of electrolytes or catabolites. Rare minor adverse events were reported. The clinical examinations and laboratory tests showed no changes before or after the experiment, suggesting that the herb was safe for acute use (Carneiro et al., 2014).

A 12-week open-label trial in patients ($n = 100$) with BPH investigated the effects of Eviprostat, a multi-herbal formula containing horsetail plus *Populus tremula*, *Pulsatilla pratensis*, and *Triticum aestivum*, two tablets TID. IPSS was decreased by 5.67 ($P < 0.001$); QOL score was decreased by 1.44 ($P < 0.001$); Q_{max} was increased by 1.70 mL/s ($P < 0.001$); Q_{avg} was increased by 1.15 mL/s ($P < 0.001$); residual urine was decreased by 5.07 mL ($P = 0.046$), and PSA was decreased by 0.129 mcg/L ($P < 0.017$). The clinical adverse event rate was 1%. The authors concluded that Eviprostat was a safe, effective, and preferable drug for treating BPH (Singh et al., 2011).

Musculoskeletal Disorders: Osteoporosis and Musculoskeletal Pain

A 2-year RCT in menopausal women ($n = 122$) not on HRT investigated horsetail extract for 80 days compared with a sequence of placebo for 40 days and then horsetail for 40 days, with Osteosil (a combination of horsetail silica 20 mg, trace minerals and omega-3 fatty acids) for 80 days, and with no treatment (control). Placebo and control groups had no change in DXA. The total body DXA carried out at baseline and after 1 year's therapy with horsetail and with Osteosil showed a sharp increase in the average densimetric values for the vertebra, and these were significantly higher in patients treated with Osteosil, with an average recovery of bone mass of around 2.3%. During the period of the study no adverse events attributable to the administration of the study drug were reported (Corletto, 1999).

A pilot study in patients ($n = 13$) who had experienced baseline persistent musculoskeletal pain for at least 4 months (mean duration 5 years) in ≥ one body parts without relief from traditional treatments investigated the efficacy of a proprietary polyherbal combination including stinging nettle, frankincense, horsetail, garlic, celery, and thiamine 350 mg BID for 14 days. The average VAS pain subscale score was 58 at baseline and 23 at 14 days ($P < 0.05$). The average VAS subscale score for functional mobility was 57 at baseline and 29 at follow-up ($P < 0.05$). No adverse effects were reported. The authors concluded that the complex of five herbs, plus vitamin B1, should be considered as a valuable alternative treatment in the management of chronic musculoskeletal pain (Hedaya, 2017).

Dermatological Disorders: Wounds and Psoriatic Nails

An RCT in postpartum nulliparous women ($n = 108$) compared horsetail 3% topical ointment with placebo for healing of episiotomy. The case and control groups had no significant differences in baseline wound healing scores (5.0 vs 4.1) and mean pain intensity scores (5.7 vs 5.3). At 5 days the adjusted mean pain score difference was -2.3, significantly in favor of the horsetail group. At 10 days the adjusted mean pain score difference was -3.8, significantly in favor of the horsetail group. Mean numbers of acetaminophen pills used in the control and horsetail groups during the 10-day period of the study were 11.6 and 6.8, respectively ($P < 0.001$). The authors concluded that horsetail ointment promoted wound healing and relieved pain following episiotomy (Asgharikhatooni et al., 2015).

A 24-week side-by-side comparison trial in patients with nail psoriasis ($n = 30$) compared a water-soluble nail lacquer containing hydroxypropyl-chitosan, horsetail, and MSM on one hand with placebo on the other hand. With the lacquer, there was a 72% reduction in pitting, a 66% reduction in leukonychia, a 63% reduction in onycholysis, and a reduction of 65% in Nail Psoriasis Severity Index score compared with baseline. No changes were observed in the untreated nails. The patients' treatment evaluation was classified as "very satisfying" or "good" by 78.6% of patients, and 75% of them decided to continue the application after the end of the study. No adverse reactions were reported (Cantoresi et al., 2009).

A subsequent 24-week RCT in patients with nail psoriasis compared the efficacy and tolerability of the nail lacquer as noted above with placebo for effects on nail psoriasis. By 16 weeks the superiority of the nail lacquer had become apparent. After 24 weeks, the clinical cure rate showed the statistically significant superiority of the nail lacquer compared with placebo in both the intention-to-treat ($P = 0.0445$) and the per protocol population ($P = 0.0437$). Analysis of the modified Nail Psoriasis Severity Index-50 showed a statistically significant clinical improvement after 12 weeks of treatment in comparison with the results obtained after 8 weeks ($P < 0.05$). The authors concluded that the nail lacquer was an effective and safe option for decreasing the signs of nail dystrophy in psoriatic patients (Cantoresi et al., 2014).

Inflammation: Rheumatoid Arthritis

An RCT in patients ($n = 60$) with rheumatoid arthritis (RA) compared horsetail with placebo for effects on inflammatory markers. Results showed that the total effective rate for reduction of TNF-α and IL-10 with horsetail and control was 80% and 17%, respectively ($P < 0.01$). Comparisons of ESR and RF for horsetail before and after treatment were significantly different ($P < 0.01$). The differences between horsetail and placebo for before and after treatment for TNF-α, IL-10, ESR, and RF were significant ($P < 0.05$ for all). The reduction in CRP from baseline was significant ($P < 0.05$), but the difference between changes for horsetail and placebo was not significant. The authors concluded that horsetail showed a safe and reliable curative effect on RA (Jiang et al., 2014).

ACTIVE CONSTITUENTS

Aerial Parts

- Carbohydrate
  - Polysaccharides: mucilage (immune stimulating, demulcent)
  - Organic acids: equisetolic acid
- Phenolic compounds
  - Phenols (caffeic acid esters): petrosin, onitin
  - Flavonoids: quercitin, gendwanin, kaempferol glycosides, luteolin (anti-inflammatory, antispasmodic, antibacterial, hepatoprotective, anti-estrogenic, antiproliferative)
    - Tannins

- Steroids
  - Steroidal saponins: equisitonin (diuretic)
  - Phytosterols: β-sitosterol (reduces GI cholesterol absorption, inhibits 5-α-reductase), campesterol, isofucosterol
- Alkaloids: nicotine, spermidine
- Mineral silica (65%) in the form of silicic acid and silicates

HORSETAIL COMMONLY USED PREPARATIONS AND DOSAGE (FOR ADULTS UNLESS OTHERWISE SPECIFIED)

The following are examples of some available formulations and ranges of dosing for commercial herbal products. See Part III Introduction "How to prescribe medicinal herbs" for further guidance on herbal advising and prescribing.

Aerial Parts

- Infusion: 2 tsp dried herb per cup TID
- Tincture of fresh stem and leaf (1:2, 25%): 2–6 mL TID
- Tincture of dried stem and leaf (1:5, 25%): 1–4 mL TID
- Powdered stem and leaf: 450 mg (1/5 tsp) BID
- Powdered stem and leaf extract: 500–1000 mg (1/8–1/4 tsp) QD
- Capsule or tablet of powdered stem and leaf extract: 440–500 mg TID
- Capsule or tablet of standardized extract (standardized to 10% silica): 500 mg QD
- Poultice: make paste with powdered stem and leaf
- *Note: Pulse dosing 4 weeks on, 1 week off. Horsetail contains the enzyme thiaminase so needs to be taken for limited periods of time or intermittently along with thiamine supplementation. Thiaminase is neutralized by alcohol, temperature, and alkalinity so tinctures, ethanolic extracts, or preparations of the herb subjected to 100°C temperatures during manufacturing are preferred for medicinal use.*

SAFETY AND PRECAUTION

Side Effects

Horsetail is generally considered safe as long as the thiaminase activity is avoided, as noted previously. The only other concern would be that the correct species of horsetail is used. *Equisetum palustre* is a distinct species of horsetail that contains toxic alkaloids and is a well-known livestock poison.

Case Reports

A case has been reported of severe hyponatremia and hypokalemia following consumption of horsetail juice.

Toxicity

Administration of horsetail for 13 weeks to rats resulted in no toxicity at all tested doses as assessed by clinical signs, weight, urinalysis, hematology, serum biochemistry, and organ weight; the NOAEL was determined to be > 3%.

A 4% horsetail powder with a cholesterol-added diet resulted in dermatitis on the neck, head, and back in 50% of the rats studied.

Pregnancy and Lactation

Insufficient human safety data. Case report of autism when mother took horsetail during pregnancy.

Disease Interactions

Avoid with impaired cardiac and kidney function, prostate cancer, children younger than 2 years, and long-term use.

Drug Interactions

- May augment effects of diuretics
- Caution with digitalis and other cardiac glycosides due to potassium loss secondary to diuretic effect
- Caution with lithium due to potential for toxicity seen with other diuretics
- Decreased efficacy of antiretrovirals has been reported

REFERENCES

Asgharikhatooni A, Bani S, Hasanpoor S, Mohammad Alizade S, Javadzadeh Y. The effect of Equisetum arvense (horse tail) ointment on wound healing and pain intensity after episiotomy: a randomized placebo-controlled trial. Iran Red Crescent Med J 2015;17(3), e25637.

Cantoresi F, Sorgi P, Arcese A, et al. Improvement of psoriatic onychodystrophy by a water-soluble nail lacquer. J Eur Acad Dermatol Venereol 2009;23(7):832–4.

Cantoresi F, Caserini M, Bidoli A, et al. Randomized controlled trial of a water-soluble nail lacquer based on hydroxypropyl-chitosan (HPCH), in the management of nail psoriasis. Clin Cosmet Investig Dermatol 2014;7:185–90.

Carneiro DM, Freire RC, Honório TC, et al. Randomized, double-blind clinical trial to assess the acute diuretic effect of Equisetum arvense (Field Horsetail) in healthy volunteers. Evid Based Complement Alternat Med 2014;760683.

Corletto F. Female climacteric osteoporosis therapy with titrated horsetail (Equisetum arvense) extract plus calcium (osteosil calcium): randomized double-blind study. Miner Ortoped Traumatol 1999;50:201–6.

Crescenti A, Puiggròs F, Colomé A, et al. Antiurolithiasic effect of a plant mixture of Herniaria glabra, Agropyron repens, Equisetum arvense and Sambucus nigra (Herbensurina®) in the prevention of experimentally induced nephrolithiasis in rats. Arch Esp Urol 2015;68(10):739–49.

Do Monte FH, dos Santos JG, Russi M, Lanziotti VM, Leal LK, Cunha GM. Antinociceptive and anti-inflammatory properties of the hydroalcoholic extract of stems from Equisetum arvense L. in mice. Pharmacol Res 2004;49(3):239–43.

Guilherme dos Santos J, Hoffmann Martins do Monte F, Marcela Blanco M, Maria do Nascimento Bispo Lanziotti V, Damasseno Maia F, Kalyne de Almeida Leal L. Cognitive enhancement in aged rats after chronic administration of Equisetum arvense L. with demonstrated antioxidant properties in vitro. Pharmacol Biochem Behav 2005;81(3):593–600.

Hedaya R. Five herbs plus thiamine reduce pain and improve functional mobility in patients with pain: a pilot study. Altern Ther Health Med 2017;23(1):14–9.

Jiang X, Qu Q, Li M, Miao S, Li X, Cai W. Horsetail mixture on rheumatoid arthritis and its regulation on TNF-α and IL-10. Pak J Pharm Sci 2014;27(6 Suppl):2019–23.

Kotwal SD, Badole SR. Anabolic therapy with Equisetum arvense along with bone mineralising nutrients in ovariectomized rat model of osteoporosis. Indian J Pharmacol 2016;48(3):312–5.

Ozay Y, Kasim Cayci M, Guzel-Ozay S, Cimbiz A, Gurlek-Olgun E, Sabri OM. Effects of Equisetum arvense ointment on diabetic wound healing in rats. Wounds 2013;25(9):234–41.

Safiyeh S, Fathallah FB, Vahid N, Hossine N, Habib SS. Antidiabetic effect of Equisetum arvense L. (Equisetaceae) in streptozotocin-induced diabetes in male rats. Pak J Biol Sci 2007;10(10):1661–6.

Singh N, Kaur S, Bedi PM, Kaur D. Anxiolytic effects of Equisetum arvense Linn. extracts in mice. Indian J Exp Biol 2011;49(5):352–6.

Soleimani S, Azarbaizani FF, Nejati V. The effect of Equisetum arvense L. (Equisetaceae) in histological changes of pancreatic beta-cells in streptozotocin-induced diabetic in rats. Pak J Biol Sci. 2007 Dec 1;10(23):4236–40.

58

LEMON BALM (*MELISSA OFFICINALIS*)
Leaf

GENERAL OVERVIEW

A prolific plant that volunteers itself readily in most gardens, lemon balm has diverse valuable benefits. It is often studied and used as a "buddy plant" in combination with a variety of other herbs for varying indications, but it can also be effective when used by itself. In 1984, the German Commission E approved the use of lemon balm leaf, prepared as an herbal infusion, dry extract, or fluid extract, for treating nervous sleeping disorders and functional gastrointestinal complaints. In addition to its anxiolytic and gastrointestinal effects, it has cognitive, anti-diabetic, and anti-thyroid effects and demonstrates antiviral efficacy against herpes simplex virus (HSV).

Clinical research indicates that lemon balm, alone or in combination formulas, may be beneficial for bruxism, benign palpitations, dyslipidemia, diabetes, functional gastrointestinal disorders, premenstrual syndrome, dysmenorrhea, female sexual dysfunction, menopause, agitation of dementia, anxiety, insomnia, depression, attention-deficit/hyperactivity disorder, and herpes simplex infection.

IN VITRO AND ANIMAL RESEARCH

In vitro and animal studies have shown lemon balm and its relatively expensive essential oil to have anti-inflammatory, antioxidant, immune-stimulating, anticonvulsant, analgesic, antibacterial, antiviral, antiretroviral, antiproliferative, antigenotoxic, and antimutagenic properties. Inhibition of MMP-2 and AChE and stimulation of the acetylcholine and GABA receptors have been demonstrated.

Antiviral effects have been specifically demonstrated against Newcastle disease virus, Semliki Forest virus, influenza virus, myxoviruses, vaccinia, HIV, and HSV. These effects are attributed to the phenolic acid and flavonoid constituents as well as the essential oils. Antifungal and antibacterial effects have also been demonstrated with lemon balm extracts. Upper respiratory anaerobic and facultative aerobic bacteria are particularly susceptible.

Mice administered lemon balm essential oil 0.015 mg/day for 6 weeks showed significantly reduced blood glucose (65%; $P < 0.05$), improved glucose tolerance, and significantly higher serum insulin levels, compared with controls. Hepatic glucokinase, hepatic and adipocyte GLUT4, PPAR-γ, PPAR-α, and SREBP-1c expression were significantly up-regulated with lemon balm, whereas hepatic G6P and PEPCK expression were down-regulated with lemon balm essential oil. The results suggested that lemon balm is hypoglycemic via enhanced glucose uptake and metabolism in the liver and adipose tissue and inhibition of gluconeogenesis in the liver. Rats with induced diabetic neuropathy showed improvement in pain scores from the essential oil of lemon balm as well as reversal of hyperglycemia.

Lemon balm extract has moderate affinity to the GABA$_A$ site. In an in vitro study of several anxiolytic plants, lemon balm exhibited the greatest inhibition of GABA-transaminase activity, while gotu kola and valerian stimulated glutamic acid decarboxylase activity and German chamomile and hops inhibited glutamic acid decarboxylase activity.

Rat studies have demonstrated that lemon balm reduces serotonin turnover and depressive behavior. In mice, lemon balm extract produced dose-dependent sedation that did not occur with administration of the essential oil. Sedative properties have been confirmed for low doses. With high doses, a peripheral analgesic activity has been demonstrated. It has also induced sleep in mice following an infrahypnotic dose of pentobarbital and potentialized the sleep induced by a hypnotic dose of pentobarbital.

In vitro studies have found that lemon balm blocks attachment of TSH and TSH antibodies to the TSH receptors, so may be beneficial for Grave's disease. In vivo studies have also shown the TSH signal is blocked from further stimulating the excessively active thyroid gland in Grave's disease. In addition to this anti-thyroid effect, a study in rat liver microsomes showed that lemon balm aqueous extract inhibited the extrathyroidal enzymatic T4-deiodination to T3. In euthyroid rats, the administration of freeze-dried extracts of lemon balm reduced pituitary and serum TSH concentrations. Serum and pituitary prolactin levels in rats were reported to be reduced by a freeze-dried extract of lemon balm at a dose of 40 mg/100 g.

Lemon balm extract has been demonstrated in vitro to promote cell cycle arrest and apoptosis of human colon carcinoma cells through generation of free radicals. It has also been shown to inhibit proliferation of lung, breast, ovarian, and prostate cancer cell lines at low doses. Citral, the chief essential oil constituent in lemon balm, has been shown to induce apoptosis in glioblastoma multiforme cells in vitro. This effect was negated by the presence of antioxidants.

HUMAN RESEARCH

Oral and Dental Disorders: Bruxism

A 2019 systematic review and meta-analysis to evaluate the efficacy of lemon balm for childhood sleep-related bruxism selected 10 studies ($n=94$) for inclusion. Hydroxyzine therapy showed the strongest efficacy (OR 10.6). Flurazepam and lemon balm therapies presented lower grades of association with decreased bruxism symptoms (Ierardo et al., 2019).

A four-phase 30-day crossover RCT in children ($n=52$) with sleep-related bruxism compared homeopathic lemon balm with homeopathic lemon balm plus *phytolacca decandra,* with *phytolacca decandra* alone, and with placebo (all homeopathic potencies were 12c). The bruxism VAS scores were reduced significantly in all groups including placebo (-2.36, -2.21, -1.44, and -1.72 with lemon balm, lemon balm plus phytolacca, phytolacca alone, and placebo, respectively). Lemon balm was superior to both phytolacca and placebo ($P=0.018$; $P=0.050$, respectively). No side effects were observed after treatments (Tavares-Silva et al., 2019).

Cardiovascular Disorders: Palpitations and Vascular Disease

A 6-week open-label, parallel-group comparative trial in healthy subjects ($n=28$) compared the effects of lemon balm tea with barley tea for effects on glycation as reflected in arterial stiffness. The lemon balm group showed significant reductions in brachial-ankle pulse wave velocity and yellow color values in forearm skin (indicating collagen glycation) compared with the barley group. In female, but not male, subjects, cheek skin elasticity was significantly improved in the lemon balm group compared with the barley group. The authors concluded that lemon balm tea had the potential to provide health benefits regarding glycation-associated tissue damage in blood vessels and skin of healthy adults (Yui et al., 2017).

A 14-day RCT in volunteers ($n=71$) compared lemon balm extract 500 mg BID with placebo for reduction in palpitations. Lemon balm reduced the frequency of palpitation episodes and significantly reduced the number of anxious patients compared with placebo ($P=0.0001$; $P=0.004$ respectively). No serious side effects were reported. The authors concluded that lemon balm extract may be safe and effective for treatment of benign palpitations (Alijaniha et al., 2015).

Cardiometabolic Disorders: Dyslipidemia and Diabetes

A 12-week RCT in patients ($n=70$) with T2DM compared lemon balm extract 700 mg/day with placebo for effects on atherogenic surrogate markers. There were significant differences in serum Apo A-I, TC/HDL-C and LDL-C/HDL-C between the two groups at the end of the study ($P < 0.05$), but not for Apo B, Apo B/Apo A-I, TG/HDL-C, ICAM-1, AST, ALT, and ALP between the study groups. There was a significant increase in Apo A-I ($P = 0.003$) and significant reduction in TG/HDL-C ($P = 0.05$) compared with initial values in the lemon balm group. The authors concluded that lemon balm could safely improve Apo A-I, Apo B/Apo A-I, and lipid ratios as key factors promoting cardiovascular disease in patients with T2DM (Asadi et al., 2018).

A 12-week RCT in patients ($n = 62$) with T2DM compared lemon balm 700 mg/day with placebo for benefits relevant to diabetes. Lemon balm showed a significant difference from baseline in HDL-C ($P = 0.009$). There were also notable differences between lemon balm and placebo in FBS ($P = 0.007$), A1C ($P = 0.002$), β-cell activity ($P = 0.05$), TG ($P = 0.04$), HDL-C ($P = 0.05$), hs-CRP ($P = 0.001$), and SBP ($P = 0.04$). TC, LDL-C, insulin, and HOMA-IR showed no significant changes between the groups. No adverse effects were observed. The authors concluded that lemon balm was safe and effective in improvement of lipid profile, glycemic control, and reduction of inflammation (Asadi et al., 2019).

A 2-month RCT in patients ($n = 58$) with hyperlipidemia compared lemon balm 1000 mg/day with placebo for metabolic effects. LDL-C and AST decreased significantly with lemon balm compared with placebo ($P = 0.02$ and 0.009, respectively). The changes in TC, FBS, HDL-C, TG, creatinine, and ALT did not show significant differences between the two groups. The authors concluded that lemon balm could be effective in lowering of LDL-C and AST levels in patients with borderline hyperlipidemia (Jandaghi et al., 2016).

An 8-week RCT in patients ($n = 80$) with chronic stable angina compared lemon balm 3 g/day with placebo for effects on biomarkers of oxidative stress, inflammation, and lipid profiles. The mean serum concentrations of TG, TC, LDL-C, MDA, and hs-CRP were lower with lemon balm than with placebo ($P < 0.01$). The mean serum concentration of paraoxonase-1 (an antiatherogenic antioxidant) and HDL-C were higher ($P < 0.001$) with lemon balm than with placebo. The authors concluded that lemon balm improves the lipid profile, MDA, hs-CRP, and paraoxonase-1 in patients with chronic stable angina (Javid et al., 2018).

Gastrointestinal Disorders: Functional Dyspepsia, Irritable Bowel Syndrome, and Infantile Colic

A 2018 systematic review on dietary interventions for infantile colic selected 15 RCTs ($n = 1121$) for inclusion. Although the studies were small and at high risk of bias across, the authors identified benefit from an extract of fennel, chamomile, and lemon balm in one study. Average crying times for the herbal combination and placebo were 76.9 min/day and 169.9 min/day, respectively, at the end of the one-week study (Gordon et al., 2018).

A 28-day RCT in infants ($n = 176$) with colic investigated Colimil Plus (a mixture of chamomile, lemon balm, and tyndallized *Lactobacillus acidophilus* HA122 compared with *Lactobacillus reuteri* DSM 17938 and with simethicone for the treatment of infantile colic. Mean daily crying time at day 28 was significantly lower with Colimil Plus (-44 min; $P < 0.001$) and *Lactobacillus reuteri* (-35 min; $P < 0.001$) when compared with simethicone. The mean difference between the former two groups was not statistically significant ($P = 0.205$). At day 28, 95% of the Colimil Plus group responded to treatment compared with 86% of the *Lactobacillus reuteri* group and 68% of the simethicone group ($P < 0.001$). The authors concluded that the combination product and the *L. reuteri* product were significantly more effective than simethicone in infantile colic (Martinelli et al., 2017).

A 1-week RCT in breastfed infants ($n = 93$) with colic investigated a polyherbal standardized extract combination of chamomile, lemon balm, and fennel compared with placebo BID. The daily average crying time with the herbal formula decreased from 201 min/day to 77 min/day. With placebo the crying time decreased from 199 min/day to 169 min/day ($P < 0.005$). Crying time reduction was observed in 85% of subjects using the herbal formula and 49% of subjects given placebo ($P < 0.005$). No side effects were reported. The authors concluded that colic in breastfed infants improved within 1 week of treatment with this polyherbal formula (Savino et al., 2005).

A 4-week RCT in patients ($n = 60$) with functional dyspepsia investigated Iberogast in two different formulations (chamomile, peppermint, caraway, licorice, lemon balm, angelica, celandine, and milk thistle with or without bitter candy tuft) compared with placebo for effects on gastrointestinal symptoms. The herbal preparations showed a clinically significant improvement in the Gastrointestinal Symptom score compared with placebo after 2 and 4 weeks of treatment ($P<0.001$). No statistically significant difference could be observed between the efficacy of two different herbal preparations ($P>0.05$), but a solid improvement of GI symptoms could be achieved earlier with the herbal preparation that contained the bitter candy tuft ($P=0.023$). The authors concluded that Iberogast and its modified formulation improved dyspeptic symptoms better than placebo and that the bitter candy tuft had an additive effect (Madisch et al., 2001).

A 12-week partial crossover RCT in patients ($n=120$) with functional dyspepsia compared STW 5-II (containing extracts from licorice, bitter candy tuft, chamomile, peppermint, caraway, and lemon balm) with placebo. Each patient received the treatment for three consecutive 4-week treatment blocks. The first two treatment blocks were fixed. For the third treatment period, medication was based upon the investigator's judgment of symptom improvement during the preceding treatment period. In patients without adequate control of symptoms, the treatment was switched, or if symptoms were controlled, the treatment was continued. During the first 4 weeks, the Gastrointestinal Symptom score decreased significantly in subjects on active treatment compared with placebo ($P<0.001$). During the second 4-week period symptoms further improved in subjects who continued on active treatment or those who were switched to active treatment, while those switched to placebo deteriorated. After 8 weeks there was complete relief of symptoms in 43% and 3% of subjects on active treatment and placebo, respectively ($P<0.001$). The authors concluded that this polyherbal preparation improved dyspeptic symptoms better than placebo (Madisch et al., 2004).

An 8-week pilot study in patients ($n=32$) with IBS compared Carmint (a combination product containing extracts of lemon balm, spearmint, and coriander) with placebo for efficacy. All patients were also given loperamide or psyllium depending on their IBS subtype. The severity and frequency of abdominal pain/discomfort were significantly lower in the herbal group than the placebo group at the end of the treatment ($P=0.016$ and $P=0.001$, respectively). Severity and frequency

of bloating were also lower with the herbal product ($P=0.02$ and $P=0.002$, respectively). The authors concluded that Carmint plus loperamide or Carmint plus psyllium may be effective in patients with IBS (Vejdani et al., 2006).

Women's Genitourinary Disorders: Premenstrual Syndrome and Dysmenorrhea

A 3-month RCT in high school girls ($n=100$) compared lemon balm 1200 mg/day with placebo throughout the menstrual cycle for effects on PMS symptoms. Lemon balm produced a significant reduction in PMS symptoms ($P<0.001$). The mean score of PMS intensity decreased progressively from 42.5 to and 13.9 at the end of 3 months ($P=0.001$) (Akbarzadeh et al., 2015).

A three-cycle RCT in women ($n=43$) with moderate-to-severe primary dysmenorrhea compared lemon balm infusion (one teabag) q8h to mefenamic acid 250 mg q8h PRN for pain relief. The intensity and duration of pain in both groups showed a significant descending trend ($P<0.001$ for both). This trend was greater in the lemon balm group in terms of pain intensity ($P=0.008$), with no significant difference in pain duration ($P=0.10$). The authors concluded that lemon balm was more effective than mefenamic acid in relieving the pain of primary dysmenorrhea (Faranak and Parvin, 2016).

Women's Genitourinary Disorders: Menopause

A 2017 review of clinical trials on herbal efficacy in menopausal symptoms used search terms menopause, climacteric, hot flushes, flashes, herb, and phytoestrogens. The authors found that passionflower, sage, lemon balm, valerian, black cohosh, fenugreek, black seed, chasteberry, fennel, evening primrose, ginkgo, alfalfa, St. John's wort, Asian ginseng, anise, licorice, red clover, and wild soybean were effective in the treatment of acute menopausal syndrome with different mechanisms. The authors concluded that medicinal plants could play a role in the treatment of acute menopausal syndrome and that further studies were warranted (Kargozar et al., 2017).

Women's Genitourinary Disorders: Hypoactive Sexual Desire Disorder

A 4-week RCT in women ($n=89$) with hypoactive sexual desire disorder (HSDD) compared lemon balm

500 mg BID with placebo. Lemon balm produced a significant improvement from baseline in desire ($P < 0.001$), arousal ($P < 0.001$), lubrication ($P < 0.005$), orgasm ($P < 0.001$), satisfaction ($P < 0.001$), pain ($P < 0.002$), and Female Sexual Functional Index total score ($P < 0.001$). The improvement with lemon balm was significantly greater than with placebo as was the willingness to continue treatment ($P < 0.001$). The authors concluded that lemon balm may be safe and effective for the improvement of HSDD in women (Darvish-Mofrad-Kashani et al., 2018).

Neurological Disorders: Dementia

A 2020 systematic review to assess the efficacy and safety of aromatherapy for people with dementia found 13 studies ($n = 708$) that met inclusion criteria. Nine of these trials focused on agitation or other behavioral and psychological symptoms of dementia (BPSD). Lemon balm alone was studied in four trials, and lavender plus lemon balm was used in one study. Lavender alone, orange, and cedar were used in other studies. Among the five trials for which the confidence in the results was moderate or low, four trials reported no significant effect on agitation and one trial reported a significant benefit of aromatherapy. The four trials that reported significant benefit from aromatherapy for BPSD had moderate or low confidence levels. Cognition was assessed in three low-confidence trials. One did not report any data and the other two trials reported no significant effect of aromatherapy on cognition. The authors concluded that there was no convincing evidence that aromatherapy was beneficial for people with dementia. However, they acknowledged many limitations to the data and recommended better design and reporting and consistency of outcome measurement in future trials (Ball et al., 2020).

A 2006 systematic review looking at herbal treatment of cognitive disorders in the elderly identified 2 individual herbs and two herbal formulations with therapeutic effects for the treatment of AD: lemon balm, sage, Yi-Gan San, and Ba Wei Di Huang Wan. Ginkgo was identified in a meta-analysis study. All five herbs were shown to be useful for cognitive impairment of AD. Lemon balm and Yi-Gan San also demonstrated usefulness in agitation attributed to sedative effects (Dos Santos-Neto et al., 2006).

A three-phase 2-week crossover RCT in agitated nursing home patients with dementia ($n = 39$) and without dementia ($n = 10$) investigated topical application of lemon balm essential oil compared with with lavender oil essential oil and with carrier oil alone once daily for effects on agitation. Lemon balm was more effective in reducing the Neuropsychiatric Inventory (NPI) agitation ($P = 0.04$) and the Cohen-Mansfield Agitation Inventory physical non-aggressive behavior score (CMAI PNAB) ($P = 0.02$) in residents without dementia. In patients with dementia, lemon balm reduced the NPI irritability to a lesser degree ($P = 0.01$). Lavender was more effective in reducing the CMAI PNAB score in patients with dementia ($P = 0.04$). The authors concluded that lemon balm reduced agitated behavior in non-demented patients, whereas lavender was more effective in patients with dementia (Watson et al., 2019).

A 4-month RCT in patients ($n = 42$) with mild to moderate Alzheimer's disease compared lemon balm extract 60 drops/day with placebo for cognitive effects. At 4 months, lemon balm produced a significantly better outcome on cognitive function than placebo (ADAS-cog; $P = 0.01$; Clinical Dementia Rating; $P < 0.0001$). There were no significant differences between the two groups in terms of observed side effects except for agitation, which was more common in the placebo group ($P = 0.03$). The authors concluded that lemon balm had value in managing mild-to-moderate AD and had a positive effect on agitation (Akhondzadeh et al., 2003).

An RCT in long term care patients ($n = 72$) with dementia and clinically significant agitation investigated lemon balm essential oil applied topically compared with placebo BID. A 30% reduction in the Cohen-Mansfield Agitation Inventory occurred in 60% of the lemon balm group and 14% of the placebo group, respectively. An overall improvement in agitation occurred in 35% of the lemon balm group and 11% of the placebo group, respectively ($P < 0.001$). Social engagement also improved more with lemon balm than with placebo ($P = 0.001$). The authors concluded that lemon balm essential oil was a safe and effective treatment for clinically significant agitation in patients with severe dementia (Ballard et al., 2002).

A 1-month RCT in 70-year-old adults ($n = 70$) with memory impairment investigated a combination of lemon balm plus frankincense tablets compared with placebo for effects on memory scales. Comparison of the two groups showed that the total scores of the Wechsler Memory Scale-Revised and the subscales, including immediate auditory, immediate memory, immediate visual, and working memory, were increased after consumption of the combination herbal product ($P < 0.0001$).The authors concluded that frankincense plus lemon balm in older adults could be beneficial for improvement of memory (Taghizadeh et al., 2018).

Psychiatric Disorders: Anxiety, Stress, and Insomnia

A 2013 systematic review looking at plants that had both pre-clinical and clinical evidence for anti-anxiety effects found 21 plants with human clinical trial evidence. Support for efficacy identified several herbs with efficacy for anxiety spectrum disorders including kava, lemon balm, chamomile, ginkgo, skullcap, milk thistle, passionflower, ashwagandha, rhodiola, echinacea, *Galphimia glauca, Centella asiatica,* and *Echium amooenum*. Acute anxiolytic activity was found for passionflower, sage, gotu kola, lemon balm, and bergamot. The review also specifically found that bacopa showed anxiolytic effects in people with cognitive decline (Sarris et al., 2013).

A 3-month RCT in female adolescents ($n = 100$) compared lemon balm 600 mg/day with placebo for effects on psychological health. The study results showed that lemon balm produced significant improvements over placebo in the Psychosomatic Symptoms score ($P < 0.001$), anxiety and sleeping disorder ($P < 0.001$), and social function disorder ($P = 0.021$). The authors concluded that lemon balm could decrease psychosomatic symptoms, sleeping disorder, anxiety, depression, and social function disorder in female adolescents (Heydari et al., 2018).

An 8-week RCT in patients ($n = 80$) with chronic stable angina compared lemon balm 3 g/day with placebo for effects on mood and sleep disturbances. The lemon balm group showed a significant reduction in scores of depression, anxiety, stress, and total sleep disturbance compared with placebo ($P < 0.05$). The authors concluded that lemon balm could decrease mood and sleep disturbances in patients with chronic stable angina (Javid et al., 2018).

A crossover RCT with washout periods in healthy volunteers ($n = 18$) compared two separate single doses of lemon balm (300 mg or 600 mg) with placebo on separate days for effects on experimental stress. Lemon balm 600 mg ameliorated the negative mood effects of the stressor battery, with significantly increased self-ratings of calmness and reduced self-ratings of alertness. In addition, a significant increase in the speed of mathematical processing, with no reduction in accuracy, was observed after ingestion of the 300 mg dose. The authors concluded that lemon balm may be able to mitigate the effects of stress (Kennedy et al., 2004).

An acutely dosed crossover RCT in healthy young volunteers ($n = 20$) compared standardized extract of lemon balm at 300 mg, 600 mg, and 900 mg with placebo for 7-day intervals for effects on cognitive performance. A sustained improvement in Accuracy of Attention following 600 mg of lemon balm and time- and dose-specific reductions in both Secondary Memory and Working Memory factors were demonstrated with lemon balm. Self-rated "calmness," was elevated at the earliest time points by the lowest dose, and "alertness" was significantly reduced at all time points following the highest dose (Kennedy et al., 2003).

An acutely dosed crossover RCT with washout periods in healthy volunteers ($n = 24$) compared a combination of lemon balm plus valerian 600 mg, 1200 mg, and 1800 mg with placebo on separate days for effects on laboratory-induced stress. The results showed that the 600 mg dose of the combination ameliorated the negative effects of the Defined Intensity Stressor Simulation (DISS) battery on ratings of anxiety. The 1800 mg dose showed an increase in anxiety with the battery. All three doses led to decrements in performance on the Stroop task module within the battery, and the two lower doses led to decrements on the overall score generated on the DISS battery (Kennedy et al., 2004).

A 15-day prospective, open-label, trial in stressed volunteers ($n = 20$) with mild-to-moderate anxiety and sleep disturbance investigated the efficacy of Cyracos, a standardized extract of lemon balm. The product reduced anxiety manifestations by 18% ($P < 0.01$), ameliorated anxiety-associated symptoms by 15% ($P < 0.01$), and lowered insomnia by 42% ($P < 0.01$). Positive response occurred in 95% of subjects with full remission in 70% for anxiety, 85% for insomnia, and 70% for both. The authors concluded that lemon balm relieved stress-related effects and that further placebo-controlled trials were warranted (Cases et al., 2011).

A 3.5-year retrospective case-control study of hospitalized psychiatric patients ($n = 3252$) evaluated an herbal extract combination of passionflower, valerian, lemon balm, and butterbur (Ze 185) compared with no additional herbal therapy to investigate whether the herbal combination would change the prescription pattern of benzodiazepines. Data showed that both treatment modalities had a comparable clinical effectiveness, but there were significantly fewer prescriptions of benzodiazepines with the herbal combination ($P = 0.006$). The authors recommended that an RCT be performed (Keck et al., 2020).

An acutely dosed RCT in healthy men ($n = 72$) investigated pre-dosing for 4 days with Ze 185, a fixed combination of valerian, passionflower, lemon balm, and butterbur, compared with pre-dosing with placebo and with a no-treatment control for effects on biological and affective responses to a standardized psychosocial stress paradigm. The stress paradigm induced significant and large cortisol and self-reported anxiety responses. Groups did not differ significantly in their salivary cortisol response to stress, but participants in the herbal group showed significantly attenuated responses in self-reported anxiety compared with placebo ($P = 0.03$) and with no treatment ($P = 0.05$). The authors suggested that the herbal combination reduced the self-reported anxiety response to stress without affecting the assumingly adaptive biological stress responses (Meier et al., 2018).

A crossover RCT in healthy volunteers ($n = 16$) compared a multi-herbal lozenge containing lavender, hops, lemon balm and oat with a placebo lozenge with respect to EEG patterns. After baseline recording each subject sucked a lozenge and repeated 2 h later. Recording was performed immediately after finishing the lozenge and in hourly intervals thereafter. Increases in $\alpha 1$, $\alpha 2$, and $\beta 1$ electrical power occurred at the electrode positions Cz, P3, T3, and T5 and these increases were even more pronounced after a second application 2 h later. The authors concluded that this herbal lozenge could lead to improved coping with psychological and emotional stress (Dimpfel et al., 2004).

A 4-week RCT in patients with insomnia investigated a combination of lemon balm 1000 mg plus *Nepeta menthoides* 400 mg QHS compared with placebo. The lemon balm group showed a significant decrease in the mean difference of the insomnia severity index scores (4.97 and 1.60 with lemon balm and placebo, respectively; $P = 0.002$) and total Pittsburgh Sleep Quality Index scores (4.14 and 1.42 with lemon balm and placebo, respectively; $P = 0.001$). The lemon balm formula also produced a significant increase in total sleep time ($P < 0.001$). The authors concluded that this herbal combination could be an alternative therapy for insomnia (Ranjbar et al., 2018).

An open-label study in children younger than 12 years ($n = 918$) with restlessness and dyssomnia assessed the efficacy and tolerability of Euvegal forte, a combined valerian-plus-lemon balm preparation. The core symptoms dyssomnia and restlessness were reduced from "moderate/severe" to "mild" or "absent" in most of the patients. Clear improvement occurred for dyssomnia in 81% and for restlessness in 70% of the patients. Both parents and investigators assessed efficacy as "very good" or "good" (60% and 68%, respectively). The tolerability of the product was "very good" or "good" in 97% of the patients. No adverse events occurred. The authors concluded that this herbal combination product was effective in the treatment of younger children with restlessness and dyssomnia and it was very well tolerated (Müller and Klement, 2006).

A one-month RCT in women ($n = 100$) aged 50–60 years with sleep disorders investigated a combination of valerian plus lemon balm compared with placebo. A significant difference was observed with reduced levels of sleep disorders in the herbal group compared with the placebo group. Sleep improvement occurred in 36% with herbal treatment and 8% with placebo. The authors concluded that this herbal combination may assist in reducing sleep disorder symptoms during menopause (Taavoni et al., 2013).

Psychiatric Disorders: Depression

An 8-week RCT in adult patients ($n = 45$) with mild-to-moderate depression (HAM-D 8-24) compared lemon balm powdered dried leaves 2 g/day with lavender powdered dried leaves 2 g/day and with fluoxetine 20 mg/day for effect on depression. At 8 weeks, all groups had a significant improvement in HAM-D and there was no significant difference between groups.

The fluoxetine group reported more insomnia, sexual dysfunction, anxiety, and decreased appetite than the lemon balm and lavender groups. Two patients in the fluoxetine group discontinued the study due to sexual dysfunction and diarrhea, respectively. The lavender and lemon balm groups reported more sedation. One patient in the lavender group discontinued the study due to drowsiness. There were no serious side effects reported. The authors conclude that lemon balm and lavender are equally effective as fluoxetine at treating mild-to-moderate depression (Araj-Khodaei et al., 2020).

A 3-month RCT in female adolescents ($n = 100$) compared lemon balm 600 mg/day with placebo for effects on psychological health. The study results showed that lemon balm produced significant improvements over placebo in the Psychosomatic Symptoms score ($P < 0.001$), anxiety and sleeping disorder ($P < 0.001$), and social function disorder ($P = 0.021$). The authors concluded that lemon balm could decrease psychosomatic symptoms, sleeping disorder, anxiety, depression, and social function disorder in female adolescents (Heydari et al., 2018).

An 8-week RCT in patients ($n = 80$) with chronic stable angina compared lemon balm 3 g/day with placebo for effects on mood and sleep disturbances. The lemon balm group showed a significant reduction in scores of depression, anxiety, stress, and total sleep disturbance compared with placebo ($P < 0.05$). The authors concluded that lemon balm could decrease mood and sleep disturbances in patients with chronic stable angina (Javid et al., 2018).

Psychiatric Disorders: Attention-Deficit/Hyperactivity Disorder and Cognitive Performance

A 2017 systematic review looking at natural products for ADHD in children selected nine RCTs ($n = 464$) that met inclusion criteria. Low evidence could be found for lemon balm, valerian, and passionflower. Limited evidence could be found for pine bark extract and ginkgo. The other herbal preparations showed no efficacy in the treatment of ADHD symptoms (Anheyer et al., 2017).

A 7-week observational study in primary school children ($n = 169$) with hyperactivity and concentration difficulties but not meeting ADHD criteria

received Sandrin, a standardized combination of valerian 640 mg and lemon balm 320 mg daily. The fraction of children having "strong/very strong" symptoms of poor ability to focus decreased from 75% to 14%, hyperactivity decreased from 61% to 13%, and impulsiveness decreased from 59% to 22%. Parent-rated social behavior, sleep, and symptom burden showed highly significant improvements. In two children, mild transient adverse drug reactions were observed. The authors concluded that children with restlessness, concentration difficulties, and impulsiveness may benefit from this formulation of valerian and lemon balm (Gromball et al., 2014).

A 2-week RCT in healthy subjects ($n = 44$) investigated a combination product containing sage, rosemary, and lemon balm compared with placebo for cognitive effects. Although there were no significant differences between treatment and placebo with respect to change from baseline for immediate or delayed word recall, the herbal combination produced significant improvements in delayed word recall for those younger than 63 years ($P < 0.0123$). No adverse effects were observed (Perry et al., 2018).

A 4-month RCT in children ($n = 120$) with newly diagnosed ADHD compared a polyherbal formula containing ashwagandha, bacopa, lemon balm, *Paeoniae alba*, *Centella asiatica*, and *Spirulina platensis* with placebo. The treatment group showed substantial, statistically significant improvement in the four TOVA subscales and overall TOVA scores, compared with no improvement in the control group. The authors concluded that the polyherbal formula improved attention, cognition, and impulse control in children with ADHD (Katz et al., 2010).

Psychiatric Disorders: Somatoform Disorders

A 2-week RCT in patients ($n = 182$) with somatoform disorders investigated Ze 185, a four-herb combination containing valerian, passionflower, lemon balm, and butterbur compared with a three-herb combination without the butterbur and with placebo. The combination containing butterbur was significantly superior to the combination without butterbur, which was superior to placebo for changes in VAS-Anxiety scale, Beck Depression Inventory, and Clinical Global Impression. In total, nine nonserious adverse events were documented, but the distribution did not differ significantly between the treatment groups. The authors concluded that the herbal preparation Ze 185 was an efficacious and safe short-term treatment in patients with somatoform disorders (Melzer et al., 2009).

Infectious Disease: Herpes Simplex Virus

An RCT in patients ($n = 66$) with recurrent HSV-1 compared a topical ointment of 1% lemon balm oil with placebo applied QID starting with prodromal symptoms and continuing 2-3 days after lesions had healed. A combined symptom score of the values for complaints, size of affected area and blisters at day 2 of therapy was formed as the primary target parameter. There was a significant difference in the values of the primary target parameter between both treatment groups: lemon balm 4.03 and placebo 4.94. The authors noted that the difference in the combined symptom score on the second day of treatment was important since patients' symptoms are usually most intensive at that time. In addition to the shortening of the healing period, the cream also appeared to prevent spreading of the infection and produce a rapid reduction of typical symptoms of herpes such as itching, tingling, burning, stabbing, swelling, tautness, and erythema (Koytchev et al., 1999).

Oncologic Disorders: Cancer Prophylaxis

A 30-day open-label trial in radiology staff ($n = 55$) who were exposed to persistent low-dose radiation at work compared lemon balm infusion (1.5 g/100 mL) BID. After 30 days there was significant improvement in plasma levels of catalase, superoxide dismutase, and glutathione peroxidase and a marked reduction in plasma DNA damage, myeloperoxidase, and lipid peroxidation. The authors concluded that lemon balm improved oxidative stress and DNA damage related to low levels of radiation (Zeraatpishe et al., 2011).

ACTIVE CONSTITUENTS

Leaf

- Phenolic compounds
  - Phenylpropanoids (antioxidant, antimutagenic, antitumor, antimicrobial): rosmarinic acid (strongly antioxidant, anti-inflammatory,

anti-HIV, antibacterial, antiallergic) caffeic acids, chlorogenic acid, metrilic acids A and B, eugenol
  - Flavonoids: luteolin (anti-inflammatory, antispasmodic, antibacterial, hepatoprotective, anti-estrogenic, antiproliferative), luteolin 7-O-β-D-glucopyranoside, apigenin 7-O-β-D-glucopyranoside, luteolin 3'-O-β-D-gluconopuranoside
    - Tannins (antiviral)
- Terpenes (anti-anxiety, carminative):
  - Monoterpenes: linalool (sedative, antispasmodic), limonene (antineoplastic, detoxifying)
  - Monoterpene glycosides
  - Sesquiterpenes: β-carophyllene, germacrene
  - Triterpenoid saponins: carnosic acid, ursolic acid (anti-HIV, anti-EBV, antiviral, androgenic, AChEI, pro-collagen, pro-ceremide, antitumor) oleanolic acid (chemoprotective, hepatoprotective)
- Aromatic compounds (anti-HSV, antiviral, antibacterial, antiprotozoal): citronellal, citral b (neral), citral a (geranial) (anxiolytic, antiviral), eugenol (antispasmodic, anesthetic, antibacterial), sabinene, β-pinene, *limonene* (antineoplastic, detoxifying), phellandrene, methyl citronellate, ocimene, citronellol, geraniol, nerol, ß-caryophyllene, ß-caryophyllene oxide, linalool (sedative, antispasmodic), ethric oil

LEMON BALM COMMONLY USED PREPARATIONS AND DOSAGE (FOR ADULTS UNLESS OTHERWISE SPECIFIED)

The following are examples of some available formulations and ranges of dosing for commercial herbal products. See Part III Introduction "How to prescribe medicinal herbs" for further guidance on herbal advising and prescribing.

Dried Aerial Parts: Oral Use

- Infusion: 2–3 tsp per cup QD-TID
- Fluid extract (1:1, 45%): 2–4 mL QD-TID
- Tincture (1:5, 45%): 2–6 mL QD-TID

- Powdered herb extract: 800–1000 mg (1/3 tsp) QD-BID
- Capsule or tablet of powdered leaf or leaf extract: 500–1000 mg QD-BID
- Capsule or tablet of standardized extract (standardized to 14% hydroxycinnamic acids and/or 3%–7% rosmarinic acid): 300–500 mg QD-BID

Dried Aerial Parts: Topical Use

- Infusion: 2–4 tsp per cup water, cool and apply with cotton balls throughout day
- Essential oil: 1 mL of lotion with 100 mg (3–4 drops) essential oil BID for agitation

Oral use in children younger than 12 years is not recommended.

SAFETY AND PRECAUTION

Side-Effects

Minor adverse effects reported in clinical trials. Unlike sedative drugs, lemon balm appears to be safe even while driving or operating machinery. However, caution is still advised for risky activities, particularly with higher doses (e.g., 900 mg).

Case Reports

One case report of withdrawal symptoms when long-term use was discontinued.

Toxicity

Oral administration of lemon balm essential oil (citronellal, 21.2%–21.8%; neral, 17.8%–18.4%; and geranial, 22.9%–23.5%) induced pathological changes in the organs of rats at doses higher than 1 g/kg. No case of overdose has been reported.

Pregnancy and Lactation

Insufficient human safety data. Lemon balm has been safely and effectively used in the treatment of infant colic and diarrhea, therefore may be safe during breastfeeding, despite no data existing on the excretion of any of its components into breastmilk.

Disease Interactions

- Thyroid disease: Caution with thyroid disease due to in vitro and in vivo effects on TSH levels, TSH binding, and reduction in deiodination of T4 to T3

- Glaucoma: Essential oil may raise intraocular pressure

Drug Interactions

- Caution with sedating drugs
- May interfere with thyroid medications
- Unclear if it interacts with antiretrovirals so best to avoid

REFERENCES

Akbarzadeh M, Dehghani M, Moshfeghy Z, Emamghoreishi M, Tavakoli P, Zare N. Effect of *Melissa* officinalis capsule on the intensity of premenstrual syndrome symptoms in high school girl students. Nurs Midwifery Stud 2015;4(2), e27001.

Akhondzadeh S, Noroozian M, Mohammadi M, Ohadinia S, Jamshidi AH, Khani M. *Melissa officinalis* extract in the treatment of patients with mild to moderate Alzheimer's disease: a double blind, randomised, placebo-controlled trial. J Neurol Neurosurg Psychiatry 2003;74(7):863–6.

Alijaniha F, Naseri M, Afsharypuor S, et al. Heart palpitation relief with *Melissa officinalis* leaf extract: double blind, randomized, placebo-controlled trial of efficacy and safety. J Ethnopharmacol 2015;164:378–84.

Anheyer D, Lauche R, Schumann D, Dobos G, Cramer H. Herbal medicines in children with attention deficit hyperactivity disorder (ADHD): a systematic review. Complement Ther Med 2017;30:14–23.

Araj-Khodaei M, Noorbala AA, Yarani R, et al. A double-blind, randomized pilot study for comparison ofMelissa officinalisL. and Lavandula angustifoliaMill. with fluoxetine for the treatment of depression. BMC Complement Med Ther 2020;20(1):207.

Asadi A, Shidfar F, Safari M, et al. Safety and efficacy of Melissa officinalis (lemon balm) on ApoA-I, Apo B, lipid ratio and ICAM-1 in type 2 diabetes patients: a randomized, double-blinded clinical trial. Complement Ther Med 2018;40:83–8.

Asadi A, Shidfar F, Safari M, et al. Efficacy of Melissa officinalis L. (lemon balm) extract on glycemic control and cardiovascular risk factors in individuals with type 2 diabetes: a randomized, double-blind, clinical trial. Phytother Res 2019;33(3):651–9.

Ball EL, Owen-Booth B, Gray A, Shenkin SD, Hewitt J, McCleery J. Aromatherapy for dementia. Cochrane Database Syst Rev 2020;8(8), CD003150.

Ballard CG, O'Brien JT, Reichelt K, Perry EK. Aromatherapy as a safe and effective treatment for the management of agitation in severe dementia: the results of a double-blind, placebo-controlled trial with *Melissa*. J Clin Psychiatry 2002;63(7):553–8.

Cases J, Ibarra A, Feuillère N, Roller M, Sukkar SG. Pilot trial of Melissa officinalis L. leaf extract in the treatment of volunteers suffering from mild-to-moderate anxiety disorders and sleep disturbances. Med J Nutrition Metab 2011;4(3):211–8.

Darvish-Mofrad-Kashani Z, Emaratkar E, Hashem-Dabaghian F, et al. Effect of *Melissa officinalis* (Lemon balm) on sexual dysfunction in women: a double- blind, randomized, placebo-controlled study. Iran J Pharm Res 2018;17(Suppl):89–100.

Dimpfel W, Pischel I, Lehnfeld R. Effects of lozenge containing lavender oil, extracts from hops, lemon balm and oat on electrical brain activity of volunteers. Eur J Med Res 2004;9(9):423–31.

Dos Santos-Neto LL, de Vilhena Toledo MA, Medeiros-Souza P, de Souza GA. The use of herbal medicine in Alzheimer's disease-a systematic review. Evid Based Complement Alternat Med 2006;3(4):441–5.

Faranak SD, Parvin N. The effect of mefenamic acid and *Melissa officinalis* on primary dysmenorrhea: a randomized clinical trial study. Int J Pharmacog Phytochem Res 2016;8(8):1286–92.

Gordon M, Biagioli E, Sorrenti M, et al. Dietary modifications for infantile colic. Cochrane Database Syst Rev 2018;10, CD011029.

Gromball J, Beschorner F, Wantzen C, Paulsen U, Burkart M. Hyperactivity, concentration difficulties and impulsiveness improve during seven weeks' treatment with valerian root and lemon balm extracts in primary school children. Phytomedicine 2014;21(8-9):1098–103.

Heydari N, Dehghani M, Emamghoreishi M, Akbarzadeh M. Effect of Melissa officinalis capsule on the mental health of female adolescents with premenstrual syndrome: a clinical trial study. Int J Adolesc Med Health 2018;25.

Ierardo G, Mazur M, Luzzi V, Calcagnile F, Ottolenghi L, Polimeni A. Treatments of sleep bruxism in children: a systematic review and meta-analysis. Cranio 2019;26:1–7.

Jandaghi P, Noroozi M, Ardalani H, Alipour M. Lemon balm: a promising herbal therapy for patients with borderline hyperlipidemia–A randomized double-blind placebo-controlled clinical trial. Complement Ther Med 2016;26:136–40.

Javid AZ, Haybar H, Dehghan P, et al. The effects of Melissa officinalis (lemon balm) in chronic stable angina on serum biomarkers of oxidative stress, inflammation and lipid profile. Asia Pac J Clin Nutr 2018;27(4):785–91.

Kargozar R, Azizi H, Salari R. A review of effective herbal medicines in controlling menopausal symptoms. Electron Phys 2017;9(11):5826–33.

Katz M, et al. A compound herbal preparation (CHP) in the treatment of children with ADHD: a randomized controlled trial. J Atten Disord 2010;14(3):281–91.

Keck ME, Nicolussi S, Spura K, Blohm C, Zahner C, Drewe J. Effect of the fixed combination of valerian, lemon balm, passionflower, and butterbur extracts (Ze 185) on the prescription pattern of benzodiazepines in hospitalized psychiatric patients-A retrospective case-control investigation. Phytother Res 2020;34(6):1436–45.

Kennedy DO, Wake G, Savelev S, et al. Modulation of mood and cognitive performance following acute administration of single doses of Melissa officinalis (Lemon balm) with human CNS nicotinic and muscarinic receptor-binding properties. Neuropsychopharmacology 2003;28(10):1871–81.

Kennedy DO, Scholey AB, Tildesley NT, Perry EK, Wesnes KA. Attenuation of laboratory-induced stress in humans after acute administration of Melissa officinalis (Lemon Balm). Psychosom Med 2004;66(4):607–13.

Koytchev R, Alken RG, Dundarov S. Balm mint extract (Lo-701) for topical treatment of recurring herpes labialis. Phytomedicine 1999;6:225–30.

Madisch A, Melderis H, Mayr G, Sassin I, Hotz J. A plant extract and its modified preparation in functional dyspepsia. Results of a double-blind placebo controlled comparative study. Z Gastroenterol 2001;39(7):511–7.

Madisch A, Holtmann G, Mayr G, et al. Treatment of functional dyspepsia with a herbal preparation. A double-blind, randomized, placebo-controlled, multicenter trial. Digestion 2004;69(1):45–52.

Martinelli M, Ummarino D, Giugliano FP, et al. Efficacy of a standardized extract of Matricariae chamomilla L., Melissa officinalis L. and tyndallized Lactobacillus acidophilus (HA122) in infantile colic: an open randomized controlled trial. Neurogastroenterol Motil 2017;29(12).

Meier S, Haschke M, Zahner C, et al. Effects of a fixed herbal drug combination (Ze 185) to an experimental acute stress setting in healthy men—an explorative randomized placebo-controlled double-blind study. Phytomedicine 2018;39:85–92.

Melzer J, Schrader E, Brattström A, Schellenberg R, Saller R. Fixed herbal drug combination with and without butterbur (Ze 185) for the treatment of patients with somatoform disorders: randomized, placebo-controlled pharmaco-clinical trial. Phytother Res 2009;23(9):1303–8.

Müller SF, Klement S. A combination of valerian and lemon balm is effective in the treatment of restlessness and dyssomnia in children. Phytomedicine 2006;13(6):383–7.

Perry NSL, Menzies R, Hodgson F, et al. A randomised double-blind placebo-controlled pilot trial of a combined extract of sage, rosemary and melissa, traditional herbal medicines, on the enhancement of memory in normal healthy subjects, including influence of age. Phytomedicine 2018;39:42–8.

Ranjbar M, Salehi A, Rezaeizadeh H, et al. Efficacy of a combination of Melissa officinalis L. and Nepeta menthoides Boiss. & Buhse on insomnia: a triple-blind, randomized placebo-controlled clinical trial. J Altern Complement Med 2018.

Sarris J, McIntyre E, Camfield DA. Plant-based medicines for anxiety disorders, part 2: a review of clinical studies with supporting preclinical evidence. CNS Drugs 2013;27(4):301–19.

Savino F, Cresi F, Castagno E, Silvestro L, Oggero R. A randomized double-blind placebo-controlled trial of a standardized extract of *Matricariae recutita, Foeniculum vulgare* and *Melissa officinalis* (ColiMil) in the treatment of breastfed colicky infants. Phytother Res 2005;19(4):335–40.

Taavoni S, Mazem Ekbatani N, Haghani H. Valerian/lemon balm use for sleep disorders during menopause. Complement Ther Clin Pract 2013;19(4):193–6.

Taghizadeh M, Maghaminejad F, Aghajani M, Rahmani M, Mahboubi M. The effect of tablet containing Boswellia serrata and Melisa officinalis extract on older adults' memory: a randomized controlled trial. Arch Gerontol Geriatr 2018;75:146–50.

Tavares-Silva C, Holandino C, Homsani F, et al. Homeopathic medicine of Melissa officinalis combined or not with Phytolacca decandra in the treatment of possible sleep bruxism in children: a crossover randomized triple-blinded controlled clinical trial. Phytomedicine 2019;58:152869.

Vejdani R, Shalmani HR, Mir-Fattahi M, et al. The efficacy of an herbal medicine, Carmint, on the relief of abdominal pain and bloating in patients with irritable bowel syndrome: a pilot study. Dig Dis Sci 2006;51(8):1501–7. Epub 2006 Jul 26.

Watson K, Hatcher D, Good A. A randomised controlled trial of Lavender (Lavandula Angustifolia) and Lemon Balm (Melissa

Officinalis) essential oils for the treatment of agitated behaviour in older people with and without dementia. Complement Ther Med 2019;42:366–73.

Yui S, Fujiwara S, Harada K, et al. Beneficial effects of lemon balm leaf extract on in vitro glycation of proteins, arterial stiffness, and skin elasticity in healthy adults. J Nutr Sci Vitaminol (Tokyo) 2017;63(1):59–68.

Zeraatpishe A, Oryan S, Bagheri MH, et al. Effects of Melissa officinalis L. on oxidative status and DNA damage in subjects exposed to long-term low-dose ionizing radiation. Toxicol Ind Health 2011;27(3):205–12.

59

LICORICE (*GLYCYRRHIZA GLABRA*)
Root

GENERAL OVERVIEW

Licorice is as close to a pharmaceutical corticosteroid as the plant kingdom gets. It has many of both the benefits and the risks of the corticosteroid class of drugs. However, unlike the pharmaceutical corticosteroids, licorice has many other constituents, particularly flavonoids, that are beneficial in numerous diseases. The physiological effects of licorice include anti-inflammatory, antioxidant, antiallergic, antimicrobial, laxative, and ulcer-healing properties. Licorice research mostly involves *Glycyrrhiza glabra*, but *G. uralensis* and *G. inflata* are two additional species that have been studied and vary somewhat in efficacy.

Since ancient times, licorice has been used for sweetening and flavoring as well as for its medicinal purposes. It has many applications in traditional herbalism including bronchitis, chest congestion, hepatitis, peptic ulcer disease, constipation, menopause, Addison's disease, general inflammation, infections, and prostate cancer. It is used in traditional Chinese medicine to detoxify and augment the effects of the other components in herbal formulations. It is used in Ayurvedic medicine as a tonic, expectorant and demulcent.

Chronic use of licorice, even in moderate doses, can lead to hypokalemia and HTN due to its mineralocorticoid activity. Some people are more sensitive to this aspect of licorice exposure, while others compensate through downregulation of aldosterone. There are numerous case reports of severe adverse reactions related to this activity of licorice. For most modern medicinal applications of licorice, a deglycyrrhizinated extract (DGL) is used to avoid the mineralocorticoid effects of glycyrrhizin (aka glycyrrhizic acid) and its metabolites. Glycyrrhizin, when ingested, is cleaved to become glycyrrhizic acid, which is subsequently converted to glycyrrhetic (AKA glycyrrhetinic) acid by gut flora. Glycyrrhetic acid is a potent inhibitor of 11β-hydroxysteroid dehydrogenase(11β-HSD) and as such performs a range of corticosteroid-like activities (11β-HSD converts mineralocorticoid-binding cortisol to biologically inactive cortisone). Salivary and serum cortisol levels have been shown to increase by 40%-50% and cortisone levels have been shown to decrease by 45% after the ingestion of 500 mg of glycyrrhetic acid, supporting the role of 11βHSD inhibition in licorice activity. In addition to inhibiting 11β-HSD, licorice demonstrates mineralocorticoid-like activity by binding directly to the mineralocorticoid receptor, adding to potentially adverse risks of mineralocorticoid-like overactivity.

Deglycyrrhizinated licorice or "DGL" is a special ethanolic extract of licorice that concentrates the flavonoids in licorice, leaving a low glycyrrhizin content. Some of the concentrated flavonoids, including glabridol and liquirtigenin, appear to have uniquely beneficial properties.

Clinical research indicates that licorice, alone or in combination formulas, may be beneficial for mucositis, pharyngitis, asthma, dyslipidemia, hepatoprotection, peptic ulcer disease (non-DGL only), functional dyspepsia, polycystic ovary syndrome, menopause, Parkinson's Disease, hyperpigmentation, and eczema.

IN VITRO AND ANIMAL RESEARCH

Preclinical studies have shown that licorice has antibacterial, antiviral, anticancer, anti-inflammatory, estrogenic, and hepatoprotective properties. A study of letrozole-induced PCOS in rats demonstrated that licorice root extract normalized the FSH/LH ratio and reversed the PCOS ovarian histological changes. Licorice aqueous extract has been shown to inhibit 25% of AChE. Pretreatment with licorice has been shown to prevent the cognitive decline in rats treated with scopolamine or diazepam. Licorice has demonstrated chemopreventive effects by promoting apoptosis, arresting G2/M and inhibiting carcinogenesis through modulation of Bcl-2/Bax, regulation of the JAK2/STAT3 signaling pathway, and modulation of the cyclin B1-CDK1 in various cell lines. Licorice has also demonstrated protective properties against chemotherapy-induced cardiotoxicity and enhanced efficacy of cyclophosphamide.

Despite the disadvantages of glycyrrhizin (aka glycyrrhizic acid) and glycyrrhetic acid, these constituents play a critical role in many of the beneficial effects of licorice as well. Glycyrrhizin is a triterpenoid 50 times sweeter than sucrose. It acts on many key cell factors resulting in its anti-inflammatory response. It has been shown to induce modulation of the PI3K signaling pathway, the antioxidant system (with ROS reduction), cytokines, and the immune system. In allergic models glycyrrhizic acid can suppress the increased level of IL-4 to restore the immune balance of TH1/TH2 cells and can attenuate the B cells producing allergen-specific IgE and IgG. It acts as a mast cell stabilizer by inhibition of mast cell degranulation and reduction of vascular permeability by inhibiting the expression of Orai1, STIM1 and TRPC1, which block extracellular Ca^2+ influxes. In addition, glycyrrhizin and glycyrrhetic acid possess many other positive effects on human health, such as antitumor, antimicrobial, antiviral, antidiabetic, immunoregulatory, and hepatoprotective activities, contributing to protection and recovery of the respiratory, cardiovascular, gastrointestinal, neurological, and endocrine systems. Glycyrrhizin led to significant reductions in blood glucose concentrations and improvement of insulin sensitivity in rats fed a high-fat diet. In addition, it improved dyslipidemia by selectively inducing LPL expression in non-hepatic tissues. Glycyrrhizin and glycyrrhetic acid are also thought to inhibit 17,20-lysase and type 5 17-β-hydroxysteroid dehydrogenase, thereby reducing the conversion of androstenedione to testosterone, particularly in the ovary. This has implications for treatment of PCOS. Glycyrrhizin along with the constituents licopyranocoumarin, licocoumarone and glycyrrhisoflavone have demonstrated MAOI activity.

An aqueous extract of licorice root was shown to inhibit SARS-COV-2 at a concentration of 2 mg/mL (typical licorice tea is concentrated at 12.5 mg/mL). The activity was attributed mainly to glycyrrhizin, which was then shown to potently inhibit the main SARS-COV-2 protease (Ghannad et al., 2014). Glycyrrhizin had previously been shown to inhibit the replication of two clinical isolates of the 2003 SARS-associated coronavirus through inhibition of adsorption, penetration, and replication. Additionally, the constituent liquiritin was found to significantly inhibit replication of SARS-CoV-2 likely by mimicking type I interferon (Zhu et al., 2020). An in silico molecular docking simulation study of licorice using two protein targets from COVID-19 (spike glycoprotein and Nonstructural Protein-15) identified two constituents with antiviral activity. Glyasperin A showed high affinity towards Non-structural Protein-15 endoribonuclease with uridine specificity. Glycyrrhizic acid showed affinity for the binding pocket of spike glycoprotein and prohibited the entry of the virus into the host cell. Further analysis indicated high binding affinity towards the respective protein receptor cavity (Orhan and Deniz, 2020). Through several mechanisms, glycyrrhizin also demonstrates antiviral activity against HAV, HBV, HCV, influenza A, VZV, parainfluenza type 2, EBV, Dengue, and Chikungunya virus.

Glycyrrhetic acid has been shown to uncouple the cardiomyocyte connexins, providing potential protection against ischemia/reperfusion damage. It also has anti-adipogenic effects in preadipocytes secondary to downregulation of PPARγ and inhibition of Akt. Glycyrrhetic acid has demonstrated antiproliferative effects via apoptosis in MCF-7 cells.

The constituent isoliquiritigenin appears to have spasmolytic properties in the lower intestines similar to papavarine. Licorice has been shown to prevent glutamate induced cell death attributed to liquiritigenin, isoliquiritigenin, and glycycoumarin, which have antagonistic binding affinities to NMDA receptors.

Isoliquiritigenin has demonstrated the ability to suppress dopamine release induced by cocaine and acts in a dose-dependent manner via $GABA_B$ receptor agonism. Isoliquiritigenin has been shown to have inhibitory effects against COX but not LOX and to inhibit aromatase. It has been shown to reduce the rate of testosterone-induced breast tumor growth in mice.

The flavonoid constituent liquiritigenin appears to be a selective $ER\beta$ agonist. Isoliquiritigenin also demonstrated estrogenic activities. Liquiritigenin showed selectivity in a competitive binding assay and isoliquiritigenin was equipotent for $ER\alpha$ and $ER\beta$ subtypes. Research done in estrogen-sensitive human cells compared the estrogenic activity of licorice against that of hops. The estrogenic activity decreased in the order hops > *G. uralensis* > *G. inflata* > *G. glabra*.

The anti-inflammatory effects of liquiritigenin were demonstrated in rats where paw edema was reduced, but with less potency than 1 mg/kg dexamethasone. Liquiritigenin cut in half the locomotion induction of 20 mg/kg cocaine and almost normalized CREB and c-Fos phosphorylation induced by cocaine in the nucleus accumbens, suggesting a role for licorice in treatment of cocaine addiction. This flavonoid has also been shown to improve learning in a mouse model of AD associated with a reduction in oligomeric $A\beta$ proteins by 77% and 65% with 10 and 30 mg/kg, respectively, and a decrease in astrocytosis in the hippocampus. It has demonstrated neuroprotective effects in scopolamine-induced mice likely via increasing expression of BDNF and phosphorylation of extracellular signal-regulated kinase and CREB in the hippocampus. Isoliquiritigenin and liquiritigenin have been shown to reduce aldose reductase. Isoliquiritigenin, liquiritigenin and licuroside have all been shown to inhibit pancreatic lipase, thus reducing intestinal absorption of lipids.

The constituent glabridin has been shown to have a high affinity for LDL and to reduce LDL oxidation in mice. It has been shown to enhance cognition with T2DM models. It activates AMPK, but not as strongly as berberine, and suppresses food intake in mice. Glabridin has been shown to have anti-inflammatory properties via inhibition of PGE2, thromboxane A2, COX, LTB4, and LOX. It inhibits NF-kB activation secondary to preventing TNF-α induced Akt and ERK activation. It has been shown to reduce microglial inflammation. It has also been shown to reduce injury-induced AChE activity, and in a stroke model it attenuated the neurological deficit. Glabridin has been shown to enhance swimming endurance in mice by 50% at 20 mg/kg, and this was associated with less exercise-induced lactate and reduced serum BUN. Glabridin and glabrene appear to be $ER\alpha$ agonists, and in the presence of estrogen glabridin reduces signaling via $ER\alpha$ by 80% (SERM) without inhibiting $ER\beta$. Glabridin and glabrene have been shown to inhibit serotonin uptake, albeit to a lesser degree than imipramine. Another constituent glabrol at 50 mg/kg has been shown in animal models to be as sedating as 10 mg/kg zolpidem and appears to be a $GABA_A$ agonist.

HUMAN RESEARCH

Ear, Nose, and Throat Disorders: Xerostomia, Mucositis, Stomatitis, and Pharyngitis

A 2019 systematic review of efficacy of licorice for prevention of postoperative sore throat found five RCTs ($n = 609$) that met inclusion criteria. Compared with non-analgesic control, topical licorice was associated with a reduced incidence ($RR = 0.44$; $P < 0.001$) and severity ($SMD = -0.69$; $P < 0.001$) of postoperative sore throat. Four trials reported adverse events, but none were related to topical licorice. The authors concluded that preoperative application of licorice appeared to be significantly more effective than non-analgesic methods for preventing postoperative sore throat (Kuriyama and Maeda, 2019).

A perioperative RCT in patients ($n = 236$) undergoing thoracic surgery requiring intubation compared licorice fluid extract 0.5 g with a solution of sugar 5 g, administered as 1-min gargles 5 min prior to intubation. Ten minutes after extubation the incidence of postoperative sore throat was 19% and 36% with licorice and sugar-water gargles, respectively ($RR = 0.54$; $P = 0.005$). The incidence decreased further in the licorice group to 10% and 21% at 1.5 h and 4 h, respectively, while the incidence was 35% and 45% in the sugar-water group, respectively ($RR = 0.31$; $P < 0.001$; and $RR = 0.48$; $P < 0.001$, respectively). The authors concluded that licorice gargling cut the incidence of post-intubation sore throat in half (Ruetzler et al., 2013).

A 10-day RCT in patients ($n = 122$) undergoing hemodialysis compared licorice mouthwash with water mouthwash and with no mouthwash for hemodialysis-associated xerostomia. Compared with no mouthwash, the water mouthwash resulted in an increase in the unstimulated salivary flow rates of 25.85×10^{-3} mL/min and 25.78×10^{-3} mL/min ($P < 0.05$ for both) at day 5 and day 10, respectively. The estimated effect size was 1.38. However, there was no significant decrease in Summated Xerostomia Inventory scores. Compared with no mouthwash, the licorice mouthwash also improved the unstimulated salivary flow rates by 114.92×10^{-3} mL/min, and 131.61×10^{-3} mL/min at day 5 and day 10, respectively ($P < 0.001$ for both), and resulted in a significant improvement in the scores for the Summated Xerostomia Inventory ($P < 0.001$). The authors concluded that licorice mouthwash improved salivary flow rate and provided subjective relief of xerostomia and may effectively relieve feelings of dry mouth in hemodialysis patients (Yu et al., 2016).

A radiation-based RCT in patients ($n = 60$) undergoing head and neck cancer radiotherapy compared licorice mucoadhesive film with triamcinolone mucoadhesive film for prevention of oral mucositis. Both licorice and triamcinolone were associated with a meaningful reduction in VAS for oral pain ($P < 0.05$). There was no difference between treatments. The authors noted that licorice mucoadhesive film was equally efficacious as, with a trend toward superiority over, triamcinolone in the management of oral mucositis during radiotherapy. The authors concluded that both triamcinolone and licorice mucoadhesive films are effective in the management of oral mucositis during radiotherapy (Ghalayani et al., 2017).

A radiation-based RCT in patients ($n = 37$) undergoing radiation for head and neck cancer compared licorice aqueous extract with placebo applied topically BID for 2 weeks for effect on oral mucositis. Significant differences were found in the maximum grade of mucositis and oral mucosal irritation between the intervention and control groups ($P < 0.001$). The authors concluded that licorice aqueous extract could decrease the severity of oral mucositis in head and neck cancer patients undergoing radiotherapy (Najafi et al., 2017).

An 8-day RCT in patients ($n = 69$) with recurrent aphthous ulcers studied an intraoral adhesive patch containing licorice root extract compared with a placebo patch administered at onset of a lesion and with no treatment. Lesion size and pain report (unstimulated and stimulated) were assessed at intervals. By the eighth day, the ulcer size for the active treatment group was significantly lower ($P < 0.05$) than for the placebo group. With treatment 81%, 63%, and 40% of subjects reported significantly less pain with licorice, placebo, and no treatment, respectively (Martin et al., 2008).

Pulmonary Disorders: Asthma

A 2016 systematic review and meta-analysis of herbal medicines showing efficacy in asthma found 29 RCTs ($n = 3001$) that met inclusion criteria. Herbal interventions used multi-herb ingredients such as licorice root, crow-dipper, astragalus, and angelica. Compared with routine pharmacotherapies alone, herbal medicines as add-on therapy improved lung function as follows: FEV1 (MD = 7.81%, $I^2 = 63\%$); PEFR (MD = 65.14 L/min, $I^2 = 21\%$); asthma control (MD = 2.47 points, $I^2 = 55\%$); reduced salbutamol usage (MD = -1.14 puffs/day, $I^2 = 92\%$); and reduced acute asthma exacerbations over one year (MD = -1.20, $I^2 = 95\%$, one study). Compared with placebo plus pharmacotherapies herbal medicines as add-on therapy improved lung function as follows: FEV1 (MD = 15.83%) and PEFR (MD = 55.20 L/min). The authors concluded that herbal medicines combined with routine pharmacotherapies improved asthma outcomes greater than pharmacotherapies alone (Shergis et al., 2016).

A 21-day RCT in patients ($n = 54$) with chronic asthma compared licorice with frankincense and with prednisolone for effect on pulmonary function. FEV1 was increased from 62% to 81% and from 61% to 72.4% with licorice and frankincense, respectively. FVC increased from 1.08 to 3.6, from 0.72 to 2.63, and from 0.05 to 2.25 with licorice, frankincense, and prednisolone, respectively. Symptomatic improvement was greater with licorice than with frankincense. The authors concluded that licorice was superior to frankincense for chronic asthma (Al-Jawad et al., 2012).

Cardiometabolic Disorders: Hyperlipidemia and Dyslipidemia

A 2010 systematic review looking at herbal medicine (including TCM formulations) for hyperlipidemia identified 53 RCTs that met criteria. There were significant decreases in TC and LDL-C after treatment with licorice as well as milk thistle, fenugreek, yarrow, guggul, Daming capsule, chunghyul-dan, garlic powder, black tea, green tea, soy drink enriched with plant sterols, *Satureja khuzestanica, Monascus purpureus,* Went rice, C. Koch, Ningzhi capsule, cherry, composite salvia dropping pill (CSDP), shanzha xiaozhi capsule, Ba-wei-wan (hachimijiogan), rhubarb stalk, *Rheum ribes,* and primrose oil. Data were conflicting for red yeast rice, garlic, and guggul. No significant adverse effect or mortality were observed with licorice and several others. The authors concluded that 22 natural products were found effective in the treatment of hyperlipidemia and that further research was warranted (Hasani-Ranjbar et al., 2010).

A 6-month open-label trial in healthy subjects investigated the antioxidant effects of licorice root ethanolic extract selecting for the isoflavane glabridin. After oral administration of licorice-root ethanol extract to healthy subjects for 6 months, the subjects' oxidative stress level as well as plasma LDL oxidation were reduced by 20%. The authors concluded that dietary consumption of licorice protected LDL from oxidation (Carmeli and Fogelman, 2009).

A 2-week ex-vivo study performed in normolipidemic humans ($n=20$) investigated the antioxidant effect of licorice root extract on LDL extracted from the study subjects. The human subjects were supplemented with 100 mg/day of licorice root for 2 weeks. Before and after treatment, LDL showed reduction in susceptibility to oxidation following licorice treatment. The same authors also studied E-deficient mice (whose LDL is highly susceptible to oxidation) using either licorice 200 mcg/day or pure glabridin 20 mcg/day for 6 weeks. The mouse study showed a substantial reduction in the susceptibility of mouse LDL to oxidation along with a reduction in the atherosclerotic lesion area (Fuhrman et al., 1997).

Cardiometabolic Disorders: Obesity

A 2018 systematic review to assess the metabolic changes after licorice consumption found 26 RCTs ($n=985$) that met inclusion criteria. The findings showed that licorice consumption significantly reduced body weight (BW) (WMD $=-0.433$ kg; $P=0.001$) and BMI (WMD $=-0.150$ kg/m^2; $P=0.001$). There was an increase in DBP (1.737 mmHg; $P<0.0001$) related to licorice consumption. The authors concluded that licorice consumption produced a reduction in BW and BMI, but that DBP was increased due to the hypernatremia caused by licorice and should therefore be avoided in hypertensive patients (Luís et al., 2018).

A pair of 8-week RCTs looked at licorice flavonoid oil (LFO) for effects on weight. The first trial was in overweight/obese subjects ($n=22$), the second trial in athletic men who ate more than their energy requirements. Both studies compared LFO with placebo. No differences of statistical significance were noted between LFO and placebo for any measured variable in Study 1 or Study 2. However, in Study 2 the subjects taking LFO experienced less overall fat gain and attenuation in the elevation in selected blood lipids. The authors concluded that LFO supplementation had little effect in overweight/obese people except for possible attenuation in body fat gain and lipid changes in response to overfeeding (Bell et al., 2011).

Gastrointestinal Disorders: Alcohol-Induced Hepatitis

A crossover RCT in healthy subjects ($n=12$) compared a proprietary glycyrrhizin product with placebo for liver response to a nightly vodka challenge for 12 days. Consumption of alcohol was dosed to achieve a blood alcohol level of 0.12%. In the placebo group, AST, ALT, and GGT significantly increased from baseline to day 12. With licorice, no statistically significant increases were observed for AST, ALT, and GGT, while ALP significantly decreased, and plasma GSH decreased compared with placebo. The authors concluded that consumption of the proprietary glycyrrhizin product during alcohol consumption may support improved liver health compared with drinking alcohol alone (Chigurupati et al., 2016).

Gastrointestinal Disorders: Heartburn and Peptic Ulcer Disease

A 30-day RCT in patients ($n=50$) with functional dyspepsia including the symptom of heartburn compared licorice extract 75 mg BID with placebo. After 30 days, heartburn score decreased by 2.12 points with licorice and 1.44 points with placebo (effect sizes 2.18 and 1.54, respectively). Licorice was generally found to be safe and well tolerated by all patients. The authors concluded that this licorice extract had significant efficacy in the management of functional dyspepsia including the symptom of heartburn (Raveendra et al., 2012).

An 8-week RCT in patients ($n = 142$) with *Helicobacter pylori* infection investigated the combination of fermented milk with *L. paracasei HP7* plus licorice compared with fermented milk alone, each given daily. Compared with baseline data, the quantitative value of urea breath tests AUC at 8 weeks was significantly reduced with licorice (from 20.8% to 16.9%; $P = 0.035$), but not with placebo ($P = 0.130$). Chronic inflammation on histology, GI symptoms, and QOL all improved significantly only with licorice ($P = 0.013$; $P = 0.049$, and $P = 0.029$, respectively). Neutrophil activity deteriorated significantly only with placebo ($P = 0.003$). No serious adverse events were observed. The authors concluded that the combination of fermented milk and licorice reduced *H. pylori* density and improved histologic inflammation (Yoon et al., 2019).

A 6-week RCT in patients ($n = 120$) with *H. pylori* compared triple therapy alone for 2 weeks with triple therapy plus licorice for 2 weeks for eradication of *H. pylori*. Peptic ulcers were documented in 30% of patients in each group. At 6 weeks, *H. pylori* eradication was documented on breath tests in 62.5% of the group receiving triple therapy alone and 83.3% of the group receiving triple therapy plus licorice. The authors concluded that addition of licorice to the triple clarithromycin-based regimen increased *H. pylori* eradication, especially in the presence of peptic ulcer disease (Hajiaghamohammadi et al., 2016).

A crossover RCT in patients with chronic gastric ulcers ($n = 38$) compared deglycyrrhizinated licorice 760 mg TID with placebo for 4 weeks and then crossed over. There was no tendency to quicker healing in either group for change of ulcer area or complete healing. Small ulcers healed more quickly than big ones. Ulcers at the angular notch healed very poorly. No side effects of treatment were observed. The authors concluded that there was no difference between deglycyrrhizinated licorice extract and placebo in healing of gastric ulcers (Engqvist et al., 1973).

A 30-day RCT in patients ($n = 47$) with chronic duodenal ulcers investigated a combination product containing deglycyrrhizinated licorice 760 mg plus frangula bark, bismuth, aluminum hydroxide gel, magnesium carbonate, and sodium bicarbonate compared with the same combination of substances but with aniseed flavoring instead of licorice. Tablets were given TID for 30 days. No advantage of deglycyrrhizinated licorice over placebo was found. There were no side effects attributable to treatment including no fluid retention, no BP elevation, and no effect on electrolytes (Feldman and Gilat, 1971).

Gastrointestinal Disorders: Functional Dyspepsia and Infantile Colic

A 30-day RCT in patients ($n = 50$) with functional dyspepsia compared licorice extract 75 mg BID with placebo. Licorice showed a significant decrease compared with placebo in total symptom scores and in the Nepean dyspepsia index on day 15 and day 30 ($P < 0.05$ for both), and there was a marked improvement in the global assessment of efficacy with licorice compared with placebo ($P < 0.05$). Licorice was generally found to be safe and well tolerated by all patients. The authors concluded that this licorice extract had significant efficacy in the management of functional dyspepsia (Raveendra et al., 2012).

A 4-week RCT in patients ($n = 60$) with functional dyspepsia studied Iberogast in two different formulations (chamomile, peppermint, caraway, licorice, lemon balm, angelica, celandine, and milk thistle with or without bitter candy tuft) compared with placebo for effects on gastrointestinal symptoms. The herbal preparations showed a clinically significant improvement in the Gastrointestinal Symptom score compared with placebo after 2 and 4 weeks of treatment ($P < 0.001$). No statistically significant difference could be observed between the efficacy of two different herbal preparations ($P > 0.05$), but a solid improvement of GI symptoms could be achieved earlier with the herbal preparation that contained the bitter candy tuft ($P = 0.023$). The authors concluded that Iberogast and its modified formulation improved dyspeptic symptoms better than placebo and that the bitter candy tuft had an additive effect (Madisch, 2001).

A 12-week partial crossover RCT in patients ($n = 120$) with functional dyspepsia compared STW 5-II (containing extracts from licorice, bitter candy tuft, chamomile, peppermint, caraway, and lemon balm) with placebo. Each patient received treatment for three consecutive 4-week treatment blocks. The first two treatment blocks were fixed. For the third treatment period, medication was based upon the investigator's judgement of symptom improvement during the preceding treatment period. In patients without adequate control of symptoms, the treatment was switched, or if symptoms were controlled, the treatment was continued. During the first 4 weeks, the gastrointestinal symptom score decreased significantly in subjects on active treatment compared with placebo ($P < 0.001$). During the second 4-week period symptoms further improved in subjects who continued on active treatment or those who were switched to active treatment, while those switched to placebo deteriorated. After 8 weeks there was complete relief of symptoms in 43% and 3% of subjects on active treatment and placebo, respectively ($P < 0.001$). The authors concluded that this polyherbal preparation improved dyspeptic symptoms better than placebo (Madisch et al., 2004).

A 1-week RCT in healthy term 2- to 8-week-old infants ($n = 68$) who had colic compared a polyherbal tea (German chamomile, vervain, licorice, fennel, and balm mint) with a placebo tea (glucose and flavoring) up to 150 mL/dose up to TID. Parents reported that colic was eliminated in 57% and 26% of the infants given active tea and placebo tea, respectively ($P < 0.01$). No adverse effects were noted in either group (Weizman et al., 1993).

Women's Genitourinary and Related Disorders: Hyperprolactinemia, Polycystic Ovary Syndrome, and Hirsutism

A 2018 meta-analysis of RCTs to evaluate the efficacy of peony and licorice decoction (PGD) for antipsychotic-induced hyperprolactinemia found five RCTs ($n = 450$) that met inclusion criteria. The PGD group showed a significantly lower serum prolactin level at the endpoint than the control group (WMD $= -32.69$ ng/mL; $P < 0.00001$, $I^2 = 97\%$). Hyperprolactinemia-related symptoms were also improved significantly in the PGD groups compared with control groups. No difference was found in the improvement of psychiatric symptoms assessed by the Positive and Negative Syndrome Scale (WMD $= -0.62$; $P = 0.49$, $I^2 = 0\%$). There were similar rates of all-cause discontinuation ($n = 330$, RR $= 0.93$; $P = 0.71$, $I^2 = 0\%$) and adverse drug reactions between the two groups. The level of evidence of primary and secondary outcomes ranged from "very low" (14.3%),

to "low" (42.8%), to "moderate" (14.3%), and to "high" (28.6%). The authors concluded that use of PGD to suppress antipsychotic-induced hyperprolactinemia was supported by existing studies and that additional high-quality studies were warranted (Zheng et al., 2018).

A two-cycle open-label RCT in healthy women ($n = 9$) assessed the effects of licorice 3.5 g/day for effects on androgen metabolism in the luteal phase. Total serum testosterone decreased from 27.8 ng/dL to 19.0 ng/dL in the first month and to 17.5 ng/dL in the second month of therapy ($P < 0.05$). It returned to pre-treatment levels after discontinuation. Androstenedione, 17OH-progesterone, and LH levels did not change significantly during treatment. Plasma renin activity and aldosterone were depressed during therapy, while BP and cortisol remained unchanged. The authors concluded that licorice could reduce serum testosterone, likely due to the block of 17-hydroxysteroid dehydrogenase and 17–20 lyase, and that licorice could be considered an adjuvant therapy for hirsutism and polycystic ovary syndrome (Armanini et al., 2004).

An RCT in women ($n = 32$) with PCOS compared spironolactone 100 mg/day alone or in combination with licorice 3.5 g/day for hormonal and metabolic effects. Mean BP was significantly reduced during spironolactone treatment, while it was unchanged with spironolactone plus licorice. Symptoms of volume depletion were reported by 20% and 0% of women with spironolactone alone and spironolactone plus licorice, respectively. The activation of the renin-aldosterone system was significantly higher with spironolactone alone compared with spironolactone plus licorice. The prevalence of metrorrhagia was lower in the combined therapy group. The authors concluded that the mineralocorticoid properties of licorice could reduce the prevalence of side effects related to spironolactone in women with PCOS (Armanini et al., 2007).

A 3-month RCT in overweight women ($n = 122$) with PCOS compared lifestyle intervention alone with lifestyle intervention plus an herbal combination of licorice, St. John's wort, peony, and cinnamon plus a separate tablet of tribulus. At 3 months, women in the combination group recorded a reduction in oligomenorrhoea by 32.9% ($P < 0.01$) compared with controls. Other significant improvements were found for

BMI ($P<0.01$); insulin ($P=0.02$); LH ($P=0.04$); BP ($P=0.01$); QOL ($P<0.01$); depression, anxiety, and stress ($P<0.01$); and pregnancy rates ($P=0.01$). The authors concluded that lifestyle combined with herbal medicines was safe and effective in women with PCOS (Arentz et al., 2017).

Women's Genitourinary Disorders: Perimenopause and Menopause

A 2017 review of clinical trials on herbal efficacy in menopausal symptoms used search terms menopause, climacteric, hot flushes, flashes, herb, and phytoestrogens. The authors found that passionflower, sage, lemon balm, valerian, black cohosh, fenugreek, black seed, chasteberry, fennel, evening primrose, ginkgo, alfalfa, St. John's wort, Asian ginseng, anise, licorice, red clover, and wild soybean were effective in the treatment of acute menopausal syndrome with different mechanisms. The authors concluded that medicinal plants could play a role in the treatment of acute menopausal syndrome and that further studies were warranted (Kargozar et al., 2017).

A 2016 systematic review of Iranian herbal medicines for menopausal hot flushes found 19 RCTs that met inclusion criteria. Overall, studies showed that licorice, anise, soy, black cohosh, red clover, evening primrose, flaxseed, sage, passionflower, chasteberry, avocado plus soybean oil, St. John's wort, and valerian could alleviate hot flushes. The authors concluded that several herbal medicines were effective in relieving hot flushes and could be seen as an alternative for women experiencing hot flushes (Ghazanfarpour et al., 2016).

A 14-week RCT in menopausal women ($n=90$) with hot flushes compared licorice extract 330 mg TID with placebo for 8 weeks. The frequency of hot flushes decreased significantly with licorice compared with placebo, and the benefit extended for 2 weeks after the administration of the capsules. The severity of hot flush also decreased with licorice as well. The authors concluded that licorice root decreased the frequency and severity of hot flushes and could be useful in menopausal women (Nahidi et al., 2012).

An 8-week RCT in menopausal women ($n=70$) with vaginal atrophy compared licorice 2% vaginal cream with placebo vaginal cream. The vaginal cell maturation Index within 65–100 in MVI category increased from the baseline of 0% to 89% and 11.4% with licorice and placebo, respectively ($P<0.001$). The difference between licorice and baseline and between licorice and placebo in the transformation of vaginal epithelial cells from parabasal cells to intermediate and superficial cells was significant ($P<0.001$). Vaginal pH also decreased significantly with licorice. The authors concluded that licorice vaginal cream could improve signs and symptoms of vaginal atrophy in postmenopausal women (Sadeghi et al., 2020).

Men's Genitourinary Disorders: Testosterone Levels

A 9-week open-label trial in healthy women ($n=15$) and men ($n=21$), some of whom had essential HTN, assessed the impact of 150 mg glycyrrhetinic acid on sex steroid production. The licorice constituent was given for 4 weeks with 5 weeks of follow-up off the licorice. Licorice induced a moderate decrease in the serum concentrations of DHEA-S in men ($P=0.002$), and the relative change in serum levels of DHEA-S differed between the genders ($P=0.03$). No significant changes were observed in the serum testosterone levels after 4 weeks in either group, and the urine excretion of androgens (etiocholanolone and androstenedione) did not change. The authors concluded that glycyrrhetinic acid in moderate doses primarily affected cortisol metabolism and only marginally androgen hormones, especially in men (Sigurjonsdottir et al., 2006).

An open-label pilot study in men ($n=7$) assessed the effect of licorice 7 g on circulating testosterone levels. The trial showed a reduction in testosterone. A subsequent study by the same leading author using licorice 7 g in a larger cohort revealed a 26% reduction in total testosterone levels ($P<0.01$) and an insignificant decrease in free testosterone. There was an increase in 17-OHP and LH. Response of the latter two hormones to stimulation with β-HCG was not affected by licorice (Armanini et al., 1999, 2003).

Another author reported two attempts to replicate the findings of decreased testosterone with moderate licorice (5.6 g with 500 mg glycyrrhizic acid), with negative findings in both cases (Josephs et al., 2001).

Neurological Disorders: Parkinson's Disease

A 6-month RCT in patients ($n = 39$) with PD (YAHR staging ≤ 3) compared oral licorice syrup with placebo syrup 5 mL BID. Each 5 mL of active syrup contained 136 mg of licorice extract with 12.14 mg glycyrrhizic acid and 136 mcg of polyphenols. At 6 weeks, total UPDRS, daily activities, and tremor were significantly improved with licorice with a considerable effect size. Significant improvements in motor and rigidity scores were observed by 4 months ($P < 0.05$). No significant changes in electrolytes, blood pressure, or blood glucose were observed during the study. The authors concluded that licorice could improve symptoms in PD patients without serious adverse events (Petramfar et al., 2020).

Dermatological Disorders: Hyperpigmentation and Eczema

A 2018 systematic review of clinical studies evaluating the use of natural products in treating hyperpigmentation found 30 clinical studies that met inclusion criteria. Several natural ingredients did show efficacy as depigmenting agents, including licorice extracts, azelaic acid, soy, lignin peroxidase, ascorbic acid iontophoresis, arbutin, ellagic acid, niacinamide, and mulberry. The authors concluded that these products showed promise for patients with hyperpigmentation disorders (Hollinger et al., 2018).

A 2017 systematic review of studies to assess the efficacy and safety of topical herbal preparations for allergic eczema found eight studies that met inclusion criteria. Only two studies that showed a positive effect were considered to have a low risk of bias across all domains; those of licorice gel and St. John's wort. In these two studies, the test product was reported to be superior to placebo, and the findings warranted further research. No meta-analysis could be performed due to heterogeneity (Thandar, 2017).

Adrenal Disorders

A dose connected RCT in patients ($n = 17$) with Addison's disease stable on cortisone acetate replacement therapy compared the effects of supplementation with licorice to that of grapefruit juice. Compared with baseline, the median AUC for serum cortisol increased with licorice (from 50,882 to 53,783; $P < 0.05$) and grapefruit juice (from 50,882 to 60,661; $P < 0.05$). Median serum cortisol levels also increased from baseline 2.6 h after licorice intake (from 186 nmol/L to 223 nmol/L; $P < 0.05$) and grapefruit juice intake (from 186 nmol/L to 337 nmol/L; $P < 0.01$). Licorice increased the median urinary cortisol/cortisone ratio from baseline (from 0.21 to 0.43; $P < 0.00001$). Grapefruit juice increased the allo-tetrahydrocortisol + tetrahydrocortisol)/tetrahydrocortisone ratio (from 0.43 to 0.55; $P < 0.05$). The authors concluded that both licorice and grapefruit juice increased cortisol available to tissues in the hours following cortisone acetate administration, and that patients and physicians should be aware of these interactions (Methlie et al., 2011).

A one-week open-label trial in male and female volunteers compared licorice-containing and non-licorice-containing confectionaries for effect on salivary steroids. In the licorice group, salivary aldosterone was decreased, while deoxycorticosterone, DHEA, and testosterone were increased. Cortisol levels increased and cortisone levels decreased, reflecting expected inhibition of 11β-HSD2 by glycyrrhetinic acid. In step 2 of the study, adrenocortical H295 cells were incubated with glycyrrhetinic acid in the presence or absence of forskolin to assess impact on free and conjugated steroids. Glycyrrhetinic acid inhibited cortisone and enhanced cortisol synthesis consistent with 11β-HSD2 inhibition. Basal and forskolin-stimulated syntheses of deoxycorticosterone and DHEA conjugates were also inhibited by glycyrrhetinic acid in a dose-dependent manner and not associated with changes in the expression of SULT 2A1 mRNA. The authors concluded that glycyrrhetinic acid increased circulating and salivary levels of unconjugated deoxycorticosterone and DHEA by inhibiting their conjugation at the source within the adrenal cortex, which may contribute to the mineralocorticoid and androgenic actions of glycyrrhetinic acid (Al-Dujaili et al., 2011).

Inflammation: Familial Mediterranean Fever

A one-month Phase II RCT of young patients ($n = 24$) with familial Mediterranean fever (FMF) compared ImmunoGuard (a standardized fixed combination of eleuthero, andrographis, schisandra, and licorice extracts) four tablets TID with placebo. The patient's self-evaluation was based on symptoms of abdominal pain, chest pain, temperature, arthritis, myalgia, and erysipelas-like erythema. All three features (duration, frequency, and severity of attacks) showed significant improvement in the ImmunoGuard group compared with placebo. In both clinical assessment and self-evaluation, the severity of attacks was found to show the most significant improvement in the herbal group. The authors concluded that both the clinical and laboratory results of the clinical study suggested that ImmunoGuard was a safe and efficacious herbal drug for the management of patients with FMF (Amaryan et al., 2003).

ACTIVE CONSTITUENTS

Root

- Phenolic compounds
  - Coumarins: liqcoumarin, glabrocoumarone A and B, herniarin (antispasmodic, antigenotoxic, antimicrobial in presence of UV light), umbelliferone (anti-inflammatory, venotonic, lymphatotonic, possibly anticoagulant, antispasmodic, antigenotoxic, hepatoprotective, antifungal), glycyrin (PPARγ activity), glycocoumarin, licofuranocoumarin, licopyranocoumarin and glabrocoumarin.
  - Flavonoids: liquiritin, liquiritigenin, rhamnoliquiritin, neoliquiritin, isoliquiritin, isoliquiritigenin, neoisoliquiritin, licuraside, glabrolide, licoflavonol, glabridin, galbrene, glabrone, shinpterocarpin, glyzarin, kumatakenin, hispaglabridin A, hispaglabridin B.
- Isoflavonoids (phytoestrogenic): formononetin, licoisoflavones A and B, glycyrrhisoflavone (tyrosinase inhitibor, MAO-I, α-glucosidase inhibitor).

- Terpenes
  - Monoterpenes: thymol (strong antimicrobial)
  - Triterpenoid saponins: glycyrrhizin (aka glycyrrhizic acid), 18-β glycyrrhetinic acid, liquiritic acid, glycyrretol, glabrolide, isoglaborlide and liquorice acid
- Aromatic compounds: β-caryophyllene oxide, decadienol, 1α, 10α-epoxyamorpha-4-ene, β-dihydroionone, thymol (strong antimicrobial), carvacrol

LICORICE COMMONLY USED PREPARATIONS AND DOSAGE (FOR ADULTS UNLESS OTHERWISE SPECIFIED)

The following are examples of some available formulations and ranges of dosing for commercial herbal products. See Part III Introduction "How to prescribe medicinal herbs" for further guidance on herbal advising and prescribing.

Before prescribing licorice, consider how much is safe and whether to recommend regular or deglycyrrhizinated licorice. It depends on the patient's risks for HTN and hypokalemia (see "Safety and Precaution/Disease interactions") and the indication for which licorice is being considered. The recommendations in the herbal literature are quite variable, so it is important to be fully aware of these considerations and proceed with caution.

It is generally stated that up to 5–15 g/day of licorice is considered safe for short-term use. In 1991, the European Union proposed a provisional figure of 100 mg/day as the upper limit for ingestion of glycyrrhizin. The Dutch Nutrition Information Bureau advised against daily glycyrrhizin consumption in excess of 200 mg. A daily oral intake of 0.2 mg/kg/day of glycyrrhizin has been estimated to be a safe dose for most healthy adults. This would be 12 mg/day of glycyrrhizin in a 60 kg person. However, in an 8-week study noted below, the NOAEL for glycyrrhizin was 2 mg/kg/day in women. Glycyrrhizin makes up 2%-25% of the total licorice content of a product depending on species and growing variables. Licorice extract is often standardized to 7%-20% glycyrrhizin. In a survey of 33 brands of licorice tea, the mean glycyrrhizin content was found to be 126 mg/L (range 2–450 mg/L). A cup of licorice tea with a volume of 250 mL could therefore be expected to contain, on average, approximately 31.5 mg of glycyrrhizin. Depending on the product purchased, calculations will be necessary. Deglycyrrhizinated licorice (DGL) up to 1800 mg/day for 4 weeks is not associated with toxicity in humans.

The bottom line is to be aware of the potential for hypertension and hypokalemia in non-DGL formulations and to monitor patients closely for these effects during the course of therapy.

Root

Not for use in children younger than 4 years. Do not use longer than 4–6 weeks without monitoring BP and electrolytes. If glycyrrhizin effects are to be avoided in patients at increased risk of HTN or hypokalemia, keep glycyrrhizin content less than 150 mg. Older women are at greater risk for complications, so monitor closely when used for menopausal complaints or use DGL, which still contains estrogenic constituents.

For Bronchitis or Sore Throat

- Infusion: 4.5 g root in 150 mL TID
- Decoction: 1–1.5 g licorice root per 150–250 mL water TID
- Fluid extract: 0.5 g per 30 mL gargled for one minute before intubation
- Lozenge: 97 mg 30 min before anesthesia
- Topical spray

For GERD or GI Ulcers

- DGL (deglycyrrhizinated) chewable tablets: 760 mg (two tablets) QAC
- Standardized fluid extract (standardized to minimum 7% glycyrrhizin): 2–5 mL TID (corresponding to 5–15 g of root daily)
- Powdered root: 5–15 g daily or 2–4 g per dose
- Powdered root extract: 500–600 mg (1/5–1/4 tsp) QD
- Capsule or tablet of standardized extract (standardized to 20% glycyrrhizin): 300–800 mg TID PC

For PCOS

Capsule or tablet of powdered root: 800–900 mg TID-QID; safer if used in conjunction with spironolactone 100 mg per day.

For Menopause

- Powdered root extract: 600 mg (1/4 tsp) QD
- Capsule or tablet of powdered root extract: 330–450 mg QD-TID
- DGL (deglycyrrhizinated) native powdered extract: 400–1600 mg TID
- Licorice 2% vaginal gel

For Atopic Eczema or Hyperpigmentation

- Licorice root 2% gel: applied TID

SAFETY AND PRECAUTION

Side Effects

In 2017 the USFDA issued an advisement that warned consumers that adults older than 40 years who eat 2 ounces of natural black licorice per day for at least 2 weeks could develop cardiac arrhythmia or other serious complications.

Eating 200 g of licorice within 45 min has been shown to make 75% of persons feel queasy and tired, the dose of which correlates with serum glycyrrhizin levels. HTN, hypertensive retinopathy, hypertensive nephropathy, lethargy, muscle pain, carpal tunnel syndrome, sodium retention, hypokalemia, adrenal crisis, cardiac arrhythmias, leukoderma, and thrombocytopenia have been reported when taken at high doses or for long periods of time.

Case Reports

A woman who only ate licorice for an undisclosed time appeared to have died from a hyperglycemic coma, mostly through interactions with the carbohydrate content of licorice.

Several reports have been made of hypertensive crisis, intracranial hemorrhage, stroke, leukoderma, hypokalemic paralysis, rhabdomyolysis, increased anorexia in anorexia nervosa, carpal tunnel syndrome, ventricular fibrillation, and hypercalcemia.

Toxicity

A significant fall in plasma potassium concentration from 4.3 to 3.5 mmol/L has been documented at the dose of $\geq$ 800 mg/day of licorice.

A 4-week study in healthy volunteers ($n = 6$) administered doses of 108, 217, 380, and 814 mg/day of glycyrrhizin to monitor for adverse effects. NOAEL based on the study report was 217 mg/day. At higher dose levels, sodium retention and depression of plasma renin and aldosterone levels were observed. Female participants were slightly more sensitive to glycyrrhizin than male participants.

A subsequent 8-week RCT in healthy females ($n = 40$) compared 0, 1, 2, or 4 mg/kg/day of pure glycyrrhizin. In this study the NOAEL for glycyrrhizinic acid was 2 mg/kg/day (Bijlsma et al., 1996).

Dosing of up to 1200 mg/day for 7 days or 1800 mg/day for 4 weeks of Licorice Flavanoid Oil (LFO) without glycyrrhizin does not appear to be associated with any serum indicators of toxicity.

Deglycyrrhizinated licorice (DGL) up to 1800 mg/day for 4 weeks is not associated with toxicity in humans.

Up to 800 mg/kg of licorice in male mice and 400 mg/kg in female mice for 90 days has demonstrated no apparent toxicity, with the next highest tested doses (1600 mg/kg in males, 800 mg/kg in females) associated with excessive anticoagulative effects.

Pregnancy and Lactation

A systematic review showed an association between heavy licorice use and early preterm births. Do not use during pregnancy. Insufficient evidence for safety with lactation.

Disease Interactions

- Sensitivities to glycyrrhizin effects: Prolonged GI transit time, diarrhea (K+ loss), advanced age, female gender, anorexia nervosa, and genetic polymorphisms resulting decreased 11-ß-HSD2
- May worsen HTN, Cushing's disease, Conn's syndrome, male hypogonadism, osteoporosis.
- Avoid in estrogen-sensitive cancers due to estrogenic activity
- Increases cortisol in patients being treated for Addison's disease

Cautionary Human Trials for HTN and Osteoporosis

A 2018 systematic review of the adverse effects of chronic licorice ingestion (at least 100 mg/day of glycyrrhizic acid) found 18 studies ($n = 337$) that met inclusion criteria. There was a statistically significant increase in mean SBP (5.45 mm Hg) and diastolic BP (3.19 mm Hg) after chronic ingestion of a product containing glycyrrhizic acid. There were significant reductions in plasma potassium (-0.33 mmol/L), plasma renin activity (-0.82 ng/mL/h), and plasma aldosterone (-173.24 pmol/L). A significant correlation was noted between daily dose of glycyrrhizic acid and SBP ($r^2 = 0.55$) and diastolic BP ($r^2 = 0.65$), but not for the other outcome measures. The authors concluded that chronic licorice ingestion was associated with an increase in BP and a drop in plasma potassium, even at modest doses (Penninkilampi et al., 2017).

A 4-week trial in healthy volunteers and patients with HTN assessed the effects of 100 g of licorice equivalent to 150 mg/day glycyrrhetinic acid to assess effects on BP. The mean increase in SBP with office measurements after 4 weeks of licorice was 3.5 mmHg ($P < 0.06$) in normotensive and 15.3 mmHg ($P = 0.003$) in hypertensive subjects ($P = 0.004$). The mean rise in DBP was 3.6 mmHg ($P = 0.01$) in normotensive and 9.3 mmHg ($P < 0.001$) in hypertensive subjects ($P = 0.03$). The difference in the effect on the BP was not significant between genders and was not dependent on age, the change in PRA, or weight. The authors concluded that patients with essential HTN were more sensitive to the inhibition of 11-ß-HSD2 by licorice than normotensive subjects, and that this inhibition caused more clinical symptoms in women than in men (Sigurjonsdottir et al., 2003).

A two-cycle open-label trial in healthy young women ($n = 9$) administered licorice (containing 7.6% glycyrrhizic acid) 3.5 g/day to measure effects on hormones and electrolytes. PTH, 25OHD, and urinary calcium increased significantly from baseline values after 2 months of therapy, while 1,25OHD and ALP did not change during treatment. All these parameters returned to pretreatment levels 1 month after discontinuation of licorice. PRA and aldosterone were depressed during therapy, while BP and plasma cortisol remained unchanged. The authors concluded that licorice could increase serum PTH and urinary calcium levels from baseline values in healthy women after only 2 months of treatment, an effect they attributed to the aldosterone-like, estrogen-like and antiandrogen activity (Mattarello et al., 2006).

Drug Interactions

- CYP: Glycyrrhizin induces CYP3A and CYP2D6. Glabridin was found to inactivate the enzymatic activities of CYP 3A4 and 2B6 and competitively inhibited 2C9
- Pgp: Inhibits P-glycoprotein, resulting in increased intracellular concentration of daunorubicin
- Anticoagulants: May increase the metabolism and clearance of warfarin
- Antihypertensives: may reduce efficacy
- β-agonists: May aggravate hypokalemia
- Cardiac glycosides: hypokalemia may increase toxicity

- Cyclosporine: Reduces the oral bioavailability of cyclosporine
- Corticosteroids: decreases clearance, increases availability
- Diuretics: May increase the risk of hypokalemia
- Insulin: May aggravate hypokalemia
- MAO-inhibitors (MAOIs): May potentiate activity of MAOIs
- Metformin: Pre-administration of licorice juice reduced the efficacy of metformin in a rat model
- Oral contraceptive use: OCs may increase sensitivity to glycyrrhizin

REFERENCES

Al-Dujaili EA, Kenyon CJ, Nicol MR, Mason JI. Liquorice and glycyrrhetinic acid increase DHEA and deoxycorticosterone levels in vivo and in vitro by inhibiting adrenal SULT2A1 activity. Mol Cell Endocrinol 2011;336(1-2):102–9.

Al-Jawad F, Al-Razzuqi R, Hashim H, Al-Bayati N. Glycyrrhiza glabra vs Boswellia carterii in chronic bronchial asthma: a comparative study of efficacy. Ind J Allergy Asthma Immunol 2012;26(1):6–8.

Amaryan G, Astvatsatryan V, Gabrielyan E, Panossian A, Panosyan V, Wikman G. Double-blind, placebo-controlled, randomized, pilot clinical trial of ImmunoGuard—a standardized fixed combination of Andrographis paniculata Nees, with Eleutherococcus senticosus Maxim, Schisandra chinensis Bail. and Glycyrrhiza glabra L. extracts in patients with familial mediterranean fever. Phytomedicine 2003;10(4):271–85.

Arentz S, Smith CA, Abbott J, Fahey P, Cheema BS, Bensoussan A. Combined lifestyle and herbal medicine in overweight women with polycystic ovary syndrome (PCOS): a randomized controlled trial. Phytother Res 2017;31(9):1330–40.

Armanini D, Bonanni G, Palermo M. Reduction of serum testosterone in men by licorice. N Engl J Med 1999;341(15):1158.

Armanini D, Bonanni G, Mattarello MJ, Fiore C, Sartorato P, Palermo M. Licorice consumption and serum testosterone in healthy man. Exp Clin Endocrinol Diabetes 2003;111(6):341–3.

Armanini D, Mattarello MJ, Fiore C, et al. Licorice reduces serum testosterone in healthy women. Steroids 2004;69(11-12):763–6.

Armanini D, Castello R, Scaroni C, et al. Treatment of polycystic ovary syndrome with spironolactone plus licorice. Eur J Obstet Gynecol Reprod Biol 2007;131(1):61–7.

Bell ZW, Canale RE, Bloomer RJ. A dual investigation of the effect of dietary supplementation with licorice flavonoid oil on anthropometric and biochemical markers of health and adiposity. Lipids Health Dis 2011;10:29.

Bijlsma J, Van Vloten P, Van Gelderen C, et al. Study into the effects of different dosages of glycyrrhizin in health female volunteers. RIVM report no. 348801004, The Netherlands: RIVM, Bilthoven; 1996.

Carmeli E, Fogelman Y. Antioxidant effect of polyphenolic glabridin on LDL oxidation. Toxicol Ind Health 2009;25(4-5):321–4.

Chigurupati H, Auddy B, Biyani M, Stohs SJ. Hepatoprotective effects of a proprietary glycyrrhizin product during alcohol consumption: a randomized, double-blind, placebo-controlled, crossover study. Phytother Res 2016;30(12):1943–53.

Engqvist A, von Feilitzen F, Pyk E, Reichard H. Double-blind trial of deglycyrrhizinated liquorice in gastric ulcer. Gut 1973;14(9):711–5.

Feldman H, Gilat T. A trial of deglycyrrhizinated liquorice in the treatment of duodenal ulcer. Gut 1971;12(6):449–51.

Fuhrman B, Buch S, Vaya J, et al. Licorice extract and its major polyphenol glabridin protect low-density lipoprotein against lipid peroxidation: in vitro and ex vivo studies in humans and in atherosclerotic apolipoprotein E-deficient mice. Am J Clin Nutr 1997;66(2):267–75.

Ghalayani P, Emami H, Pakravan F, Nasr IM. Comparison of triamcinolone acetonide mucoadhesive film with licorice mucoadhesive film on radiotherapy-induced oral mucositis: a randomized double-blinded clinical trial. Asia Pac J Clin Oncol 2017;13(2):e48–56.

Ghannad MS, et al. The effect of aqueous extract of Glycyrrhiza glabra on Herpes Simplex Virus 1. Jundishapur J Microbiol 2014;7(7), e11616.

Ghazanfarpour M, Sadeghi R, Abdolahian S, Latifnejad RR. The efficacy of Iranian herbal medicines in alleviating hot flashes: a systematic review. Int J Reprod Biomed (Yazd) 2016;14(3):155–66.

Hajiaghamohammadi A, Zargar A, Oveisi S, Samimi R, Reisian S. To evaluate of the effect of adding licorice to the standard treatment regimen of Helicobacter pylori. Braz J Infect Dis 2016;20.

Hasani-Ranjbar S, Nayebi N, Moradi L, Mehri A, Larijani B, Abdollahi M. The efficacy and safety of herbal medicines used in the treatment of hyperlipidemia; a systematic review. Curr Pharm Des 2010;16(26):2935–47.

Hollinger JC, Angra K, Halder RM. Are natural ingredients effective in the management of hyperpigmentation? a systematic review. J Clin Aesthet Dermatol 2018;11(2):28–37.

Josephs RA, Guinn JS, Harper ML, Askari F. Liquorice consumption and salivary testosterone concentrations. Lancet 2001;358(9293):1613–4.

Kargozar R, Azizi H, Salari R. A review of effective herbal medicines in controlling menopausal symptoms. Electron Phys 2017;9(11):5826–33.

Kuriyama A, Maeda H. Topical application of licorice for prevention of postoperative sore throat in adults: a systematic review and meta-analysis. J Clin Anesth 2019;54:25–32.

Luís Â, Domingues F, Pereira L. Metabolic changes after licorice consumption: a systematic review with meta-analysis and trial sequential analysis of clinical trials. Phytomedicine 2018;39:17–24.

Madisch A, Holtmann G, Mayr G, et al. Treatment of functional dyspepsia with a herbal preparation. A double-blind, randomized, placebo-controlled, multicenter trial. Digestion 2004;69(1):45–52.

Madisch A, Melderis H, Mayr G, Sassin I, Hotz J. A plant extract and its modified preparation in functional dyspepsia. Results of a double-blind placebo controlled comparative study. Z Gastroenterol 2001 Jul;39(7):511-7.

Martin MD, Sherman J, van der Ven P, Burgess J. A controlled trial of a dissolving oral patch concerning glycyrrhiza (licorice) herbal extract for the treatment of aphthous ulcers. Gen Dent 2008;56(2):206–10.

Mattarello MJ, Benedini S, Fiore C, et al. Effect of licorice on PTH levels in healthy women. Steroids 2006;71(5):403–8.

Methlie P, Husebye EE, Hustad S, Lien EA, Løvås K. Grapefruit juice and licorice increase cortisol availability in patients with Addison's disease. Eur J Endocrinol 2011;165(5):761–9.

Nahidi F, Zare E, Mojab F, Alavi-majd H. Effects of licorice on relief and recurrence of menopausal hot flashes. Iran J Pharm Res 2012;11(2):541–8.

Najafi S, Koujan SE, Manifar S, Kharazifard MJ, Kidi S, Hajheidary S. Preventive effect of glycyrrhiza glabra extract on oral mucositis in patients under head and neck radiotherapy: a randomized clinical trial. J Dent (Tehran) 2017;14(5):267–74.

Orhan IE, Deniz FS. Natural products as potential leads against coronaviruses: could they be encouraging structural models against SARS-CoV-2? Nat Prod Bioprospect 2020;10(4):171–86.

Penninkilampi R, Eslick EM, Eslick GD. The association between consistent licorice ingestion, HTN and hypokalaemia: a systematic review and meta-analysis. J Hum Hypertens 2017;29.

Petramfar P, Hajari F, Yousefi F, Azadi S, Hamedi A. Efficacy of oral administration of licorice as an adjunct therapy on improving the symptoms of patients with Parkinson's disease, A randomized double blinded clinical trial. J Ethnopharmacol 2020;247:112–26.

Raveendra KR, Jayachandra, Srinivasa V, et al. An extract of *Glycyrrhiza glabra* (GutGard) alleviates symptoms of functional dyspepsia: a randomized, double-blind, placebo-controlled study. Evid Based Complement Alternat Med 2012;216970.

Ruetzler K, Fleck M, Nabecker S, et al. A randomized, double-blind comparison of licorice vs sugar-water gargle for prevention of postoperative sore throat and postextubation coughing. Anesth Analg 2013;117(3):614–21.

Sadeghi M, Namjouyan F, Cheraghian B, Abbaspoor Z. Impact of Glycyrrhiza glabra (licorice) vaginal cream on vaginal signs and symptoms of vaginal atrophy in postmenopausal women: a randomized double-blind controlled trial. J Tradit Complement Med 2020;10(2):110–5.

Shergis JL, Wu L, Zhang AL, Guo X, Lu C, Xue CC. Herbal medicine for adults with asthma: a systematic review. J Asthma 2016;53(6):650–9.

Sigurjonsdottir HA, Manhem K, Axelson M, Wallerstedt S. Subjects with essential HTN are more sensitive to the inhibition of 11 β-HSD by liquorice. J Hum Hypertens 2003;17(2):125–31.

Sigurjonsdottir HA, Axelson M, Johannsson G, Manhem K, Nystrom E, Wallerstedt S. Liquorice in moderate doses does not affect sex steroid hormones of biological importance although the effect differs between the genders. Horm Res 2006;65(2):106–10.

Thandar Y. Topical herbal medicines for atopic eczema: a systematic review of randomized controlled trials. Br J Dermatol 2017;176(2):330–43.

Weizman Z, Alkrinawi S, Goldfarb D. Efficacy of herbal tea preparation in infantile colic. J Pediatr 1993;122(650):652.

Yoon JY, Cha JM, Hong SS, et al. Fermented milk containing Lactobacillus paracasei and Glycyrrhiza glabra has a beneficial effect in patients with Helicobacter pylori infection: a randomized, double-blind, placebo-controlled study. Medicine (Baltimore) 2019;98(35), e16601.

Yu IC, Tsai YF, Fang JT, Yeh MM, Fang JY, Liu CY. Effects of mouthwash interventions on xerostomia and unstimulated whole saliva flow rate among hemodialysis patients: a randomized controlled study. Int J Nurs Stud 2016;63:9–17.

Zheng W, Cai DB, Li HY, et al. Adjunctive Peony-Glycyrrhiza decoction for antipsychotic-induced hyperprolactinaemia: a meta-analysis of randomised controlled trials. Gen Psychiatr 2018;31(1), e100003.

Zhu, et al. An artificial intelligence system reveals liquiritin inhibits SARS-CoV-2 by mimicking type I interferon. bioRxiv 2020.05.02.074021. https://doi.org/10.1101/2020.05.02.074021.

60

MACA (*LEPIDIUM MEYENII*)
Root

GENERAL OVERVIEW

People of the Andes have used maca root traditionally for more than 2000 years for nutrition, cognition, and fertility. The root comes mainly in three different colors—black, red, and yellow—each of which imparts different benefits. Red maca is the rarest of the three colors and provides the most antioxidants. Studies have shown it to be effective against prostate cancer. Black maca or "natural Viagra" has been shown to significantly increase sperm count and sperm motility in men and to reduce stress and fatigue, increase memory and learning ability, and work as a natural antidepressant. Red maca and to a lesser degree black maca have shown positive effects on bone structure. Yellow maca has shown a moderate effect on sperm count and sex drive, while red maca had no such effect.

Maca's popularity has spread throughout the world as an aphrodisiac for both men and women. It may be particularly useful for this benefit at higher altitudes. Unlike other adaptogenic herbs, maca does not appear to work through raising testosterone. Yet it has been shown to increase sperm production and counteract benign prostatic hyperplasia (BPH) in men. Conflicting research shows variable effects of maca on estrogenic activity, yet it has consistently been shown to ameliorate perimenopausal and menopausal symptoms in women. It is also neuroprotective and osteoprotective.

Clinical research indicates that maca, alone or in combination formulas, may be beneficial for menopause, menopausal sexual dysfunction, erectile dysfunction, male infertility, and general wellness at high altitudes.

IN VITRO AND ANIMAL RESEARCH

Research in male rodents showed increased sexual behavior, but findings have been mixed. Maca (particularly black and yellow maca) has been shown to increase sperm count and motility in normal rats, in rats with a variety of induced pathologies, and in normal bulls. In mice, guinea pigs, and trout, maca (particularly red maca) has been shown to improve embryo quality and/or offspring quantity.

Maca appears to have a dose-dependent effect on estrogen levels. When maca was given to ovariectomized rats at 0.5 g/kg and 1.25 g/kg of dry root extract for 28 weeks, the results showed that the lower dose preserved bone mineral density nonsignificantly relative to control, while the higher dose increased femur diameter and calcium content. The higher dose also increased uterine weight, indicating estrogenic effects. In other research, red and black maca were protective of bone architecture in ovariectomized rats, without estrogenic effects on uterine weight. Higher doses of maca have been shown to have proliferative effects on MCF-7 breast cancer cells, while lower doses do not.

With respect to prostate health, red maca has been shown to be effective in reducing prostatic hyperplasia in rodents. Research has suggested that this effect is due to the benzyl glucosinolate in red maca. Research has shown that an extract delivering 0.1 mg benzyl glucosinolate was more effective in suppressing prostatic weight gain than 0.1 mg finasteride and that 0.1 g/kg and 0.5 g/kg of red maca (0.64% benzyl glucosinolate content) were more effective than 0.6 mg/kg of finasteride in suppressing prostate growth without influencing seminal vesicle weight or testosterone levels, suggesting that the mechanism of action is downstream of DHT conversion.

Black maca improved memory and learning in memory-impaired mice (memory impairment induced by either alcohol or scopolamine); red and yellow maca did not.

HUMAN RESEARCH

Women's Genitourinary Disorders: Perimenopause and Menopause

A 2011 systematic review assessing maca and human sexual function selected four clinical trials that met inclusion criteria. These RCTs tested the effects of maca on menopausal symptoms in healthy perimenopausal, early postmenopausal, and late postmenopausal women. Using the Kupperman Menopausal Index and the Greene Climacteric Score, all RCTs demonstrated favorable effects of maca. However, the authors concluded that there was limited evidence for the effectiveness of maca as a treatment for menopausal symptoms (Lee et al., 2011).

A 4-month crossover RCT in *perimenopausal* women ($n = 20$) compared gelatinized maca root 500 mg BID for 2 months with placebo. With maca, significant alleviation of the negative physiological and psychological symptoms of perimenopause occurred in 74%-87% of the women. The maca group demonstrated a significant increase in estradiol, with a decrease in LH, T3, cortisol, and ACTH. Levels remained steady for FSH and progesterone. In addition, there was a highly significantly reduction in BMI. The authors noted a transient placebo effect. A second part of this study involved *postmenopausal* women ($n = 34$) who were also crossed over between gelatinized maca root 500 mg BID for 2 months and placebo for 2 months. Estradiol increased from baseline with maca ($P < 0.05$) and there were significant reductions in FSH, T3, ACTH, cortisol, and BMI ($P < 0.05$ for all). Menopausal symptoms as measured by the Greene Menopausal Score and the Kupperman Index showed alleviation ($P < 0.001$) (Meissner et al., 2006).

A 12-week crossover RCT in postmenopausal women ($n = 29$) compared maca 3.3 g/day with placebo for effects on hormones, blood pressure, and general well-being. The authors found no differences between maca and placebo in estradiol, FSH, TSH, SHBG, glucose, lipid profiles, and serum cytokines. However, there were significant decreases in DBP and depression (based on Women's Health Questionnaire and Utian Quality of Life Scale) (Stojanovska et al., 2015).

A 12-week crossover RCT in postmenopausal women ($n = 14$) compared maca 3.5 g/day with placebo for effects on sexual function and hormones. No differences from baseline in estradiol, FSH, LH, or SHBG occurred in either group. The Greene Climacteric Scale revealed significant reductions psychological symptoms, including the subscales for anxiety and depression and sexual dysfunction after maca consumption compared with both baseline and placebo ($P < 0.05$). The authors concluded that there is preliminary evidence that maca reduces psychological symptoms, including anxiety and depression, and lowers measures of sexual dysfunction in postmenopausal women independent of estrogenic and androgenic activity (Brooks et al., 2008).

Women's Genitourinary Disorders: Female Sexual Dysfunction

A 2018 systematic review to evaluate the effectiveness of phytoestrogens for sexual disorders and dyspareunia in women found that the phytoestrogens isolated from maca as well as French maritime pine bark, fennel, and fenugreek significantly improved sexual function, whereas the phytoestrogens isolated from Korean red ginseng, flaxseed, red clover, and soy did not lead to significant effects on sexual function (Najafi and Ghazanfarpour, 2018).

A 2010 systematic review assessing the clinical evidence for or against the effectiveness of the maca as a treatment for sexual dysfunction selected four RCTs that met inclusion criteria. Two RCTs suggested a significant positive effect of maca on sexual dysfunction or sexual desire in healthy menopausal women or healthy adult men, respectively, while the other RCT failed to show any effects in healthy cyclists but did show improved self-rated desire compared with baseline and placebo. One RCT assessing the effects of maca in patients with erectile dysfunction showed significant effects. The authors concluded that there is limited evidence for the effectiveness of maca in improving sexual function (Shin et al., 2010).

A pilot study in remitted depressed outpatients (*n* = 20) with SSRI-induced sexual dysfunction compared maca 1.5 g/day with maca 3 g/day. The higher-dose group had a significant improvement in Arizona Sexual Experience Scale scores (from 22.8 to 16.9; $P = 0.028$) and in Massachusetts General Hospital Sexual Function Questionnaire scores (from 24.1 to 17.0; $P = 0.017$). This benefit was not apparent with the lower dose. However, libido improved in both groups. Maca was well tolerated. The authors concluded that maca root may alleviate SSRI-induced sexual dysfunction with a dose-related effect. Maca may also have a beneficial effect on libido (Dording et al., 2008).

A 12-week RCT in women (*n*=45) with antidepressant-induced sexual dysfunction compared maca 1500 mg BID with placebo. Sexual dysfunction scores from the Arizona Sexual Experience Scale (ASEX) and Massachusetts General Hospital Sexual Function Questionnaire (MGH-SFQ) showed remission in 9.5% with maca and 4.8% with placebo based on an ASEX score of < 10, and in 30% with maca and 20% with placebo based on an MGH-SFQ score < 12. The higher remission rates were noted in postmenopausal women but not premenopausal women (Dording et al., 2015).

Men's Genitourinary Disorders: Male Sexual Dysfunction and Infertility

A 2018 systematic review to evaluate the efficacy of herbal medicines for erectile dysfunction (ED) identified 24 RCTs (*n*=2080) for inclusion. Among these, five investigated ginseng (*n*=399), three investigated saffron (*n*=397), and two investigated tribulus (*n*=202). Twelve studies investigated combinations of herbs and or supplements. Ginseng significantly improved erectile function (IIEF-5 score: 140 with ginseng, 96 with placebo; SMD = 0.43; $P < 0.01$). *Pinus pinaster* and maca showed very preliminary positive results, and saffron and tribulus produced mixed results. Adverse events were recorded in 19 of 24 trials, with no significant differences between placebo and verum in placebo-controlled studies. The authors concluded that there was encouraging evidence to suggest that ginseng may be an effective herbal treatment for ED (Borrelli et al., 2018).

A 2016 systematic review to assess the effectiveness of maca for improving semen quality selected five studies that met inclusion criteria. One RCT found favorable effects of maca on sperm mobility in infertile men. The two other RCTs showed positive effects of maca on several semen quality parameters in healthy men. The two open-label studies also suggested favorable effects of maca on semen quality. The authors concluded that there is suggestive evidence for the effectiveness of maca for improving semen quality (Lee et al., 2016).

A 12-week RCT in men (*n* = 50) with mild erectile dysfunction compared maca 2400 mg/day with placebo. The IIEF-5 and the Satisfaction Profile (SAT-P) were followed. There was an increase in IIEF-5 scores in both maca and placebo groups ($P < 0.05$ for both). However, patients taking maca experienced a more significant increase than those taking placebo (1.6 vs 0.5; $P < 0.001$). Improvement in psychological performance-related SAT-P scores improved more with maca than with placebo (+9 vs +6; $P < 0.05$). Physical and social performance-related SAT-P scores improved significantly in the maca group alone (+7 and +7 respectively; $P < 0.05$ for both) (Zenico et al., 2009).

A 6-month study in healthy men (*n* = 57) studied maca 1.5 g/day to or maca 3 g/day compared with placebo. With both doses of maca there was an increase in sexual desire in 24%, 40%, and 40% of men at 4, 8, and 12 weeks, respectively. The increase from baseline was significant ($P < 0.01$). With placebo there was an increase in sexual desire in 16%, 0%, and 0% of men at 4, 8, and 12 weeks, respectively. The difference between the maca and placebo groups became significant at 8 and 12 weeks. There was no influence on testosterone or estradiol levels or HAM-D or HAM-A scores. The authors concluded that maca at both 1.5 g/day and 3 g/day improved sexual desire independently of mood or hormone levels (Gonzales et al., 2002).

A 4-month RCT in healthy men (*n*=9) compared maca 1.5 g/day with maca 3 g/day for effects on semen parameters. Treatment with maca resulted in increased seminal volume, sperm count per ejaculate, motile sperm count, and sperm motility. Serum hormone levels were not modified with maca. There was no difference between dosages with respect to the increase in sperm count. The authors concluded that maca improves sperm production and motility unrelated to sex hormones (Gonzales et al., 2001a).

A 12-week pilot study in healthy men ($n = 56$) aged 21–56 compared maca 1.5 g/day and maca 3 g/day with placebo for effects on reproductive hormone levels. Compared with baseline and placebo, maca had no effect on LH, FSH, prolactin, 17-α hydroxyprogesterone, testosterone, or 17-β estradiol (Gonzales et al., 2003).

A 12-week RCT in male volunteers ($n = 20$) aged 20–40 years compared maca 1.75 g/day with placebo for effects on semen and hormone levels. Sperm concentration and motility showed rising trends compared with placebo even though levels of hormones did not change significantly after 12 weeks of trial. The authors concluded that maca may possess fertility enhancing properties in men (Melnikovova et al., 2015).

Disorders of Vitality: General Wellness and Resilience

A study of adults ($n = 50$) 35-75 years old in the Peruvian Andes compared the health status of those who regularly consumed maca root ($n = 27$) compared with those who did not. Maca was associated with higher health status scores, fewer fractured bones, lower signs of chronic mountain sickness, lower BMI, and lower SBP. Compared with nonconsumers, the maca consumers also had lower values for serum testosterone and IL-6 levels and higher serum estradiol levels. Differences were more marked comparing highest users with lowest users of maca. Liver and kidney function, lipid profiles, and glycemic function of users did not differ between groups (Gonzales et al., 2013).

A 12-week RCT in volunteers ($n = 175$) living at sea level or high altitude compared health effects of red or black maca 3 g/day with placebo for effect on quality of life. At low and high altitudes, both red and black maca resulted similarly in improvement in mood, energy, and HRQOL, and reduced chronic mountain sickness (CMS) scores. Effects on mood, energy, and CMS scores were better with red maca. Black maca and, in smaller doses, red maca reduced hemoglobin levels only in high altitude subjects who had elevated hemoglobin. Black maca reduced blood glucose levels. Both forms of maca at both elevations showed good acceptability and did not show serious adverse effects (Gonzales-Arimborgo et al., 2016).

ACTIVE CONSTITUENTS

Research comparing the constituents of maca grown in different regions showed that maca grown in China had higher levels of glucosinolates, while maca grown in Peru had higher levels of imidazole alkaloids.

Root

- Carbohydrates
  - Organic acids: methyltetrahydro-β-carboline-3-carboxylic acid (CNS activity)
- Lipids
  - Fatty acids: macaenes, macamides
  - Alkamides (immunomodulatory, anti-inflammatory)
- Amino acid derivatives
  - Amino acids: arginine, histidine, phenylalanine, threonine, and tyrosine
  - Glucosinolates (antiproliferative, apoptotic): glucoalyssin, glucosinalbin, glucoaubrietin, benzyl glucosinolate (red maca suppresses prostatic hyperplasia) glucotropaeolin, m-methoxyglucotropaeolin, and p-methoxyglucotropaeolin
- Steroids
  - Phytosterols: β-sitosterol (reduces GI cholesterol absorption, inhibits 5-α-reductase), campesterol
- Alkaloids: macaridine, lepidine A, lepidine B, methyltetrahydro-β-carboline, macamides (octadecenamides)
- Aromatic compounds: phenyl acetonitrile, benzaldehyde, 3-methoxyphenylacetonitrile

MACA COMMONLY USED PREPARATIONS AND DOSAGE (FOR ADULTS UNLESS OTHERWISE SPECIFIED)

The following are examples of some available formulations and ranges of dosing for commercial herbal products. See Part III Introduction "How to prescribe medicinal herbs" for further guidance on herbal advising and prescribing.

Root

- Tincture (1:3, 50%): 1 mL TID
- Powdered root extract: 1 g (1/3 tsp) in beverage QD-TID

■ Capsule or tablet of powdered root: 500-1000 mg QD-TID with food

Specific Uses

■ *Red maca for BPH*
■ *Black maca for memory impairment or cognitive enhancement*
■ *Black or yellow maca for improvement of sperm quality and quantity*

SAFETY AND PRECAUTION

Side Effects

Glucosinolates can cause goiter if taken in excess combined with a low-iodine diet. Though this is documented to occur with other glucosinolate-rich foods, it is not known if maca causes goiter.

Toxicity

The data are limited. Maca has been reported in the scientific literature to have a low degree of acute oral toxicity in animals and low cellular toxicity in vitro. Rats tolerate up to 5 g/kg without adverse effects. Human trials have shown maca has been well tolerated up to 3 g per day. The traditional method of boiling up to 20 g of maca to make into juice has not currently been associated with toxicity.

Pregnancy and Lactation

Insufficient human safety data. In mice, 1 g/kg lyophilized maca resulted in increased litter size and no fetal abnormalities.

Disease Interactions

Avoid use in women with breast cancer and other estrogen-sensitive cancers due to variable evidence for stimulation of breast cancer cells and increases in estradiol levels.

Drug Interactions

■ There are no reported preclinical or clinical drug interaction data for maca. Use with caution.

REFERENCES

Borrelli F, Colalto C, Delfino DV, Iriti M, Izzo AA. Herbal dietary supplements for erectile dysfunction: a systematic review and meta-analysis. Drugs 2018;78(6):643–73.

Brooks NA, et al. Beneficial effects of Lepidium meyenii (Maca) on psychological symptoms and measures of sexual dysfunction in postmenopausal women are not related to estrogen or androgen content. Menopause 2008.

Dording CM, et al. A double-blind, randomized, pilot dose-finding study of maca root (L. meyenii) for the management of SSRI-induced sexual dysfunction. CNS Neurosci Ther 2008.

Dording CM, Schettler PJ, Dalton ED, et al. A double-blind placebo-controlled trial of maca root as treatment for antidepressant-induced sexual dysfunction in women. Evid Based Complement Alternat Med 2015;2015:949036.

Gonzales GF, Cordova A, Gonzales C, et al. *Lepidium meyenii* (maca) improved semen parameters in adult men. Asian J Androl 2001;3:301–3.

Gonzales GF, Cordova A, Vega K, et al. Effect of Lepidium meyenii (maca) on sexual desire and its absent relationship with serum testosterone levels in adult healthy men. Andrologia 2002;34:367–72.

Gonzales GF, Córdova A, Vega K, et al. Effect of *Lepidium meyenii* (maca), a root with aphrodisiac and fertility-enhancing properties, on serum reproductive hormone levels in adult healthy men. J Endocrinol 2003;176:163–8.

Gonzales GF, Gasco M, Lozada-Requena I. Role of maca (*Lepidium meyenii*) consumption on serum interleukin-6 levels and health status in populations living in the Peruvian Central Andes over 4000m of altitude. Plant Foods Hum Nutr 2013;68(4):347–51.

Gonzales-Arimborgo C, Yupanqui I, Montero E, et al. Gonzales "Acceptability, safety, and efficacy of oral administration of extracts of black or red Maca (*Lepidium meyenii*) in adult human subjects: a randomized, double-blind, placebo-controlled study". Pharmaceuticals (Basel) 2016;9(3):49.

Lee MS, Shin BC, Yang EJ, Lim HJ, Ernst E. Maca (Lepidium meyenii) for treatment of menopausal symptoms: a systematic review. Maturitas 2011;70(3):227–33.

Lee MS, Lee HW, You S, Ha KT. The use of maca (Lepidium meyenii) to improve semen quality: a systematic review. Maturitas 2016;92:64–9.

Meissner HO, Reich-Bilinska H, Mscisz A, Kedzia B. Therapeutic effects of pre-gelatinized Maca (Lepidium Peruvianum Chacon) used as a non-hormonal alternative to HRT in peri-menopausal women—Clinical Pilot Study. Int J Biomed Sci 2006;2(2):143–59.

Melnikovova I, Fait T, Kolarova M, Fernandez EC, Milella L. Effect of Lepidium meyenii Walp. on semen parameters and serum hormone levels in healthy adult men: a double-blind, randomized, placebo-controlled pilot study. Evid Based Complement Alternat Med 2015;324369.

Najafi NM, Ghazanfarpour M. Effect of phytoestrogens on sexual function in menopausal women: a systematic review and meta-analysis. Climacteric 2018;21(5):437–45.

Shin BC, Lee MS, Yang EJ, Lim HS, Ernst E. Maca (*L. meyenii*) for improving sexual function: a systematic review. BMC Complement Altern Med 2010;10:44.

Stojanovska L, et al. Maca reduces BP and depression, in a pilot study in postmenopausal women. Climacteric 2015.

Zenico T, et al. Subjective effects of Lepidium meyenii (Maca) extract on well-being and sexual performances in patients with mild erectile dysfunction: a randomised, double-blind clinical trial. Andrologia 2009.

61

MILK THISTLE (*SILYBUM MARIANUM*)

Seeds, Flower Heads

GENERAL OVERVIEW

Milk thistle has a reputation as a liver savior. It has been used successfully in cases of acetaminophen overdose and amanita mushroom poisoning due to its ability to block and remove toxins from and promote regeneration of hepatocytes. In one multicenter study it cut death from amanita poisoning roughly in half. It has also been shown to reduce hepatic fibrosis. However, numerous studies have cast into doubt its efficacy in reducing morbidity and mortality associated with hepatitis C and alcoholic hepatitis. More recent interest has developed for the use of milk thistle in diabetes and dyslipidemia where good evidence supports its efficacy. It has been studied alone and in combination with an herbal source of berberine for diabetes and dyslipidemia, as milk thistle enhances absorption of berberine. Silymarin (a combination of constituents) and silybin (a constituent in silymarin that can be given intravenously) have undergone extensive research.

Clinical research indicates that milk thistle, alone or in combination formulas, may be beneficial for hyperlipidemia, dyslipidemia, diabetes, acute and chronic hepatitis, diabetic nephropathy, lactation, benign prostatic hyperplasia, obsessive-compulsive disorder, vitiligo, acne, iron overload, radiation dermatitis and mucositis, and chemotherapy-induced hand-foot syndrome.

IN VITRO AND ANIMAL RESEARCH

Several of the constituents of milk thistle have been shown to have antioxidant, anti-inflammatory and anticancer effects. Research has shown that milk thistle or its constituents are able to inhibit lipid peroxidation, enhance Phase I liver detoxification and glucuronidation, maintain glutathione levels and inhibit neutrophil migration. Silymarin may also be useful against liver carcinogenesis by negatively affecting the activity of mast cells, a source of MMPs, which are involved in invasion and angiogenesis.

Silybin inhibits gluconeogenesis and glucose-6-phosphate hydrolysis in perfused hepatocytes, but it does not seem to have significant effects in the fructose cycle. Silybin appears to increase the viability of pancreatic β-cells by inhibiting fibrillation, improving oligomerization, and decreasing β-cell cytotoxicity of human islet amyloid polypeptide. Isosylibin A was identified as the first PPAR-γ flavonoglycan agonist. Milk thistle has been shown to competitively inhibit cellular GLUT-4 uptake of glucose. Silybin inhibits aldose reductase in tissues susceptible to accumulation of sorbitol. In vitro studies have shown silybin to protect nerve tissue from high glucose concentrations. In a rat model of diabetes, silymarin has been shown to reduce glucose, normalize insulin and A1C levels, and preserve renal function. Treating animals on a high-fat diet with silybin resulted in significantly lower BW, decreased visceral fat-to-total BW ratio, and reduced insulin resistance compared with the control group.

Milk thistle reduces TC, raises HDL-C, and reduces the cholesterol concentration in bile through increased bile volume, so it may be effective in reducing cholelithiasis. Silymarin alters the structure of the cell membrane of hepatocytes in such a way as to prevent penetration of liver toxins. Silymarin also increases ribosomal protein synthesis via nucleolar polymerase A, thereby promoting regeneration of hepatocytes. A constituent of silymarin, silybin appears to have steroid-like activity in its ability to bind to polymerase I, stimulating enzyme activity. Milk thistle has been shown to reduce conversion of hepatic stellate cells into myofibroblasts, thereby preventing hepatic fibrosis. Silymarin has been shown in mice to produce a downregulation of extracellular matrix proteins such as collagen after thioacetamide exposure.

Silymarin has demonstrated marked suppression of Aβ-protein fibril formation and neurotoxicity in PC12 cells in vitro. In vivo studies have indicated a significant reduction in brain Aβ deposition and improvement in behavioral abnormalities in amyloid precursor protein transgenic mice that had been preventively treated with a powdered diet containing 0.1% silymarin for 6 months. The silymarin-treated APP mice showed less anxiety than the vehicle-treated APP mice in association with a decline in Aβ oligomer production induced by silymarin intake.

Patients with gout may benefit from milk thistle as silymarin has been shown to inhibit xanthine oxidase with equal efficacy to allopurinol. It may also be useful for psoriasis due to its ability to inhibit cAMP phosphodiesterase and leukotriene synthesis, both of which are overactive in psoriasis.

Studies in rats demonstrated that silymarin reduced cisplatin-induced kidney damage without diminishing its antitumor activity. In other animal studies, milk thistle appears to reduce the growth rate of hepatocellular carcinoma tumors providing there was no alcohol exposure. Silymarin demonstrated estrogenic activity with mild proliferative effects in rat uteri.

HUMAN RESEARCH

Cardiometabolic Disorders: Hyperlipidemia, Dyslipidemia, and Diabetes

A 2010 systematic review looking at herbal medicine (including TCM formulations) for hyperlipidemia identified 53 RCTs that met criteria. There were significant decreases in TC and LDL-C after treatment with milk thistle as well as licorice, fenugreek, yarrow, guggul, Daming capsule, chunghyul-dan, garlic powder, black tea, green tea, soy drink enriched with plant sterols, *Satureja khuzestanica*, *Monascus purpureus*, Went rice, C. Koch, Ningzhi capsule, cherry, composite salvia dropping pill (CSDP), shanzha xiaozhi capsule, Ba-wei-wan (hachimijiogan), rhubarb stalk, *Rheum ribes*, and primrose oil. Data were conflicting for red yeast rice, garlic, and guggul. No significant adverse effects or mortality were observed with licorice and several others. The authors concluded that 22 natural products were found effective in the treatment of hyperlipidemia and that further research was warranted (Hasani-Ranjbar et al., 2010).

A 45-day RCT in patients (n = 40) with T2DM compared silymarin 140 mg TID with placebo for effects on glycemia and lipids. Compared with placebo, silymarin led to significant reductions in fasting blood sugar, serum insulin, HOMA-IR, TG, and TG/HDL-C by 11%, 14.3%, 25.9%, 23.7%, and 27.7% respectively. There was also a significant 6.8% increase in HDL-C and a 5.6% increase in quantitative insulin sensitivity check index with silymarin compared with placebo (P < 0.05). TC and LDL-C concentrations significantly decreased with silymarin compared with baseline, by 7.9% (P = 0.001) and 7% (P = 0.02), respectively. The authors concluded that silymarin supplementation may improve glycemic indices and lipid profiles in patients with T2DM (Ebrahimpour Koujan et al., 2015).

A 4-month RCT in T2DM patients (n = 51) compared silymarin 200 mg TID plus conventional therapy with placebo plus conventional therapy. The results showed a significant decrease in A1C, FBS, TC, LDL-C, TG, AST, and ALT levels in silymarin-treated patients compared with baseline and with placebo. The authors concluded that silymarin had a beneficial effect on improving glycemic profile in patients with T2DM (Huseini et al., 2006).

A 6-month RCT in euglycemic dyslipidemic patients (n = 137) with previous adverse events to statins at high doses compared a half-dose of statin plus placebo with a half-dose of statin plus Berberol (a combination of *Berberis aristata* 588 mg plus milk thistle 105 mg), one tablet during lunch and dinner. The lipid profile did not significantly change after 6 months with the reduction of statin dosage and the introduction of the herbal combination, while it worsened in the placebo group (+23.4 mg/dL for TC, +19.6 mg/dL for LDL-C, +23.1 mg/dL for TG with placebo compared with the herbal combination). The herbal combination reduced FBG (−9 mg/dL), insulin (−0.7 μU/mL), and

HOMA-IR (− 0.35) levels compared with baseline and with placebo. The authors concluded that this herbal combination could be added to lower-dose statins in patients not tolerating high-dose statins (Derosa et al., 2015).

A multi-phase RCT in patients (*n* = 102) with dyslipidemia studied Berberol (a combination of *Berberis aristata* 588 mg plus milk thistle 105 mg) BID for 3 months compared with placebo, given after a 6-month run-in period of diet and physical activity. The treatments were then interrupted for 2 months (washout period), and then restarted for an additional 3-month period. The herbal combination reduced TC, TG, and LDL-C, and increased HDL-C after 3 months. The lipid profile worsened during the 2-month interruption, and it improved again when treatment was resumed. During the glucagon stimulation test, the herbal combination produced a greater increase of C-peptide levels and a lesser increase in glycemia compared with placebo and baseline. No patients had serious adverse events in either group. The authors concluded that Berberol was safe and effective in improving lipid profiles and insulin secretion in euglycemic dyslipidemic patients (Derosa et al., 2013b).

A 12-week RCT in diabetic patients (*n* = 50) with dyslipidemia despite statin therapy studied a combination of aloe, black seed, fenugreek, garlic, milk thistle, and psyllium (one sachet BID) plus conventional therapy compared with conventional therapy alone. Each sachet contained 300 mg of aloe leaf gel, 1.8 g of black seed, 300 mg of garlic, 2.5 g of fenugreek seed, 1 g of psyllium seed, and 500 mg of milk thistle seed. The levels of serum TG, TC, LDL-C, and A1C, but not FBS, showed a significant in-group improvement in the intervention group. Renal and hepatic transaminases were unchanged with the herbal compound. The authors concluded that this herbal compound was a safe and effective adjunctive treatment in lowering serum lipids in diabetic patients with uncontrolled dyslipidemia (Ghorbani et al., 2019).

A 40-day Phase I open-label clinical trial in diabetic patients (*n* = 30) with uncontrolled hyperglycemia and dyslipidemia despite standard therapy compared a polyherbal formulation containing garlic, aloe, black seed, psyllium, fenugreek, and milk thistle one sachet BID in addition to their usual medications. The herbal formula significantly decreased FBG from 162 mg/dL

to 146 mg/dL and A1C from 8.4% to 7.7%. LDL-C decreased significantly from 138 mg/dL to 108 mg/dL, and TG decreased from 203 mg/dL to 166 mg/dL. There were no changes in liver function, kidney function, or hematologic parameters. The authors concluded that the formulation was safe and effective in lowering blood glucose and serum lipids in patients with advanced-stage T2DM. After consumption of the herbal combination, two patients complained of mild nausea, and two patients reported diarrhea (Zarvandi et al., 2017).

Cardiometabolic Disorders: Diabetes

(See studies above for trials addressing both lipids and glycemia)

A 2013 systematic review to assess the glucose lowering effects of medicinal plants identified 18 human studies that met inclusion criteria. Among the RCTs, the best results in glycemic control were found with milk thistle as well as with aloe, nettle, *Citrullus colocynthus*, *Plantago ovata*, and *Rheum ribes* (Rashidi et al., 2013).

A 2011 systematic review and meta-analysis regarding herbs for glycemic control in diabetics identified nine RCTs (*n* = 487) that met inclusion criteria. In addition to milk thistle, fenugreek and sweet potato significantly improved glycemia, whereas cinnamon did not. The pooled mean differences in A1C were − 1.92% (*P* = 0.008, − 1.13% (*P* = 0.03), and − 0.3% (*P* = 0.02) for milk thistle, fenugreek, and sweet potato, respectively. The values for FBS were − 38.05 mg/dL (*P* = 0.009) for milk thistle. The authors concluded that supplementation with milk thistle, fenugreek, and/or sweet potato may improve glycemic control in T2DM (Suksomboon et al., 2011).

In a separate report of the study by Derosa reported in the "Cardiometabolic Disorders: Hyperlipidemia, Dyslipidemia and Diabetes" section (Derosa et al., 2013a), the same study design found that Berberol (the herbal combination of *Berberis aristata* plus milk thistle 588 mg/105 mg) BID for 3 months decreased fasting plasma insulin and HOMA-IR compared with baseline and with placebo. Retinol-binding protein-4 and resistin decreased and adiponectin increased after 3 months of the herbal product. The positive effects disappeared during the washout period and reappeared after resumption of the product. The authors concluded that this herbal combination improved insulin resistance and adipocytokine levels (Derosa et al., 2013a).

A 12-month open, controlled study in insulin-treated diabetics ($n=60$) with alcoholic cirrhosis compared investigated silymarin 600 mg/day plus standard therapy compared with standard therapy alone for effects on glycemic control and oxidation. FBS, mean daily blood glucose levels, daily glucosuria, and A1C levels had decreased by 4 months of treatment in the silymarin group ($P<0.01$). Fasting insulin levels and mean exogenous insulin requirements decreased with silymarin ($P<0.01$), but insulin levels increased, and insulin dosing was unchanged in the control group ($P<0.05$). Basal and glucagon-stimulated C-peptide levels decreased with silymarin ($P<0.01$) and increased in the control group. MDA levels decreased in the silymarin group ($P<0.01$). The authors concluded that silymarin may reduce lipoperoxidation of cell membranes and insulin resistance (Velussi et al., 1993).

An open-label trial in T2DM patients ($n=69$) with suboptimal glycemic control compared the glycemic effect of adding to standard therapy either an extract of Berberis aristata (standardized to 85% berberine corresponding to 1000 mg/day of berberine), or Berberol (a fixed combination of Berberis aristata plus an extract of milk thistle, standardized to >60% silymarin, for a total intake of 1000 mg/day of berberine and 210 mg/day of silymarin). Both treatments similarly improved fasting glucose, TC, LDL-C, TG, and liver enzyme levels, whereas A1C values were reduced to a greater extent by the fixed combination. The authors explained that berberine, an isoquinoline alkaloid widely used to improve the glucose and lipid profiles of patients with hypercholesterolemia, metabolic syndrome, and T2DM, is limited by its poor oral bioavailability due to the P-glycoprotein in enterocytes. Silymarin is a P-glycoprotein antagonist. The herbal product Berberol was formulated to address the bioavailability issue. The association of the two herbs was demonstrated to be more effective than berberine alone in reducing A1C when administered at the same dose and in the form of standardized extracts (Di Pierro et al., 2012).

A 6-month RCT in patients ($n=85$) with T1DM investigated the glycemic effects of Berberol one tablet at lunch and dinner compared with placebo. There was a reduction of total insulin consumption in the herbal group, compared with both baseline and placebo. The herbal group also used less insulin at meals and at bedtime. There was a decrease of FBG and PPG with the herbal combination compared with both baseline and placebo. A1C decreased in the herbal group compared with baseline, but not compared with placebo. There was a decrease of TC, TG, and LDL-C and an increase of HDL-C with the herbal combination, both compared with baseline and with placebo. The authors concluded that the addition of Berberis aristata and milk thistle to insulin therapy in T1DM patients led to a reduction of the insulin dose needed to achieve adequate glycemic control (Derosa et al., 2016).

A 3-month RCT in patients ($n=60$) with T2DM studied an herbal blend containing milk thistle, nettle, and frankincense compared with placebo for glycemic control. The mean FBS, A1C, and TG with the herbal combination were significantly less than with placebo after 3 months of the intervention. The authors concluded that there was a potential antihyperglycemic and TG-lowering effect of the herbal formulation, while it did not have any significant cholesterol or BP-lowering effect (Khalili et al., 2017).

A 45-day RCT in T2DM patients ($n=40$) who were stable on medication compared silymarin 140 mg TID with placebo for antioxidant and anti-inflammatory effects. Silymarin supplementation significantly increased SOD, glutathione peroxidase activity, and TAC by 12.85%, 30.32%, and 8.43%, respectively, compared with placebo, ($P<0.05$). There were significant reductions in hs-CRP levels and MDA concentration by 27% and 12%, respectively, compared with placebo ($P<0.05$ for both). There were no reported adverse effects or symptoms with the silymarin supplementation. The authors concluded that silymarin supplementation improved the measured antioxidant indices and decreased hs-CRP in T2DM patients (Ebrahimpour-Koujan et al., 2018).

Gastrointestinal Disorders: Liver Disease

With a body of conflicting literature for benefits in liver disease, human studies have suggested that milk thistle reduces death due to alcohol-induced cirrhosis (one positive and one negative study). Several studies have shown benefit from milk thistle for both acute and chronic viral hepatitis. It may be more effective for HBV than for HCV. One study of silymarin showed that at least 420 mg was necessary to improve outcomes in viral hepatitis. For amanita mushroom poisoning, a preparation of the silybin fraction is available from Germany as an IV drip for such acute cases.

A 2019 systematic review assessing the efficacy of silymarin to prevent anti-TB drug-induced liver toxicity identified five RCTs ($n = 1198$) that met inclusion criteria. Overall, silymarin significantly reduced the occurrence of anti-TB drug-induced liver injury at week 4 (RR = 0.33). In addition, silymarin exerted a protective effect on liver function in patients undergoing anti-TB drug therapy (SMD = −0.15; $P < 0.001$; SMD = −0.14; $P = 0.001$; SMD = −0.12; $P = 0.008$ for ALT, AST, and ALP, respectively). Silymarin groups had similar adverse events as placebo groups. The authors concluded that prophylactic therapy with silymarin is associated with a noticeably reduced risk of development of anti-TB drug-induced liver injury 4 weeks after initiation and improved liver function in patients on these drugs (Tao et al., 2019).

A 2017 systematic review with meta-analysis evaluating the effects of silymarin in patients with liver diseases identified 17 RCTs that met criteria for review and six that met criteria for meta-analysis (out of 10,904 publications). In the meta-analysis, the results indicated silymarin produced a reduction of 0.26 IU/mL in ALT levels and 0.53 IU/mL in AST levels, both being statistically significant but not clinically relevant. There was no significant change in GGT levels. The authors concluded that silymarin minimally reduced serum ALT and AST levels (de Avelar et al., 2017).

A 2017 systematic review and meta-analysis to evaluate the efficacy of silymarin for NAFLD identified eight RCTs ($n = 587$) that met inclusion criteria. The results showed that silymarin reduced AST and ALT levels more significantly than the control group (MD = −6.57 IU/L for AST; $P = 0.0002$; MD = −9.16 IU/L for ALT; $P = 0.01$). When silymarin was used alone the significant differences persisted (MD = −5.44 for AST; $P = 0.002$; MD = −5.08 for ALT; $P = 0.003$). The authors concluded that silymarin had positive efficacy to reduce transaminases in NAFLD patients (Zhong et al., 2017).

A 2014 systematic review to assess efficacy of silymarin or silibinin in chronic HCV infection found five RCTs ($n = 389$) that met inclusion criteria. Serum HCV RNA relatively but insignificantly decreased in patients treated with silymarin compared with those treated with placebo ($P = 0.09$). Meta-analysis of patients treated with silymarin indicated that the changes in HCV RNA were similar to placebo ($P = 0.19$). Silymarin's effect on ALT did not differ from that of placebo ($P = 0.45$). Improvements in quality-of-life (Short Form-36) in both silymarin and placebo recipients were impressive but relatively identical (0 = 0.09). The authors concluded that silymarin was well tolerated in chronic HCV infection, but there was no evidence of benefit based on intermediate endpoints (ALT and HCV RNA) (Yang et al., 2014).

A 2008 systematic review to evaluate the therapeutic effect of silymarin in toxic liver disease found 19 studies that met inclusion criteria for meta-analysis. The authors found that the clinical evidence for a therapeutic effect of silymarin in toxic liver disease was scarce. There was no evidence of favorable influence on the evolution of viral hepatitis, particularly hepatitis C. With alcoholic liver disease, AST was reduced in the silymarin-treated groups ($P = 0.01$), while ALP was not. In liver cirrhosis, mostly alcoholic, total mortality was 16.1% with silymarin and 20.5% with placebo (N.S.); liver-related mortality was 10% with silymarin and 17.3% with placebo ($P = 0.01$). The authors concluded that it would be reasonable to employ silymarin as a supportive element in the therapy of *Amanita phalloides* poisoning and liver cirrhosis (Saller et al., 2008).

A 2005 systematic review on efficacy of milk thistle in liver disease from alcoholism and/or HBV or HCV identified 13 RCTs ($n = 915$) that met inclusion criteria. Milk thistle, compared with placebo or with no intervention, for a median duration of 6 months had no significant effects on all-cause mortality (RR = 0.78), complications of liver disease, or liver histology. Liver-related mortality was significantly reduced by milk thistle in all trials (RR = 0.50) but not in high-quality trials (RR = 0.57). Milk thistle was not associated with a significantly increased risk of adverse events. The authors concluded that based on the higher-quality trials, milk thistle did not seem to significantly influence the course of patients with liver disease due to alcohol, HBV, or HCV (Rambaldi et al., 2005).

A 2005 systematic review to evaluate the efficacy of milk thistle for chronic HBV and HCV found four trials in patients with HCV, one in patients with HBV and two with unspecified chronic viral hepatitis. However, only one trial exclusively studied patients with HCV, and none involved patients with only HBV. Silymarin treatment resulted in a decrease in serum transaminases compared with baseline in four studies and compared with placebo in one study. The authors concluded that silymarin compounds were likely to decrease serum transaminases in patients with chronic viral hepatitis but did not appear to affect viral load or liver histology (Mayer et al., 2005).

A study in HCV patients ($n = 16$) who were nonresponders to full-dose pegylated interferon/ribavirin assessed the effects of silybin 10 mg/kg/day IV for 7 days along with PegIFN-RBV starting on day 8. HCV-RNA declined by 1.32 log ($P < 0.001$) but increased again after the infusion period despite PegIFN-RBV. A second study ($n = 20$) investigated the effects of different doses of IV silybin: 5, 10, 15, or 20 mg/kg/day for 14 days along with the PegIFN-RBV starting on day 8. The viral load decrease was dose dependent (log drop after 7 days on silybin: 0.55 at 5 mg/kg, 1.41 at 10 mg/kg, 2.11 at 15 mg/kg, and 3.02 at 20 mg/kg ($P < 0.001$). The viral load decreased further after 7 days combined with PegIFN-RBV (1.63 at 5 mg/kg, 4.16 at 10 mg/kg, 3.69 at 15 mg/kg, and 4.85 at 20 mg/kg ($P < 0.001$). Viral load became undetectable in seven patients on 15 or 20 mg/kg of silybin at week 12. Besides mild gastrointestinal symptoms, IV silybin was well tolerated. The authors concluded that IV silybin was well tolerated and showed antiviral effects against HCV in nonresponders (Ferenci et al., 2008).

A 24-week open-label study in patients ($n = 55$) with HCV assessed the effects of silymarin 650 mg/day. Compared with baseline, ALT declined from 109 to 70 ($P < 0.001$) and AST declined from 99 to 60 ($P = 0.004$). After the treatment, nine patients became HCV-RNA negative ($P = 0.004$). Liver fibrosis markers improved in the fibrosis group ($P = 0.015$) and quality of life was improved ($P < 0.001$). The authors concluded that silymarin 650 mg/day for 6 months improved serum HCV-RNA titer, ALT, AST, hepatic fibrosis, and QOL in patients with chronic HCV (Kalantari et al., 2011).

A 3-week RCT in patients ($n = 57$) with acute viral hepatitis compared silymarin, 140 mg TID with placebo for effects on liver enzymes. Elevations in bilirubin and AST resolved significantly faster with silymarin, with a trend for greater regression of ALT. The number of patients having attained normal values after 3 weeks of treatment was greater in the silymarin group than in the placebo group. The authors concluded that the use of silymarin in acute viral hepatitis could lead to an accelerated regression in pathological values, thus supporting its use in the treatment of this disease (Magliulo et al., 1978).

An 8-week RCT in patients ($n = 105$) diagnosed with acute hepatitis compared silymarin 140 mg TID with a vitamin placebo for 4 weeks with respect to effects on course of disease. Patients taking silymarin had a quicker resolution of symptoms related to biliary retention (dark urine; $P = 0.013$; jaundice; $P = 0.02$; and scleral icterus; $P = 0.043$). ALT and AST were not significantly reduced. No adverse events were noted. The authors concluded that silymarin produced earlier improvement in subjective and clinical markers of biliary excretion in the setting of acute hepatitis (El-Kamary et al., 2009).

A two-year RCT in alcoholics ($n = 200$) with histologically or laparoscopically proven liver cirrhosis compared silymarin 150 mg TID with placebo for impact on time to death and progression to liver failure. By 2 years, death had occurred in 15 and 14 of the patients receiving silymarin and placebo, respectively. Silymarin did not have any significant effect on the course of the disease. The authors concluded that silymarin had no effect on survival or clinical course in alcoholics with liver cirrhosis (Parés et al., 1998).

A 6-month RCT in patients ($n = 36$) with chronic alcoholic liver disease compared silymarin (Legalon) with placebo for effects on liver function tests, procollagen III peptide levels, and liver histology. During silymarin treatment bilirubin, AST, and ALT were normalized, while GGT activity and procollagen III peptide levels decreased. The changes were significant. With placebo, GGT decreased significantly but to a lesser extent than with silymarin. There was a significant difference between groups. The histological alterations showed an improvement in the silymarin group, while it remained unchanged in the placebo group. The authors concluded that silymarin exerted hepatoprotective activity and was able to improve liver functions in alcoholic patients (Feher et al., 1990).

A four-year RCT in patients ($n = 170$) with cirrhosis of varying etiologies and at varying stages compared silymarin 140 mg TID with placebo for effect on outcomes of cirrhosis (the mean observation period was 41 months). By the end of the observation period, death had occurred in 37 and 24 patients with placebo and silymarin, respectively. Deaths due to liver disease were 31 and 18 with placebo and silymarin, respectively. The four-year survival rate was 39% and 58% with placebo and silymarin, respectively ($P = 0.036$). Analysis of subgroups indicated that treatment was effective in patients with alcoholic cirrhosis ($P = 0.01$) and in patients initially rated Child-Pugh Class A ($P = 0.03$). No side effects of drug treatment were observed (Ferenci et al., 1989).

A 50-week Phase II multi-center RCT was performed in patients ($n = 78$) with NASH without cirrhosis and with NAFLD Activity Score (NAS) ≥ 4 per biopsy site. The study evaluated a proprietary blend of silymarin (Legalon) 420 mg or 700 mg TID compared with placebo for 48 weeks to assess the safety and efficacy of higher doses of silymarin in this group of patients. After 48–50 weeks, 4/27 (15%) with the 700 mg dose, 5/26 (19%) with the 420 mg dose, and 3/25 (12%) with placebo reached the primary endpoint, which was histological improvement ≥ 2 points in NAS ($P = 0.79$), indicating no benefit from silymarin in the intention-to-treat analysis. Review by a central pathologist demonstrated that fibrosis stage improved most in the placebo group, although not significantly different from other groups. There were no significant differences in adverse events among the treatment groups. The authors concluded that the effect of silymarin in patients with NASH remained inconclusive and that further studies were needed (Navarro et al., 2019).

A 6-month RCT in patients ($n = 72$) with NAFLD compared 3 months of silymarin BID with a baseline of 3 months of a restricted diet. SteatoTest, ALT, AST, and GGT were significantly reduced with silymarin ($P < 0.001$). Hepatorenal brightness ratio, as an index of hepatic steatosis, significantly decreased with silymarin ($P < 0.05$). The authors concluded that silymarin was effective in reducing biochemical, inflammatory, and ultrasonic indices of hepatic steatosis (Cacciapuoti et al., 2013).

A 3-month RCT in patients ($n = 60$) receiving chronic psychotropic drug therapy compared silymarin 800 mg/day with placebo, with or without psychotropic drugs, for ability to prevent psychotro-

pic drug-induced liver damage. Based on measurements of MDA levels and liver enzymes, the data showed that silymarin reduced the lipoperoxidative hepatic damage that occurs during treatment with butyrophenones or phenothiazines and that increased lipoperoxidation may contribute to psychotropic drug-induced hepatotoxicity (Palasciano et al., 1994).

Biliary lipid composition was assayed in patients with gallstones ($n = 4$) and patients s/p cholecystectomy before and after silymarin 420 mg/day for 30 days or placebo to determine effects on bile composition. In both groups, biliary cholesterol concentrations were reduced after silymarin treatment and the bile saturation index significantly decreased accordingly. These data suggest that a silymarin-induced reduction of biliary cholesterol concentration might, at least in part, be due to a decreased synthesis of liver cholesterol (Nassuato et al., 1991).

Gastrointestinal Disorders: Functional Dyspepsia

A 4-week RCT in patients ($n = 60$) with functional dyspepsia compared Iberogast in two different formulations (chamomile, peppermint, caraway, licorice, lemon balm, angelica, celandine and milk thistle with or without bitter candy tuft) with placebo for effects on gastrointestinal symptoms The herbal preparations showed a clinically significant improvement in the Gastrointestinal Symptom score compared with placebo after 2 and 4 weeks of treatment ($P < 0.001$). No statistically significant difference could be observed between the efficacy of two different herbal preparations ($P > 0.05$), but a solid improvement of GI symptoms could be achieved earlier with the herbal preparation that contained the bitter candy tuft ($P = 0.023$). The authors concluded that Iberogast and its modified formulation improved dyspeptic symptoms better than placebo and that the bitter candy tuft had an additive effect (Madisch et al., 2001).

Renal Disorders: Diabetic Nephropathy

A 3-month RCT in T2DM patients ($n = 60$) with macroalbuminuria despite treatment with maximum dose of a renin-angiotensin inhibitor for more than 6 months and eGFR > 30 mL/min compared silymarin 140 mg TID with placebo. Although UACR decreased in both groups, this decrement was significantly greater with silymarin compared with placebo; mean difference in change in UACR between the two groups was −347 mg/g. Urinary levels of TNF-α and urinary and serum levels of MDA also decreased significantly with silymarin compared with placebo. The authors concluded that silymarin reduced urinary excretion of albumin, TNF-α, and MDA in patients with diabetic nephropathy and may be considered as a novel addition to the anti-diabetic nephropathy armamentarium (Fallahzadeh et al., 2012).

Women's Disorders: Lactation

A 63-day RCT in lactating women ($n = 50$) compared micronized silymarin 420 mg/day with placebo for effects on lactation. Women on silymarin had an 86% increase in daily milk production compared with 32% for the placebo group. Compliance and tolerability were good. The authors concluded that silymarin was a safe and effective herbal product for improvement of daily milk production in healthy women after delivery (Di Pierro et al., 2008).

Women's Genitourinary Disorders: Perimenopause and Menopause

A 12-week RCT in women ($n = 80$) with menopausal hot flushes compared milk thistle 400 mg/day with placebo. With milk thistle hot flush frequency and severity decreased from 4.32/day to 1.31/day and from 5.25/day to 1.62/day, respectively ($P < 0.001$), and these effects were significantly better than the effects of placebo ($P < 0.001$). Significant decreases in Green Climacteric Scale and the Hot Flash Related Daily Interference Scale scores were also detected with milk thistle compared with placebo after 4, 8, and 12 weeks ($P < 0.001$). The authors concluded that milk thistle could decrease frequency and severity of hot flushes significantly (Saberi et al., 2020).

A 3-month RCT in premenopausal and post-menopausal women ($n = 50$) compared Phyto-Female Complex (American ginseng, black cohosh, dong quai, milk thistle, red clover, and chasteberry) with placebo BID for effect on menopausal symptoms. The women receiving Phyto-Female Complex reported a significantly superior mean reduction in menopausal symptoms with the herbal complex than with placebo. The effect of treatment improvements in menopausal symptoms increased over time; by 3 months there was a 73% decrease in hot flushes and a 69% reduction of night sweats as well as a decrease in hot flush intensity and a significant improvement in sleep quality. Hot flushes ceased completely in 47% and 19% of women with the herbal product and placebo, respectively. There were no changes in findings on vaginal ultrasonography or levels of estradiol, FSH, liver enzymes, or TSH in either group. The authors concluded that Phyto-Female Complex was safe and effective for the relief of hot flushes and sleep disturbances in pre- and postmenopausal women, at least for 3 months' use (Rotem and Kaplan, 2007).

A pilot RCT in healthy premenopausal women ($n = 40$) investigated a combination botanical supplement (dandelion, schisandra, turmeric, rosemary, milk thistle, and *Cynara scolymus*) compared with dietary changes (three servings/d crucifers or dark leafy greens, 30 g/day fiber, 1–2 L/d of water, and limiting caffeine and alcohol consumption to one serving per week) and with placebo for hormonal effects. During the early follicular phase, compared with placebo, the polyherbal product decreased DHEA (−13.2%; $P = 0.02$), DHEA-S (−14.6%; $P = 0.07$), androstenedione (−8.6%; $P = 0.05$), and estrone-sulfate (−12.0%; $P = 0.08$). When comparing dietary changes with placebo, no statistically significant differences were observed. There were no substantial effects on estrone-sulfate, total estradiol, free estradiol, testosterone, SHBG, insulin, IGF-I, or leptin. The authors concluded that early-follicular phase androgens were decreased with the polyherbal product (Greenlee et al., 2007).

An RCT in premenopausal women ($n = 47$) and post-menopausal women ($n = 49$) compared a combination product (containing schisandra plus lignan, indole-3-carbinol, calcium glucarate, milk thistle, and stinging nettle) with placebo for effects on estrogen metabolism and carcinogenic byproducts. In pre-menopausal women, treatment supplementation resulted in a significant increase ($P < 0.05$) in urinary 2-OHE concentrations and in the 2:16α-OHE ratio. In post-menopausal women, treatment supplementation resulted in a significant increase in urinary 2-OHE concentrations. In pre- and post-menopausal women combined, treatment supplementation produced a significant increase in urinary 2-OHE concentration and a trend ($P = 0.074$) toward an increased 2:16α-OHE ratio. The authors concluded that the mixture in question significantly increased estrogen C-2 hydroxylation, which may reduce estrogen-related cancer risk (Laidlaw et al., 2010).

Men's Genitourinary Disorders: Benign Prostatic Hyperplasia

A 6-month RCT in male patients ($n = 55$) with BPH and LUTS investigated a combination of selenium 240 μg plus silymarin 570 mg QD compared with placebo. The resulting changes in IPSS score, urodynamic parameters, maximal flow, average flow, bladder volume, residual volume, total PSA, and serum selenium levels showed statistically significant differences between treatment and control groups ($P < 0.05$). There was a significant reduction in PSA in the selenium-silymarin group but no effect on blood testosterone level. Overall, the treatment was well tolerated with no adverse effects (Vostalova et al., 2013).

Psychiatric Disorders: Anxiety and Obsessive–Compulsive Disorder

A 2013 systematic review looking at plants that had both pre-clinical and clinical evidence for anti-anxiety effects found 21 plants with human clinical trial evidence. Support for efficacy identified several herbs with efficacy for anxiety spectrum disorders including kava, lemon balm, chamomile, ginkgo, skullcap, milk thistle, passionflower, ashwagandha, rhodiola, echinacea, *Galphimia glauca*, *Centella asiatica*, and *Echium amooenum*. Acute anxiolytic activity was found for passionflower, sage, gotu kola, lemon balm, and bergamot. The review also specifically found that bacopa showed anxiolytic effects in people with cognitive decline (Sarris et al., 2013).

A 2012 systematic review of studies using CAM, self-help, and lifestyle interventions for treatment of OCD and trichotillomania (TTM) identified 14 studies that met inclusion criteria. In OCD, tentative evidentiary support was found for mindfulness meditation ($D = 0.63$), electroacupuncture ($D = 1.16$), and kundalini yoga ($D = 1.61$), although the studies were methodologically weak. Better-designed studies revealed positive results for glycine ($D = 1.10$), milk thistle (insufficient data for calculating D), and borage ($D = 1.67$). A rigorous study showed that *N*-acetylcysteine ($D = 1.31$) was effective in TTM while

"movement decoupling" also demonstrated efficacy ($D = 0.94$) (Sarris et al., 2012).

An 8-week RCT in patients ($n = 35$) with OCD compared milk thistle extract 600 mg/day with fluoxetine 30 mg/day for efficacy. The results showed no significant difference between the extract and fluoxetine in the treatment of OCD. There was also no significant difference between the two groups in terms of observed side effects (Sayyah et al., 2010).

Dermatological Disorders: Acne, Vitiligo, and Radiation Dermatitis

An 8-week RCT in patients ($n = 56$) with acne vulgaris compared silymarin 70 mg TID with *N*-acetylcysteine 600 mg BID, with selenium 100 μg BID, and with placebo for effects on lesions and oxidation markers. The study included a control group of healthy volunteers ($n = 28$). Administration of each of the antioxidants to patients with acne vulgaris significantly reduced serum MDA and increased serum GSH compared with pre-treatment values. IL-8 and the number of inflammatory lesions were significantly reduced in patients with acne compared with placebo. Silymarin and placebo reduced lesions from 19.6 to 9.1 and from 19.2 to 17.1, respectively ($P < 0.05$). The authors concluded that silymarin, *N*-acetylcysteine, and selenium had beneficial effects in patients with acne vulgaris based on clinical improvement that strongly and positively correlated with improvement in biochemical data (Sahib et al., 2012).

An RCT in patients ($n = 34$) with vitiligo studied phototherapy plus oral silymarin compared with phototherapy plus placebo. The mean of the vitiligo severity index score showed a statistically significant decrease in both groups at the end of the study ($P < 0.05$), but the decrease in patients who received silymarin was greater than in those who received placebo. The authors concluded that milk thistle might be a useful adjunct to phototherapy in patients with vitiligo (Jowkar et al., 2019).

A 4-week study in healthy volunteers ($n = 20$) assessed the effects of a cream containing palmitoyl peptides, milk thistle seed oil, vitamin E, and other functional ingredients applied BID on facial wrinkles to assess effects on elasticity, dermal density, and skin tone. Crow's feet wrinkles were decreased 6% after 2 weeks of the cream and 14% after 4 weeks compared with baseline. Skin elasticity increased 7% after 2 weeks and 9% after 4 weeks. Dermal density was increased 17% after 2 weeks and 28% after 4 weeks. Skin brightness was increased 1.7% after 2 weeks and 2% after 4 weeks, and erythema was decreased 10% after 2 weeks and 22% after 4 weeks. There were no abnormal skin responses from the participants during the trial period. The authors concluded that this combination product skin cream had effects on the improvement of facial wrinkles, elasticity, dermal density, and skin tone (Hahn et al., 2016).

Disorders of Vitality: Hangover

A 2017 systematic review to evaluate herbs for hangover benefit selected six studies for analysis. Of the interventions, the use of polysaccharide-rich extract of eleuthero, red ginseng anti-hangover drink, Korean pear juice, KSS formula (pith of citrus tangerine, tanaka, ginger root, and brown sugar), and After-Effect (borage oil, fish oil, vitamins B1, B6, and C, magnesium, milk thistle, and prickly pear) were associated with a significant improvement of hangover symptoms, particularly tiredness, nausea/vomiting, and stomachache ($P < 0.05$) (Jayawardena et al., 2017).

Autoimmune Disorders: Rheumatoid Arthritis

A 90-day non-randomized single-arm clinical trial in patients ($n = 44$) with stable RA investigated the effects of a silymarin tablet (Livergol) added to a standard drug regimen for RA on inflammatory markers. Disease activity score was reduced from 3.02 to 2.3 after addition of silymarin ($P < 0.001$). The authors postulated that the mechanism of the benefit could be due to the results of its anti-inflammatory and antioxidative properties (Shavandi et al., 2017).

Hematologic Disorders: Iron Overload

A 2016 review of the literature assessing the potential effects of silymarin on controlling the complications induced by iron overload in patients with β-thalassemia determined that silymarin may be useful as an adjuvant for improving multiple organ dysfunctions (Kazazis et al., 2016).

A 3-month RCT in patients ($n = 59$) with β-thalassemia compared silymarin 140 mg TID plus deferoxamine with placebo plus deferoxamine for effects on iron over-load. Silymarin produced significant improvement in liver ALP and RBC GSH levels compared with placebo. Silymarin also produced greater reductions in serum ferritin levels, but the difference did not reach statistical significance by 3 months. The authors concluded that silymarin in combination with deferoxamine can be safely and effectively used in the treatment of iron-loaded patients (Gharagozloo et al., 2013).

A 9-month RCT in patients ($n = 97$) with iron over-load from β-thalassemia compared deferoxamine plus silymarin (Legalon) with deferoxamine plus placebo for effects on iron-chelating activity. With silymarin, serum ferritin levels decreased significantly from 3028 to 1972 ng/mL and serum iron, TIBC, hepcidin, and soluble transferrin receptor were significantly reduced. No significant change in serum ferritin was observed in the patients receiving placebo (from 2249 to 2016 ng/mL). A significant improvement in liver function tests was observed with silymarin compared with placebo. The authors concluded that silymarin was effective at reducing iron overload in patients when used in conjunction with deferoxamine and that therapeutic effects of silymarin on a background of deferoxamine suggested the potential effectiveness of silymarin alone in reducing body iron burden (Moayedi et al., 2013).

A crossover RCT in patients ($n = 10$) with hemochromatosis investigated the effects of 200 mL of water compared with silybin 140 mg plus 200 mL of and with 200 mL of tea following a vegetarian meal containing 12.9 mg iron. Consumption of silybin with the meal resulted in a reduction in the postprandial increase in serum iron compared with water and tea (1726 vs 2988 vs 2099, respectively; $P < 0.05$). The authors concluded that silybin had the potential to reduce iron absorption (Hutchinson et al., 2010).

Oncologic Disorders: Radiation Dermatitis, Radiation Mucositis, and Hand-Foot Syndrome

A 5-week RCT in patients ($n = 40$) undergoing radiation for breast cancer compared silymarin 1% gel with placebo applied to chest wall skin QD for effects on radiodermatitis occurrence. The median National Cancer Institute Common Terminology for Adverse Events and Radiation Therapy Oncology Group scores were significantly lower in the silymarin group at the end of the third to fifth weeks ($P < 0.05$). The scores increased significantly in both placebo and silymarin groups during radiotherapy, but there was a delay in radiodermatitis development and progression in the silymarin group. The authors concluded that prophylactic administration of silymarin gel could reduce the severity of radiodermatitis and delay its occurrence (Karbasforooshan et al., 2019).

A 9-week pilot RCT in patients ($n = 40$) undergoing chemotherapy with capecitabine for GI cancer compared silymarin gel 1% with placebo gel applied to palms and soles BID during chemotherapy for prevention of capecitabine-induced hand-foot syndrome (palmar-plantar erythrodysesthesia). The median WHO hand-foot syndrome scores were significantly lower in silymarin group at the end of the ninth week ($P < 0.05$). The scores increased significantly in both placebo and silymarin groups during chemotherapy, but there was a delay for hand-foot syndrome development and progression in the silymarin group. The authors concluded that prophylactic administration of silymarin topically could significantly reduce the severity of capecitabine-induced hand-foot syndrome (Elyasi et al., 2017).

A 6-week RCT in patients ($n = 27$) with head and neck cancer compared silymarin 140 mg TID with placebo for prevention of radiotherapy-induced mucositis. The median World Health Organization and National Cancer Institute Common Terminology Criteria scores were significantly lower in the silymarin group at the end of the first to sixth weeks ($P < 0.05$). The scores increased significantly in both placebo and silymarin groups during radiotherapy, but there was a delay for mucositis development and progression in silymarin group. The authors concluded that prophylactic administration of silymarin tablets could significantly reduce the severity of radiotherapy-induced mucositis and delay its occurrence in patients with head and neck cancer (Elyasi et al., 2016).

Oncologic Disorders: Lung Cancer and Acute Lymphoblastic Leukemia

A case study in two patients with brain metastases from NSCLC who had failed to respond to whole brain radiation and chemotherapy investigated the response to administration of a silibinin-based nutraceutical Legasil. Each Legasil capsule contains 210 mg of Eurosil 85 (60% of silibinin isoforms). The treatment was titrated from two capsules up to 3–5 capsules as tolerated. After 4–8 weeks of Legasil monotherapy, the patients showed clinical improvement. Brain MRIs revealed a considerable decrease in the volume of the lesions and the extent of the edema and mass effect. Cognitive performance improved and the patients were able to initiate second-line chemotherapy (Bosch-Barrera et al., 2016).

A 56-day RCT in children ($n = 50$) with ALL and hepatic toxicity compared milk thistle with placebo. At day 56, but not at day 28, the milk thistle group had a significantly lower AST ($P = 0.05$) and a trend toward a significantly lower ALT ($P = 0.07$). Although not significantly different, chemotherapy doses were reduced in 61% of the milk thistle group compared with 72% of the placebo group. In vitro experiments had revealed no antagonistic interactions between milk thistle and vincristine or L-asparaginase in CCRF-CEM cells. A modest synergistic effect was observed with vincristine. The authors concluded that in children with ALL and liver toxicity, milk thistle was associated with a trend toward reductions in liver toxicity and did not antagonize the effects of chemotherapy (Ladas et al., 2010).

ACTIVE CONSTITUENTS

Seeds

- Lipids
  - Fatty acids: linoleic, oleic, palmitic acids
- Amino acid derivatives
  - Amino acids: betaine (trimethylglycine; gastric acidification)
- Phenolic compounds
  - Flavonoids: quercetin (anti-inflammatory, antioxidant, hypotensive, antidiabetic, antispasmodic, neuroprotective, XO inhibition, antibacterial, anticancer), kaempferol (anti-inflammatory, antidepressant, strengthens capillaries), apigenin (anti-inflammatory, antioxidant, antihistamine, hypotensive, anti-serotonin release, GABA agonism, antispasmodic, antibacterial, chemopreventive, antineoplastic, ERB)
    - Flavonolignans—silymarin complex (antioxidant, anti-inflammatory, hepatoprotective, hepatoregenerative, nephroprotective, inhibit H_2O_2 and TNF-α, reduce MDA

levels thereby increasing NOS levels, inhibit endosomal trafficking of virions, arrest G1 and S phases of cell cycle, suppresse EGFR-induced expression of CD44 and EGFR in breast cancer cells, and inhibit Notch signaling pathway): silybin—aka silibinin (hypoglycemic, hepatoregenerative, potent antibacterial activity against G+), silydianin, silychristine, silyhermin, taxifolin, isosilybin, neosilyhermin A and B dehydrosilybin, desoxy-silydianin, and silybinomer

- Steroids
  - Phytosterols: cholesterol, campesterol, stigmasterol, β-sitosterol (reduces GI cholesterol absorption, inhibits 5-α-reductase)

MILK THISTLE COMMONLY USED PREPARATIONS AND DOSAGE (FOR ADULTS UNLESS OTHERWISE SPECIFIED)

The following are examples of some available formulations and ranges of dosing for commercial herbal products. See Part III Introduction "How to prescribe medicinal herbs" for further guidance on herbal advising and prescribing.

Fruit (Flowering Head and Seeds)

- Infusion: not recommended due to poor water solubility
- Dried fruit: 12–15 g ground and eaten (for general health purposes)
- Tincture: (1:1, 70%): 0.7 mL (700 mg) BID-QID
- Powdered standardized extract (standardized to 80% silymarin): 250 mg (1/8 tsp) QD
- Capsule or tablet of powdered (4:1) extract: 250 mg (equivalent to 1000 mg herb) QD-BID
- Capsule or tablet of standardized extract (standardized to 80% silymarin content): 100–300 mg TID to deliver 420–600 mg per day of silymarin

Improvement will take 8–12 weeks.

SAFETY AND PRECAUTION

Side Effects

Possible mild laxative effect at high doses (> 1500 mg/d). Rare mild allergic reactions.

Case Reports

A patient experienced intermittent sweating, nausea, vomiting, diarrhea, abdominal pain, weakness, and collapse that resolved after discontinuation of milk thistle supplementation.

A 25-year-old man developed a severe case of epistaxis, which may have been due to self-medication with aspirin, garlic, and milk thistle.

A man on warfarin had an increase in his therapeutic INR when using a "liver detox" supplement that contained milk thistle.

Toxicity

At high doses, silybin can elevate bilirubin and liver enzymes.

Pregnancy and Lactation

Insufficient human data. However, milk thistle has been used historically for pregnant women with cholestatic pruritis and no adverse effects have been reported.

Disease Interactions

May augment effects of hypoglycemic drugs.

Drug Interactions

- CYP: Inhibits CYP3A4 substrates (data are conflicting). Silybin A inhibits CYP2C9. Silybin B inhibits CYP3A4/5.
- UGT: Modulates UGT enzymes.
- Has limited protein binding to albumin site I; may displace site I drugs such as warfarin.
- May increase levels of raloxifene.
- Milk thistle has been studied with numerous chemotherapeutic drugs and has not been found to reduce efficacy of those studied. In vitro synergy has been demonstrated with cisplatin and doxorubicin.
- May reduce levels of antiretrovirals.

A three-period RCT in healthy volunteers ($n = 16$) compared milk thistle with a control group while receiving initial dosing of indinavir to determine the possible effects of milk thistle on drug levels. There were no significant between-group differences. The mean AUC of indinavir decreased by 4.4% from phase 1 to phase 2 in the active group ($P = 0.78$) and by 17.3% in phase 3 ($P = 0.25$). The mean AUC decreased by 21.5% from phase 1 to phase 2 in the control group

($P = 0.2$) and by 38.5% at phase 3 ($P = 0.01$). The authors concluded that indinavir levels were not reduced significantly in the presence of milk thistle (Mills et al., 2005).

REFERENCES

Bosch-Barrera J, Sais E, Cañete N, et al. Response of brain metastasis from lung cancer patients to an oral nutraceutical product containing silibinin. Oncotarget 2016;7(22):32006–14.

Cacciapuoti F, Scognamiglio A, Palumbo R, Forte R, Cacciapuoti F. Silymarin in NAFLD. World J Hepatol 2013;5(3):109–13.

de Avelar CR, Pereira EM, de Farias Costa PR, de Jesus RP, de Oliveira LPM. Effect of silymarin on biochemical indicators in patients with liver disease: systematic review with meta-analysis. World J Gastroenterol 2017;23(27):5004–17.

Derosa G, Bonaventura A, Bianchi L, et al. Effects of *Berberis aristata/Silybum marianum* association on metabolic parameters and adipocytokines in overweight dyslipidemic patients. J Biol Regul Homeost Agents 2013a;27(3):717–28.

Derosa G, Bonaventura A, Bianchi L, et al. *Berberis aristata/Silybum marianum* fixed combination on lipid profile and insulin secretion in dyslipidemic patients. Expert Opin Biol Ther 2013b;13(11):1495–506.

Derosa G, Romano D, D'Angelo A, Maffioli P. *Berberis aristata* combined with *Silybum marianum* on lipid profile in patients not tolerating statins at high doses. Atherosclerosis 2015;239(1):87–92.

Derosa G, D'Angelo A, Maffioli P. The role of a fixed *Berberis aristata/Silybum marianum* combination in the treatment of type 1 diabetes mellitus. Clin Nutr 2016;35(5):1091–5.

Di Pierro F, Callegari A, Carotenuto D, Tapia MM. Clinical efficacy, safety and tolerability of BIO-C (micronized Silymarin) as a galactagogue. Acta Biomed 2008;79(3):205–10.

Di Pierro F, et al. Pilot study on the additive effects of berberine and oral type 2 diabetes agents for patients with suboptimal glycemic control. Diabetes Metab Syndr Obes 2012;5:213–7.

Ebrahimpour Koujan S, Gargari BP, Mobasseri M, Valizadeh H, Asghari-Jafarabadi M. Effects of *Silybum marianum* (L.) Gaertn. (silymarin) extract supplementation on antioxidant status and hs-CRP in patients with type 2 diabetes mellitus: a randomized, triple-blind, placebo-controlled clinical trial. Phytomedicine 2015;22(2):290–6.

Ebrahimpour-Koujan S, Gargari BP, Mobasseri M, Valizadeh H, Asghari-Jafarabadi M. Lower glycemic indices and lipid profile among type 2 diabetes mellitus patients who received novel dose of *Silybum marianum* (L.) Gaertn. (silymarin) extract supplement: a triple-blinded randomized controlled clinical trial. Phytomedicine 2018;44:39–44.

El-Kamary SS, Shardell MD, Abdel-Hamid M, et al. A randomized controlled trial to assess the safety and efficacy of silymarin on symptoms, signs and biomarkers of acute hepatitis. Phytomedicine 2009;16(5):391–400.

Elyasi S, Hosseini S, Niazi Moghadam MR, Aledavood SA, Karimi G. Effect of oral silymarin administration on prevention of radiotherapy induced mucositis: a randomized, double-blinded, placebo-controlled clinical trial. Phytother Res 2016 Nov;30(11):1879–85.

Elyasi S, Shojaee FSR, Allahyari A, Karimi G. Topical silymarin administration for prevention of capecitabine-induced hand-foot syndrome: a randomized, double-blinded, placebo-controlled clinical trial. Phytother Res 2017;31(9):1323–9.

Fallahzadeh MK, Dormanesh B, Sagheb MM, et al. Effect of addition of silymarin to renin-angiotensin system inhibitors on proteinuria in type 2 diabetic patients with overt nephropathy: a randomized, double-blind, placebo-controlled trial. Am J Kidney Dis 2012;60(6):896–903.

Feher J, et al. Hepatoprotective activity of silymarin therapy in patients with chronic alcoholic liver disease. Orv Hetil 1990;130:51.

Ferenci P, Dragosics B, Dittrich H, et al. Randomized controlled trial of silymarin treatment in patients with cirrhosis of the liver. J Hepatol 1989;9:105–13.

Ferenci P, Scherzer TM, Kerschner H, et al. Silibinin is a potent antiviral agent in patients with chronic hepatitis C not responding to pegylated interferon/ribavirin therapy. Gastroenterology 2008;135(5):1561–7.

Gharagozloo M, Karimi M, Amirghofran Z. Immunomodulatory effects of silymarin in patients with β-thalassemia major. Int Immunopharmacol 2013;16(2):243–7.

Ghorbani A, Zarvandi M, Rakhshandeh H. A randomized controlled trial of a herbal compound for improving metabolic parameters in diabetic patients with uncontrolled dyslipidemia. Endocr Metab Immune Disord Drug Targets 2019;6.

Greenlee H, Atkinson C, Stanczyk FZ, Lampe JW. A pilot and feasibility study on the effects of naturopathic botanical and dietary interventions on sex steroid hormone metabolism in premenopausal women. Cancer Epidemiol Biomarkers Prev 2007;16(8):1601–9.

Hahn HJ, Jung HJ, Schrammek-Drusios MC, et al. Instrumental evaluation of anti-aging effects of cosmetic formulations containing palmitoyl peptides, *Silybum marianum* seed oil, vitamin E and other functional ingredients on aged human skin. Exp Ther Med 2016;12(2):1171–6.

Hasani-Ranjbar S, Nayebi N, Moradi L, Mehri A, Larijani B, Abdollahi M. The efficacy and safety of herbal medicines used in the treatment of hyperlipidemia; a systematic review. Curr Pharm Des 2010;16(26):2935–47.

Huseini HF, Larijani B, Heshmat R, et al. The efficacy of *Silybum marianum* (L.) Gaertn. (silymarin) in the treatment of type II diabetes: a randomized, double-blind, placebo-controlled, clinical trial. Phytother Res 2006;20(12):1036–9.

Hutchinson C, Bomford A, Geissler CA. The iron-chelating potential of silybin in patients with hereditary haemochromatosis. Eur J Clin Nutr 2010;64(10):1239–41.

Jayawardena R, Thejani T, Ranasinghe P, Fernando D, Verster JC. Interventions for treatment and/or prevention of alcohol hangover: systematic review. Hum Psychopharmacol 2017;32(5). https://doi.org/10.1002/hup.2600.

Jowkar F, Godarzi H, Parvizi MM. Can we consider silymarin as a treatment option for vitiligo? A double-blind controlled randomized clinical trial of phototherapy plus oral Silybum marianum product vs phototherapy alone. J Dermatolog Treat 2019;2:1–5.

Kalantari H, Shahshahan Z, Hejazi SM, Ghafghazi T, Sebghatolahi V. Effects of *Silybum marianum* on patients with chronic hepatitis C. J Res Med Sci 2011 Mar;16(3):287–90.

Karbasforooshan H, Hosseini S, Elyasi S, Fani Pakdel A, Karimi G. Topical silymarin administration for prevention of acute radiodermatitis in breast cancer patients: a randomized, double-blind, placebo-controlled clinical trial. Phytother Res 2019 Feb;33(2):379–86.

Kazazis CE, Evangelopoulos AA, Kollas A, et al. Potential effects of silymarin and its flavonolignan components in patients with β-thalassemia major: a comprehensive review in 2015. Adv Pharmacol Sci 2016;2016, 3046373.

Khalili N, Fereydoonzadeh R, Mohtashami R, Mehrzadi S, Heydari M, Huseini HF. Silymarin, Olibanum, and Nettle, A mixed herbal formulation in the treatment of type II diabetes: a randomized, double-blind, placebo-controlled, clinical trial. J Evid Based Complementary Altern Med 2017 Oct;22(4):603–8.

Ladas EJ, Kroll DJ, Oberlies NH, et al. A randomized, controlled, double-blind, pilot study of milk thistle for the treatment of hepatotoxicity in childhood acute lymphoblastic leukemia (ALL). Cancer 2010;116(2):506–13.

Laidlaw M, Cockerline CA, Sepkovic DW. Effects of a breast-health herbal formula supplement on estrogen metabolism in pre- and post-menopausal women not taking hormonal contraceptives or supplements: a randomized controlled trial. Breast Cancer (Auckl) 2010;4:85–95.

Madisch A, Melderis H, Mayr G, Sassin I, Hotz J. A plant extract and its modified preparation in functional dyspepsia. Results of a double-blind placebo controlled comparative study. Z Gastroenterol 2001;39(7):511–7.

Magliulo E, Gagliardi B, Fiori GP. Results of a double-blind study on the effect of silymarin in the treatment of acute viral hepatitis, carried out at two medical centres. Med Klin 1978;73:1060–5.

Mayer KE, Myers RP, Lee SS. Silymarin treatment of viral hepatitis: a systematic review. J Viral Hepat 2005;12(6):559–67.

Mills E, Wilson K, Clarke M, et al. Milk thistle and indinavir: a randomized controlled pharmacokinetics study and meta-analysis. Eur J Clin Pharmacol 2005;61(1):1–7.

Moayedi B, Gharagozloo M, Esmaeil N, Maracy MR, Hoorfar H, Jalaeikar M. A randomized double-blind, placebo-controlled study of therapeutic effects of silymarin in β-thalassemia major patients receiving desferrioxamine. Eur J Haematol 2013 Mar;90(3):202–9.

Nassuato G, Iemmolo RM, et al. Effect of silibinin on biliary lipid composition. Experimental and clinical study. J Hepatol 1991;12:290–5.

Navarro VJ, Belle SH, D'Amato M, et al. Silymarin in non-cirrhotics with non-alcoholic steatohepatitis: a randomized, double-blind, placebo controlled trial. PLoS One 2019;14(9):e0221683.

Palasciano G, Portinascasa P, Palmieri V, et al. The effect of silymarin on plasma levels of malondialdehyde in patients receiving long-term treatment with psychotropic drugs. Curr Ther Res 1994;S5:S37–45.

Parés A, Planas R, Torres M, et al. Effects of silymarin in alcoholic patients with cirrhosis of the liver: results of a controlled, double-blind, randomized and multicenter trial. J Hepatol 1998;28(4):615–21.

Rambaldi A, Jacobs BP, Iaquinto G, Gluud C. Milk thistle for alcoholic and/or hepatitis B or C liver diseases – a systematic cochrane hepato-biliary group review with meta-analyses of randomized clinical trials. Am J Gastroenterol 2005;100(11):2583–91.

Rashidi AA, Mirhashemi SM, Taghizadeh M, Sarkhail P. Iranian medicinal plants for diabetes mellitus: a systematic review. Pak J Biol Sci 2013;16(9):401–11.

Rotem C, Kaplan B. Phyto-female complex for the relief of hot flushes, night sweats and quality of sleep: randomized, controlled, double-blind pilot study. Gynecol Endocrinol 2007;23(2):117–22.

Saberi Z, Gorji N, Memariani Z, Moeini R, Shirafkan H, Amiri M. Evaluation of the effect of *Silybum marianum* extract on menopausal symptoms: a randomized, double-blind placebo-controlled trial. Phytother Res 2020;34:3359–66. https://doi.org/10.1002/ptr.6789.

Sahib A, Al-Anbari H, Salih M, Abdullah F. Effects of oral antioxidants on lesion counts associated with oxidative stress and inflammation in patients with papulopustular acne. J Clin Exp Dermatol Res 2012;3:5.

Saller R, Brignoli R, Melzer J, Meier R. An updated systematic review with meta-analysis for the clinical evidence of silymarin. Forsch Komplementmed 2008;15(1):9–20.

Sarris J, Camfield D, Berk M. Complementary medicine, self-help, and lifestyle interventions for obsessive compulsive disorder (OCD) and the OCD spectrum: a systematic review. J Affect Disord 2012;138(3):213–21.

Sarris J, McIntyre E, Camfield DA. Plant-based medicines for anxiety disorders, part 2: a review of clinical studies with supporting preclinical evidence. CNS Drugs 2013 Apr;27(4):301–19.

Sayyah M, Boostani H, Pakseresht S, Malayeri A. Comparison of *Silybum marianum* (L.) Gaertn. with fluoxetine in the treatment of obsessive-compulsive disorder. Prog Neuropsychopharmacol Biol Psychiatry 2010;34(2):362–5.

Shavandi M, Moini A, Shakiba Y, et al. Silymarin (Livergol®) decreases disease activity score in patients with rheumatoid arthritis: a non-randomized single-arm clinical trial. Iran J Allergy Asthma Immunol 2017;16(2):99–106.

Suksomboon N, Poolsup N, Boonkaew S, Suthisisang CC. Meta-analysis of the effect of herbal supplement on glycemic control in type 2 diabetes. J Ethnopharmacol 2011;137(3):1328–33.

Tao L, Qu X, Zhang Y, Song Y, Zhang SX. Prophylactic therapy of Silymarin (Milk thistle) on antituberculosis drug-induced liver injury: a meta-analysis of randomized controlled trials. Can J Gastroenterol Hepatol 2019;2019:3192351.

Velussi M, Cernigoi AM, Viezzoli L, Dapas F, Caffau C, Zilli M. Silymarin reduces hyperinsulinemia, malondialdehyde levels, and daily insulin need in cirrhotic diabetic patients. Curr Therap Res 1993;53(5):533–45.

Vostalova J, Vidlar A, Ulrichova J, Vrbkova J, Simanek V, Student V. Use of selenium-silymarin mix reduces lower urinary tract symptoms and prostate specific antigen in men. Phytomedicine 2013;21(1):75–81.

Yang Z, Zhuang L, Lu Y, Xu Q, Chen X. Effects and tolerance of silymarin (milk thistle) in chronic hepatitis C virus infection patients: a meta-analysis of randomized controlled trials. Biomed Res Int 2014;2014, 941085.

Zarvandi M, Rakhshandeh H, Abazari M, Shafiee-Nick R, Ghorbani A. Safety and efficacy of a polyherbal formulation for the management of dyslipidemia and hyperglycemia in patients with advanced-stage of type-2 diabetes. Biomed Pharmacother 2017;89:69–75.

Zhong S, Fan Y, Yan Q, et al. The therapeutic effect of silymarin in the treatment of nonalcoholic fatty disease: a meta-analysis (PRISMA) of randomized control trials. Medicine (Baltimore) 2017;96(49), e9061.

62

MOTHERWORT (*LEONURUS CARDIACA*)
Above-Ground Parts

GENERAL OVERVIEW

The common and Latin names for this plant reveal its two main uses. Put in simple terms, it promotes menses and calms the cardiovascular system. It is another useful herb for the treatment of anxiety spectrum disorders and for palpitations related to hyperthyroidism. It has been used for centuries for arrhythmias and in the postpartum period to promote uterine tone and breast milk production. It is traditionally used to treat hypertension especially when accompanied by anxiety. It may be useful for amenorrhea of certain etiologies. Although motherwort has traditionally been thought to stimulate absent or diminished menses, it has not been studied clinically for this use.

Clinical trials with this herb are few, and some trials involve intravenous or intramyometrial injections. Clinical research indicates that motherwort, alone or in combination formulas, may be beneficial for cardiovascular disease, postpartum hemorrhage, and mood disorders, but further research is warranted.

IN VITRO AND ANIMAL RESEARCH

In laboratory research motherwort has been shown to have sedative, anxiolytic, antibacterial, antifungal, hypothyroid, diaphoretic, cardiotonic, antiatherosclerotic, antiarrhythmic, negative chronotropic, vasodilating, hypotensive, hepatic, laxative, antispasmodic, oxytocic, and emmenagogic properties. It has demonstrated phytoestrogenic properties. The labdane diterpenoids in motherwort have demonstrated anti-inflammatory, antiplatelet, and anti-cholinesterase effects.

A study in various mammals fed with a high-fat diet compared the constituent leonurine with atorvastatin. TC and TG were significantly reduced by leonurine and atorvastatin. By day 150 there was a 24% reduction in TC with leonurine, and a similar reduction with atorvastatin. In addition, leonurine suppressed gene expression for fatty acid synthesis in the liver in Apo E$-/-$ mice on a high-fat diet (Suguro et al., 2018). In a rabbit atherosclerotic model, leonurine dose-dependently ameliorated the progression of atherosclerotic lesions and vascular dysfunction accompanied by the suppression of inflammatory factors and oxidative stress (Zhang et al., 2012).

A refined extract of motherwort applied intracoronary in isolated rabbit myocardium was shown to act on multiple electrophysiological targets. Leonurine has been shown to inhibit vascular smooth muscle tone, probably via inhibition of calcium influx and the release of intracellular calcium. In a rat model of chronic myocardial ischemia and an H9c2 cardiac myocyte model of oxidative stress, leonurine significantly improved myocardial function as evidenced by decreased LVEDP. It was shown to have potent antiapoptotic effects after chronic myocardial ischemia mediated by activating the PI3K/Akt signaling pathway through gene upregulation (Liu et al., 2010a). In another rat myocardial ischemia model, leonurine was found to decrease plasma LDH and CK levels as well as infarct size. The gene for SOD was significantly upregulated resulting in an increase in SOD activity and a decrease in lipid peroxidation (Liu et al., 2010b).

Research on the effects of leonurine on nephrotoxicity in mice demonstrated that leonurine protected against LPS-induced AKI, improved animal survival, and maintained redox balance. These benefits were accompanied by the downregulation of TNF-α, IL-1, IL-6, IL-8, and KIM-1 expression and by the inhibition of the phosphorylation of IκBα and p65 translocalization. These results suggested that leonurine may suppress NF-κB activation and inhibit pro-inflammatory cytokine production via decreasing cellular ROS production (Xu et al., 2014).

Chronic ingestion of a methanol extract of motherwort by mice was associated with a decrease in formation of hyperplastic alveolar nodules and markedly suppressed the development of mammary cancers originating from these nodules. However, the development of pregnancy-dependent mammary tumors (PDMT) and mammary cancers originating from PDMT was enhanced. The incidence of uterine adenomyosis was also inhibited in the mice. The excretion of carcinogenic factors was increased (Nagasawa et al., 1990). The alkaloids leonurine and stachydrine have been shown to be uterotonic (hence motherwort's use following childbirth).

Extracts of motherwort have demonstrated GABA receptor binding. Leonurine exhibits 5-HT 3A inhibition, suggesting potential for anti-emetic action. Ethanolic extract of motherwort produced a significant antinociceptive effect in the first and second phases of formalin, hot plate, and tail flick tests, suggesting that motherwort possesses central and peripheral antinociceptive actions (Rezaee-Asl et al., 2014). In a rat model of ischemic stroke, pretreatment with leonurine reduced brain infarct volume, improved neurological deficit, increased activities of SOD and glutathione peroxidase, and decreased levels of the lipid peroxidation marker MDA. Leonurine also inhibited mitochondrial ROS production and ATP biosynthesis (Loh et al., 2010).

HUMAN RESEARCH

Cardiovascular Disorders: Hyperviscosity of Blood

A 15-day study in patients ($n = 105$) assessed the blood viscosity effects of motherwort 10 mL/day in 250 mL D5W given IV. The experimental and clinical study indicated that motherwort had a favorable clinical impact and an effective improvement of hemorheology. A decrease in blood viscosity and fibrinogen volume and an increase in the deformability of RBCs, a shorting of the time of RBC electrophoresis, and an increase in antiplatelet aggregation occurred in 95% of cases (Zou et al., 1989).

Women's Genitourinary Disorders: Uterine Tone and Post-Partum Hemorrhage

A 2018 systematic review to assess the impact of motherwort injection alone or combined with oxytocin for preventing postpartum hemorrhage in pregnant women with C-section found 46 RCTs ($n = 7359$) that met inclusion criteria. Compared with oxytocin, both motherwort injection and motherwort injection combined with oxytocin had significantly lower blood loss within 2 h (MD = −21.81 and MD = −53.04, respectively); lower blood loss within 24 h (MD = −25.44 and MD = −67.81, respectively); and lower risk of adverse events (OR = 0.40 and OR = 0.50, respectively). Motherwort injection combined with oxytocin also decreased the risk of postpartum hemorrhage (OR 0.22). The authors concluded that motherwort injection appeared to have efficacy and safety in pregnant women with C-section (Chen and Kwan, 2001).

A study in normal fertile women ($n = 121$) compared the uterotonic effects of an oral dose of motherwort 30 g via decoction with ergonovine 0.2 mg IM and with water (control). There was an increase in intra-uterine pressure in 41.3%, 61%, and 2.7% of subjects with motherwort, ergonovine, and water, respectively. The increase in intra-uterine pressure with motherwort ranged from 150% to more than 300% of spontaneous activity. There were no observable side effects apart from diuresis (Chan et al., 1983).

An RCT in women ($n = 440$) undergoing C-section compared (1) intrauterine injection of motherwort 40 mg during C/S and 20 mg IM Q12h X 3 following C/S, (2) intrauterine injection of motherwort 40 mg plus oxytocin 10 U during C/S and motherwort 20 mg IM Q 12 h × 3 after C/S, and (3) intrauterine injection of oxytocin 10 U and 10 U IV during C/S and oxytocin 10 U IM Q12h X 3 after C/S. The mean amount of intraoperative blood loss with groups 1, 2, and 3 were 368 mL, 255 mL, and 269 mL, respectively ($P < 0.01$). Postpartum, no significant difference between groups was noted for blood loss. The amount of blood loss postpartum at 24 h for groups 1, 2, and 3 were 480 mL, 361 mL, and 381 mL, respectively ($P < 0.01$). The incidence of postpartum hemorrhage for groups 1, 2, and 3 was 32.0%, 11.1%, and 18.8%, respectively. The authors concluded that it was safe and efficacious to combine motherwort injection and oxytocin to prevent postpartum hemorrhage during or after caesarian delivery (Lin et al., 2009).

Psychiatric Disorders: Anxiety, Insomnia and Depression

A 28-day open-label study in hypertensive patients ($n = 50$) with anxiety and sleep disorders assessed the effect of motherwort oil extract 1200 mg/day. Positive effects of motherwort on psycho-emotional status and BP in patients with stage 1 HTN were observed 1 week earlier than in patients with stage 2 HTN. A large improvement in the symptoms of anxiety and depression was observed in 32% of patients, a moderate improvement in 48%, and a weak improvement in 8%; 12% of patients did not respond to therapy. Side effects were minimal in all groups. The authors concluded that motherwort oil extract was a potentially effective therapeutic agent for patients with HTN and concurrent psychoneurological disorders (Shikov et al., 2011).

A 10-day open-label study in anxious young subjects compared the effects of melatonin 0.75 mg with those of motherwort tincture each given HS. There was a significant decrease in the thresholds of retinal brightness sensitivity and improvement in emotional state in anxious young subjects with melatonin. Analogous changes were less pronounced after the treatment with motherwort tincture. The authors concluded that there may be a relationship between the limitation of anxiety and the improvement of visual sensitivity (Ovanesov et al., 2006).

ACTIVE CONSTITUENTS

Aerial Parts

- Phenolic compounds
  - Phenylpropanoids (antioxidant, antimutagenic, antitumor, antimicrobial): chlorogenic acid (antioxidant)
  - Flavonoids: hyperoside (antioxidant, anti-inflammatory, antiproliferative, apoptotic, hepatoprotective, nephroprotective, anti-osteoporotic), orientin, rutin (antioxidant,

anti-inflammatory, antidiabetic, nephroprotective, anti-osteoporotic, antispasmodic, neuroprotective, anti-anxiety), apigenin (anti-inflammatory, antioxidant, antihistamine, hypotensive, anti-serotonin release, GABA agonism, antispasmodic, antibacterial, chemopreventive, antineoplastic, ERB), kaempferol (anti-inflammatory, antidepressant, strengthens capillaries), quercitin, vitexin (antioxidant, anti-inflammatory, hepatoprotective, estrogen-β agonism, anti-hyperalgesic, antiarthritis, neuroprotective, antidepressant, dopaminergic, serotonergic, anti-cancer)
    - Tannins
- Terpenes
  - Monoterpenes
    - Iridoid glycosides (negative chronotropic, hypotensive, antiseptic, nervine, antispasmodic): lavandulifolioside, leonosides-A
  - Diterpenes: labdane diterpenoids (block conversion of estradiol to estrone)
  - Triterpenoid saponins: ursolic acid (anti-HIV, anti-EBV, antiviral, androgenic, AChEI, pro-collagen, pro-ceremide, antitumor)
- Steroids
  - Phytosterols and steroidal glycosides: β-sitosterone, ergosterols
- Alkaloids: leonurine (mostly in *L. japonicus*; CNS sedative, oxytocic, uterotonic, vascular relaxant, hypotensive), betonicine (hemostatic, antibacterial), stachydrine (anticancer, provascular, hypoglycemic), betaine (gastric acidification), trigonelline (hypoglycemic, hypolipidemic, hypotensive, neuroprotective, antimigraine, sedative, memory-improving, antipyretic, antibacterial, antiviral, antitumor)

MOTHERWORT COMMONLY USED PREPARATIONS AND DOSAGE (FOR ADULTS UNLESS OTHERWISE SPECIFIED)

The following are examples of some available formulations and ranges of dosing for commercial herbal products. See Part III Introduction "How to prescribe medicinal herbs" for further guidance on herbal advising and prescribing.

Dried Aerial Parts

- Infusion: 1 tsp. per cup TID
- Tincture (1:5, 40%–60%): 1–2 mL BID-QID
- Powdered (5:1) extract: 1 tsp. BID
- Capsule or tablet of powdered herb extract: 200–500 mg QD-TID

SAFETY AND PRECAUTION

Side Effects

No adverse effects expected within recommended doses. Abdominal pain, cramping, diarrhea, drowsiness, and hypotension may occur with higher doses. Topical application may cause photosensitivity.

Toxicity

An excess of 3 g in a single dose may cause diarrhea, uterine bleeding, and gastritis.

Pregnancy and Lactation

Insufficient human data. Should be avoided. May cause preterm labor or miscarriage. However, it has been used traditionally during parturition to control postpartum bleeding.

Disease Interactions

Uterotonic effects may result in increased uterine bleeding in some women with menorrhagia.

Drug Interactions

- Theoretically may interact with heart and cardiovascular drugs.
- May increase effects of sedating drugs.

REFERENCES

Chan WC, Wong YC, Kong YC, Chun YT, Chang HT, Chan WF. Clinical observation on the uterotonic effect of I-mu Ts'ao (*Leonurus artemisia*). Am J Chin Med 1983;11(1–4):77–83.

Chen CX, Kwan CY. Endothelium-independent vasorelaxation by leonurine, a plant alkaloid purified from Chinese motherwort. Life Sci 2001;68(8):953–60.

Lin JH, Lin QD, Liu XH, et al. Multi-center study of motherwort injection to prevent postpartum hemorrhage after caesarian section. Zhonghua Fu Chan Ke Za Zhi 2009;44(3):175–8.

Liu C, Guo W, Shi X, Kaium MA, Gu X, Zhu YZ. Leonurine-cysteine analog conjugates as a new class of multifunctional anti-myocardial ischemia agent. Eur J Med Chem 2011;46(9):3996–4009.

Liu X, Pan L, Gong Q, Zhu Y. Leonurine (SCM-198) improves cardiac recovery in rat during chronic infarction. Eur J Pharmacol 2010a;649(1–3):236–41.

Liu X, Pan LL, Chen PF, Zhu ZH. Leonurine improves ischemia-induced myocardial injury through antioxidant activity. Phytomedicine 2010b;17(10):753–9.

Loh KP, Qi J, Tan BK, Liu XH, Wei BG, Zhu YZ. Leonurine protects middle cerebral artery occluded rats through antioxidant effect and regulation of mitochondrial function. Stroke 2010;41(11):2661–8.

Nagasawa H, Onoyama T, Suzuki M, Hibino A, Segawa T, Inatomi H. Effects of motherwort (*Leonurus sibiricus* L) on preneoplastic and neoplastic mammary gland growth in multiparous GR/A mice. Anticancer Res 1990;10(4):1019–23.

Ovanesov KB, Ovanesova IM, Arushanian EB. Effects of melatonin and motherwort tincture on the emotional state and visual functions in anxious subjects. Eksp Klin Farmakol 2006;69(6):17–9.

Rezaee-Asl M, Sabour M, Nikoui V, Ostadhadi S, Bakhtiarian A. The study of analgesic effects of *Leonurus cardiaca* L. in mice by formalin, tail flick and hot plate tests. Int Sch Res Notices 2014;2014, 687697.

Shikov AN, Pozharitskaya ON, Makarov VG, Demchenko DV, Shikh EV. Effect of *Leonurus cardiaca* oil extract in patients with arterial HTN accompanied by anxiety and sleep disorders. Phytother Res 2011;25(4):540–3.

Suguro R, Chen S, Yang D, et al. Anti-hypercholesterolemic effects and a good safety profile of SCM-198 in animals: from ApoE knockout mice to rhesus monkeys. Front Pharmacol 2018;9:1468.

Xu D, Chen M, Ren X, Ren X, Wu Y. Leonurine ameliorates LPS-induced acute kidney injury via suppressing ROS-mediated NF-κB signaling pathway. Fitoterapia 2014;97:148–55.

Zhang Y, Guo W, Wen Y, et al. SCM-198 attenuates early atherosclerotic lesions in hypercholesterolemic rabbits via modulation of the inflammatory and oxidative stress pathways. Atherosclerosis 2012;224(1):43–50.

Zou QZ, Bi RG, Li JM, et al. Effect of motherwort on blood hyperviscosity. Am J Chin Med 1989;17(1–2):65–70.

63

PASSIONFLOWER (*PASSIFLORA INCARNATA*)
(Flowering Vine)

GENERAL OVERVIEW

Passionflower is another promising arrow in the quiver of herbal options for anxiety and insomnia. Some research has shown passionflower to have comparable efficacy to benzodiazepines with fewer side effects. According to archeological evidence, human use of passionflower began in the late Archaic period (3500–800 BCE) in North America. Its name is traced back to 1605 CE when the plant was given as a gift to Pope Paul V who observed that the flower's corona was similar crown of thorns from the crucifixion of Jesus, the three styles being the nails of the cross, the three-lobed leaves being the spear, and the five anthers representing the marks of the five wounds.

A relative to *Passiflora incarnata*, purple passionflower (*P. edulis*) has evidence for osteoarthritis and diabetes from the fruit peel. The studies for *P. edulis* are included below.

Clinical research indicates that passionflower, alone or in combination formulas, may be beneficial for menopause, anxiety including perioperative anxiety, insomnia, attention-deficit/hyperactivity disorder, and opiate withdrawal.

IN VITRO AND ANIMAL RESEARCH

In vitro and animal studies show passionflower to have anti-inflammatory, anti-asthmatic, antitussive, glucose-lowering, anticonvulsant, sedative, and anti-anxiety effects. Streptozotocin-induced diabetic mice were given passionflower extract 100 and 200 mg/kg

for 15 days. There was a significant reduction in FBS, urine glucose, OGTT, serum lipid profile, and BW compared with non-treated and drug-treated mice. Histopathological studies of the pancreas showed regeneration of cells that were earlier necrosed by streptozotocin (Gupta et al., 2012). The constituent in passionflower known as chrysin has demonstrated aromatase inhibiting activity.

At least three studies in mice have demonstrated reduction in seizure frequency and severity. In vitro research has demonstrated that passionflower induces dose-dependent direct GABA$_A$ currents in hippocampal slices attributed to the GABA found to be a prominent ingredient of passionflower extract. Anticonvulsant effects against pentylenetetrazole-induced seizures were seen in mice given passionflower extract. Delayed onset and reduced duration of seizures and post-ictal mobility occurred, and at the dose of 0.4 mg/kg, seizure and mortality protection were 100%. Brain levels of serotonin and norepinephrine were retained (in contrast to the reduction with benzodiazepines). Antagonists flumazenil and naloxone did not suppress anticonvulsant effects of passionflower (Singh et al., 2012).

The antidepressant effects of a combination of St. John's wort and passionflower were compared with those of St. John's wort alone in a mouse model. Passionflower significantly enhanced the pharmacological potency of St. John's wort. The authors concluded that anti-depressive therapeutic effects of St. John's wort were possible with lower doses, when combined with passionflower (Fiebich et al., 2011).

HUMAN RESEARCH

Women's Genitourinary Disorders: Menopause

A 2017 review of clinical trials on herbal efficacy in menopausal symptoms used search terms menopause, climacteric, hot flushes, flashes, herb, and phytoestrogens. The authors found that passionflower, sage, lemon balm, valerian, black cohosh, fenugreek, black seed, chasteberry, fennel, evening primrose, ginkgo, alfalfa, St. John's wort, Asian ginseng, anise, licorice, red clover, and wild soybean were effective in the treatment of acute menopausal syndrome with different mechanisms. The authors concluded that medicinal plants could play a role in the treatment of acute menopausal syndrome and that further studies were warranted (Kargozar et al., 2017).

A 2016 systematic review to assess effectiveness of Iranian herbal medicine for menopausal hot flushes found 19 RCTs that met inclusion criteria. Overall, studies showed that passionflower, anise, licorice, soy, black cohosh, red clover, evening primrose, flaxseed, sage, chasteberry, St. John's wort, valerian, and avocado plus soybean oil could alleviate hot flushes. The authors concluded that herbal medicines had efficacy in alleviating hot flushes (Ghazanfarpour et al., 2016).

A 6-week RCT in menopausal women ($n = 59$) compared passionflower with St. John's wort for efficacy on menopausal symptoms. The average scores of menopausal symptoms in the two treatment groups showed significant decreases throughout the third and sixth weeks of the study ($P < 0.05$). There was no statistically significant difference between the two groups ($P > 0.05$) (Fahami et al., 2010).

Musculoskeletal Disorders: Osteoarthritis

A 2-month RCT in patients ($n = 33$) with OA compared passion fruit (*P. edulis*) peel extract (PFP) 150 mg/day with placebo. In the PFP group, at 60 days, there were significant reductions of 18.6%, 18%, 19.6%, and 19.2% in pain, stiffness, physical function, and composite WOMAC scores, respectively, whereas, in the placebo group, the WOMAC scores increased in every category. The results of this study indicate that PFP could substantially alleviate osteoarthritis symptoms. The authors postulated that the beneficial effect of PFP

may be due to its antioxidant and anti-inflammatory properties (Farid et al., 2010).

Psychiatric Disorders: Anxiety and Perioperative Anxiety

A 2018 systematic review to identify single-herb medicines that may warrant further study for treatment of anxiety and depression in cancer patients found 100 studies involving 38 botanicals that met inclusion criteria. Among herbs most studied ($\geq$ six randomized controlled trials each), passionflower, lavender, and saffron produced benefits comparable to standard anxiolytics and antidepressants. Black cohosh, chamomile, and chasteberry were also promising. Overall, 45% of studies reported positive findings with fewer adverse effects when compared with conventional medications. The authors concluded that saffron, black cohosh, chamomile, chasteberry, lavender, and passionflower appeared useful in mitigating anxiety or depression with favorable risk-benefit profiles compared with standard treatments, and these botanicals may benefit cancer patients by minimizing medication load and accompanying side effects (Yeung et al., 2018).

A 2013 systematic review looking at plants that had both pre-clinical and clinical evidence for anti-anxiety effects found 21 plants with human clinical trial evidence. Support for efficacy identified several herbs with efficacy for anxiety spectrum disorders including passionflower, kava, lemon balm, chamomile, ginkgo, skullcap, milk thistle, ashwagandha, rhodiola, echinacea, *Galphimia glauca*, *Centella asiatica*, and *Echium amooenum*. Acute anxiolytic activity was found for passionflower, sage, gotu kola, lemon balm, and bergamot. The review also specifically found that bacopa showed anxiolytic effects in people with cognitive decline (Sarris et al., 2013).

A 2010 systematic review and meta-analysis of CAM therapies for anxiety identified 24 studies ($n = 2619$) that investigated five different CAM monotherapies and eight different combination treatments that met the inclusion criteria. Of the randomized controlled trials reviewed, 71% showed a positive direction of evidence. Any reported side effects were mild to moderate. The reviewers concluded that nutritional and herbal supplementation were effective methods for treating anxiety and anxiety-related conditions without the risk of serious side effects; strong evidence existed for the use of herbal supplements containing extracts of passionflower or kava and combinations of L-lysine and L-arginine as treatments for anxiety symptoms and disorders. Magnesium-containing supplements and other herbal combinations appeared promising but needed more research, and St. John's wort monotherapy had insufficient evidence (Lakhan and Vieira, 2010).

A 2010 review to evaluate effectiveness of herbal medicines for generalized anxiety disorder (GAD) found that kava had an unequivocal anxiolytic effect. Isolated studies with passionflower, valerian, ginkgo, chamomile, and *Galphimia glauca* showed a potential use for anxious diseases. Ginkgo and chamomile showed an effect size (Cohen's d = 0.47 to 0.87) similar to or greater than standard anxiolytics drugs (benzodiazepines, buspirone, and antidepressants, d = 0.17 to 0.38) (Faustino et al., 2010).

A 2007 systematic review of studies on passionflower for anxiety spectrum disorders identified two studies (n = 198) that met inclusion criteria. One study showed a lack of difference in efficacy between benzodiazepines and passionflower. Dropout rates were similar between the two interventions. Although the findings from one study suggested an improvement in job performance in favor of passionflower and one study showed a lower rate of drowsiness as a side effect with passionflower compared with mexazolam, neither of these findings reached statistical significance. The authors concluded that more research was warranted (Miyasaka et al., 2007).

A 4-week RCT in patients (n = 36) with a *DSM-IV* diagnosis of GAD investigated passionflower extract 45 drops/day plus placebo tablet compared with oxazepam 30 mg/day plus placebo drops. Both treatments were effective in reducing anxiety with no significant difference between the two protocols at the end of trial. Oxazepam showed a rapid onset of action. On the other hand, significantly more problems relating to impairment of job performance were encountered in subjects given oxazepam. The authors concluded that passionflower was an effective drug for managing GAD with a low incidence of impairment of job performance compared with oxazepam (Akhondzadeh et al., 2001).

An acutely dosed RCT in patients (n = 40) undergoing bilateral extraction of their mandibular third molars compared passionflower 260 mg with midazolam 15 mg given orally 30 min before surgery. More than 70% of the volunteers responded that they felt calm or a little anxious under both protocols. However, 20% of the participants given midazolam reported amnesia (not remembering anything at all), while none in the passionflower group reported interference with memory formation. The authors concluded that passionflower showed an anxiolytic effect equivalent to midazolam and was safe and effective in promoting conscious sedation for molar extraction (Dantas et al., 2017).

An acutely dosed RCT in patients (n = 63) with moderate, high, and severe anxiety who were to undergo periodontal treatment studied pre-treatment with passionflower compared with placebo and with no treatment for effects on anxiety. Anxiety levels on a VAS changed from 12.1 to 8.5, 12.0 to 10.5, and 11.7 to 11.2 for passionflower, placebo, and control respectively (P < 0.0001 for passionflower when compared pre- and post-treatment and when compared with placebo and control groups) (Kaviani et al., 2013).

An acutely dosed RCT in patients (n = 60) who were scheduled for spinal anesthesia compared passionflower with placebo given 30 min prior to anesthesia to assess the effect on anxiety just prior to the spinal injection. There was a statistically significant difference between the two groups for the increase in State Anxiety Inventory score obtained just before spinal anesthesia when compared with baseline. There was no statistically significant difference in psychomotor function from the baseline for either group. The authors concluded that preoperative administration of passionflower suppressed the increase in anxiety before spinal anesthesia without changing psychomotor function, sedation level, or hemodynamics (Aslanargun et al., 2012).

An acutely dosed RCT in patients (n = 52) about to undergo surgery compared passionflower 1000 mg with melatonin 6 mg given orally 1 h before surgery for effects on postoperative pain and anxiety. The mean score of pain upon discharge from post-anesthesia care was 27.63 and 25.37 with melatonin and passionflower, respectively, but there were no significant differences between groups in pain VAS (P > 0.05). The anxiety scores decreased significantly from pre- to post-operative periods with both drugs (P = 0.001), but sedation scores were higher with melatonin comparing pre- and post-op periods ($P = 0.003$ vs 0.008). Regarding cognitive testing, only passionflower showed a significant difference between pre- and post-op periods ($P = 0.03$). The authors concluded that surgical premedication with passionflower reduced anxiety similar to melatonin but caused more cognitive impairment (Rokhtabnak et al., 2016).

An acutely dosed RCT in patients ($n = 60$) scheduled for outpatient surgery compared passionflower 500 mg with placebo given 90 min before surgery. The anxiety scores were significantly lower in the passionflower group than in the control group ($P < 0.001$). There were no significant differences in psychological variables in the post-anesthesia care unit, and recovery of psychomotor function was comparable in both groups. The authors concluded that passionflower as a surgical premedication reduced anxiety without inducing sedation (Movafegh et al., 2008).

An acutely dosed RCT in healthy men ($n = 72$) investigated pre-dosing for 4 days with Ze 185, a fixed combination of valerian, passionflower, lemon balm, and butterbur, compared with pre-dosing with placebo and with a no-treatment control for effects on biological and affective responses to a standardized psychosocial stress paradigm. The stress paradigm induced significant and large cortisol and self-reported anxiety responses. Groups did not differ significantly in their salivary cortisol response to stress, but participants in the herbal group showed significantly attenuated responses in self-reported anxiety compared with placebo ($P = 0.03$) and with no treatment ($P = 0.05$). The authors suggested that the herbal combination reduced the self-reported anxiety response to stress without affecting the assumingly adaptive biological stress responses (Meier et al., 2018).

A 3.5-year retrospective case-control study of hospitalized psychiatric patients ($n = 3252$) evaluated an herbal extract combination of passionflower, valerian, lemon balm, and butterbur (Ze 185) compared with no additional herbal therapy to investigate whether the herbal combination would change the prescription pattern of benzodiazepines. Data showed that both treatment modalities had a comparable clinical effectiveness, but there were significantly fewer prescriptions of benzodiazepines with the herbal combination ($P = 0.006$). The authors recommended that an RCT be performed (Keck et al., 2020).

A 28-day RCT in patients ($n = 182$) with adjustment disorder with anxious mood investigated Euphytose, a polyherbal product containing hawthorn, passionflower, valerian, *Ballota*, *Cola*, and *Paullinia* (the combination being theoretically both calming and stimulating) compared with placebo, two tablets TID, for effects on anxiety. Comparing the two groups, 42.9% and 25.3% of the herbal and placebo groups, respectively, had a HAM-A score of less than 10 by day 28 ($P = 0.012$). The authors noted that from day 7 to day 28 there was a significant difference ($P = 0.042$) between the groups, indicating that Euphytose was better than placebo in the treatment of adjustment disorder with anxious mood (Bourin et al., 1997).

Psychiatric Disorders: Insomnia

A 2-week RCT in patients ($n = 110$) with insomnia compared the effects of passionflower extract with placebo for effects on polysomnographic sleep parameters. Total sleep time (TST) was increased with passionflower and decreased with placebo (23.05 min and -0.16 min, respectively; $P = 0.049$). Sleep efficiency and wake after sleep onset significantly improved with passionflower, but there was no difference compared with the placebo group. The authors concluded that passionflower had positive effects on objective sleep parameters including TST (Lee et al., 2020).

A 2-week RCT in patients ($n = 91$) with primary insomnia investigated NSF-3, an herbal combination containing valerian, hops, and passionflower one tablet QHS compared with zolpidem 10 mg QHS. There was a significant improvement in total sleep time, sleep latency, number of nightly awakenings, and insomnia severity index scores in both groups. No statistically significant difference was observed between the groups. Epworth Sleepiness scores did not change significantly over the study period. Mild adverse events were reported in 12 herbal subjects and 16 zolpidem subjects. The authors concluded that this combination of valerian, passionflower, and hops was a safe and effective short-term alternative to zolpidem for primary insomnia (Maroo et al., 2013).

A crossover RCT in volunteers ($n = 41$) compared passionflower tea with placebo tea for sleep and anxiety effects. Ten participants also underwent overnight PSG on the last night of each treatment period to validate reports on sleep diaries. Sleep quality on sleep diaries showed a significantly better rating for passionflower compared with placebo ($P < 0.01$). The authors concluded that the consumption of a low dose of passionflower, in the form of tea, yielded short-term subjective sleep benefits for healthy adults with mild fluctuations in sleep quality (Ngan and Conduit, 2011).

Psychiatric Disorders: Attention-Deficit/Hyperactivity Disorder

A 2017 systematic review to assess efficacy of herbal therapies for ADHD in children found nine RCTs ($n = 464$) that met inclusion criteria. Seven different herbs were tested in the treatment of ADHD symptoms. Low evidence could be found for lemon balm, valerian, and passionflower. Limited evidence could be found for pine bark extract and gingko. The other herbal preparations showed no efficacy in the treatment of ADHD symptoms (Anheyer et al., 2017).

An 8-week RCT in children ($n = 34$) with a *DSM-IV* diagnosis of ADHD compared passionflower 0.04 mg/kg/day with methylphenidate 1 mg/kg/day, each given as BID dosing. No significant differences were observed between passionflower and methylphenidate on the Parent and Teacher Rating Scale scores over the course of the trial. Both treatment groups demonstrated significant clinical benefit over the period of treatment as assessed by both parents and teachers. Decreased appetite and anxiety/nervousness were observed more often in the methylphenidate group. The authors concluded that passionflower may be a therapeutic agent for the treatment of ADHD, with a tolerable side-effect profile (Akhondzadeh et al., 2005).

Psychiatric Disorders: Somatoform Disorder

A 2-week RCT in patients ($n = 182$) with somatoform disorders investigated Ze185, a four-herb combination containing valerian, passionflower, lemon balm, and butterbur, compared with a three-herb combination without the butterbur, and with placebo. The combination containing butterbur was significantly superior to the combination without butterbur, which was superior to placebo for changes in VAS-Anxiety scale, Beck Depression Inventory, and Clinical Global Impression. In total, nine non-serious adverse events were documented, but the distribution did not differ significantly between the treatment groups. The authors concluded

that the herbal preparation Ze185 was an efficacious and safe short-term treatment in patients with somatoform disorders (Melzer et al., 2009).

Psychiatric Disorders: Alcohol and Opiate Withdrawal

A 14-day RCT in patients ($n = 65$) with opiate addiction who were undergoing withdrawal studied clonidine 0.8 mg/day plus placebo drops compared with clonidine 0.8 mg/day plus passionflower 60 drops, each divided into TID dosing. The severity of the opiate withdrawal syndrome was measured on days 0, 1, 2, 3, 4, 7, and 14 using the Short Opiate Withdrawal Scale. Both protocols were equally effective in treating the physical symptoms of withdrawal syndromes. However, the passionflower group showed a significant superiority over clonidine alone in the management of psychological symptoms. The authors concluded that passionflower extract may be an effective adjuvant agent in the management of opiate withdrawal (Akhondzadeh et al., 2011).

A 15-day open-label pilot trial in patients ($n = 32$) hospitalized for alcohol detoxification investigated the effect of an herbal combination (black seed, saffron, passionflower, cocoa seed, and radish) given TID. The herbal combination was associated with a significantly reduced percentage of patients with hyperhidrosis ($r = 0.815$; $P < 0.001$), a reduction in serum liver enzymes by 50%–80% ($P < 0.05$), and a normalization of appetite ($r = 0.777$; $P < 0.001$). Quality of life measured by Befindlichkeits-Skala improved from 28.3 to 15.6 ($P < 0.001$). The product was rated as good to excellent by 84.4% of patients. The authors concluded that there was potential for use of this herbal combination in patients undergoing alcohol withdrawal and that further studies were warranted (Mansoor et al., 2018).

ACTIVE CONSTITUENTS

There are two chemotypes resulting in variability of the flavonoid content. Those high in swertisin are low in shaftoside and isoshaftoside.

- Carbohydrates
  - Disaccharides: maltol
  - Polysaccharides: arabinoglucan (immunomodulating)

- Amino acid derivatives
  - amino acids: gamma-aminobutyric acid (GABA)
- Phenolic compounds
  - Coumarins: scopoletin (anti-inflammatory, α-glucosidase inhibitor, AChE inhibitor, neuroprotective, antipsychotic, melanogenic, anticancer), gamma-pyrone derivatives (activation of GABA receptors)
  - Flavonoids: chrysin, isovitexin (hepatoprotective, anticarcinogenic, apoptotic, antistapyholcoccal), isoshaftoside, shaftoside, isorientin, swertisin, vitexin (antioxidant, anti-inflammatory, hepatoprotective, estrogen-β agonism, anti-hyperalgesic, anti-arthritis, neuroprotective, antidepressant, dopaminergic, serotonergic, anticancer), rutin (antioxidant, anti-inflammatory, antidiabetic, nephroprotective, anti-osteoporotic, antispasmodic, neuroprotective, anti-anxiety)
  - Alkaloids: harman, harmaline (reversible MAO-A inhibition, muscle-relaxant, sedative)

PASSIONFLOWER COMMONLY USED PREPARATIONS AND DOSAGE (FOR ADULTS UNLESS OTHERWISE SPECIFIED)

The following are examples of some available formulations and ranges of dosing for commercial herbal products. See Part III Introduction "How to prescribe medicinal herbs" for further guidance on herbal advising and prescribing.

Dried Flower and Leaf

- Infusion: 1/2–1 tsp. per cup up to TID or HS prn insomnia
- Fluid extract (1:1, 25%): 1/2–2 mL up to TID or HS prn insomnia
- Tincture (1:5, 40%–70%): 0.7–4 mL up to QID or HS prn insomnia
- Powdered extract: 1 g (1/3 tsp) QD prn
- Capsule or tablet of powdered extract: 0.04 mg/kg per day for ADHD; 500–1000 mg for acute dosing
- Capsule or tablet of 4:1 extract 250 mg (equivalent to 1000 mg of passionflower): 250 mg QD-QID
- Capsule or tablet of standardized extract (standardized to at least 3.5% flavonoids or vitexin): 250–700 mg QD-BID prn

SAFETY AND PRECAUTION

Side-Effects

Dizziness, sedation, ataxia, impaired cognition, and allergic reactions have been reported.

Case Reports

A 34-year-old female developed severe nausea, vomiting, drowsiness, prolonged QTc, and episodes of nonsustained ventricular tachycardia following self-administration of passionflower at therapeutic doses. She required hospital admission for cardiac monitoring and intravenous fluid therapy.

A man with GAD who self-medicated with valerian and passionflower while he was on lorazepam developed tremor, dizziness, throbbing, and muscular fatigue. An additive or synergistic effect was suspected to have produced these symptoms. The active principles of valerian and passionflower might increase the inhibitory activity of benzodiazepines binding to the GABA receptors, causing severe secondary effects.

Toxicity

Large doses are potentially cardiotoxic (can prolong QTc). Acute and chronic administration of high doses of passionflower extract exhibited no adverse effects or toxicity to mice, rats, or dogs. No adverse effects on the biochemical and hematological parameters or toxicity were found in rats administered up to 2000 mg/kg of aqueous extract of *P. edulis* for 7 days.

Pregnancy and Lactation

Avoid due to possible uterine contractions and aromatase inhibiting activity. A study in pregnant rats found that passionflower extract up to 300 mg/kg throughout pregnancy did not influence bodyweight or food intake, post-implantation loss, litter size, litter weight, or physical development or behavior of pups. However, sexual behavior was disrupted in adult male pups exposed to the high dose (but not at 30 mg/kg). Only 3 out of 11 pups were sexually competent. This behavioral disruption was not accompanied by alterations in plasma testosterone levels, reproductive-related organs, and glands weights or sperm count. The authors hypothesized that aromatase inhibition may be involved in the observed effect (Bacchi et al., 2013).

Disease Interactions

Hypothyroidism: the constituent vitexin in high doses has been shown to reduce thyroid hormone in rats.

Drug Interactions

- May potentiate CNS depressants.
- Drugs that prolong the QT interval (e.g., azithromycin, dasatinib, fingolimod): The pharmacologic profile of passionflower suggests prolonged QT interval with large doses, and it is not known whether passionflower may have added cardiac effects with these medications.
- St. John's wort potency is increased by passionflower.

REFERENCES

Akhondzadeh S, Kashain L, Mobaseri M, Hosseini SH, Nikzad S, Khani M. Passionflower in the treatment of opiates withdrawal: a double-blind randomized controlled trial. J Clin Pharm Ther 2001;26:369–73.

Akhondzadeh S, Mohammadi MR, Momeni F. *Passiflora incarnata* in the treatment of attention-deficit hyperactivity disorder in children and adolescents. Therapy 2005;2(4):609–14.

Akhondzadeh S, Naghavi HR, Vazirian M, Shayeganpout A, Rashidi H, Khan M. Passionflower in the treatment of generalized anxiety: a pilot double-blind randomized controlled trial with oxazepam. J Clin Pharm Ther 2011;26:363–7.

Anheyer D, Lauche R, Schumann D, Dobos G, Cramer H. Herbal medicines in children with attention deficit hyperactivity disorder (ADHD): a systematic review. Complement Ther Med 2017;30:14–23.

Aslanargun P, Cuvas O, Dikmen B, Aslan E, Yuksel MU. *Passiflora incarnata* Linneaus as an anxiolytic before spinal anesthesia. J Anesth 2012;26:39–44.

Bacchi AD, Ponte B, Vieira ML, de Paula JC, Mesquita SF, Gerardin DC, Moreira EG, et al. Developmental exposure to *Passiflora incarnata* induces behavioural alterations in the male progeny. Reprod Fertil Dev 2013;25(5):782–9.

Bourin M, Bougerol T, Guitton B, Broutin E. A combination of plant extracts in the treatment of outpatients with adjustment disorder with anxious mood: controlled study vs placebo. Fundam Clin Pharmacol 1997;11:127–32.

Dantas LP, de Oliveira-Ribeiro A, de Almeida-Souza LM, Groppo FC. Effects of passiflora incarnata and midazolam for control of anxiety in patients undergoing dental extraction. Med Oral Patol Oral Cir Bucal 2017;22(1):e95–e101.

Fahami F, Asali Z, Aslani A, Fathizadeh N. A comparative study on the effects of *Hypericum perforatum* and passionflower on the menopausal symptoms of women referring to Isfahan city health care centers. Iran J Nurs Midwifery Res 2010;15(4):202–7.

Farid R, Rezaieyazdi Z, Mirfeizi Z, et al. Oral intake of purple passion fruit peel extract reduces pain and stiffness and improves physical function in adult patients with knee osteoarthritis. Nutr Res 2010;30(9):601–6.

Faustino TT, Almeida RB, Andreatini R. Medicinal plants for the treatment of generalized anxiety disorder: a review of controlled clinical studies. Braz J Psychiatry 2010;32(4):429–36.

Fiebich BL, Knörle R, Appel K, Kammler T, Weiss G, et al. Pharmacological studies in an herbal drug combination of St. John's wort (*Hypericum perforatum*) and passionflower (*Passiflora incarnata*): *In vitro* and *in vivo* evidence of synergy between Hypericum and Passiflora in antidepressant pharmacological models. Fitoterapia 2011;82(3):474–80.

Ghazanfarpour M, Sadeghi R, Abdolahian S, Latifnejad RR. The efficacy of Iranian herbal medicines in alleviating hot flushes: a systematic review. Int J Reprod Biomed (Yazd) 2016;14(3):155–66.

Gupta RK, Kumar D, Chaudhary AK, Maithani M, Singh R. Antidiabetic activity of *Passiflora incarnata* Linn. in streptozotocin-induced diabetes in mice. J Ethnopharmacol 2012;139(3):801–6.

Kargozar R, Azizi H, Salari R. A review of effective herbal medicines in controlling menopausal symptoms. Electron Physician 2017;9(11):5826–33.

Kaviani N, Tavakoli M, Tabanmehr M, Havaei R. The efficacy of *Passiflora incarnata* linnaeus in reducing dental anxiety in patients undergoing periodontal treatment. J Dent (Shiraz) 2013;14(2):68–72.

Keck ME, Nicolussi S, Spura K, Blohm C, Zahner C, Drewe J. Effect of the fixed combination of valerian, lemon balm, passionflower, and butterbur extracts (Ze 185) on the prescription pattern of benzodiazepines in hospitalized psychiatric patients – a retrospective case-control investigation. Phytother Res 2020;34(6):1436–45.

Lakhan SE, Vieira KF. Nutritional and herbal supplements for anxiety and anxiety-related disorders: systematic review. Nutr J 2010;9:42.

Lee J, Jung HY, Lee SI, Choi JH, Kim SG. Effects of *Passiflora incarnata* Linnaeus on polysomnographic sleep parameters in subjects with insomnia disorder: a double-blind randomized placebo-controlled study. Int Clin Psychopharmacol 2020;35(1):29–35.

Mansoor K, Qadan F, Hinum A, et al. An open prospective pilot study of a herbal combination "relief" as a supportive dietetic measure during alcohol withdrawal. Neuro Endocrinol Lett 2018;39(1):1–8.

Maroo N, Hazra A, Das T. Efficacy and safety of a polyherbal sedative-hypnotic formulation NSF-3 in primary insomnia in comparison with zolpidem: a randomized controlled trial. Indian J Pharmacol 2013;45(1):34–9.

Meier S, Haschke M, Zahner C, et al. Effects of a fixed herbal drug combination (Ze 185) to an experimental acute stress setting in healthy men – an explorative randomized placebo-controlled double-blind study. Phytomedicine 2018;39:85–92.

Melzer J, Schrader E, Brattström A, Schellenberg R, Saller R. Fixed herbal drug combination with and without butterbur (Ze 185) for the treatment of patients with somatoform disorders: randomized, placebo-controlled pharmaco-clinical trial. Phytother Res 2009;23(9):1303–8.

Miyasaka LS, Atallah AN, Soares BG. Passiflora for anxiety disorder. Cochrane Database Syst Rev 2007;1, CD004518.

Movafegh A, Alizadeh R, Hajimohamadi F, Esfehani F, Nejatfar M. Preoperative oral *Passiflora incarnata* reduces anxiety in ambulatory surgery patients: a double-blind, placebo-controlled study. Int Anesth Res Soc 2008;106(6):1728–32.

Ngan A, Conduit R. A double-blind, placebo-controlled investigation of the effects of *Passiflora incarnata* (passionflower) herbal tea on subjective sleep quality. Phytother Res 2011;25(8):1153–9.

Rokhtabnak F, Ghodraty MR, Kholdebarin A, et al. Comparing the effect of preoperative administration of melatonin and *Passiflora incarnata* on postoperative cognitive disorders in adult patients undergoing elective surgery. Anesth Pain Med 2016;7(1):e41238.

Sarris J, McIntyre E, Camfield DA. Plant-based medicines for anxiety disorders, part 2: a review of clinical studies with supporting preclinical evidence. CNS Drugs 2013;27(4):301–19.

Singh B, Singh D, Goel RK. Dual protective effect of *Passiflora incarnata* in epilepsy and associated post-ictal depression. J Ethnopharmacol 2012;139(1):273–9.

Yeung KS, Hernandez M, Mao JJ, Haviland I, Gubili J. Herbal medicine for depression and anxiety: a systematic review with assessment of potential psycho-oncologic relevance. Phytother Res 2018;32(5):865–91.

64

PEPPERMINT (*MENTHA PIPERITA*)
Leaf

GENERAL OVERVIEW

Peppermint is commonly employed as an oil (essential oil), although the whole leaf, including the aqueous extract peppermint tea, is also effective for many overlapping applications. Peppermint is the first herb to try for abdominal pain related to irritable bowel syndrome (IBS) due to its relaxing effect on the smooth muscles of the entire GI tract from esophagus to colon. It reduces spasms during endoscopic GI procedures. It is useful for various causes of nausea, but evidence is mixed for its efficacy with postoperative nausea. Peppermint the plant is a hybrid of water mint and spearmint. Note that spearmint (*Mentha spicata*) has been included in the research below for its use with hirsutism, and there may be some overlap in this regard with peppermint. Peppermint contains a high amount of the essential oil constituent menthol, which is its chief bioactive ingredient. High concentrations of menthol have demonstrated carcinogenicity in mice, but recommended dosing in humans is far below this level. Enteric-coated peppermint oil tends to avoid the upper GI side effects (mostly heartburn) when the intention is to treat IBS.

Clinical research indicates that peppermint, alone or in combination formulas, may be beneficial for gastric hypermotility, nausea and vomiting, functional dyspepsia, irritable bowel syndrome, infantile colic, pruritus gravidarum, nipple fissures, tension headache, cognitive performance, hirsutism, and athletic performance.

IN VITRO AND ANIMAL RESEARCH

Peppermint has smooth muscle relaxing properties. It has been shown in animal research to potently reduce the small and large intestinal contractility caused by acetylcholine and histamine. It may decrease gastric motility due to its antispasmodic effects. It also demonstrates smooth muscle relaxant properties in the trachea and sphincter of Oddi and increases bile secretion in rats. Pretreatment with peppermint essential oil has been shown to protect mouse liver and kidney from CCl4-induced toxicity through antioxidant and anti-inflammatory mechanisms.

Peppermint essential oil is stimulating, enhancing cognition and attention but not memory. The essential oil has demonstrated antioxidant properties. The dominant constituent menthol has calcium-channel blocking properties. Peppermint has been shown to reduce circulating testosterone by 23% in rats. Spearmint reduced it by 51%. Spearmint contains more carvone than peppermint, which may account for the difference. Peppermint has demonstrated virucidal activity against HSV-1 and HSV-2, Newcastle disease, vaccinia, Semliki Forest virus, and West Nile virus. It has been shown to have similar potency to gentamicin against Gram-positive bacteria and lesser potency than gentamicin against Gram-negative bacteria. Peppermint essential oil has demonstrated antifungal effects against 11 different fungi. It has shown some cancer prevention properties, protecting animal lungs against tobacco and animal testicles against radiation. It shows antitumorigenic properties against several human cancer cell lines. Menthol has been reported to induce PC-3 prostate cancer cell death in vitro by activating JNK.

HUMAN RESEARCH

Oral and Dental Disorders

A 5-day RCT in patients ($n = 80$) studied an oral moisturizing gel containing aloe and peppermint compared with a placebo gel for effects on mouth dryness and plaque development. By the third day, the mean oral health score was significantly better in the treatment group than in the placebo group ($P = 0.0001$), and by the fifth day, the mean score of mouth dryness in the intervention group was significantly lower than the placebo group ($P = 0.0001$). The authors concluded that this combination gel was useful for relieving mouth dryness, preventing dental plaque formation, and improving oral health, and thus may be used for improving oral care outcomes in ICUs (Atashi et al., 2018).

Gastrointestinal Disorders: Gastric Motility, Nausea, and Vomiting

A crossover RCT in healthy volunteers compared the effect of encapsulated peppermint oil 182 mg with placebo on intragastric pressure measurements before and during continuous intragastric infusion of a nutrient drink. In the fasting state, intragastric pressure and motility of the proximal stomach decreased significantly with peppermint administration compared with placebo ($P < 0.0001$ and $P < 0.05$, respectively). There was also a difference in appetite scores, which were reduced with peppermint. These differences disappeared when the intragastric infusion of a nutrient drink occurred. The authors concluded that peppermint oil reduces intragastric pressure, proximal phasic contractility, and appetite with little effect on gastric sensitivity, tone, accommodation, and nutrient tolerance (Papathanasopoulos et al., 2013).

An RCT in women ($n = 35$) who had undergone C-section compared peppermint inhaled aromatherapy with placebo aromatherapy and with standard anti-emetic therapy (ondansetron or promethazine), each administered PRN nausea postoperatively. The nausea levels of participants in the peppermint spirits group were significantly lower than those of participants in the other groups 2 and 5 min after the initial intervention. The authors concluded that peppermint essential oil inhalation may be useful in the treatment of postoperative nausea (Lane et al., 2012).

A four-night RCT in pregnant women ($n = 60$) with nausea and vomiting of pregnancy investigated four drops of peppermint in water placed at the bedside QHS compared with four drops of normal saline in water at the bedside. During the 4-day intervention, the severity of nausea showed a decreasing trend (especially by the fourth night) with peppermint and an increasing trend with placebo. The severity of nausea within 7 days after the intervention had a decreasing trend in both groups; however, the intensity was insignificantly lower with peppermint. The severity of nausea and vomiting did not differ between the two groups in 7 days before and after intervention. Intensity of vomiting did not differ between groups (Pasha et al., 2012).

A perioperative RCT in patients ($n = 60$) following cardiac surgery evaluated pre-extubation nebulizer aromatherapy with peppermint essential oil compared with a control group for effects on postoperative nausea and vomiting. With the intervention and control groups the frequency of nausea was 0.63 and 1.46, respectively; nausea duration was 3.78 min and 7.97 min, respectively; nausea severity was 2.43 and 4.61, respectively; and frequency of vomiting episodes in the first 4 h after extubation was 0.17 and 0.73, respectively ($P < 0.05$). The authors concluded that peppermint essential oil inhalation was beneficial for reducing nausea and vomiting after open-heart surgery, and its use was recommended (Maghami et al., 2020).

Gastrointestinal Disorders: Functional Dyspepsia

An RCT in patients ($n = 223$) with non-ulcer dyspepsia compared two different preparations of a fixed combination of peppermint oil and caraway oil (enteric-coated capsules of 90 mg peppermint oil plus 50 mg caraway oil and an enteric-soluble formulation of 36 mg peppermint oil plus 20 mg caraway oil). There was a statistically significant decline in pain intensity from beginning to end of therapy with both the enteric-coated and soluble formulations (-3.6 and -3.3 points, respectively; $P < 0.001$). Equivalent efficacy of both preparations was demonstrated ($P < 0.001$). Regarding "pain frequency," the efficacy of the enteric-coated preparation was significantly better ($P = 0.04$). Both preparations were well tolerated. Despite the higher dose, the adverse event "eructation with peppermint taste" was less frequent in the group treated with the enteric-coated formula (Friese and Köhler, 1999).

A 28-day RCT in patients ($n = 96$) with functional dyspepsia compared a fixed combination of peppermint and caraway oils (90/50 mg) with placebo. On day 29, the average intensity of pain was reduced by 40% and 22% from baseline with peppermint/caraway oil and placebo, respectively. Pressure, heaviness, and fullness were reduced by 43% and 22% with the combination oil and placebo, respectively. Improvement was rated as much or very much improved in 67% and 21% of the oil combination and placebo groups, respectively. The authors concluded that there was good tolerability and a favorable risk–benefit ratio of the peppermint/caraway combination product for the treatment of functional dyspepsia (May et al., 2000).

A 12-week partial crossover RCT in patients ($n = 120$) with functional dyspepsia studied STW 5-II (containing extracts from peppermint, licorice, bitter candy tuft, chamomile, caraway, and lemon balm) compared with placebo. Each patient received the treatment for 3 consecutive 4-week treatment blocks. The first two treatment blocks were fixed. For the third treatment period, medication was based upon the investigator's judgment of symptom improvement during the preceding treatment period. In patients without adequate control of symptoms, the treatment was switched, or if symptoms were controlled, the treatment was continued. During the first 4 weeks, the Gastrointestinal Symptom score decreased significantly in subjects on active treatment compared with placebo ($P < 0.001$). During the second 4-week period symptoms further improved in subjects who continued on active treatment or those who were switched to active treatment, while those switched to placebo deteriorated. After 8 weeks there was complete relief of symptoms in 43% and 3% of subjects on active treatment and placebo, respectively ($P < 0.001$). The authors concluded that this polyherbal preparation improved dyspeptic symptoms better than placebo (Madisch et al., 2004).

A 4-week RCT in patients ($n = 120$) with functional dyspepsia studied a fixed combination preparation consisting of peppermint oil and caraway oil BID compared with the prokinetic agent cisapride 10 mg TID (*taken off the market in 2000 for prolonged QT interval*). Mean reduction of pain was 4.62 points and 4.6 points with the peppermint combination and cisapride, respectively ($P = 0.021$). Pain frequency was reduced by 4.65 and 4.16 points with the peppermint combination and cisapride, respectively ($P = 0.0034$). Comparable results were attained with both treatments in the Dyspeptic Discomfort Score, which included the other dyspeptic symptoms as well as intestinal and extraintestinal autonomic symptoms, in the prognosis as appraised by the physician, and in the CGI scales. Results were also similar between groups in *Helicobacter pylori*-positive patients and patients with initially intense epigastric pain. The authors concluded that the peppermint-caraway oil combination preparation appeared to be comparable to cisapride and provided an effective means for treatment of functional dyspepsia (Madisch et al., 1999).

A 4-week RCT in patients ($n = 60$) with functional dyspepsia investigated Iberogast in two different formulations (peppermint, chamomile, caraway, licorice, lemon balm, angelica, celandine, and milk thistle with or without bitter candy tuft) compared with placebo for effects on gastrointestinal symptoms. The herbal preparations showed a clinically significant improvement in the Gastrointestinal Symptom score compared with placebo after 2 and 4 weeks of treatment ($P < 0.001$). No statistically significant difference could be observed between the efficacy of the two different herbal preparations ($P > 0.05$), but a solid improvement of GI symptoms could be achieved earlier with the herbal preparation that contained the bitter candy tuft ($P = 0.023$). The authors concluded that Iberogast and its modified formulation improved dyspeptic symptoms better than placebo and that the bitter candy tuft had an additive effect (Madisch et al., 2001).

Gastrointestinal Disorders: Irritable Bowel Syndrome and Infantile Colic

A 2019 systematic review to assess the efficacy of peppermint oil for IBS found 12 RCTs ($n = 835$) that met inclusion criteria. The RR for global symptom improvement and reduction of abdominal pain for peppermint oil and placebo were 2.39 and 1.78, respectively ($P < 0.00001$ for each). Overall, there were no differences in the reported adverse effects. The NNT with peppermint oil to prevent one patient from having persistent symptoms was three for global symptoms and four for abdominal pain. The authors concluded that peppermint oil was shown to be a safe and effective therapy for pain and global symptoms in adults with IBS (Alammar et al., 2019).

A 2014 systematic review assessing the efficacy of peppermint oil for IBS found nine RCTs ($n = 726$) that met inclusion criteria. Peppermint oil was found to be significantly superior to placebo for global improvement of IBS symptoms (RR = 2.23) and improvement in abdominal pain (RR = 2.14). Although peppermint oil patients were significantly more likely to experience an adverse event, such events were mild and transient in nature. The most reported adverse event was heartburn. The authors concluded that peppermint oil was a safe and effective short-term treatment for IBS (Khanna et al., 2014).

A 2009 systematic review to assess the efficacy of fiber, antispasmodics, and peppermint oil for IBS found 12 studies that met inclusion criteria, four of which involved peppermint oil ($n = 392$) and revealed a decreased risk of persistent symptoms (RR = 0.43). Fiber and antispasmodics also demonstrated a decreased risk of persistent symptoms (RR = 0.87 and RR = 0.68, respectively). The authors concluded that fiber, antispasmodics, and peppermint oil were all more effective than placebo for IBS (Ford et al., 2008).

A 6-week RCT in patients ($n = 74$) diagnosed with diarrhea-dominant IBS compared peppermint oil with placebo TID. By the sixth week, abdominal pain scores were improved with peppermint oil compared with placebo (4.94 and 6.15, respectively; $P < 0.001$). But 2 weeks after the end of treatment the pain score again increased in the peppermint group (6.09). Other symptoms and quality of life did not improve significantly. The authors concluded that peppermint oil provided transient relief of abdominal pain in diarrhea predominant IBS, but other symptoms were not affected (Alam et al., 2013).

A 1-month RCT in patients ($n = 110$) with IBS symptoms compared Colpermin, a pH-dependent enteric-coated peppermint oil, with placebo TID-QID AC. In the peppermint and placebo groups, respectively, there was reduced severity of abdominal pain in 79% and 43%; reduced abdominal distention in 83%

and 29%; reduced stool frequency in 83% and 32%; fewer borborygmi in 73% and 31%; and less flatulence in 79% and 22%. One patient on Colpermin experienced heartburn (because of chewing the capsules) and one developed a mild transient skin rash (Liu et al., 1997).

An 8-week RCT in patients ($n = 57$) with IBS, for whom SIBO and celiac disease had been excluded, compared peppermint oil two enteric-coated capsules BID with placebo for 4 weeks. By the fourth week there was more than a 50% reduction of total IBS symptom score in 75% and 38% of the peppermint and placebo groups, respectively ($P < 0.009$). The total IBS score decreased significantly from baseline to the fourth and eighth week of follow-up in the peppermint group (2.19, 1.07, 1.60, respectively), but there was no change from baseline with placebo. The authors concluded that a 4-week treatment with peppermint oil improved abdominal symptoms in patients with irritable bowel syndrome (Cappello et al., 2007).

An 8-week RCT in patients ($n = 90$) with IBS compared Colpermin, a pH-dependent enteric-coated peppermint oil, with placebo TID. The number of subjects free from abdominal pain or discomfort by the eighth week was 14 and 6 with peppermint and placebo, respectively ($P < 0.001$). The severity of abdominal pain was also reduced significantly, and quality of life was significantly improved in the peppermint group compared with controls. There was no significant adverse reaction. The authors concluded that this enteric-coated peppermint oil preparation was effective and safe as a therapeutic agent in patients with IBS suffering from abdominal pain or discomfort (Merat et al., 2010).

A 2-week RCT in children ($n = 42$) with IBS compared pH-dependent, enteric-coated peppermint oil capsules with placebo. After 2 weeks, 75% of those receiving peppermint oil had reduced severity of pain associated with IBS. The authors concluded that peppermint oil may be used as a therapeutic agent during the symptomatic phase of IBS (Kline et al., 2001).

An 8-week RCT in patients ($n = 190$) with IBS compared the efficacy of small-intestinal-release peppermint oil 182 mg, ileocolonic-release peppermint oil 182 mg, and placebo for reduction of IBS symptoms. Abdominal pain response ($\geq 30\%$ improvement) occurred in 46.8%, 41.3%, and 34.4% of patients in the small-intestinal-release, ileocolonic-release, and placebo groups, respectively ($P = 0.170$ and $P = 0.385$ for the two treatment groups vs placebo, respectively). Overall relief occurred in 9.7%, 1.6%, and 4.7% of the two treatment groups and placebo, respectively (n.s.). However, the small-intestinal-release formulation of peppermint oil did produce greater improvements than placebo in secondary outcomes of abdominal pain ($P = 0.016$), discomfort ($P = 0.020$), and IBS severity ($P = 0.020$). Mild AEs were more common in both peppermint oil groups ($P < 0.005$). The authors concluded that neither small-intestinal-release nor ileocolonic-release peppermint oil produced statistically significant reductions in abdominal pain response or overall symptom relief, but that the small-intestinal-release peppermint oil did reduce abdominal pain, discomfort, and IBS severity (Weerts et al., 2020).

A 1-month RCT in children 4–13 years of age ($n = 120$) with functional abdominal pain studied Colpermin, a pH-dependent enteric coated peppermint oil, compared with Lactol (*Bacillus coagulans* plus fructooligosaccharides) and with placebo. Improvement in pain duration and frequency was better in both active groups ($P = 0.001$ and $P = 0.001$ for pain and frequency, respectively, with Colpermin; and $P = 0.12$ and $P = 0.001$ for pain and frequency, respectively, with Lactol). Pain severity decreased over placebo with Colpermin ($P = 0.0001$) but did not reach significance with Lactol ($P = 0.373$). The authors concluded that pH-dependent peppermint oil was superior to placebo for decreasing severity, duration, and frequency of abdominal pain in functional GI disorders (Asgarshirazi et al., 2015).

A 7-day crossover RCT in infants ($n = 30$) with colic compared peppermint with simethicone. At the end of the study, episodes of colic fell from 3.9 to 1.6 and crying duration decreased from 192 min to 111 min per day with similar reductions seen in both groups. All mothers reported decreased frequency and duration of episodes of colic and there were no differences between peppermint and simethicone. The authors concluded that peppermint could be useful for infantile colic (Alves et al., 2012).

Gastrointestinal Disorders: Scope-Induced Spasm

A non-randomized prospective study in patients ($n = 8269$) undergoing esophagogastroduodenoscopy (EGD) compared peppermint oil with hyoscine butyl bromide, with glucagon, and with control for antispasmodic effects. Overall, the antispasmodic scores (score 1–5 where 5 indicates no spasm) were 4.024 and 4.063 with peppermint and hyoscine, respectively (no significant difference). In patients older than 70 years, the scores were 4.025 and 4.063 for peppermint and hyoscine, respectively (no difference). However, in the patients younger than 70 years, the scores were 3.923 and 4.062 for peppermint and hyoscine, respectively, indicating a significant superiority of hyoscine ($P < 0.001$). In the older group, peppermint had better scores than glucagon (4.073 vs 3.797; $P < 0.05$). The authors concluded that peppermint oil was useful as an antispasmodic during EGD, especially in elderly patients (Imagawa et al., 2012).

A single-application RCT in patients ($n = 87$) scheduled for EGD compared intra-procedural gastric mucosal spraying of L-menthol 160 mg with placebo for effects on gastric peristalsis. Gastric peristalsis was completely suppressed in 35.6% and 7.1% of patients in the L-menthol and placebo groups, respectively ($P < 0.001$). No or mild peristalsis at the completion of endoscopy occurred in 77.8% of patients in the L-menthol group and only 1 of 35 patients in this group had minor peristalsis interfere with the intragastric examination (Hiki et al., 2011).

An RCT in patients ($n = 100$) undergoing EGD studied the gastric dynamic effects of hyoscine-*N*-butylbromide administered IM plus a placebo solution administered intraluminally endoscopically compared with a placebo solution administered IM plus a peppermint oil solution administered intraluminally. The change in diameter of the pyloric ring before and after administration was significantly larger with peppermint oil than with hyhoscine-*N*-butylbromide injection. The change in diameter between maximally and minimally opened pyloric ring states was significantly smaller with peppermint. The time until disappearance of the contraction ring in the gastric antrum was shorter with peppermint (97.1 s vs 185.9 s; $P < 0.0001$). No significant side effects were associated with peppermint, while hyoscine produced dry mouth, blurred vision, and urinary retention. The authors concluded that peppermint oil solution given intraluminally during EGD can be used as an antispasmodic agent with superior efficacy and fewer side effects than hyoscine-N-butylbromide administered by intramuscular injection (Hiki et al., 2003).

A single-dose RCT in adult patients ($n = 65$) undergoing colonoscopy compared Colpermin, a pH-dependent enteric-coated peppermint oil, with placebo given 4h prior to the procedure. Duration time was shorter for both total procedure and cecal intubation with peppermint than with placebo. Scores for colonic spasm and pain were significantly lower and endoscopist satisfaction was higher with peppermint. Patients in the peppermint group were more willing to repeat colonoscopy in the future. The authors concluded that enteric-coated peppermint was beneficial in terms of procedure time, colon spasm, endoscopist satisfaction, and patient perception (Shavakhi et al., 2012).

An RCT in patients ($n = 48$) undergoing screening colonoscopy compared peppermint oil with placebo for procedural efficacy. During the procedure, 50 mL of either solution was directly injected through the scope once the cecum was reached. Mean total colonoscopy time with peppermint and placebo was 17.8 min and 21.9 min, respectively ($P = 0.07$). Mean cecal intubation time with peppermint and placebo was 7.2 min and 10.3 min, respectively ($P = 0.04$). Complete absence of bowel spasticity was observed among 58.3% and 45.8% of patients in the peppermint oil and placebo groups, respectively ($P = 0.05$). More than 75% of bowel was visualized in 83% of patients in both groups ($P = 0.56$). Mean ADR was 45.8% and 37.5% with peppermint and placebo, respectively ($P = 0.56$). The authors concluded that topical peppermint oil reduced bowel spasticity and could result in better visualization of the bowel during screening colonoscopy (Shah et al., 2019).

Musculoskeletal Disorders: Musculoskeletal Pain Syndromes

A 4-week RCT in patients ($n = 60$) with neck pain and a Neck Disability Index score > 10% investigated a 3% concentration cream composed of four essential oils (marjoram, black pepper, lavender, and peppermint) compared with an unscented cream, each applied 2 g to the neck QD. Pressure pain threshold scores for the left and right upper trapezius improved (2.96 and 2.88, respectively) with the essential oil cream. The Neck Disability Index also showed significant improvement with the active cream ($P = 0.02$). Motion analysis system values before and after the intervention showed significant improvement of the 10 motion areas in the experimental group. VAS scores improved significantly for both groups ($P < 0.05$). The authors concluded that the essential oil cream in this study could be used to improve neck pain (Ou et al., 2014).

Neurological Disorders: Tension and Migraine Headache

A 2020 systematic review to assess herbal treatments for acute and prophylactic treatment of migraine headaches found 19 trials that met inclusion criteria, including studies of feverfew, butterbur, curcumin, menthol/peppermint oil, coriander, citron, Damask rose, chamomile, and lavender. Overall, there was positive, albeit limited evidence for butterbur, and mixed findings for feverfew. There were positive, preliminary findings on curcumin, citron, and coriander as a prophylactic treatment for migraine, and the use of menthol and chamomile as an acute treatment. High risk for bias was noted in many of the studies. The authors concluded that several herbal medicines, via their multifactorial physiological influences, may enhance the treatment of migraine and that further high-quality research was warranted (Lopresti et al., 2020).

An RCT in patients ($n = 120$) with migraine headaches compared the efficacy of two drops of intranasal lidocaine 4%, peppermint 1.5% essential oil, or placebo, applied abortively. Repeat dosing was given after 15 min PRN. Patients rated the impact of the intervention as "strong" in 41.5%, 42.1%, and 4.9% of the lidocaine, peppermint, and placebo groups, respectively ($P < 0.001$). In 31.7%, 44.7%, and 7.3% of the lidocaine, peppermint, and placebo groups, respectively, the headache was relieved 5 min after intranasal drops ($P < 0.01$). The subsequent headache frequency showed a significant decrease from baseline in all three study groups ($P < 0.0001$) with no difference between groups. The authors concluded that nasal application of peppermint oil and lidocaine produced similar strong reductions in the intensity and frequency of headache and relieved the majority of patients' pain (Rafieian-Kopaei et al., 2019).

An RCT in patients ($n = 41$) with tension headaches studied 10% peppermint oil in ethanol compared with traces of peppermint oil in ethanol (placebo), each with or without acetaminophen. Four headache episodes per patient were treated in a double-blind, randomized crossover design. Each headache attack was treated by the administration of two capsules of the oral medication (1000 mg of acetaminophen or placebo) and the cutaneous application across the forehead and temples of the oil preparation (peppermint oil or placebo solution). Compared with the application of placebo, the 10% peppermint oil solution significantly reduced the clinical headache intensity at 15 min ($P < 0.01$) and this reduction continued over the 1-h observation period. Acetaminophen was also superior to placebo ($P < 0.01$). There was no significant difference between the efficacy of 1000 mg of acetaminophen and 10% peppermint oil solution. Simultaneous application of 1000 mg of acetaminophen and 10% peppermint oil produced an additive effect, which was not statistically significant. The patients reported no adverse events. The authors concluded that 10% peppermint oil in ethanol alleviated tension-type headaches (Göbel et al., 1996).

An RCT in healthy subjects ($n = 32$) with headache compared peppermint oil, eucalyptus oil and ethanol applied in various combinations topically to the forehead and temples. The combination of peppermint and ethanol produced a significant analgesic effect with a reduction in sensitivity to headache. The combination of peppermint oil, eucalyptus oil, and ethanol increased cognitive performance and had a muscle-relaxing and mental-relaxing effect but had little influence on pain sensitivity. The authors concluded that these essential oils could exert significant effects associated with the pathophysiology of headaches (Gobel et al., 1994).

Neurological Disorders: Postherpetic Neuralgia

A case of a 76-year-old woman whose post-zoster pain that had been resistant to standard therapies was reported. The patient was instructed to apply neat (nondiluted) peppermint oil (containing 10% menthol) to her skin. This resulted in an almost immediate improvement in her pain. This pain relief persisted for 4–6 h after application of the oil. During 2 months of follow-up she had only a minor side effects, with continuing analgesia (Davies et al., 2002).

Psychiatric Disorders: Cognitive Performance

An acutely dosed crossover RCT in young adults ($n = 24$) compared single doses of 50 μL or 100 μL of encapsulated peppermint essential oil to a matched placebo on psychological functioning. The higher dose of peppermint improved performance on the Rapid Visual Information Processing task at 1- and 3-h postdose, and both doses attenuated fatigue and improved performance of Serial 3 Subtraction at 3 h. The authors concluded that peppermint essential oil with high levels of menthol/menthone beneficially modulated performance on demanding cognitive tasks (Kennedy et al., 2018).

An acutely dosed RCT in volunteers ($n = 144$) compared diffusion of peppermint with diffusion of ylang-ylang and with no essential oil for effects on cognitive performance and mood. Using the Cognitive Drug Research battery, peppermint was found to enhance memory, whereas ylang-ylang impaired it and slowed processing speed. Peppermint increased alertness. Ylang-ylang decreased alertness and increased calmness. The authors concluded that the aromas of essential oils can produce significant and idiosyncratic effects on both subjective and objective measures of human behavior (Moss et al., 2008).

Psychiatric Disorders: Tobacco Addiction

A two-week RCT in smoker volunteers ($n = 24$) investigated the effects of peppermint on nicotine metabolism (conversion to cotinine). The two groups were administered a peppermint drink TID for 1 week followed by no peppermint and no menthol cigarettes for 1 week, and this was compared with the same treatments in reverse order (no peppermint/menthol for 1 week, then peppermint drink for 1 week). Mean nicotine/cotinine ratio during the peppermint drink period for all participants was higher than that during the off-menthol period (1.327 and 0.993, respectively; $P < 0.0001$). The authors concluded that the peppermint drink reduced the conversion of nicotine to cotinine. By extension, menthol cigarettes may reduce metabolism of nicotine (Ghazi et al., 2011).

Dermatological Disorders: Pressure Ulcers, Pruritus Gravidarum, Nipple Fissures, and Hirsutism (Spearmint)

An RCT in ICU patients ($n = 150$) with head trauma evaluated peppermint gel TID for up to 14 days applied to high-risk pressure points compared with a placebo gel for prevention of pressure injuries. The incidence rate of pressure injuries (Stage I or greater) was 22.8% and 77% in the intervention and placebo groups, respectively ($P < 0.001$). The sacrum was the most common site for pressure injuries. The authors concluded that peppermint gel had a preventive effect on pressure injuries in head trauma ICU patients (Babamohamadi et al., 2019).

A 2-week RCT in pregnant women ($n = 96$) with pruritus gravidarum investigated peppermint oil 0.5% in sesame oil compared with placebo oil applied BID. The severity of the itch showed a significant reduction with peppermint compared with placebo ($P = 0.003$). The authors concluded that peppermint oil could be effective in reducing the severity of pruritus gravidarum (Akhavan Amjadi et al., 2012).

An RCT in primiparous breastfeeding women ($n = 196$) compared peppermint water with expressed breast milk for prevention of nipple pain and cracks. Nipple and areola cracks occurred in 9% and 27% of women in the peppermint and breast milk groups, respectively ($P < 0.01$). Women who used the peppermint water were less likely to have a cracked nipple than women who did not use peppermint water (RR = 3.6). Nipple pain was less in the peppermint water group than the expressed breast milk group (OR = 5.6; $P < 0.005$). The authors concluded that peppermint water was effective in the prevention of nipple pain and damage in breastfeeding women (Sayyah Melli et al., 2007).

A 14-day RCT in primiparous breast-feeding women ($n = 110$) studied menthol essence four drops compared with breast milk four drops applied to the nipple and areola after each feeding. The difference in mean intensity of pain and nipple fissure before treatment (8.55), and at day 10 (4.26) and day 14 (1.32) was significant with the menthol essence ($P < 0.001$). Nipple discharge occurrence decreased in the menthol group from 75% at baseline to 31% and 15% at days 10 and 14, respectively ($P < 0.001$) (Akbari et al., 2014).

A 6-week RCT in primiparous breastfeeding women ($n = 216$) compared a peppermint gel with a lanolin gel and with a neutral ointment applied daily for 14 days for effects on nipple soreness. At serial follow-up visits, nipple cracking was less with peppermint than with lanolin or placebo (df = 6; $P = 0.01$). Relative risk of nipple cracking was less for peppermint than for lanolin (RR = 1.85 and 2.41 for peppermint and lanolin, respectively). The author concluded that peppermint gel may have an application in breastfeeding women in prevention of nipple cracks (Melli et al., 2007).

A study of women ($n = 21$) with hirsutism, 12 with PCOS and 9 with idiopathic hirsutism, assessed the effect on testosterone levels of spearmint tea one cup daily for 5 days in the follicular phase of the cycle. After treatment with spearmint teas, there was a significant decrease in free testosterone and increase in LH, FSH, and estradiol. There were no significant decreases in total testosterone or DHEA-S levels. The authors concluded that spearmint could be an alternative to antiandrogenic treatment for mild hirsutism (Akdogan et al., 2004).

A 30-day RCT in women ($n = 42$) with hirsutism compared spearmint tea BID with placebo tea for effects on hormones and degree of hirsutism. Free and total testosterone levels were significantly reduced over the 30-day period in the spearmint tea group ($P < 0.05$). LH and FSH levels increased ($P < 0.05$). Subjective assessments of hirsutism were significantly improved in the spearmint tea group ($P < 0.05$). There was, however, no significant reduction in the objective Ferriman-Gallwey ratings of hirsutism between the two trial groups over the trial duration ($P = 0.12$). The authors concluded that the preliminary findings were encouraging, but the study duration was not long enough, and a much longer future study was proposed (Grant, 2010).

Disorders of Vitality: Athletic Performance

An acutely dosed RCT in healthy male university students ($n = 30$) compared oral peppermint oil with no treatment for effects on physical performance and pulmonary function. At 5 min after the dose, peppermint compared with control showed an increase in grip force (36.1%), standing vertical jump (7.0%), standing long jump (6.4%), FEV1 (35.1%), PIF (66.4%), and PEF (65.1%). However, after 1 h, only PIF continued to show a significant increase with peppermint compared with baseline and with the control group. The authors concluded that peppermint may produce an improvement in spirometrics via effects on bronchial smooth muscle tonicity with or without affecting the lung surfactant (Meamarbashi and Rajabi, 2014).

A 10-day open-label study in healthy male students ($n = 12$) assessed the effect of consumption of 500 mL of mineral water containing 0.05 mL of peppermint essential oil on exercise parameters. There were significant pre-to-post improvements in FVC (4.57 vs 4.79; $P < 0.001$), PEF (8.50 vs 8.87; $P < 0.01$), PIF (5.71 vs 6.58; $P < 0.005$), time to exhaustion (664 s vs 830 s; $P < 0.001$), work (78.3 KJ vs 118.7 KJ; $P < 0.001$), and power (114.3 KW vs 139.4 KW; $P < 0.001$). There were also significant differences in VO_2 (2.74 L/min vs 3.03 L/min; $P < 0.001$) and VCO_2 (3.08 L/min vs 3.73 L/min; $P < 0.001$). The authors concluded that peppermint essential oil improved exercise performance, gas analysis, spirometry, BP, and respiratory rate in young male students, possibly via relaxation of bronchial smooth muscles, increases in ventilation and brain oxygen concentration, and decreases in the blood lactate level (Meamarbashi, 2013).

Infectious Diseases: Upper Respiratory Infection

A 3-day RCT in patients ($n = 60$) with URI symptoms compared a throat spray containing essential oils of peppermint, rosemary, *Eucalyptus citriodora*, *E. globulus*, and *Origanum syriacum* with placebo spray, each applied five times a day. Improvement in symptom severity 20 min following the spray use was greater with the essential oil than with placebo ($P = 0.019$). There was no difference in symptom severity between the two groups after three days of treatment ($P = 0.042$). The authors concluded that application of these five aromatic plants produced significant and immediate improvement in symptoms of upper respiratory ailment but that the effect was not significant after 3 days of treatment (Ben-Arye et al., 2011).

Oncologic Disorders: Chemotherapy-Induced Nausea and Vomiting

An RCT in cancer patients ($n = 200$) undergoing chemotherapy and on usual anti-emetic therapy compared the addition of encapsulated spearmint essential oil two drops, with encapsulated peppermint essential oil two drops, with placebo and with a control group for effect on chemo-induced nausea and vomiting. The additional treatments were given 30 min before chemo and repeated every 4 h for two doses. There was a significant reduction in the intensity and number of

emetic events in the first 24 h with spearmint and peppermint ($P < 0.05$) when compared with placebo and the control group. No adverse effects were reported. The cost of treatment was reduced when essential oils were used. The authors concluded that spearmint and peppermint essential oils were safe and effective as well as cost-effective in chemo-induced nausea and vomiting (Tayarani-Najaran et al., 2013).

ACTIVE CONSTITUENTS

- Carbohydrates
  - Polysaccharides (antitumor): glucuronic acid, galacturonic acid, glucose, galactose, arabinose
- Phenolic compounds
  - Phenylpropanoids (antioxidant, antimutagenic, antitumor, antimicrobial): caffeic acid, chlorogenic acid, rosmarinic acid
  - Flavonoids: luteolin (anti-inflammatory, antispasmodic, antibacterial, hepatoprotective, anti-estrogenic, antiproliferative), hesperidin, rutin (antioxidant, anti-inflammatory, antidiabetic, nephroprotective, anti-osteoporotic, antispasmodic, neuroprotective, anti-anxiety)
    - Tannins
- Terpenes
  - Monoterpenes: menthol (carminative, antispasmodic): see aromatic compounds
  - Triterpenes: α-amyrin
  - Tetraterpenes/Carotenoids: *a*- and *b*-carotenes
- Aromatic compounds: menthol (up to 50% of the oil content, carminative, antispasmodic), menthone (20%–30%), cineole (2%–13%), pulegone (1%–11%), menthyl acetate, menthofuran, limonene

PEPPERMINT COMMONLY USED PREPARATIONS AND DOSAGE (FOR ADULTS UNLESS OTHERWISE SPECIFIED)

The following are examples of some available formulations and ranges of dosing for commercial herbal products. See Part III Introduction "How to prescribe medicinal herbs" for further guidance on herbal advising and prescribing.

Leaf

Do not use internally or around the face in infants and young children due to potential for bronchospasm, tongue spasms, possibility of respiratory arrest.

For Dyspepsia

- Infusion of dried leaf: 1 tsp per cup TID prn.
- Tincture of dried leaf (1:5, 40%–75%): 1–5 mL TID AC.
- Powdered extract: 700 mg (1/3 tsp) BID.
- Capsule or tablet of peppermint leaf: 700 mg TID.
- Essential oil: 3–5 drops mixed with 3–5 drops caraway oil added to water TID AC.

For IBS

- 1–2 enteric-coated capsules containing 0.1–0.2 mL (100-200 mg) of peppermint oil BID to TID (1 capsule for children weighing 60–100 lbs).
- Essential oil (therapeutic grade): 3–5 drops in water TID AC (is as effective and EC capsules but more likely to cause heartburn due to relaxation of the lower esophageal sphincter).

pH-dependent and enteric coated peppermint oil preparations release the oil in the small bowel to minimize the relaxation of the LES.

For Tension or Mixed Headaches

Peppermint essential oil 3–5 drops in 3–5 mL base oil (like olive oil, grapeseed oil, almond oil) applied to the temples at the onset of the headache and every 30–60 min PRN.

SAFETY AND PRECAUTION

Side Effects

Heartburn, anal burning, blurred vision, nausea, and vomiting have been reported. Allergic reactions may occur with topical use. Large doses may reduce sperm maturation.

Peppermint oil should not be used internally or on or near the face in infants and young children due to potential for bronchospasm, tongue spasms, and respiratory arrest.

Toxicity

The LD_{50} of peppermint oil in rats is 4400 mg/kg, which is approximately 300 mL/kg as an estimated human equivalent.

Peppermint has been shown in large doses to cause seizures in rats. The maximum recommended human oral dose of peppermint oil is 1.2 mL, which is 116× less than the lowest seizure-inducing dose in rats.

Pugelone has been shown to be carcinogenic and to produce cyst-like lesions in the brains of rats (*pugelone content of peppermint varies between sites of cultivation and age of leaves, with older leaves having considerably less pugelone*). Excessive doses have been associated with interstitial nephritis and acute renal failure.

Pregnancy and Lactation

Avoid essential oil in pregnancy due to anti-androgen and emenegogic effects. There is insufficient data to assess its safety during lactation. The small amount of peppermint in over-the-counter medications, topical preparations, and herbal teas is likely safe in pregnant and lactating women and in young children.

Disease Interactions

- Due to LES relaxation avoid in patients with GERD or hiatal hernia (or cautiously use enteric coated capsules).
- Due to choleretic effect avoid in patients with cholelithiasis or cholecystitis.

Drug Interactions

- CYP: Inhibits CYP1A2/2C8/2C9/2C19/2D6 and 3A4 enzymes.
- May increase bioavailability of felodipine.
- May increase or decrease levels of cyclosporine.
- Can decrease dermal absorption of 5-fluorouracil.
- May increase levels of simvastatin.

REFERENCES

Akbari SA, Alamolhoda SH, Baghban AA, Mirabi P. Effects of menthol essence and breast milk on the improvement of nipple fissures in breastfeeding women. J Res Med Sci 2014;19(7):629–33.

Akdogan M, Ozguner M, Kocak A, Oncu M, Cicek E. Effects of peppermint teas on plasma testosterone, follicle-stimulating hormone, and luteinizing hormone levels and testicular tissue in rats. Urology 2004;64(2):394–8.

Akhavan Amjadi M, Mojab F, Kamranpour SB. The effect of peppermint oil on symptomatic treatment of pruritus in pregnant women. Iran J Pharm Res 2012;11(4):1073–7.

Alam MS, Roy PK, Miah AR, et al. Efficacy of peppermint oil in diarrhea predominant IBS—a double blind randomized placebo—controlled study. Mymensingh Med J 2013;22(1):27–30.

Alammar N, Wang L, Saberi B, et al. The impact of peppermint oil on the irritable bowel syndrome: a meta-analysis of the pooled clinical data. BMC Complement Altern Med 2019;19:21.

Alves JG, de Brito RC, Cavalcanti TS. Effectiveness of Mentha piperita in the treatment of infantile colic: a crossover study. Evid Based Complement Alternat Med 2012;981:352.

Asgarshirazi M, Shariat M, Dalili H. Comparison of the effects of pH-dependent peppermint oil and synbiotic lactol (*Bacillus coagulans* + fructooligosaccharides) on childhood functional abdominal pain: a randomized placebo-controlled study. Iran Red Crescent Med J 2015;17(4), e23844.

Atashi V, Yazdannik A, Mahjobipoor H, Ghafari S, Bekhradi R, Yousefi H. The effects of Aloe vera-peppermint (Veramin) moisturizing gel on mouth dryness and oral health among patients hospitalized in intensive care units: a triple-blind randomized placebo-controlled trial. J Res Pharm Pract 2018;7(2):104–10.

Babamohamadi H, Ansari Z, Nobahar M, Mirmohammadkhani M. The effects of peppermint gel on prevention of pressure injury in hospitalized patients with head trauma in neurosurgical ICU: a double-blind randomized controlled trial. Complement Ther Med 2019;47:102223.

Ben-Arye E, Dudai N, Eini A, Torem M, Schiff E, Rakover Y. Treatment of upper respiratory tract infections in primary care: a randomized study using aromatic herbs. Evid Based Complement Alternat Med 2011;690346.

Cappello G, Spezzaferro M, Grossi L, Manzoli L, Marzio L. Peppermint oil (Mintoil) in the treatment of irritable bowel syndrome: a prospective double blind placebo-controlled randomized trial. Dig Liver Dis 2007;39(6):530–6.

Davies SJ, Harding LM, Baranowski AP. A novel treatment of postherpetic neuralgia using peppermint oil. Clin J Pain 2002;18(3):200–2.

Ford AC, Talley NJ, Spiegel BM, et al. Effect of fibre, antispasmodics, and peppermint oil in the treatment of irritable bowel syndrome: systematic review and meta-analysis. BMJ 2008;337:a2313.

Friese J, Köhler S. Peppermint oil-caraway oil fixed combination in non-ulcer dyspepsia comparison of the effect of 2 Galenical preparations. Pharmazie 1999;54(3):210–5.

Ghazi AM, Salhab AS, Arafat TA, Irshaid YM. Effect of mint drink on metabolism of nicotine as measured by nicotine to cotinine ratio in urine of Jordanian smoking volunteers. Nicotine Tob Res 2011;13(8):661–7.

Göbel H, Fresenius J, Heinze A, Dworschak M, Soyka D. Effectiveness of Oleum Menthae piperitae and paracetamol in therapy of tension headache. Nervenarzt 1996;67(8):672–81.

Gobel H, Schmidt G, Soyka D. Effect of peppermint and eucalyptus oil preparations on neurophysiological and experimental algesimetric headache parameters. Cephalalgia 1994;14(3):228–34. discussion 182.

Grant P. Spearmint herbal tea has significant anti-androgen effects in polycystic ovarian syndrome. A randomized controlled trial. Phytother Res 2010;24(2):186–8.

Hiki N, Kaminishi M, Yasuda K, et al. Antiperistaltic effect and safety of L-menthol sprayed on the gastric mucosa for upper GI endoscopy: a phase III, multicenter, randomized, double-blind, placebo-controlled study. Gastrointest Endosc 2011;73(5):932–41.

Hiki N, Kurosaka H, Tatsutomi Y, et al. Peppermint oil reduces gastric spasm during upper endoscopy: a randomized, double-blind, double-dummy controlled trial. Gastrointest Endosc 2003;57(4):475–82.

Imagawa A, Hata H, Nakatsu M, et al. Peppermint oil solution is useful as an antispasmodic drug for esophagogastroduodenoscopy, especially for elderly patients. Dig Dis Sci 2012;57(9):2379–84.

Kennedy D, Okello E, Chazot P, et al. Volatile terpenes and brain function: investigation of the cognitive and mood effects of Mentha × Piperita L. essential oil with in vitro properties relevant to central nervous system function. Nutrients 2018;10(8), E1029.

Khanna R, MacDonald JK, Levesque BG. Peppermint oil for the treatment of irritable bowel syndrome: a systematic review and meta-analysis. J Clin Gastroenterol 2014;48(6):505–12.

Kline RM, Kline JJ, Di Palma J, Barbero GJ. Enteric-coated, pH-dependent peppermint oil capsules for the treatment of irritable bowel syndrome in children. J Pediatr 2001;138(1):125–8.

Lane B, Cannella K, Bowen C, et al. Examination of the effectiveness of peppermint aromatherapy on nausea in women post C-section. J Holist Nurs 2012;30(2):90–104. quiz 105–6.

Liu JH, Chen GH, Yeh HZ, Huang CK, Poon SK. Enteric-coated peppermint-oil capsules in the treatment of irritable bowel syndrome: a prospective, randomized trial. J Gastroenterol 1997;32(6):765–8.

Lopresti A, Smith S, Drummond P. Herbal treatments for migraine: a systematic review of randomized-controlled studies. Phytother Res 2020;34(10):2493–517.

Madisch A, Heydenreich C, Wieland V, Hufnagel R, Hotz J. Treatment of functional dyspepsia with a fixed peppermint oil and caraway oil combination preparation compared with cisapride. A multicentre, reference-controlled double-blind equivalence study. Arzneimittelforschung 1999;49(11):925–32.

Madisch A, Holtmann G, Mayr G, et al. Treatment of functional dyspepsia with a herbal preparation. A double-blind, randomized, placebo-controlled, multicenter trial. Digestion 2004;69(1):45–52.

Madisch A, Melderis H, Mayr G, Sassin I, Hotz J. A plant extract and its modified preparation in functional dyspepsia. Results of a double-blind placebo controlled comparative study. Z Gastroenterol 2001;39(7):511–7.

Maghami M, Afazel MR, Azizi-Fini I, Maghami M. The effect of aromatherapy with peppermint essential oil on nausea and vomiting after cardiac surgery: a randomized clinical trial. Complement Ther Clin Pract 2020;40:101199.

May B, Köhler S, Schneider B. Efficacy and tolerability of a fixed combination of peppermint oil and caraway oil in patients suffering from functional dyspepsia. Aliment Pharmacol Ther 2000;14(12):1671–7.

Meamarbashi A, Rajabi A. The effects of peppermint on exercise performance. J Int Soc Sports Nutr 2013;10(1):15.

Meamarbashi A. Instant effects of peppermint essential oil on the physiological parameters and exercise performance. Avicenna J Phytomed 2014;4(1):72–8.

Melli MS, Rashidi MR, Nokhoodchi A, et al. A randomized trial of peppermint gel, lanolin ointment, and placebo gel to prevent nipple crack in primiparous breastfeeding women. Med Sci Monit 2007;13(9):CR406–411.

Merat S, Khalili S, Mostajabi P, et al. The effect of enteric-coated, delayed-release peppermint oil on irritable bowel syndrome. Dig Dis Sci 2010;55(5):1385–90.

Moss M, Hewitt S, Moss L, Wesnes K. Modulation of cognitive performance and mood by aromas of peppermint and ylang-ylang. Int J Neurosci 2008;118(1):59–77.

Ou MC, Lee YF, Li CC, Wu SK. The effectiveness of essential oils for patients with neck pain: a randomized controlled study. J Altern Complement Med 2014;20(10):771–9.

Papathanasopoulos A, Rotondo A, Janssen P, et al. Effect of acute peppermint oil administration on gastric sensorimotor function and nutrient tolerance in health. Neurogastroenterol Motil 2013;25(4):e263–71.

Pasha H, Behmanesh F, Mohsenzadeh F, Hajahmadi M, Moghadamnia AA. Study of the effect of mint oil on nausea and vomiting during pregnancy. Iran Red Crescent Med J 2012;14(11):727–30.

Rafieian-Kopaei M, Hasanpour-Dehkordi A, Lorigooini Z, Deris F, Solati K, Mahdiyeh F. Comparing the effect of intranasal lidocaine 4% withpeppermintessential oil drop 1.5% on migraine attacks: a double-blind clinical trial. Int J Prev Med 2019;10:121.

Sayyah Melli M, Rashidi MR, Delazar A, et al. Effect of peppermint water on prevention of nipple cracks in lactating primiparous women: a randomized controlled trial. Int Breastfeed J 2007;2:7.

Shah I, Baffy NJ, Horsley-Silva JL, Langlais BT, Ruff KC. Peppermint oil to improve visualization in screening colonoscopy: a randomized controlledclinical trial. Gastroenterol Res 2019;12(3):141–7.

Shavakhi A, Ardestani SK, Taki M, Goli M, Keshteli AH. Premedication with peppermint oil capsules in colonoscopy: a double-blind placebo-controlled randomized trial study. Acta Gastroenterol Belg 2012;75(3):349–53.

Tayarani-Najaran Z, Talasaz-Firoozi E, Nasiri R, Jalali N, Hassanzadeh M. Antiemetic activity of volatile oil from *Mentha spicata* and Mentha × piperita in chemotherapy-induced nausea and vomiting. Ecancermedicalscience 2013;7:290.

Weerts ZZRM, Masclee AAM, Witteman BJM, et al. Efficacy and safety ofpeppermint oil in a randomized, double-blind trial of patients with irritable bowel syndrome. Gastroenterology 2020;158(1):123–36.

RHODIOLA (*RHODIOLA ROSEA*)
Root

GENERAL OVERVIEW

Although rhodiola is sometimes referred to as "Arctic ginseng," it was not included in the ginseng group due to considerable differences in chemical constituents. Among other traditional uses of this herb, the Vikings used it for physical strength and endurance. It also has traditional and modern usage as an anti-fatigue adaptogen. Rhodiola is a useful herb for "stressed out, burned out and wimped out" conditions. One might also use it for a short-term physical or mental competitive edge under stressful circumstances.

Clinical research indicates that rhodiola, alone or in combination formulas, may be beneficial for ischemic heart disease, premature ejaculation, anxiety, depression, cognitive performance, xeroderma, stress, burnout, chronic fatigue, athletic performance, chemo-induced myocarditis, and immune suppression.

IN VITRO AND ANIMAL RESEARCH

Rhodiola (particularly *R. rosea*) has been extensively studied in Russia. It has been shown to protect the nervous system, heart, and liver and to produce antimutagenic and anticancer effects. Rhodiola has been shown to protect tissue against ischemia and to enhance physical endurance. It decreases CRP and lactate and reduces reperfusion arrhythmias in ischemic myocardium via increases in β-endorphins and enkephalin. In mice made to swim to their limit, rhodiola increased ATP and creatine phosphate in muscle and brain mitochondria. A chief constituent of rhodiola, salidroside has been shown in rats to decrease age-related immune se-

nescence. Non-mammalian animal studies have shown a 20% increase in lifespan from rhodiola. Rhodiola has been shown to improve thyroid, thymus, adrenal, and sexual functions. The herb appears to be anti-estrogenic as it is a competitive inhibitor of estrogen receptor binding and increases metabolism of estradiol.

There are numerous in vitro and animal studies showing that rhodiola can create both a stimulating and a sedating effect on the central nervous system, depending on dosage. In small and medium doses rhodiola stimulates CNS dopamine, norepinephrine, and serotonin and produces nicotinic cholinergic effects. It increases the permeability of the blood–brain barrier to precursors of dopamine and serotonin. Rhodiola has also been shown to reduce cortisol. Rhodiola shows promise for cognitive performance through reversal of the blockade of acetylcholine ascending pathways in the brain.

In rats, rhodiola inhibits tumor growth and reduces metastasis of three cancer cell lines (adenocarcinoma, lymphosarcoma, and lung carcinoma). Salidroside induces cell-cycle arrest and apoptosis of breast cancer cells independent of the estrogen receptor. Animal studies have shown that rhodiola decreases toxicity and enhances efficacy of cyclophosphamide, daunorubicin, and doxorubicin.

HUMAN RESEARCH

Cardiovascular Disorders: Coronary Artery Disease/Ischemic Heart Disease

A 2014 systematic review to evaluate the efficacy and safety of rhodiola in treating ischemic heart disease either as a sole agent or in combination with routine Western medicine (RWM) found 13 studies ($n=1672$) that met inclusion criteria. The rhodiola formulations used alone or in combination with RWM demonstrated a positive effect on both improvement of symptoms and ECG. Subgroup analysis of rhodiola compared with other Chinese herbal medicines (CHMs), rhodiola compared with RWM, and rhodiola plus RWM compared with RWM alone demonstrated improvements in symptoms (OR = 1.51, 2.64, and 5.63, respectively), and improvements in ECGs (OR = 1.33, 3.11, 2.27, respectively). Overall, the effectiveness of rhodiola formulations was greater compared with medicines in control groups, with statistically significant differences observed both in symptomatic improvement (OR = 2.40; $P < 0.0001$) and ECG improvement (OR = 1.48; $P < 0.01$). The authors concluded that rhodiola may have a positive effect on treating ischemic heart disease alone and in combination with RWM (Yu et al., 2014).

A 2014 systematic review to assess the efficacy of rhodiola for chronic stable angina found seven RCTs ($n=662$) that met inclusion criteria. Compared with conventional Western medicine treatment, the addition of oral rhodiola improved angina (OR = 2.49) but not ECG (OR = 1.25). Addition of IV rhodiola to conventional medicine improved angina (OR = 4.86) and ECG and reduced the whole blood viscosity but not serum fibrinogen and D-dimer levels. The authors concluded that addition of rhodiola to routine treatment in patients with chronic stable angina could further improve patients' symptoms, and IV rhodiola could increase the ECG improvement rate and reduce adverse reactions (Chu et al., 2014).-

Women's Genitourinary Disorders: Amenorrhea and Menopause

An unpublished but frequently described Soviet study in women with amenorrhea ($n=40$) investigated the effect of rhodiola 100 mg BID 2 weeks on and 2 weeks off. Of the women in the study, 25 resumed normal menses and 11 became pregnant. In those with normal menses, the mean length of the uterine cavity increased from 5.5 cm to 7.0 cm. It has been postulated that these results may be due to the competitive estrogen receptor binding activity of rhodiola.

A 12-week RCT in women ($n=220$) with menopausal complaints compared two capsules daily of either black cohosh 6.5 mg, black cohosh 500 mg, a combination of black cohosh and rhodiola (Menopause Relief EP), or placebo. The menopause symptom relief effects of the combination formula were significantly superior in all tests to the effects of either dose of black cohosh alone and placebo after 6 and 12 weeks. There was no statistically significant difference between the effects of the two doses of black cohosh. The combination formula significantly improved the QOL index in patients, compared with the other groups, mainly due to the beneficial effects on the emotional and health domains. The authors concluded that black cohosh was more effective in combination with rhodiola for relief of menopausal symptoms, particularly psychological symptoms (Pkhaladze et al., 2020).

Men's Genitourinary Disorders: Premature Ejaculation

A 90-day open-label Phase I - II trial in patients ($n=91$) with lifelong premature ejaculation assessed the tolerability and efficacy of EndEP, a combination of rhodiola, folic acid, biotin, and zinc administered QD. A statistically significant difference was detected between the mean intravaginal ejaculation latency time at baseline and after treatment (73.6 s and 102.3 s, respectively; $P < 0.001$). Improvement in the control of ejaculation was reported by 60% of the patients. Very few adverse events were reported (4.4%). The authors concluded that this combination formula including rhodiola significantly improved ejaculatory control and the quality of sexual life in patients affected by lifelong premature ejaculation, with a low rate of adverse events (Cai et al., 2016).

Psychiatric Disorders: Anxiety

A 2013 systematic review looking at plants that had both pre-clinical and clinical evidence for anti-anxiety effects found 21 plants with human clinical trial evidence. Support for efficacy identified several herbs with efficacy for anxiety spectrum disorders including rhodiola, kava, lemon balm, chamomile, ginkgo, skullcap, milk thistle, passionflower, ashwagandha, echinacea, *Galphimia glauca*, *Centella asiatica*, and *Echium amooenum*. Acute anxiolytic activity was found for passionflower, sage, gotu kola, lemon balm, and bergamot. The review also specifically found that bacopa showed anxiolytic effects in people with cognitive decline (Sarris et al., 2011, 2013).

A 2-week RCT in patients ($n = 80$) with mild anxiety studied rhodiola 200 mg BID compared with no treatment. Self-reported mood and cognitive measures were repeated four times over the study period. Relative to the controls, the experimental group demonstrated a significant reduction in self-reported anxiety, stress, anger, confusion, and depression at 14 days and a significant improvement in total mood. No relevant differences in cognitive performance between the groups were observed. The authors noted that the changes appeared gradually and were specific to certain psychological measures, making placebo effect less likely (Cropley et al., 2015).

A 10-week pilot study in patients ($n = 10$) with a diagnosis of GAD, investigated rhodiola 340 mg/ day for effects on anxiety scales. There was a significant decrease in mean HAM-A scores at the endpoint ($P = 0.01$). Adverse events were generally mild or moderate in severity, the most common being dizziness and dry mouth. The authors concluded that significant improvement in GAD symptoms was found with rhodiola and noted that the HAM-A score reduction was similar to that found in clinical trials (Bystritsky et al., 2008).

Psychiatric Disorders: Depression

A 2011 systematic review to evaluate herbal medicines, other than St. John's wort, in the treatment of mild-to-moderate depression found nine trials that met inclusion criteria. Six of the studies involved saffron. Individual trials investigating lavender, *Echium amoenum*, and rhodiola were also included. Saffron showed good efficacy. Lavender was found to be less effective than imipramine, but the combination of lavender and imipramine was significantly more effective than imipramine alone. Rhodiola was also found to significantly improve depressive symptoms when compared with placebo. The authors concluded that several herbs showed promise in the management of mild-to-moderate depression (Dwyer et al., 2011).

A 2011 systematic review to assess the efficacy of rhodiola for any condition found 11 RCTs that met inclusion criteria. Six trials investigated the effects of rhodiola on physical performance, four on mental performance, and two in patients diagnosed with mental health conditions. The authors concluded that rhodiola may have beneficial effects on physical performance, mental performance, and certain mental health conditions (Hung et al., 2011).

A 2011 systematic review of herbal antidepressant, anxiolytic, and hypnotic psychopharmacology and applications in depression, anxiety, and insomnia found 66 studies involving 11 herbs. St John's wort had a high level of evidence of efficacy for depression and kava had high level evidence for anxiety. Several studies provided preliminary positive evidence of antidepressant effects for rhodiola, saffron, and *Echium amoenum*, and anxiolytic activity for chamomile, ginkgo, passionflower, *E. amoenum*, and skullcap (Sarris et al., 2011, 2013).

A 6-week phase-III RCT in patients ($n = 89$) with mild-moderate depression studied a standardized extract of rhodiola 340 mg QD compared with the same extract given BID and with placebo given BID. Overall depression, insomnia, emotional instability, and somatization, but not self-esteem, improved significantly with both doses of rhodiola but not with placebo. HAM-D score decreased from 24.5 to 16.0 ($P < 0.0001$) with the lower dose and from 23.8 to 16.7 with the higher dose. Mean BDI scores decreased from 12.2 to 7.1 with the lower dose and from 10.4 to 4.8 with the higher dose. The placebo group showed no improvement in HAM-D scores. The authors concluded that the standardized extract of rhodiola showed antidepressive potency in patients with mild-to-moderate depression when administered in dosages of either 340 or 680 mg/day over a 6-week period (Darbinyan et al., 2000, 2007).

A 12-week Phase II RCT in patients ($n = 57$) with mild-moderate depression compared rhodiola with sertraline and with placebo. Modest but statistically non-significant reductions were observed for HAM-D, BDI, and CGI-C scores for all treatment conditions with no significant difference between groups ($P = 0.79$, $P = 0.28$, and $P = 0.17$, respectively). The declines in HAM-D scores with sertraline, rhodiola, and placebo were -8.2, -5.1, and -4.6, respectively. The improvement over placebo for sertraline was greater than for rhodiola (OR = 1.90 and OR = 1.39, respectively), adverse events occurred in 63%, 30%, and 17% with sertraline, rhodiola, and placebo, respectively. The authors concluded that although rhodiola produced less antidepressant effect than sertraline, it was better tolerated (Mao et al., 2014).

A 6-week observational study in adults ($n = 45$) with mild-to-moderate depression investigated the effects of a combination of rhodiola 154 mg plus saffron 15 mg two tablets per day. After 6 weeks, HAM-D scores decreased by 58%, from 13.6 to 5.6; $P < 0.0001$. Score improvement was reported in 85% of patients. A sustained significant drop in Hospital Anxiety and Depression Scale scores was also observed at 2 weeks. There was a significant improvement in the Clinical Global Impression for both physicians and patients. Safety was excellent, and no serious adverse effects were recorded. The authors concluded that the combination of rhodiola and saffron could be useful for the management of mild-moderate depression and could improve depressive and anxiety symptoms (Bangratz et al., 2018).

A 12-week RCT in patients ($n = 100$) with mild-to-moderate major depressive disorder (MDD) randomized patients into three groups to compare efficacy. One group received sertraline plus two placebo pills, the second group received sertraline plus two rhodiola capsules (600 mg/day), and the third received sertraline plus one placebo and one rhodiola capsule (300 mg/day). Although statistically significant reductions were observed for HAM-D, BDI, and CGI scores for all treatment groups, the declines in HAM-D, BDI, and CGI scores were significantly greater in the second group compared with the first and third groups. The authors concluded that the rhodiola demonstrated anti-depressive potency in patients with depression when administered in dosages of either 300 mg/day or 600 mg/day, with the higher dose being more efficacious (Gao et al., 2020).

Psychiatric Disorders: Cognitive Performance

A 2011 systematic review to assess the efficacy of rhodiola for any condition found 11 RCTs that met inclusion criteria. Six trials investigated the effects of rhodiola on physical performance, four on mental performance, and two in patients diagnosed with mental health conditions. The authors concluded that rhodiola may have beneficial effects on physical performance, mental performance, and certain mental health conditions (Hung et al., 2011).

An acutely dosed RCT in volunteers ($n = 112$) investigated a combination of ginkgo plus rhodiola compared with each herb alone and with placebo for effects on psychomotor vigilance task and short-term working memory accuracy. The herbal combination improved the psychomotor vigilance task performance and low-to-moderate working memory accuracy ($P < 0.01$), while there was no improvement with placebo ($P > 0.05$). The combined effect of rhodiola plus ginkgo led to a more significant effect on psychomotor vigilance task performance, all levels of short-term working memory accuracy, and critical fusion versus flicker ($P < 0.01$), with the improvement being greater than either herb used alone (Al-Kuraishy, 2015).

A 20-day RCT in foreign students ($n = 40$) during a stressful examination period compared a standardized extract of rhodiola 432 mg with placebo taken during a 20-day exam period. The most significant improvements in the herbal group were seen in physical fitness, mental fatigue, and neuro-motor tests ($P < 0.01$). The self-assessment of the general well-being was also significantly better with rhodiola ($P < 0.05$). No significant difference was seen in the correction of text tests or neuro-muscular tapping tests. The authors concluded that rhodiola gave significant results but that the dose level was probably suboptimal (Spasov et al., 2000a,b).

A single-dose RCT in cadets ($n = 161$) with fatigue and stress investigated a dose of standardized extract of rhodiola 432 mg two capsules or three capsules compared with placebo for cognitive effects. Both doses of rhodiola had anti-fatigue index mean values of 1.03 and 1.01, with two and three capsules, respectively, while the anti-fatigue index value was 0.90 with placebo ($P < 0.001$). No significant difference between the two dosage groups was observed (Shevtsov et al., 2003).

A pilot RCT in stressed-out adults ($n = 40$) studied the effects of a single dose of ADAPT-232 (a standardized combination of rhodiola, schisandra, and eleuthero) compared with placebo on cognitive attention, speed, and accuracy while performing stressful cognitive tasks. The results showed a significant difference ($P < 0.05$) in attention, speed, and accuracy between the two treatment groups with superiority in the herbal treatment group. No serious side effects were reported, although a few minor adverse events, such as sleepiness and cold extremities, were observed in both treatment groups (Aslanyan et al., 2010).

Dermatological Disorders: Xeroderma

A 28-day RCT in volunteers (*n* = 124) with sensitive skin compared a rhodiola-L-carnosine cream with a placebo cream BID. The test cream produced in vivo protective effects in skin barrier function as measured by a reduction in transepidermal water loss. There was a positive subjective response with respect to skin dryness and skin comfort sensation and reduction of discomfort after a stinging challenge (Dieamant Gde et al., 2008).

Disorders of Vitality: Stress, Burnout, and Chronic Fatigue

A 2012 systematic review to evaluate the efficacy and safety of rhodiola for physical and mental fatigue found 11 studies that met inclusion criteria. Two of six trials examining physical fatigue in healthy populations found rhodiola to be effective as did three of five RCTs evaluating rhodiola for mental fatigue. The authors concluded that the research on this topic was conflicting (Ishaque et al., 2012).

A 6-week crossover RCT in young healthy physicians (*n* = 56) on call at night compared a standardized extract of rhodiola with placebo for effects on fatigue during night duty. A statistically significant improvement in cognitive testing was observed in the treatment group during the first 2-week period. No side effects were reported for either treatment noted. The authors concluded that rhodiola may reduce general fatigue under certain stressful conditions (Darbinyan et al., 2000, 2007).

A 4-week Phase III RCT in patients (*n* = 60) suffering from stress-related fatigue compared a standardized extract of rhodiola 576 mg/day with placebo. Significant post-treatment improvements were observed for both groups in Pines' burnout scale, mental health (SF-36), Montgomery-Asberg depression rating scale, and several Conners' computerized continuous performance test II (CCPT II) indices of attention. When the two groups were compared, significant effects of the rhodiola extract were observed compared with placebo in Pines' burnout scale and the CCPT II indices. Pre- and post-treatment cortisol responses to awakening stress were significantly different between treatment and placebo groups. The authors concluded that administration of rhodiola standardized extract had an anti-fatigue effect that increased mental performance and decreased cortisol response to awakening stress in burned-out patients with fatigue (Olsson et al., 2009).

A 12-week open-label exploratory study in patients (*n* = 118) with burnout investigated rhodiola 400 mg/day on measures on burnout. Clinical outcomes were assessed by the German version of the Maslach Burnout Inventory, Burnout Screening Scales I and II, Sheehan Disability Scale, Perceived Stress Questionnaire, Number Connection Test, Multidimensional Mood State Questionnaire, Numerical Analogue Scales for different stress symptoms and impairment of sexual life, Patient Sexual Function Questionnaire, and the Clinical Global Impression Scales. Most of the outcome measures showed clear improvement starting after 1 week of treatment and continuing further up to the end of the study. The incidence of adverse events was low (Kasper and Dienel, 2017).

A 4-week open-label trial in patients (*n* = 101) with life stress symptoms investigated the effects of a standardized rhodiola extract 200 mg BID on stress symptoms. Assessments were made with the Numerical Analogue Scales of Subjective Stress Symptoms, Perceived Stress Questionnaire, Multidimensional Fatigue Inventory 20, Numbers Connecting Test, Sheehan Disability Scale, and Clinical Global Impressions. Starting at 3 days and continually improving, all tests showed clinically relevant improvements of stress symptoms, disability, functional impairment, and overall therapeutic effect. Adverse events were mostly of mild intensity and no serious adverse events were reported. The authors concluded that rhodiola standardized extract at a dose of 200 mg BID for 4 weeks is safe and effective in improving life stress symptoms to a clinically relevant degree (Edwards et al., 2012).

An 8-week open-label pilot study in patients (*n* = 100) with prolonged or chronic fatigue symptoms assessed the efficacy of a standardized extract of rhodiola 200 mg, two tablets per day, for fatigue. The greatest change in measurements of fatigue was observed after 1 week of treatment with continued decline and statistically significant improvement at week 8. Most adverse events were mild and not related to the study drug. The authors concluded that this standardized extract of rhodiola may be safe and effective in subjects suffering from prolonged or chronic fatigue (Lekomtseva et al., 2017).

Disorders of Vitality: Athletic performance

A 2011 systematic review to assess the efficacy or effectiveness of rhodiola for any condition found 11 RCTs that met inclusion criteria. Six trials investigated the effects of rhodiola on physical performance, four on mental performance, and two in patients diagnosed with mental health conditions. The authors concluded that rhodiola may have beneficial effects on physical performance, mental performance, and certain mental health conditions (Hung et al., 2011).

A crossover RCT in healthy males ($n = 10$) compared rhodiola 3 mg/kg with placebo dosed just prior to a 30-minute submaximal cycling performance for the effect on substrate utilization, mood state, rated perceived exertion, and exercise affect. Perceived exertion was significantly lower at 30 minutes into exercise with rhodiola than with placebo ($P = 0.003$). Rhodiola produced higher post-exercise perceptions of arousal ($P = 0.05$) and pleasure ($P = 0.003$) than did placebo. Mood state scores for vigor were also higher with rhodiola than with placebo ($P = 0.008$). There were no significant differences in energy expenditure, carbohydrate, or fat oxidation between conditions ($P > 0.05$). The authors concluded that rhodiola favorably influenced perceived exertion and exercise attitude without changing energy expenditure or substrate utilization (Duncan and Clarke, 2014).

A 3-day RCT in physically active female college students ($n = 11$) investigated rhodiola 1500 mg/day plus an acute pre-exercise dose of 500 mg compared with daily and acute dosing of placebo. With anaerobic exercise, rhodiola was associated with higher mean watts ($P = 0.017$), mean anaerobic capacity ($P = 0.025$), mean anaerobic power ($P = 0.03$), mean peak watts ($P = 0.029$), and mean total work ($P = 0.017$). However, mean fatigue index ($P = 0.094$) did not differ between groups. The authors concluded that rhodiola supplementation enhanced anaerobic exercise performance and may possess ergogenic benefits (Ballmann et al., 2019).

A 4-week crossover RCT in trained male athletes ($n = 14$) compared rhodiola with placebo for effects on physical performance as well as on the redox status. Rhodiola produced statistically significant reductions in plasma-free fatty acid levels. Blood lactate and plasma CK levels were also significantly lower ($P < 0.05$) with rhodiola than with placebo. The authors concluded that chronic rhodiola was able to reduce lactate and muscle damage after an exhaustive exercise session and that it seemed to ameliorate fatty acid consumption, suggesting adaptogenic effects on exercise (Parisi et al., 2010).

A two-phase RCT in healthy volunteers ($n = 24$) studied a standardized extract of rhodiola 200 mg compared with placebo given one hour before physical exercise with washout and crossover in phase 1. This was followed by an RCT in subjects ($n = 12$) who underwent episodic administration of rhodiola or placebo as in phase 1 with an additional 4-week daily administration of rhodiola or placebo at the same dose between challenges. In phase 1, rhodiola increased time to exhaustion from 16.8 min to 17.2 min ($P < 0.05$). VO2$_{peak}$ and VCO2 peak increased from 51 to 53 mL/min/kg and from 60 to 63.5 mL/min/kg, respectively ($P < 0.05$ for both). Pulmonary ventilation tended to increase more with rhodiola than with placebo ($P = 0.07$). In phase 2 the 4-week intake of rhodiola did not alter any of the variables. The authors concluded that acute rhodiola intake could improve endurance exercise capacity in young healthy volunteers and that the response was not altered by prior daily 4-week rhodiola intake (De Bock et al., 2004).

Infectious Disease: Pneumonia

A 10-15-day RCT in patients ($n = 60$) with pneumonia investigated the efficacy of ADAPT-232 (a standardized combination of eleuthero, schisandra, and rhodiola) BID plus standard treatment with cefazolin, bromhexine, and theophylline compared with standard treatment plus placebo. The mean duration of treatment with antibiotics required to bring about recovery from the acute phase of the disease was 2 days shorter with the herbal product than with placebo. Compared with the placebo group, patients in the herbal group scored higher in QOL domains at the beginning of the rehabilitation period, and improvement was significantly higher on the fifth day after clinical convalescence. The authors concluded that adjuvant therapy with ADAPT-232 had a positive effect on the recovery of patients with pneumonia (Narimanian et al., 2005).

Oncologic Disorders: Chemotherapy-Induced Myocarditis, Chemotherapy-Induced Immune Suppression, Bladder Carcinoma

A chemotherapy-based RCT in patients ($n = 60$) with breast cancer compared the rhodiola constituent salidroside 600 mg/day with placebo starting 1 week before chemotherapy for myocardial protection from chemotherapy. At growing cumulative doses of epirubicin, the echocardiographic strain rate normalized only with salidroside. At epirubicin 300 mg/m^2 the strain rates of salidroside and placebo were 1.66/s and 1.32/s ($P < 0.05$). At epirubicin 400 mg/m^2 the respective strain rates were 1.68/s and 1.40/s ($P < 0.05$). A significant increase in plasma concentrations of ROS was found with placebo but remained unchanged with salidroside. The authors concluded that salidroside could provide a protective effect on epirubicin-induced early left ventricular regional systolic dysfunction in patients with breast cancer (Zhang et al., 2010, 2012).

An open-label trial in patients ($n = 12$) with superficial bladder carcinoma (T1G1-2) administered oral rhodiola extract, resulting in improved characteristics of urothelial tissue integration, parameters of leukocyte integrins, and T-cell immunity. The average frequency of relapses for these patients decreased twofold, although statistical differences were not significant (Bocharova et al., 1995).

A 4-week RCT in stage III-IV ovarian cancer patients ($n = 28$) investigated the immunological effects of AdMax (eleuthero, rhodiola, schisandra, and *Rhaponticum carthamoides*) 270 mg/day compared with a control group for 4 weeks. Patients were treated with a dose of cisplatin 75 mg/m^2 and cyclophosphamide 600 mg/m^2, and labs were followed up at 4 weeks. In patients who took AdMax following chemotherapy, the mean numbers of CD3, CD4, CD5, and CD8 were increased compared with those who did not take the herbal combination. Also, the mean amounts of IgG and IgM were increased in the herbal group compared with control. The authors concluded that the combination of extracts from adaptogenic plants may boost suppressed immunity in ovarian cancer patients subject to chemotherapy (Kormosh et al., 2006).

ACTIVE CONSTITUENTS

- Phenolic compounds
  - Phenylethanols: tyrosol, salidroside, viridoside (antioxidant, stimulant, adaptogenic, antiviral, anti-inflammatory, anticarcinogenic, antiapoptotic, antifibtrotic)
  - Phenolic acids: gallic acid
  - Phenylpropanoids (antioxidant, antimutagenic, antitumor, antimicrobial): chlorogenic acid (antioxidant), hydroxycinnamic acid, "rosavins" (unique to the *R. rosea* species) including rosarin rosavin, rosin (stimulant, adaptogenic)
  - Flavonoids: rodiolin, rodionin, rodiosin, acetylrodalgin, tricin, catechins, proanthocyanidins (antioxidant, antilipemic)
- Terpenes
  - Monoterpenes: rosiridol, rosaridin
- Steroids
  - Phytosterols: daucosterol, β-stiosterol

RHODIOLA COMMONLY USED PREPARATIONS AND DOSAGE (FOR ADULTS UNLESS OTHERWISE SPECIFIED)

The following are examples of some available formulations and ranges of dosing for commercial herbal products. See Part III Introduction "How to prescribe medicinal herbs" for further guidance on herbal advising and prescribing.

Root

- Tincture (1:5, 50%): 1 mL BID-TID 30 min AC for 10-60 days; shorter for asthenia, longer for depression
- Powdered root extract (standardized to 3% rosavin): 400 mg (1/8 tsp) BID
- Capsule or tablet of standardized root extract (standardized to 3% rosavins and 1% salidroside): 250-500 mg QD-BID for treatment dosing. Prophylactic dosing against fatigue is 50 mg per day. Acute pre-stressor dosing is 200 mg.

Note about standardization: If standardized to less rosavin, higher dosing can be used. For preliminary dosing, calculate to roughly 3-6 mg rosavins per day. Although rosavins are now the accepted marker for genetically pure R. rosea (and its extracts), they are not necessarily the only pharmacologically active ingredients responsible for the efficacy observed in clinical studies. In fact, precise identification of the compounds responsible for the numerous health benefits of rhodiola remains to be confirmed.

Use lower dose if chronic administration. Limit continuous use to 4 months due to lack of research on longer use. May resume continuous use following "herb holiday." For single use prior to athletic or other performance, a higher dose may be used. In anticipation of a stressful event, begin dosing days to weeks prior to the stressor and continue through the stress.

Efficacy based on dosing shows a bell-shaped curve, so doses > 680 mg will have diminishing returns. Doses as low as 50 mg are effective for preventing fatigue. Lower doses are more stimulating and higher doses are more sedating.

SAFETY AND PRECAUTION

Side Effects

There are no definite side effects, but rhodiola may cause dizziness and dry mouth. It may be activating for patients with anxiety. Also, it may cause insomnia and vivid dreams, so it is best to avoid at bedtime.

Case Reports

- A woman added rhodiola to her SSRI antidepressant resulting in a tachyarrhythmia.
- Suspected serotonin syndrome in a 68-year-old woman on paroxetine.

Toxicity

An ethanol extract from the roots of rhodiola 10–316 mg/kg was orally administered to mice and revealed a significant reduction in exploratory behavior and in the number of rearings and head dippings, but no change in sedative-hypnotic and anticonvulsant response. It showed no toxicity.

Pregnancy and Lactation

Insufficient human safety data.

Disease Interactions

Due to activating effects, avoid in acute mania and use caution with history of mania (theoretical).

Drug Interactions

- CYP: Inhibits CYP3A4. Modestly inhibits CYP2C9
- Pgp: Inhibits P-glycoprotein
- Case reports and theoretical potential for interactions with other antidepressants
- MAO activity: although this activity may not be clinically significant, caution with antidepressants, antihypertensives, CNS stimulants
- Research demonstrated decreased metabolism of losartan

REFERENCES

Al-Kuraishy HM. Central additive effect of Ginkgo biloba and Rhodiola rosea on psychomotor vigilance task and short-term working memory accuracy. J Intercult Ethnopharmacol 2015;5(1):7–13.

Aslanyan G, Amroyan E, Gabrielyan E, Nylander M, Wikman G, Panossian A. Double-blind, placebo-controlled, randomised study of single dose effects of ADAPT-232 on cognitive functions. Phytomedicine 2010;17(7):494–9.

Ballmann CG, Maze SB, Wells AC, Marshall MM, Rogers RR. Effects of short-term Rhodiola rosea (golden root extract) supplementation on anaerobic exercise performance. J Sports Sci 2019;37(9):998–1003.

Bangratz M, Ait Abdellah S, Berlin A, et al. A preliminary assessment of a combination of rhodiola and saffron in the management of mild-moderate depression. Neuropsychiatr Dis Treat 2018;14:1821–9.

Bocharova OA, Matveev BP, Baryshnikov AI, Figurin KM, Serebriakova RV, Bodrova NB. The effect of a Rhodiola rosea extract on the incidence of recurrences of a superficial bladder cancer (experimental clinical research). Urol Nefrol (Mosk) 1995;2:46–7.

Bystritsky A, Kerwin L, Feusner JD. A pilot study of Rhodiola rosea (Rhodax) for generalized anxiety disorder (GAD). J Altern Complement Med 2008;14(2):175–80.

Cai T, Verze P, Massenio P, et al. Rhodiola rosea, folic acid, zinc and biotin (EndEP) is able to improve ejaculatory control in patients affected by lifelong premature ejaculation: Results from a phase I-II study. Exp Ther Med 2016;12(4):2083–7. Epub 2016 Aug 12.

Chu JF, Wu GW, Zheng GH, et al. A system review of randomized controlled trials on treating chronic stable angina by rhodiola. Zhongguo Zhong Xi Yi Jie He Za Zhi 2014;34(8):940–6.

Cropley M, Banks AP, Boyle J. The effects of Rhodiola rosea L. extract on anxiety, stress, cognition and other mood symptoms. Phytother Res 2015;29(12):1934–9.

Darbinyan V, Kteyan A, Panossian A, Gabrielian E, Wikman G, Wagner H. Rhodiola rosea in stress induced fatigue—a double blind crossover study of a standardized extract SHR-5 with a repeated low-dose regimen on the mental performance of healthy physicians during night duty. Phytomedicine 2000;7(5):365–71.

Darbinyan V, Aslanyan G, Amroyan E, Gabrielyan E, Malmström C, Panossian A. Clinical trial of Rhodiola rosea L. extract SHR-5 in the treatment of mild to moderate depression. Nord J Psychiatry 2007;61(5):343–8.

De Bock K, Eijnde BO, Ramaekers M, et al. Acute Rhodiola rosea intake can improve endurance exercise performance. Int J Sport Nutr Exerc Metab 2004;14(3):298–307.

Dieamant Gde C, Velazquez Pereda Mdel C, Eberlin S, Nogueira C, Werka RM, Queiroz ML. Neuroimmunomodulatory compound for sensitive skin care: *in vitro* and clinical assessment. J Cosmet Dermatol 2008;7(2):112–9.

Duncan MJ, Clarke ND. The effect of acute Rhodiola rosea ingestion on exercise heart rate, substrate utilisation, mood state, and perceptions of exertion, arousal, and pleasure/displeasure in active men. J Sports Med (Hindawi Publ Corp) 2014;2014:563043.

Dwyer AV, Whitten DL, Hawrelak JA. Herbal medicines, other than St. John's Wort, in the treatment of depression: a systematic review. Altern Med Rev 2011;16(1):40–9.

Edwards D, Heufelder A, Zimmermann A. Therapeutic effects and safety of Rhodiola rosea extract WS° 1375 in subjects with life-stress symptoms—results of an open-label study. Phytother Res 2012;26(8):1220–5.

Gao L, Wu C, Liao Y, Wang J. Antidepressants effects of Rhodiola capsule combined with sertraline for major depressive disorder: a randomized double-blind placebo-controlled clinical trial. J Affect Disord 2020;265:99–103.

Hung SK, Perry R, Ernst E. The effectiveness and efficacy of Rhodiola rosea L.: a systematic review of randomized clinical trials. Phytomedicine 2011;18(4):235–44.

Ishaque S, Shamseer L, Bukutu C, Vohra S. Rhodiola rosea for physical and mental fatigue: a systematic review. BMC Complement Altern Med 2012;12:70.

Kasper S, Dienel A. Multicenter, open-label, exploratory clinical trial with Rhodiola rosea extract in patients suffering from burnout symptoms. Neuropsychiatr Dis Treat 2017;13:889–98.

Kormosh N, Laktionov K, Antoshechkina M. Effect of a combination of extract from several plants on cell-mediated and humoral immunity of patients with advanced ovarian cancer. Phytother Res 2006;20(5):424–5.

Lekomtseva Y, Zhukova I, Wacker A. Rhodiola rosea in subjects with prolonged or chronic fatigue symptoms: results of an open-label clinical trial. Complement Med Res 2017;24(1):46–52.

Mao JJ, Li QS, Soeller I, Xie SX, Amsterdam JD. Rhodiola rosea therapy for major depressive disorder: a study protocol for a randomized, double-blind, placebo-controlled trial. J Clin Trials 2014;4:170.

Narimanian M, Badalyan M, Panosyan V, et al. Impact of Chisan° (ADAPT-232) on the quality-of life and its efficacy as an adjuvant in the treatment of acute non-specific pneumonia. Phytomedicine 2005;12:723–9.

Olsson EM, von Schéele B, Panossian AG. A randomised, double-blind, placebo-controlled, parallel-group study of the standardised extract shr-5 of the roots of Rhodiola rosea in the treatment of subjects with stress-related fatigue. Planta Med 2009;75(2):105–12.

Parisi A, Tranchita E, Duranti G, et al. Effects of chronic Rhodiola Rosea supplementation on sport performance and antioxidant capacity in trained male: preliminary results. J Sports Med Phys Fitness 2010;50(1):57–63.

Pkhaladze L, Davidova N, Khomasuridze A, Shengelia R, Panossian A. *Actaea racemosa* L. is more effective in combination with *Rhodiola rosea* L. for relief of menopausal symptoms: a randomized, double-blind, placebo-controlled study. Pharmaceuticals (Basel) 2020;13(5):102.

Sarris J, Panossian A, Schweitzer I, Stough C, Scholey A. Herbal medicine for depression, anxiety and insomnia: a review of psychopharmacology and clinical evidence. Eur Neuropsychopharmacol 2011;21(12):841–60.

Sarris J, McIntyre E, Camfield DA. Plant-based medicines for anxiety disorders, part 2: a review of clinical studies with supporting preclinical evidence. CNS Drugs 2013;27(4):301–19.

Shevtsov VA, Zholus BI, Shervarly VI, et al. A randomized trial of 2 different doses of a SHR-5 Rhodiola rosea extract vs placebo and control of capacity for mental work. Phytomedicine 2003;10(2-3):95–105.

Spasov AA, Mandrikov VB, Mironova IA. The effect of the preparation rhodiosin on the psychophysiological and physical adaptation of students to an academic load. Eksp Klin Farmakol 2000a;63(1):76–8.

Spasov AA, Wikman GK, Mandrikov VB, Mironova IA, Neumoin VV. A double-blind, placebo-controlled pilot study of the stimulating and adaptogenic effect of Rhodiola rosea SHR-5 extract on the fatigue of students caused by stress during an examination period with a repeated low-dose regimen. Phytomedicine 2000b;7(2):85–9.

Yu L, Qin Y, Wang Q, et al. The efficacy and safety of Chinese herbal medicine, Rhodiola formulation in treating ischemic heart disease: a systematic review and meta-analysis of randomized controlled trials. Complement Ther Med 2014;22(4):814–25.

Zhang L, Yu H, Zhao X, et al. Neuroprotective effects of salidroside against β-amyloid-induced oxidative stress in SH-SY5Y human neuroblastoma cells. Neurochem Int 2010;57(5):547–55.

Zhang H, Shen WS, Gao CH, Deng LC, Shen D. Protective effects of salidroside on epirubicin-induced early left ventricular regional systolic dysfunction in patients with breast cancer. Drugs R D 2012;12(2):101–6.

66

SAFFRON (*CROCUS SATIVUS*)
Stigma, Petal

GENERAL OVERVIEW

Saffron has been a rising star in research and recognition of its multiple beneficial effects. It is currently second only to St. John's wort in the volume of research performed for antidepressant effects. The name of this herb is derived from the Arabic word "za-faran" meaning "be yellow." Saffron formulations have historically used the tiny stigma of the blossoms of *Crocus sativus*, so you can imagine how labor intensive and wasteful, not to mention expensive, it may be as a source of medicine. Yet it has some remarkable properties that may warrant such apparently profligate use of a plant. Saffron stigma is commonly used as a culinary spice in Middle Eastern dishes. It has been used in traditional Persian medicine for cataracts, kidney stones, sexual dysfunction, stomachache, insomnia, and depression.

Fortunately, recent research has demonstrated that the entire blossom of saffron contains good medicine, so it may with good conscience be added to the list of useful herbs. Saffron petal, previously considered a byproduct, contains several active constituents including anthocyanins, flavonoids, glycosides, alkaloids, and kaempferol. The pharmacological properties of saffron petal include antibacterial, antispasmodic, immunomodulatory, antitussive, antidepressant, antinociceptive, hepatoprotective, reno-protective, antihypertensive, antidiabetic, and antioxidant activity. Accordingly, saffron petal may be used as an alternative or supplementary medicine in several diseases (Hosseini et al., 2018b).

Clinical research indicates that saffron, alone or in combination formulas, may be beneficial for gingivitis, burning mouth syndrome, asthma, ischemic heart disease, dyslipidemia, diabetes, obesity, premenstrual syndrome, menopause, labor induction, male and female sexual dysfunction, fibromyalgia, stroke recovery, cognitive impairment, dementia, anxiety, OCD, depression, attention-deficit/hyperactivity disorder, and addiction disorders.

IN VITRO AND ANIMAL RESEARCH

In vitro research has demonstrated antispasmodic, antitussive, expectorant, hypolipidemic, memory enhancing, neuroprotective, antinociceptive, antidepressant, anxiolytic, anticonvulsant, and anticancer effects with saffron. The herb also has antibacterial, antiseptic, and antifungal properties. The methanolic extract of saffron petal showed antibacterial activity against *Staphylococcus aureus, Bacillus cereus, Salmonella typhi, Escherichia coli,* and *Shigella dysenteriae.*

With its high carotenoid content, saffron stigma extract given orally at 1 mg/kg to rats exposed to continuous bright light prevented retinal damage similar to 1 mg/kg β-carotene. Supplementation for 10 days was more protective than 2-5 days for light-induced retinal damage. Saffron has also been shown in rodents to prevent selenite-induced cataract formation. With respect to UV radiation to skin, a cream containing 8% dried and powdered saffron demonstrated a superior SPF to an 8% homosalate solution.

In asthma models, guinea pigs who drank water containing a 70% ethanolic extract of saffron or the constituent safranal alone developed improved histamine levels and pathological signs of asthma. The guinea pigs also showed a decreased tracheal response to methacholine. Saffron also decreased nitric oxide and nitrite levels (*iNOS activity has been shown to be increased in asthma and plays a role in cellular damage*). Saffron petal extract has shown smooth muscle relaxant activity in rat vas deferens and guinea pig ileum through antiadrenergic and antimuscarinic activity. In an anesthetized rat model, aqueous and ethanolic extracts of saffron petal reduced BP, which correlated with effects on peripheral resistance.

Saffron extract given to rats on a high-fat diet decreased TC, TG, LDL-C, LDL/HDL, ALT, AST, and ALP while increasing HDL-C. The levels of leptin and insulin were reduced by saffron extracts. In STZ-diabetic rats, saffron petal reduced FBS, urine volume, and BUN, and it improved the histological damages induced by STZ. The aqueous extract of saffron petal after CCl4 or acetaminophen liver toxicity reduced ALT and AST as well as liver lesions. A rat study demonstrated that both saffron and silymarin (from milk thistle) decreased AST, ALT, MDA, and bilirubin levels in a model of cisplatin-induced liver toxicity.

Another constituent class, crocins have been show in vitro to attenuate the formation of Aβ protein fibrils in a concentration-dependent manner. Trans-crocin-4 is likely the major active ingredient to produce this effect through antioxidant properties.

In rat research, standard doses of saffron are not associated with sedation, but higher intraperitoneal injections have produced sleepiness. Anxiolytic properties have been demonstrated with intraperitoneal injections in mice at up to 80 mg/kg, with higher doses up to 560 mg/kg losing this property. The anxiolytic effect appeared to be comparable to 3 mg/kg of diazepam and is attributed to the crocins. Crocins have also demonstrated the ability to reverse a chemically induced model of OCD in rats.

Antidepressant activity of aqueous and ethanolic extracts of saffron stigma, safranal, and crocin were investigated in mice in a forced swimming test. The immobility time was reduced by saffron stigma (0.8 g/kg), safranal (0.15-0.5 mL/kg) and crocin (50-600 mg/kg). Safranal and both extracts of stigma increased swimming time. In another rodent study, immobility time in a forced swimming test was reduced by crocin. Crocins were shown in a rat model to hinder

5-HT_{2c} signaling due to antagonism of the serotonin receptor agonist. Antidepressant activity of crocin may also be related to an increase of the CREB, VGF, and BDNF. In mice and rats, the antidepressant activity of kaempferol, an active compound of saffron petal, was compared with fluoxetine as a positive control and was found to reduce immobility time similar to fluoxetine.

Saffron and its constituent safranal have shown preventive effects on serum inflammatory markers in sensitized guinea pigs. Ethanolic and aqueous extracts of saffron have demonstrated anti-nociceptive effects against chemical-induced pain in mice. The ethanolic extract reduced chronic inflammation but not acute inflammation.

Prostate cancer cells were induced to undergo apoptosis when incubated with safranal, while nonmalignant cells failed to undergo apoptosis under similar incubation parameters. · Crocetin has been demonstrated in vitro to bind to DNA and form adducts in various cancerous lines (HeLa, A-549, and VA-13) and normal cells.

HUMAN RESEARCH

The human research on saffron and its constituents crocin and safranal seems to be fraught with inconsistencies. Some of this appears to be dose related. The evidence for cardiometabolic benefits is mixed, as is the evidence for sexual dysfunction. Saffron appears to have a modest effect for lowering blood glucose, TG, and appetite. The psychiatric benefits are supported by compelling evidence, particularly for depression.

Ophthalmological Disorders: Macular Degeneration, Diabetic Maculopathy, and Glaucoma

A 6-month crossover RCT in adults ($n = 100$) with mild/moderate age-related macular degeneration (ARMD) and vision greater than 20/70 in at least one eye compared saffron 20 mg/day with placebo for 3 months, followed by crossover for another 3 months. Saffron as compared with placebo improved the mean best-corrected visual acuity (BCVA) by 0.69 letters ($P = 0.001$) and decreased mean-pooled multifocal electroretinogram (mfERG) latency by 0.17 ms ($P = 0.04$). The subset of participants on AREDS supplements showed a mean BCVA improvement of 0.73 letters ($P = 0.006$) and mean-pooled mfERG response density improvement of 2.8% ($P = 0.038$). There was no significant difference in adverse event occurrence. The authors concluded that saffron modestly improved visual function in patients with ARMD including those already on eye supplements (Broadhead et al., 2019).

A six-month crossover RCT in patients ($n = 25$) with early ARMD compared oral saffron 20 mg/day with placebo for 3 months then crossed over for another 3 months. With saffron, the focal electroretinograms (fERGs) were increased in amplitude compared with baseline and with placebo (mean change after saffron, 0.25 log μV; mean change after placebo, −0.003 log μV; $P < 0.01$). With saffron, fERG thresholds were decreased compared with baseline and with placebo (mean change after saffron, −0.26 log units; mean change after placebo, 0.0003 log units). The authors concluded that short-term saffron improved retinal flicker sensitivity in early ARMD (Falsini et al., 2010).

A 12-month open-label trial in patients ($n = 33$) with early ARMD who were screened for complement factor H (CFH) and age-related maculopathy susceptibility ARMS-2 polymorphisms investigated the effects of oral saffron 20 mg/day over an average period of 11 months of treatment. After 3 months of supplementation, mean focal electroretinogram (fERG) amplitude and sensitivity improved significantly over baseline ($P < 0.01$) and these changes were stable throughout the follow-up period. No significant differences in clinical and fERG improvements were observed across different CFH or ARMS2 genotypes. The authors concluded that the functional effect of saffron in patients with ARMD was not related to the major risk genotypes of the disease (Marangoni et al., 2013).

A 3-month Phase II RCT in patients ($n = 60$; 101 eyes) with diabetic maculopathy refractory to conventional therapy (including macular photocoagulation and intravitreal injection of anti-VEGF agent with or without steroid) compared crocin 5 mg/day and crocin 15 mg/day with placebo. Crocin 15 mg/day compared with placebo was associated with decreases in A1C ($P = 0.024$) and central macular thickness ($P = 0.005$) and improvement in best corrected visual acuity ($P = 0.012$). While the lower dose produced improvements in the measured parameters, the difference from placebo was not statistically significant. The authors concluded that crocin had short-term benefit for the treatment of refractory diabetic maculopathy (Sepahi et al., 2018).

A 2-month RCT in patients ($n = 34$ eyes) with stable primary open-angle glaucoma on timolol and dorzolamide drops compared oral saffron aqueous extract 30 mg/day with placebo in addition to existing eye medication for 1 month, followed by a 1-month washout. After 3 weeks of saffron or placebo, the IOPs changed from 12.9 to 10.9 and from 14.0 to 13.5, respectively ($P = 0.013$). By 4 weeks, IOPs were 10.6 and 13.8 with saffron and placebo, respectively ($P = 0.001$). At the end of the washout period, IOPs were 12.9 and 14.2 with saffron and placebo, respectively ($P = 0.175$). None of the patients experienced side effects during the study and wash-out period. The authors concluded that oral aqueous saffron extract exerted an ocular hypotensive effect in primary open-angle glaucoma (Jabbarpoor Bonyadi et al., 2014).

Oral and Dental Disorders: Gingivitis and Burning Mouth Syndrome

A 1-month RCT in patients ($n = 22$) with generalized marginal gingivitis investigated a toothpaste containing an aqueous extract of saffron stigma compared with a placebo toothpaste. With saffron there was a significant difference for reduction in gingival index and bleeding on probing index compared with placebo ($P < 0.05$). The differences between pocket depth and plaque index were not statistically significant. The authors concluded that saffron-containing toothpaste might have a positive effect on some gingival indices in patients with gingivitis (Forouzanfar et al., 2016).

An 11-week RCT in patients ($n = 47$) with burning mouth syndrome compared crocin with citalopram. The VAS for burning mouth as well as HAM-D and HAM-A questionnaires were improved significantly with crocin. The authors concluded that crocin could be considered for treatment of burning mouth syndrome in patients with concurrent anxiety and/or depression (Pakfetrat et al., 2019).

Pulmonary Disorders: Asthma

An 8-week RCT in patients ($n = 80$) with mild and moderate allergic asthma compared saffron 100 mg/day with placebo for effects on spirometry, inflammation, and anti-HSP70 (*a risk factor for asthma*).

Compared with placebo saffron reduced the hs-CRP ($P < 0.001$) and anti-HSP70 ($P < 0.001$) concentrations. Spirometry showed a significant increase in FEV1, FVC, FEV1/FVC, and FEF 25-75 with saffron compared with placebo ($P < 0.05$). The authors concluded that saffron improved some spirometric measurements and reduced anti-HSP70 and hs-CRP in patients with allergic asthma (Hosseini et al., 2018a)

An 8-week RCT in patients ($n = 80$) with mild-to-moderate asthma compared saffron 100 mg/day with placebo. Saffron improved the frequency of daytime dyspnea, nocturnal dyspnea, use of rescue inhaler, and activity limitation compared with placebo ($P < 0.001$). In addition, saffron significantly reduced SBP, DBP, TG, and LDL-C. Eosinophils and basophils were also reduced in the saffron group ($P = 0.06$ and $P = 0.05$, respectively). The authors concluded that saffron may be an effective and safe option to improve clinical symptoms in allergic asthma, but they cautioned about unknown long-term side effects (Zilaee et al., 2019).

Cardiovascular Disorders: Coronary Artery Disease/Ischemic Heart Disease

An 8-week RCT in patients ($n = 84$) with CAD compared crocin 30 mg/day with saffron aqueous extract 30 mg/day and with placebo for impacts on atherosclerosis-related gene expression and inflammatory markers. Compared with the placebo group, gene expression of SIRT1 and AMPK increased significantly in the crocin group ($P = 0.001$), and the expression of LOX1 and NF-κB decreased significantly ($P = 0.016$ and 0.004, respectively). Serum ox-LDL levels decreased significantly in the crocin group ($P = 0.002$). MCP-1 levels decreased in both crocin and saffron groups ($P = 0.001$). The authors concluded that crocin may have beneficial effects in CAD patients by increasing the gene expression of SIRT1 and AMPK and decreasing the expression of LOX1 and NF-κB (Abedimanesh et al., 2019).

Cardiometabolic Disorders: Hyperlipidemia and Dyslipidemia

A 2019 systematic review and meta-analysis to investigate the effects of saffron on lipid profiles found 14 RCTs that met inclusion criteria. There was a significant reduction in TC and TG following saffron intervention (WMD = −6.36 mg/dL and WMD = −5.37 mg/dL, respectively). There was no significant effect on weight and LDL-C. A meta-regression analysis showed that long-term saffron intervention could increase HDL-C. The authors concluded that saffron had some benefits on TC, HDL, and TG compared with placebo (Rahmani et al., 2019).

A 2019 systematic review of the effect of saffron supplementation on serum concentrations of lipid and glucose profiles found six studies that met inclusion criteria. Pooled analysis showed a significant reduction in TG (WMD = −8.93 mg/dL; $P = 0.02$) and TC levels (WMD = −5.72 mg/dL; $P = 0.03$), a significant increase in HDL-C (WMD = 2.7 mg/dL; $P = 0.03$) and no significant effect on LDL-C (WMD = −2.30 mg/dL; $P = 0.63$) and FBS levels (WMD = −5.30 mg/dL; $P = 0.51$). The authors concluded that there were significant reductions in TC and TG and an increase in HDL-C with saffron but no significant influences on FBG or LDL-C (Asbaghi et al., 2019).

A 6-week open label trial in volunteers ($n = 20$) with and without CAD investigated the effect of saffron 50 mg dissolved in 100 mL of milk BID for effects on oxidation. There was a constant decrease in lipoprotein oxidation susceptibility from a mean of 66.4 to 38.3 in the 10 healthy individuals and from 76.0 to 48.8 in the 10 patients with CAD ($P < 0.001$ for both). The authors concluded that saffron had potential as an antioxidant (Verma and Bordia, 1998).

A 3-month RCT in patients ($n = 64$) with T2DM compared saffron 30 mg/day with placebo for effects on inflammation. After 3 months of treatment, IL-6 and TNF-α increased significantly in both groups ($P < 0.05$) with no significant difference between groups. Total antioxidant capacity, MDA, hs-CRP, and IL-10 did not change significantly in either group compared with baseline. Homocysteine decreased significantly in the control group. The authors concluded that saffron demonstrated no improvement in homocysteine, antioxidant status, or inflammatory biomarkers in patients with T2DM (Shahbazian et al., 2019).

A 4-week RCT in patients ($n = 40$) with severe depression investigated saffron 30 mg/day plus fluoxetine 20 mg/day compared with placebo plus fluoxetine 20 mg/day for effects on homocysteine levels and depression. With fluoxetine plus saffron there was a significant reduction from baseline in homocysteine levels ($P < 0.04$). There was no change in homocysteine with placebo plus fluoxetine. Based on baseline and follow-up BDI values, both groups showed improvement in depression and there was no significant difference between groups. The authors concluded that saffron had beneficial effects on depression and homocysteine levels in patients with major depression (Jelodar et al., 2018).

A 3-month RCT in patients ($n = 64$) with T2DM compared saffron 30 mg/day with placebo in addition to an oral antidiabetic drug regimen. With saffron, FBG, A1C, TC, LDL-C, and LDL/HDL ratio decreased significantly over baseline ($P < 0.0001$). The mean differences between saffron and placebo for FBG, TC, LDL-C, and LDL/HDL were significant ($P < 0.0001$). A1C, HDL-C, TG, and anthropometric indices showed no significant differences between groups (Moravej Aleali et al., 2019).

A 12-week open-label trial in adults ($n = 44$) with metabolic syndrome investigated the effects of saffron 100 mg/day on metabolic markers. Saffron resulted in lower levels of TC, LDL-C, TG, FBS, and hs-CRP ($P < 0.05$ for all). TG decreased from 148 to 101 ($P = 0.003$). Proinflammatory cytokine reduction was also noted for IL-6 and EGF. The authors concluded that saffron may promote beneficial effects in patients with metabolic syndrome via impact on serum cytokines and reducing TG and LDL-C/TC (Kermani et al., 2017).

Cardiometabolic Disorders: Diabetes, Metabolic Syndrome, and Obesity

A 2020 systematic review and meta-analysis to review the saffron effects on WC, FPG, and A1C concentrations found nine studies ($n = 595$) that met inclusion criteria. Saffron was associated with significant reductions in WC (WMD: -2.18 cm) and FPG (WMD: -6.54 mg/dL). FPG levels decreased significantly when the intervention duration was longer than 12 weeks (WMD: -10.24 mg/dL). There was no significant effect on A1C levels (WMD: -0.13%) following saffron intervention. The authors concluded that saffron led to beneficial effects on WC and FPG (Rahmani et al., 2020).

A 2019 meta-analysis aiming to summarize the clinical evidence regarding the use of saffron and its constituents on cardiovascular risk factors found 10 studies ($n = 622$) that met inclusion criteria. Pooling of results showed significant effects of saffron on DBP (-1.2 mmHg; $I^2 = 0\%$), BW (-1.29 kg; $I^2 = 70\%$), and WC (-1.68 cm; $I^2 = 51\%$). Subgroup analysis based on quality of studies showed a significant reduction in FBG in high quality studies (-10.1 mg/dL; $I^2 = 0\%$). Meta-analysis did not reveal any significant change in lipid profile, fasting insulin, SBP, or BMI following saffron consumption. The authors concluded that saffron might be beneficial in several outcomes associated with cardiovascular disease (Pourmasoumi et al., 2019).

An 8-week RCT in patients ($n = 54$) with T2DM compared saffron with placebo BID plus routine antidiabetic medication. Both groups had similar baseline FBS. FBS significantly decreased with saffron to 129 mg/dL compared with 154 mg/dL with placebo ($P < 0.001$). There were no statistical differences in other metabolic parameters such as serum lipids, blood pressure, and A1C ($P > 0.01$). The authors concluded that saffron hydroalcoholic extract may improve glycemic control in T2DM but had no significant effect on other aspects of diabetic control (Milajerdi et al., 2018a).

A 12-week RCT in patients ($n = 105$) with metabolic syndrome compared saffron 100 mg/day with placebo and with a control group for impact on antibodies against heat shock proteins 17, 60, 65, and 70. At 12 weeks, saffron produced a significant decrease in antiHSP 27 and 70 levels. The authors concluded that saffron can improve some markers of autoimmunity against HSPs in patients with metabolic syndrome, which may explain part of the anti-atherosclerotic effect of saffron (Shemshian et al., 2014).

An 8-week RCT in patients ($n = 44$) with metabolic syndrome compared crocin 30 mg/day with placebo. With crocin there was a 28% increase over baseline in plasma CETP ($P = 0.013$), but the difference between crocin and placebo was not significant. The percent changes in TC ($P = 0.702$), TG ($P = 0.080$), LDL-C ($P = 0.986$), HDL-C ($P = 0.687$), and FBS ($P = 0.614$) did not differ significantly between groups. The authors concluded that although crocin supplements increased the serum CETP in patients with metabolic syndrome, this change was not significant between treatment and placebo groups (Javandoost et al., 2017).

An 8-week RCT in middle-aged patients ($n = 84$ patients) with CAD compared saffron aqueous extract 30 mg/day with crocin 30 mg/day and with placebo for effects on weight. With saffron and crocin, anthropometric variables improved after 8 weeks. Reductions in BMI, WC, and fat mass values with saffron were significantly greater than with crocin ($P < 0.001$). Mean dietary intake decreased significantly from baseline with both saffron and crocin ($P < 0.001$ and $P = 0.046$, respectively) and was unchanged with placebo. Appetite also decreased significantly with saffron and crocin ($P < 0.001$ and $P = 0.029$, respectively). The authors concluded that there was an indication of anti-obesity effects with saffron and crocin in patients with CAD, with saffron having superiority over crocin for some parameters (Abedimanesh et al., 2017).

An 8-week RCT in patients ($n = 75$) with prediabetes compared saffron 15 mg/day with placebo for glycemic effects. With saffron, FBS decreased from a baseline of 118 mg/dL to 109 mg/dL; A1C decreased from a baseline of 5.8% to 5.7%; and diphenylpycrylhydrazyl (*a measure of free radical scavenging activity*) increased from a baseline of 11% to 13.5% ($P < 0.005$ for all). No significant changes in anthropometric measures, lipid profile, and renal markers were observed after saffron intake compared with placebo. The authors concluded that saffron could improve glycemic and antioxidant indices in overweight/obese individuals with prediabetes (Karimi-Nazari et al., 2019).

An 8-week RCT in healthy, mildly overweight women ($n = 60$) studied Satiereal, a high-dose saffron extract of 176.5 mg/day compared with placebo for effects on appetite and weight. The mean snacking frequency was significantly decreased with the saffron extract compared with placebo ($P < 0.05$). With the saffron extract there was a significantly greater BW reduction than with placebo ($P < 0.01$). Other anthropometric dimensions and vital signs remained almost unchanged in both groups. No subject withdrawal attributable to side effects was reported throughout the trial. The authors concluded that this saffron extract produced a reduction of snacking and created a satiating effect that could contribute to BW loss (Gout et al., 2010).

A 12-week RCT in patients ($n = 80$) with T2DM compared saffron 100 mg/day with placebo for effects on BP, liver, and kidneys. With saffron there was a significant reduction over placebo in SBP ($P < 0.005$). There were no differences between groups in changes to DBP, liver enzymes, creatinine, BUN, 24-h urine albumin, dietary intake, or activity levels. The authors concluded that saffron improved SBP, but did not improve DBP, nephropathy indices, or liver functions in patients with T2DM. In a separate analysis and publication, it was noted that saffron resulted in significant decreases in WC and MDA compared with placebo ($P < 0.001$ for both). Serum fasting insulin, FBS, A1C, HOMA-IR, lipid profile, hs-CRP, TNF-α, and total antioxidant capacity did not differ significantly between groups. The authors concluded that saffron had beneficial effects on WC and MDA levels but did not influence several other cardiometabolic risk markers in patients with T2DM (Ebrahimi et al., 2019a,b).

An 8-week RCT in patients ($n = 60$) with T2DM compared saffron 100 mg/day with placebo for effects on glycemia and inflammation. FBG levels decreased more with saffron than with placebo (to 130.93 mg/dL and 135.13 mg/dL, respectively; $P = 0.012$). TNF-α decreased to 114.4 and 140.9 with saffron and placebo, respectively ($P < 0.001$). Saffron was associated with a downregulation of the expressions of TNF-α ($P = 0.035$) and IL-6 mRNA levels ($P = 0.014$). The authors concluded that saffron modulated glucose levels and inflammation in T2DM patients through decreasing the expression of inflammatory mediators (Mobasseri et al., 2020).

A 12-week RCT in patients ($n = 66$) diagnosed with schizophrenia who were on olanzapine 5-20 mg daily but were without metabolic syndrome compared saffron aqueous extract 30 mg/day with crocin 30 mg/day and with placebo for risk of development of metabolic syndrome. Time-treatment interaction showed a significant difference in FBS with both saffron and crocin compared with placebo ($P = 0.004$). Saffron prevented reaching the criteria of metabolic syndrome (zero patients) compared with crocin (9.1%) and placebo (27.3%) as early as week 6. The authors concluded that saffron could prevent metabolic syndrome in schizophrenics taking olanzapine (Fadai et al., 2014).

Women's Genitourinary Disorders: Premenstrual Syndrome

A 2011 systematic review evaluating the effects of herbal medicine for PMS found 17 RCTs that met inclusion criteria and selected 10 of them for analysis, of which four trials ($n = 500$) studied chasteberry. Chasteberry was reported to consistently ameliorate PMS better than placebo. Single trials also supported the use of either ginkgo or saffron. Evening primrose oil and St. John's wort did not differ from placebo. None of the herbs was associated with major health risks, although the reduced number of tested patients did not allow definitive conclusions on safety (Dante and Facchinetti, 2011).

A four-cycle RCT in women aged 20-45 years ($n = 50$) with PMS compared saffron 15 mg BID with placebo given for the third and fourth menstrual cycles. Based on Daily Symptom Report scores and HAM-D scores, saffron was found to be effective in relieving symptoms of PMS. Positive response (defined as 50% reduction in severity of symptoms) occurred in 76% with saffron and 8% with placebo ($P < 0.0001$, NNT = 1.47). There was a significant effect of saffron on Total Daily Symptom Ratings ($P < 0.0001$). The authors concluded that saffron was effective in the treatment of PMS (Agha-Hosseini et al., 2008).

An acutely dosed open label trial in healthy women ($n = 35$) assessed the salivary hormonal effect of 20 min of exposure to saffron aroma. Saffron odor significantly decreased cortisol levels and increased 17-β estradiol levels in both follicular and luteal phases. State-Trait Anxiety Inventory scores decreased in the follicular and luteal phases. The authors concluded that saffron aroma produced physiological and psychological effects in women, and saffron aroma may play a role in the treatment of PMS, dysmenorrhea, and irregular menstruation (Fukui et al., 2011).

Women's Genitourinary Disorders: Menopause

A 6-week RCT in post-menopausal women ($n = 60$) with hot flushes compared saffron 30 mg/day with placebo. Results were based on scores for the Hot Flush Related Daily Interference Scale (HFRDIS) and HAM-D. General linear model repeated measures at 3 and 6 weeks demonstrated significant effect for time × treatment interaction on the HFRDIS score [F $(3,162) = 10.41$; $P = 0.0001$] and HAM-D score [F $(3,162) = 5.48$; $P = 0.001$]. Frequency of adverse events was not significantly different between the two groups. The authors concluded that saffron was a safe and effective treatment in improving hot flushes and de-

pressive symptoms in post-menopausal women and may provide a non-hormonal alternative for treatment of hot flushes (Kashani et al., 2018).

Women's Genitourinary Disorders: Prepartum Cervical Ripening

An acutely dosed RCT in pregnant women ($n = 50$) who were 39-41 weeks EGA with Bishop's score < 4 compared saffron 250 mg with placebo for effect on cervical ripening. Bishop's scores were similar between groups at baseline ($P = 0.792$) and at 12 hours ($P = 0.159$), but significantly higher with saffron at 20-24 hours ($P = 0.029$) and just after onset of active uterine contractions ($P = 0.003$). In the saffron group, there was no cesarean section and one meconium staining of the fetus, while there were three cesarean sections and four meconium stainings, in the placebo group. There was no statistically significant difference between the groups in terms of the timing of the onset of spontaneous active uterine contractions, the duration of the first and second stages of labor, the need for delivery augmentation, and Apgar scores ($P > 0.05$). No adverse events were reported. The authors concluded that saffron could increase cervical readiness in term pregnancy but that more research was needed to assess its effect on delivery and neonatal outcomes (Sadi et al., 2016).

Men's Genitourinary Disorders: Male Infertility

A 2018 systematic review and meta-analysis to determine saffron effectiveness and safety in male infertility problems found six trials that met inclusion criteria. In one study conducted on sperm parameters, the mean percentage of sperm with normal morphology and sperm motility were increased ($P < 0.001$ for both). Quantitative analysis showed that saffron had a significantly positive effect on all dimensions of Erectile Function questionnaire: Erectile function (MD = 5.36; $P = 0.00$); Orgasmic Function (MD = 1.12; $P = 0.007$); Overall Satisfaction (MD = 1.23; $P = 0.005$); Satisfaction with Intercourse (MD = 2.18; $P = 0.00$); and Sexual Desire (MD = 0.78; $P = 0.00$). The result of subgroup analysis based on dimensions of Erectile Function questionnaire showed statistically significant differences among subgroups ($P = 0.00$). The authors concluded that saffron had a positive effect on erectile dysfunction but that there were contradictory results about semen parameters (Maleki-Saghooni et al., 2018).

A 26-week RCT in infertile men ($n = 260$) with oligoasthenoteratozoospermia (OAT) compared saffron 60 mg/day with placebo for changes in semen parameters and total seminal plasma antioxidant capacity. At the end of the trial, mean motility was 25.7% with saffron and 24.9% with placebo; normal sperm morphology was 18.7% with saffron and 18.4% with placebo; mean sperm density was 20.5% with saffron and 21.4% with placebo ($P = 0.1$ for all). Saffron also did not improve total seminal plasma antioxidant capacity, compared with baseline ($P = 0.1$) and with placebo subjects ($P = 0.1$). The authors concluded that saffron did not appear to improve semen parameters in infertile men with idiopathic OAT (Safarinejad et al., 2011).

An open-label trial in infertile men ($n = 52$) whose problem could not be solved surgically investigated the effects of saffron 50 mg in milk 3x/week on several semen parameters. After treatment, the mean percentage of sperm with normal morphology increased from 26.5% to 33.9% ($P < 0.001$); the mean percentage of sperm with Class A motility increased from 5.3% to 11.8% ($P < 0.001$); Class B and C motilities increased from 10.1% and 19.8% to 17.9% and 25.3%, respectively ($P < 0.001$ for both). No significant increase was detected in sperm count ($P = 0.30$). The authors concluded that saffron had positive effects on sperm morphology and motility but did not increase sperm count in infertile men (Heidary et al., 2008).

Male and Female Sexual Dysfunction

A 2019 systematic review and meta-analysis to evaluate the effect of saffron on sexual dysfunction and its subscales among men and women found five studies ($n = 173$) that met inclusion criteria. The analysis showed a statistically significant positive effect of saffron on sexual dysfunction (SMD = 0.811) and its subscales (SMD = 0.493). There was heterogeneity among the studies ($Q = 9.981$, df = 4; $P = 0.041$, $I^2 = 59.92\%$). There was no evidence of publication bias. The authors concluded that in general saffron was proven effective in improving sexual dysfunction and its subscales (Ranjbar and Ashrafizaveh, 2019).

A 2018 systematic review to evaluate the efficacy of saffron for erectile dysfunction (ED) found three RCTs involving saffron ($n = 397$) out of a total of 24 RCTs on the subject of herbal treatments for ED (other herbs studied included ginseng, tribulus,

Pinus pinaster, and maca). Ginseng significantly improved erectile function (IIEF-5 score: 140 with ginseng, 96 with placebo; SMD = 0.43; $P < 0.01$; $I^2 = 0$). *P. pinaster* and maca showed very preliminary positive results, and saffron and tribulus produced mixed results. Adverse events were recorded in 19 of 24 trials, with no significant differences between placebo and verum in placebo-controlled studies. The authors concluded that ginseng may be an effective herbal treatment for ED and that preliminary promising results have been generated for the other herbal formulations (Borrelli et al., 2018).

A 1-month RCT in diabetic men ($n = 50$) with erectile dysfunction compared a 1% saffron gel with placebo gel applied 30 min prior to intercourse for effects on ED. Changes from baseline to 1 month in the IIEF Questionnaire showed that saffron gel significantly improved ED compared with placebo ($P < 0.001$). The authors concluded that saffron could be considered a treatment option for diabetic men with ED (Mohammadzadeh-Moghadam et al., 2015).

A 4-week RCT in men ($n = 36$) with MDD stabilized on fluoxetine but with sexual impairment compared saffron 15 mg BID with placebo. Outcomes were based on the IIEF scale measured at baseline, week 2, and week 4. The effect of time–treatment interaction on the total score was significant [F (1.444, 40.434) = 6.154; $P = 0.009$]. By week 4, saffron resulted in significantly greater improvements in erectile function ($P < 0.001$), intercourse satisfaction domains ($P = 0.001$), and total scores ($P < 0.001$) than the placebo group. The effect of saffron did not differ significantly from placebo for orgasmic function ($P = 0.095$), overall satisfaction ($P = 0.334$), and sexual desire ($P = 0.517$). Normal erectile function (score > 25 on erectile function domain) was achieved in 60% and 7% of the saffron and placebo groups, respectively ($P = 0.005$). Final depressive symptoms scores were similar between the two groups. Frequency of side effects were similar between the two groups. The authors concluded that saffron was a tolerable and efficacious treatment for fluoxetine-related ED (Modabbernia et al., 2012).

A 4-week RCT in women ($n = 38$) with MDD stabilized on fluoxetine 40 mg/day but with sexual dysfunction compared saffron 30 mg/day with placebo for effects on fluoxetine-induced sexual dysfunction. Outcomes were based on the Female Sexual Function

Index (FSFI). Two-factor repeated measure analysis of variance showed a significant effect of time–treatment interaction [F (1.580, 50.567) = 5.366; $P = 0.012$] and treatment for FSFI total score [F (1,32) = 4.243; $P = 0.048$]. Patients in the saffron group experienced significantly more improvement in total FSFI ($P < 0.001$) and domains for arousal ($P = 0.028$), lubrication ($P = 0.035$), and pain ($P = 0.016$) but not in desire ($P = 0.196$), satisfaction ($P = 0.206$), or orgasm ($P = 0.354$). Frequency of side effects was similar between the two groups. The authors concluded that saffron may safely and effectively improve some of the fluoxetine-induced sexual problems including arousal, lubrication, and pain (Kashani et al., 2013).

An open-label trial in men ($n = 20$) with ED investigated the effects of saffron 200 mg/day for 10 days on penile tumescence. The 15-question IIEF scores increased from 22.1 to 39.2 after treatment ($P < 0.001$). There was a statistically significant improvement in tip rigidity and tip tumescence as well as base rigidity and base tumescence. The authors concluded that saffron showed a positive effect on sexual function with increased number and duration of erectile events seen in patients with ED after 10 days (Shamsa et al., 2009).

Musculoskeletal Disorders: Chronic Musculoskeletal Pain/Fibromyalgia

An 8-week RCT in patients ($n = 46$) with fibromyalgia compared saffron 15 mg with duloxetine 30 mg, given daily for 1 week then BID for 7 weeks for effects on seven different disease-related scales. No significant difference was detected for any of the scales in terms of score changes from baseline to the endpoint between the two groups (Mean score changes: −4.26 to 2.37; $P = 0.182$-0.900) nor in terms of time–treatment interactions ($P = 0.209$-0.964). The authors concluded that saffron and duloxetine demonstrated comparable efficacy in the treatment of fibromyalgia (Shakiba et al., 2018).

Neurological Disorders: Stroke

A 3-month RCT in patients ($n = 39$) with acute ischemic stroke investigated saffron 200 mg/day plus routine care compared with routine care alone (control) starting at stroke onset and continuing for 3 months. Based on the NIH Stoke Scale, the severity of stroke

during the first 4 days was significantly lower in the saffron-treated group than in the control group ($P < 0.05$). Compared with the levels on the first day, serum NSE and s100 levels were significantly decreased and BDNF concentration was increased in the saffron-treated group on the fourth day. At the end of the 3-month follow-up period, the mean Barthel index (*for ADLs*) was significantly higher in the saffron-treated group than in the control group ($P < 0.001$). The authors concluded that short and long-term use of saffron had neuroprotective effects following acute ischemic stroke (Asadollahi et al., 2019).

A 4-day RCT in patients ($n = 40$) with acute ischemic stroke compared routine care alone with routine care plus saffron 200 mg BID for effects on oxidation and clinical status. The severity of stroke, based on the National Institute of Health Stroke Scale scores, was significantly reduced after 4 days in the saffron group. On the fourth day after ischemic stroke onset, antioxidant enzymes activities, GSH, and TAC levels were higher and MDA levels were lower with saffron compared with the control group. The severity of stroke was negatively correlated with the levels of GSH and TAC and positively correlated with MDA level. The authors concluded that saffron had modulatory effects on ischemic-induced oxidative stress due to its free radical scavenging and antioxidant properties (Gudarzi et al., 2020).

Neurological Disorders: Cognitive Impairment

A 12-week RCT in patients ($n = 76$) with on-pump CABG, who had Wechsler Memory Scale (WMS) score > 70 and age < 70 years, compared saffron 15 mg BID with placebo. No significant differences in mean total score changes from baseline for WMS-Revised, MMSE, or subscales of Hospital Anxiety and Depression Scale were present between saffron and placebo groups. The authors concluded that saffron did not appear to provide any benefit in treatment of CABG-related neuropsychiatric conditions (Moazen-Zadeh et al., 2018).

Neurological Disorders: Dementia

A 22-week Phase II RCT in adults ($n = 54$) with mild-to-moderate Alzheimer's disease (AD) compared saffron 30 mg/day with donepezil 10 mg/day.

Based on the change in the ADAS-cognitive subscale and Clinical Dementia Rating Scale-Sums of Boxes scores saffron was found to be as effective as donepezil in the treatment of mild-to-moderate AD after 22 weeks. The frequency of adverse events was similar between groups except for vomiting, which occurred significantly more frequently in the donepezil group. The authors concluded that there was a possible therapeutic effect of saffron for mild-to-moderate AD (Akhondzadeh et al., 2010b).

A 12-month RCT in patients ($n = 68$) with moderate-to-severe AD (MMSE 8-14) compared saffron 30 mg/day with memantine 20 mg/day. There were no significant differences between the two groups in the Severe Cognitive Impairment Rating Scale score changes ($P = 0.38$) and FAST ($P = 0.87$) from baseline to the endpoint. The frequency of adverse events was not significantly different between the two groups. The authors concluded that 1 year of saffron was comparable to memantine in reducing cognitive decline in patients with moderate-to-severe AD (Farokhnia et al., 2014).

A 16-week RCT in patients ($n = 46$) with probable AD compared saffron 30 mg/day with placebo. After 16 weeks, the ADAS-cog score with saffron was significantly better than placebo (F = 4.12, df = 1; $P = 0.04$). The Clinical Dementia Rating Scale-sums of boxes score was also significantly better with saffron (F = 4.12, df = 1; $P = 0.04$). There were no significant differences between the two groups in terms of observed adverse events. The authors concluded that saffron was both safe and effective for mild-to-moderate AD, at least in the short term (Akhondzadeh et al., 2010a).

A 12-month RCT in patients ($n = 35$) with amnesic and multi-domain mild cognitive impairment (aMCImd) compared saffron with no treatment. By 12 months the patients on saffron had improved MMSE scores ($P = 0.015$), while the control group deteriorated. MRI, EEG, and event-related brain potential showed improvement in specific domains with saffron. The authors concluded that saffron was a good choice for management for aMCImd (Tsolaki et al., 2016).

An 8-week RCT in patients ($n = 60$) with major neurocognitive disorder on anti-dementia medications compared a combination of saffron, sedge, and astragalus in honey with placebo. At one month, the Addenbrooke's Cognitive Examination scores changed from baseline of 32.2 to 38.8 with saffron and from 22.1 to 22.6 with placebo ($P = 0.007$). The Geriatric Depression Scale score changed from 14.6 to 12.9 and to 12.2 at baseline, 4 weeks, and 8 weeks, respectively, with saffron and from 14.5 to 14.3 to 14.4, respectively, with placebo ($P = 0.945$; $P = 0.465$; $P = 0.224$). The authors concluded that the herbal combination of sedge, saffron, and astragalus in honey in patients with major neurocognitive disorder could help improve cognitive and depressive scores (Akouchekian et al., 2018).

A 2-month RCT in elderly patients ($n = 30$) with MMSE scores 20-27 and self-perceived cognitive decline compared a combination of bacopa, L-theanine, saffron, copper, B vitamins, and vitamin D with placebo. MMSE and Perceived Stress Questionnaire Index significantly improved with the herbal combination, both compared with baseline and compared with placebo. Both groups experienced a significant improvement in the Self-rating Depression Scale scores. The authors concluded that this herbal combination produced significant improvements in the cognitive functions tested (Cicero et al., 2017).

Psychiatric Disorders: Anxiety and OCD

A 2020 systematic review and meta-analysis to assess the effects of saffron on mental health parameters and CRP levels found 21 trials that met inclusion criteria. Consumption of saffron resulted in significant reductions in BDI (WMD: −4.86), BAI (WMD: −5.29), and Pittsburgh Sleep Quality Index (PSQI) (WMD: −2.22). Saffron did not affect HAM-D or HAM-A scores or CRP levels. The authors concluded that saffron reduced BDI, BAI, and PSQI scores (Ghaderi et al., 2020).

A 2019 systematic review and meta-analysis to investigate the effect of saffron supplementation on depression and anxiety selected 23 studies that met inclusion criteria.

Saffron had a large positive effect size when compared with placebo for depressive symptoms ($g = 0.99$; $P < 0.001$) and anxiety symptoms ($g = 0.95$; $P < 0.006$). Saffron also had a large positive effect size when used as an adjunct to antidepressants for depressive symptoms ($g = 1.23$; $P = 0.028$). The authors concluded that saffron could be an effective intervention for symptoms of depression and anxiety, but they also found evidence of publication bias and lack of diversity (Marx et al., 2019).

A 2018 systematic review to identify single-herb medicines that may warrant further study for treatment of anxiety and depression in cancer patients found 100 studies involving 38 botanicals that met inclusion criteria. Among herbs most studied ($\geq$ six RCTs each), lavender, passionflower, and saffron produced benefits comparable to standard anxiolytics and antidepressants. Black cohosh, chamomile, and chasteberry were also promising. Overall, 45% of studies reported positive findings with fewer adverse effects compared with conventional medications. The authors concluded that saffron, black cohosh, chamomile, chasteberry, lavender, and passionflower appeared useful in mitigating anxiety or depression with favorable risk-benefit profiles compared with standard treatments, and these botanicals may benefit cancer patients by minimizing medication load and accompanying side effects (Yeung et al., 2018).

A 4-week RCT in patients ($n = 128$) with low mood, stress, anxiety, and impaired sleep, but not diagnosed with depression, compared a standardized stigma extract of saffron (affron) 28 mg/day or 22 mg/day with placebo. Negative mood and symptoms related to stress and anxiety decreased significantly with the 28 mg/day dose, with a significant difference between 28 mg/day and placebo on the Total Mood Disturbance scale ($P < 0.001$, $d = -1.10$), but there was no significant treatment effect at the 22 mg/day dose. The authors concluded that affron increased mood, reduced anxiety, and managed stress without side effects (Kell et al., 2017).

A 12-week RCT in patients ($n = 60$) with anxiety and depression compared saffron 50 mg BID with placebo. Based on changes in BDI and BAI scores at 6 and 12 weeks, saffron supplements had a significant beneficial effect compared with placebo at 12 weeks ($P < 0.001$). The authors concluded that saffron appeared to have a significant impact in the treatment of anxiety and depression with rare side effects (Mazidi et al., 2016).

An 8-week RCT in patients ($n = 54$) with mild-to-moderate comorbid depression and anxiety (CDA) and T2DM compared saffron 30 mg/day with placebo. Based on measurements HAM-D, HAM-A, and Pittsburgh Sleep Quality Index and Satisfaction with Life Scale, mild-to-moderate CDA, anxiety, and sleep disturbance, but not depression alone, were relieved significantly with saffron ($P < 0.05$) but not with placebo. Dietary intake, physical activity, and changes in life satisfaction did not differ significantly between groups. The authors concluded that saffron had a beneficial effect on mild-to-moderate CDA in patients with T2DM (Milajerdi et al., 2018b).

An 8-week RCT in teenagers ($n = 80$) with mild-to-moderate anxiety or depression compared saffron (affron) 14 mg BID with placebo. Outcomes were based on youth and parent versions of the Revised Child Anxiety and Depression Scale (RCADS). Based on youth self-reports, saffron was associated with greater improvements in overall internalizing symptoms ($P = 0.049$), separation anxiety ($P = 0.003$), social phobia ($P = 0.023$), and depression ($P = 0.016$). Total internalizing scores decreased by an average of 33% with saffron and 17% with placebo ($P = 0.029$). With parental reports, mean improvements in RCADS scores were greater with saffron (40% vs 26%) ($P = 0.026$), but no other significant differences were identified. The herb was well tolerated and there was a trend toward reduced headaches in participants on the active treatment. The authors concluded that this standardized saffron extract improved anxious and depressive symptoms in youth with mild-to-moderate symptoms, at least from the perspective of the adolescent (Lopresti et al., 2018).

A 10-week RCT in patients ($n = 50$) with mild-to-moderate OCD compared saffron 30 mg/day with fluvoxamine 100 mg/day. General linear repeated measures at 2, 4, 6, 8, and 10 weeks demonstrated no significant effect for time-treatment interaction on the Yale-Brown Obsessive-Compulsive Scale (Y-BOCS) total scores [F (2.42, 106.87) = 0.70; $P = 0.52$], obsession Y-BOCS subscale scores [F (2.47, 108.87) = 0.77; $P = 0.49$], and compulsion Y-BOCS subscale scores [F (2.18, 96.06) = 0.25; $P = 0.79$]. Frequency of adverse events was not significantly different between the two groups. The authors concluded that saffron was as effective as fluvoxamine in the treatment of patients with mild-to-moderate OCD (Esalatmanesh et al., 2017).

Psychiatric Disorders: Insomnia

A 28-day RCT in patients ($n = 63$) with insomnia compared a standardized saffron extract (Affron) 14 mg BID with placebo to assess sleep-enhancing effects of the supplement. Saffron was associated with greater improvements than placebo in the Insomnia Severity Index total score ($P=0.017$), the Restorative Sleep Questionnaire total score ($P=0.029$), and the Pittsburgh Sleep Diary sleep quality ratings ($P=0.014$). There were no reported adverse effects. The authors concluded that saffron was associated with improvements in sleep quality in people with insomnia (Lopresti et al., 2020).

Psychiatric Disorders: Depression

A 2020 systematic review and meta-analysis to assess the effects of saffron on mental health parameters and CRP levels found 21 trials that met inclusion criteria. Consumption of saffron resulted in significant reductions in BDI (WMD: -4.86), BAI (WMD: -5.29), and Pittsburgh Sleep Quality Index (PSQI) (WMD: -2.22). Saffron did not affect HAM-D or HAM-A scores or CRP levels. The authors concluded that saffron reduced BDI, BAI, and PSQI scores (Ghaderi et al., 2020).

A 2019 systematic review and meta-analysis to investigate the effect of saffron supplementation on depression and anxiety selected 23 studies that met inclusion criteria. Saffron had a large positive effect size when compared with placebo for depressive symptoms ($g=0.99$; $P<0.001$) and anxiety symptoms ($g=0.95$; $P<0.006$). Saffron also had a large positive effect size when used as an adjunct to antidepressants for depressive symptoms ($g=1.23$; $P=0.028$). The authors concluded that saffron could be an effective intervention for symptoms of depression and anxiety, but they also found evidence of publication bias and lack of diversity (Marx et al., 2019).

A 2019 systematic review and meta-analysis of the efficacy of saffron in mild-to-moderate depression found 11 RCTs that met inclusion criteria for qualitative analysis, nine of which were pooled for statistical analysis. The authors found that saffron had a significant effect on the severity of depression and was significantly more effective than placebo ($g=0.891$; $P=0.001$) and was non-inferior to tested antidepressant drugs ($g=-0.246$; $P=0.053$) (Tóth et al., 2019).

A 2019 systematic review to evaluate the effectiveness of saffron compared with placebo and with fluoxetine in the treatment of depressed patients found eight studies that met inclusion criteria. Saffron was superior to placebo (SMD $=-0.86$) and was comparable to fluoxetine (SMD $=0.11$). The authors concluded that saffron was comparable to fluoxetine for depression (Khaksarian et al., 2019).

A 2018 systematic review to determine the efficacy and safety of saffron in the treatment of MDD in comparison with placebo and synthetic antidepressants included seven RCTs for meta-analysis. The overall quality of the included studies was rated as moderate. Saffron showed more improvements in depression symptoms when compared with placebo (SMD $=-1.22$; $P=0.001$) and it was as effective as synthetic antidepressants (SMD $=0.16$ $P=0.44$). Moderate heterogeneity was present mostly due to treatment dose and duration, types of synthetic antidepressants, and outcome measures. The authors concluded that saffron was effective in the treatment of MDD and had comparable efficacy with synthetic antidepressants. Saffron was also a safe drug without serious adverse events (Yang et al., 2018).

A 2018 systematic review to identify single-herb medicines that may warrant further study for treatment of anxiety and depression in cancer patients found 100 studies involving 38 botanicals that met inclusion criteria. Among herbs most studied ($\geq$ six RCTs each), lavender, passionflower, and saffron produced benefits comparable to standard anxiolytics and antidepressants. Black cohosh, chamomile, and chasteberry were also promising. Overall, 45% of studies reported positive findings with fewer adverse effects compared with conventional medications. The authors concluded that saffron, black cohosh, chamomile, chasteberry, lavender, and passionflower appeared useful in mitigating anxiety or depression with favorable risk-benefit profiles compared with standard treatments, and these botanicals may benefit cancer patients by minimizing medication load and accompanying side effects (Yeung et al., 2018).

A 2014 expanded systematic review of the RCTs on saffron and depression, detailing dosages, extract sources, standardizations, safety profile, and treatment duration, identified six studies for review. In the placebo-comparison trials, saffron had large treatment effects and had similar efficacy to synthetic antidepressant drugs. Review of in vivo and in vitro research suggested that the antidepressant effects of saffron may be due to its serotonergic, antioxidant, anti-inflammatory, neuro-endocrine, and neuroprotective effects (Lopresti and Drummond, 2014).

A 2013 meta-analysis of RCTs examining the effects of saffron supplementation on symptoms of depression among participants with MDD found five RCTs that met inclusion criteria. A large effect size was found for saffron supplementation compared with placebo in treating depressive symptoms (ES = 1.62; $P < 0.001$), revealing that saffron supplementation significantly reduced depression symptoms compared with placebo. A null effect size was evidenced between saffron supplementation and the antidepressant groups (ES = −0.15) indicating that both treatments were similarly effective in reducing depression symptoms. The mean Jadad score was 5, indicating high quality of trials. The authors concluded that trials indicate saffron can improve symptoms of depression in adults with MDD (Hausenblas et al., 2013).

A 2011 systematic review to evaluate herbal medicines, other than St. John's wort, in the treatment of depression found nine trials that met inclusion criteria. Investigation of saffron stigma occurred in three trials and saffron petals were investigated in two trials. Saffron stigma and petals were compared in another trial. Other herbs studied were lavender, *Echium amoenum*, and rhodiola. Saffron stigma was found to be significantly more effective than placebo and equally as effective as fluoxetine and imipramine. Saffron petal was significantly more effective than placebo and was found to be equally effective as fluoxetine and saffron stigma. Lavender was found to be less effective than imipramine, but the combination of lavender and imipramine was significantly more effective than imipramine alone. When compared with placebo, *E. amoenum* was found to significantly decrease depression scores at week 4 but not week 6. Rhodiola was also found to significantly improve depressive symptoms when compared with placebo. The authors concluded that several herbal medicines showed promise in the management of mild-to-moderate depression (Dwyer et al., 2011).

An 8-week RCT in patients ($n = 160$) with persistent depression currently on medication investigated adjunctive treatment with saffron (affron) 14 mg BID compared with placebo. The scores on the clinician-rated Montgomery- Åsberg Depression Rating Scale (MADRS) were reduced by 41% and 21% with saffron and placebo, respectively ($P = 0.001$). However, scores on the self-rated MADRS decreased

27% and 26% with saffron and placebo, respectively ($P = 0.831$). Saffron was associated with a greater reduction in adverse effects of antidepressants ($P = 0.019$), although this was non-significant after covarying for baseline values ($P = 0.449$). Quality of life improved in both groups with no significant between-group differences ($P = 0.638$). The authors concluded that adding saffron to antidepressants was associated with a greater improvement in depressive symptoms as perceived by clinicians but not by self-report (Lopresti et al., 2019).

A 6-week RCT in patients ($n = 40$) with MDD compared saffron 30 mg BID with placebo. At 6 weeks, saffron had a significantly better outcome than placebo on the HAM-D (F = 18.89, df = 1; $P < 0.001$). There were no significant differences between groups for observed side effects. The authors concluded that saffron was efficacious in the treatment of mild-to-moderate depression (Akhondzadeh et al., 2005).

A 6-week RCT in patients ($n = 40$) with mild-to-moderate MDD compared saffron petal extract 30 mg/day with placebo to assess the efficacy of saffron petal in the treatment of depression. At 6 weeks, saffron petal produced a significantly better outcome on HAM-D than placebo (F = 16.87, df = 1; $P < 0.001$). There were no significant differences between groups in terms of observed side effects. The authors concluded that the petal of saffron was effective in the treatment of mild to moderate depression (Moshiri et al., 2006).

A 4-week RCT in patients ($n = 40$) with MDD compared an average-dosed SSRI plus either crocin 30 mg/day or placebo. Based on BDI, BAI, the General Health Questionnaire (GHQ), and Mood Disorder Questionnaire, there were significant improvements in scores with crocin compared with placebo ($P < 0.0001$). The average of decreases in BDI, BAI, and GHQ scores were 17.6, 12.7, and 17.2, respectively with crocin and 6.15, 2.6, and 10.3, respectively, with placebo. The authors concluded that crocin was efficacious in depression and could be given in the treatment of MDD patients (Talaei et al., 2015).

An 8-week pilot RCT in patients ($n = 40$) with MDD compared saffron 15 mg BID with fluoxetine 10 mg BID. Based on HAM-D scores, saffron was found to have similar efficacy to fluoxetine (F = 0.03, df = 1; $P = 0.84$). Remission rate was 25% in both groups. Side effects were similar between groups. The authors concluded that saffron had antidepressant effects as born out in other studies (Akhondzadeh Basti et al., 2007.

A 6-week RCT in patients ($n = 40$) with mild-to-moderate depression compared saffron 30 mg/day with fluoxetine 20 mg/day. Saffron was found have similar efficacy to fluoxetine in the treatment of mild-to-moderate depression (F = 0.13, df = 1; $P = 0.71$). Side effects did not differ significantly between groups. The authors concluded that saffron was effective in in the treatment of mild-to-moderate depression (Noorbala et al., 2005).

A 6-week RCT in patients ($n = 30$) with mild-to-moderate MDD compared saffron 30 mg/day with imipramine 100 mg/day. Based on HAM-D scores, saffron showed similar efficacy to imipramine (F = 2.91, df = 1; $P = 0.09$). In the imipramine group, anticholinergic effects and sedation were observed more often. The authors concluded that saffron may be of therapeutic benefit in the treatment of mild-to-moderate depression (Akhondzadeh et al., 2004).

A 6-week RCT in patients ($n = 66$) with MDD accompanied by anxious distress compared saffron 30 mg/day with citalopram 40 mg/day. Patients who received either saffron or citalopram showed significant improvement in scores of the HAM-D ($P < 0.001$ in both groups) and HAM-A ($P < 0.001$ in both groups). Comparison of score changes between the two groups showed no significant difference ($P = 0.984$). Frequency of side effects was not significantly different between the two groups. The authors concluded that saffron was potentially efficacious and tolerable as treatment for MDD with anxious distress (Ghajar et al., 2017).

A 12-week RCT in patients ($n = 60$) with anxiety and depression compared saffron 50 mg BID with placebo. Based on changes in BDI and BAI scores at 6 and 12 weeks, saffron supplements had a significant beneficial effect compared with placebo at 12 weeks ($P < 0.001$). The authors concluded that saffron appeared to have a significant impact in the treatment of anxiety and depression with rare side effects (Mazidi et al., 2016).

An 8-week RCT in patients ($n = 54$) with mild-to-moderate comorbid depression and anxiety (CDA) and T2DM compared saffron 30 mg/day with placebo. Based on measurements HAM-D, HAM-A, and

Pittsburgh Sleep Quality Index and Satisfaction with Life Scale, mild-to-moderate CDA, anxiety, and sleep disturbance, but not depression alone, were relieved significantly with saffron ($P < 0.05$) but not with placebo. Dietary intake, physical activity, and changes in life satisfaction did not differ significantly between groups. The authors concluded that saffron had a beneficial effect on mild-to-moderate CDA in patients with T2DM (Milajerdi et al., 2018b).

An 8-week RCT in teenagers ($n = 80$) with mild-to-moderate anxiety or depression compared saffron (affron) 14 mg BID with placebo. Outcomes were based on youth and parent versions of the Revised Child Anxiety and Depression Scale (RCADS). Based on youth self-reports, saffron was associated with greater improvements in overall internalizing symptoms ($P = 0.049$), separation anxiety ($P = 0.003$), social phobia ($P = 0.023$), and depression ($P = 0.016$). Total internalizing scores decreased by an average of 33% with saffron and 17% with placebo ($P = 0.029$). With parental reports, mean improvements in RCADS scores were greater with saffron (40% vs 26%) ($P = 0.026$), but no other significant differences were identified. The herb was well tolerated and there was a trend toward reduced headaches in participants on the active treatment. The authors concluded that this standardized saffron extract improved anxious and depressive symptoms in youth with mild-to-moderate symptoms, at least from the perspective of the adolescent (Lopresti et al., 2018).

A 6-week RCT in postpartum women ($n = 64$) with mild-to-moderate postpartum depression compared saffron 15 mg BID with fluoxetine 20 mg BID. There was no significant effect for time–treatment interaction on HAM-D score between the two groups [F (4.90, 292.50) = 1.04; $P = 0.37$]. Complete response ($\geq 50\%$ reduction in HAM-D) occurred in 41% with saffron and 50% with fluoxetine, and the difference between groups was not significant ($P = 0.61$). Frequency of adverse events was also not significantly different between groups. The authors concluded that saffron was a safe alternative medication for improving postpartum depression (Kashani et al., 2017).

An 8-week RCT in breastfeeding women ($n = 60$) with postpartum depression and a maximum score of 29 on the BDI-II compared saffron 15 mg BID with placebo. The mean BDI-II scores decreased from

20.3 to 8.4 with saffron ($P < 0.0001$) and from 19.8 to 15.1 with placebo ($P < 0.01$). The difference between groups was significant. Remission occurred in 96% with saffron and 43% with placebo ($P < 0.01$). The complete response rates were 66% with saffron and 6% with placebo. The authors concluded that saffron was more effective than placebo in breastfeeding mothers with mild postpartum depression (Tabeshpour et al., 2017).

A 6-week RCT in older patients ($n = 50$) with MDD compared saffron 60 mg/day with sertraline 100 mg/day. Based on serial HAM-D scores at baseline, 2, 4, and 6 weeks, symptoms of depression decreased over time, with no advantages or disadvantages for saffron or sertraline. The authors concluded that both saffron and sertraline had potential to significantly decrease symptoms of depression in older patients (Ahmadpanah et al., 2019).

A 6-week RCT in patients ($n = 40$) with mild-to-moderate depression and CAD and who had undergone percutaneous coronary intervention within the previous 6 months compared saffron 30 mg/day with fluoxetine 40 mg/day. Based on HAM-D scores at 3 and 6 weeks, no significant difference was detected between groups ($P = 0.62$), and remission and response rates were not significantly different ($P = 1.00$ and $P = 0.67$; respectively). There was no significant difference between two groups in the frequency of adverse events during this trial. The authors concluded that short-term therapy with saffron showed similar efficacy to fluoxetine in patients with mild-to-moderate depression and recent PCI (Shahmansouri et al., 2014).

A 12-week RCT in women ($n = 73$) with BMI $\geq$ 25 and mild-to-moderate depression compared saffron 15 mg BID with placebo. Mean BDI-II scores decreased significantly with saffron compared with placebo (-8.4 vs -3.9; $P = 0.007$). There was no significant effect of saffron on food craving. Patients in the saffron group showed fewer side effects. The authors concluded that saffron was not effective at reducing food craving but was effective at reducing depression in overweight patients with mild-to-moderate depression (Akhondzadeh et al., 2020).

An 8-week RCT in patients ($n = 34$) with metabolic syndrome compared crocin 30 mg/day with placebo for effects on mood and oxidation balance. Based on before and after BDI scores, the degree of depression decreased significantly in the crocin group ($P = 0.005$) but not in the placebo group ($P > 0.05$), and the difference between the two groups was statistically significant ($P = 0.013$). No significant relationship was observed between changes in depression symptoms and changes in oxidation balance ($P > 0.05$). The authors concluded that this dose of crocin reduced symptoms of depression in patients with metabolic syndrome independently of its effect on oxidation balance (Jam et al., 2017).

An 8-week RCT in patients ($n = 57$) with HIV/AIDS recovering from methamphetamine abuse compared saffron 30 mg/day with placebo. Based on BDI-II scores, saffron was superior to placebo in reducing depression ($P < 0.05$). The authors concluded that saffron, through serotonin and dopamine pathways, helped reduce depression among recovered consumers of methamphetamine living with HIV/AIDS (Jalali and Hashemi, 2018).

A 12-week RCT in patients ($n = 123$) with MDD compared curcumin 250 mg BID with curcumin 500 mg BID, with curcumin 250 mg plus saffron 15 mg BID, and with placebo. The active drug treatments (combined) were associated with significantly greater improvements in depressive symptoms compared with placebo ($P = 0.031$), and superior improvements in STAI-state ($P < 0.001$) and STAI-trait scores ($P = 0.001$). Active treatments also had greater efficacy in people with atypical depression compared with placebo (response rates of 65% and 35%, respectively; $P = 0.012$). No differences were found between the differing doses of curcumin or the curcumin-saffron combination. The authors concluded that low and high doses of curcumin and combined curcumin-saffron were effective in reducing depressive and anxious symptoms in people with MDD (Lopresti and Drummond, 2017).

A 4-week RCT in patients ($n = 40$) with severe depression studied saffron 30 mg/day plus fluoxetine 20 mg/day compared with placebo plus fluoxetine for effects on homocysteine levels and depression. With fluoxetine plus saffron there was a significant reduction from baseline in homocysteine levels ($P < 0.04$). There was no change in homocysteine with placebo plus fluoxetine. Based on baseline and follow-up BDI values, both groups showed improvement in depression and there was no significant difference between groups. The authors concluded that saffron had beneficial effects on depression and homocysteine levels in patients with major depression (Jelodar et al., 2018).

A 6-week observational study in adults ($n=45$) with mild-to-moderate depression investigated the effects of a combination of rhodiola 154 mg plus saffron 15 mg two tablets per day. After 6 weeks, HAM-D scores decreased by 58%, from 13.6 to 5.6; $P < 0.0001$. Score improvement was reported in 85% of patients. A sustained significant drop in Hospital Anxiety and Depression Scale scores was also observed at 2 weeks. There was a significant improvement in the Clinical Global Impression for both physicians and patients. Safety was excellent and no serious adverse effects were recorded. The authors concluded that the combination of rhodiola and saffron could be useful for the management of mild-moderate depression and could improve symptoms of depression and anxiety (Bangratz et al., 2018).

Psychiatric Disorders: Attention-Deficit/Hyperactivity Disorder

A 6-week RCT in children 7-17 years old ($n=54$) with ADHD compared saffron 20-30 mg/day (based on weight) with methylphenidate 20-30 mg/day (based on weight). General linear model repeated measures showed no significant difference between the two groups on Parent and Teacher Rating Scale scores (F=0.749, df=1.317; $P=0.425$, and F=0.249, df=1.410; $P=0.701$, respectively). There were no significant differences between saffron and methylphenidate with respect to changes in Teacher ADHD Rating Scale and Parent ADHD Rating Scale scores from baseline to the study end ($P=0.731$ and $P=0.883$, respectively). The frequency of adverse effects was similar between groups. The authors concluded that short-term therapy with saffron was as effective as methylphenidate for ADHD in children (Baziar et al., 2019).

Psychiatric Disorders: Addiction Disorders

A 12-week RCT in opiate addicted patients ($n=60$) undergoing methadone maintenance treatment compared crocin 30 mg/day with placebo. Compared with the placebo group, crocin resulted in a significant improvement in craving scores ($P=0.03$) and withdrawal symptoms scores ($P=0.01$). Crocin did not affect cognitive function parameters. The authors concluded that crocin for patients undergoing MMT for opiate addiction had beneficial effects on craving and withdrawal symptoms score but did not affect the cognitive function parameters (Abbaszadeh-Mashkani et al., 2020).

An 8-week RCT in patients ($n=44$) in an addiction treatment center studied methadone plus saffron 30 mg once a week compared with methadone plus placebo once a week. Per protocol, methadone was reduced by 5 mg each week in both groups. With saffron, loss of appetite decreased to 50% of participants after one month and to 31.8% at the end of the second month, whereas there was no change in the placebo group. With saffron, rhinorrhea decreased from 40% at baseline to 27% at the end of the second month, whereas it increased from 59% to 63% with placebo. Diarrhea decreased from 50% to 40% after 2 months, while it increased from 36% to 63% with placebo. Myalgia decreased from 64% to 9% with saffron, while it increased from 40% to 68% with placebo. Temptation decreased from 59% to 50% with saffron but no decrease occurred with placebo. Overall, saffron plus methadone had greater efficacy in reducing symptoms of withdrawal ($P < 0.001$). The authors concluded that saffron alleviated the symptoms of withdrawal syndrome in patients undergoing maintenance treatment for opioid addiction and could be used in combination with methadone for this purpose (Nemat Shahi et al., 2017).

A 15-day open-label pilot trial in patients ($n=32$) hospitalized for alcohol detoxification investigated the effect of an herbal combination (saffron, passionflower, cocoa seed, radish, and black seed) given TID. The herbal combination was associated with a significantly reduced percentage of patients with hyperhidrosis ($r=0.815$; $P < 0.001$), a reduction in serum liver enzymes by 50%-80% ($P < 0.05$), and a normalization of appetite ($r=0.777$; $P < 0.001$). Quality of life measured by Befindlichkeits-Skala improved from 28.3 to 15.6 ($P < 0.001$). The product was rated as "good to excellent" by 84.4% of patients. The authors concluded that there was potential for use of this herbal combination in patients undergoing alcohol withdrawal and that further studies were warranted (Mansoor et al., 2018).

Disorders of Vitality: Physical Stamina

A 10-day RCT in nonactive male college students ($n = 39$) compared saffron 300 mg/day with indomethacin 75 mg/day and with placebo given 1 week before and 3 days after eccentric exercise to determine effect on muscle soreness and muscle enzymes. CK and LDH concentrations were significantly decreased with saffron ($P < 0.0001$). There was no decline in maximum isometric and isotonic forces after eccentric exercise with saffron, but a significant decline in the isometric force was observed with placebo ($P < 0.0001$). No pain was reported in the saffron group, whereas the indomethacin group experienced pain before 72 h ($P < 0.001$). The authors concluded that 10-days of saffron had a preventive effect on delayed-onset muscle soreness (Meamarbashi and Rajabi, 2015).

Immune Disorders: Immune Function and Autoimmune Disorders

A 12-week RCT in patients ($n = 66$) with active RA compared saffron 100 mg/day with placebo to determine the effect of saffron on clinical outcomes and metabolic profiles. With saffron and placebo, respectively, the changes in number of tender joints were -1.38 and 0.10 ($P < 0.001$), the changes in number of swollen joints were -2.12 and 0.63 ($P < 0.001$), the changes in VAS for pain intensity were -18.36 and -2.33 ($P < 0.001$), and changes in disease activity score (DAS28) were -0.75 and 0.26 ($P < 0.001$). Physician Global Assessment was significantly improved ($P = 0.002$), and ESR significantly improved compared with placebo after intervention (24.06 vs 32.00, $P = 0.028$). Saffron produced a reduction in hsCRP compared with baseline values (from 12.0 to 8.82, $P = 0.004$). TNF-α, IFN-γ, and MDA were decreased, and TAC was increased, but the differences between the two groups were not significant. The authors concluded that saffron could improve clinical outcomes in patients with RA (Hamidi et al., 2020).

A 6-week RCT in healthy men ($n = 89$) compared saffron stigma extract 100 mg/day with placebo for 6 weeks with respect to effects on the blood serum levels of IgG, IgM, IgA, C(3) and C(4), counts and percentages of white blood cells, platelets, neutrophils, eosinophils, basophils, lymphocytes and monocytes, creatinine, AST, and ALT. After 3 weeks, saffron increased the IgG level and decreased the IgM level compared with baseline and placebo ($P < 0.01$), decreased the basophil % and platelet counts compared with baseline, and increased the monocyte % compared with placebo ($P < 0.05$). These parameters returned to the baseline levels by 6 weeks. Saffron did not have any significant effects on the other parameters. No adverse effects were reported. The authors concluded that subchronic daily use of saffron 100 mg/day had temporary immunomodulatory activities without any adverse effects (Kianbakht and Ghazavi, 2011).

A 12-week RCT in patients ($n = 105$) with metabolic syndrome compared saffron 100 mg/day with placebo and with a control group for impact on antibodies against heat shock proteins 17, 60, 65, and 70. At 12 weeks, saffron produced a significantly decrease in AntiHSP 27 and 70 levels. The authors concluded that saffron could improve some markers of autoimmunity against HSPs in patients with metabolic syndrome, which may explain part of the antiatherosclerotic effect of saffron (Shemshian et al., 2014).

A 4-month RCT in patients ($n = 40$) with OA compared a proprietary crocin supplement (Krocina) with placebo for effects on immune parameters. Crocin was associated with significant decreases in CRP ($P < 0.05$) and Th 17 cells. Crocin was associated with an increase in Tregs ($P = 0.02$) and the Treg/Th17 ratio. IL-17 decreased with crocin and increased with placebo ($P < 0.05$). CD8+ T cells decreased with placebo ($P < 0.05$). The disease VAS decreased significantly in both groups ($P < 0.05$). The authors concluded that Krocina had immunoregulatory effects on patients with OA, ameliorating the disease (Poursamimi et al., 2020).

Oncologic Disorders: Cancer-Related Mood Disorders and Liver Metastases

A 2018 systematic review to identify single-herb medicines that may warrant further study for treatment of anxiety and depression in cancer patients found 100 studies involving 38 botanicals that met inclusion criteria. Among herbs most studied ($\geq$ six RCTs each), lavender, passionflower, and saffron produced benefits comparable to standard anxiolytics and antidepressants. Black cohosh, chamomile, and chasteberry were also promising. Overall, 45% of studies reported positive findings with fewer adverse effects compared with conventional medications. The authors concluded that saffron, black cohosh, chamomile, chasteberry, laven-der, and passionflower appeared useful in mitigating anxiety or depression with favorable risk-benefit pro-files compared with standard treatments, and these botanicals may benefit cancer patients by minimizing medication load and accompanying side effects (Yeung et al., 2018).

A chemotherapy based RCT in cancer patients ($n = 13$) with liver metastases and on chemotherapy investigated saffron 50 mg BID during chemotherapy (six 3-week courses) compared with placebo during chemotherapy. Of the four saffron-treated patients who continued the study to completion, one patient showed partial response (> 30% reduction in longest diameter of lesion on contrast CT scan), one patient showed com-plete response (elimination of lesion), one patient re-mained stable, and one patient progressed. Of the three remaining placebo-treated patients, two were stable and one progressed. Death occurred in two patients in the placebo group and one patient in the saffron group. The authors concluded that saffron might be useful in can-cer patients with liver metastases but that further inves-tigations were required (Hosseini et al., 2015).

ACTIVE CONSTITUENTS

Stigma

- Phenolic compounds
  - Flavonoids
    - Aanthocyanins
- Terpenes
  - Monoterpene glycoside: pirocrocin (antioxi-dant, antineoplastic, bitter principle)
  - Tetraterpene/carotenoids (water soluble): crocin (antioxidant, antineoplastic, anti-inflammatory, anti-atherosclerotic, hypotensive, neuropro-tective, antidepressant, anti-OCD), crocetin (antioxidant, retinoprotective, hypolipidemic, anti-atherosclerotic, insulin-sensitizing, neuro-protective, antineoplastic)
  - Tetraterpene/Carotenoids (fat soluble): zeaxanthin
- Aromatic compounds:
  - Aldehydes (from drying): safranal (antioxi-dant, hypotensive, anticonvulsant, antineo-plastic, antidepressant)
  - Monoterpene aldehydes: safranol and hydroxysafranol

Petal

- Carbohydrates
  - Organic acids: 3-hydroxy-γ-butyrolactone
  - Glycosides: kinsenoside (pancreatoprotec-tive, hepatoprotective), goodyeroside A (hepatoprotective)
- Phenolic compounds
  - Phenolic acids: protocatechuic acid
  - Flavonoids
    - Flavonoles: kaempferol (anti-inflammatory, antidepressant, strengthens capillaries), and kaempferol 7-O-â-D-glucopyranoside (strongly antioxidant), kaempferol 3-O-3 sophoroside,
    - Anthocyanins
- Terpenes
  - Monoterpenes
    - Crocusatins (antityrosinase): crocusatin-J, 4-dihydroxybutyric acid, crocusatin-K, crocusatin-L, and 4-hydroxy3,5,5-trimethylcyclohex-2-enone (antityrosinase activity)
  - Tetraterpene/Carotenoids (stimulate granula-tion tissue): crocin (antioxidant, antineoplastic, anti-inflammatory, anti-atherosclerotic, hypo-tensive, neuroprotective, antidepressant, anti-OCD), crocetin (antioxidant, retinoprotective, hypolipidemic, anti-atherosclerotic, insulin-sensitizing, neuroprotective, antineoplastic)
- Alkaloids

SAFFRON COMMONLY USED PREPARATIONS AND DOSAGE (FOR ADULTS UNLESS OTHERWISE SPECIFIED)

The following are examples of some available formu-lations and ranges of dosing for commercial herbal products. See Part III Introduction "How to prescribe medicinal herbs" for further guidance on herbal advis-ing and prescribing.

Stigma and Petals

- Capsule or tablet of whole ground stigmas: 15 mg QD
- Capsule or tablet of powdered extract of stigma or petals: 15 mg BID (mostly studied and generally

recommended) up to 200 mg per day (for short-term treatment)

- Capsule or tablet of standardized extract (standardized to 3–10% crocins or 0.3–2% safranal): 15–88.5 mg QD-BID
- Saffron essential oil: aromatherapy diffusion for 20 min per day
- Saffron 1% topical gel: for ED

SAFETY AND PRECAUTION

Side Effects

Saffron appears to be well tolerated acutely at normal doses (30 mg/day), whereas larger doses for more prolonged periods (6 months) can induce adverse effects. An overview of systematic reviews of herb safety placed saffron in the "minor adverse effects" category. Doses larger than 200 mg and chronic use of > 60 mg/day in humans have been associated with decreased appetite and decreases in WBC, RBC platelet counts, and BP, which, although statistically significant, where not of large enough magnitude to be considered adverse. Pro-glycation properties with saffron have been demonstrated in mice.

Case Reports

Abnormal uterine bleeding was reported in two women at doses of 200-400 mg.

Toxicity

Doses of 1200–2000 mg of saffron in humans can acutely cause symptoms such as nausea, vomiting, diarrhea, and bleeding.

A 7-day RCT in healthy volunteers ($n = 60$) compared the effect of saffron tablets 200 mg or 400 mg with placebo for effects on fibrinogen and bleeding. There was no difference between groups for plasma levels of fibrinogen, factor VII, C and S protein, PT, and PTT. Statistical analysis showed no difference between groups for any of investigated factors. The authors concluded that saffron at 200 mg and 400 mg for 1 week did not have an impact on the coagulant and anticoagulant systems (Ayatollahi et al., 2014).

In rat research saffron petal extract at doses of 0, 75, 150, 225, and 450 mg/kg for 14 days demonstrated no difference between treated groups and control groups in hematological parameters such as RBCs, hgb, hct,

and platelets. Saffron petal increased IgG at a dose of 75 mg/kg in comparison with other groups. According to toxicological studies, toxicity of the stigma is greater than toxicity of the petal. The LD50 values of saffron stigma and petal in mice were 1.6 g/kg and 6 g/kg, respectively. In a sub-acute toxicity study, saffron stigma was injected IP at doses of 0.16, 0.32, and 0.48 g/kg, while petal was administered at doses of 1.2, 2.4, and 3.6 g/kg for 2 weeks. This study reported that saffron petal and stigma extracts reduced BW, hgb, hct, and erythrocytes. Pathological examination showed the stigma did not cause damage in different organs significantly, while liver and lung injuries were observed in animals that received saffron petal.

Pregnancy and Lactation

Avoid during pregnancy. There was a report that a continuous dosage > 10 g saffron was enough to cause abortion. Associated with skeletal malformations in mice.

Some studies in lactating women with postpartum depression show beneficial effects, but long-term consequences have not been studied. High doses in lactating mice produced adverse effects in neonatal kidneys.

Disease Interactions

Saffron is to be avoided in chronic liver disease, hypermagnesemia, polycythemia, and a genetic condition of dystonia/parkinsonism due to its reportedly high manganese content.

Drug Interactions

- Crocin decreases CYP1A2, CYP2B, CYP2C11 and CYP3A enzymes.
- Safranal increases CYP2B, CYP2C11 and CYP3A enzymes.

REFERENCES

Abbaszadeh-Mashkani S, Hoque SS, Banafshe HR, Ghaderi A. The effect of crocin (the main active saffron constituent) on the cognitive functions, craving, and withdrawal syndrome in opioid patients under methadone maintenance treatment. Phytother Res 2020;19.

Abedimanesh N, Bathaie SZ, Abedimanesh S, Motlagh B, Separham A, Ostadrahimi A. Saffron and crocin improved appetite, dietary intakes and body composition in patients with coronary artery disease. J Cardiovasc Thorac Res 2017;9(4):200–8.

Abedimanesh N, Motlagh B, Abedimanesh S, Bathaie SZ, Separham A, Ostadrahimi A. Effects of crocin and saffron aqueous extract on gene expression of SIRT1, AMPK, LOX1, NF-κB, and MCP-1 in patients with coronary artery disease: a randomized placebo-controlled clinical trial. Phytother Res 2019;3.

Agha-Hosseini M, Kashani L, Aleyaseen A, et al. Crocus sativus L. (saffron) in the treatment of premenstrual syndrome: a double-blind, randomised and placebo-controlled trial. BJOG 2008;115(4):515–9.

Ahmadpanah M, Ramezanshams F, Ghaleiha A, Akhondzadeh S, Sadeghi Bahmani D, Brand S. Crocus Sativus L. (saffron) vs sertraline on symptoms of depression among older people with major depressive disorders-a double-blind, randomized intervention study. Psychiatry Res 2019;282:112613.

Akhondzadeh Basti A, Moshiri E, Noorbala AA, Jamshidi AH, Abbasi SH, Akhondzadeh S. Comparison of petal of Crocus sativus L. and fluoxetine in the treatment of depressed outpatients: a pilot double-blind randomized trial. Prog Neuropsychopharmacol Biol Psychiatry 2007;31(2):439–42.

Akhondzadeh S, Fallah-Pour H, Afkham K, Jamshidi AH, Khalighi-Cigaroudi F. Comparison of Crocus sativus L. and imipramine in the treatment of mild to moderate depression: a pilot double-blind randomized trial [ISRCTN45683816]. BMC Complement Altern Med 2004;4:12.

Akhondzadeh S, Tahmacebi-Pour N, Noorbala AA, et al. Crocus sativus L. in the treatment of mild to moderate depression: a double-blind, randomized and placebo-controlled trial. Phytother Res 2005;19(2):148–51.

Akhondzadeh S, Sabet MS, Harirchian MH, et al. Saffron in the treatment of patients with mild to moderate Alzheimer's disease: a 16-week, randomized and placebo-controlled trial. J Clin Pharm Ther 2010a;35(5):581–8.

Akhondzadeh S, Shafiee Sabet M, Harirchian MH, et al. A 22-week, multicenter, randomized, double-blind controlled trial of Crocus sativus in the treatment of mild-to-moderate Alzheimer's disease. Psychopharmacology (Berl) 2010b;207(4):637–43.

Akhondzadeh S, Mostafavi SA, Keshavarz SA, Mohammadi MR, Hosseini S, Eshraghian MR. A placebo controlled randomized clinical trial of Crocus sativus L. (saffron) on depression and food craving among overweight women with mild to moderate depression. J Clin Pharm Ther. 2020 Feb;45(1):134-143.

Akouchekian S, Omranifard V, Maracy MR, Pedram A, Zefreh AA. Efficacy of herbal combination of sedge, saffron, and Astragalus honey on major neurocognitive disorder. J Res Med Sci 2018;23:58.

Asadollahi M, Nikdokht P, Hatef B, et al. Protective properties of the aqueous extract of saffron (Crocus sativus L.) in ischemic stroke, randomized clinical trial. J Ethnopharmacol 2019;238:111833.

Asbaghi O, Soltani S, Norouzi N, Milajerdi A, Choobkar S, Asemi Z. The effect of saffron supplementation on blood glucose and lipid profile: a systematic review and meta-analysis of randomized controlled trials. Complement Ther Med 2019;47:102158.

Ayatollahi H, Javan AO, Khajedaluee M, Shahroodian M, Hosseinzadeh H. Effect of Crocus sativus L. (saffron) on coagulation and anticoagulation systems in healthy volunteers. Phytother Res 2014;28(4):539–43.

Bangratz M, Ait Abdellah S, Berlin A, et al. A preliminary assessment of a combination of rhodiola and saffron in the management of mild-moderate depression. Neuropsychiatr Dis Treat 2018;14:1821–9.

Baziar S, Aqamolaei A, Khadem E, et al. Crocus sativus L. vs methylphenidate in treatment of children with attention-deficit/hyperactivity disorder: a randomized, double-blind pilot study. J Child Adolesc Psychopharmacol 2019;29(3):205–12.

Borrelli F, Colalto C, Delfino DV, Iriti M, Izzo AA. Herbal dietary supplements for erectile dysfunction: a systematic review and meta-analysis. Drugs 2018;78(6):643–73.

Broadhead GK, Grigg JR, McCluskey P, Hong T, Schlub TE, Chang AA. Saffron therapy for the treatment of mild/moderate age-related macular degeneration: a randomised clinical trial. Graefes Arch Clin Exp Ophthalmol 2019;257(1):31–40.

Cicero AF, Bove M, Colletti A, et al. Short-term impact of a combined nutraceutical on cognitive function, perceived stress and depression in young elderly with cognitive impairment: a pilot, double-blind, randomized clinical trial. J Prev Alzheimers Dis 2017;4(1):12–5.

Dante G, Facchinetti F. Herbal treatments for alleviating premenstrual symptoms: a systematic review. J Psychosom Obstet Gynaecol 2011;32(1):42–51.

Dwyer AV, Whitten DL, Hawrelak JA. Herbal medicines, other than St. John's Wort, in the treatment of depression: a systematic review. Altern Med Rev 2011;16(1):40–9.

Ebrahimi F, Aryaeian N, Pahlavani N, et al. The effect of saffron (Crocus sativus L.) supplementation on blood pressure, and renal and liver function in patients with type 2 diabetes mellitus: a double-blinded, randomized clinical trial. Avicenna J Phytomed 2019a;9(4):322–33.

Ebrahimi F, Sahebkar A, Aryaeian N, et al. Effects of saffron supplementation on inflammation and metabolic responses in type 2 diabetic patients: a randomized, double-blind, placebo-controlled trial. Diabetes Metab Syndr Obes 2019b;12:2107–15.

Esalatmanesh S, Biuseh M, Noorbala AA, et al. Comparison of saffron and fluvoxamine in the treatment of mild to moderate obsessive-compulsive disorder: a double blind randomized clinical trial. Iran J Psychiatry 2017;12(3):154–62.

Fadai F, Mousavi B, Ashtari Z, et al. Saffron aqueous extract prevents metabolic syndrome in patients with schizophrenia on olanzapine treatment: a randomized triple blind placebo-controlled study. Pharmacopsychiatry 2014;47(4-5):156–61.

Falsini B, Piccardi M, Minnella A, et al. Influence of saffron supplementation on retinal flicker sensitivity in early age-related macular degeneration. Invest Ophthalmol Vis Sci 2010;51(12):6118–24.

Farokhnia M, Shafiee Sabet M, Iranpour N, et al. Comparing the efficacy and safety of Crocus sativus L. with memantine in patients with moderate to severe Alzheimer's disease: a double-blind randomized clinical trial. Hum Psychopharmacol 2014;29(4):351–9.

Forouzanfar A, Mokhtari MR, Kamalinezhad M, Babayian M, Tavakoli-Kakhki M, Lotfalizadeh MH. Evaluation of toothpaste containing aqueous saffron stigma extract on gingival indices in patients with marginal generalized plaque-induced gingivitis. Iran J Med Sci 2016;41(3 Suppl):S31.

Fukui H, Toyoshima K, Komaki R. Psychological and neuroendocrinological effects of odor of saffron (Crocus sativus). Phytomedicine 2011;18(8-9):726–30.

Ghaderi A, Asbaghi O, Reiner Ž, et al. The effects of saffron (Crocus sativus L.) on mental health parameters and C-reactive protein:

a meta-analysis of randomized clinical trials. Complement Ther Med 2020;48:102250.

Ghajar A, Neishabouri SM, Velayati N, et al. Crocus sativus L. vs citalopram in the treatment of major depressive disorder with anxious distress: a double-blind, controlled clinical trial. Pharmacopsychiatry 2017;50(4):152–60.

Gout B, Bourges C, Paineau-Dubreuil S. Satiereal, a Crocus sativus L extract, reduces snacking and increases satiety in a randomized placebo-controlled study of mildly overweight, healthy women. Nutr Res 2010;30(5):305–13.

Gudarzi S, Jafari M, Pirzad Jahromi G, Eshrati R, Asadollahi M, Nikdokht P. Evaluation of modulatory effects of saffron (Crocus sativus L.) aqueous extract on oxidative stress in ischemic stroke patients: a randomized clinical trial. Nutr Neurosci. 2020 Nov 5:1-10.

Hamidi Z, Aryaeian N, Abolghasemi J, et al. The effect of saffron supplement on clinical outcomes and metabolic profiles in patients with active rheumatoid arthritis: a randomized, double-blind, placebo-controlled clinical trial. Phytother Res 2020;34(7):1650–8.

Hausenblas HA, Saha D, Dubyak PJ, Anton SD. Saffron (Crocus sativus L.) and major depressive disorder: a meta-analysis of randomized clinical trials. J Integr Med 2013;11(6):377–83.

Heidary M, Vahhabi S, Reza Nejadi J, et al. Effect of saffron on semen parameters of infertile men. Urol J 2008;5(4):255–9.

Hosseini A, Mousavi SH, Ghanbari A, et al. Effect of saffron on liver metastases in patients suffering from cancers with liver metastases: a randomized, double blind, placebo-controlled clinical trial. Avicenna J Phytomed 2015;5(5):434–40.

Hosseini SA, Zilaee M, Shoushtari MH, Ghasemi DM. An evaluation of the effect of saffron supplementation on the antibody titer to heat-shock protein (HSP) 70, hs-CRP and spirometry test in patients with mild and moderate persistent allergic asthma: a triple-blind, randomized placebo-controlled trial. Respir Med 2018a;145:28–34.

Hosseini A, Razavi B, Hosseinzadeh H. Saffron (*Crocus sativus*) petal as a new pharmacological target: a review. Iran J Basic Med Sci 2018b;21(11):1091–9.

Jabbarpoor Bonyadi MH, Yazdani S, Saadat S. The ocular hypotensive effect of saffron extract in primary open angle glaucoma: a pilot study. BMC Complement Altern Med 2014;14:399.

Jalali F, Hashemi SF. The effect of saffron on depression among recovered consumers of methamphetamine living with HIV/AIDS. Subst Use Misuse 2018;53(12):1951–7.

Jam IN, Sahebkar AH, Eslami S, et al. The effects of crocin on the symptoms of depression in subjects with metabolic syndrome. Adv Clin Exp Med 2017;26(6):925–30.

Javandoost A, Afshari A, Nikbakht-Jam I, et al. Effect of crocin, a carotenoid from saffron, on plasma cholesteryl ester transfer protein and lipid profile in subjects with metabolic syndrome: a double blind randomized clinical trial. ARYA Atheroscler 2017;13(5):245–52.

Jelodar G, Javid Z, Sahraian A, Jelodar S. Saffron improved depression and reduced homocysteine level in patients with major depression: a randomized, double-blind study. Avicenna J Phytomed 2018;8(1):43–50.

Karimi-Nazari E, Nadjarzadeh A, Masoumi R, et al. Effect of saffron (Crocus sativus L.) on lipid profile, glycemic indices and an-

tioxidant status among overweight/obese prediabetic individuals: a double-blinded, randomized controlled trial. Clin Nutr Espen 2019;34:130–6.

Kashani L, Raisi F, Saroukhani S, et al. Saffron for treatment of fluoxetine-induced sexual dysfunction in women: randomized double-blind placebo-controlled study. Hum Psychopharmacol 2013;28(1):54–60.

Kashani L, Eslatmanesh S, Saedi N, et al. Comparison of saffron vs fluoxetine in treatment of mild to moderate postpartum depression: a double-blind, randomized clinical trial. Pharmacopsychiatry 2017;50(2):64–8.

Kashani L, Esalatmanesh S, Eftekhari F, et al. Efficacy of Crocus sativus (saffron) in treatment of major depressive disorder associated with post-menopausal hot flushes: a double-blind, randomized, placebo-controlled trial. Arch Gynecol Obstet 2018;297(3):717–24.

Kell G, Rao A, Beccaria G, Clayton P, Inarejos-García AM, Prodanov M. affron a novel saffron extract (Crocus sativus L.) improves mood in healthy adults over 4 weeks in a double-blind, parallel, randomized, placebo-controlled clinical trial. Complement Ther Med 2017;33:58–64.

Kermani T, Zebarjadi M, Mehrad-Majd H, et al. Anti-inflammatory effect of Crocus sativus on serum cytokine levels in subjects with metabolic syndrome: a randomized, double-blind, placebo-controlled trial. Curr Clin Pharmacol 2017;12(2):122–6.

Khaksarian M, Behzadifar M, Behzadifar M, et al. The efficacy of *Crocus sativus* (Saffron) vs placebo and fluoxetine in treating depression: a systematic review and meta-analysis. Psychol Res Behav Manag 2019;12:297–305.

Kianbakht S, Ghazavi A. Immunomodulatory effects of saffron: a randomized double-blind placebo-controlled clinical trial. Phytother Res 2011;25(12):1801–5.

Lopresti AL, Drummond PD. Saffron (Crocus sativus) for depression: a systematic review of clinical studies and examination of underlying antidepressant mechanisms of action. Hum Psychopharmacol 2014;29(6):517–27.

Lopresti AL, Drummond PD. Efficacy of curcumin, and a saffron/curcumin combination for the treatment of major depression: a randomised, double-blind, placebo-controlled study. J Affect Disord 2017;207:188–96.

Lopresti AL, Drummond PD, Inarejos-García AM, Prodanov M. Affron, a standardised extract from saffron (Crocus sativus L.) for the treatment of youth anxiety and depressive symptoms: a randomised, double-blind, placebo-controlled study. J Affect Disord 2018;232:349–57.

Lopresti AL, Smith SJ, Hood SD, Drummond PD. Efficacy of a standardised saffron extract (affron®) as an add-on to antidepressant medication for the treatment of persistent depressive symptoms in adults: a randomised, double-blind, placebo-controlled study. J Psychopharmacol 2019;33(11):1415–27.

Lopresti AL, Smith SJ, Metse AP, Drummond PD. Effects of saffron on sleep quality in healthy adults with self-reported poor sleep: a randomized, double-blind, placebo-controlled trial. J Clin Sleep Med 2020;16(6):937–47.

Maleki-Saghooni N, Mirzaeii K, Hosseinzadeh H, Sadeghi R, Irani M. A systematic review and meta-analysis of clinical trials on saffron (*Crocus sativus*) effectiveness and safety on erectile dysfunction and semen parameters. Avicenna J Phytomed 2018;8(3):198–209.

Mansoor K, Qadan F, Hinum A, et al. An open prospective pilot study of a herbal combination "Relief" as a supportive dietetic measure during alcohol withdrawal. Neuro Endocrinol Lett 2018;39(1):1–8.

Marangoni D, Falsini B, Piccardi M, et al. Functional effect of Saffron supplementation and risk genotypes in early age-related macular degeneration: a preliminary report. J Transl Med 2013;11:228.

Marx W, Lane M, Rocks T, et al. Effect of saffron supplementation on symptoms of depression and anxiety: a systematic review and meta-analysis. Nutr Rev 2019. pii: nuz023.

Mazidi M, Shemshian M, Mousavi SH, et al. A double-blind, randomized and placebo-controlled trial of Saffron (Crocus sativus L.) in the treatment of anxiety and depression. J Complement Integr Med 2016;13(2):195–9.

Meamarbashi A, Rajabi A. Preventive effects of 10-day supplementation with saffron and indomethacin on the delayed-onset muscle soreness. Clin J Sport Med 2015;25(2):105–12.

Milajerdi A, Jazayeri S, Hashemzadeh N, et al. The effect of saffron (Crocus sativus L.) hydroalcoholic extract on metabolic control in type 2 diabetes mellitus: a triple-blinded randomized clinical trial. J Res Med Sci 2018a;23:16.

Milajerdi A, Jazayeri S, Shirzadi E, et al. The effects of alcoholic extract of saffron (Crocus satious L.) on mild to moderate comorbid depression-anxiety, sleep quality, and life satisfaction in type 2 diabetes mellitus: a double-blind, randomized and placebo-controlled clinical trial. Complement Ther Med 2018b;41:196–202.

Moazen-Zadeh E, Abbasi SH, Safi-Aghdam H, et al. Effects of saffron on cognition, anxiety, and depression in patients undergoing coronary artery bypass grafting: a randomized double-blind placebo-controlled trial. J Altern Complement Med 2018;24(4):361–8.

Mobasseri M, Ostadrahimi A, Tajaddini A, et al. Effects of saffron supplementation on glycemia and inflammation in patients with type 2 diabetes mellitus: a randomized double-blind, placebo-controlled clinical trial study. Diabetes Metab Syndr 2020;14(4):527–34.

Modabbernia A, Sohrabi H, Nasehi AA, et al. Effect of saffron on fluoxetine-induced sexual impairment in men: randomized double-blind placebo-controlled trial. Psychopharmacology (Berl) 2012;223(4):381–8.

Mohammadzadeh-Moghadam H, Nazari SM, Shamsa A, et al. Effects of a topical saffron (Crocus sativus L) gel on erectile dysfunction in diabetics: a randomized, parallel-group, double-blind, placebo-controlled trial. J Evid Based Complement Altern Med 2015;20(4):283–6.

Moravej Aleali A, Amani R, Shahbazian H, Namjooyan F, Latifi SM, Cheraghian B. The effect of hydroalcoholic Saffron (Crocus sativus L.) extract on fasting plasma glucose, A1C, lipid profile, liver, and renal function tests in patients with type 2 diabetes mellitus: a randomized double-blind clinical trial. Phytother Res 2019;33(6):1648–57.

Moshiri E, Basti AA, Noorbala AA, Jamshidi AH, Hesameddin Abbasi S, Akhondzadeh S. Crocus sativus L. (petal) in the treatment of mild-to-moderate depression: a double-blind, randomized and placebo-controlled trial. Phytomedicine 2006;13(9-10):607–11.

Nemat Shahi M, Asadi A, Behnam Talab E, Nemat SM. The impact of saffron on symptoms of withdrawal syndrome in patients undergoing maintenance treatment for opioid addiction in sabzevar Parish in 2017. Adv Med 2017;1079132.

Noorbala AA, Akhondzadeh S, Tahmacebi-Pour N, Jamshidi AH. Hydro-alcoholic extract of Crocus sativus L. vs fluoxetine in the treatment of mild to moderate depression: a double-blind, randomized pilot trial. J Ethnopharmacol 2005;97(2):281–4.

Pakfetrat A, Talebi M, Dalirsani Z, Mohajeri A, Zamani R, Ghazi A. Evaluation of the effectiveness of crocin isolated from saffron in treatment of burning mouth syndrome: a randomized controlled trial. Avicenna J Phytomed 2019;9(6):505–16.

Pourmasoumi M, Hadi A, Najafgholizadeh A, Kafeshani M, Sahebkar A. Clinical evidence on the effects of saffron (Crocus sativus L.) on cardiovascular risk factors: a systematic review meta-analysis. Pharmacol Res 2019;139:348–59.

Poursamimi J, Shariati-Sarabi Z, Tavakkol-Afshari J, Mohajeri SA, Ghoryani M, Mohammadi M. Immunoregulatory effects of krocina, a herbal medicine made of crocin, on osteoarthritis patients: a successful clinical trial in Iran. Iran J Allergy Asthma Immunol 2020;19(3):253–63.

Rahmani J, Manzari N, Thompson J, et al. The effect of saffron on weight and lipid profile: a systematic review, meta-analysis, and dose-response of randomized clinical trials. Phytother Res 2019;33(9):2244–55.

Rahmani J, Bazmi E, Clark C, Hashemi Nazari SS. The effect of Saffron supplementation on waist circumference, HA1C, and glucose metabolism: a systematic review and meta-analysis of randomized clinical trials. Complement Ther Med 2020;49:102298.

Ranjbar H, Ashrafizaveh A. Effects of saffron (Crocus sativus) on sexual dysfunction among men and women: a systematic review and meta-analysis. Avicenna J Phytomed 2019;9(5):419–27.

Sadi R, Mohammad-Alizadeh-Charandabi S, Mirghafourvand M, Javadzadeh Y, Ahmadi-Bonabi A. Effect of saffron (Fan Hong Hua) on the readiness of the uterine cervix in term pregnancy: a placebo-controlled randomized trial. Iran Red Crescent Med J 2016;18(10), e27241.

Safarinejad MR, Shafiei N, Safarinejad S. A prospective double-blind randomized placebo-controlled study of the effect of saffron (Crocus sativus Linn.) on semen parameters and seminal plasma antioxidant capacity in infertile men with idiopathic oligoasthenoteratozoospermia. Phytother Res 2011;25(4):508–16.

Sepahi S, Mohajeri SA, Hosseini SM, et al. Effects of crocin on diabetic maculopathy: a placebo-controlled randomized clinical trial. Am J Ophthalmol 2018;190:89–98.

Shahbazian H, Moravej Aleali A, Amani R, et al. Effects of saffron on homocysteine, and antioxidant and inflammatory biomarkers levels in patients with type 2 diabetes mellitus: a randomized double-blind clinical trial. Avicenna J Phytomed 2019;9(5):436–45.

Shahmansouri N, Farokhnia M, Abbasi SH, et al. A randomized, double-blind, clinical trial comparing the efficacy and safety of Crocus sativus L. with fluoxetine for improving mild to moderate depression in post percutaneous coronary intervention patients. J Affect Disord 2014;155:216–22.

Shakiba M, Moazen-Zadeh E, Noorbala AA, et al. Saffron (Crocus sativus) vs duloxetine for treatment of patients with fibromyalgia: a randomized double-blind clinical trial. Avicenna J Phytomed 2018;8(6):513–23.

Shamsa A, Hosseinzadeh H, Molaei M, Shakeri MT, Rajabi O. Evaluation of Crocus sativus L. (saffron) on male erectile dysfunction: a pilot study. Phytomedicine 2009;16(8):690-3.

Shemshian M, Mousavi SH, Norouzy A, et al. Saffron in metabolic syndrome: its effects on antibody titers to heat-shock proteins 27, 60, 65 and 70. J Complement Integr Med 2014;11(1):43-9.

Tabeshpour J, Sobhani F, Sadjadi SA, et al. A double-blind, randomized, placebo-controlled trial of saffron stigma (Crocus sativus L.) in mothers suffering from mild-to-moderate postpartum depression. Phytomed 2017;36:145-52.

Talaei A, Hassanpour Moghadam M, Sajadi Tabassi SA, Mohajeri SA. Crocin, the main active saffron constituent, as an adjunctive treatment in major depressive disorder: a randomized, double-blind, placebo-controlled, pilot clinical trial. J Affect Disord 2015;174:51-6.

Tóth B, Hegyi P, Lantos T, et al. The efficacy of saffron in the treatment of mild to moderate depression: a meta-analysis. Planta Med 2019;85(1):24-31.

Tsolaki M, Karathanasi E, Lazarou I, et al. Efficacy and safety of Crocus sativus L. in patients with mild cognitive impairment: one year single-blind randomized, with parallel groups, clinical trial. J Alzheimers Dis 2016;54(1):129-33.

Verma SK, Bordia A. Antioxidant property of Saffron in man. Indian J Med Sci 1998;52(5):205-7.

Yang X, Chen X, Fu Y, et al. Comparative efficacy and safety of *Crocus sativus* L. for treating mild to moderate major depressive disorder in adults: a meta-analysis of randomized controlled trials. Neuropsychiatr Dis Treat 2018;14:1297-305.

Yeung KS, Hernandez M, Mao JJ, Haviland I, Gubili J. Herbal medicine for depression and anxiety: a systematic review with assessment of potential psycho-oncologic relevance. Phytother Res 2018;32(5):865-91.

Zilaee M, Hosseini SA, Jafarirad S, et al. An evaluation of the effects of saffron supplementation on the asthma clinical symptoms and asthma severity in patients with mild and moderate persistent allergic asthma: a double-blind, randomized placebo-controlled trial. Respir Res 2019;20(1):39.

ST. JOHN'S WORT (*HYPERICUM PERFORATUM*)
Flowering Buds and Tops

GENERAL OVERVIEW

St. John's wort (SJW) is probably the best-known medicinal herb on the market. It has been one of the most extensively studied herbs, with its chief constituents hyperforin and hypericin being the focus of most research. At the time of this writing, the American Botanical Council lists 238 clinical trials for this herb. Despite its popularity, its application is tempered by lukewarm clinical results and a plethora of adverse drug and herb interactions. It is known for its antidepressant properties, but it is also quite useful as a neuroprotective, antineuralgic, and antiviral herb. It has been shown to have comparable efficacy to pharmaceutical antidepressants for mild-to-moderate depression, but the findings are mixed. It has some evidence for efficacy with premenstrual syndrome and with perimenopausal and menopausal symptoms. Although SJW can cause photosensitization, it also has dermatological applications, including topical use for sunburn and eczema. One of the main constituents, hyperforin, provides anti-inflammatory, antioxidant, antitumor, neurotrophic, and antibacterial properties.

Clinical research indicates that SJW, alone or in combination formulas, may be beneficial for premenstrual syndrome, polycystic ovary syndrome, perimenopause and menopause, depression, eczema, and psoriasis.

IN VITRO AND ANIMAL RESEARCH

In vitro studies have shown that SJW inhibits serotonin, norepinephrine, and dopamine reuptake by neurons. The mechanism is thought to be due to activation of sodium uptake in nonselective cation channels thereby preventing neurotransmitter reuptake. MAO inhibiting properties, while present, are not significant in vivo at standard doses. The constituent hyperforin may stimulate the development and function of oligodendrocytes, which could be a mechanism for its effect in depression. Hyperforin also demonstrates antiangiogenic activity and suppresses lymph angiogenesis via cell cycle arrest and apoptosis. It has also been shown to reverse P-glycoprotein and breast cancer resistance protein activity in some cancer cell lines and to have anti-metastatic properties.

The other well-studied chief constituent of SJW, hypericin, has been shown to suppress voltage-dependent calcium channel and MAPK activity and to trigger glutamate release. Hypericin also causes phototoxicity via oxygen-dependent intracellular pH reduction and mediation by the TNF-related apoptosis-inducing ligand receptor system. SJW extract has been shown to inhibit COMT, while hypericin alone does not.

Preclinical animal studies have demonstrated the ability of low doses of SJW dry extracts to induce antinociception, providing relief from acute and chronic hyperalgesic states. Research in mice has shown that its antinociceptive activity can be blocked by naloxone. It can potentiate the effects of morphine. A single large dose of SJW in otherwise normal rats increased extracellular dopamine in the prefrontal cortex by 40% with an associated decrease in dopamine metabolites. Mild elevations of serotonin have been noted in the prefrontal cortex of rats given a standardized extract of SJW.

569

A cream of SJW demonstrated strong free radical scavenging activity in keratinocytes irradiated with solar simulated radiation. Similar effects were noted in ex vivo application to porcine ear skin. When given intraperitoneally to mice that were injected with cancer cells, hyperforin reduced inflammatory infiltration, neovascularization, and number of experimental metastases.

HUMAN RESEARCH

Women's Genitourinary Disorders: Premenstrual Syndrome and Polycystic Ovary Syndrome

A four-cycle RCT crossover study in women ($n = 36$) with mild PMS compared SJW 900 mg/day with placebo for two menstrual cycles then crossed over for another two cycles. SJW resulted in improved physical and behavioral symptoms over placebo ($P < 0.05$) but did not provide significant benefit over placebo for mood or pain-related symptoms. There were no differences in serum measurements of FSH, LH, estradiol, progesterone, prolactin, testosterone, or inflammatory cytokines (Canning et al., 2010).

A 3-month RCT in overweight women ($n = 122$) with PCOS compared lifestyle intervention alone with lifestyle intervention plus an herbal combination of licorice, SJW, peony, and cinnamon plus a separate tablet of tribulus. At 3 months, women in the combination group recorded a reduction in oligomenorrhoea by 32.9% ($P < 0.01$) compared with controls. Other significant improvements were found for BMI ($P < 0.01$), insulin ($P = 0.02$), LH ($P = 0.04$), BP ($P = 0.01$), QOL ($P < 0.01$), depression, anxiety, and stress ($P < 0.01$), and pregnancy rates ($P = 0.01$). The authors concluded that lifestyle combined with herbal medicines was safe and effective in women with PCOS (Arentz et al., 2017).

Women's Genitourinary Disorders: Perimenopause and Menopause

A 2020 systematic review was undertaken to evaluate the benefits of isopropanolic extracts of black cohosh alone or in combination with SJW in breast cancer patients with anti-estrogen-induced menopausal symptoms. Most breast cancer survivors receiving anti-estrogen therapy experienced reductions in climacteric symptoms with black cohosh with or without SJW. Some studies indicated that tamoxifen's interference potential could be countered by using higher doses of either herbal regimen. No estrogen-like effects on breast tissue or on hormones were seen. Patients using black cohosh alone or combined with SJW had significantly increased recurrence-free survival rates compared with non-users. These results were noted by the authors to have been substantiated by experimental data demonstrating antiproliferative and anti-invasive effects of black cohosh in breast cancer cells and enhancement of the antineoplastic effects of tamoxifen. SJW was noted to exhibit no clinically relevant interaction potential. The authors concluded that isopropanolic extracts of black cohosh with or without SJW may offer a safe non-hormonal therapeutic option for breast cancer survivors receiving endocrine therapy (Ruan et al., 2019).

A 2017 review of clinical trials on herbal efficacy in menopausal symptoms used search terms menopause, climacteric, hot flushes, flashes, herb, and phytoestrogens. The authors found that passionflower, sage, lemon balm, valerian, black cohosh, fenugreek, black seed, chasteberry, fennel, evening primrose, ginkgo, alfalfa, SJW, Asian ginseng, anise, licorice, red clover, and wild soybean were effective in the treatment of acute menopausal syndrome with different mechanisms. The authors concluded that medicinal plants could play a role in the treatment of acute menopausal syndrome and that further studies were warranted (Kargozar et al., 2017).

A 2016 systematic review to assess effectiveness of Iranian herbal medicine for menopausal hot flushes found 19 RCTs that met inclusion criteria. Overall, studies showed that passionflower, anise, licorice, soy, black cohosh, red clover, evening primrose, flaxseed, sage, chasteberry, SJW, valerian, and avocado plus soybean oil could alleviate hot flushes. The authors concluded that herbal medicines had efficacy in alleviating hot flushes (Ghazanfarpour et al., 2016).

A 2012 systematic review assessed efficacy of black cohosh, SJW, chasteberry, and vitamins as monotherapy or in combination for menopausal symptoms. The combination of black cohosh and SJW was found to show an improvement of climacteric complaints in comparison with placebo. However, the combination of SJW and chasteberry showed no significant difference in the treatment of menopausal symptoms (Laakmann et al., 2012).

A 2006 systematic review looking at herbs and supplements for menopausal mood disorders found that five of seven trials of SJW showed benefit for mild-to-moderate depression. One RCT of ginseng in postmenopausal women reported improvements in mood and anxiety. All three RCTs of ginkgo found no effect on depression. Kava significantly reduced anxiety in four of eight RCTs. Black cohosh significantly reduced depression and anxiety in all studies reviewed. The authors concluded that SJW and black cohosh appeared to be the most useful in alleviating mood and anxiety changes during menopause, that ginseng may be effective but required more research, and that kava held promise for decreasing anxiety in peri- and postmenopausal women (Geller and Studee., 2006).

A 2-month RCT in postmenopausal women ($n = 80$) compared SJW 270–330 mg TID with placebo for effect on hot flushes, menopausal symptoms, and depression. The frequency and intensity of hot flushes and Kupperman Index scores significantly decreased with SJW compared with placebo ($P < 0.001$). The intensity of depression significantly decreased with SJW compared with placebo. By 2 months, depression was present in 20% and 94.3% of the SJW and placebo groups, respectively ($P < 0.001$). The authors concluded that SJW could reduce hot flushes, menopausal symptoms, and depression in postmenopausal women (Eatemadnia et al., 2019).

A 3-month RCT in women ($n = 47$) with perimenopausal symptoms, including three or more hot flushes a day, compared SJW 900 mg TID with placebo. Hot flush frequency after 12 weeks was -2.3 with SJW and -1.0 with placebo ($P = 0.11$). Hot flush scores were -3.8 with SJW and -1.8 with placebo ($P = 0.10$). Women in the SJW group reported significantly better quality of life ($P = 0.01$) and significantly fewer sleep problems ($P = 0.05$) compared with placebo (Al-Akoum et al., 2009).

A 6-week RCT in menopausal women ($n = 59$) compared SJW with passionflower for efficacy on menopausal symptoms. The average scores of menopausal symptoms in the two treatment groups showed significant decreases throughout the third and the sixth weeks of study ($P < 0.05$). There was no statistically significant difference between the two groups ($P > 0.05$) (Fahami et al., 2010).

An 8-week RCT in perimenopausal and postmenopausal women ($n = 100$) compared SJW extract with placebo for climacteric complaints. Both groups responded to the interventions, and the within-group differences in frequency, duration, and severity of hot flushes were statistically significant ($P < 0.05$). The decrease from baseline in frequency of hot flushes with SJW was significant by week 4 and week 8 ($P = 0.005$ and $P < 0.001$, respectively). The difference in duration of hot flushes between groups was not significant by week 4 ($P = 0.27$) but reached significance by week 8 ($P < 0.001$). The decrease in the severity of flushes with SJW was also more evident by the fourth and eighth weeks ($P = 0.004$ and $P < 0.001$, respectively). The authors concluded that SJW could be used as an effective treatment for the vasomotor symptoms of perimenopause and postmenopause (Abdali et al., 2010).

A 16-week RCT in women ($n = 301$) with menopausal complaints and psychological symptoms compared a combination of SJW plus black cohosh with placebo. The mean Menopause Rating Scale score decreased by 50% (from 0.46 to 0.23) with the herbal product and by 19.6% (from 0.46 to 0.37) with placebo. The HAM-D total score decreased by 41.8% (from 18.9 to 11.0 points) with the herbal product and by 12.7% (from 18.9 to 16.5) with placebo. The treatment was significantly ($P < 0.001$) superior to placebo in both measures. The authors concluded that this fixed combination of black cohosh and SJW was superior to placebo in alleviating menopausal complaints including related psychological aspects (Uebelhack et al., 2006).

A 16-week RCT in perimenopausal women ($n = 14$) studied a combination of chasteberry plus SJW given BID compared with placebo for effects on PMS symptoms. PMS scores were measured on the Abrahams Menstrual Symptoms Questionnaire, comprising the sub-clusters of PMS-A (anxiety), PMS-D (depression), PMS-H (hyperhydration), and PMS-C (cravings). The herbal combination resulted in a greater reduction than placebo in total PMS-like scores ($P = 0.02$), the PMS-D cluster ($P = 0.006$), the PMS-C clusters ($P = 0.027$), the PMS-A cluster ($P = 0.003$), and the PMS-H cluster ($P = 0.002$). Results of trend analyses showed significant beneficial effects across the five phases for total PMS and all subscales with the herb but not with placebo. The authors concluded that chasteberry plus SJW had a potential clinical application in PMS-like symptoms in perimenopausal women (van Die et al., 2009).

Psychiatric Disorders: Depression

A 2016 systematic review to evaluate the severity-based efficacy and safety of SJW in adults with MDD compared with placebo and with active comparator found 35 RCTs ($n = 6993$) that met inclusion criteria. Eight studies investigated a SJW extract that combined 0.3% hypericin and 1%-4% hyperforin and showed that SJW was associated with more treatment responders than placebo (RR = 1.53; $I^2 = 79\%$). Compared with patients using antidepressants, SJW participants were less likely to experience adverse events (OR: 0.67), with no difference in treatment effectiveness (RR = 1.01) in mild and moderate depression. The authors concluded that SJW monotherapy for mild and moderate depression was superior to placebo in improving depression symptoms and not significantly different from antidepressant medication. However, heterogeneity and a lack of research on severe depression reduced the quality of the evidence (Apaydin et al., 2016).

A 2014 systematic review of an herbal combination product Shuganjieyu (SJW and eleuthero) for treatment of depressive disorder identified seven RCTs ($n = 595$) for inclusion. Shuganjieyu capsule was superior to placebo in terms of response rate (RR = 2.42; $P = 0.0001$), remission rate (RR = 4.29; $P = 0.004$), mean change from baseline in the HAM-D17 scores (MD = -4.17; $P < 0.00001$), and mean change from baseline in the Chinese medicine syndrome score scale (MD = -6.00; $P < 0.00001$). When added to venlafaxine, Shuganjieyu produced a greater response rate (RR = 1.56; $P < 0.00001$) and greater mean change from baseline in HAM-D17 score and Chinese medicine syndrome score scale (MD = -0.74; $P = 0.0002$) than venlafaxine alone. The authors concluded that Shuganjieyu was superior to placebo for depressive disorder in terms of overall treatment of effectiveness and safety, and that both response rate and remission rate in patients treated with the combination of Shuganjieyu plus venlafaxine were significantly greater than in those treated with venlafaxine alone (Zhang et al., 2014)

A 2009 meta-analysis compared the efficacy and tolerability of SJW with SSRIs. Thirteen RCTs met inclusion criteria. Analysis concluded that SJW did not differ from SSRIs according to efficacy and adverse events in MDD. However, the risk for withdrawal due to side effects was less with SJW than with SSRIs (RR = 0.53; $P = 0.004$) (Rahimi et al., 2009).

A 2008 systematic review on the efficacy of SJW for depression found 29 trials ($n = 5489$) that met inclusion criteria. Nine larger trials showed that SJW was superior to placebo for combined effects (RR = 1.28). In nine smaller trials SJW was also superior (RR = 1.87). Compared with tri- or tetracyclic antidepressants and SSRIs respectively, RRs were 1.02 and 1.00. Patients given SJW extracts dropped out of trials due to adverse effects less frequently than those given older antidepressants (OR = 0.24) and those given SSRIs (OR = 0.53). The authors concluded that SJW extracts tested in the included trials were superior to placebo in patients with major depression, were similarly effective as standard antidepressants, and had fewer side effects than standard antidepressants (Linde et al., 2008).

In a mildly depressed subset ($n = 217$) of 1200 patients included in two trials of SJW and depression, patients who received 600, 900, or 1200 mg/day of SJW extract compared with placebo for 6 weeks showed a decrease in HAM-D total score by averages of 10.8 (600 mg), 9.6 (900 mg), and 10.7 (1,200 mg) compared with a 6.8-point decrease with placebo. This corresponded to average relative decreases of 49%-57% for SJW and 36% for placebo. The rates of patients with a 50% or greater decrease in HAM-D scores were 73%, 64%, 71%, and 37% for the three doses of SJW and placebo, respectively. Remission at the end of treatment was 57%, 33%, 62%, and 25% with the three doses of SJW and placebo, respectively (Kasper et al., 2008a,b).

A 26-week RCT in patients ($n = 426$) with a history of recurrent moderate-to-severe depression, who responded with 50% or greater improvement in HAM-D scores after 6 weeks, studied maintenance therapy with SJW 300 mg TID compared with placebo for relapse. Relapse occurred in 18.1% of SJW patients and 25.7% of placebo patients. Average time to relapse was 177 days with SJW and 163 days with placebo. Adverse event rates were similar between groups. The authors concluded that SJW could be an option for long-term maintenance therapy for prophylaxis of recurrent depression (Kasper et al., 2010).

A 12-week RCT in patients ($n=135$) with MDD compared SJW 900 mg/day with fluoxetine 20 mg/day and with placebo. After 12 weeks mean HAMD-17 scores with SJW, fluoxetine, and placebo were 10.2, 13.3, and 12.6, respectively ($P<0.03$ and $P=0.096$ for difference between SJW or fluoxetine and placebo, respectively). There was also a trend toward higher rates of remission (defined as HAMD-17 < 8) with SJW than with fluoxetine or placebo (38%, 30%, and 21%, respectively). Overall, SJW appeared to be safe and well tolerated. The authors concluded that SJW was more effective than fluoxetine and showed a trend toward superiority over placebo (Fava et al., 2005).

A 6-week non-inferiority RCT in patients ($n=388$) with moderate depression compared SJW 900 mg/day with citalopram 20 mg/day and with placebo. From almost identical baseline values of 22, the HAM-D score was reduced to 10.3, 10.3, and 13.0 with SJW, citalopram, and placebo, respectively. The therapeutic equivalence of SJW to citalopram ($P<0.0001$) and the superiority of SJW over placebo ($P<0.0001$) was demonstrated. At the end of treatment 54%, 56%, and 39% of patients with SJW, citalopram and placebo, respectively were assessed as therapy responders. Significantly more adverse events with "certain," "probable," or "possible" relation to study medication were documented in the citalopram group (53%) compared with SJW (17%) and placebo (30%). In most cases, the investigators assessed the tolerability of SJW, citalopram, and placebo as "good" or "very good." The authors concluded that SJW was non-inferior to citalopram, and both compounds were superior to placebo. There was better safety and tolerability of SJW compared with citalopram (Gastpar et al., 2006).

A 6-week RCT in patients with moderate depression responsive to treatment compared a standardized extract of SJW 900 mg with citalopram 20 mg. From this study, a group of responders ($n=154$) were randomized to SJW, citalopram, or placebo to evaluate duration of response and relapse/recurrence. In total, 19.5% of the 154 responders were diagnosed with a relapse: 14/54 in the citalopram group, 8/54 in the SJW group, and 8/46 in the placebo group. No difference in the severity of relapse could be observed. The duration of response was 1755 days with citalopram, 1817 days with SJW, and 802 days for placebo. The author concluded that SJW was more efficient in lowering the relapse and recurrence rates in treatment responders when compared with citalopram and placebo (Singer et al., 2011).

A 26-week RCT in patients ($n=124$) with MDD who showed initial response to therapy compared SJW 900-1500 mg with sertraline 50-100 mg and with placebo. At 26 weeks, HAM-D scores were 6.6 with SJW, 7.1 with sertraline, and 5.7 with placebo, a non-significant difference ($P=0.61$). This effect was similar on the other outcomes of BDI, CGI-severity, CGI-improvement, and intention-to-treat analyses. The author concluded that while there was an equivocal outcome between treatments at 26 weeks, both SJW and sertraline were therapeutically effective with a pronounced "placebo effect" impeding a significant result (Sarris and Kavanagh, 2009). (*Note: a 6-month study of depression will be misleadingly affected by the high spontaneous remission rate at 6 months.*)

A 1-year open-label study in patients ($n=440$) with mild-to-moderate depression investigated SJW 500 mg/day with respect to safety and efficacy. Adverse events were reported in 49% of patients, but only 6% were thought to be possibly or probably related to treatment, the most common being GI and skin complaints. The long-term intake of up to 1 year did not result in any changes in clinical chemistry, ECG, or BMI. Mean HAM-D scores decreased steadily from 20.58 at baseline to 12.07 at week 26 and to 11.18 at week 52. Mean CGI scores decreased from 3.99 to 2.20 at week 26 and 2.19 at week 52. The authors concluded that SJW was a safe and effective way to treat mild-to-moderate depression over long periods of time (Brattström, 2009).

Dermatological Disorders: Eczema and Psoriasis

A 2017 systematic review of studies to assess the efficacy and safety of topical herbal preparations for allergic eczema found eight studies that met inclusion criteria. Only two studies that showed a positive effect were considered to have a low risk of bias across all domains: those of licorice gel and SJW. In each of these two studies, the test product was reported to be superior to placebo and the findings warranted further research. No meta-analysis could be performed due to heterogeneity (Thandar et al., 2017).

A half-body, single-blinded case series of patients ($n = 10$) with plaque-type psoriasis compared SJW ointment with placebo-vehicle on opposite sides of the body BID for 4 weeks. There was a significant reduction in erythema, scaling, and thickness with SJW compared with placebo ($P = 0.01$, 0.004, and 0.04 respectively) (Najafizadeh et al., 2012).

Another intraindividual study in patients ($n = 20$) with mild-to-moderate plaque-type psoriasis compared SJW cream with placebo for immunohistochemical changes in the skin. Compared with placebo, TNF-α concentrations in dermis, endothelial cells, and dendrite cells were significantly reduced ($P = 0.014$, 0.033, and 0.014, respectively) in lesions treated with SJW cream. Erythema, scaling, and thickness were significantly less ($P = 0.014$, 0.004, and 0.003, respectively) with SJW and there were also significant improvements in clinical and histological features of SJW-treated lesions ($P < 0.05$). The authors concluded that SJW ointment could help decrease PASI scores and TNFα levels in psoriatic tissue and that its efficacy was probably related to its effect on lowering cytokines, including TNFα (Mansouri et al., 2017).

A 4-week half-body RCT in patients ($n = 21$) with mild-to-moderate atopic dermatitis compared a cream containing a 5% SJW to the affected areas on one side of the body, and a vehicle cream to the other side BID. The SJW cream was significantly superior to the vehicle at all clinical visits (days 7, 14, 28) ($P < 0.05$). The SJW cream showed a trend of better antibacterial activity ($P = 0.064$). Skin tolerance and cosmetic acceptability was good or excellent in both groups. The authors concluded that SJW cream was significantly superior to the vehicle in the topical treatment of mild-to-moderate atopic dermatitis (Schempp et al., 2000).

Infectious Disease: Herpes Simplex Virus

A 14-day open-label clinical trial in patients ($n = 149$) with HSV-1 and HSV-2 lesions studied single applications of Dynamiclear (a topical combination of SJW plus copper sulfate) compared with 5% acyclovir. The odds of being affected by symptoms of acute pain, erythema, and vesiculation were 1.8, 2.4, and 4.4 times greater, respectively, in the acyclovir group in comparison to the SJW-copper group. The odds of being affected by burning and stinging sensation were 1.9 times greater in the acyclovir group. The authors concluded that the SJW-copper formulation was well tolerated and effective for HSV-1 and HSV-2 lesions even after a single application (Clewell et al., 2012).

ACTIVE CONSTITUENTS

- Amino acid derivatives
  - Amino acids
- Phenolic compounds
  - Phenylpropanoids (antioxidant, antimutagenic, antitumor, antimicrobial): chlorogenic acid, caffeic acid, p-coumaric acid, ferulic acid
  - Xanthones (MAO-I): norathyriol
  - Flavonoids: EGCG, rutin (antioxidant, anti-inflammatory, antidiabetic, nephroprotective, anti-osteoporotic, antispasmodic, neuroprotective, anti-anxiety), hyperoside (antioxidant, anti-inflammatory, antiproliferative, apoptotic, hepatoprotective, nephroprotective, anti-osteoporotic), isoquercetin, quercetin (anti-inflammatory, antioxidant, hypotensive, antidiabetic, antispasmodic, neuroprotective, XO inhibition, antibacterial, anticancer)
    - ▫ Proanthocyanidins: oligomeric procyanidines
  - Napthodianthrones: hypericin (antibiotic, antiviral, nonspecific kinase inhibitor, MAO-I), pseudohypericin, protohypericin, protopseudohypericin
  - Phloroglucinols (major psychoactive component; reuptake inhibition of DA, serotonin, NE, GABA, glutamate; stimulates IL-8): hyperforin, adhyperforin

SJW COMMONLY USED PREPARATIONS AND DOSAGE (FOR ADULTS UNLESS OTHERWISE SPECIFIED)

The following are examples of some available formulations and ranges of dosing for commercial herbal products. See Part III Introduction "How to prescribe medicinal herbs" for further guidance on herbal advising and prescribing.

Flower and Leaf

- Infusion of dried flowering herb: 1–2 tsp per cup TID
- Fluid extract (1:1, 25%): 2–4 mL TID

- Tincture of dried flowering herb (1:5, 40%–75%): 1–4 mL TID
- Tincture of fresh flowering herb (1:1.5, 70%): 0.7 mL (467 mg) BID-QID
- Capsule or tablet of powdered aerial parts: 700 mg BID
- Capsule or tablet of standardized extract (standardized to 0.3% hypericin or 0.5% hyperforin): 250–450 mg BID-TID
- Topical cream (standardized to 1.5% hyperforin or 5% SJW): applied TID

SAFETY AND PRECAUTION

Side Effects

May cause photosensitivity or subacute neuropathy with UV exposure or radiation therapy. While hypericin has been shown to be photosensitizing in high doses orally, it does not appear to produce more than mild photosensitivity with topical application in skin types II and III. In vitro research indicates hypericin has potential for oxidative damage to retinal epithelium. Other reported side effects include headache, nausea, abdominal discomfort, constipation, dizziness, confusion, sedation, sleep disturbances, fatigue, dry mouth, and anticoagulant effects.

Case Reports

Prolonged and involuntary facial muscle contractions, diffuse erythroderma, transplant rejection, mania, post-anesthetic hypotension, drug-induced hepatitis, mania, serotonin syndrome, intense neuralgia, sexual dysfunction, life-threatening immunosuppression, and withdrawal symptoms have been reported.

Toxicity

A 22-year-old man who had taken 1000 mg/day of flowering herbs of SJW had severe hematologic toxicity, with conditions involving bone marrow necrosis. Sperm motility is inhibited by high concentrations of SJW.

Pregnancy and Lactation

Avoid. Animal research shows conflicting results. No human data for lactation safety.

While one study (see below) is reassuring with respect to major malformations, it was small and warrants larger trials before it can be deemed safe during pregnancy. The toxicity of SJW administered to female rats during organogenesis did not seem to be toxic with 36 mg/kg/day administered in 0.5 mL of saline. Further studies using 36-144 mg/kg/day in pregnant rats also showed no difference from placebo in neonatal development and memory of the exposed pups. In another animal study, two doses of SJW extract, 100 mg/kg/day and 1000 mg/kg found severe histological damage in the livers and kidneys of animals euthanized postnatally on days 0 and 21. The lesions were more severe with the higher dose and in animals that were breastfed for 21 days. Renal and hepatic damage was evident also with the lower dose and in animals that were only exposed to SJW during breastfeeding.

A study prospectively collected and followed subjects taking SJW ($n = 54$) and compared them to a matched group of pregnant women taking other pharmacologic therapy for depression and a third group of healthy women, not exposed to any known teratogens ($n = 108$). The rates of major malformations were statistically similar across the three groups, with 5%, 4%, and 0% in the SJW group, disease comparator group, and healthy group, respectively ($P = 0.26$). The live birth and prematurity rates were also not different among the three groups (Moretti et al., 2009).

Disease Interactions

- Caution in surgical conditions due to potential anticoagulant effects.
- May worsen macular degeneration.
- May increase risk for mania in patients with bipolar mood disorder.

Drug Interactions

- CYP: Induces CYP450 3A4 and CYP 2C9 substrate drugs: indinavir, ritonavir, nevirapine, cyclosporin, tacrolimus, diltiazem, nifedipine, irinotecan, imatinib, docetaxel, warfarin (effect may last up to 3 weeks after stopping SJW).
- Pgp: Induces P-glycoprotein substrate drugs: digoxin, talinolol, and fexofenadine.
- UGT: Modulates UGT substrates. May increase the side effects of drugs such as acetaminophen.
- Lowers plasma levels and efficacy of simvastatin, rosuvastatin and atorvastatin (pravastatin not affected); proton pump inhibitors; oral

contraceptives; opiates; many antimicrobials; cyclosporin A; many antineoplastic drugs; zolpidem; alprazolam; clozapine and theophylline.

- Increases effects of (and toxicity of) tolbutamide, antiplatelets, methotrexate, pegylated interferon α.
- Potential for serotonin syndrome when taken in combination with SSRIs, TCAs, heterocyclic antidepressants, triptans this needs to be treated as a separate item.
- Although animal research has shown that SJW potentiates the effects of morphine, human research is lacking. However, it has been demonstrated that SJW decreases serum concentrations and effects of oxycodone.
- Numerous documented interactions with conventional drugs should preclude its use while undergoing chemotherapy, radiation therapy, antiretroviral therapy, immunosuppressive therapy, and anticoagulant therapy. Caution and close monitoring when used with many other drugs.

A pharmacokinetics RCT in healthy volunteers ($n = 16$) studied the impact of SJW on fentanyl infusions. The subjects received fentanyl fixed-dose infusions and individually tailored target-controlled infusions on separate days, before and after 30 days of SJW 300 mg TID or placebo control. Clearance before and after SJW was 1.13 L/min 1.24 L/min, respectively. This was not statistically different from clearance before and after placebo, which was 0.96 L/min and 1.12 L/min, respectively. SJW also did not affect fentanyl pharmacodynamics as measured by pupil constriction after fixed dose and tailored fentanyl infusions. EC50 was 1.1 ng/mL and 1.4 ng/mL before and after SJW, respectively, and was 1.2 ng/mL and 1.4 ng/mL before and after placebo, respectively. Effect site equilibration time was 12.8 min and 11.3 min before and after SJW, respectively and was 11.4 min and 11.1 min before and after placebo, respectively. SJW had no influence on analgesia, cognitive performance, or somatic cognitive-affective effects of fentanyl. The authors concluded that SJW did not alter fentanyl pharmacokinetics, pharmacodynamics, or clinical effects, suggesting no effect on hepatic clearance or blood-brain barrier efflux, and that patients taking SJW would likely not respond differently to IV fentanyl for anesthesia or analgesia (Loughren et al., 2020).

In a Phase I, open-label study in healthy volunteers ($n = 20$) a low-hyperforin SJW extract (Ze 117) was investigated for drug interactions with several drugs. No pharmacokinetic interactions of Ze 117 were observed for CYP1A2, CYP2B6, CYP2C9, CYP2C19, CYP3A4, and P-glycoprotein. AUC and peak plasma concentration of the used probe drugs showed 80%-125%. bioequivalence between the probe drug alone and the probe drug plus Ze 117. Ze 117 weakly increased dextromethorphan AUC ratio but not the corresponding metabolic ratio. The authors concluded that Ze 117 did not show clinically relevant pharmacokinetic interactions with important CYPs and P-glycoprotein (Zahner et al., 2019).

REFERENCES

Abdali K, Khajehei M, Tabatabaee HR. Effect of St John's wort on severity, frequency, and duration of hot flushes in premenopausal, perimenopausal and postmenopausal women: a randomized, double-blind, placebo-controlled study. Menopause 2010;17(2):326–31.

Al-Akoum M, Maunsell E, Verreault R, Provencher L, Otis H, Dodin S. Effects of Hypericum perforatum (St. John's wort) on hot flushes and quality of life in perimenopausal women: a randomized pilot trial. Menopause 2009;16(2):307–14.

Apaydin EA, Maher AR, Shanman R, Booth MS, Miles JN, Sorbero ME, Hempel S. A systematic review of St. John's wort for major depressive disorder. Syst Rev 2016 Sep 2;5(1):148.

Arentz S, Smith CA, Abbott J, Fahey P, Cheema BS, Bensoussan A. Combined Lifestyle and Herbal Medicine in Overweight Women with Polycystic Ovary Syndrome (PCOS): A Randomized Controlled Trial. Phytother Res 2017;31(9):1330–40.

Brattström A. Long-term effects of St. John's wort (Hypericum perforatum) treatment: a 1-year safety study in mild to moderate depression. Phytomedicine 2009;16(4):277–83.

Canning S, Waterman M, Orsi N, Ayres J, Simpson N, Dye L. The efficacy of Hypericum perforatum (St John's wort) for the treatment of premenstrual syndrome: a randomized, double-blind, placebo-controlled trial. CNS Drugs 2010;24(3):207–25.

Clewell A, Barnes M, Endres JR, Ahmed M, Ghambeer DK. Efficacy and tolerability assessment of a topical formulation containing copper sulfate and hypericum perforatum on patients with herpes skin lesions: a comparative, randomized controlled trial. J Drugs Dermatol 2012;11(2):209–15.

Eatemadnia A, Ansari S, Abedi P, Najar S. The effect of Hypericum perforatum on postmenopausal symptoms and depression: a randomized controlled trial. Complement Ther Med 2019;45:109–13.

Fahami F, Asali Z, Aslani A, Fathizadeh N. A comparative study on the effects of Hypericum Perforatum and passionflower on the menopausal symptoms of women referring to Isfahan city health care centers. Iran J Nurs Midwifery Res 2010;15(4):202–7.

Fava M, Alpert J, Nierenberg AA, et al. A Double-blind, randomized trial of St John's wort, fluoxetine, and placebo in major depressive disorder. J Clin Psychopharmacol 2005;25(5):441–7.

Gastpar M, Singer A, Zeller K. Comparative efficacy and safety of a once-daily dosage of hypericum extract STW3-VI and citalopram in patients with moderate depression: a double-blind, randomised, multicentre, placebo-controlled study. Pharmacopsychiatry 2006;39(2):66–75.

Geller SE, Studee L. Contemporary alternatives to plant estrogens for menopause. Maturitas 2006 Nov 1;55(Suppl 1):S3–13. Suppl 1.

Ghazanfarpour M, Sadeghi R, Abdolahian S, Latifnejad Roudsari R. The efficacy of Iranian herbal medicines in alleviating hot flashes: A systematic review. Int J Reprod Biomed 2016 Mar;14(3):155–66.

Kargozar R, Azizi H, Salari R. A review of effective herbal medicines in controlling menopausal symptoms. Electron Physician 2017;9(11):5826–33.

Kasper S, Volz HP, Moller HJ, et al. Continuation and long-term maintenance treatment with Hypericum extract WS 5570 after recovery from an acute episode of moderate depression—a double-blind, randomized, placebo controlled long-term trial. Eur Neuropsychopharmacol 2008a;18(11):803–13.

Kasper S, Gastpar M, Müller WE, et al. Efficacy of St. John's wort extract WS 5570 in acute treatment of mild depression: a reanalysis of data from controlled clinical trials. Eur Arch Psychiatry Clin Neurosci 2008b;258(1):59–63.

Kasper S, Caraci F, Forti B, Drago F, Aguglia E. Efficacy and tolerability of Hypericum extract for the treatment of mild to moderate depression. Eur Neuropsychopharmacol 2010;20(11):747–65.

Laakmann E, Grajecki D, Doege K, zu Eulenburg C, Buhling KJ. Efficacy of Cimicifuga racemosa, Hypericum perforatum and Agnus castus in the treatment of climacteric complaints: a systematic review. Gynecol Endocrinol 2012;28(9):703–9.

Linde K, Berner MM, Kriston L. St John's wort for major depression. Cochrane Database Syst Rev 2008;4, CD000448.

Loughren MJ, Kharasch ED, Kelton-Rehkopf MC, Syrjala KL, Shen DD. Influence of St. John's Wort on intravenous fentanyl pharmacokinetics, pharmacodynamics, and clinical effects: a randomized clinical trial. Anesthesiology 2020;132(3):491–503.

Mansouri P, Mirafzal S, Najafizadeh P, Safaei-Naraghi Z, Salehi-Surmaghi MH, Hashemian F. The impact of topical Saint John's Wort (Hypericum perforatum) treatment on tissue TNF-α levels in plaque-type psoriasis: a pilot study. J Postgrad Med 2017;63(4):215–20.

Moretti ME, Maxson A, Hanna F, Koren G. Evaluating the safety of St. John's Wort in human pregnancy. Reprod Toxicol 2009;28(1):96–9.

Najafizadeh P, Hashemian F, Mansouri P, Farshi S, Surmaghi MS, Chalangari R. The evaluation of the clinical effect of topical St Johns wort (Hypericum perforatum L.) in plaque type psoriasis vulgaris: a pilot study. Australas J Dermatol 2012;53(2):131–5.

Rahimi R, Nikfar S, Abdollahi M. Efficacy and tolerability of Hypericum perforatum in major depressive disorder in comparison with selective serotonin reuptake inhibitors: a meta-analysis. Prog Neuropsychopharmacol Biol Psychiatry 2009;33(1):118–27.

Ruan X, Mueck A, Beer A-M, Naser B, Pickartz S. Benefit-risk profile of black cohosh (isopropanolic *Cimicifuga racemosa* extract) with and without St John's wort in breast cancer patients. Climacteric 2019;22(4):339–47.

Sarris J, Kavanagh DJ. Kava and St. John's Wort: current evidence for use in mood and anxiety disorders. J Altern Complement Med 2009;15(8):827–36.

Schempp CM, Lüdtke R, Winghofer B, Simon JC. Effect of topical application of Hypericum perforatum extract (St. John's wort) on skin sensitivity to solar simulated radiation. Photodermatol Photoimmunol Photomed 2000;16(3):125–8.

Singer A, Schmidt M, Hauke W, Stade K. Duration of response after treatment of mild to moderate depression with Hypericum extract STW 3-VI, citalopram and placebo: a reanalysis of data from a controlled clinical trial. Phytomedicine 2011;18(8-9):739–42.

Thandar Y, Gray A, Botha J, Mosam A. Topical herbal medicines for atopic eczema: a systematic review of randomized controlled trials. Br J Dermatol 2017 Feb;176(2):330–43.

Uebelhack R, Blohmer JU, Graubaum HJ, Busch R, Gruenwald J, Wernecke KD. Black cohosh and St. John's wort for climacteric complaints: a randomized trial. Obstet Gynecol 2006 Feb;107(2 Pt 1):247–55.

van Die MD, Bone KM, Burger HG, Reece JE, Teede HJ. Effects of a combination of Hypericum perforatum and Vitex agnus-castus on PMS-like symptoms in late-perimenopausal women: findings from a subpopulation analysis. J Altern Complement Med 2009 Sep;15(9):1045–8.

Zahner C, Kruttschnitt E, Uricher J, et al. No clinically relevant interactions of St. John's Wort extract Ze 117 low in hyperforin with cytochrome P450 enzymes and P-glycoprotein. Clin Pharmacol Ther 2019;106(2):432–40.

Zhang X, Kang D, Zhang L, Peng L. Shuganjieyu capsule for major depressive disorder (MDD) in adults: a systematic review. Aging Ment Health 2014;18(8):941–53.

68

SAW PALMETTO (*SERENOA REPENS*)
Fruit

GENERAL OVERVIEW

Saw palmetto is one of the more widely recognized and utilized herbs for men's health, particularly for disorders of the prostate. It has been well studied, but the findings have been conflicting, particularly with a Cochrane review that indicated it was no better than placebo. Nevertheless, in vitro and animal research indicates that it has constituents that should be efficacious in diseases of the prostate, and it continues to be included in herbal blends for prostatic health. Hexanic extracts of saw palmetto have been studied in the preponderance of more recent research, and this research has more convincingly demonstrated the herb's efficacy in benign prostatic hyperplasia (BPH). Hexane is present in volatile fractions of several fruits and vegetables. It is used instead of alcohol to extract the constituents from the berries of saw palmetto, a process also used for processing canola oil and other foods. Saw palmetto may also be beneficial for women with polycystic ovary syndrome and hirsutism, but its use in women with childbearing potential should occur with great caution (see "Safety and Precaution").

Clinical research indicates that saw palmetto, alone or in combination formulas, may be beneficial for benign prostatic hyperplasia, acute and chronic prostatitis, and androgenic alopecia.

IN VITRO AND ANIMAL RESEARCH

Hexanic extracts of saw palmetto have been shown in vitro and in animal studies to have anti-inflammatory, anti-androgenic, and antiproliferative activity. These extracts have been shown to decrease prostaglandin and leukotriene production and decrease B lymphocyte infiltrates, IL-1β, and TNF-α. The berries have been shown to inhibit COX and 5-LOX, resulting in anti-inflammatory properties. A saw palmetto extract was found to inhibit growth of normal prostate cells and increase their sensitivity to radiation in vitro, but it did not affect malignant prostate cancer cells. Hexanic liposterolic extracts of saw palmetto have been shown to reduce tissue uptake of testosterone and DHT by more than 40% and to reduce conversion of testosterone to DHT via 5-α-reductase inhibition. Saw palmetto also appears to have estrogen-receptor blocking activity in the prostate and antispasmodic and anti-inflammatory activities in the bladder. Other in vitro research has demonstrated that saw palmetto decreases MCP-1 and VCAM-1 expression in human prostate and vascular cells, respectively. Other in vitro studies have shown that components of saw palmetto have α-1 adrenergic blocking activity. However, when rats were given a supercritical CO_2 extract over 4 weeks, they showed an increase in binding of prazosin to α-1 adrenergic receptors, suggesting a chronic adaptation.

Oleic acid and lauric acid from saw palmetto have muscarinic receptor blocking activity. These two fats also block the binding of calcium channel blockers and are likely the active constituents in saw palmetto that block 5-α-reductase activity. Studies have also demonstrated inhibition of the prolactin receptor on ovarian cells. In human prostate carcinoma cells, downregulation of inflammatory-related genes and activation of NF-κB pathway has been demonstrated.

HUMAN RESEARCH

Systematic reviews demonstrate conflicting evidence for this herb. Some of the difference in efficacy appears to be related to the method of extraction with hexanic extracts (which are higher in phytosterols) showing the most positive results.

Men's Genitourinary Disorders: Benign Prostatic Hyperplasia

A 2020 systematic review and meta-analysis to evaluate the efficacy and safety of saw palmetto combined with an α-blocker compared with α-blocker monotherapy in the treatment of BPH found seven trials ($n = 1009$) that met inclusion criteria. Compared with the patients treated with α-blocker monotherapy, those treated with α-blocker plus saw palmetto showed significant decreases in total IPSS, sub-IPSS in the storage and voiding stages, QOL, and PSA levels ($P < 0.05$ for all). With the addition of saw palmetto, there was also an increase in Q_{max} ($P = 0.04$), but no statistically significant differences in the prostate volume or PVR. The authors concluded that saw palmetto extract combined with α-blockers was safe and more efficacious than α-blocker monotherapy in the treatment of BPH (Zong et al., 2019).

A 2018 systematic review and meta-analysis of hexanic extracts of saw palmetto 320 mg/day selected 27 RCTs and prospective observational studies in patients with BPH with lower urinary tract symptoms (LUTS). Compared with placebo, the saw palmetto extracts were associated with 0.64 fewer voids/night ($P < 0.001$) and an additional mean increase in Q_{max} of 2.75 mL/s. When compared with α-blockers, the saw palmetto extracts showed similar improvements on IPSS and improvements in Q_{max}. When compared with 5-α-reductase inhibitors, the saw palmetto extracts showed similar efficacy on IPSS after 6 months of treatment. Overall data showed saw palmetto hexanic extracts provided a mean 5.73-point improvement in IPSS from baseline. There were no adverse effects on sexual function and no clinically relevant effect on PSA. Prostate volume decreased slightly. The beneficial effects appeared to extend to the 447 patients who were treated for ≥ 1 year. Gastrointestinal disorders were the most frequently reported side effect, with a mean incidence of 3.8% (Vela-Navarrete et al., 2018).

A 2017 systematic review investigated the efficacy of saw palmetto at a dose of 320 mg/day for the treatment of LUTS. Of the RCTs conducted for up to 6 months, a benefit was seen in three of three RTCs with ethanolic extraction, in eight of nine RTCs with hexanic extraction, and in one of two RCTs with CO_2 extraction. When the RCTs were conducted for more than 6 months, the benefits were less impressive. There were two of four RCTs with hexanic extraction and in one of two RTCs with CO_2 extraction that showed benefit. The one longer RCT with an ethanolic extract did not show positive results (Görne et al., 2017).

A 2016 systematic review focused on Permixon, a hexanic extract of saw palmetto, for efficacy in BPH. Twelve RCTs met inclusion criteria. Permixon was significantly more effective than placebo in reducing the number of nocturnal voids (WMD = -0.31; $P = 0.03$) and increasing Q_{max} (WMD = 3.37; $P < 0.0001$). Overall adverse events and withdrawal were similar with Permixon and placebo. Permixon was as effective as tamsulosin monotherapy and short-term therapy with finasteride in improving IPSS (WMD = 1.15; $P = 0.32$) and Q_{max} (WMD = -0.16; $P = 0.48$). The combination of Permixon and tamsulosin was more effective than Permixon monotherapy in relieving LUTS (WMD = 0.31; $P < 0.01$) but not for improving Q_{max} (WMD = 0.10). With regard to adverse effects, Permixon had a limited impact on ejaculatory dysfunction compared with tamsulosin (0.5% and 4%, respectively; $P = 0.007$). Decreased libido and impotence occurred in 2.2% and 1.5%, respectively, with saw palmetto and 3% and 2.8%, respectively, with finasteride. The authors concluded that Permixon decreased nocturnal voids and Q_{max} compared with placebo and had efficacy in relieving LUTS similar to tamsulosin and short-term finasteride and that it had a favorable safety profile with a very limited impact on sexual function, which was significantly affected by all other drugs used to treat LUTS/BPH (Novara et al., 2016).

A 2014 post hoc evaluation of BPH looked at four published RCTs ($n = 922$) on PRO 160/120, a fixed-dose herbal combination of saw palmetto 160 mg plus stinging nettle root 120 mg, compared with placebo (two studies), compared with finasteride (one study) and compared with tamsulosin (one study). In the pooled analysis of placebo-controlled trials, nocturnal voids improved by 0.8 (29%) with PRO 160/120 compared with 0.6 (18%) with placebo ($P = 0.015$). Responder rate to the herbal product compared with placebo was 69% and 52%, respectively ($P = 0.003$). Most responders improved by one void/night. There were no differences between PRO 160/120 and finasteride or tamsulosin regarding absolute improvement of nocturnal voids or response rates. The authors concluded that PRO 160/120 significantly improved nocturnal voiding frequency compared with placebo and was similar to tamsulosin and finasteride (Oelke et al., 2014).

A 2012 systematic review assessing the effect of saw palmetto for BPH LUTS selected 17 RCTs ($n = 2008$) that met inclusion criteria. Trial lengths ranged from 4 to 72 weeks. In a meta-analysis of three high-quality long-to-moderate term trials ($n = 661$), saw palmetto was no better than placebo in reducing LUTS based on the AUASI/IPSS or Q_{max}. One long-term dose escalation trial (72 weeks) found double and triple doses of saw palmetto did not improve AUASI compared with placebo and the proportions of clinical response were nearly identical. Long-term, saw palmetto was no better than placebo in improving nocturia in one high-quality study ($P = 0.19$). Pooled analysis of nine short-term Permixon trials showed a reduction in the frequency of nocturia (WMD = -0.79 times/night), although there was evidence of heterogeneity. The authors concluded that saw palmetto did not improve LUTS or Q_{max} compared with placebo in men with BPH, even at double and triple the usual dose but that adverse events were generally mild and comparable to placebo (MacDonald et al., 2012).

A 1-year study of men ($n = 70$) with symptomatic BPH studied saw palmetto ethanolic extract compared with no treatment for effect on prostate size, PSA, and uroflowmetry. The patients in the saw palmetto group showed a statistically significant increment of the Q_{max} and Q_{avg} as well as reduction of PVR relative to the control group ($P < 0.05$) with differences more pronounced in those men with prostate volume > 40 mL. The mean IPSS score was significantly reduced in the treatment group ($P < 0.01$) (Saidi et al., 2017).

A 24-week multicenter RCT in patients ($n = 354$) with BPH LUTS compared saw palmetto extract 320 mg with placebo. Statistically significant improvement in the peak urinary flow, IPSS, quality of life score, four-item male sexual function questionnaire score, and IIEF score were observed in the saw palmetto group compared with those in the placebo group ($P < 0.05$). Adverse events occurred in 1.2% and 1.9% of placebo and saw palmetto groups, respectively (Ye et al., 2019).

A 2-year RCT in patients ($n = 427$) between the ages of 50 and 80 years with LUTS (IPSS score ≥ 12, $Q_{max} \leq 15$ mL/s, and PVR < 100 mL) investigated a combination of saw palmetto plus selenium and lycopene compared with tadalafil 5 mg daily for 6 months. Median change in IPSS was -3 in both groups ($P < 0.01$), IPSS quality of life was -2 in both groups ($P < 0.05$), and Q_{max} was $+2$ in both groups ($P < 0.01$). An increase of Q_{max} by ≥ 3 points occurred in 39% of saw palmetto group and 27% of tadalafil group ($P < 0.01$). Adverse events were reported by 1.4% of patients in the saw palmetto group and 7.8% of patients in the tadalafil group ($P < 0.05$). The authors concluded that treatment with saw palmetto plus selenium and lycopene was not inferior to tadalafil 5 mg for improving IPSS and Q_{max} in men with LUTS (Morgia et al., 2013, 2014, 2018).

A 24-month open-label study in patients ($n = 120$) with BPH and mild or moderate LUTS, Q_{max} volume ≥ 150 mL, PSA < 4 ng/mL, and PVR < 150 mL, investigated the effect of saw palmetto 320 mg/day. Statistically significant improvements in the IPSS (5.5 points), QOL (1.8 points), Q_{max} (5.6 mL/s), IIEF (6.4 points), and reduction in residual urinary volume were observed by 24 months, and the mean prostate volume at was reduced from 39.8 mL to 36 mL. The authors concluded that long-term treatment with 320 mg of saw palmetto was beneficial for BPH (Sinescu et al., 2011).

A 6-month open-label RCT in men ($n = 1713$) with an IPPS score ≥ 8 compared α-blocker alone, 5-α-reductase inhibitor alone, saw palmetto alone, or dual combinations of α-blockers with the other two classes. There were no clinically significant differences between the treatment groups, and all showed significant improvement over watchful waiting ($P < 0.05$). Saw palmetto showed similar efficacy to the other two treatments both as monotherapy and in combination with α-blockers (Vela-Navarrete et al., 2018).

A 12-month open-label RCT in patients ($n = 140$) with BPH compared tamsulosin 0.2 mg/day alone or in conjunction with saw palmetto 320 mg/day.

Storage symptoms improved significantly more with the combination treatment compared with tamsulosin alone at 12 months (-1.7 and -0.8, respectively; $P=0.028$). IPSS scores decreased similarly between groups, and changes in other parameters were similar between groups (Ryu et al., 2015).

A 12–20-month matched-pair study in patients ($n=186$) with BPH compared silodosin monotherapy with silodosin plus a hexanic liposterolic extract of saw palmetto. Mean IPSS scores were significantly lower in patients treated with the addition of saw palmetto ($P=0.002$). The combined-therapy group more frequently than the silodosin monotherapy group achieved a greater than three-point improvement in IPSS scores (69.9% and 30.1%, respectively; $P=0.001$) and a 25% improvement in IPSS from baseline (68.8% and 31.2%, respectively; $P<0.001$) (Boeri et al., 2017).

A 48-week extended RCT in elderly men ($n=257$) with BPH and LUTS studied PRO 160/12, a fixed combination of 160 mg saw palmetto and 120 mg nettle root given BID, compared with placebo for 24 weeks. Double-blind treatment was followed by an open control period of 24 weeks during which all patients were administered PRO 160/120. Reduction of IPSS after the first 24 weeks was six points and four points with the herbal product and placebo, respectively ($P=0.003$). This applied to obstructive as well as to irritative symptoms and to patients with moderate or severe symptoms at baseline. The patient's quality of life was also significantly better with PRO 160/120 in comparison with placebo. During the second 24-week period, patients who were switched from placebo to the herbal product showed a marked improvement in LUTS ($P=0.01$) compared with those who had been treated with PRO 160/120 in the initial phase. The tolerability of PRO 160/120 was comparable to the placebo. The authors concluded that PRO 160/120 was superior to placebo in attenuating LUTS as assessed by IPSS. It improved obstructive and irritative symptoms and was effective in patients with moderate and severe symptoms. Tolerance of the plant extract was good (Lopatkin et al., 2007).

An open-label 96-week extension of the above RCT in men ($n=219$) with BPH and LUTS assessed the long-term efficacy and tolerability of PRO 160/120, a fixed combination of 160 mg saw palmetto and 120 mg nettle root given BID for an additional 48-week follow-up period. Between baseline (of the original study) and end of observation (week 96) the total IPSS was reduced by 53% ($P<0.001$), peak and average urinary flow increased by 19% ($P<0.001$), and residual urine volume decreased by 44% ($P=0.03$). The incidence of adverse events during follow-up was 1/1181 treatment days with only one event being possibly due to the herbal product. The authors concluded that treatment with PRO 160/120 provided a clinically relevant benefit over a period of 96 weeks (Lopatkin et al., 2005).

A 48-week RCT in elderly men ($n=543$) with BPH studied PRO 160/120, a fixed combination of 160 mg saw palmetto and 120 mg nettle root given BID, compared with finasteride given QD. Urinary flow rate increased 1.9 mL/s and 2.4 mL/s with the herbal product and finasteride, respectively ($P=0.52$). Urinary flow rate increased and micturition time decreased similarly with both treatments. The IPSS decreased from 11.3 to 8.2 and 6.5 after 24 and 48 weeks, respectively, with the herbal product. IPSS decreased from 11.8 to 8.0 and 6.2 at 24 and 48 weeks, respectively, with finasteride. Quality of life improved from 7.5 to 4.3 and from 7.7 to 4.1 with the herbal product and finasteride, respectively. Fewer adverse events occurred with the herbal product, particularly with respect to diminished ejaculation volume, erectile dysfunction, and headache (Sökeland and Albrecht, 1997).

From the above study, a subgroup analysis of 431 patients with small prostates compared with large prostates was undertaken. The subgroups with small prostates (≤ 40 mL) showed similar improvements in urinary flow rates, with mean values of 1.8 mL/s with PRO 160/120 and 2.7 mL/s with finasteride. The mean values for the subgroups with prostates of > 40 mL were similar, at 2.3 and 2.2 mL/s, respectively. There were improvements in IPSS in both treatment groups, with no statistically significant differences. The subgroup analysis showed slightly better results for voiding symptoms in the patients with prostates of > 40 mL. The safety analysis showed that more patients in the finasteride group reported adverse events. The authors concluded that the efficacies of PRO 160/120 and finasteride were equivalent and unrelated to prostate volume. However, PRO 160/120 had better tolerability than finasteride (Sökeland, 2000).

A 60-week RCT in elderly men ($n=140$) with BPH and LUTS and an IPSS ≥ 13 investigated Prostagutt

Forte, a combination of saw palmetto 160 mg plus nettle root 120 mg given BID, compared with tamsulosin 0.4 mg QD. The total IPSS was reduced by a median of nine points in both groups. The IPSS score was ≤ 7 points at endpoint ("responders") in 32.4% of the patients in the herbal group and 27.9% in the tamsulosin group (test for non-inferiority of the herb: $P = 0.034$; non-inferiority margin 10%). Both drugs were well tolerated, with one adverse event in 1514 treatment days for the herbal product and one event in 1164 days for tamsulosin. The authors concluded that the fixed combination of saw palmetto and stinging nettle was non-inferior to tamsulosin 0.4 mg in the treatment of LUTS caused by BPH (Engelmann et al., 2006).

A 12-week RCT in men ($n = 99$) with BPH compared 500 mg/day of 3% β-sitosterol-enriched saw palmetto oil, 500 mg/day of nonenriched saw palmetto oil, and placebo for effects on BPH and androgen deficiency. Subjects treated with β-sitosterol-enriched saw palmetto oil showed significant decreases from baseline, as compared with placebo, in IPSS, Aging Male Symptoms, and Androgen Deficiency in the Aging Male scores along with reduced PVR ($P < 0.001$), PSA ($P < 0.01$), and 5α-reductase. Q_{max} and Q_{avg} ($P < 0.001$) as well as free T increased significantly with the enhanced formulation compared with placebo. The authors concluded that β-sitosterol-enriched saw palmetto oil was superior to conventional saw palmetto oil for BPH and androgen deficiency treatment (Sudeep et al., 2020).

Men's Genitourinary Disorders: Acute and Chronic Prostatitis

A 6-month study in patients ($n = 97$) with BPH and biopsy-proven prostatic inflammation compared a hexanic extract of saw palmetto 320 mg/day with no treatment. The second biopsy at 6 months with saw palmetto showed a decrease in the mean inflammation grading and aggressiveness grading score from 1.55 and 1.55 at baseline to 0.79 ($P = 0.001$) and 0.87 ($P = 0.001$), respectively. In the control group the mean inflammation grading and mean aggressiveness grading scores changed from 1.44 and 1.09 at baseline to 1.23 (P=0.09) and 0.89 (P=0.74), respectively. The mean decrease in all inflammation scores was statistically greater in the saw palmetto patients compared with controls. The authors concluded that this hexanic extract of saw palmetto reduced prostatic inflammation histologically and immunohistochemically (Gravas et al., 2018).

A 12-week study men ($n = 54$) with chronic inflammatory non-bacterial prostatitis who were treated with saw palmetto extract 320 mg/day resulted in the NIH-Chronic Prostatitis Symptom Index and IPSS scores decreasing from 27.6 to 18.6 and from 20.4 to 10.9, respectively ($P < 0.01$ for both). The average urinary flow rate improved from 8.05 to 12.05 mL/s ($P < 0.01$), maximum urinary flow rate improved from 14.2 to 21.3 mL/s ($P < 0.01$), residual urine volume decreased from 46.1 to 14.5 mL ($P < 0.01$), maximum urethral closure pressure fell from 76.5 to 65.3 cm H_2O ($P < 0.01$), mean urinary volume increased from 124.6 to 285.9 mL ($P < 0.01$), urination frequency fell from 16.9 to 8.9 ($P < 0.01$), and nocturia frequency fell from 8.9 to 3.1 ($P < 0.01$). No apparent adverse reactions were observed in any of the patients (Shao et al., 2017).

A 14-day RCT in patients ($n = 34$) with acute prostatitis studied Prostagutt Forte, an herbal combination of saw palmetto 160 mg plus stinging nettle root 120 mg BID, along with ciprofloxacin 500 mg BID for 14 days plus diclofenac 50 mg QHS for 7 days compared with ciprofloxacin plus diclofenac without the herbal product. Patients receiving add-on herbal product experienced a pronounced and significant decrease of WBCs in prostatic secretions, a decrease in prostate volume per transrectal ultrasound, and more rapid reductions of hyperthermia and severity of bladder outlet obstruction (Pul'bere and Avdoshin, 2012).

An RCT in men ($n = 100$) with symptoms and color doppler indicative of prostatitis studied levofloxacin 500 mg/day for 10 days plus Prostamev Plus (a combination of saw palmetto 320 mg, bromelain, and nettle) given daily for 2 months compared with levofloxacin (same regimen) plus saw palmetto 320 mg/day for 2 months, compared with sensitivity-based antibiotic treatment for 10 days plus the polyherbal formula for 2 months, and compared with sensitivity-based antibiotic treatment for 10 days plus saw palmetto for 2 months. The groups treated with antibiotic plus Prostamev Plus achieved better improvements of IPSS, urinary flow and sexual life compared with the groups treated with antibiotic plus saw palmetto alone (Marzano et al., 2015).

A 36-week RCT in patients ($n = 120$) with chronic bacterial prostatitis and recurrent infections due to *Escherichia coli* and *Enterococcus faecalis* evaluated treatment with 24 weeks of daily Bifiprost (a combination of cranberry, goji, and probiotics) plus saw palmetto 320 mg compared with 24 weeks of saw palmetto 320 mg monotherapy, each group having received appropriate antibiotic treatment with subsequently negative cultures. At 24 and 36 weeks, the patients in the Bifiprost group experienced a significantly greater reduction in episodes of prostatitis than the patients in the saw palmetto monotherapy group. There was also a significant difference in the mean NIH-CPSI scores between the two groups at 24 and 36 weeks. At 12 weeks of treatment, the mean NIH-CPSI score was reduced in both groups compared with baselines, but no significant differences were seen between groups; nor was there a difference in reduction of episodes of prostatitis between groups at this time point. The authors concluded that combining Bifiprost and saw palmetto 320 mg improved the prevention of episodes of CBP due to Enterobacteriaceae and ameliorated prostatitis-related symptoms after 6 months of therapy, with continued benefit extending 3 months beyond the end of therapy (Chiancone et al., 2019).

A 6-month RCT in patients ($n = 143$) with chronic bacterial prostatitis investigated prulifloxacin 600 mg/day for 14 days plus ProstaMEV (a combination of saw palmetto and nettle) plus FlogMEV (a combination of quercetin and curcumin) compared with the same prulifloxacin regimen without the additional herbs and supplements. 1 month after treatment, 89.6% and 27% of patients who had received prulifloxacin+ProstaMEV+FlogMEV and prulifloxacin alone, respectively, were recurrence-free ($P < 0.0001$). Significant differences were found between groups in terms of symptoms and QOL ($P < 0.0001$ for both). 6 months after treatment, no patients in the combination group had recurrence of disease, whereas two patients in the antibiotic-alone group did. Results on the NIH Chronic Prostatitis Symptom Index and IPSS demonstrated statistically significant differences between groups ($P < 0.001$ for both). The authors concluded that the association of saw palmetto, nettle, quercetin, and curcumin was able to improve the clinical efficacy of prulifloxacin in patients affected by CBP (Cai et al., 2009).

A 6-week RCT in men ($n = 63$) with chronic prostatitis/chronic pelvic pain syndrome investigated Deprox 500 (a flower pollen extract plus vitamins) compared with Permixon (a hexane extract of saw palmetto 320 mg) one or two tablets/day of each. The mean score variation for IPSS was -12.7 in the Deprox 500 group and -7.8 in the Permixon group ($P = 0.0005$). The IPSS/NIH-Chronic Prostatitis Symptom Index (NIH-CPSI) changed by -17.3 in the Deprox 500 group and -13.6 in the Permixon group ($P = 0.0016$). The mean score of the symptoms portion of the NIH-CPSI questionnaire changed by -11.5 in the Deprox 500 group and -9.02 Permixon group ($P = 0.009321$). In patients with HTN, the mean IPSS score variation was -14.3 in the Deprox 500 group and -9.02 in the Permixon group. The authors concluded that in patients with CP/CPPS, Deprox 500 improved IPSS and NIH-CPSI scores up to 74.5% and 84.5% respectively (Macchione et al., 2018).

Dermatological Disorders: Androgenic alopecia

A 24-month open-label study in men ($n = 100$) with androgenic alopecia compared saw palmetto 320 mg/day with finasteride 1 mg/day for 24 months. The saw palmetto group showed increased hair growth in 38% (only at the vertex), while the finasteride group showed increased hair growth in 68% (both frontal and vertex). The latter was more effective with more advanced alopecia. It appears finasteride is a better choice for male-pattern hair loss, but saw palmetto may be an option for some men who develop sexual dysfunction or headache from finasteride (Rossi et al., 2012).

ACTIVE CONSTITUENTS

- Carbohydrates
  - Polysaccharides
  - Alcohols
- Lipids
  - Fatty acids (likely responsible for the majority of beneficial effects: 5-α-reductase inhibition, α-blocking): lauric acid, oleic acid, capric acid, caprylic acid, caproic acid, myristic acid
- Phenolic compound:
  - Flavonoids: isoquercetin, kaempferol (anti-inflammatory, antidepressant, strengthens capillaries), rutin (antioxidant, anti-inflammatory, antidiabetic, nephroprotective, anti-osteoporotic, antispasmodic, neuroprotective, anti-anxiety)

- Terpenes
- Steroids
  - Phytosterols: β-sitosterol (reduces GI cholesterol absorption, inhibits 5-α-reductase) and its glycosides, campesterol, stigmasterol

SAW PALMETTO COMMONLY USED PREPARATIONS AND DOSAGE (FOR ADULTS UNLESS OTHERWISE SPECIFIED)

The following are examples of some available formulations and ranges of dosing for commercial herbal products. See Part III Introduction "How to prescribe medicinal herbs" for further guidance on herbal advising and prescribing.

Dried Berry

- Decoction: 2–4 tsp per cup TID.
- Fluid extract (1:1, 60%): 0.6–1.5 mL TID.
- Tincture (1:5, 50%–70%): 1–2 mL TID.
- Powdered berry extract: 500 mg (1/5 tsp) QD-BID.
- Capsule or tablet of powdered berry: 450–900 mg BID-QID.
- Capsule or tablet of powdered berry extract: 160-200 mg BID
- Capsule or tablet of standardized hexanic extract (standardized to 80%–95% liposterolic compounds): 160–320 mg QD-BID, ideally with food.

Standardized hexanic extracts or combination formulas with extracts of stinging nettle, pumpkin seed, and others may be more effective.

SAFETY AND PRECAUTION

Side-Effects

Generally, saw palmetto is well tolerated. Minor side effects include gastrointestinal symptoms (abdominal pain, nausea, diarrhea), fatigue, headache, decreased libido, and rhinitis.

Case Reports

- Two case reports of pancreatitis.
- Two case reports of hot flushes in preadolescent teens.
- One case report of rhabdomyolysis.

Toxicity

The Complementary and Alternative Medicine for Urological Symptoms trial of 369 men with lower urinary tract symptoms due to BPH found no evidence of toxicity from ethanolic saw palmetto extract administered up to three times the clinical dose during an 18-month period.

Pregnancy and Lactation

Category X in pregnancy due to anti-androgen effects. Lactation effects unknown.

(Note possibility of reduction in efficacy of oral contraceptive pills).

Disease Interactions

Caution is advised with recent intraocular lens replacement. One study showed a slight increased risk of floppy iris syndrome.

There are concerns with prostate cancer monitoring and effect on PSA. However, in one large study, a saw palmetto extract did not affect serum PSA more than placebo, even at high doses. A large epidemiologic study did not find associations with the use of saw palmetto and reduced risk of prostate cancer.

Drug Interactions

- CYP: Inhibits CYP450 3A4, 2D6, and 2C8, 2C9.
- UGT: Inhibits UGT enzymes.
- Anticoagulants, antiplatelets: Saw palmetto may have additive anticoagulant effects.
- NSAIDs: Saw palmetto may have increase the risk of side effects with these drugs due to anti-inflammatory effects.
- MAOI's: Saw palmetto contains tyramine.
- Oral contraceptives: possibly less effective with saw palmetto.

REFERENCES

Boeri L, Capogrosso P, Ventimiglia E, et al. Clinically meaningful improvements in LUTS/BPH severity in men treated with silodosin plus hexanic extract of Serenoa repens or silodosin alone. Sci Rep 2017;7(1):15179.

Cai T, Mazzoli S, Bechi A, et al. Serenoa repens associated with Urtica dioica (ProstaMEV) and curcumin and quercitin (FlogMEV) extracts are able to improve the efficacy of prulifloxacin in bacterial prostatitis patients: results from a prospective randomised study. Int J Antimicrob Agents 2009;33(6):549–53.

Chiancone F, Carrino M, Meccariello C, Pucci L, Fedelini M, Fedelini P. The use of a combination of *Vaccinium Macracarpon, Lycium barbarum L.* and Probiotics (Bifiprost) for the prevention of chronic bacterial prostatitis: a double-blind randomized study. Urol Int 2019;103(4):423–6.

Engelmann U, Walther C, Bondarenko B, Funk P, Schläfke S. Efficacy and safety of a combination of sabal and urtica extract in lower urinary tract symptoms. A randomized double-blind study vs tamsulosin. Arzneimittelforschung 2006;56(3):222–9.

Görne RC, Wegener T, Kelber O, Feistel B, Reichling J. Randomized double-blind controlled clinical trials with herbal preparations of *Serenoa repens* fruits in treatment of lower urinary tract symptoms: an overview. Wien Med Wochenschr 2017;167(7–8):177–82.

Gravas S, Samarinas M, Zacharouli K, et al. The effect of hexanic extract of Serenoa repens on prostatic inflammation: results from a randomized biopsy study. World J Urol 2018;19.

Lopatkin N, Sivkov A, Walther C, et al. Long-term efficacy and safety of a combination of sabal and urtica extract for lower urinary tract symptoms—a placebo-controlled, double-blind, multicenter trial. World J Urol 2005;23(2):139–46.

Lopatkin N, Sivkov A, Schläfke S, Funk P, Medvedev A, Engelmann U. Efficacy and safety of a combination of Sabal and Urtica extract in lower urinary tract symptoms—long-term follow-up of a placebo-controlled, double-blind, multicenter trial. Int Urol Nephrol 2007;39(4):1137–46.

Macchione N, Bernardini P, Piacentini I, Mangiarotti B, Del Nero A. Flower pollen extract in association with vitamins (Deprox 500*) vs Serenoa repens in chronic prostatitis/chronic pelvic pain syndrome: a comparative analysis of 2 different treatments. Antiinflamm Antiallergy Agents Med Chem 2018;28.

MacDonald R, Tacklind JW, Rutks I, et al. Serenoa repens monotherapy for benign prostatic hyperplasia (BPH): an updated Cochrane systematic review. BJU Int 2012;109(12):1756–61.

Marzano R, Dinelli N, Ales V, Bertozzi MA. Effectiveness on urinary symptoms and erectile function of Prostamev plus* vs only extract Serenoa repens. Arch Ital Urol Androl 2015;87(1):25–7.

Morgia G, Cimino S, Favilla V, et al. Effects of Serenoa repens, selenium and lycopene (Profluss*) on chronic inflammation associated with benign prostatic hyperplasia: results of "FLOG" (Flogosis and Profluss in Prostatic and Genital Disease), a multicentre Italian study. Int Braz J Urol 2013;39(2):214–21.

Morgia G, Russo GI, Voce S, et al. Serenoa repens, lycopene and selenium vs tamsulosin for the treatment of LUTS/BPH. An Italian multicenter double-blinded randomized study between single or combination therapy (PROCOMB trial). Prostate 2014;74(15):1471–80.

Morgia G, Vespasiani G, Pareo RM, et al. Serenoa repens + selenium + lycopene vs tadalafil 5 mg for the treatment of lower urinary tract symptoms secondary to benign prostatic obstruction: a Phase IV, non-inferiority, open-label, clinical study (SPRITE study). BJU Int 2018;122(2):317–25.

Novara G, Giannarini G, Alcaraz A, et al. Efficacy and safety of hexanic lipidosterolic extract of Serenoa repens (Permixon) in the treatment of lower urinary tract symptoms due to benign prostatic hyperplasia: systematic review and meta-analysis of randomized controlled trials. Eur Urol Focus 2016;2(5):553–61.

Oelke M, Berges R, Schläfke S, Burkart M. Fixed-dose combination PRO 160/120 of sabal and urtica extracts improves nocturia in men with LUTS suggestive of BPH: re-evaluation of four controlled clinical studies. World J Urol 2014;32(5):1149–54.

Pul'bere SA, Avdoshin VP. Combined therapy using phytopreparation prostagutt forte in patients with acute prostatitis. Urologia 2012;5:53–54, 56.

Rossi A, Mari E, Scarno M, et al. Comparitive effectiveness of finasteride vs Serenoa repens in male androgenetic alopecia: a two-year study. Int J Immunopathol Pharmacol 2012;25(4):1167–73.

Ryu YW, Lim SW, Kim JH, et al. Comparison of tamsulosin plus Serenoa repens with tamsulosin in the treatment of benign prostatic hyperplasia in Korean men: 1-year randomized open label study. Urol Int 2015;94(2):187–93.

Saidi S, Stavridis S, Stankov O, Dohcev S, Panov S. Effects of Serenoa repens alcohol extract on benign prostate hyperplasia. Pril (Makedon Akad Nauk Umet Odd Med Nauki) 2017;38(2):123–9.

Shao YP, Xue HL, Shen BX, Ding LC, Chen ZS, Wei ZQ. Saw palmetto fruit extract improves LUTS in type IIIA prostatitis patients. Zhonghua Nan Ke Xue 2017;23(5):417–21.

Sinescu I, Geavlete P, Multescu R, et al. Long-term efficacy of Serenoa repens treatment in patients with mild and moderate symptomatic benign prostatic hyperplasia. Urol Int 2011;86(3):284–9.

Sökeland J. Combined sabal and urtica extract compared with finasteride in men with benign prostatic hyperplasia: analysis of prostate volume and therapeutic outcome. BJU Int 2000;86(4):439–42.

Sökeland J, Albrecht J. Combination of Sabal and Urtica extract vs finasteride in benign prostatic hyperplasia (Aiken stages I to II). Comparison of therapeutic effectiveness in a one-year double-blind study. Urologe A 1997;36(4):327–33.

Sudeep HV, Thomas JV, Shyamprasad K. A double blind, placebo-controlled randomized comparative study on the efficacy of phytosterol-enriched and conventional saw palmetto oil in mitigating benign prostate hyperplasia and androgen deficiency. BMC Urol 2020;20(1):86.

Vela-Navarrete R, Alcaraz A, Rodríguez-Antolín A, et al. Efficacy and safety of a hexanic extract of Serenoa repens (Permixon) for the treatment of lower urinary tract symptoms associated with benign prostatic hyperplasia (LUTS/BPH): systematic review and meta-analysis of randomised controlled trials and observational studies. BJU Int 2018.

Ye Z, Huang J, Zhou L, et al. Efficacy and safety of Serenoa repens extract among patients with benign prostatic hyperplasia in China: a multicenter, randomized, double-blind, placebo-controlled trial. Urology 2019. pii: S0090–4295(19)30236–5.

Zong HT, Wang XY, Wang T, Zhou X, Zhang Y. Efficacy and safety of Serenoa repens extract combined with alpha-receptor blocker in the treatment of benign prostatic hyperplasia. Zhonghua Nan Ke Xue 2019 Jun;25(6):553–8.

69

SCHISANDRA/SCHIZANDRA (*SCHISANDRA CHINENSIS*)
Fruit

GENERAL OVERVIEW

Not as well studied in humans as most other adaptogenic herbs, schisandra has been used in traditional Chinese medicine for a host of afflictions. The list includes coughs and wheezing, liver diseases, stomach disorders, excessive sweating, and generalized stress. Siberian hunters used the herb to improve stamina and night vision and to reduce hunger and thirst. Preclinical studies have shown some unique effects on amyloid precursor protein, which warrants study in humans.

Clinical research indicates that schisandra, often in combination with other herbs, may be beneficial for congestive heart failure, diabetes, obesity, hepatitis, polycystic ovary syndrome, menopause, cognitive performance, physical stamina, pneumonia, renal xenograft rejection, familial Mediterranean fever, and estrogen-dependent cancer prevention.

IN VITRO AND ANIMAL RESEARCH

In vitro studies have shown that schisandra has anti-inflammatory, antioxidant, cardiotonic, hypoglycemic, neuroprotective, anti-anxiety, sedative, astringent, adaptogenic, energy-enhancing, antimicrobial, immune-enhancing, and anticancer activity. It protects against the sequelae of myocardial infarction and stroke in mice likely via nitric oxide pathways. It improves insulin sensitivity in mice and is hepatoprotective against various toxins.

Schisandra has been shown to enhance sildenafil-induced relaxation of rabbit penile corpus cavernosum, showing potential suitability for patients not completely responding to sildenafil. Schisandra enhances endurance and metabolism. It improves cognition, enhancing brain cholinergic activity. A study of a mouse model of AD found that intragastric infusion of schisandra total lignans produced improved cognition and stamina and ameliorated neurodegeneration in the hippocampus of mice. In addition to antioxidant effects, the research showed that the lignans decreased the activity of β-secretase 1, a crucial protease in the pathway to making amyloid precursor protein, which is under current focus in the pharmaceutical industry's quest for a cure for Alzheimer's disease (AD). In a mouse restraint model of anxiety, oral administration of schisandra lignans extract 100 and 200 mg/kg/day for 8 days reduced the level of stress-induced anxious behavior, brain MAO levels, and plasma cortisol levels, suggesting that the extract reversed stress-induced anxiety via modulation of a hyperactive HPA axis.

Schisandra was one of the four traditional Chinese medicines, out of the 40 tested, that exhibited the strongest inhibitory activities against all fungal strains tested. Combinations with *Punica granatum* and/or *Melaphis chinensis* were synergistic for antifungal activity. Schisandra protects against doxorubicin-induced cardiotoxicity and has been shown to reverse the Pgp-mediated multidrug resistance that cancer cells develop to doxorubicin, vincristine, and paclitaxel. Schisandronic acid has been shown to inhibit entry of HCV into hepatocytes.

HUMAN RESEARCH

Cardiovascular Disorders: Congestive Heart Failure

A 2011 systematic review looking at the traditional Chinese medicine (TCM) formula Shengmai (also called Shen-Mai-San, containing schisandra, ginseng, and *Liriope spicata*) as a complementary treatment for heart failure in China selected six RCTs ($n=440$) that met inclusion criteria. Compared with usual treatment alone, Shengmai plus usual treatment in five trials indicated an improvement in NYHA classification (RR = 0.37). Other possible benefits included improved EF, CO, stroke volume, exercise test, and ratio of peak early-to-late diastolic filling velocity. Only one RCT with 40 patients compared Shengmai with placebo, and improvements were seen in stroke volume, health, cardiac indexes, and myocardial contractility. The authors concluded that Shen-Mai alone or in addition to usual treatment could be beneficial for heart failure compared with placebo or with usual treatment alone (Zheng et al., 2011).

Cardiometabolic Disorders: Diabetes and Obesity

A 12-week RCT in obese women ($n=28$) compared schisandra fruit extract with placebo for metabolic and gut flora effects. Although the values did not differ significantly between the two groups, schisandra tended to show a greater decrease than placebo in WC, fat mass, FBS, TG, AST, and ALT. *Bacteroides* and *Bacteroidetes* were both increased with schisandra and showed a negative correlation with fat mass, AST, and ALT. *Ruminococcus* was decreased by schisandra and showed a negative correlation with HDL-C and FBS (Song et al., 2015).

Gastrointestinal Disorders: Hepatitis

A 5-month RCT in subjects ($n=40$) with borderline elevations in ALT and AST compared schisandra plus sesamin (a sesame seed lignan) with placebo for effects on hepatic health. The schisandra product reduced the levels of ALT and AST, increased antioxidant capacity, and decreased the values of thiobarbituric acid-reactive substances (indicators of oxidation), total free radicals, and SO radicals in the plasma. The activities of GSH peroxidase and reductase in the erythrocytes were significantly increased. In addition, the lag time for LDL oxidation was increased. The authors concluded that the schisandra-sesamin compound had effects of antioxidation and improving liver function (Chiu et al., 2013).

A study in patients ($n=32$) infected with HBV assessed the effects of schisandra on immune-hematologic parameters. The circulating monocyte count significantly dropped after 2 weeks of therapy while WBCs, neutrophils, and lymphocytes were unchanged. The authors concluded that the reduction in circulating monocytes may reduce the self-inflicted host immune-mediated hepatocellular damage, a possible explanation for schisandra's hepatoprotective effect demonstrated in animal research (Yip et al., 2007).

Women's Genitourinary Disorders: Polycystic Ovary Syndrome and Menopause

A pilot RCT in healthy premenopausal women ($n=40$) studied a combination botanical supplement (dandelion, schisandra, turmeric, rosemary, milk thistle, and *Cynara scolymus*) compared with dietary changes (three servings/day of crucifers or dark leafy greens, 30 g/day of fiber, 1-2 L/day of water, and limiting caffeine and alcohol consumption to one serving per week) and with placebo for hormonal effects. During the early follicular phase, compared with placebo, the polyherbal product decreased DHEA (-13.2%; $P=0.02$), DHEA-S (-14.6%; $P=0.07$), androstenedione (-8.6%; $P=0.05$), and estrone-sulfate (-12.0%; $P=0.08$). When comparing dietary changes with placebo, no statistically significant differences were observed. There were no substantial effects on estrone-sulfate, total estradiol, free estradiol, testosterone, SHBG, insulin, IGF-I, or leptin. The authors concluded that early-follicular phase androgens were decreased with the polyherbal product (Greenlee et al., 2007).

A 12-week RCT in women ($n=36$) with menopausal symptoms compared schisandra 196 mg BID with placebo given for 6 weeks. The Kupperman Index decreased by 21.6% and 41.2% at the 6- and 12-week visits, respectively, with schisandra, and 12.6% and 27.2%, respectively, with placebo. Schisandra produced roughly 50% reductions in hot flushes, sweating, and palpitations. Estradiol serum levels were slightly increased with schisandra, but the change was not statistically significant when compared with placebo (Park and Kim, 2016).

Psychiatric Disorders: Cognitive Performance

A pilot study in the form of an RCT in stressed-out adults ($n = 40$) investigated a single dose of ADAPT-232 (a standardized combination of rhodiola, schisandra, and eleuthero) compared with placebo for effects on cognitive attention, speed, and accuracy while performing stressful cognitive tasks. The results showed a significant difference ($P < 0.05$) in attention, speed, and accuracy between the two treatment groups with superiority in the herbal treatment. No serious side effects were reported, although a few minor adverse events such as sleepiness and cold extremities were observed in both treatment groups (Aslanyan et al., 2010).

Disorders of Vitality: Physical Stamina

An 8-day RCT in athletes ($n = 109$) undergoing heavy physical exercise studied the adaptive effects of standardized schisandra 182 mg BID compared with standardized *Bryonia alba* tablets and with placebo. Initially those in the treatment group showed an increase in NO and cortisol that correlated with improvement in physical performance compared with placebo. At the completion of heavy physical exercise there was no increase in salivary NO and cortisol in the athletes given the herbs, whereas athletes treated with placebo showed increased salivary NO. The authors concluded that the salivary NO test could be used for the evaluation of both physical loading and the stress protective effect of adaptogens (Panossian et al., 1999).

A 12-week RCT in healthy postmenopausal women ($n = 45$) compared schisandra 1000 mg/day with placebo for effects on quadriceps muscle strength (QMS) and lactate at rest. After 12 weeks of schisandra, QMS was significantly increased ($P < 0.001$) and lactate levels at rest were significantly decreased ($P < 0.05$). The authors concluded that schisandra extract may help improve QMS and decrease lactate levels at rest in postmenopausal women (Park et al., 2020).

Infectious Disease: Pneumonia

A 10-15-day RCT in patients ($n = 60$) with pneumonia investigated ADAPT-232 (a standardized combination

of schisandra, rhodiola, and eleuthero) given BID plus standard treatment with cefazolin, bromhexine, and theophylline compared with the standard treatment plus placebo. The mean duration of treatment with antibiotics required to bring about recovery from the acute phase of the disease was 2 days shorter with the herbal product compared with placebo. Patients in the herbal group scored higher than the placebo group in QOL domains at the beginning of the rehabilitation period, and significantly higher on the fifth day after clinical convalescence. The authors concluded that adjuvant therapy with ADAPT-232 had a positive effect on the recovery of patients with pneumonia (Narimanian et al., 2005)

Immune Disorders: Renal Xenograft Rejection

In the first of a two-phase trial in renal transplant patients ($n = 12$) who were high-dose users of tacrolimus (*CYP3A5*1* allele carriers, CYP3A5 expressers), schisandra tablets were administered to assess the impact on tacrolimus dosing. The average individual increment in dose-adjusted C_0, C_{max}, and $AUC_{0-12\ hour}$ of tacrolimus were 198.8%, 111.0%, and 126.1%, respectively ($P < 0.01$), while the average individual reduction in tacrolimus daily dose was 40.9% ($P < 0.01$). Part II of the study (RCT) in renal transplant patients ($n = 32$) investigated schisandra plus guided dosing of tacrolimus compared with standard dosing of tacrolimus alone. Besides a reduced tacrolimus dose requirement ($P < 0.01$), a more accurate tacrolimus initial dose characterized by lower incidence of out-of-range C_0 after initial dose ($P < 0.01$) and fewer dose changes ($P < 0.01$) occurred with schisandra. No significant differences in acute rejection rate and serum creatinine levels were observed between the two groups. The authors concluded that schisandra plus *CYP3A5* genotype-guided tacrolimus dosing was a promising therapy for CYP3A5 expressers in the early post-transplant stage (Li et al., 2017).

Inflammation: Familial Mediterranean Fever

A one-month Phase II RCT of young patients ($n = 24$) with familial Mediterranean fever (FMF) compared ImmunoGuard (a standardized fixed combination of eleuthero, andrographis, schisandra, and licorice extracts) four tablets TID with placebo. The patient's self-evaluation was based on symptoms of abdominal pain, chest pain, temperature, arthritis, myalgia, and erysipelas-like erythema. All three features (duration, frequency, and severity of attacks) showed significant improvement in the ImmunoGuard group compared with placebo. In both clinical assessment and self-evaluation, the severity of attacks was found to show the most significant improvement in the herbal group. The authors concluded that both the clinical and laboratory results of the study suggested that ImmunoGuard was a safe and efficacious herbal drug for the management of patients with FMF (Amaryan et al., 2003).

Oncologic Disorders: Prophylaxis

An RCT in premenopausal women ($n = 47$) and post-menopausal women ($n = 49$) studied a combination product containing schisandra, HMR lignan, indole-3-carbinol, calcium glucarate, milk thistle, and stinging nettle compared with placebo for effects on estrogen metabolism and carcinogenic byproducts. In premenopausal women, treatment supplementation resulted in a significant increase ($P < 0.05$) in urinary 2-OHE concentrations and in the 2:16α-OHE ratio. In post-menopausal women, treatment supplementation resulted in a significant increase in urinary 2-OHE concentrations. In pre and post-menopausal women combined, treatment supplementation produced a significant increase in urinary 2-OHE concentration and a trend ($P = 0.074$) toward an increased 2:16α-OHE ratio. The authors concluded that the mixture in question significantly increased estrogen C-2 hydroxylation, which may reduce estrogen-related cancer risk (Laidlaw et al., 2010).

Oncologic Disorders: Cancer-Related Quality of Life and Immunity

A 9-day RCT in gastric cancer patients ($n = 58$) investigated parenteral Shen-Mai (also called Shengmai, a TCM formula containing schisandra, ginseng, and *Liriope spicata*) alone compared with enteral nutrition alone and with a combination of Shen-Mai plus parenteral nutrition for impact on postoperative fatigue. Conditions of recovery, postoperative mood, and sleep quality were better, and postoperative fatigue was reduced more significantly, in the combined treatment group than in the other two groups ($P < 0.05$).

Additionally, pre-albumin, CD3, CD4, and CD4/CD8 were significantly higher with combined treatment ($P < 0.05$). The authors concluded that combining Shen-Mai with enteral nutrition could improve mood, sleep, and postoperative fatigue through improved nutritional status and immune function, thus speeding up the recovery of patients (Dong et al., 2010).

A 4-week RCT in patients with cancer undergoing chemotherapy or radiotherapy investigated Shen-Mai-San (also called Shengmai San, a TCM formula containing schisandra, ginseng, and *Liriope spicata*) compared with placebo for quality of life. Based on measurements using the European Organization for Research and Treatment of Cancer Quality of Life questionnaire, Shen-Mai-San was found to be effective in treating cancer-related fatigue. This supported the TCM approach to addressing Qi and Yin deficiency in the face of chemotherapy or radiotherapy for cancer (Lo et al., 2012).

A 4-week RCT in stage III-IV ovarian cancer patients ($n = 28$) investigated the immunological effects of AdMax (a combination of schisandra, eleuthero, rhodiola, and *Rhaponticum carthamoides*) 270 mg/day compared with a control group for 4 weeks. Patients were treated with a dose of cisplatin 75 mg/m^2 and cyclophosphamide 600 mg/m^2, and labs were followed-up at 4 weeks. In patients who took AdMax following chemotherapy, the mean numbers of CD3, CD4, CD5, and CD8 cells were increased compared with those who did not take the herbal combination. Also, the mean amounts of IgG and IgM were increased in the herbal group compared with the control group. The authors concluded that the combination of extracts from adaptogenic plants may boost the suppressed immunity in ovarian cancer patients who were subjected to chemotherapy (Kormosh et al., 2006).

ACTIVE CONSTITUENTS

- Carbohydrates
  - Polysaccharides (induce apoptosis, anti-hepatic cancer, increase IL-2 and TNF-α): SCP, SCPP11
- Phenolic compounds
  - Lignans in seeds of fruit (promote regeneration of hepatocytes, restore glutathione, block

NF-kB and MAPK signaling, promote Pgp and total protein kinase C function/expression, immunomodulating, PPARγ activating, α-glucosidase inhibiting, antiproliferative, weakly estrogenic): schisandrins A-C, γ-schisandrin, schisandrols, deoxyschizandrin, gomisins, pregomisin, schisantherins, α-iso-cubebenol (anti-inflammatory); α-iso-cubebene

- Flavonoids
  - Anthocyanins (antioxidant): cyanidin-3-O-xylosylrutinoside (Cya-3-O-xylrut)
- Terpenes
  - Triterpenoids: nigranoic acid (anti-HIV); schisandronic acid; preschisanartanin, schindilactone A-C, schintrilactone A-B, lancifodilactone C, henridilactone D, micrandilactone B, wuweizidilactone A-F, micrantherin A

SCHISANDRA COMMONLY USED PREPARATIONS AND DOSAGE (FOR ADULTS UNLESS OTHERWISE SPECIFIED)

The following are examples of some available formulations and ranges of dosing for commercial herbal products. See Part III Introduction "How to prescribe medicinal herbs" for further guidance on herbal advising and prescribing.

Berry

- Infusion of dried berry: 1-2 tsp per cup BID
- Tincture of dried berry (1:5, 95%): 1–4 mL up to TID
- Capsule or tablet of powdered berry: 580–1000 mg BID
- Standardized powdered berry extract (standardized to > 1% schisandrins): 1000 mg (1/3 tsp) QD
- Capsule or tablet of 10:1 extract standardized to 6% schisandrin: 250 mg TID

SAFETY AND PRECAUTION

Side Effects

Rare abdominal upset, decreased appetite, and skin rash.

Toxicity

- Toxicity of oral dose in mice occurs at a dose of 3.6 g/kg of schisandra *seed (not berry).*

- The ethanolic extract of the fruit was non-toxic in dogs.
- The lignan constituent schisandrin injected into mice was able to induce convulsions at 175 mg/kg and paresis at 350 mg/kg; however, no deaths occurred.
- Schisandrin B 0.125–2 g/kg is hepatotoxic in mice.

Pregnancy and Lactation

Avoid. May stimulate uterine contractions. Slightly estrogenic. No data for lactation.

Disease Interactions

Due to weak estrogenic activity in some studies, it should be used with caution if at all in patients with estrogen-sensitive cancers.

Drug Interactions

- CYP: Variably inhibits or induces CYP enzymes depending on extraction method, dose, and duration. (*Bottom line is to cautiously monitor for interactions in either direction.*)
- Pgp: Schisandra can inhibit P-glycoprotein activity and interfere with the metabolism of certain drugs (may also be beneficial for reducing multidrug resistance of certain cells and organisms)
- UGT: Inhibits the activities of UGT1A1, 1A3, 1A9, and 2B7
- Warfarin: May reduce warfarin levels
- Decreases metabolism and increases bioavailability of tacrolimus

REFERENCES

Amaryan G, Astvatsatryan V, Gabrielyan E, Panossian A, Panosyan V, Wikman G. Double-blind, placebo-controlled, randomized, pilot clinical trial of ImmunoGuard—a standardized fixed combination of Andrographis paniculata Nees, with Eleutherococcus senticosus Maxim, Schizandra chinensis Bail. and Glycyrrhiza glabra L. extracts in patients with Familial Mediterranean Fever. Phytomedicine 2003;10(4):271–85.

Aslanyan G, Amroyan E, Gabrielyan E, Nylander M, Wikman G, Panossian A. Double-blind, placebo-controlled, randomised study of single dose effects of ADAPT-232 on cognitive functions. Phytomedicine 2010;17(7):494–9.

Chiu HF, Chen TY, Tzeng YT, Wang CK. Improvement of liver function in humans using a mixture of schisandra fruit extract and sesamin. Phytother Res 2013;27(3):368–73.

Dong QT, Zhang XD, Yu Z. Integrated Chinese and Western medical treatment on postoperative fatigue syndrome in patients with gastric cancer. Zhongguo Zhong Xi Yi Jie He Za Zhi 2010;30(10):1036–40.

Greenlee H, Atkinson C, Stanczyk FZ, Lampe JW. A pilot and feasibility study on the effects of naturopathic botanical and dietary interventions on sex steroid hormone metabolism in premenopausal women. Cancer Epidemiol Biomarkers Prev 2007;16(8):1601–9.

Kormosh N, Laktionov K, Antoshechkina M. Effect of a combination of extract from several plants on cell-mediated and humoral immunity of patients with advanced ovarian cancer. Phytother Res 2006;20(5):424–5.

Laidlaw M, Cockerline CA, Sepkovic DW. Effects of a breast-health herbal formula supplement on estrogen metabolism in pre- and post-menopausal women not taking hormonal contraceptives or supplements: a randomized controlled trial. Breast Cancer (Auckl) 2010;4:85–95.

Li J, Chen S, Qin X, et al. Wuzhi tablet (*Schisandra sphenanthera* extract) is a promising tacrolimus-sparing agent for renal transplant recipients who are CYP3A5 expressers: a two-phase prospective study. Drug Metab Dispos 2017;45(11):1114–9.

Lo LC, Chen CY, Chen ST, Chen HC, Lee TC, Chang CS. Therapeutic efficacy of traditional Chinese medicine, Shen-Mai San, in cancer patients undergoing chemotherapy or radiotherapy: study protocol for a randomized, double-blind, placebo-controlled trial. Trials 2012;13:232.

Narimanian M, Badalyan M, Panosyan V, et al. Impact of Chisan (ADAPT-232) on the quality-of-life and its efficacy as an adjuvant in the treatment of acute non-specific pneumonia. Phytomedicine 2005;12(10):723–9.

Panossian AG, Oganessian AS, Ambartsumian M, Gabrielian ES, Wagner H, Wikman G. Effects of heavy physical exercise and adaptogens on nitric oxide content in human saliva. Phytomedicine 1999;6(1):17–26.

Park JY, Kim KH. A randomized, double-blind, placebo-controlled trial of Schisandra chinensis for menopausal symptoms. Climacteric 2016;19(6):574–80.

Park J, Han S, Park H. Effect of Schisandra chinensis extract supplementation on quadriceps muscle strength and fatigue in adult women: a randomized, double-blind, placebo-controlled trial. Int J Environ Res Public Health 2020;17(7):2475.

Song MY, Wang JH, Eom T, Kim H. Schisandra chinensis fruit modulates the gut microbiota composition in association with metabolic markers in obese women: a randomized, double-blind placebo-controlled study. Nutr Res 2015;35(8):655–63.

Yip AY, Loo WT, Chow LW. Fructus Schisandrae (Wuweizi) containing compound in modulating human lymphatic system—a Phase I minimization clinical trial. Biomed Pharmacother 2007;61(9):588–90.

Zheng H, Chen Y, Chen J, Kwong J, Xiong W. Shengmai (a traditional Chinese herbal medicine) for heart failure. Cochrane Database Syst Rev 2011;2, CD005052.

70

SKULLCAP/SCULLCAP (*SCUTELLARIA BAICALENSIS, SCUTELLARIA LATERIFLORA*)
Above-Ground Parts

GENERAL OVERVIEW

Skullcap comes in two varieties: Chinese (*baicalensis*) and American (*lateriflora*). Because the two varieties vary in chief constituents, they have distinct activities and should not be used interchangeably. However, they do appear to share many of the most active constituents (particularly baicalin, baicalein, wogonin, and oroxylin A) and further studies may reveal that their applications have some overlap. The root has the most activity in Chinese skullcap, and the aerial parts are thought to be most medicinal in American skullcap. Chinese skullcap flowers truly look like hoods from medieval times, hence the name. American skullcap, as the Latin name implies, has blossoms that just shoot straight sideways without all the delicate convolutions of their Chinese cousin. While there is a paucity of human evidence for skullcap, it has a long and wide history of use, herbalists love it, and it has been subjected to a fair amount of animal research, mostly in China. It appears regularly on patients' herbal lists and in popular polyherbal products.

American skullcap has been most commonly used to treat anxiety and insomnia, often in combination with other sedating herbs. Chinese skullcap is used in combination with other herbs to treat bronchitis, atherosclerosis, hepatitis, hepatic cirrhosis, inflammation, epilepsy, headaches, neurodegeneration, and cancer.

Clinical trials have indicated that Chinese skullcap may be beneficial for allergic rhinitis, attention-deficit/hyperactivity disorder, pneumonia, and chemotherapy-induced bone marrow suppression; American skullcap may be beneficial for anxiety and mood disturbance.

IN VITRO AND ANIMAL RESEARCH

American skullcap has been shown to have anticonvulsant and cognition-enhancing properties in animals. Its constituents show numerous positive effects on the brain.

In research on Chinese skullcap and cardiovascular health, pre-dosing with Chinese skullcap extract in a myocardial infarction model in mice resulted in reduction of infarct size. In diabetic research, streptozotocin-induced diabetic rats treated with Chinese skullcap and those treated with metformin plus skullcap had elevated SOD, catalase, and GSH peroxidase levels (all being hepatic antioxidants) as well as reduced plasma and hepatic lipid peroxide concentrations. The metformin plus skullcap group had significant elevations of insulin levels and reductions of TG and TC levels compared with either skullcap or metformin alone. The findings suggested that Chinese skullcap enhanced the antidiabetic effect of metformin in STZ-induced diabetic rats by improving antioxidant status (Waisundara et al., 2008).

Chinese skullcap administration resulted in an increase in cholinergic neurons and enhanced the survival of a hippocampal progenitor cell line, HiB5, and its differentiation to cholinergic cells. The NMDA receptor also was increased, and activated microglia were decreased, indicating neuroprotection (Zhuang et al., 2013).

Studies of experimental cerebral hypoperfusion in Wister rats given Chinese skullcap extract after carotid artery occlusion or LPS infusion showed a reduction in memory impairments in the treated rats.

The pathological changes in the neurons of rat hippocampus and cortex were also attenuated. These findings suggest that skullcap may be beneficial for the prevention or treatment of vascular dementia (Hwang et al., 2011).

Chinese skullcap demonstrated a strong dose-dependent growth inhibition and COX-2 inhibition of the most common human cancer cells. It produced a 66% reduction in tumor mass in mice with head and neck squamous cell cancer. The whole herb was more effective than its isolated flavonoid baicalein. In mice with experimental lung carcinoma, Chinese skullcap potentiated the antimetastatic effect of cyclophosphamide. Combined treatment with cyclophosphamide and Chinese skullcap modulated cytotoxic activity of NK cells and peritoneal macrophages during tumor growth.

Numerous flavonoids from Chinese skullcap (the 2'-OH flavones) exhibited potent GABA-receptor-binding affinity. Baicalin, a major constituent of Chinese skullcap, shows GABA subtype selectivity through the α-2- and α-3-containing GABA receptor subtypes.

Baicalin was shown to suppress BW gain and reduce visceral fat mass in rats fed a high-fat diet. In the same rats, baicalin significantly decreased the elevated serum cholesterol, free fatty acids, and insulin concentrations as well as TNF-α caused by the diet. It reduced hepatic lipid accumulation, enhanced the phosphorylation of AMPK and acetyl-CoA carboxylase, and down-regulated genes involved in lipogenesis. These findings suggested that baicalin might have beneficial effects on the development of hepatic steatosis and obesity-related disorders by targeting hepatic AMPK (Guo et al., 2009).

In rats exposed to cigarette smoke, baicalin treatment markedly reduced the inflammatory effects of smoke in a dose-dependent manner, likely through inhibition of the NF-κB pathway. Baicalin is a potent eNOS inducer even at low doses. Maternal baicalin treatment has been shown to increase the pulmonary surfactant phospholipids of fetal rat lungs and increase maternal serum growth hormone. Topical baicalin has been shown to mitigate against UVB-induced DNA damage to skin.

In a study of relapsing and remitting experimental autoimmune encephalomyelitis, baicalin caused an increase in IL-4 and inhibited IFN-γ and the proliferation of mononuclear cells in a concentration-dependent manner. The results suggest that baicalin might be useful in the treatment of multiple sclerosis (Zeng et al., 2007).

Baicalin's activity against Gram-positive bacteria is likely due to its binding of α-hemolysin binding sites, inhibiting heptamer formation and consequent cell lysis. It prevents alveolar epithelial cell injury in the presence of *Staphylococcus aureus*. In an in vivo study baicalin protected mice from *S. aureus* pneumonia. Baicalin has been shown to inhibit HIV-1 infection and replication, at least in part by inhibiting recombinant HIV-1/RT.

Baicalein, another one of the active principles of Chinese skullcap, interacts with GABA receptors. Both baicalein and baicalin significantly reduce anxious behavior in mice, an effect that is antagonized by co-administration with flumazenil but not by the 5-HT(1A) receptor antagonist pindolol, suggesting that the anxiolytic-like effect of baicalein or baicalin may be mediated through activation of the benzodiazepine binding site of $GABA_A$ receptors (Liao et al., 2003).

Baicalein prolonged influenza survival times and rates in mice. Lung consolidation and viral titers were reduced in dose-dependent manners. Baicalein has effects on macrophages via suppression of NF-kB activation. Baicalein has demonstrated activity against proliferation of pulmonary artery smooth muscle cells, suggesting a possible role for pulmonary artery HTN.

A study examining the effects of baicalin, baicalein, and Chinese skullcap extract against noise-induced hearing loss in a mouse model found that the skullcap extract significantly reduced threshold shift, central auditory function damage, and cochlear function deficits, suggesting that skullcap may protect auditory function in noise-induced hearing loss, and that the active constituent may be the flavonoid, baicalein (Kang et al., 2010).

Administration of oroxylin A, another major flavonoid in skullcap, in a dose-dependent and time-dependent manner increased the number of BrdU-incorporating cells in the hippocampus, indicating cell proliferation and suggesting that increased neurogenesis induced by oroxylin A could be associated with positive effects on cognitive processing. Oroxylin A has been shown to alleviate

ADHD-like behaviors in a rat model of ADHD. A derivative of oroxylin A, compound 7-7 (5,7-dihydroxy-6-methoxy-4'-phenoxyflavone) showed inhibition of dopamine reuptake comparable to methylphenidate and did not influence norepinephrine reuptake unlike atomoxetine. Compound 7-7 reduced hyperactivity, inattention, and impulsivity in the rat model. Repeated treatment with compound 7-7 failed to elicit addictive behavior in rats (dela Peña et al., 2013).

Oroxylin A has been found to inhibit GABA at the benzodiazepine site, opposing the actions of baicalein and wogonin. This action appears to increase NMDA activity supporting neurogenesis. Oroxylin A has been shown to improve cognition in healthy young rodents. One study showed oroxylin A dramatically attenuated the memory impairment induced by bilateral carotid artery occlusion in mice, and this effect may be mediated by reductions in activated microglia and increases in BDNF expression and CREB phosphorylation (Kim et al., 2006).

Wogonin, another skullcap constituent, possesses anxiolytic and neuroprotective activities. Wogonin significantly blocks convulsion induced by pentylenetetrazole and electroshock but not convulsion induced by strychnine. Mice treated with wogonin did not show signs of sedation or myorelaxation. Studies have indicated that the anticonvulsive effects produced by wogonin are mediated by GABAergic neurons. Wogonin has also been shown to be strongly anti-inflammatory and gastroprotective against ethanol.

Scutellarin, a constituent of American skullcap, has demonstrated mild sedative and antispasmodic properties in animal research. It has demonstrated a moderate affinity to the benzodiazepine site in rat brains. In a study of extracts of American skullcap aerial parts (flowers, leaves, stems) and its flavonoids baicalin, scutellarin, wogonin, lateriflorein, ikonnikoside I and dihydrobaicalin, all had high affinity for the 5HT7 receptor (Zhang et al., 2009).

With respect to skullcap's cancer effects, baicalin, baicalein, and wogonin have been shown to induce apoptosis in liver cancer cell lines via G1 phase arrest and G2/M accumulation. Baicalin has also been shown in higher doses to cause apoptosis in leukemia-derived T cells and to inhibit angiogenesis, but in lower doses it promotes angiogenesis. Baicalein has demonstrated antiproliferative effects on pancreatic cancer cells.

Scutellarin has been shown to induce apoptosis in ovarian and breast cancer cells. Wogonin demonstrates anti-metastatic activity in human gallbladder carcinoma cells via inhibition of mobility and invasion activity and suppression of MMP and ERK 1/ 2. It also upregulates maspin, a metastasis suppressor protein.

HUMAN RESEARCH

Allergic Disorders: Allergic Rhinitis

An ex-vivo study in healthy patients ($n = 12$) incubated their nasal mucosal cells with tissue culture medium, skullcap, and/or eleuthero and/or vitamin C and stimulated with anti-IgE for 30 min and 6 h to imitate the allergic early and late phases. Additionally, *S. aureus* superantigen B stimulation for 6 h was used to imitate T-cell activation. The combination of skullcap and eleuthero had a more potent suppressive effect on the release of PGD2, histamine, and IL-5 than skullcap alone. The combination also resulted in a significant inhibition of the *S. aureus* superantigen B-induced cytokines comparable to or superior to fluticasone propionate. Vitamin C increased ciliary beat frequency but had no anti-inflammatory effects. The authors concluded that the combination of skullcap and eleuthero may be able to significantly block allergic early- and late-phase mediators and substantially suppress the release of proinflammatory, Th1-, Th2-, and Th17-derived cytokines (Zhang et al., 2012).

Cardiometabolic Disorders: Diabetes

A 20-week crossover RCT in patients ($n = 17$) with T2DM compared Chinese skullcap 3.52 g/day with placebo, each in addition to metformin for effects on of T2D and changes in the gut microbiota composition. The initial treatment session was 8 weeks, with a 4-week washout period before crossing over treatments for another 8 weeks. Glucose tolerance was improved with skullcap greater than with placebo ($P < 0.05$). The relative RNA expression of TNF-α was significantly reduced after with skullcap compared with placebo ($P < 0.05$). Gut colonization with *Lactobacillus* and *Akkermansia* was increased with skullcap. Three patients in the skullcap group and one in the placebo group demonstrated a mild increase above the normal range in liver enzymes. Those subjects had a different baseline gut microbial composition than the other subjects. The authors concluded that skullcap given adjunctively to metformin may improve glucose tolerance and inflammation and influence gut microbes beneficially in patients with T2DM (Shin et al., 2020).

Psychiatric Disorders: Anxiety

A 2013 systematic review looking at plants that had both pre-clinical and clinical evidence for anti-anxiety effects found 21 plants with human clinical trial evidence. Support for efficacy identified several herbs with efficacy for anxiety spectrum disorders including American skullcap, kava, lemon balm, chamomile, ginkgo, milk thistle, passionflower, ashwagandha, rhiodola, echinacea, *Galphimia glauca*, *Centella asiatica*, and *Echium amooenum*. Acute anxiolytic activity was found for passionflower, sage, gotu kola, lemon balm, and bergamot. The review also specifically found that bacopa showed anxiolytic effects in people with cognitive decline (Sarris et al., 2013).

A 2-week RCT in healthy volunteers ($n = 43$) compared American skullcap 350 mg TID with placebo for effects on mood. With skullcap, total mood disturbance decreased significantly from baseline ($P < 0.001$), whereas there was no change with placebo. The authors noted that skullcap enhanced global mood without reducing energy or cognition (Brock et al., 2014).

Psychiatric Disorders: Attention-Deficit/ Hyperactivity Disorder

A 3-month RCT in children ($n = 100$) with minimal brain dysfunction studied a polyherbal TCM formula containing Chinese skullcap, astragalus, *Bupleurum chinense*, *Codonopsis pilosula*, *Ligustrum lucidum*, *Lophatherum gracile* and thread of ivory. compared with methylphenidate 5–15 mg BID for one month for cognitive affects. In the polyherbal group, 23/80 cases were cured (clinical symptoms were gone for 6 months of observation), 46/80 cases were improved, and 11/80 cases were unchanged. With methylphenidate, 6/20 cases were cured, 12/20 cases were improved, and 2/20 cases were unchanged. The herbal formula was found to have similar efficacy to methylphenidate but with less side effects (Zhang and Huang, 1990).

Infectious Disease: Pneumonia

A 1-week RCT in patients ($n = 60$) with pulmonary infection (mainly nosocomial pneumonia) compared Chinese skullcap injection with piperacillin injection for recovery from infection. Total effective rates were 73.3% and 76.7% in each group with skullcap and piperacillin, respectively. X-ray abnormalities disappeared or became smaller in the same timeframe (16.1 days for each group). Fungal infections were identified in 4/30 and 0/30 patients with piperacillin and skullcap, respectively (Lu, 1990).

Oncologic Disorders: Chemotherapy-Induced Bone Marrow Suppression

A study in patients ($n = 88$) with lung cancer undergoing chemotherapy assessed the hemopoietic effect of adding Chinese skullcap to chemotherapy. Administration of the herb was accompanied by intensification of bone-marrow erythropoiesis and granulocytopoiesis and an increase in the content of circulating erythroid and granulomonocytic colony-forming units (Gol'dberg et al., 1997).

ACTIVE CONSTITUENTS

- Amino acid derivatives
  - Amino acids: GABA, glutamine
- Phenolic compounds
  - Dihydropyranocoumarins: scuteflorin A, scuteflorin B
  - Flavonoids *(Both American and Chinese skullcap contain the following constituents to varying degrees and are thought to be the active principles for most of the herbs' actions)*: scutellarin (esp. Chinese), scutellarein, baicalin, baicalein, wogonin, lateriflorin (American), oroxylin A, dihydrochrysin (American), dihydrooroxylin A, chrysin, decursin (American), neobaicalein (Chinese), viscidulins (Chinese), apigenin (anti-inflammatory, antioxidant, antihistamine, hypotensive, anti-serotonin release, GABA agonism, antispasmodic, antibacterial, chemopreventive, antineoplastic, ERB), luteolin (anti-inflammatory, antispasmodic, antibacterial, hepatoprotective, anti-estrogenic, antiproliferative), carthamidin (Chinese)
- Terpenes
  - Triterpenoid saponins: pomolic acid; ursolic acid (anti-HIV, anti-EBV, antiviral, androgenic, AChEI, pro-collagen, pro-ceremide, antitumor)

- Steroids
  - Phytosterols: β-sitosterol (reduces GI cholesterol absorption, inhibits 5-α-reductase), daucosterol

SKULLCAP COMMONLY USED PREPARATIONS AND DOSAGE (FOR ADULTS UNLESS OTHERWISE SPECIFIED)

The following are examples of some available formulations and ranges of dosing for commercial herbal products. See Part III Introduction "How to prescribe medicinal herbs" for further guidance on herbal advising and prescribing.

Chinese Skullcap—Root

- Infusion of dried root: 1-2 tsp per cup TID
- Tincture of fresh root (1:2; 50–95%): 1–2 mL TID
- Capsule or tablet of powdered root: 400–500 mg BID-TID
- Baicalin: 500 mg QD

American Skullcap—Aerial Parts

- Infusion of dried herb: 1-2 tsp per cup TID
- Tincture of fresh herb (1:2; 50–95%): 1–2 mL TID
- Tincture of dried herb (1:5; 45%): 1–2 mL TID
- Capsule or tablet of powdered aerial parts: 850–1200 mg QD

SAFETY AND PRECAUTION

Side Effects

Possible sedation. Use with caution when alertness is critical.

Case Reports

An elderly woman who began taking Move Free Advanced for arthritis (contains glucosamine, chondroitin, Chinese skullcap, and black catechu) presented with cholestasis and hepatitis, which significantly improved after discontinuation of the supplement. She resumed taking the supplement and again suffered from hepatotoxicity.

Toxicity

In the 1970s, reports of liver damage from American skullcap emerged with a resultant decline in use of the herb. Subsequent analysis indicated that the cause of the hepatotoxicity was adulteration of the herb with germander (*Teucrium*), which contains pyrrolizidine alkaloids.

High doses of the American skullcap tincture may cause giddiness, confusion, twitching, irregular heartbeat, and seizures.

The maximal tolerated dose of the aqueous extracts of Chinese skullcap in mice was 72 g/kg and the LD_{50} of 80% ethanol extracts was 39.6 g/kg. Hepatotoxicity occurred when the dose was as high as 2500 mg/kg per day.

At 1000 mg/kg/day baicalin had no observed adverse effects.

Wogonin offered a wide margin of safety and had no organ toxicity for a continuous intravenous administration in dogs. The LD_{50} value of the mouse was 286 mg/kg after IV injection of wogonin.

Pregnancy and Lactation

Although animal research is reassuring there is insufficient human data. Baicalin has been shown to have weak embryotoxicity.

Drug Interactions

- CYP: Wogonin inhibits CYP1A2, CYP 2C19
- Pgp: Oroxylin A inhibits P-glycoprotein.
- SLC transporters: Baicalein, baicalin, and wogonin inhibit uptake of specific substrates mediated by essential SLC transporters
- May increase effects of anticoagulants and antiplatelet drugs
- Reduces absorption of cyclosporine May interact with paclitaxel
- May increase the antiviral activity of lamivudine

REFERENCES

Brock C, Whitehouse J, Tewfik I, Towell T. American skullcap (Scutellaria lateriflora): a randomised, double-blind placebo-controlled crossover study of its effects on mood in healthy volunteers. Phytother Res 2014;28(5):692–8.

dela Peña IC, Young Yoon S, Kim Y, Park H, Man Kim K, Hoon Ryu J, Young Shin C, Hoon Cheong J. 5,7-Dihydroxy-6-methoxy-4'-phenoxyflavone, a derivative of oroxylin A improves attention-deficit/hyperactivity disorder (ADHD)-like behaviors in spontaneously hypertensive rats. Eur J Pharmacol. 2013 Sep 5;715(1-3):337–44.

Gol'dberg VE, Ryzhakov VM, Matiash MG, et al. Dry extract of Scutellaria baicalensis as a hemostimulant in antineoplastic chemotherapy in patents with lung cancer. Eksp Klin Farmakol 1997;60(6):28–30.

Guo HX, et al. Long-term baicalin administration ameliorates metabolic disorders and hepatic steatosis in rats given a high-fat diet.
Acta Pharmacol Sin 2009.

Hwang YK, et al. Effects of Scutellaria baicalensis on chronic cerebral hypoperfusion-induced memory impairments and chronic
lipopolysaccharide infusion-induced memory impairments. J
Ethnopharmacol 2011.

Kang TH, Hong BN, Park C, Kim SY, Park R. Effect of baicalein from
Scutellaria baicalensis on prevention of noise-induced hearing
loss. Neurosci Lett 2010;469(3):298–302.

Kim DH, Jeon SJ, Son KH, Jung JW, Lee S, Yoon BH, Choi JW,
Cheong JH, Ko KH, Ryu JH. Effect of the flavonoid, oroxylin A, on
transient cerebral hypoperfusion-induced memory impairment
in mice. Pharmacol Biochem Behav. 2006 Nov;85(3):658–68.

Liao JF, Hung WY, Chen CF. Anxiolytic-like effects of baicalein and
baicalin in the Vogel conflict test in mice. Eur J Pharmacol. 2003
Mar 19;464(2-3):141–6.

Lu Z. Clinical comparative study of intravenous piperacillin sodium
or injection of scutellaria compound in patients with pulmonary
infection. Zhong Xi Yi Jie He Za Zhi 1990;10(7):413–5. 389.

Sarris J, McIntyre E, Camfield DA. Plant-based medicines for anxiety disorders, part 2: a review of clinical studies with supporting
preclinical evidence. CNS Drugs 2013;27(4):301–19.

Shin NR, Gu N, Choi HS, Kim H. Combined effects of Scutellaria
baicalensis with metformin on glucose tolerance of patients with
type 2 diabetes via gut microbiota modulation. Am J Physiol
Endocrinol Metab 2020;318(1):E52–61.

Waisundara VY, et al. Scutellaria baicalensis enhances the antidiabetic activity of metformin in streptozotocin-induced diabetic
Wistar rats. Am J Chin Med 2008.

Zeng Y, Song C, Ding X, Ji X, Yi L, Zhu K. Baicalin reduces the severity of experimental autoimmune encephalomyelitis. Braz J Med
Biol Res 2007;40(7):1003–10.

Zhang H, Huang J. Preliminary study of traditional Chinese medicine treatment of minimal brain dysfunction: analysis of 100
cases. Zhong Xi Yi Jie He Za Zhi 1990;10(5):278–9. 260.

Zhang N, Van Crombruggen K, Holtappels G, Bachert C. A herbal composition of Scutellaria baicalensis and Eleutherococcus senticosus
shows potent anti-inflammatory effects in an ex vivo human mucosal
tissue model. Evid Based Complement Alternat Med 2012;673145.

Zhang Z, Lian XY, Li S, Stringer JL. Characterization of chemical
ingredients and anticonvulsant activity of American skullcap
(Scutellaria lateriflora). Phytomedicine. 2009 May;16(5):485–93.

Zhuang PW, et al. Baicalin regulates neuronal fate decision in neural
stem/progenitor cells and stimulates hippocampal neurogenesis
in adult rats. CNS Neurosci Ther 2013.

71

STINGING NETTLE/NETTLES/ NETTLE (*URTICA DIOICA, URTICA URENS*)
Leaf, Root

GENERAL OVERVIEW

The leaves and root of stinging nettle/nettles have distinct medical uses. The leaves are used more for allergic and diabetic issues and the roots more for prostate issues. Nettle has been used traditionally all over the globe for pretty much you name it. *Urere*, the root of its Latin name means "to burn," referring to the burning pain upon contact with the hairs on its leaves. The burning or stinging sensation is due to the histamine and formic acid in the leaves. This stinging property is lost when the plant is dried or extracted. The leaves also contain acetylcholine and serotonin. The root is often combined with herbs such as *Pygeum* and saw palmetto for treatment of benign prostatic hyperplasia (BPH). Herbalists recommend it during pregnancy for anemia and pruritic urticarial papules and plaques of pregnancy.

Clinical research indicates that stinging nettle *leaf*, alone or in combination formulas, may be beneficial for allergic rhinitis, hypertension, dyslipidemia, diabetes, and osteoarthritis.

Clinical research indicates that stinging nettle *root*, alone or in combination formulas, may be beneficial for menopause, benign prostatic hyperplasia, acute and chronic prostatitis, and estrogen-sensitive cancer prophylaxis.

IN VITRO AND ANIMAL RESEARCH

In vitro studies of stinging nettle show antagonist and inverse agonist activity against H1 receptors and inhibition of COX-1, COX2, and prostaglandin D2 synthase, all resulting in a reduction in inflammation.

Nettle also inhibits mast cell tryptase. Various other in vitro and in vivo studies have demonstrated antioxidant, anti-inflammatory, antilipidemic, platelet-aggregating, cardiovascular, diuretic, vasoconstrictive, hepatoprotective, antiulcer, gastrointestinal, analgesic, anesthetic, immunomodulatory, antibacterial, central depressive, endocrine, anti-anemic, and chemopreventive properties. Nettle leaves have insulin secretagogue, PPAR-γ agonistic, and α-glucosidase inhibitory effects. Animal studies have shown nettle to have renal sparing and hepatoprotective properties and to have efficacy in colitis. Nettle has also been shown to reduce testosterone-induced prostatic hyperplasia in rodents and has demonstrated antiproliferative effects in human prostate cancer cells. It has also shown protective effects against cisplatin-induced toxicity.

HUMAN RESEARCH

Allergic Disorders: Allergic rhinitis

A 1-week RCT in patients ($n=98$) with allergic rhinitis compared a freeze-dried nettle leaf preparation 300 mg/day with placebo taken PRN for allergy symptoms. Most patients found that the herb was comparable in efficacy to whatever allergy medicine they had been using, and 48% of them found the herb to be more efficacious than the drug (Mittman, 1990).

Cardiovascular Disorders: Hypertension

A 16-week RCT in patients ($n=29$) with mild HTN compared stinging nettle leaves with *Mentha longifolia*, with *Viola odorata* (300 mg/day for each), and with placebo for antihypertensive effects. The trial revealed dose- and duration-dependent significant reductions in SBP, DBP, and MAP of subjects treated with stinging nettle, *M. longifolia*, or *V. odorata*. The authors concluded that there is some evidence for the ethnopharmacological use of these plants for mild HTN (Samaha et al., 2019).

Cardiometabolic Disorders: Dyslipidemia and Diabetes

A 2020 systematic review and meta-analysis to assess the effect of stinging nettle leaf on glycemic parameters in T2DM found eight RCTs ($n = 401$) that met inclusion criteria. The results of the meta-analysis revealed a significant reduction with stinging nettle in FBS (WMD: -18.01 mg/dL; $P < 0.001$; $I^2 = 94.6\%$), but no significant reduction in insulin levels (WMD: 0.83; $P = 0.13$; $I^2 = 89.4\%$), HOMA-IR (WMD: -0.22; $P = 0.49$; $I^2 = 69.2\%$), or A1C (WMD: -0.77%; $P = 0.12$, $I^2 = 83.0\%$). The authors concluded that stinging nettle may be effective in controlling FBS for T2DM patients (Ziaei et al., 2020).

A 2013 systematic review of herbs having antidiabetic activity identified 18 human trials and 67 animal trials involving 62 plants. Among the RCTs, the best results for glycemic control were found with stinging nettle, aloe, milk thistle, *Citrullus colocynthis*, *Plantago ovata*, *and Rheum ribes*. The authors noted that most of the plants studied for antidiabetic activity showed promising results. However, efficacy and safety of plants used in the treatment of diabetes were deemed insufficient (Rashidi et al., 2013).

A 3-month RCT in patients ($n = 92$) with T2DM investigated nettle leaf extract 500 mg TID for 3 months compared with placebo, each combined with conventional oral antihyperglycemic drugs. Nettle lowered FBS, two-hour PPG, and A1C significantly greater than placebo ($P < 0.001$; $P = 0.009$, and $P = 0.006$, respectively). There were no significant effects on liver enzymes or blood pressure. The authors concluded that nettle may safely improve glycemic control in T2DM patients needing insulin therapy (Kianbakht et al., 2013).

An 8-week RCT in women ($n = 50$) with T2DM studied nettle leaf hydro-alcoholic extract (tincture) 5 mL TID compared with placebo for effects on lipids, liver enzymes, and NO levels. FBG, TG, and ALT levels significantly decreased with nettle compared with placebo ($P < 0.01$; $P < 0.5$, and $P < 0.05$, respectively). HDL, NO, and SOD levels significantly increased with nettle compared with placebo ($P < 0.05$; $P < 0.01$, and $P < 0.05$, respectively). The authors concluded that nettle leaf extract may decrease risk factors of cardiovascular disease and other complications of T2DM (Amiri Behzadi et al., 2016).

An 8-week RCT in patients ($n = 50$) with T2DM studied 100 mg/kg nettle extract divided TID compared with placebo. After 8 weeks, IL-6 and hs-CRP showed a significant decrease in the intervention group compared with the control group ($P < 0.05$). The authors concluded that nettle extract had decreasing effects on IL-6 and hs-CRP in patients with T2DM after 8 weeks of intervention (Namazi et al., 2011)

An 8-week RCT in patients ($n = 60$) with T2DM compared nettle 100 mg/kg/day with placebo. The mean reduction of FBS from baseline was 20.2 mg/dL and -0.7 mg/dL with nettle and placebo, respectively ($P = 0.14$). The mean plasma insulin level was 2.5 mU/l and 0.2 mU/l with nettle and placebo, respectively ($P = 0.003$), showing a significant increase in insulin concentration with nettle. The mean IR was 0.3 and 0.1 with nettle and placebo, respectively ($P = 0.01$), demonstrating a significant decrease in IR with nettle. The mean difference from baseline of β% (β cell function) was -24.2% and 1.2% with nettle and placebo, respectively ($P = 0.003$), indicating improved β-cell function. The mean difference from baseline of S% (insulin sensitivity) was -54.7% and 1.1% with nettle and placebo, respectively ($P = 0.009$), indicating improved insulin sensitivity. The authors concluded that nettle did not have significant effect on FBS but did have a significant effect on insulin resistance indices (Khajeh-Mehrizi et al., 2014).

A 12-week unblinded prospective study in patients ($n = 119$) with T2DM investigated the efficacy of SR2004, a combination of stinging nettle plus dandelion, cinnamon, tarragon, and *Morus alba*, as add-on therapy for glycemic and lipid response. At 12 weeks, A1C decreased from 9% to 7.1% (22% reduction; $P < 0.0001$), mean BG decreased from 211 mg/dL to 133 mg/dL (37% reduction; $P < 0.0001$), mean TC decreased from 213 to 185 mg/dL (13% reduction; $P < 0.01$), and mean serum TG decreased from 266 to 160 mg/dL (a reduction of 40% from baseline;

$P < 0.001$). Of the 13 patients requiring insulin at baseline, five were able to get off insulin and five reduced their daily insulin requirements by at least 30%. No response was noted in 12% of patients. Clinical observations included improvements in vasculopathy, including reversal of established retinopathic changes in two patients. No major adverse effects were observed, with minor abdominal symptoms reported in 16 patients (16%). The authors concluded that this herbal combination reduced A1C, glucose, and lipids with good tolerability (Chatterji and Fogel, 2018).

Women's Genitourinary Disorders: Perimenopause and Menopause

An 11-week RCT in postmenopausal women ($n = 72$) with hot flushes studied stinging nettle 450 mg/day for 7 weeks plus 11 sessions of acupuncture compared with stinging nettle plus sham acupuncture, compared with placebo plus acupuncture, and compared with sham acupuncture plus placebo. At 7 and 11 weeks the median hot flush score decreased by 20.2 and 21.1 with combination therapy. It decreased by 19 and 17.3 with stinging nettle alone, by 14.6 and 20.8 with acupuncture alone, and by 1.6 and 1 with placebo ($P < 0.0001$ and $P < 0.0001$, respectively, for difference between treatment groups and placebo, with no significant difference between the three treatment groups). At 7 weeks, the mean QOL score improved with combined therapy by 42.6, with stinging nettle alone by 40.7, with acupuncture alone by 37.8, and with placebo by 9.8 ($P = 0.001$ for any treatment compared with placebo, and there was no significant difference between treatment groups). The authors concluded that stinging nettle decreased menopausal hot flushes and increased quality of life similar to acupuncture and better than placebo in postmenopausal women, with no significant advantage to combining therapies (Kargozar et al., 2019).

Men's Genitourinary Disorders: Benign Prostatic Hyperplasia

A 2016 systematic review and meta-analysis to assess the efficacy and safety of stinging nettle root for BPH found five studies ($n = 1128$) that met inclusion criteria. Meta-analysis found favorable results with stinging nettle for IPSS ($SMD = -10.47$; $P = 0.007$); Qmax ($SMD = 4.37$; $P = 0.002$), and prostate volume

($SMD = -3.63$; $P < 0.00001$). The authors concluded that stinging nettle was more effective than placebo or controls for LUTS symptoms in BPH. Safety assessment of PSA ($SMD = -0.08$; $P = 0.31$) showed that PSA levels were unaffected in both groups (Men et al., 2016).

An 18-month extended RCT in men ($n = 620$) with BPH compared stinging nettle root extract with placebo for 6 months. At the end of the 6-month trial, unblinding allowed patients who initially received the placebo to be switched to nettle. Both groups continued the medication for up to 18 months. At the end of the initial 6-month trial, 81% and 16% of patients in the nettle and placebo groups, respectively, reported improved LUTS ($P < 0.001$). The IPSS decreased from 19.8 to 11.8 with nettle and from 19.2 to 17.7 with placebo ($P = 0.002$). Peak flow rates improved by 8.2 mL/s with nettle and by 3.4 mL/s for placebo ($P < 0.05$). PVR decreased from 73 to 36 mL with nettle ($P < 0.05$). No appreciable change was seen in the placebo group. Serum PSA and testosterone levels were unchanged in both groups. Prostate size decreased from 40.1 cc to 36.3 cc with nettle ($P < 0.001$), whereas there was no change with placebo. At the 18-month follow-up, only patients who continued therapy had favorable treatment variables. No side effects were identified in either group. The authors concluded that nettle had beneficial effects in symptomatic BPH (Safarinejad, 2005).

A 1-year RCT in patients ($n = 246$) with BPH compared stinging nettle root extract 459 mg/day with placebo. The IPSS decreased on average from 18.7 to 13.0 with nettle and from 18.5 to 13.8 with placebo ($P = 0.0233$). The median Q_{max} increased by 3.0 mL/s and 2.9 mL/s with nettle and placebo, respectively (N.S.). Residual urine volume changed from 35.5 mL to 20.0 mL with nettle and from 40.0 mL to 21.0 mL with placebo. Adverse events were seen with 29 and 38 of nettle and placebo patients, respectively. UTIs were seen in 3 and 10 of nettle and placebo patients, respectively. The authors concluded that treatment with this dose of nettle root was a safe therapeutic option for BPH, especially for reducing irritative symptoms and BPH-associated complications (Schneider and Rübben, 2004).

An 8-week RCT in patients ($n = 100$) with BPH compared stinging nettle 300 mg two capsules BID with placebo. The averages of AUA scores significantly improved over baseline from 26.5 to 2.1 ($P=0.000$) with nettle, while the placebo group showed no change (27.8 before and after treatment; $P=1.0$). No side effects were reported by the patients at the end of the study. The authors concluded that nettle had a better effect in relieving clinical symptoms in patients with BPH compared with placebo (Ghorbanibirgani et al., 2013).

A 9-week RCT in patients ($n=50$) with BPH compared stinging nettle root extract with placebo. Sex hormone binding globulin decreased significantly over baseline ($P=0.0005$) with nettle. Micturition volume and maximal urinary flow increased significantly over baseline with nettle. Residual volume did not change significantly (Vontobel et al., 1985).

A 6-month RCT in men who were candidates for surgery for BPH-induced LUTS investigated Pluvio, a combination of stinging nettle root, avocado, and soy oil, compared with no treatment. A marked benefit in terms of quality of life, measured by IPSS, uroflow, residual urine, and nocturia, was observed in the treated group compared with the control group. PSA and prostate volume were not significantly affected. No noteworthy adverse events were observed. The authors concluded that this nettle preparation was highly effective for the treatment of LUTS in BPH patients, and it was without the negative side effects (Bercovich and Saccomanni, 2010).

A post hoc evaluation looked at four published RCTs ($n=922$) on PRO 160/120, a fixed-dose herbal combination of saw palmetto 160 mg plus stinging nettle root 120 mg, compared with placebo (two studies), with finasteride (one study), and with tamsulosin (one study). In the pooled analysis of placebo-controlled trials, nocturnal voids improved by 0.8 (29%) with PRO 160/120 compared with 0.6 (18%) with placebo ($P=0.015$). Responder rates to the herbal product and placebo were 69% and 52%, respectively ($P=0.003$). Most responders improved by one void/night. There were no differences between PRO 160/120 and finasteride or tamsulosin regarding absolute improvement of nocturnal voids or response rates. The authors concluded that PRO 160/120 significantly improved nocturnal voiding frequency compared with placebo and was similar to tamsulosin and finasteride (Oelke et al., 2014).

A 48-week extended RCT in elderly men ($n=257$) with BPH and LUTS studied PRO 160/120, a fixed combination of 160 mg saw palmetto and 120 mg nettle root BID, compared with placebo for 24 weeks. Double-blind treatment was followed by an open control period of 24 weeks during which all patients were administered PRO 160/120. Reduction of IPSS after the first 24 weeks was six points and four points with the herbal product and placebo, respectively ($P=0.003$). This applied to obstructive as well as to irritative symptoms, and to patients with moderate or severe symptoms at baseline. The patients' quality of life was also significantly better under PRO 160/120 compared with placebo. During the second 24-week period, patients who were switched from placebo to the herbal product showed a marked improvement in LUTS ($P=0.01$) compared with those who had been treated with PRO 160/120 in the initial phase. The tolerability of PRO 160/120 was comparable to that of placebo. The authors concluded that PRO 160/120 was superior to placebo in attenuating LUTS as assessed by IPSS. It improved obstructive and irritative symptoms and was effective in patients with moderate and severe symptoms. Tolerance of the plant extract was good (Lopatkin et al., 2005).

An open-label 96-week extension of the above RCT in men ($n=219$) with BPH and LUTS assessed the long-term efficacy and tolerability of PRO 160/120, given for an additional 48-week follow-up period. Between baseline (of the original study) and end of observation (week 96) the total IPSS was reduced by 53% ($P<0.001$), peak and average urinary flow increased by 19% ($P<0.001$), and residual urine volume decreased by 44% ($P=0.03$). The incidence of adverse events during follow-up was one per 1181 treatment days with only one event being possibly due to the herbal product. The authors concluded that treatment with PRO 160/120 provided a clinically relevant benefit over a period of 96 weeks (Lopatkin et al., 2007).

A 48-week RCT in elderly men ($n=543$) with BPH studied PRO 160/120, containing 160 mg of saw palmetto and 120 mg of nettle root BID, compared with finasteride QD. Urinary flow rate increased 1.9 mL/s and 2.4 mL/s with the herbal product and finasteride, respectively ($P=0.52$). Urinary flow rate increased and micturition time decreased similarly with both treatments. The IPSS decreased from 11.3 to 8.2 and 6.5 after 24 and 48 weeks, respectively, with the herbal product. IPSS decreased from 11.8 to 8.0 and 6.2 at 24 and 48 weeks, respectively, with finasteride. Quality of life improved from 7.5 to 4.3 and from 7.7 to 4.1 with the herbal product and finasteride, respectively. Fewer adverse events occurred with the herbal product, particularly with respect to diminished ejaculation volume, erectile dysfunction, and headache (Sökeland and Albrecht, 1997).

From the above study, a subgroup analysis of 431 patients with small prostates or large prostates was undertaken. The subgroups with small prostates (≤40 mL) showed similar improvements in urinary flow rates, with mean values of 1.8 mL/s with PRO 160/120 and 2.7 mL/s with finasteride. The means of values for the subgroups with prostates of >40 mL were similar, at 2.3 mL/s and 2. 2 mL/s, respectively. There were improvements in the IPSS in both treatment groups, with no statistically significant differences. The subgroup analysis showed slightly better results for voiding symptoms in the patients with large prostates. The safety analysis showed that more patients in the finasteride group reported adverse events. The authors concluded that the efficacy of both PRO 160/120 and finasteride was equivalent and unrelated to prostate volume. However, PRO 160/120 had better tolerability than finasteride (Sökeland, 2000).

A 60-week RCT in elderly men (n = 140) with BPH and LUTS and an IPSS ≥ 13 investigated Prostagutt Forte, a combination of saw palmetto 160 mg plus nettle root 120 mg given BID, compared with tamsulosin 0.4 mg QD. The total IPSS was reduced by a median of nine points in both groups. The IPSS score was ≤ seven points at endpoint ("responders") in 32.4% of the patients in the herbal group and 27.9% in the tamsulosin group (test for non-inferiority of the herb: P = 0.034; non-inferiority margin 10%). Both drugs were well tolerated, with one adverse event in 1514 treatment days for the herbal product and one event in 1164 days for tamsulosin. The authors concluded that the fixed combination of saw palmetto and stinging nettle was non-inferior to tamsulosin 0.4 mg in the treatment of LUTS caused by BPH (Engelmann et al., 2006).

A 6-month RCT in patients (n = 49) with BPH and IPSS scores ≥ 12 investigated a combination of 25 mg *Pygeum africanum* extract plus 300 mg stinging nettle

root extract compared with placebo. IPSS decreased 21.6% with the herbal combination and 19.7% with placebo (N.S.) improved 9.3% with the herbal combination and 6% with placebo (N.S.). QOL improved increased 17.2% with the herbal combination and 13.3% with placebo (P = 0.463, N.S.). The authors concluded that this combination of herbal extracts produced clinical and urodynamic effects similar to placebo in a group of BPH patients (Melo et al., 2002).

Men's Genitourinary Disorders: Acute and Chronic Prostatitis

A 14-day RCT in patients (n = 34) with acute prostatitis studied Prostagutt Forte, an herbal combination of saw palmetto 160 mg plus stinging nettle root 120 mg BID, along with ciprofloxacin 500 mg BID for 14 days plus diclofenac 50 mg QHS for 7 days compared with ciprofloxacin plus diclofenac without the herbal product. Patients receiving add-on herbal product experienced a pronounced and significant decrease of WBCs in prostatic secretions, a decrease in prostate volume per transrectal ultrasound, and more rapid reductions of hyperthermia and severity of bladder outlet obstruction (Pul'bere and Avdoshin, 2012).

An RCT in men (n = 100) with symptoms and color doppler indicative of prostatitis studied levofloxacin 500 mg/day for 10 days plus Prostamev Plus (a combination of saw palmetto, bromelain, and stinging nettle root) given daily for 2 months compared with levofloxacin (same regimen) plus saw palmetto 320 mg/day for 2 months, compared with sensitivity-based antibiotic treatment for 10 days plus the polyherbal formula for 2 months, and compared with sensitivity-based antibiotic treatment for 10 days plus saw palmetto for 2 months. The groups treated with Prostamev Plus achieved better improvements of both IPSS, urinary flow and sexual life compared with the groups treated with saw palmetto alone (Marzano et al., 2015).

A 6-month RCT in patients (n = 143) with chronic bacterial prostatitis investigated prulifloxacin 600 mg/day for 14 days plus ProstaMEV (a combination of saw palmetto and stinging nettle root) plus FlogMEV (a combination of quercetin and curcumin) compared with the same prulifloxacin regimen without the additional herbs and supplements. One month after treatment, 89.6% and 27% of patients who had received prulifloxacin plus the supplements and prulifloxacin alone, respectively, were recurrence-free ($P < 0.0001$). Significant differences were found between groups in terms of symptoms and QOL ($P < 0.0001$ for both). Six months after treatment, no patients in the combination group had recurrence of disease, while two patients in the antibiotic-alone group did. Results on the NIH Chronic Prostatitis Symptom Index and IPSS demonstrated statistically significant differences between groups ($P < 0.001$ for both). The authors concluded that the association of saw palmetto, nettle, quercetin, and curcumin was able to improve the clinical efficacy of prulifloxacin in patients affected by CBP (Cai et al., 2009).

Musculoskeletal Disorders: Osteoarthritis

A 3-month RCT in patients ($n = 81$) with OA of the knee or hip using NSAIDs or analgesics regularly studied Phytalgic, a combination of nettle leaf with fish oil and vitamin E, compared with placebo. After 3 months of treatment, the mean use of acetaminophen-equivalent analgesics was 6.5 and 16.5 tablets/week with the supplement and placebo, respectively ($P < 0.001$). The mean use of NSAIDs was 0.4 and 1.0 doses/day with the supplement and placebo, respectively ($P = 0.02$). Mean WOMAC scores for pain, stiffness, and function were (86.5, 41.4, and 301.6, respectively) and (235.3, 96.3, and 746.5, respectively) with supplement and placebo, respectively ($P < 0.001$). The authors concluded that Phytalgic appeared to decrease the need for analgesics and NSAIDs and improve the symptoms of osteoarthritis (Jacquet et al., 2009).

A 12-week RCT in patients ($n = 92$) with knee OA investigated 40 mL/day of a polyherbal formula composed of rosehip juice concentrate, nettle leaf extract, devil's claw root extract, and vitamin D compared with placebo. During the study, the mean WOMAC and quality of life scores significantly improved in both groups. The mean pre-post change of the WOMAC pain score was 29.87 in the polyherbal group and 10.23 in the placebo group ($P < 0.001$). The polyherbal product was significantly superior to placebo for both physical and mental quality of life. There was a trend towards reduced analgesic consumption with the polyherbal product compared with placebo. In the final efficacy evaluation, physicians and patients rated the polyherbal product superior to placebo ($P < 0.001$ for both). The product was well tolerated. The authors

concluded that the polyherbal product demonstrated excellent efficacy for knee OA (Moré et al., 2017).

A crossover RCT in patients ($n = 27$) with OA pain in the first or second MCP joints compared topical nettle leaf with topical placebo (white deadnettle leaf) each applied for 1 week with a 5-week washout period. After one week's treatment with nettle, score reductions on both VAS for pain and health assessment questionnaire for disability were significantly greater than with placebo ($P = 0.026$ and $P = 0.0027$, respectively) (Randall et al., 2000).

Oncologic Disorders: Estrogen-Dependent Cancer Prophylaxis

An RCT in premenopausal women ($n = 47$) and postmenopausal women ($n = 49$) studied a combination product containing schisandra, HMR lignan, milk thistle, stinging nettle, indole-3-carbinol, and calcium glucarate compared with placebo for effects on estrogen metabolism and carcinogenic byproducts. In pre-menopausal women, treatment supplementation resulted in a significant increase ($P < 0.05$) in urinary 2-OHE concentrations and in the 2:16α-OHE ratio. In post-menopausal women, treatment supplementation resulted in a significant increase in urinary 2-OHE concentrations. In pre- and post-menopausal women combined, treatment supplementation produced a significant increase in urinary 2-OHE concentration and a trend ($P = 0.074$) toward an increased 2:16α-OHE ratio. The authors concluded that the mixture in question significantly increased estrogen C-2 hydroxylation, which may reduce estrogen-related cancer risk (Laidlaw et al., 2010).

ACTIVE CONSTITUENTS

Leaf

- Carbohydrates
  - Organic acids: ascorbic acid
- Phenolic compounds
  - Phenylpropanoids: caffeic acid, chlorogenic acid
  - Flavonoids: glucosides and rutinosides of isorhamnetin, kaempferol (anti-inflammatory, antidepressant, strengthens capillaries), and quercetin (anti-inflammatory, antioxidant, hypotensive, antidiabetic, antispasmodic,

neuroprotective, XO inhibition, antibacterial, anticancer), isoquercetin, rutin (antioxidant, anti-inflammatory, antidiabetic, nephroprotective, anti-osteoporotic, antispasmodic, neuroprotective, anti-anxiety)
  □ Tannins
  □ Anthocyanins: pelargondin (antioxidant, anti-inflammatory, antineoplastic
  ■ Quinones: glucoquinone
- ■ Terpenes: carotenes
- ■ Silica

Hairs

- ■ Carbohydrates
  - ■ Organic acids: formic acid, oxalic acid, tartaric acid, malic acid, acetic acid
- ■ Amino acid derivatives: histamine, serotonin
- ■ Phenolic compounds
  - ■ Phenylpropanoids (antioxidant, antimutagenic, antitumor, antimicrobial): caffeoylmalic acid

Root

- ■ Carbohydrates
  - ■ Polysaccharides
- ■ Lipids
  - ■ Fatty acids
- ■ Amino acid derivatives: isolectins
- ■ Phenolic compounds
  - ■ Polyphenols
  - ■ Phenylpropanoids
  - ■ Coumarin: scopoletin
  - ■ Lignans: secoisolariciresinol (binds SHBG)
  - ■ Flavonoids: tannins
- ■ Steroids
- ■ Phytosterols: β-sitosterol (reduces GI cholesterol absorption, inhibits 5-α-reductase)

STINGING NETTLE COMMONLY USED PREPARATIONS AND DOSAGE (FOR ADULTS UNLESS OTHERWISE SPECIFIED)

The following are examples of some available formulations and ranges of dosing for commercial herbal products. See Part III Introduction "How to prescribe medicinal herbs" for further guidance on herbal advising and prescribing.

For Allergies or Glycemic Control—Use Dried Leaf

- ■ Infusion: 2-3 tbsp per cup TID
- ■ Tincture of dried leaf (1:5, 50%): 2–5 mL TID
- ■ Capsule or tablet of powdered leaf: 225–900 mg BID-TID
- ■ Freeze-dried leaf: 300–600 mg QD-BID

For BPH—Use Root

- ■ Powdered root extract: 750 mg (1/3 tsp) QD-BID
- ■ Capsule or tablet of powdered root: 500 mg QD
- ■ Capsule or tablet of standardized powdered root extract (standardized to 0.8% sterols): 250—500 QD-BID.

SAFETY AND PRECAUTION

Side Effects

Generally, stinging nettle is well tolerated with rare ADRs in clinical trials. Transient contact irritation may occur with fresh leaves.

Case Reports

Hypoglycemia, gynecomastia, and galactorrhea have been reported in case reports. Gynecomastia in a man and hyperestrogenism in a woman in Turkey were attributed to ingestion of nettle herbal tea.

A 17-day-old infant presented to ER with a generalized urticaria. The infant's mother reported having applied water boiled with stinging nettle onto her nipples twice a day for 2 days to heal her nipple cracks.

Toxicity

The LD50 of an aqueous extract of stinging nettle, when injected, is 1.72 g/kg bodyweight; and is 1.93 g/kg for root extract. Oral administration up to 1.31 g/kg in rats has been well tolerated.

Pregnancy and Lactation

Avoid due to possible effects on sex hormones. Insufficient data for lactation.

Drug Interactions

- ■ CYP: Inhibits cytochrome P450.
- ■ May augment effects of diuretics and hypotensives.

- May augment effects of hypoglycemic drugs.
- Root contains coumarins: caution with anticoagulants.

REFERENCES

Amiri Behzadi A, Kalalian-Moghaddam H, Ahmadi AH. Effects of Urtica dioica supplementation on blood lipids, hepatic enzymes and nitric oxide levels in type 2 diabetic patients: a double blind, randomized clinical trial. Avicenna J Phytomed 2016;6(6):686–95.

Bercovich E, Saccomanni M. Analysis of the results obtained with a new phytotherapeutic association for LUTS vs control [corrected]. Urologia 2010;77(3):180–6.

Cai T, Mazzoli S, Bechi A, et al. Serenoa repens associated with Urtica dioica (ProstaMEV) and curcumin and quercitin (FlogMEV) extracts are able to improve the efficacy of prulifloxacin in bacterial prostatitis patients: results from a prospective randomised study. Int J Antimicrob Agents 2009;33(6):549–53.

Chatterji S, Fogel D. Study of the effect of the herbal composition SR2004 on hemoglobin A1C, fasting blood glucose, and lipids in patients with type 2 diabetes mellitus. Integr Med Res 2018;7(3):248–56.

Engelmann U, Walther C, Bondarenko B, Funk P, Schläfke S. Efficacy and safety of a combination of sabal and urtica extract in lower urinary tract symptoms. A randomized double-blind study vs tamsulosin. Arzneimittelforschung 2006;56(3):222–9.

Ghorbanibirgani A, Khalili A, Zamani L. The efficacy of stinging nettle (urtica dioica) in patients with benign prostatic hyperplasia: a randomized double-blind study in 100 patients. Iran Red Crescent Med J 2013;15(1):9–10.

Jacquet A, Girodet PO, Pariente A, Forest K, Mallet L, Moore N. Phytalgic, a food supplement, vs placebo in patients with osteoarthritis of the knee or hip: a randomised double-blind placebo-controlled clinical trial. Arthritis Res Ther 2009;11(6):R192.

Kargozar R, Salari R, Jarahi L, et al. Urtica dioica in comparison with placebo and acupuncture: a new possibility for menopausal hot flushes: a randomized clinical trial. Complement Ther Med 2019;44:166–73.

Khajeh-Mehrizi R, Mozaffari-Khosravi H, Ghadiri-Anari A, Dehghani A. The effect of Urtica dioica extract on glycemic control and insulin resistance indices in patients with type 2 diabetes: a randomized double-blind clinical trial. Iran J Diab Obes 2014;6(4):149–55.

Kianbakht S, Khalighi-Sigaroodi F, Dabaghian FH. Improved glycemic control in patients with advanced type 2 diabetes mellitus taking Urtica dioica leaf extract: a randomized double-blind placebo-controlled clinical trial. Clin Lab 2013;59(9-10):1071–6.

Laidlaw M, Cockerline CA, Sepkovic DW. Effects of a breast-health herbal formula supplement on estrogen metabolism in pre- and post-menopausal women not taking hormonal contraceptives or supplements: a randomized controlled trial. Breast Cancer (Auckl) 2010;4:85–95.

Lopatkin N, Sivkov A, Walther C, et al. Long-term efficacy and safety of a combination of sabal and urtica extract for lower urinary tract symptoms—a placebo-controlled, double-blind, multicenter trial. World J Urol 2005;23(2):139–46.

Lopatkin N, Sivkov A, Schläfke S, Funk P, Medvedev A, Engelmann U. Efficacy and safety of a combination of Sabal and Urtica extract in lower urinary tract symptoms—long-term follow-up of a placebo-controlled, double-blind, multicenter trial. Int Urol Nephrol 2007;39(4):1137–46.

Marzano R, Dinelli N, Ales V, Bertozzi MA. Effectiveness on urinary symptoms and erectile function of Prostamev Plus* vs only extract Serenoa repens. Arch Ital Urol Androl 2015;87(1):25–7.

Melo EA, Bertero EB, Rios LA, Mattos Jr D. Evaluating the efficiency of a combination of Pygeum africanum and stinging nettle (Urtica dioica) extracts in treating benign prostatic hyperplasia (BPH): double-blind, randomized, placebo-controlled trial. Int Braz J Urol 2002;28(5):418–25.

Men C, Wang M, Aiyireti M, Cui Y. The efficacy and safety of Urtica dioica in treating benign prostatic hyperplasia: a systematic review and meta-analysis. Afr J Tradit Complement Alternat Med 2016;13(2):143.

Mittman P. Randomized, double-blind study of freeze-dried Urtica dioica in the treatment of allergic rhinitis. Planta Med 1990;56(1):44–7.

Moré M, Gruenwald J, Pohl U, Uebelhack R. A Rosa canina—Urtica dioica—Harpagophytum procumbens/zeyheri combination significantly reduces gonarthritis symptoms in a randomized, placebo-controlled double-blind study. Planta Med 2017;83(18):1384–91.

Namazi N, Esfanjani AT, Heshmati J, Bahrami A. The effect of hydro alcoholic Nettle (Urtica dioica) extracts on insulin sensitivity and some inflammatory indicators in patients with type 2 diabetes: a randomized double-blind control trial. Pak J Biol Sci 2011;14(15):775–9.

Oelke M, Berges R, Schläfke S, Burkart M. Fixed-dose combination PRO 160/120 of sabal and urtica extracts improves nocturia in men with LUTS suggestive of BPH: re-evaluation of four controlled clinical studies. World J Urol 2014;32(5):1149–54.

Pul'bere SA, Avdoshin VP. Combined therapy using phytopreparation prostagutt forte in patients with acute prostatitis. Urologia 2012;5. 53-54,56.

Randall C, Randall H, Dobbs F, Hutton C, Sanders H. Randomized controlled trial of nettle sting for treatment of base-of-thumb pain. J R Soc Med 2000;93(6):305–9.

Rashidi AA, Mirhashemi SM, Taghizadeh M, Sarkhail P. Iranian medicinal plants for diabetes mellitus: a systematic review. Pak J Biol Sci 2013;16(9):401–11.

Safarinejad MR. Urtica dioica for treatment of benign prostatic hyperplasia: a prospective, randomized, double-blind, placebo-controlled, crossover study. J Herb Pharmacother 2005;5(4):1–11.

Samaha AA, Fawaz M, Salami A, Baydoun S, Eid AH. Antihypertensive indigenous lebanese plants: ethnopharmacology and a clinical trial. Biomolecules 2019;9(7).

Schneider T, Rübben H. Stinging nettle root extract (Bazoton-uno) in long term treatment of benign prostatic syndrome (BPS). Results of a randomized, double-blind, placebo controlled multi-center study after 12 months. Urologe A 2004;43(3):302–6.

Sökeland J. Combined sabal and urtica extract compared with finasteride in men with benign prostatic hyperplasia: analysis of prostate volume and therapeutic outcome. BJU Int 2000;86(4):439–42.

Sökeland J, Albrecht J. Combination of Sabal and Urtica extract vs finasteride in benign prostatic hyperplasia (Aiken stages I to II). Comparison of therapeutic effectiveness in a one-year double-blind study. Urologe A 1997;36(4):327–33.

Vontobel HP, Herzog R, Rutishauser G, Kres H. Results of a double-blind study of the efficacy of ERU* capsules in the conservative treatment of benign prostatic hyperplasia. Urologe 1985;24:49–51.

Zhu Y, Ge XD, Shi Y, Guo JH, Liu ZJ, Zeng QQ. Efficacy and safety of № i empirical prescription for chronic prostatitis in the treatment of type III refractory chronic prostatitis. Zhonghua Nan Ke Xue 2018;24(7):640–4.

Ziaei R, Foshati S, Hadi A, et al. The effect of nettle (*Urtica dioica*) supplementation on the glycemic control of patients with type 2 diabetes mellitus: a systematic review and meta-analysis. Phytother Res 2020;34(2):282–94.

72

TRIBULUS (*TRIBULUS TERRESTRIS*)
Fruit, Above-Ground Parts, Root

GENERAL OVERVIEW

It is not unusual for middle-aged and older male patients to seek information about tribulus from their integrative primary care providers due to its reputation with respect to both sexual and athletic performance. While tribulus is best known for its aphrodisiac properties, it also has potential for use in several other disorders. It has evidence in favor of benefits for sexual dysfunction and evidence against its use as an athletic or testosterone booster. Both the root and fruit of the plant have been used medicinally in traditional Chinese medicine and Ayurvedic medicine for their phytochemical attribute. Tribulus may have cardiometabolic benefits for both men and women. Because this herb's target symptoms render it more prone to overdosing, it is important to educate patients about its potential toxicities (see "Safety and Precaution").

Clinical research indicates that tribulus, alone or in combination formulas, may be beneficial for hypertension, coronary artery disease, hyperlipidemia, diabetes, polycystic ovary syndrome, and male and female sexual dysfunction; however, it does not improve athletic performance or bodybuilding.

IN VITRO AND ANIMAL RESEARCH

Tribulus has demonstrated diuretic, aphrodisiac, anti-urolithic, immunomodulatory, antihypertensive, antihyperlipidemic, antidiabetic, hepatoprotective, anticancer, anthelmintic, antibacterial, analgesic, and anti-inflammatory properties. Tribulus has demonstrated pro-erectile effects in rabbits following 8 weeks

of treatment at varying doses. This effect appears to be due to an increase in release of nitric oxide from the endothelium and nitregeric nerve synapses. Similarly, a dose-dependent improvement in sexual behavior and an increase in testosterone levels were observed in rats with an extract of the dried fruits, more so with chronic administration. Tribulus also exhibited protective effects against cadmium-induced testicular damage, apparently through antioxidant and chelating activities. In fish, the male population rose with tribulus treatment. Protodioscin, a major saponin in tribulus, appears to increase conversion of testosterone into DHT, thereby stimulating sex drive as well as hematopoiesis and muscle development.

The saponins in tribulus are also thought to be responsible for the demonstrated reductions in serum glucose, postprandial glucose, triglycerides, and cholesterol in mice. They have been shown to inhibit gluconeogenesis and glucosidase and aldose reductase activity. The hypolipidemic activity is ascribed to an increase in lipoprotein lipases in muscles preferentially over adipose tissue. Tribulus has also been shown in animal research to produce coronary artery dilation and improve endothelial function. One constituent, tribulosin, has been shown to protect against ischemia-reperfusion injury through protein kinase C activation. Tribulus fruits have ACE inhibitory effects in vitro. Antihypertensive activity has been demonstrated in rats.

Tribulus has demonstrated hepatoprotective activity against acetaminophen-induced toxicity in fish. It has antispasmodic activity in rabbit jejunum. In research related to traditional use of tribulus for nephrolithiasis, the herb has shown a dose-dependent protection against deposition of calculogenic material around a glass bead. Research has revealed that tribulus extract is able to inhibit nucleation and growth of the calcium oxalate crystals and to have a cytoprotective role. Tribulus also exhibits glycolate oxidase (GOX) inhibition, another mechanism for blocking stone development. Two constituents, quercetin and kaempherol, were found to be non-competitive and competitive inhibitors of GOX, respectively. Tribulus has been shown to have diuretic activity due to nitrates, potassium salts, and essential oils. In guinea pigs, an aqueous extract in oral dose of 5 g/kg, produced greater diuresis than comparable dosing of furosemide, with a potassium-sparing bonus. Increased smooth muscle tonicity has also been demonstrated in the urinary tract, another potentially beneficial mechanism for nephrolithiasis.

Tribulus has been shown in vitro to inhibit COX-2, iNOS, TNF-α, and IL-4, mechanisms accounting for its anti-inflammatory activity that has been demonstrated in rats. In mice it has shown a non-opioid analgesic activity that is less than morphine but greater than ASA. Tribulus is part of a combination product that is used for depression in Ayurvedic medicine. It has produced antidepressant and anxiolytic activity in mice. One constituent, harmine, possesses MAO inhibiting activity.

The root appears to be more chemopreventive than the fruit. Tribulus blocks liver cancer cell proliferation and induces apoptosis. It also prevents the glutathione depletion of radiation, thereby providing protection against radiation.

HUMAN RESEARCH

Cardiovascular Disorders: Hypertension and Coronary Artery Disease

A 4-week RCT in patients with mild-to-moderate HTN ($n=75$) compared tribulus whole plant 1 g TID with tribulus fruit 1 g TID and with placebo for BP effects. With tribulus, both whole plant and fruit, there was a gradual reduction in BP with a reduction in SBP of 18 mmHg and in DBP of 9 mmHg. This was associated with a significant increase in urine volume. There was also a reduction in TC by about 10%, being greater with the whole plant. The placebo group had negligible reductions in their readings (Murthy, 2000).

A study in patients ($n=406$) with CAD investigated the "saponin" from tribulus compared with a positive control Yufen Ningxin Pian (A TCM product traditionally used to relieve spasms, alleviate pain, and ameliorate blood flow). The authors reported a total efficacious rate of 82.3% for remission of angina pectoris with tribulus and 67.2% with the positive control ($P<0.05$). ECG improvement was reported in 52.7% and 35.8% with tribulus and control, respectively. The authors concluded that tribulus improved coronary circulation (Wang et al., 1990).

Cardiometabolic Disorders: Hyperlipidemia and Diabetes

A 3-month RCT in women ($n=98$) with T2DM compared tribulus 1000 mg/day with placebo for effects on glycemia and lipids. The tribulus group showed a significant lowering of TC, LDL-C, and glucose compared with placebo ($P<0.05$). A1C decreased from 8.16% to 7.67% with tribulus and increased from 7.33% to 7.50% with placebo. No significant difference was observed for TG or HDL-C. The authors concluded that tribulus had promising hypoglycemic effects in women with T2DM (Samani et al., 2016).

Women's Genitourinary Disorders: Polycystic Ovary Syndrome

A 3-month RCT in overweight women ($n=122$) with PCOS compared lifestyle intervention alone with lifestyle intervention plus an herbal combination of licorice, St. John's wort, peony, and cinnamon plus a separate tablet of tribulus. At 3 months, women in the combination group recorded a reduction in oligomenorrhoea by 32.9% ($P<0.01$) compared with controls. Other significant improvements were found for BMI ($P<0.01$); insulin ($P=0.02$); LH ($P=0.04$); BP ($P=0.01$); QOL ($P<0.01$); depression, anxiety, and stress ($P<0.01$); and pregnancy rates ($P=0.01$). The authors concluded that lifestyle combined with herbal medicines was safe and effective in women with PCOS (Arentz et al., 2014).

Genitourinary Disorders: Male and Female Sexual Dysfunction

A 2018 systematic review to evaluate the efficacy of herbal medicines for erectile dysfunction (ED) identified 24 RCTs ($n=2080$) for inclusion. Among these, five investigated ginseng ($n = 399$), three investigated saffron ($n = 397$), and two investigated tribulus ($n = 202$). Twelve studies investigated combinations of herbs and or supplements. Ginseng significantly improved erectile function (IIEF-5 score: 140 with ginseng, 96 with placebo; SMD $= 0.43$; $P < 0.01$). *Pinus pinaster* and maca showed very preliminary positive results, and saffron and tribulus produced mixed results. Adverse events were recorded in 19 of 24 trials, with no significant differences between placebo and verum in placebo-controlled studies. The authors concluded that there was encouraging evidence to suggest that ginseng may be an effective herbal treatment for ED (Borrelli et al., 2018).

A 2016 systematic review to assess the impact of tribulus on sexual dysfunction analyzed phytochemical and pharmacological studies in humans and animals. It found an important role for tribulus in treating ED and sexual desire problems; however, the androgen-enhancing properties were determined to be unlikely. The authors noted emerging evidence that the efficacy of tribulus was related to endothelium and nitric oxide-dependent mechanisms (Neychev and Mitev, 2016).

A 12-week Phase IV RCT in males ($n = 180$) with mild or moderate ED with or without hypoactive sexual desire disorder studied Tribestan, an extract of tribulus standardized to furostanol saponins $>$ 112.5 mg per 250 mg tablet, two tablets TID PC compared with placebo. The IIEF Questionnaire and Global Efficacy Question (GEQ) were followed. The IIEF score improved significantly with tribulus compared with placebo ($P < 0.0001$). A statistically significant difference between tribulus and placebo was found for Intercourse Satisfaction ($P = 0.0005$), Orgasmic Function ($P = 0.0325$), Sexual Desire ($P = 0.0038$), and Overall Satisfaction ($P = 0.0028$). GEQ responses were also significantly favored tribulus ($P < 0.0001$). Adverse events were similar between groups and therapy was well tolerated (Kamenov et al., 2017).

A 3-month RCT in aging males ($n = 70$) with ED, LUTS, and partial androgen deficiency compared tribulus TID with placebo for effects on ED and LUTS. With tribulus there were significant elevations in both total testosterone (from 2.2 to 2.7; $P < 0.001$) and the IIEF-5 (from 10.7 to 16.1; $P < 0.001$). The mean of the total PSA increased with tribulus from 1.4 to 1.7

($P = 0.007$), but there was no associated worsening of LUTS based on stable scores of the IPSS. The authors concluded that tribulus was effective in elevating testosterone levels and improving sexual function in patients who suffered from ED with partial androgen deficiency (GamalEl Din et al., 2019).

An RCT in premenopausal women ($n = 40$) with hypoactive sexual desire (HSDD) compared tribulus with placebo for effects on sexual function and serum levels of testosterone. Tribulus led to improvements in total FSFI scores ($P < 0.001$) and the domains "desire" ($P < 0.001$), "sexual arousal" ($P = 0.005$), "lubrication" ($P = 0.001$), "orgasm" ($P < 0.001$), "pain" ($P = 0.030$), and "satisfaction" ($P = 0.001$), whereas treatment with placebo did not improve the scores for the "lubrication" and "pain." The scale for Quality of Sexual Function scores improved with tribulus for "desire" ($P = 0.012$), "sexual arousal/lubrication" ($P = 0.002$), "pain" ($P = 0.031$), "orgasm" ($P = 0.004$), and "satisfaction" ($P = 0.001$), whereas placebo was not associated with improvement in these domains. Tribulus was associated with increases in both free and bioavailable testosterone ($P = 0.046$ and $P < 0.048$, respectively). The authors concluded that tribulus may be a safe alternative for the treatment of premenopausal women with HSDD, and that its efficacy may be due to an increase in testosterone levels (Vale et al., 2018).

A 4-week RCT in younger women ($n = 67$) with HSDD compared tribulus 7.5 mg/day with placebo. The tribulus group experienced significant improvement in their total Female Sexual Function Index (FSFI) score ($P < 0.001$) and the desire ($P < 0.001$), arousal ($P = 0.037$), lubrication ($P < 0.001$), satisfaction ($P < 0.001$), and pain ($P = 0.041$) domains of FSFI. Frequency of side effects was similar between the two groups. The authors concluded that tribulus could safely and effectively improve desire in women with HSDD (Akhtari et al., 2014).

In contrast, a 30-day RCT in healthy men ($n = 30$) with ED compared tribulus 400 mg BID with placebo for effects on ED. The mean IIEF score was 13.2 and 15.3 before and after treatment, respectively, with tribulus, and 11.6 and 13.6 before and after treatment, respectively, with placebo. The difference between tribulus and placebo was not significant. The changes in total testosterone were also not significantly different (Santos et al., 2014).

An 8-week RCT in postmenopausal women ($n = 60$) compared tribulus extract syrup (0.5 mg/dL, 0.7 mg/dL, or 0.9 mg/dL) with placebo syrup for effects on sexual satisfaction. Sexual satisfaction was calculated based on Larsson questionnaire. The mean sexual satisfaction scores increased with Tribulus (from 25.4 to 37.5; $P < 0.001$) and increased insignificantly with placebo (from 35.2 to 36.3; $P = 0.197$). The authors concluded that Tribulus syrup increased sexual satisfaction in postmenopausal women (Tadayon et al., 2018).

A 2-month exploratory, prospective, non-controlled, observational study in postmenopausal women ($n = 29$) with sexual dysfunction as defined by a Female Sexual Function Index (FSFI) score < 25.83 assessed the effects of Libicare, a polyherbal product containing fenugreek, tribulus, ginkgo, and *Temera diffusa*, two tablets daily. FSFI mean score showed a significant increase from 20.15 at baseline to 25.03 after treatment ($P = 0.0011$). The FSFI score was increased in 86% of the subjects. All FSFI domains, except dyspareunia, showed significant increases. The highest increase was observed in the desire domain ($P = 0.0004$). A significant increase in testosterone level occurred in roughly half of the subjects, from 0.41 to 0.50 pg/mL. A significant decrease in SHBG level occurred in 95% of subjects from 85 to 73 nmol/L ($P = 0.0001$). The authors concluded that this polyherbal formula provided a significant improvement in sexual function and related hormone levels (Palacios et al., 2019).

Disorders of Vitality: Athletic Performance and Bodybuilding

A 2014 systematic review to assess the effect of tribulus on testosterone levels in humans and animals selected 11 studies that met the inclusion criteria. The authors found that trials varied in duration, dosage, and supplementation with tribulus as sole or combined treatment, rendering meta-analysis impossible. A limited number of animal studies displayed a significant increase in serum testosterone levels after tribulus administration, but this effect was only noted in humans when it was part of a combined supplement administration. The authors concluded that evidence to date suggests that tribulus is ineffective for increasing testosterone levels in humans. The nitric oxide release effect of tribulus may offer a plausible explanation for the observed physiological responses to tribulus supplementation, independent of the testosterone level (Qureshi et al., 2014).

A 5-week RCT in preseason male rugby players ($n = 22$) compared tribulus 450 mg/day with placebo with respect to the effects on strength, fat-free mass, and the urinary T/E ratio. After 5 weeks of training, strength and fat-free mass increased significantly without any between-group differences. No between-group differences were noted in the urinary T/E ratio. It was concluded that tribulus did not produce the large gains in strength or lean muscle mass that many manufacturers claim can be experienced within 5-28 days. Furthermore, tribulus did not alter the urinary T/E ratio and would not place an athlete at risk of testing positive based on the World Anti-Doping Agency's urinary T/E ratio limit of 4:1 (Rogerson et al., 2007).

A 4-week RCT in healthy young men ($n = 21$) compared tribulus 20 mg/kg/day with tribulus 10 mg/kg/day and with placebo for effects on steroidal hormone levels. There was no significant difference between the tribulus and placebo groups in serum testosterone, androstenedione, or LH ($P > 0.05$ for all). All results were within the normal range. The authors concluded that tribulus steroid saponins possess neither direct nor indirect androgen-increasing properties (Neychev and Mitev, 2005).

An 8-week RCT in resistance-trained male athletes ($n = 15$) compared tribulus 3.2 mg/kg/day with placebo for body composition and exercise performance. There were no changes in BW, percentage fat, total body water, dietary intake, or mood states in either group. Muscle endurance as determined by the maximal number of repetitions at 100%-200% of BW increased for the bench and leg press exercises in the placebo group ($P < 0.05$), while the tribulus group experienced an increase in leg press strength only ($P < 0.05$). The authors concluded that tribulus did not enhance body composition or exercise performance in resistance-trained males (Antonio et al., 2000).

A 20-day open-label study in athletes investigated tribulus one capsule TID with respect to effects on physical power in various energy producing zones: anaerobic alactic muscular power and anaerobic alactic glycolytic power. These zones were reported to be significantly increased. Testosterone levels increased significantly during the first 10 days only. There were significant increases in CK, with a steady decline in creatinine, BUN, cholesterol, and bilirubin. There was no change in RBCs, Hgb, or platelets (Milasius et al., 2009).

An open-label study in female volunteers ($n = 2$) assessed the effects of tribulus 500 mg TID for 2 days on androgenic hormones. They found that the short-term treatment with tribulus showed no impact on the endogenous testosterone metabolism of the two subjects (Saudan et al., 2008).

ACTIVE CONSTITUENTS

Root

- Phenolic compounds:
  - Flavonoids: kaempferol (anti-inflammatory, antidepressant, strengthens capillaries), kaempferol-3-glucoside, kaempferol-3-rutinoside, tribuloside caffeoyl derivatives, quercetin glycosides
    - Glycosides: quercetin 3-*O*-glycoside, quercetin 3-*O*-rutinoside, and kaempferol 3-*O*-glycoside
    - Tannins
- Terpenes
  - Triterpenes: α-amyrin
  - Triterpenoid saponins: tigogenin, neotigogenin, gitogenin, neogitogenin, hecogenin, neohecogenin
- Steroids
  - Steroidal saponins: protodioscin (up to 45% of dry extract), pseudoprotodioscin, protogracillin, diosgenin, chlorogenin, ruscogenin, sarsasapogenin, protodibestin, tribestin (aphrodisiac)
  - Steroids: β-sitosterol (reduces GI cholesterol absorption, inhibits 5-α-reductase), stigmasterols, tribulosin
- Alkaloids: harmane, norharmane, tribulusterine

Dried Fruit

- Amino acid derivatives: aurantiamide acetate
- Phenolic compounds
  - Phenylpropanoids (antioxidant, antimutagenic, antitumor, antimicrobial): N-p-coumaroyltyramine, terrestriamide, tribulusamides A-D, terrestribisamide
- Steroids
  - Steroidal saponins: terrestroside A and B, terrestrinin B, terrestroneoside A, chloromaloside, hecogenin

- Phytosterols: tribulosin (cardioprotective); β-sitosterol (reduces GI cholesterol absorption, inhibits 5-α-reductase), 25R-spirost-4-en-3, 12-dione
- Alkaloid: tribulusterine

TRIBULUS COMMONLY USED PREPARATIONS AND DOSAGE (FOR ADULTS UNLESS OTHERWISE SPECIFIED)

The following are examples of some available formulations and ranges of dosing for commercial herbal products. See Part III Introduction "How to prescribe medicinal herbs" for further guidance on herbal advising and prescribing.

Fruit and Root

- Capsule or tablet of whole herb powder: 500-1500 mg QD
- Capsule or tablet of standardized extract (standardized to 45%-60% saponins): 250-500 mg QD-BID for libido (5 mg/kg of saponins)

SAFETY AND PRECAUTION

Side Effects

Rarely minor stomach cramps, GERD, insomnia, and menstrual irregularity may occur. Nephrotoxicity is possible (See "Case reports" and "Toxicity").

Case Reports

A case report was made of hepatorenal syndrome in one young man who drank 2 L/day of a tribulus decoction for 2 days.

A 21-year-old man with light tobacco and moderate alcohol history reported a benign left breast nodule that coincided with consumption of a tribulus product, but causation could not be clearly ascribed to the product.

A 41-year-old man taking an herbal combination of tribulus, oat, and Asian ginseng was hospitalized with a massive pulmonary embolism. The same combination was associated with three case reports of acute coronary syndrome.

Toxicity

Hepatitis, nephrotoxicity, neurotoxicity, and hepatorenal syndrome have been reported in animals feeding on tribulus. A study in diabetic rats given a hydroalcoholic extract of tribulus at 50 mg/kg showed histological damage to distal tubules and collecting ducts along with reductions in serum creatinine, cystatin c, and β-2 microglobulin. Glomerular function and the renal cortex seemed unaffected. Protein/albumin normalized suggesting an increase in GFR.

A 28-day oral toxicology test of 500 mg/kg lyophilized dry fruit extract in rats (80 mg/kg human dose) failed to establish any toxic signs. An LD50 study found that the LD50 of a basic lyophilized extract from both aerial parts and root of tribulus was 813 mg/kg, translating to a dose of 118-143 mg/kg for humans.

Pregnancy and Lactation

No data; concern about DHT blockade and male fetal development. Avoid.

Disease Interactions

- Caution with estrogen-sensitive cancers due to estrogenic activity of water extracts.
- Non-aqueous extraction methods have demonstrated anti-estrogen activity.
- Caution with gallbladder disease as steroidal saponins have been associated with gallstones.

Drug Interactions

- May interact with antihypertensives (additive effects), digoxin and nitrates.

REFERENCES

Akhtari E, Raisi F, Keshavarz M, et al. Tribulus terrestris for treatment of sexual dysfunction in women: randomized double-blind placebo—controlled study. Daru 2014;22(1):40.

Antonio J, Uelmen J, Rodriguez R, Earnest C. The effects of Tribulus terrestris on body composition and exercise performance in resistance-trained males. Int J Sport Nutr Exerc Metab 2000;10(2):208–15.

Arentz S, Abbott JA, Smith CA, Bensoussan A. Herbal medicine for the management of polycystic ovary syndrome (PCOS) and associated oligo/amenorrhoea and hyperandrogenism; a review of the laboratory evidence for effects with corroborative clinical findings. BMC Complement Altern Med 2014;14:511.

Borrelli F, Colalto C, Delfino DV, Iriti M, Izzo AA. Herbal dietary supplements for erectile dysfunction: a systematic review and meta-analysis. Drugs 2018;78(6):643–73.

GamalEl Din SF, Abdel Salam MA, Mohamed MS, et al. Tribulus terrestris versus placebo in the treatment of erectile dysfunction and lower urinary tract symptoms in patients with late-onset hypogonadism: a placebo-controlled study. Urologia 2019;86(2):74–8.

Kamenov Z, Fileva S, Kalinov K, Jannini EA. Evaluation of the efficacy and safety of Tribulus terrestris in male sexual dysfunction-A prospective, randomized, double-blind, placebo-controlled clinical trial. Maturitas 2017;99:20–6.

Milasius K, Dadeliene R, Skernevicius J. The influence of the Tribulus terrestris extract on the parameters of the functional preparedness and athletes' organism homeostasis. Fiziol Zh 2009;55(5):89–96.

Murthy AR. Antihypertensive effect of Gokshura (Tribulus terrestris Linn.). Ancient Sci Life 2000;XIX(3&4).

Neychev VK, Mitev VI. The aphrodisiac herb Tribulus terrestris does not influence the androgen production in young men. J Ethnopharmacol 2005;101(1-3):319–23.

Neychev V, Mitev V. Pro-sexual and androgen enhancing effects of Tribulus terrestris L.: fact or fiction. J Ethnopharmacol 2016;179:345–55.

Palacios S, Soler E, Ramírez M, Lilue M, Khorsandi D, Losa F. Effect of a multi-ingredient-based food supplement on sexual function in women with low sexual desire. BMC Womens Health 2019;19(1):58.

Qureshi A, Naughton DP, Petroczi A. A systematic review on the herbal extract Tribulus terrestris and the roots of its putative aphrodisiac and performance enhancing effect. J Diet Suppl 2014;11(1):64–79.

Rogerson S, Riches CJ, Jennings C, Weatherby RP, Meir RA, Marshall-Gradisnik SM. The effect of five weeks of Tribulus terrestris supplementation on muscle strength and body composition during preseason training in elite rugby league players. J Strength Cond Res 2007;21(2):348–53.

Samani NB, Jokar A, Soveid M, Heydari M, Mosavat SH. Efficacy of the hydroalcoholic extract of Tribulus terrestris on the serum glucose and lipid profile of women with diabetes mellitus: a double-blind randomized placebo-controlled clinical trial. J Evid Based Complement Altern Med 2016;21(4). NP91-7.

Santos Jr CA, Reis LO, Destro-Saade R, Luiza-Reis A, Fregonesi A. Tribulus terrestris vs placebo in the treatment of erectile dysfunction: A prospective, randomized, double blind study. Actas Urol Esp 2014;38(4):244–8.

Saudan C, Baume N, Emery C, Strahm E, Saugy M. Short term impact of Tribulus terrestris intake on doping control analysis of endogenous steroids. Forensic Sci Int 2008;178(1):e7–10.

Tadayon M, Shojaee M, Afshari P, Moghimipour E, Haghighizadeh MH. The effect of hydro-alcohol extract ofTribulusterrestris on sexual satisfaction in postmenopause women: a double-blind randomized placebo-controlled trial. J Family Med Prim Care 2018;7(5):888–92.

Vale FBC, Zanolla Dias de Souza K, Rezende CR, Geber S. Efficacy of Tribulus terrestris for the treatment of premenopausal women with hypoactive sexual desire disorder: a randomized double-blinded, placebo-controlled trial. Gynecol Endocrinol 2018;34(5):442–5.

Wang B, Ma L, Liu T. 406 cases of angina pectoris in coronary heart disease treated with saponin of Tribulus terrestris. Zhong Xi Yi Jie He Za Zhi 1990;10(2):85–7. 68.

TURMERIC (*CURCUMA LONGA*)
Root

GENERAL OVERVIEW

Having a 4000-to-6000-year history of medicinal use, the root of turmeric gains its fame from its most active and well-studied phenolic constituents curcumin and related curcuminoids. There have been more than 5600 studies involving curcumin, with increased interest in the past decade. Most of the research cited in this chapter is related to curcumin. However, whole turmeric may be a preferable way to ingest curcumin in most conditions due to the other but lesser researched constituents that have demonstrated activities that act uniquely, additively, or synergistically with curcumin. For example, studies have indicated that the turmerones, present in turmeric can enhance the bioavailability of curcumin, which by itself has extremely limited bioavailability. Studies of curcumin-free turmeric components have demonstrated many beneficial activities including anti-inflammatory, anticancer, and antidiabetic activities. Some of these constituents include turmerin, turmerone, elemene, furanodiene, curdione, bisacurone, cyclocurcumin, calebin A, and germacrone. Elemene is approved in China for the treatment of cancer.

Turmeric should come to mind when there is a need to address inflammatory conditions or to institute primary or secondary cancer prevention, but as the research indicates, it is a protean botanical with much of its activity attributed to its underlying potent anti-inflammatory properties. It is essential to add a little piperine (from black pepper) to any turmeric preparation, particularly curcumin, to allow for adequate absorption. Other bio-enhancements are available to increase absorption but have not been proven to be better than turmeric combined with piperine.

Clinical research indicates that turmeric or curcumin, alone or in combination formulas, may be beneficial for anterior uveitis, oral lichen planus, gingivitis, dental pain, periodontal health, oral submucous fibrosis, asthma, endothelial dysfunction, hyperlipidemia, dyslipidemia, diabetes, metabolic syndrome, obesity, nonalcoholic fatty liver disease, iron overload, hepatotoxicity, gallbladder dyskinesis, peptic ulcer disease, functional dyspepsia, ulcerative colitis, diabetic nephropathy, lupus nephritis, lactational mastitis, cervical intraepithelial neoplasia, chronic prostatitis, osteoarthritis, musculoskeletal pain, migraine headaches, degenerative brain disorders, depression, psoriasis, inflammation, rheumatoid arthritis, radiation-induced mucositis, hand-foot syndrome, and colorectal cancer.

IN VITRO AND ANIMAL RESEARCH

Curcumin has demonstrated the following anti-inflammatory mechanisms: downregulation of COX-2 via suppression of NF-κB; downregulation of LOX, iNOS, and mitogen-activated and Janus kinases; inhibition of TNF-α, IL-1, -2, -6, -8, and -12; inhibition of monocyte chemoattractant protein; inhibition of PPAR-γ; and inhibition of migration inhibitory protein. Turmeric has antibacterial, fungistatic, and wound-healing properties.

With potential benefits to the cardiovascular system, in addition to its strong antioxidant and anti-inflammatory properties, curcumin has antiplatelet properties and reduces TC, TG, and LDL-C lipid peroxidation. The inhibition of platelet aggregation by turmeric constituents is thought to be via its potentiation of prostacyclin synthesis and inhibition of thromboxane synthesis. Turmeric lowers histamines by increasing adrenal cortisol production.

Sodium curcuminate, a salt of curcumin, exerts choleretic effects by increasing biliary excretion of bile salts, cholesterol, and bilirubin as well as increasing bile solubility, therefore possibly preventing and treating cholelithiasis. The hepatoprotective effects of curcumin may occur via MMP-13 induction and TGF-α inhibition as well as via antiapoptotic and anti-necrotic mechanisms. In animal research, turmeric has been shown to protect and support GI functions through anti-inflammatory mechanisms and improvement of secretion of gastrin, secretin, bicarbonate, gastric wall mucus, and pancreatic enzymes. It inhibits intestinal spasms and stress or chemical-induced ulcer formation. In in vivo studies, curcumin was shown to effectively prevent the esophageal mucosal damage induced by acute reflux esophagitis. Although curcumin was less potent than lansoprazole in the inhibition of acid reflux esophagitis, it was found to be superior to lansoprazole in the inhibition of mixed acid-bile reflux-induced esophagitis. This protective mechanism has been attributed to the antioxidant nature of curcumin.

In vitro curcumin has been shown to prevent formation and increase dissolution of amyloid plaque. In animal studies, the constituent turmerone has been shown to stimulate neural stem cells. Curcumin and its analogues have been shown in vitro to inhibit HIV infection and replication. Curcuminoids are inhibitors of HIV protease and integrase. Curcumin also inhibits transactivation of the HIV1-LTR genome, interleukins, TNF-α, NF-κB, COX-2, and various HIV-associated kinases including tyrosine kinase, PAK1, MAPK, PKC, and CDK. In addition, curcumin enhances the effect of conventional therapeutic drugs and minimizes their side effects.

Turmeric has demonstrated activity against a wide variety of viruses by interfering with pathways controlling penetration and cellular signaling. It interacts with more than 30 viral proteins, including DNA polymerase and protein kinase (Wen et al., 2007). It has been shown to inhibit ACE-2 receptors and may thus prevent SARS-CoV-2 attachment. It also forms a stable complex with the SARS-CoV-2 main protease (Orhan and Deniz, 2020).

Turmeric demonstrates several anticancer activities including inhibition of carcinogen activation, stimulation of carcinogen detoxification, suppression of pro-inflammatory signaling, inhibition of Stat-3 pathway, downregulation of β-catenin expression, induction of cancer cell apoptosis cell cycle arrest, inhibition of angiogenesis and metastasis, and modulation of oncogenes and tumor suppressor genes. Turmeric's antioxidant activity and increase of GSH levels are also thought to play a role in its anticancer activity. Curcumin has been found to inhibit cell growth in prostate, colon cancer, breast, GI, GU, lung, leukemia, lymphoma, ovarian, pancreatic, melanoma and sarcoma cells. Curcumin has been shown with isoflavones to synergistically suppress PSA production in prostate cells through anti-androgen effects. Curcumin has been shown to reduce glutathione S-transferase activity, PGE2 production, and levels of M1G in vitro, all indicative of potential preventive use in colorectal cancer.

HUMAN RESEARCH

General Health Benefits

A 2018 overview of systematic reviews for turmeric or curcumin found 22 systematic reviews that met inclusion criteria. Most of the reviews were rated as being of high quality. There was some evidence that curcumin-containing nutraceuticals could exert systemic antioxidant actions, anti-inflammatory actions in arthritis and IBD, lipid level normalization, cardiovascular risk mitigation, and benefits for skin disease. Cautious preliminary positive results were reported for depressive disorders. No efficacy was observed in Alzheimer's disease patients. Curcumin-containing nutraceuticals appear to be safe, as assessed by the adverse events reported in 12 SRs (Pagano et al., 2018).

Ophthalmological Disorders: Anterior Uveitis

A 12-month RCT in patients ($n=106$) with anterior uveitis of different etiologies (autoimmune, herpetic, and miscellaneous) investigated Norflo, a curcumin-phosphatidylcholine complex, plus traditional treatment compared with traditional treatment alone. The number of relapses was reduced ($P < 0.001$) with the addition of the curcumin supplement for all types of uveitis. The supplement was well tolerated and reduced eye discomfort and objective findings in more than 80% of patients after a few weeks of treatment. The authors concluded that curcumin held promise for relapsing inflammatory eye diseases such as anterior uveitis (Allegri et al., 2010).

A 12-week RCT in patients ($n = 32$) with chronic anterior uveitis compared curcumin 375 mg TID alone in PPD-negative patients with curcumin plus antitubercular medication in PPD-positive patients. The patients in both the groups started improving after 2 weeks of treatment, with response in 100% of patients with curcumin alone and 86% of patients with curcumin plus antitubercular medication. After 3 years of follow-up, recurrence rate was 55% with curcumin alone and 36% with curcumin plus antitubercular medication. Loss of vision due to various ocular complications occurred in 22% of patients with curcumin alone and 21% of patients with curcumin plus antitubercular medication. The authors noted that the efficacy of curcumin and recurrences following treatment were comparable to corticosteroid therapy (Lal et al., 1999).

Oral and Dental Disorders

A 2019 systematic review to evaluate the existing evidence for the safety of curcumin in treating oral lichen planus found nine studies ($n = 259$) that met inclusion criteria including six RCTs, two pilot clinical trials, and one case report. Seven studies showed statistically significant differences from baseline in pain severity and clinical appearance of oral lesions after extended treatment with curcumin ($P < 0.05$). Three trials showed no statistically significant differences between curcumin and corticosteroids in pain severity and clinical appearance of oral lesions. The authors concluded that curcumin was a safe adjunctive treatment to reduce pain, burning, and lesions in oral lichen planus (Lv et al., 2019).

A 2016 comprehensive review to summarize and evaluate the evidence on the efficacy of turmeric compared with chlorhexidine in the prevention and treatment of gingivitis found five studies that met inclusion criteria, and all five studies showed that both turmeric

and chlorhexidine significantly decreased plaque index and gingival index. The authors concluded that both chlorhexidine and turmeric could be used as adjuncts to mechanical means in preventing and treating gingivitis (Stoyell et al., 2016).

A 12-week RCT in patients ($n = 40$) with oral lichen planus compared a topical curcumin mucoadhesive paste with topical corticosteroids. The lesion sizes, pain severities, and changes in classification of the lesions improved over baseline in both groups ($P < 0.05$). There were no significant differences in response between curcumin and corticosteroids ($P > 0.05$). The authors concluded that topical curcumin was safe and effective in the treatment of oral lichen planus lesions (Nosratzehi et al., 2018).

A 2-week RCT in patients ($n = 20$) with oral lichen planus compared curcuminoids 2000 mg TID with placebo for efficacy and safety. The changes from baseline for curcumin and placebo, respectively, in median numerical rating scale were -22% and 0%. Changes for erythema were -17% and 0%, changes for ulceration were -14% and 0%, and changes for total Modified Oral Mucositis Index (MOMI) scores were -24 and -3.2. The changes from baseline were not significant with placebo but were significant with curcuminoids. Curcuminoids performed significantly better than placebo for erythema ($P = 0.05$) and total MOMI score ($P = 0.03$) and in the proportion showing improvement in the numerical rating scale (0.8 and 0.3, respectively; $P = 0.02$). The authors concluded that curcuminoids at the dose given were well tolerated and possibly efficacious in oral lichen planus (Chainani-Wu et al., 2012).

An acutely dosed RCT in patients ($n = 90$) who were post-surgical extraction of impacted third molars compared curcumin with mefenamic acid. Pain evaluation was performed immediately after the anesthesia effect disappeared and an hour after each participant took their first, second, and third doses of drugs. Participants in both groups experienced significantly less pain compared with their initial pain level ($P < 0.01$). However, there was significantly less pain with curcumin than with mefenamic acid ($P < 0.01$). The authors concluded that curcumin was effective in treating acute inflammatory pain in post-surgical removal of impacted third molars (Maulina et al., 2018).

A 6-month RCT in children ($n = 45$) undergoing pulpotomy of primary molar teeth compared formocresol (control), propolis extract, turmeric gel, and calcium hydroxide for clinical pulp response and radiographic signs. A comparable clinical and radiographic success rate was seen with all experimental groups compared with the formocresol group. The authors concluded that, given safety concerns of formocresol, the other materials tested could be considered as promising alternatives to formocresol in pediatric endodontic treatment (Hugar et al., 2017).

An acutely dosed RCT in patients ($n = 178$) who had undergone oral and maxillofacial surgery and had dry sockets studied a turmeric dressing plus mustard oil compared with zinc oxide eugenol (ZOE) dressing. There was significant reduction in pain, inflammation, and discomfort after both turmeric and ZOE dressing. Wound healing was faster with turmeric/mustard than with ZOE dressing ($P < 0.05$). Turmeric was well tolerated (Lone et al., 2018).

A study in patients ($n = 30$) who were undergoing root canal treatment investigated turmeric ethanolic extract compared with green tea ethanolic extract and with sodium hypochlorite for antibacterial effectiveness. The most commonly isolated bacteria included *Porphyromonas* sp., *Bacteroides fragilis*, *Peptostreptococcus*, and *Staphylococcus aureus*. Sodium hypochlorite and turmeric showed good antibacterial effect against most of the isolated bacteria. There was no significant difference in antibacterial effect between sodium hypochlorite and turmeric, while green tea was significantly inferior to both sodium hypochlorite and turmeric ($P < 0.001$ for both). The authors concluded that the turmeric irrigant showed promise at eradicating the predominant micro-organisms while avoiding the side effects of sodium hypochlorite (Dhariwal et al., 2016).

A 3-month RCT in patients ($n = 40$) with oral submucous fibrosis studied turmeric plus black pepper compared with black seed. With turmeric and black seed, respectively, mouth-opening improved by 3.85 mm and 3.6 mm ($P < 0.01$), and maximum mouth opening was 8 mm and 7 mm. Burning sensation decreased by 88% and 79% with turmeric and black seed, respectively ($P < 0.01$). SOD levels improved by 0.62 U/mL and 0.74 U/mL with turmeric and black seed, respectively ($P < 0.5$). The authors concluded that both turmeric with black pepper and black seed improved mouth opening, burning sensation, and SOD levels in patients with submucous fibrosis (Pipalia et al., 2016).

Pulmonary Disorders: Asthma

A 6-month RCT in children and adolescents with persistent asthma compared turmeric 30 mg/kg/day with placebo. Overall, both groups experienced reduced frequency of symptoms and interference with normal activity, but no differences were found between the two treatment groups. However, patients receiving turmeric experienced less frequent nighttime awakenings, less frequent use of SABAs, and better disease control after 3 and 6 months. The authors concluded that turmeric led to better disease control than placebo in patients with persistent asthma (Manarin et al., 2019).

Cardiovascular Disorders: Endothelial Dysfunction and Coronary Artery Disease

An 8-week RCT in healthy adults ($n = 59$) compared curcumin 50 mg with curcumin 200 mg and with placebo for effects on endothelial function. Flow-mediated dilation was improved by 3% over placebo with high-dose curcumin ($P = 0.032$) and by 1.7% over placebo with low-dose curcumin ($P = 0.23$). The authors concluded that curcumin may decrease the risk of cardiovascular disease (Oliver et al., 2016).

An 8-week RCT in postmenopausal women ($n = 32$) studied daily curcumin compared with moderate aerobic training and with a control group for effects on flow-mediated dilation as an indicator of endothelial function. Flow-mediated dilation increased significantly and equally in the curcumin and exercise groups, whereas no changes were observed in the control group. The authors concluded that curcumin and aerobic exercise training could increase flow-mediated dilation in postmenopausal women and therefore improve endothelial function (Akazawa et al., 2012).

An acutely dosed RCT in healthy sedentary young men ($n = 14$) compared curcumin with placebo given before exercise for effects of exercise on endothelial function. Brachial artery flow-mediated dilation significantly decreased following eccentric exercise in the placebo group ($P < 0.05$), but acute supplementation with curcumin before exercise nullified this change.

The change in FMD before and after eccentric exercise between the placebo and curcumin groups was significantly different ($P < 0.05$). The authors concluded that curcumin could attenuate the decrease in endothelial function following eccentric exercise (Choi et al., 2019).

A 3-month RCT in patients ($n = 136$) with T2DM compared turmeric with placebo for effect on arterial stiffness and endothelial dysfunction. After 3 months, turmeric produced significant reduction from baseline in carotid-femoral pulse wave velocity ($P = 0.002$), left brachial-ankle pulse wave velocity ($P = 0.001$), aortic augmentation pressure ($P = 0.007$), aortic augmentation index ($P = 0.007$), and aortic augmentation index at a heart rate of 75 ($P = 0.018$) compared with placebo. The authors concluded that 3 months of turmeric significantly decreased arterial stiffness compared with placebo in patients with T2DM (Srinivasan et al., 2019).

A perioperative RCT in patients ($n = 121$) undergoing CABG compared curcuminoids 4 g/day with placebo beginning 3 days before surgery and continuing 5 days postoperatively for effect on subsequent MI incidence. Incidence of in-hospital MI was decreased from 30.0% in the placebo group to 13.1% in the curcuminoid group (AHR = 0.35; $P = 0.038$). Postoperative CRP, MDA, and BNP levels were also lower in the curcuminoid group than in the placebo group. The authors concluded that curcuminoids significantly decreased MI associated with CABG, possibly due to the antioxidant and anti-inflammatory effects of curcuminoids (Wongcharoen et al., 2012).

Cardiometabolic Disorders: Hyperlipidemia and Dyslipidemia

A 2019 systematic review and meta-analysis to evaluate the effects of turmeric and curcuminoids on lipids in patients with metabolic syndrome found 12 RCTs for TG, 14 RCTs for TC, 13 RCTs for LDL-C, and 16 RCTs for HDL-C that met inclusion criteria. The analysis showed that turmeric and curcuminoids could lower blood TG by − 19.1 mg/dL ($P = 0.003$), TC by − 11.4 mg/dL ($P < 0.0001$), and LDL-C by − 9.83 mg/dL ($P = 0.002$) and could increase HDL-C by 1.9 mg/dL ($P = 0.02$). The authors concluded that turmeric and curcuminoids could significantly modulate blood lipids in adults with metabolic diseases (Yuan et al., 2019).

A 2019 systematic review and meta-analysis to determine and clarify the impact of curcuminoids on serum lipid levels found 20 RCTs ($n = 1427$) that met inclusion criteria. Meta-analysis suggested a significant and duration-independent decrease in plasma concentrations of TG (WMD = − 21.36 mg/dL; $P < 0.001$), and an elevation in plasma HDL-C levels (WMD = 1.42 mg/dL; $P = 0.046$). There were no significant changes in levels of LDL-C (WMD = − 5.82 mg/dL; $P = 0.253$) and TC (WMD = − 9.57 mg/dL; $P = 0.098$) (Simental-Mendía et al., 2019).

A 2017 systematic review and meta-analysis to assess the efficacy and safety of turmeric and curcumin for lowering blood lipids in patients at risk of CVD found seven studies ($n = 649$) that met inclusion criteria. Turmeric and curcumin significantly reduced serum LDL-C (SMD = − 0.340; $P < 0.0001$) and TG (SMD = − 0.214; $P = 0.007$) compared with controls. In patients with metabolic syndrome, TC levels were reduced (SMD = − 0.934; $P < 0.0001$). Serum HDL-C levels were not obviously improved. Turmeric and curcumin appeared safe and no serious adverse events were reported in any of the included studies. The authors concluded that turmeric and curcumin could protect patients at risk of CVD through improving serum lipid levels (Qin et al., 2017).

A 2017 systematic review to evaluate polyphenol-rich interventions to attenuate cardiovascular disease risk factors in hemodialysis patients found 12 studies that met inclusion criteria. Polyphenol-rich interventions included soy, cocoa, pomegranate, grape, and turmeric. Polyphenol-rich interventions significantly improved DBP (MD = − 5.62 mmHg; $P = 0.0001$), TG (MD = − 26.52 mg/dL; $P = 0.01$), and myeloperoxidase (MD = − 90.10; $P = 0.0001$). The authors concluded that there was support for the use of polyphenol-rich interventions for improving cardiovascular risk markers in hemodialysis patients (Marx et al., 2017).

Cardiometabolic Disorders: Diabetes, Metabolic Syndrome, and Obesity

A 2019 systematic review to assess the effect of curcumin or turmeric on metabolic factors in patients with metabolic syndrome identified seven trials that met inclusion criteria. The results showed significant improvements of FBG ($P = 0.01$), TG ($P < 0.001$), HDL-C

($P = 0.003$), and DBP ($P = 0.007$) levels. Curcumin was not associated with a significant change in WC measurement ($P = 0.6$) or SBP level ($P = 0.269$). The authors concluded that curcumin improved some components of metabolic syndrome (Azhdari et al., 2019).

A 2019 systematic review with meta-analysis to assess the effects of curcumin or turmeric on BW, BMI, and WC in patients with NAFLD found eight RCTs ($n = 449$) that met inclusion criteria. Overall, the meta-analysis did not show any beneficial effect of turmeric or curcumin supplementation on BW (WMD = -0.54 kg; $P = 0.56$), BMI (WMD = -0.21 kg/m^2; $P = 0.39$), or WC (WMD = -0.88 cm; $P = 0.54$). Subgroup analysis based on participants' baseline BMI, type of intervention, and study duration did not show any significant association in all subgroups. The authors concluded that turmeric or curcumin supplementation had no significant effect on BW, BMI, or WC in patients with NAFLD (Jafarirad et al., 2019).

A 2018 systematic review and meta-analysis to evaluate whether supplementation with turmeric extract, curcuminoids and/or isolated curcumin was effective in decreasing FBS in adults found 11 studies that met inclusion criteria. In the overall analysis, turmeric, curcuminoids, and curcumin all led to a decrease in FBS (-8.88 mg/dL; $P = 0.005$) and A1C (-0.54; $P = 0.049$). Baseline FBS was an important covariate. HOMA-IR was not significantly decreased (-1.26; $P = 0.31$). The authors concluded that isolated curcumin and combined curcuminoids were both effective in lowering the FBS concentrations of individuals with some degree of dysglycemia, but not in non-diabetic individuals. Isolated curcumin led to significant decreases in A1C compared with placebo (de Melo, 2018).

A 2017 systematic review and meta-analysis to evaluate the effect of curcumin on leptin levels found four trials that met inclusion criteria. Meta-analysis showed a significant decrease in plasma leptin concentrations following curcumin treatment (SMD = -0.69; $P = 0.003$). The authors concluded that curcumin supplementation was associated with a decrease in leptin levels, a potential mechanism for the metabolic effects of curcumin (Atkin et al., 2017).

An 8-week RCT in patients ($n = 80$) with hyperlipidemia and T2DM compared turmeric 2100 mg/day with placebo. The turmeric group showed significant decreases in BW, TG, and LDL-C compared with baseline ($P < 0.05$). BMI, TG, and TC decreased significantly with turmeric compared with placebo ($P < 0.05$). The authors concluded that turmeric improved some fractions of the lipid profile and decreased BW in hyperlipidemic patients with T2DM but had no significant effect on glycemic status, CRP, or total antioxidant capacity (Adab et al., 2019).

A 10-week RCT in patients ($n = 44$) with T2DM compared curcumin 1500 mg/day with placebo. TG levels at baseline and at 10 weeks were 124 and 109, respectively, with curcumin ($P < 0.05$). At 10 weeks, hs-CRP was 2.9 and 3.4 with curcumin and placebo, respectively ($P < 0.05$), and adiponectin was 64 and 63 with curcumin and placebo ($P < 0.05$). The authors concluded that curcumin consumption could reduce diabetic complications through decreasing TG levels and inflammation (Adibian et al., 2019).

A 12-week RCT in patients ($n = 118$) with T2DM studied curcumin 1000 mg plus 10 mg of piperine (to enhance absorption) QD compared with placebo for effects on adiponectin, leptin, and ghrelin. Between-group comparison of the magnitude of changes showed serum levels of leptin ($P < 0.001$), TNF-α ($P < 0.001$), and leptin/adiponectin ratios ($P < 0.001$) to be significantly reduced, while serum adiponectin levels were elevated with curcumin over placebo ($P = 0.032$). Changes in serum ghrelin levels did not differ between the study groups ($P = 0.135$). The authors concluded that curcumin increased adiponectin and reduced leptin and leptin/adiponectin levels independent of weight change. They postulated this may reflect a decrease in TNF-α levels (Panahi et al., 2017).

A 10-week RCT in overweight patients ($n = 53$) with T2DM compared curcumin 1500 mg TID with placebo for effects on anthropometric indices, glycemic control, and oxidative stress. With curcumin and placebo, respectively, mean weight changed by -0.64 and 0.19 ($P < 0.05$), WC changed by -1.2 and -0.43 ($P < 0.05$), and FBS changed by -7 and 3 ($P < 0.05$). There were no differences for A1C, MDA, total antioxidant capacity, HOMA-IR, and pancreatic β cell function. The authors concluded that this dose of curcumin had positive effects in reducing FBS and weight in patients with T2DM (Hodaei et al., 2019).

A 4-week RCT in diabetic patients ($n = 60$) on metformin investigated continued treatment with metformin (no change) compared with metformin plus turmeric 2 g/day to investigate the effect of turmeric as an adjuvant to anti-diabetic therapy. The FBS decreased from baseline of 111 to 102 mg/dL with metformin ($P=0.008$) and from 116 to 95 mg/dL with adjuvant turmeric; $P<0.001$). A1C levels decreased from baseline of 7.8% to 7.5% with metformin ($P=0.054$) and from 7.9% to 7.4% with adjuvant turmeric ($P=0.044$) Turmeric was also associated with a reduction in MDA (0.51 μmol/L; $P<0.05$), LDL-C (113.2 mg/dL; $P<0.01$), non-HDL-C (138.3 mg/dL; $P<0.05$), LDL/HDL ratio (3.01; $P<0.01$), and hs-CRP (3.4 mg/dL; $P<0.05$). Total antioxidant status improved (511 μmol/L; $P<0.05$). The author concluded that turmeric as an adjuvant to metformin in diabetics had a beneficial effect on blood glucose, oxidative stress, and inflammation (Selvi et al., 2015).

A 12-week RCT in patients ($n=46$) with NAFLD compared turmeric 500 mg, six capsules per day, with placebo for effects on glycemic regulation. Turmeric consumption decreased serum levels of glucose, insulin, HOMA-IR, and leptin 1.2%, 17.7%, 19.5%, and 21.3%, respectively, compared with placebo ($P<0.05$ for all). Changes in weight, BMI, and liver enzymes were not significantly different between groups. The authors concluded that turmeric improved glucose regulation and leptin levels and may be useful to control NAFLD complications (Navekar et al., 2017).

An 8-week RCT in males ($n=250$) with metabolic syndrome studied turmeric 2.4 g/day compared with black seed 1.5 g/day, with a combination of black seed 900 mg plus turmeric 1.5 g/day, and with placebo. At 4 weeks, compared with baseline, black seed and turmeric individually and in combination showed improvement in BMI, WC, and percent body fat. In addition, the combination lowered FBS and LDL-C compared with placebo. At 8 weeks black seed reduced lipids and FBS, turmeric reduced LDL-C and CRP, and the combination improved all of the above. Compared with placebo, the combination reduced percent body fat, FBS, TC, TG, LDL-C, and CRP in addition to raising HDL-C. The authors concluded that turmeric and black seed improved all parameters of metabolic syndrome when co-administered at lower doses (Amin et al., 2015).

An 8-week polyherbal combination (turmeric, gymnema, *Salacia oblonga*, *Tinospora cordifolia*, *Emblica offinalis*, and *Moringa phytosperma gaertn*)

was given to patients ($n=89$) newly diagnosed with T2DM and healthy age-matched volunteers ($n=50$) at a total dose of 1000 mg/day. Significant improvements were seen in fasting and postprandial glucose, A1C, TC, HDL-C, LDL-C, and TG. There were no adverse effects on liver or kidney function. The authors concluded that short-term supplementation of this polyherbal combination attenuated hyperglycemia and acted as a hypolipidemic agent in patients with diabetes (Kurian et al., 2014).

Gastrointestinal Disorders: Liver Disease and Hepatotoxicity

A 2019 systematic review and meta-analysis to assess the efficacy of turmeric or curcumin on transaminases in NAFLD selected six RCTs that met inclusion criteria. Results from pooled analysis revealed that turmeric or curcumin supplementation reduced ALT (MD = −7.31 UL/L; $P=0.014$) and AST (MD = −4.68 UL/L; $P=0.026$). These significant reductions in serum concentrations of ALT and AST were observed only in studies lasting less than 12 weeks. The authors concluded that turmeric or curcumin might have a favorable effect on ALT and AST in patients with NAFLD (Goodarzi et al., 2019).

A 2019 systematic review to assess the effects of turmeric or curcumin in NAFLD found five RCTs that met inclusion criteria. Trials were small, short, and heterogeneous. Three of the four trials with turmeric or curcumin compared with their own baseline showed significant reductions in ALT, AST, and NAFLD severity grade. Two of the four placebo-controlled trials had significant mean difference reductions in ALT and AST for turmeric or curcumin compared with placebo while two out of three of these trials found significant reductions in NAFLD severity grade. Only one trial used turmeric instead of a curcumin extract and this trial did not demonstrate any differences in ALT, AST, or NAFLD severity between the turmeric and placebo groups. The authors concluded that curcumin extract was promising for reducing ALT, AST, and NAFLD severity (White and Lee, 2019).

A 2019 systematic review to assess the effects of turmeric or curcumin in NAFLD found four RCTs ($n=228$) that met inclusion criteria. There was a trend toward significant reductions of ALT in the subgroup receiving ≥ 1000 mg/day of curcumin (−11.36 IU/L).

There was a significant reduction of AST in studies with 8 weeks of administration (-9.22IU/L). The authors concluded that higher doses of turmeric or curcumin may have favorable effects on NAFLD (Mansour-Ghanaei et al., 2019).

A 3-month pilot RCT in patients ($n = 70$) with liver cirrhosis compared curcumin 1000 mg/day with placebo for the effects of curcumin supplementation in patients with liver cirrhosis. By 3 months, Model for End-stage Liver Disease (MELD) scores and Child-Pugh scores decreased significantly in the curcumin group: MELD(i) (from 15.55 to 12.41; $P < 0.001$), MELD (from 15.31 to 12.03; $P < 0.001$), MELD-Na (from 15.97 to 13.55; $P = 0.001$), and Child-Pugh (from 7.17 to 6.72; $P = 0.051$). The same measurements showed significant increases in the placebo group. Significant differences between the two groups were observed in MELD(i), MELD, MELD-Na, and Child-Pugh scores only after 3 months of intervention ($P < 0.001$ for all). The authors concluded that curcumin showed beneficial effects in decreasing disease activity scores and severity of cirrhosis in patients with cirrhosis (Nouri-Vaskeh et al., 2020).

A 12-week RCT in patients ($n = 92$) with NAFLD and BMI 25–40 compared turmeric 3 g/day with chicory seed 9 g/day, with turmeric 3 g/day plus chicory seed 9 g/day, and with placebo. Significant decreases were observed in BMI and WC with chicory alone or in combination with turmeric compared with placebo ($P < 0.05$). Serum ALP level decreased significantly with turmeric plus chicory combined ($P < 0.05$). HDL-C levels increased with turmeric and with turmeric plus chicory to a greater extent than with placebo ($P < 0.05$). TG/HDL-C and LDL-C/HDL-C ratios decreased significantly with turmeric alone and combined with chicory compared with placebo ($P < 0.05$). The authors concluded that turmeric and chicory seed supplementation could be useful in management of NAFLD risk factors (Ghaffari et al., 2019).

A 12-week RCT in patients ($n = 68$) with β-thalassemia major compared curcumin 500 mg BID with placebo for effect on iron overload. Compared with baseline, curcumin significantly reduced serum levels of free iron (from 2.83 to 2.22 μmol/L; $P = 0.001$), ALT (from 42.86 to 40.60 U/L; $P = 0.018$), and AST (from 49.45 to 46.30 U/L; $P = 0.002$) at 12 weeks. Compared with placebo, curcumin significantly reduced levels of free iron

(2.55 vs 2.22 μmol/L; $P = 0.026$), ALT (45.01 vs 40.60 U/L; $P = 0.004$), and AST (50.99 vs 46.30 U/L; $P = 0.009$) at 12 weeks. The authors concluded that curcumin alleviated iron burden and liver dysfunction in patients with β-thalassemia major (Mohammadi et al., 2018).

An 8-week RCT in patients ($n = 55$) with NAFLD compared curcuminoids 500 mg/day with placebo for effects on disease and inflammation. Curcuminoids were associated with a decrease in weight compared with placebo ($P = 0.016$), and they improved the severity of NAFLD findings on ultrasound ($P = 0.002$). The curcuminoids were associated with improved serum concentrations of TNF-α ($P = 0.024$), MCP-1 ($P = 0.008$), and EGF ($P = 0.0001$). The authors concluded that curcumin could improve serum levels of inflammatory cytokines in subjects with NAFLD and that this might may play a role in the anti-steatotic effects of curcuminoids (Saberi-Karimian et al., 2020).

A 6-month RCT in patients ($n = 528$) on quadruple-then-triple anti-tuberculous treatment compared curcumin-enriched turmeric 500 mg BID plus *Tinospora cordifolia* 500 mg BID (another Ayurvedic herb used for liver disease) for hepatotoxicity. Hepatotoxicity developed in 2 of 316 patients with the herbs and in 27 of 192 patients in the control group ($P < 0.0001$). The treatment group also showed a decrease in ESR compared with the control group. The authors concluded that the herbal formulation prevented hepatotoxicity significantly and improved the disease outcome as well as patient compliance without any toxicity or side effects (Adhvaryu et al., 2008).

Gastrointestinal Disorders: Gallbladder Dysfunction

An acutely dosed RCT in healthy volunteers compared curcumin 20 mg with placebo for gallbladder volume. The gallbladder volume was reduced by 12% and 30% at 30 min and 2 h following curcumin administration ($P < 0.001$), whereas the gallbladder initially contracted by 10% at 30 min with placebo and thereafter relaxed (-18% by 2 h) (Rasyid and Lelo, 1999).

Gastrointestinal Disorders: Peptic Ulcer Disease and Functional Dyspepsia

A 14-day RCT in patients with PUD investigated *Helicobacter pylori* eradication triple therapy with clarithromycin, amoxicillin, and pantoprazole plus curcumin 500 mg/day compared with the same triple therapy plus placebo. The Hong Kong dyspepsia index score decreased by 12.9 and 9.6 points with curcumin and placebo, respectively ($P < 0.001$). Dyspepsia resolved during treatment in 27.6% and 6.7% of patients with curcumin and placebo, respectively ($P = 0.042$). Urea breath test showed equal rates of eradication of *H. pylori* with curcumin and placebo (73.3%). The authors concluded that adding curcumin to standard triple therapy for *H. pylori* improved dyspepsia symptoms but did not enhance eradication of *H. pylori* (Khonche et al., 2016).

A 12-week Phase II clinical trial in patients ($n = 45$) with dyspepsia investigated the effect of turmeric 600 mg five times daily. Of the original 45 patients, 25 were endoscopically proven to have duodenal or gastric ulcers. In these 25 patients, by 4 weeks, 48% of ulcers had healed. By 8 weeks, 18/25 patients had healed their ulcers (13 duodenal and five gastric ulcers). By 12 weeks, 19/25 patients had healed (one additional duodenal ulcer). In the remaining 20 patients who did not have ulcers but had erosions, inflammation, or lesion-free dyspepsia, the abdominal pain and discomfort subsided in the first and second weeks (Prucksunand et al., 2001).

A 60-day open-label study in patients ($n = 311$) with functional dyspepsia investigated the effect of the combination product Cynarepa (dandelion, rosemary, artichoke leaf, and turmeric) on a 10-point scale. The herbal formula resulted in steadily increasing improvement in functional dyspepsia symptoms. A 50% reduction in the total scores of all symptoms was recorded in 38% of patients at 30 days and in 79% at 60 days. At 60 days, TC, LDL-C, and TG levels had decreased by 6%–8% over baseline values ($P \le 0.001$); AST, ALT, and GGT concentrations had diminished by 13–20 U/L ($P < 0.01$) in patients with relatively elevated baseline values (Sannia, 2010).

Gastrointestinal Disorders: Inflammatory Bowel Disease

A 2020 systematic review and meta-analysis to assess the efficacy of curcumin as adjuvant therapy in UC found seven studies ($n = 380$) for inclusion. Clinical remission with curcumin was greater than with placebo (pooled OR = 2.9, $I^2 = 45\%$, $P = 0.002$). Clinical response with curcumin was greater than with placebo

(pooled OR = 2.6, $I^2 = 74\%$, $P = 0.001$). Endoscopic response/remission was greater with curcumin than with placebo (pooled OR = 2.3, $I^2 = 35.5\%$, $P = 0.01$). The authors concluded that the addition of curcumin to mesalamine was associated with roughly threefold better odds of a clinical response over placebo (mesalamine alone), with minimal side effects (Chandan et al., 2020).

A 2020 systematic review of RCTs and prior conflicting meta-analyses was performed to re-evaluate whether turmeric could still be considered in the therapeutic approach for patients with Crohn's disease and ulcerative colitis. They found promising results with the use of curcumin for both UC and CD patients. The authors noted that the findings for curcumin in CD and UC patients were challenging to evaluate due to small sample size, variability in dose and formulation, treatment duration, and route of administration (Goulart et al., 2020).

A 2018 systematic review and meta-analysis to explore the role of curcumin in endoscopic remission of ulcerative colitis found three RCTs ($n = 142$) that met inclusion criteria. Use of curcumin plus mesalamine was associated with increased odds of clinical remission (pooled OR: 6.78, $P = 0.042$). Clinical improvement, endoscopic remission, and improvement rate also trended higher in the curcumin group compared with placebo. The authors concluded that there were higher clinical remission rates when curcumin was used in combination with mesalamine in patients with UC, and that curcumin may decrease healthcare burden and morbidity associated with UC (Iqbal et al., 2018).

A 2017 systematic review to determine whether curcumin as adjuvant therapy could induce or maintain remission in patients with ulcerative colitis found three RCTs that met inclusion criteria. Curcumin was significantly more effective than placebo in all RCTs. The authors concluded that curcumin had the potential to induce and maintain remission in UC patients with no serious side effects and that the efficacy of curcumin could be explained by its anti-inflammatory properties, which inhibit the NF-kB pathway (Simadibrata et al., 2017).

A 6-month RCT in patients ($n = 89$) with quiescent ulcerative colitis studied curcumin 1 g BID plus sulfasalazine or mesalamine compared with placebo plus sulfasalazine or mesalamine. Relapse of disease occurred in 4.65% and 20.5% of patients on turmeric plus drugs and drugs alone, respectively ($P = 0.04$). Recurrence rates investigated with intention to treat showed a significant difference between curcumin and placebo ($P = 0.049$). Curcumin also improved both clinical activity index ($P = 0.038$) and endoscopic index ($P = 0.0001$). The authors concluded that curcumin appeared to be a promising and safe medication for maintaining remission in patients with quiescent UC (Hanai et al., 2006).

An 8-week pilot study in patients ($n = 45$) with distal ulcerative colitis of mild-to-moderate severity studied a standardized curcumin preparation enema (NCB-02) 140 mg in 20 mL water plus oral 5-ASA compared with a placebo enema plus oral 5-ASA. Response to treatment (a reduction in the Ulcerative Colitis Diseases Activity Index by three points) was observed in 56.5% and 36.4% of the curcumin and placebo groups, respectively ($P = 0.175$). Clinical remission was observed in 43.4% and 22.7% of the curcumin and placebo groups, respectively ($P = 0.14$). Improvement on endoscopy was noted in 52.2% and 36% of the curcumin and placebo groups, respectively ($P = 0.29$). Per protocol analysis of clinical response was 92.9% and 50% with curcumin and placebo, respectively ($P = 0.01$). Per protocol analysis of clinical remission was 71.4% and 31.3%, with curcumin and placebo, respectively ($P = 0.03$), and analysis of improvement on endoscopy was 85.7% and 50%, with curcumin and placebo, respectively ($P = 0.04$). The authors concluded that use of this standardized curcumin enema tended to result in greater improvements in disease activity compared with placebo in patients with mild-to-moderate distal UC (Singla et al., 2014).

Renal Disorders: Diabetic Nephropathy and Lupus Nephritis

A 3-month RCT in patients ($n = 24$) with relapsing or refractory biopsy-proven lupus nephritis compared turmeric 500 mg TID with placebo. With turmeric there was a significant decrease in proteinuria from baseline at 1, 2, and 3 months (954.2, 448.8, 235.9, and 260.9 mg/24 h, respectively). Furthermore, SBP and hematuria decreased significantly from baseline with turmeric. Placebo did not exert any statistically significant effect on measured variables. No adverse

effect related to turmeric supplementation was observed during the trial. The authors concluded that short-term turmeric supplementation could decrease proteinuria, hematuria, and SBP in patients with relapsing or refractory lupus nephritis and could safely be used as an adjuvant (Khajehdehi et al., 2011, 2012).

A 2-month RCT in patients ($n = 40$) with T2DM and nephropathy compared turmeric 500 mg TID with placebo for effects on serum and urinary TGF-β, IL-8, TNF-α, and proteinuria. Urinary protein decreased from 4328 to 2354 mg/24 h and from 4695 to 4169 mg/24 h with turmeric and placebo respectively ($P < 0.001$ and $P = 0.43$, respectively). Serum levels of TGF-β and IL-8 and urinary levels of IL-8 also decreased significantly from baseline with turmeric. No adverse effects related to turmeric supplementation were observed during the trial. The authors concluded that short-term turmeric supplementation could attenuate proteinuria, TGF-β, and IL-8 in patients with overt type 2 diabetic nephropathy and could be administered as a safe adjuvant therapy for these patients (Khajehdehi et al., 2012).

Women's Disorders: Lactational mastitis

A 3-day RCT in breastfeeding women ($n = 63$) with mastitis studied curcumin topical cream, two pumps TID for 3 days compared with a topical moisturizer. Compared with the moisturizer, curcumin was associated with significantly lower scores for tension, erythema, and pain after 72 h of treatment ($P < 0.001$ for all parameters) and a lower rate of moderate ($P = 0.019$) and mild ($P = 0.002$) mastitis. The authors concluded that topical curcumin decreased the markers of lactational mastitis within 72 hours of administration without side effects (Afshariani et al., 2014).

Women's Genitourinary Disorders: Cervical Intraepithelial Neoplasia

A 12-week trial in women ($n = 21$) with persistent LSIL following antimicrobial therapy (if indicated) assessed the effect of NBFR-03, a supercritical turmeric oil extract, 0.2 g orally BID for 12 weeks. At 12 weeks, pap smears, colposcopy, clinical biochemistry, urinalysis, and assessment of serum IL-6 were repeated. No patient progressed to a higher-grade lesion. Regression to atypia, ASCUS, or an inflammatory pattern occurred in 16/21; three persisted as LSIL, one discontinued early because of itching, and one did not start. None developed any significant abnormality clinically or biochemically. Micrometry showed a significant reduction in nuclear diameter and nucleocytoplasmic ratio after treatment ($P < 0.02$ and $P < 0.05$, respectively). Serum IL-6 levels showed a significant decline (Joshi et al., 2016).

A 36-month follow-up of the above study was undertaken in 18 of the subjects as well as 10 case controls who had received only standard therapy with targeted antimicrobials. None of the curcumin-treated patients developed HSIL or cancer. All 15 of those who showed regression in the initial phase of the trial remained free of LSIL from 6 to 36 months following turmeric treatment. LSIL recurred in one patient at 10 months, and this regressed to mild atypia after eight more weeks of turmeric oil. In the control group, persistence of LSIL occurred in 5/10 cases up to 36 months. The authors concluded that addition of turmeric to standard treatment was beneficial for LSIL management (Joshi et al., 2011).

Women's Genitourinary Disorders: Polycystic Ovary Syndrome

A pilot RCT in healthy premenopausal women ($n = 40$) studied a combination botanical supplement (turmeric, dandelion, schisandra, rosemary, milk thistle, and *Cynara scolymus*) compared with dietary changes (three servings per day of crucifers or dark leafy greens, 30 g/day of fiber, 1-2 L/day of water, and limiting caffeine and alcohol consumption to one serving per week) and with placebo for hormonal effects. During the early follicular phase, compared with placebo, the polyherbal product decreased DHEA (-13.2%; $P = 0.02$), DHEA-S (-14.6%; $P = 0.07$), androstenedione (-8.6%; $P = 0.05$), and estrone-sulfate (-12.0%; $P = 0.08$). When comparing dietary changes with placebo, no statistically significant differences were observed. There were no substantial effects on estrone-sulfate, total estradiol, free estradiol, testosterone, SHBG, insulin, IGF-I, or leptin. The authors concluded that early-follicular phase androgens were decreased with the polyherbal product (Greenlee et al., 2007).

Men's Genitourinary Disorders: Chronic Prostatitis and Prostate-Specific Antigen

A 3-month Phase II clinical trial in patients ($n = 60$) with chronic prostatitis/chronic pelvic pain syndrome type III compared rectal suppositories of curcumin 350 mg plus calendula 80 mg QD with placebo suppositories. The curcumin group had a significant improvement in NIH-Chronic Prostatitis Symptoms Index (from 20.5 to 15; $P < 0.01$), IIEF-5 (from 18.5 to 22; $P < 0.01$), Premature Ejaculation Diagnostic Tool (from 11 to 5.5; $P < 0.01$), peak flow (from 14 to 16.8; $P < 0.01$), and VAS (from 7.5 to 1.0; $P < 0.01$), with all changes being significantly different from the placebo group. The authors concluded that there was clinical efficacy with a combined curcumin and calendula suppository in patients with CP/CPPSIII (Morgia et al., 2017).

A 30-day open-label study in patients ($n = 50$) with a first PSA over 4 ng/mL or a PSA velocity > 0.75 mL/year compared turmeric extract BID to assess the effect on the total and free PSA. Baseline and 30-day PSA values were 6.84 ng/mL and 4.65 ng/mL, respectively ($P < 0.0001$). Free/total PSA ratio was 16.85 and 19.68 at baseline and 30 days, respectively ($P < 0.0036$). The authors concluded that turmeric extract lowered PSA after 30 days but that the PSA reduction did not assist in excluding prostate cancer through free/total PSA determination (Fabiani et al., 2018).

Musculoskeletal Disorders: Arthritis, Osteoarthritis, and Musculoskeletal Pain

A 2018 systematic review looked at trials comparing curcuminoids (from turmeric) or frankincense formulations with placebo or NSAIDs for OA. The authors included 11 RCTs ($n = 1009$) and found that both curcuminoid and frankincense formulations were statistically significantly more effective than placebo for pain relief and functional improvement. There were no significant differences between curcuminoids or frankincense and placebo in safety outcomes. Curcuminoids showed no statistically significant differences in efficacy outcomes compared with NSAIDs; patients receiving curcuminoids were significantly less likely to experience gastrointestinal adverse events. No RCTs compared frankincense against approved NSAIDs (Bannuru et al., 2018).

A 2018 systematic review to investigate the efficacy and safety of dietary supplements for patients with osteoarthritis found 69 studies that met inclusion criteria. Of the 20 supplements investigated, seven (collagen hydrolysate, passion fruit peel extract, turmeric, curcumin, frankincense, pycnogenol and L-carnitine) demonstrated large and clinically important effects for pain reduction and improved function at short term (effect size > 0.80). Another six (undenatured type II collagen, avocado soybean unsaponifiables, MSM, diacerein, glucosamine, and chondroitin) revealed statistically significant improvements in pain and function but were of unclear clinical importance. Only green-lipped mussel extract and undenatured type II collagen had clinically important effects on pain and function at medium term. For long-term pain reduction, there were no supplements identified with clinically important effects. Chondroitin demonstrated statistically significant but not clinically important structural benefits. There were no differences between supplements and placebo for safety outcomes, except for diacerein. The authors concluded that supplements provided moderate and clinically meaningful treatment effects on pain and function in patients with hand, hip, or knee osteoarthritis at short term, although the quality of evidence was very low (Liu et al., 2018).

A 2016 systematic review and meta-analysis to evaluate the efficacy of turmeric extracts and curcumin for treating arthritis symptoms found eight RCTs that met selection criteria. Pain was reduced with turmeric or curcumin compared with placebo on the VAS in three trials (MD = − 2.04; $P < 0.00001$). Meta-analysis of four other studies showed a decrease of WOMAC with turmeric or curcumin treatment (MD = − 15.36; $P = 0.009$). There was no significant mean difference in PVAS between turmeric or curcumin and pain medicine in meta-analysis of five studies. The authors concluded that there was support for the efficacy of turmeric extract (about 1000 mg/day of curcumin) in the treatment of arthritis (Daily et al., 2016).

A three-month RCT in patients (n=150) with knee OA compared low and high doses of bio-optimized (enhanced absorption) turmeric with placebo. Low and high doses of turmeric showed a greater decrease of Patient Global Assessment of Disease Activity scores compared with placebo. Levels of sColl2-1 (a biomarker of cartilage degradation) were present in placebo and low-dose, but not high-dose turmeric, but these levels decreased to similar levels as the study progressed. Pain reduction at day 90 with low- and high-dose turmeric (− 29.5 mm and − 36.5 mm, respectively) was greater than with placebo (− 8 mm; $P = 0.018$). The global Knee Injury and Osteoarthritis Outcome Score significantly decreased overtime, but changes were comparable across treatment arms. The ratio of patients with adverse events related to the product was similar in the placebo and treatment groups, but the number of adverse events linked to the product was higher in the high-dose turmeric group compared with the placebo ($P = 0.012$). The authors concluded that bio-optimized turmeric was safe and well tolerated, that there was a rapid reduction in pain, and that there were positive trends for reduction in disease activity and levels of a cartilage degeneration biomarker (Henrotin et al., 2019).

A 4-month RCT in patients (n = 160) with knee OA compared a turmeric extract with placebo along with a standard drug regimen in both groups. Improvements in WOMAC and VAS scores were significantly greater with turmeric than with placebo. Levels of IL-1β, ROS, and MDA were also significantly improved ($P < 0.05$). The authors concluded that turmeric brought clinical improvement in patients with knee OA likely due to reduction in inflammation and oxidative stress (Srivastava et al., 2016).

A 60-day RCT in patients (n = 50) with knee OA studied Curene, a bioavailable formulation of turmeric, 500 mg QD compared with placebo. The reduction from baseline in WOMAC total and subscale scores and the VAS score resulted in statistically significant difference when compared with placebo. Curene was also found to be safe and well tolerated as there was no incidence of treatment related adverse events. The authors concluded that this bioavailable form of turmeric safely produced significant and clinically meaningful reductions in pain and stiffness and improvement in physical functioning in patients with knee OA (Panda et al., 2018).

A four-week RCT in patients (n = 367) with knee OA compared turmeric 1500 mg/day with ibuprofen 1200 mg/day for pain reduction. The mean of all WOMAC scores at weeks 0, 2, and 4 compared with baseline showed significant improvement in both groups. The mean differences of WOMAC total, WOMAC pain, and WOMAC function scores at week 4 with turmeric extracts were noninferior to those with ibuprofen ($P = 0.010$, $P = 0.018$, and $P = 0.010$, respectively), except for the WOMAC stiffness subscale, which showed a trend toward significance ($P = 0.060$). The number of events of abdominal pain or discomfort was significantly higher with ibuprofen than with turmeric ($P=0.046$). Satisfaction with treatment occurred in 97% of patients, with self-rated global improvement in two-thirds of patients. The authors concluded that turmeric was as effective as ibuprofen for knee OA with fewer GI adverse events (Kuptniratsaikul et al., 2014).

A 28-day RCT in patients ($n=140$) with knee OA evaluated a curcuminoid complex 500 mg plus diclofenac 50 mg BID compared with the same dose of diclofenac alone. Both treatment groups showed improvement in the Knee Injury and OA Outcome score (KOOS) at 14 and 28 days. Patients receiving the curcuminoid complex plus diclofenac showed significantly superior improvement in KOOS subscales for pain and quality of life ($P<0.001$) when compared with diclofenac alone. Rescue analgesics were required in 3% of the curcuminoid group and 17% of the diclofenac-alone group. H2 blockers were required by 6% and 28% of the curcuminoid and diclofenac-alone groups, respectively ($P<0.001$). AEs occurred in 13% and 38% of the curcuminoid and diclofenac-alone groups, respectively ($P<0.001$). Patient's and physician's global assessment of therapy favored curcuminoid complex plus diclofenac. The authors concluded that the combination of curcuminoid complex and diclofenac showed a greater improvement in pain and functional capacity with better tolerability than diclofenac alone and could be a better alternative treatment option in symptomatic management of knee OA (Shep et al., 2020).

A 12-week RCT in patients ($n=30$) with knee OA studied turmeric 350 mg plus frankincense 150 mg BID compared with celecoxib for safety and efficacy. In the herbal group 85.7% and 21.4% of the subjects were in the moderate/severe category at baseline and at 12 weeks, respectively. In the celecoxib group, 78.57% and 50% of patients were in the moderate/severe category at baseline and 12 weeks, respectively. Statistically significant improvements in the proportion of individuals scoring a walking distance of > 1000 m were observed within the two groups over a period of 12 weeks. In the herbal group, 92.8% of subjects could walk > 1000 m compared with 85.7% in the celecoxib group following treatment, with the difference between groups being non-significant. Joint-line tenderness decreased more with the herbal product than with the drug. Crepitus and tenderness decreased signifi-

cantly and equally in both groups. The treatment was well tolerated and did not produce any adverse effect in patients (Kizhakkedath, 2013).

A pilot study in patients ($n=42$) with acute or chronic degenerative arthritis of the spine or limbs investigated AINAT, a combination of turmeric, devil's claw, and bromelain, 650 mg 2 capsules TID for acute pain and BID for chronic pain. The VAS pain score for acute pain decreased from 69.1 mm to 42 mm at 15 days, and for chronic pain the VAS score decreased from 68.0 mm to 37.8 mm at 60 days. This reduction of pain, as a percentage as well as an absolute value, corresponded to the required definition of minimum clinically important improvement (MCII), particularly in patients with chronic joint pain. At the endpoint, most of the patients in both groups reached the level of pain defined as patient acceptable symptom state (PASS). No withdrawals occurred due to treatment side effects. The authors concluded that acute and chronic joint pain improvement was clinically relevant with this herbal combination which may be a safe alternative to NSAIDs in patients with DJD (Conrozier et al., 2014).

A 32-week RCT in patients ($n=90$) with OA studied an Ayurvedic combination containing turmeric, ashwagandha, frankincense, and ginger compared with placebo. The mean reduction in pain VAS for the herbal combination and placebo, respectively, was 2.7 and 1.3 at week 16. At week 32 the pain VAS reduction for the herbal combination and placebo, respectively, was 2.8 and 1.8 ($P<0.05$). The improvements in the WOMAC scores at week 16 and week 32 were also significantly superior ($P<0.01$) with the combination herbal product. Both groups reported mild adverse events without any significant difference between groups (Chopra et al., 2004).

Musculoskeletal Disorders: Postoperative Pain

A perioperative RCT in patients ($n=60$) undergoing laparoscopic gynecologic surgery studied a curcuminoid extract 250 mg QID on postoperative days 1-3 compared with a control group for postoperative pain. The median VAS score 24 h after surgery was 3 in the intervention group and 4.5 in the control group ($P=0.001$). The median VAS at 72 h after surgery was 1 in the intervention group and 2 in the control group ($P<0.001$). The authors concluded that curcuminoids could be an effective supplement to reduce pain severity postoperatively following laparoscopic gynecologic surgery (Phoolcharoen et al., 2019).

A 6-month RCT in patients with full-thickness supraspinatus tendon tear undergoing arthroscopy investigated Tendisulfur, a combination of frankincense and turmeric, compared with placebo starting 3 weeks before surgery. At week 1 postoperatively, the overall pain scores were significantly lower with the herbal product than with placebo ($P = 0.0477$), and at week 2 the scores continued to be lower but not significantly so with the herbal product ($P = 0.0988$). Thereafter the pain scores were not different between groups. The authors concluded that this herbal combination, added to standard analgesics, was beneficial for postoperative rotator cuff pain, alleviating short-term and partially mid-term pain (Merolla et al., 2015).

Neurological Disorders: Migraine Headaches

A 2-month RCT in patients ($n = 74$) with episodic migraine headaches investigated omega-3 fatty acids compared with nano-curcumin, with a combination of the two, and with placebo for expression of COX-2 and iNOS in peripheral monocytes and serum. The results showed that omega-3 fatty acids and nano-curcumin reinforced each other's effects in the downregulation of COX-2 and iNOS mRNA and serum levels. In addition, the combination of significantly reduced the frequency, severity, and duration of headaches ($P < 0.05$). The authors concluded that this combination of supplements could be considered for migraine prevention (Abdolahi et al., 2019).

Neurological Disorders: Neurodegenerative Diseases

A 2019 systematic review to assess the impact of curcumin on serum BDNF levels found four RCTs ($n = 139$) that met inclusion criteria. Curcumin supplementation dose and duration ranged from 200 to 1820 mg/day and 8 to 12 weeks, respectively. Curcumin supplementation significantly increased serum BDNF levels (WMD = 1789 pg/mL; $P < 0.01$). Subgroup analysis showed that sex, mean age of participants, curcumin dosage, and trial duration were potential sources of heterogeneity. The authors concluded that

the significant positive impact of curcumin supplementation on BDNF levels indicated its potential use for neurological disorders that are associated with low BDNF levels (Sarraf et al., 2019).

Psychiatric Disorders: Anxiety and Depression

A 2017 systematic review and meta-analysis to assess the efficacy of turmeric, curcumin, or curcuminoids for depression found six trials ($n = 377$) that met inclusion criteria. In patients with depression, the pooled SMD from baseline for HAM-D scores was -0.344 ($P = 0.002$). Significant anti-anxiety effects were also reported in three of the trials. The authors concluded that curcumin appeared to be safe, well tolerated, and efficacious among depressed patients (Ng et al., 2017).

A 2016 systematic review and meta-analysis to assess the antidepressant effect of curcumin in patients with major depressive disorders found six RCTs that met inclusion criteria. Curcumin was associated with a significantly higher reduction in depression symptoms (SMD = -0.34; $P = 0.002$). Curcumin had the highest effect in middle-aged patients (SMD = -0.36; $P = 0.002$), for longer duration of treatment (SMD = -0.40; $P = 0.001$), and at higher doses (SMD = -0.36; $P = 0.002$). Conventional curcumin-piperine formulas were as effective as newer "bio-optimized" formulations. The authors concluded that there was supporting evidence that curcumin reduces depressive symptoms in patients with major depression (Al-Karawi et al., 2016).

A 12-week RCT in patients ($n = 123$) with major depressive disorder compared curcumin 250 mg BID with curcumin 500 mg BID, with curcumin 250 mg BID plus saffron 15 mg BID, and with placebo. Combined depressive symptom score improvements of the active drug treatments were significantly greater than placebo ($P = 0.031$). The Spielberger State-Trait Anxiety Inventory also showed greater improvements with active drug treatments than with placebo ($P < 0.001$) and superior improvements in STAI-state ($P < 0.001$). Active drug treatments had greater efficacy in people with atypical depression compared with the remainder of patients (response rates of 65% and 35% respectively; $P = 0.012$). No differences were found between the differing doses of curcumin and the curcumin plus saffron combination. The authors concluded that different doses of curcumin with or without saffron were effective in reducing depression and anxiety symptoms in patients with MDD (Lopresti and Drummond, 2017).

A 6-week RCT in patients ($n = 60$) with MDD compared curcumin 1000 mg/day with fluoxetine 20 mg/day and with a combination of the two for safety and efficacy. The proportion of responders as measured by the HAM-D17 scale was 62.5%, 64.7%, and 77.8% with curcumin, fluoxetine, and the combination, respectively, a nonsignificant difference ($P = 0.58$). The mean change in HAM-D17 score at the end of 6 weeks was comparable in all three groups ($P = 0.77$). Curcumin was well tolerated by all the patients. The authors concluded that curcumin may be used safely and effectively in patients with MDD who lack suicidal ideation or psychotic disorders (Sanmukhani et al., 2014).

Dermatological Disorders: Psoriasis

A 2016 systematic review to examine the evidence for the use of both topical and ingested turmeric or curcumin to modulate skin health and function found 18 studies that met inclusion criteria: nine studied ingestion, eight studied topical application, and one studied both ingested and topical application of turmeric or curcumin. Statistically significant improvement in skin disease severity in the turmeric or curcumin treatment groups compared with control groups was present in 10 studies. Skin conditions examined include acne, alopecia, atopic dermatitis, facial photoaging, oral lichen planus, pruritus, psoriasis, radiodermatitis, and vitiligo. The authors concluded that there was evidence that turmeric and curcumin products and supplements, both oral and topical, may provide therapeutic benefits for skin health (Vaughn et al., 2016).

A 9-week RCT in patients ($n = 40$) with mild-to-moderate scalp psoriasis compared turmeric tonic BID with placebo applied topically. Compared with the placebo, turmeric tonic significantly reduced the erythema, scaling and induration of lesions, and quality of life was improved ($P < 0.05$). The authors concluded that turmeric tonic applied to the scalp was beneficial and could be considered as a treatment for scalp psoriasis (Bahraini et al., 2018).

A 10-week RCT in patients ($n = 21$) with moderate to severe plaque psoriasis compared a turmeric extract plus real or simulated visible light phototherapy to

affected areas while the rest of the body surface was treated with UVA radiation. No patients in the real light therapy group showed "moderate" or "severe" plaques after the treatment, in contrast to the patients in the simulated light therapy group ($P < 0.01$). Lesions within the experimental area showed a response in 81% of the patients in the real light therapy group and 30% of the patients in the simulated light therapy group. The authors concluded that moderate to severe plaque psoriasis should show a therapeutic response to orally administered turmeric if activated with visible light phototherapy (Carrion-Gutierrez et al., 2015).

A 9-week left-right comparison RCT in patients ($n = 40$) with mild-to-moderate plaque psoriasis compared a novel topical turmeric microemulgel preparation with placebo for efficacy. The results showed improvement in clinical and quality of life parameters with turmeric compared with placebo. Mean PASI scores decreased from 3.6 to 1.4 and from 3.5 to 3.2 with turmeric and placebo, respectively ($P < 0.05$). The reported side effects were minor. The authors concluded that the turmeric microemulgel may well be considered as an alternative or as add-on therapy for patients with plaque psoriasis (Sarafian et al., 2015).

Inflammation

A 2019 systematic review to assess the impact of turmeric or curcumin on inflammatory markers found 19 RCTs that met inclusion criteria, including patients with rheumatic diseases, advanced chronic kidney disease with hemodialysis, metabolic syndrome, and cardiovascular diseases. Turmeric was the intervention in five RCTs ($n = 356$) and curcumin or curcuminoids in 14 RCTs ($n = 988$). In comparison with controls, turmeric or curcumin did not reach statistical significance in decreasing levels of CRP (MD $= -2.71$ mg/L; $P = 0.08$), hs-CRP (MD $= -1.44$ mg/L; $P = 0.06$), IL-1β (MD $= -4.25$ pg/mL; $P = 0.36$), IL-6 (MD $= -0.71$ pg/mL; $P = 0.15$), and TNF-α (MD $= -1.23$ pg/mL; $P = 0.18$). There were no differences between turmeric and curcumin interventions. The authors concluded that turmeric or curcumin did not decrease several inflammatory markers in patients with chronic inflammatory diseases (White et al., 2019).

A 2016 systematic review and meta-analysis to evaluate the efficacy of curcuminoids on IL-6 levels found nine RCTs that were eligible for meta-analysis.

There was a significant reduction of circulating IL-6 concentrations following curcuminoid supplementation (WMD = -0.60 pg/mL; $P = 0.011$), and there was a significant association between the IL-6-lowering activity and baseline IL-6 concentration (slope: -0.51; $P = 0.005$). Dose and duration of curcuminoid treatment did not alter the finding. The authors concluded that curcumin has a significant effect of lowering IL-6 levels, more so in patients with higher degrees of systemic inflammation (Derosa et al., 2016).

A 2016 systematic review and meta-analysis to evaluate the efficacy of curcumin supplementation on circulating levels of TNF-α found eight RCTs that met criteria for meta-analysis. There was a significant reduction of circulating TNF-α concentrations following curcumin supplementation (WMD = -4.69 pg/mL; $P < 0.001$). The effect size was robust and there was no association with dose or duration of curcumin treatment. The authors concluded that curcumin had a significant effect in lowering TNF-α concentration (Sahebkar et al., 2016).

A 12-week RCT in middle-aged and elderly overweight adults ($n = 90$) with preHTN/mild HTN compared turmeric hot water extract 900 mg tablets with placebo for anti-inflammatory effects. Compared with the placebo group, the turmeric group had significantly lower serum levels of CRP, TNF-α, IL-6, soluble VCAM-1, glucose, A1C, and TG as well as higher serum levels of HDL-C. The turmeric group also showed significant improvement of Short-Form Health Survey scores (for general health, vitality, mental health, and mental summary component) and Profile of Mood State scores for positive mood states (vigor-activity and friendliness). The authors concluded that turmeric hot water extract could ameliorate chronic low-grade inflammation, thus contributing to the improvement of associated metabolic disorders and general health (Uchio et al., 2019).

Autoimmune Disorders: Rheumatoid Arthritis

A 90-day RCT in patients ($n = 35$) with active RA compared curcumin 250 mg BID with curcumin 500 mg BID (each in a novel turmeric matrix) and with placebo for impact on disease activity. Both low and high doses of curcumin produced statistically significant changes in clinical symptoms and reductions in ESR, CRP, and RF values compared with placebo. The authors concluded that curcumin in a novel turmeric matrix

had analgesic and anti-inflammatory effects in the management of RA at a dose as low as 250 mg BID (Amalraj et al., 2017).

Oncologic Disorders: Mucositis and Hand-Foot Syndrome

A 2019 systematic review to evaluate the effect of turmeric or curcumin topical gel or mouthwash in oral mucositis in cancer patients undergoing chemo and/or radiotherapy included four randomized and one nonrandomized clinical trial in the analysis. Patients treated with turmeric or curcumin experienced reduced grade of mucositis, pain, erythema intensity, and ulcerative area. The authors concluded that topical application of turmeric or curcumin may be effective in controlling signs and symptoms of oral mucositis (Normando et al., 2019).

A 6-week open-label pilot study in patients ($n = 40$) who were initiating treatment with capecitabine for breast or GI cancers investigated turmeric 2 g BID for the prevention of capecitabine-induced hand-foot syndrome (HFS). After the first cycle of capecitabine treatment, 27.5% patients developed HFS with 10% having grade 2 HFS. There were no correlations between the inflammatory markers tested and HFS. The authors concluded that turmeric produced lower rates and grades of HFS when added to capecitabine therapy (Scontre et al., 2018).

Oncologic Disorders: Colorectal Cancer and Pancreatic Cancer

A Phase IIa open-label RCT in patients ($n = 28$) with metastatic colorectal cancer investigated FOLFOX (folinic acid/5-fluorouracil/oxaliplatin chemotherapy) compared with FOLFOX plus curcumin 2 g/day to assess safety, efficacy, quality of life, neurotoxicity, curcuminoids, and C-X-C-motif chemokine ligand 1 (implicated in melanoma pathogenesis). Addition of daily oral curcumin to FOLFOX chemotherapy was safe and tolerable (primary outcome). Similar adverse event profiles were observed for both arms. In the intention-to-treat population, progression-free median survival was 171 and 291 days for FOLFOX alone and FOLFOX plus curcumin, respectively. Median overall survival was 200 and 502 days for FOLFOX alone FLOFOX plus curcumin, respectively. There was no significant difference between arms for quality of life ($P = 0.248$) or neurotoxicity ($P = 0.223$). Curcumin glucuronide was detectable at concentrations > 1.00 pmol/mL in 15 of 18 patients receiving the combination. Curcumin did not significantly alter CXCL1 over time ($P = 0.712$). The authors concluded that curcumin was a safe and tolerable adjunct to FOLFOX in patients with metastatic colorectal cancer (Howells et al., 2019).

A Phase I and Phase II trial in patients ($n = 21$) with pancreatic cancer who were gemcitabine-resistant investigated the safety and feasibility of combination therapy using curcumin 8 g/day with gemcitabine-based chemotherapy. No dose-limiting toxicities were observed in the Phase I study and oral curcumin 8 g/day was selected as the recommended dose for the Phase II study. No patients were withdrawn from this study because of the intolerability of curcumin, which met the primary endpoint of the Phase II study. Median survival time after initiation of curcumin was 161 days, and 1-year survival was 19%. The authors concluded that combination therapy using oral curcumin 8 g/day with gemcitabine-based chemotherapy was safe and feasible in patients with pancreatic cancer and warrants further investigation into its efficacy (Kanai et al., 2011).

A clinical trial in patients ($n = 17$) with advanced pancreatic cancer assessed the activity and feasibility of combining oral curcumin 8 g/day with gemcitabine 1000 mg/m^2 IV weekly for 3 of 4 weeks. Intractable abdominal fullness or pain caused five of the patients to stop curcumin, and two patients to reduce the dose to 4 g/day. In the remaining 11 patients, partial response occurred in one patient (9%); stable disease occurred in four patients (36%) and disease progression occurred in 6 (55%). Time to tumor progression was 1-12 months and overall survival was 1–24 months, with a median of 5 months. The authors concluded that low tolerance of the high dose of curcumin required to achieve systemic effect may be an obstacle for use of curcumin in this setting (Epelbaum et al., 2010).

ACTIVE CONSTITUENTS

- Amino acid deriviatives: turmerin (antioxidant, anti-mutagen)
  - Glucosinolates: *p*-tolymethylcarbinol (increases gastrin, secretin, bicarbonate, pancreatic enzyme secretion)

- Phenolic compounds
  - Phenylpropanoids
    - Curcuminoids (weakly estrogenic, neuroprotective, hepatoprotective, digestive bitter, choleretic, anti-inflammatory, antioxidant, immunomodulatory, antiproliferative, chemopreventive, antineoplastic): curcumin, cyclocurcumin, calebin A, bisdemethoxycurcumin, demethoxycurcumin
- Terpenes
  - Sesquiterpenes: zingiberene (carminative), elemene
- Aromatic compounds (anti-inflammatory, anticancer): zingiberene, turmerones (increase absorption of curcumin), atlantone, elemene, furanodiene, curdione, bisacurone, curcumenone, curcumenol, germacrone

TURMERIC COMMONLY USED PREPARATIONS AND DOSAGE (FOR ADULTS UNLESS OTHERWISE SPECIFIED)

The following are examples of some available formulations and ranges of dosing for commercial herbal products. See Part III Introduction "How to prescribe medicinal herbs" for further guidance on herbal advising and prescribing.

Root

- Stir-fried root added to food per recipe (the oils in the root enhance bioavailability of curcumin)
- Tincture of turmeric root (1:4, 70%): 0.5 to 1.5 mL TID
- Standardized powdered extract (standardized to 95% curcumin): 1000 mg (1/2 tsp) QD
- Capsule or tablet of standardized extract of turmeric root (50-500 mg of which is standardized to 95% curcuminoids with added piperine): 300-1000 mg QD-TID
- Curcumin 1500 mg plus piperine 60 mg QD (Adding piperine (from black pepper) is important to reduce the rapid hepatic and intestinal glucuronidation and excretion of curcumin. In one human study after a dose of 2 g curcumin alone, serum levels were either undetectable or extremely low. Concomitant administration of piperine 20 mg produced an increase in bioavailability of 2000%.

■ Golden Milk: Whisk 1 cup coconut milk, a dash of cinnamon, 1/2–1 tsp turmeric powder, 1/2 tsp ginger powder or cardamom, 1 T honey, and 1/4 tsp black peppercorns in a small saucepan; bring to a low boil. Reduce heat and simmer until flavors have melded, about 10 min.

SAFETY AND PRECAUTION

Side Effects

Topical use may cause contact dermatitis. An overview of systematic reviews found only mild adverse effects from turmeric (Posadzki et al., 2013).

Case Reports

■ Transient elevations in hepatic transaminases and hepatotoxicity have been reported.
■ A physician taking high doses for arthritis developed iron deficiency. (Turmeric binds iron in the gut.)
■ A woman developed a reversible yellow discoloration of the skin after taking 500 mg/day of curcumin for 4 months.

Toxicity

No significant toxicity has been reported following either acute or chronic administration of turmeric extracts at standard doses. At extremely high doses (100 mg/kg), curcumin may be ulcerogenic and is toxic to human dermal fibroblasts. A study in mice showed that higher doses thought to be cancer preventive were hepatotoxic.

A study in humans given curcumin 6 g/day for 4-7 weeks did not show toxic effects.

Pregnancy

Considered safe in culinary use. Avoid large doses as may cause uterine contractions. No data for breastfeeding.

Disease Interactions

Caution with cholelithiasis or biliary obstruction due to increase in bile flow.

Drug Interactions

■ CYP: Inhibits CYPP450
■ Pgp: Inhibits P-glycoprotein

■ Antagonistic to ranitidine
■ May increase levels of midazolam, celiprolol, verapamil, tacrolimus, acetaminophen, ibuprofen, aspirin
■ Generally, avoid with chemotherapy as has been shown to interact with chemotherapy drugs like cyclophosphamide and doxorubicin. May inhibit antitumor action of cyclophosphamide. Inhibits apoptosis of several chemotherapeutic drugs. However, has also been shown to have synergism in vitro for glioblastoma, breast cancer, and several other cancers. Further studies are warranted.
■ May increase risk of bleeding with anticoagulants/antiplatelets. However, one clinical trial was reassuring in this regard.

A crossover RCT in healthy volunteers ($n = 25$) compared turmeric alone, turmeric plus aspirin, angelica alone, angelica plus aspirin, Asian ginseng alone, and Asian ginseng plus aspirin for anticoagulation effects. Each phase lasted 3 weeks with a 2-week washout between phases. In 5/24 subjects on turmeric, 2/24 subjects on angelica, and 1/23 subjects on Asian ginseng there was an inhibition in arachidonic-acid induced platelet aggregation. Combination of these herbal products with aspirin respectively did not further aggravate platelet inhibition caused by aspirin. None of the herbs impaired PT/APTT or thrombin generation. There was no significant bleeding manifestation. The authors concluded that there was good evidence for lack of bleeding risks with turmeric, angelica, and Asian ginseng used alone or in combination with aspirin (Fung et al., 2017).

REFERENCES

Abdolahi M, Jafarieh A, Sarraf P, et al. The neuromodulatory effects of ω-3 fatty acids and nano-curcumin on the COX-2/iNOS network in migraines: a clinical trial study from gene expression to clinical symptoms. Endocr Metab Immune Disord Drug Targets 2019;19(6):874–84.

Adab Z, Eghtesadi S, Vafa MR, et al. Effect of turmeric on glycemic status, lipid profile, hs-CRP, and total antioxidant capacity in hyperlipidemic type 2 diabetes mellitus patients. Phytother Res 2019;33(4):1173–81.

Adhvaryu M, Reddy N, Vakharia B. Prevention of hepatotoxicity due to anti tuberculosis treatment: a novel integrative approach. World J Gastroenterol 2008;14(30):4753–62.

Adibian M, Hodaei H, Nikpayam O, Sohrab G, Hekmatdoost A, Hedayati M. The effects of curcumin supplementation on high-sensitivity C-reactive protein, serum adiponectin, and lipid profile in patients with type 2 diabetes: a randomized, double-blind, placebo-controlled trial. Phytother Res 2019;33(5):1374–83.

Afshariani R, Farhadi P, Ghaffarpasand F, Roozbeh J. Effectiveness of topical curcumin for treatment of mastitis in breastfeeding women: a randomized, double-blind, placebo-controlled clinical trial. Oman Med J 2014;29(5):330–4.

Akazawa N, Choi Y, Miyaki A, et al. Curcumin ingestion and exercise training improve vascular endothelial function in postmenopausal women. Nutr Res 2012;32(10):795–9.

Al-Karawi D, Al Mamoori DA, Tayyar Y. The role of curcumin administration in patients with major depressive disorder: mini meta-analysis of clinical trials. Phytother Res 2016;30(2):175–83.

Allegri P, Mastromarino A, Neri P. Management of chronic anterior uveitis relapses: efficacy of oral phospholipidic curcumin treatment. Long-term follow-up. Clin Ophthalmol 2010;4:1201–6.

Amalraj A, Varma K, Jacob J, et al. A novel highly bioavailable curcumin formulation improves symptoms and diagnostic indicators in rheumatoid arthritis patients: a randomized, double-blind, placebo-controlled, two-dose, three-arm, and parallel-group study. J Med Food 2017;20(10):1022–30.

Amin F, Islam N, Anila N, Gilani AH. Clinical efficacy of the co-administration of turmeric and black seeds (Kalongi) in metabolic syndrome—a double blind randomized controlled trial—TAK-MetS trial. Complement Ther Med 2015;23(2):165–74.

Atkin SL, Katsiki N, Derosa G, Maffioli P, Sahebkar A. Curcuminoids lower plasma leptin concentrations: a meta-analysis. Phytother Res 2017;31(12):1836–41.

Azhdari M, Karandish M, Mansoori A. Metabolic benefits of curcumin supplementation in patients with metabolic syndrome: a systematic review and meta-analysis of randomized controlled trials. Phytother Res 2019;33(5):1289–301.

Bahraini P, Rajabi M, Mansouri P, Sarafian G, Chalangari R, Azizian Z. Turmeric tonic as a treatment in scalp psoriasis: a randomized placebo-control clinical trial. J Cosmet Dermatol 2018;17(3):461–6.

Bannuru RR, Osani MC, Al-Eid F, Wang C. Efficacy of curcumin and Boswellia for knee osteoarthritis: systematic review and meta-analysis. Semin Arthritis Rheum 2018;48(3):416–29.

Carrion-Gutierrez M, Ramirez-Bosca A, Navarro-Lopez V, et al. Effects of Curcuma extract and visible light on adults with plaque psoriasis. Eur J Dermatol 2015;25(3):240–6.

Chainani-Wu N, Madden E, Lozada-Nur F, Silverman Jr S. High-dose curcuminoids are efficacious in the reduction in symptoms and signs of oral lichen planus. J Am Acad Dermatol 2012;66(5):752–60.

Chandan S, Mohan BP, Chandan OC, et al. Curcumin use in ulcerative colitis: is it ready for prime time? A systematic review and meta-analysis of clinical trials. Ann Gastroenterol 2020;33(1):53–8.

Choi Y, Tanabe Y, Akazawa N, Zempo-Miyaki A, Maeda S. Curcumin supplementation attenuates the decrease in endothelial function following eccentric exercise. J Exerc Nutrition Biochem 2019;23(2):7–12.

Chopra A, Lavin P, Patwardhan B, Chitre D. A 32-week randomized, placebo-controlled clinical evaluation of RA-11, an ayurvedic drug, on osteoarthritis of the knees. J Clin Rheumatol 2004;10(5):236–45.

Conrozier T, Mathieu P, Bonjean M, Marc JF, Renevier JL, Balblanc JC. A complex of 3 natural anti-inflammatory agents provides relief of osteoarthritis pain. Altern Ther Health Med 2014;20(Suppl 1):32–7.

Daily JW, Yang M, Park S. Efficacy of turmeric extracts and curcumin for alleviating the symptoms of joint arthritis: a systematic review and meta-analysis of randomized clinical trials. J Med Food 2016;19(8):717–29.

de Melo ISV, Dos Santos AF, Bueno NB. Curcumin or combined curcuminoids are effective in lowering the fasting blood glucose concentrations of individuals with dysglycemia: Systematic review and meta-analysis of randomized controlled trials. Pharmacol Res. 2018 Feb;128:137–44.

Derosa G, Maffioli P, Simental-Mendía LE, Bo S, Sahebkar A. Effect of curcumin on circulating interleukin-6 concentrations: a systematic review and meta-analysis of randomized controlled trials. Pharmacol Res 2016;111:394–404.

Dhariwal NS, Hugar SM, Harakuni S, Sogi S, Assudani HG, Mistry LN. A comparative evaluation of antibacterial effectiveness of sodium hypochlorite, Curcuma longa, and Camellia sinensis as irrigating solutions on isolated anaerobic bacteria from infected primary teeth. J Indian Soc Pedod Prev Dent 2016;34(2):165–71.

Epelbaum R, Schaffer M, Vizel B, et al. Curcumin and gemcitabine in patients with advanced pancreatic cancer. Nutr Cancer 2010;62(8):1137–41.

Fabiani A, Morosetti C, Filosa A, et al. Effect on prostatic specific antigen by a short time treatment with a Curcuma extract: a real life experience and implications for prostate biopsy. Arch Ital Urol Androl 2018;90(2):107–11.

Fung FY, Wong WH, Ang SK, et al. A randomized, double-blind, placebo- controlled study on the anti-haemostatic effects of Curcuma longa, Angelica sinensis and Panax ginseng. Phytomedicine 2017;32:88–96.

Ghaffari A, Rafraf M, Navekar R, Sepehri B, Asghari-Jafarabadi M, Ghavami SM. Turmeric and chicory seed have beneficial effects on obesity markers and lipid profile in non-alcoholic fatty liver disease (NAFLD). Int J Vitam Nutr Res 2019;24:1–10.

Goodarzi R, Sabzian K, Shishehbor F, Mansoori A. Does turmeric/curcumin supplementation improve serum alanine aminotransferase and aspartate aminotransferase levels in patients with NAFLD? A systematic review and meta-analysis of randomized controlled trials. Phytother Res 2019;33(3):561–70.

Goulart RA, Barbalho SM, Lima VM, et al. Effects of the use of Curcumin on ulcerative colitis and Crohn's disease: a systematic review. J Med Food 2020;5.

Greenlee H, Atkinson C, Stanczyk FZ, Lampe JW. A pilot and feasibility study on the effects of naturopathic botanical and dietary interventions on sex steroid hormone metabolism in premenopausal women. Cancer Epidemiol Biomarkers Prev 2007;16(8):1601–9.

Hanai H, Iida T, Takeuchi K, et al. Curcumin maintenance therapy for ulcerative colitis: randomized, multicenter, double-blind, placebo-controlled trial. Clin Gastroenterol Hepatol 2006;4(12):1502–6.

Henrotin Y, Malaise M, Wittoek R, et al. Bio-optimized Curcuma longa extract is efficient on knee osteoarthritis pain: a double-blind multicenter randomized placebo controlled three-arm study. Arthritis Res Ther 2019;21(1):179.

Hodaei H, Adibian M, Nikpayam O, Hedayati M, Sohrab G. The effect of curcumin supplementation on anthropometric indices, insulin resistance and oxidative stress in patients with type 2 diabetes: a randomized, double-blind clinical trial. Diabetol Metab Syndr 2019;11:41.

Howells LM, Iwuji COO, Irving GRB, et al. Curcumin combined with FOLFOX chemotherapy is safe and tolerable in patients with metastatic colorectal cancer in a randomized phase IIa trial. J Nutr 2019;149(7):1133–9.

Hugar SM, Kukreja P, Hugar SS, Gokhale N, Assudani H. Comparative evaluation of clinical and radiographic success of formocresol, propolis, turmeric gel, and calcium hydroxide on pulpotomized primary molars: a preliminary study. Int J Clin Pediatr Dent 2017;10(1):18–23.

Iqbal U, Anwar H, Quadri AA. Use of curcumin in achieving clinical and endoscopic remission in ulcerative colitis: a systematic review and meta-analysis. Am J Med Sci 2018;356(4):350–6.

Jafarirad S, Mansoori A, Adineh A, Panahi Y, Hadi A, Goodarzi R. Does turmeric/curcumin supplementation change anthropometric indices in patients with non-alcoholic fatty liver disease? a systematic review and meta-analysis of randomized controlled trials. Clin Nutr Res 2019;8(3):196–208.

Joshi JV, Paradkar PH, Jagtap SS, Agashe SV, Soman G, Vaidya AB. Chemopreventive potential and safety profile of a Curcuma longa extract in women with cervical low-grade squamous intraepithelial neoplasia. Asian Pac J Cancer Prev 2011;12(12):3305–11.

Joshi JV, Jagtap SS, Paradkar PH, et al. Cytologic follow up of low-grade squamous intraepithelial lesions in pap smears after integrated treatment with antimicrobials followed by oral turmeric oil extract. J Ayurveda Integr Med 2016;7(2):109–12.

Kanai M, Yoshimura K, Asada M, et al. A phase I/II study of gemcitabine-based chemotherapy plus curcumin for patients with gemcitabine-resistant pancreatic cancer. Cancer Chemother Pharmacol 2011;68(1):157–64.

Khajehdehi P, Pakfetrat M, Javidnia K, et al. Oral supplementation of turmeric attenuates proteinuria, transforming growth factor-β and interleukin-8 levels in patients with overt type 2 diabetic nephropathy: a randomized, double-blind and placebo-controlled study. Scand J Urol Nephrol 2011;45(5):365–70.

Khajehdehi P, Zanjaninejad B, Aflaki E, et al. Oral supplementation of turmeric decreases proteinuria, hematuria, and SBP in patients suffering from relapsing or refractory lupus nephritis: a randomized and placebo-controlled study. J Ren Nutr 2012;22(1):50–7.

Khonche A, Biglarian O, Panahi Y, et al. Adjunctive therapy with curcumin for peptic ulcer: a randomized controlled trial. Drug Res (Stuttg) 2016;66(8):444–8.

Kizhakkedath R. Clinical evaluation of a formulation containing Curcuma longa and Boswellia serrata extracts in the management of knee osteoarthritis. Mol Med Rep 2013;8(5):1542–8.

Kuptniratsaikul V, Dajpratham P, Taechaarpornkul W, et al. Efficacy and safety of Curcuma domestica extracts compared with ibuprofen in patients with knee osteoarthritis: a multicenter study. Clin Interv Aging 2014;9:451–8.

Kurian GA, Manjusha V, Nair SS, Varghese T, Padikkala J. Short-term effect of G-400, polyherbal formulation in the management of hyperglycemia and hyperlipidemia conditions in patients with type 2 diabetes mellitus. Nutrition 2014;30(10):1158–64.

Lal B, Kapoor AK, Asthana OP, et al. Efficacy of curcumin in the management of chronic anterior uveitis. Phytother Res 1999;13(4):318–22.

Liu X, Machado GC, Eyles JP, Ravi V, Hunter DJ. Dietary supplements for treating osteoarthritis: a systematic review and meta-analysis. Br J Sports Med 2018;52(3):167–75.

Lone PA, Ahmed SW, Prasad V, Ahmed B. Role of turmeric in management of alveolar osteitis (dry socket): a randomised clinical study. J Oral Biol Craniofac Res 2018;8(1):44–7.

Lopresti AL, Drummond PD. Efficacy of curcumin, and a saffron/curcumin combination for the treatment of major depression: a randomised, double-blind, placebo-controlled study. J Affect Disord 2017;207:188–96.

Lv KJ, Chen TC, Wang GH, Yao YN, Yao H. Clinical safety and efficacy of curcumin use for oral lichen planus: a systematic review. J Dermatolog Treat 2019;30(6):605–11.

Manarin G, Anderson D, Silva JME, et al. Curcuma longa L. ameliorates asthma control in children and adolescents: a randomized, double-blind, controlled trial. J Ethnopharmacol 2019;238:111882.

Mansour-Ghanaei F, Pourmasoumi M, Hadi A, Joukar F. Efficacy of curcumin/turmeric on liver enzymes in patients with non-alcoholic fatty liver disease: a systematic review of randomized controlled trials. Integr Med Res 2019;8(1):57–61.

Marx W, Kelly J, Marshall S, Nakos S, Campbell K, Itsiopoulos C. The effect of polyphenol-rich interventions on cardiovascular risk factors in haemodialysis: a systematic review and meta-analysis. Nutrients 2017;9(12). pii: E1345.

Maulina T, Diana H, Cahyanto A, Amaliya A. The efficacy of curcumin in managing acute inflammation pain on the post-surgical removal of impacted third molars patients: a randomised controlled trial. J Oral Rehabil 2018;45(9):677–83.

Merolla G, Dellabiancia F, Ingardia A, Paladini P, Porcellini G. Co-analgesic therapy for arthroscopic supraspinatus tendon repair pain using a dietary supplement containing Boswellia serrata and Curcuma longa: a prospective randomized placebo-controlled study. Musculoskelet Surg 2015;99(Suppl 1):S43–52.

Mohammadi E, Tamaddoni A, Qujeq D, et al. An investigation of the effects of curcumin on iron overload, hepcidin level, and liver function in β-thalassemia major patients: a double-blind randomized controlled clinical trial. Phytother Res 2018;32(9):1828–35.

Morgia G, Russo GI, Urzì D, et al. A phase II, randomized, single-blinded, placebo-controlled clinical trial on the efficacy of Curcumina and Calendula suppositories for the treatment of patients with chronic prostatitis/chronic pelvic pain syndrome type III. Arch Ital Urol Androl 2017;89(2):110–3.

Navekar R, Rafraf M, Ghaffari A, Asghari-Jafarabadi M, Khoshbaten M. Turmeric supplementation improves serum glucose indices and leptin levels in patients with NAFLDs. J Am Coll Nutr 2017;36(4):261–7.

Ng QX, Koh SSH, Chan HW, Ho CYX. Clinical use of curcumin in depression: a meta-analysis. J Am Med Dir Assoc 2017;18(6):503–8.

Normando AGC, de Menêses AG, de Toledo IP, et al. Effects of turmeric and curcumin on oral mucositis: a systematic review. Phytother Res 2019;33(5):1318–29.

Nosratzehi T, Arbabi-Kalati F, Hamishehkar H, Bagheri S. Comparison of the effects of curcumin mucoadhesive paste and local corticosteroid on the treatment of erosive oral lichen planus lesions. J Natl Med Assoc 2018;110(1):92–7.

Nouri-Vaskeh M, Malek Mahdavi A, Afshan H, Alizadeh L, Zarei M. Effect of curcumin supplementation on disease severity in patients with liver cirrhosis: a randomized controlled trial. Phytother Res 2020;34(6):1446–54.

Oliver JM, Stoner L, Rowlands DS, et al. Novel form of Curcumin improves endothelial function in young, healthy individuals: a double-blind placebo controlled study. J Nutr Metab 2016;2016:1089653.

Orhan IE, Deniz FS. Natural products as potential leads against coronaviruses: could they be encouraging structural models against SARS-CoV-2? Nat Prod Bioprospect 2020;10(4):171–86.

Pagano E, Romano B, Izzo AA, Borrelli F. The clinical efficacy of curcumin-containing nutraceuticals: an overview of systematic reviews. Pharmacol Res 2018;134:79–91.

Panahi Y, Khalili N, Sahebi E, et al. Curcuminoids plus piperine modulate adipokines in type 2 diabetes mellitus. Curr Clin Pharmacol 2017;12(4):253–8.

Panda SK, Nirvanashetty S, Parachur VA, Mohanty N, Swain T. A randomized, double blind, placebo controlled, parallel-group study to evaluate the safety and efficacy of Curene® vs placebo in reducing symptoms of knee OA. Biomed Res Int 2018;2018:5291945.

Phoolcharoen N, Oranratanaphan S, Ariyasriwatana C, Worasethsin P. Efficacy of curcuminoids for reducing postoperative pain after laparoscopic gynecologic surgery: a pilot randomized trial. J Complement Integr Med 2019. pii://j/jcim.ahead-of-print/jcim-2018-0224/jcim-2018-0224.xml.

Pipalia PR, Annigeri RG, Mehta R. Clinicobiochemical evaluation of turmeric with black pepper and nigella sativa in management of oral submucous fibrosis-a double-blind, randomized preliminary study. Oral Surg Oral Med Oral Pathol Oral Radiol 2016;122(6):705–12.

Posadzki P, Watson LK, Ernst E. Adverse effects of herbal medicines: an overview of systematic reviews. Clin Med (Lond) 2013;13(1):7–12.

Prucksunand C, Indrasukhsri B, Leethochawalit M, Hungspreugs K. Phase II clinical trial on effect of the long turmeric (Curcuma longa Linn) on healing of peptic ulcer. Southeast Asian J Trop Med Public Health 2001;32(1):208–15.

Qin S, Huang L, Gong J, et al. Efficacy and safety of turmeric and curcumin in lowering blood lipid levels in patients with cardiovascular risk factors: a meta-analysis of randomized controlled trials. Nutr J 2017;16(1):68.

Rasyid A, Lelo A. The effect of curcumin and placebo on human gall-bladder function: an ultrasound study. Aliment Pharmacol Ther 1999;13(2):245–9.

Saberi-Karimian M, Keshvari M, Ghayour-Mobarhan M, et al. Effects of curcuminoids on inflammatory status in patients with non-alcoholic fatty liver disease: a randomized controlled trial. Complement Ther Med 2020;49:102322.

Sahebkar A, Cicero AF, Simental-Mendía LE, Aggarwal BB, Gupta SC. Curcumin downregulates human TNF-α levels: a systematic review and meta-analysis of randomized controlled trials. Pharmacol Res 2016;107:234–42.

Sanmukhani J, Satodia V, Trivedi J, et al. Efficacy and safety of curcumin in major depressive disorder: a randomized controlled trial. Phytother Res 2014;28(4):579–85.

Sannia A. Phytotherapy with a mixture of dry extracts with hepato-protective effects containing artichoke leaves in the management of functional dyspepsia symptoms. Minerva Gastroenterol Dietol 2010;56(2):93–9.

Sarafian G, Afshar M, Mansouri P, Asgarpanah J, Raoufinejad K, Rajabi M. Topical turmeric microemulgel in the management of plaque psoriasis: a clinical evaluation. Iran J Pharm Res 2015;14(3):865–76.

Sarraf P, Parohan M, Javanbakht MH, Ranji-Burachaloo S, Djalali M. Short-term curcumin supplementation enhances serum brain-derived neurotrophic factor in adult men and women: a systematic review and dose-response meta-analysis of randomized controlled trials. Nutr Res 2019;69:1–8.

Scontre VA, Martins JC, de Melo Sette CV, et al. Curcuma longa (Turmeric) for prevention of capecitabine-induced hand-foot syndrome: a pilot study. J Diet Suppl 2018;15(5):606–12.

Selvi N, Sridhar MG, Swaminathan RP, Sripradha R. Efficacy of turmeric as adjuvant therapy in type 2 diabetic patients. Indian J Clin Biochem 2015;30(2):180–6.

Shep D, Khanwelkar C, Gade P, Karad S. Efficacy and safety of combination of curcuminoid complex and diclofenac versus diclofenac in knee osteoarthritis: a randomized trial. Medicine (Baltimore) 2020;99(16), e19723.

Simadibrata M, Halimkesuma CC, Suwita BM. Efficacy of Curcumin as adjuvant therapy to induce or maintain remission in ulcerative colitis patients: an evidence-based clinical review. Acta Med Indones 2017;49(4):363–8.

Simental-Mendía LE, Pirro M, Gotto Jr AM, et al. Lipid-modifying activity of curcuminoids: a systematic review and meta-analysis of randomized controlled trials. Crit Rev Food Sci Nutr 2019;59(7):1178–87.

Singla V, Pratap Mouli V, Garg SK, et al. Induction with NCB-02 (curcumin) enema for mild-to-moderate distal ulcerative colitis—a randomized, placebo-controlled, pilot study. J Crohns Colitis 2014;8(3):208–14.

Srinivasan A, Selvarajan S, Kamalanathan S, Kadhiravan T, Prasanna Lakshmi NC, Adithan S. Effect of Curcuma longa on vascular function in native Tamilians with type 2 diabetes mellitus: a randomized, double-blind, parallel arm, placebo-controlled trial. Phytother Res 2019;33(7):1898–911.

Srivastava S, Saksena AK, Khattri S, Kumar S, Dagur RS. Curcuma longa extract reduces inflammatory and oxidative stress biomarkers in osteoarthritis of knee: a four-month, double-blind, randomized, placebo-controlled trial. Inflammopharmacology 2016;24(6):377–88.

Stoyell KA, Mappus JL, Gandhi MA. Clinical efficacy of turmeric use in gingivitis: a comprehensive review. Complement Ther Clin Pract 2016;25:13–7.

Uchio R, Muroyama K, Okuda-Hanafusa C, Kawasaki K, Yamamoto Y, Murosaki S. Hot water extract of Curcuma longa L. improves serum inflammatory markers and general health in subjects with overweight or PreHTN/Mild HTN: a randomized, double-blind, placebo-controlled trial. Nutrients 2019;11(8).

Vaughn AR, Branum A, Sivamani RK. Effects of turmeric (Curcuma longa) on skin health: a systematic review of the clinical evidence. Phytother Res 2016;30(8):1243–64.

Wen C-C, Kuo Y-H, Jan J-T, et al. Specific plant terpenoids and lignoids possess potent antiviral activities against severe acute respiratory syndrome coronavirus. J Med Chem 2007;50:4087–95.

White CM, Lee JY. The impact of turmeric or its curcumin extract on NAFLD: a systematic review of clinical trials. Pharm Pract (Granada) 2019;17(1):1350.

White CM, Pasupuleti V, Roman YM, Li Y, Hernandez AV. Oral turmeric/curcumin effects on inflammatory markers in chronic inflammatory diseases: a systematic review and meta-analysis of randomized controlled trials. Pharmacol Res 2019;146:104280.

Wongcharoen W, Jai-Aue S, Phrommintikul A, et al. Effects of curcuminoids on frequency of acute myocardial infarction after coronary artery bypass grafting. Am J Cardiol 2012;110(1):40–4.

Yuan F, Dong H, Gong J, et al. A systematic review and meta-analysis of randomized controlled trials on the effects of turmeric and curcuminoids on blood lipids in adults with metabolic diseases. Adv Nutr 2019;10(5):791–802.

74

UMCKALOABO/SOUTH AFRICAN GERANIUM (*PELARGONIUM SIDOIDES*)
Root

. . . .

GENERAL OVERVIEW

Umckaloabo or South African geranium has been used traditionally for bronchitis, asthma, general sickness, fatigue, menstrual disorders, and tuberculosis. It is likely the best herb for acute bronchitis, pure and simple. It improves not only the cough but also the other symptoms that tend to accompany an episode of acute bronchitis such as headache, fever, fatigue, and rhinorrhea, most likely due to its efficacy against the underlying pathophysiology of bronchitis.

An aqueous ethanolic extract of umckaloabo (EPs 7630) has been widely studied and marketed for ENT and respiratory disorders. The elucidated mechanisms underlying the beneficial effects of umckaloabo in bronchitis include immunomodulatory and cytoprotective effects, inhibition of interactions between pathogens and host cells, and an increase of ciliary beat frequency in the respiratory tract. By similar mechanisms umckaloabo appears effective for the common cold.

Clinical research indicates that umckaloabo, alone or in combination formulas, may be beneficial for reactive airways, chronic obstructive pulmonary disease, upper respiratory infections, pharyngitis, acute sinusitis, acute bronchitis, and immune function.

IN VITRO AND ANIMAL RESEARCH

Preclinical research on umckaloabo has focused on antimicrobial and immunostimulatory effects and mucociliary transport. Umckaloabo has been shown to increase the ciliary beat frequency of the mucociliary system of human nasal epithelium by 133% at 100 μg/mL.

Umckaloabo has demonstrated a selective immunomodulatory effect on infected macrophages and an increase in production of TNF-α, IL-1α, and IL-12. It has been shown to induce MAPK-dependent proinflammatory cytokines in human monocytes and modulate their production of mediators that lead to an increase of acute phase protein production in the liver and neutrophil generation in the bone marrow. The herb has been shown to increase the generation of Th17 and Th22 cells. Macrophages infected with bacteria and incubated with low concentrations of umckaloabo have demonstrated enhanced phagocytosis and bactericidal activity, and neutrophils have demonstrated enhanced bactericidal activity as well in the presence of the herb. Umckaloabo has also been shown to increase the number of phagocytosing and burst-active peripheral blood phagocytes exposed to candida albicans with enhanced intracellular killing. Gallic acid extracted from umckaloabo has demonstrated decreased intracellular survival of *Leishmania donovani* amastigotes within murine macrophages through macrophage production of TNF-α and iNOS.

Umckaloabo has shown a wide range of antimicrobial activity, with particular efficacy against enveloped viruses. EPs 7630, an ethanolic extract of umckaloabo, was tested for effects on replication of a panel of respiratory viruses. At concentrations up to 100 mcg/mL it was shown to interfere with replication of seasonal Influenza A virus strains (H1N1, H3N2), RSV, human coronavirus, parainfluenza virus, and coxsackie virus but did not affect replication of avian influenza A virus (H5N1), adenovirus, or rhinovirus (Michaelis et al., 2007).

Umckaloabo has been shown to prevent attachment of HSV 1 and 2 when the viruses were pretreated with the plant extract and when the extract was added during the adsorption phase. In contrast, acyclovir demonstrated antiviral activity only during intracellular replication. EPs 7630 has been shown to have potent anti-HIV-1 activity. It protects peripheral mononuclear cells and macrophages from infection with various X4 and R5 tropic HIV-1 strains and blocks the attachment of HIV-1 particles to target cells.

Umckaloabo appears to have low-to-moderate direct antibacterial capabilities against a spectrum of Gram-negative and Gram-positive bacteria. Herbal extracts were investigated against three Gram-positive bacteria (*S. aureus*, *S. pneumoniae*, and β-hemolytic *Streptococcus* 1451) and five Gram-negative bacteria (*E. coli*, *K. pneumoniae*, *P. mirabilis*, *P. aeruginosa*, *H. influenzae*). MICs varied with the preparation of the extracts and microorganisms tested, from about 0.6 mg/mL for aqueous extracts to more than 10 mg/mL for crude preparations. The herb has also demonstrated activity against *S. pooni*, *B. cereus*, *P. mirabilis*, and all tested *Staphylococcus* strains including *S. aureus*. at MICs of 2.5-7.25 mg/mL. EPs 7630 at 12.5 mg/mL has been noted ex vivo to inhibit 96% of *M. tuberculosis* growth.

While the bioactive constituents of umckaloabo have demonstrated numerous direct and indirect antimicrobial effects, they may act primarily by interference with microbial binding to host cell receptors, inhibition of key enzymes, and production of antimicrobial effector molecules such as nitric oxide and interferons by the host cells. Proanthocyanidins appear to be responsible for the anti-adhesive principle, particularly those with pyrogallol B-ring elements of their flavanyl units.

Effects of umckaloabo on cellular bacterial adhesion have been assessed in several studies. For group A streptococcus, EPs 7630 reduced bacterial adhesion to human laryngeal cells by up to 46% in a concentration-dependent manner. Umckaloabo has also demonstrated in vitro and in situ anti-adhesive properties against *H. pylori*. with 77%-91% inhibition of adhesion in gastric epithelial cells. No direct bacterial cytotoxicity was demonstrated against *H. pylori*.

Umckaloabo appears to have anticancer effects. In osteosarcoma cells the ethanolic extract was shown to augment. IFN-β production by up to 200%. Strong activity of umckaloabo tincture was demonstrated in leukemic cells, being significantly better than the positive control 5-fluorouracil. The tincture arrested Jurkat cells at the G0/G1 phase of the cell cycle and increased the apoptotic cells from 9% to 21% and cell lethality from 4% to 17%, suggesting that umckaloabo tincture had cancer cell type-specific antiproliferative effects and may be a source of novel anticancer molecules (Pereira et al., 2016).

HUMAN RESEARCH

The majority of human trials utilized the umckaloabo formulation EPs 7630, a 1x homeopathic preparation from the roots of Pelargonium sidoides (1:8-10; ethanol 11%).

Pulmonary Disorders: Asthma and Chronic Obstructive Pulmonary Disease

A 24-week RCT in patients ($n = 200$) with moderate-to-severe COPD compared EPs 7630 30 drops TID with placebo for impact on exacerbation frequency. Median time to exacerbation was significantly prolonged with the umckaloabo formulation compared with placebo (57 and 43 days, respectively; $P = 0.005$). With umckaloabo there were also fewer exacerbations, less patients with antibiotic use, improved quality of life, higher patient satisfaction, and less days of inability to work. The incidence of minor GI adverse events was higher with umckaloabo. The authors concluded that there was statistically significant and clinically relevant superiority over placebo of add-on therapy with umckaloabo and good long-term tolerability in patients with moderate to severe COPD (Matthys et al., 2013).

A 5-day open-label trial in asthmatic children ($n = 61$) with URIs compared umckaloabo with controls (no treatment) to assess effects on viral-triggered asthma attacks. There were significant differences in cough frequency, nasal congestion, and asthma attacks between the groups ($P < 0.05$ for all). There were no significant differences between groups for fever and muscle aches. The authors concluded that umckaloabo may prevent asthma attacks during URIs (Tahan and Yaman, 2013).

Infectious Disease: Upper Respiratory Infections, Pharyngitis, and Acute Sinusitis

A 2018 systematic review assessing the evidence for herbal therapy for respiratory tract infection in children found six trials involving umckaloabo that met inclusion criteria. Umckaloabo, when compared with placebo, demonstrated efficacy (RR = 2.56; $P < 0.01$; $I^2 = 38\%$) and safety (RR = 1.06; $P = 0.9$; $I^2 = 72\%$) in treating RTI symptoms. The authors concluded that umckaloabo had moderate evidence of efficacy and safety in treatment of RTIs in children (Anheyer et al., 2018).

A 2013 systematic review of umckaloabo for the treatment of acute respiratory infections in children and adults found eight trials that met inclusion criteria. Three trials ($n = 746$) showed effectiveness for most outcomes with the liquid preparation but not with tablets. Three other trials ($n = 819$ children) showed similar results for acute bronchitis in children. One study in patients with sinusitis ($n = 103$ adults) showed significant treatment effects (complete resolution at day 21; RR = 0.43). One study of the common cold demonstrated efficacy after 10 days, but not 5 days. The study quality was rated as moderate for all studies. Adverse events were more common with umckaloabo, but none were serious. The authors concluded that umckaloabo may be effective in relieving symptoms of acute bronchitis in adults and children and sinusitis in adults (Timmer et al., 2013).

A 6-day RCT in children ($n = 143$) with tonsillopharyngitis and negative strep screens compared umckaloabo 20 drops TID with placebo. The decrease in Tonsillopharyngitis Severity Score from baseline to day 4 was 7.1 points and 2.5 points with umckaloabo and placebo, respectively ($P < 0.0001$). Adverse events did not appear to be related to umckaloabo. The authors concluded that umckaloabo was superior to placebo for treatment of non-strep pharyngitis in children and shortened duration of illness by at least 2 days (Bereznoy et al., 2003).

A 10-day RCT in adults ($n = 103$) with cold symptoms for 24-48 h compared umckaloabo 30 drops TID with placebo. From baseline to day 5, the mean Sum of Symptom Intensity Differences improved by 14.6 points and 7.6 points with umckaloabo and placebo,

respectively ($P < 0.0001$). The mean cold intensity score (CIS) decreased by 10.4 points and 5.6 points with umckaloabo and placebo, respectively. Clinical cure (CIS = 0) at day 10 occurred in 78.8% and 31.4% of patients with umckaloabo and placebo, respectively ($P < 0.0001$). The mean duration of inability to work was 6.9 days and 8.2 days with umckaloabo and placebo, respectively ($P = 0.0003$). Adverse events were nonserious and occurred in 2/52 and 1/51 patients with umckaloabo and placebo, respectively. All patients in the active treatment group judged the subjective tolerability of umckaloabo as "good" or "very good." The authors concluded that umckaloabo was an effective treatment for the common cold and was well tolerated (Lizogub et al., 2007).

A 22-day RCT in patients ($n = 103$) with radiographically proven acute rhinosinusitis of ≥ 7 days duration compared EPs 7630 60 drops TID with placebo. The mean decrease in the Sinusitis Symptoms Severity score was 5.5 points and 2.5 points with umckaloabo and placebo, respectively ($P < 0.00001$). This result was confirmed by all secondary parameters indicating a more favorable course of the disease and a faster recovery with umckaloabo. The authors concluded that this umckaloabo formulation was well tolerated and to superior to placebo in the treatment of acute rhinosinusitis of presumably bacterial origin (Bachert et al., 2009)

A 10-day RCT in adults ($n = 104$) with cold symptoms present for 24-48 h compared a high dose (60 drops TID) of an umckaloabo proprietary extract with placebo for efficacy. From baseline to day 5, the mean cold intensity score decreased by 11.2 points in the umckaloabo group and by 6.3 points in the placebo group. After 10 days, 90.4% of the group receiving the active medication and 21.2% of the control group were clinically cured ($P < 0.0001$). With umckaloabo and placebo, participants' inability to work lasted 6.4 days and 8.3 days, respectively ($P < 0.0001$). Complete recovery or major improvement at day 5 was significantly greater with umckaloabo than with placebo ($P < 0.0001$). Mild-to-moderate adverse events, all nonserious, occurred in 15.4% with umckaloabo and 5.8% with placebo. The authors concluded that umckaloabo was an effective, well-tolerated, and safe treatment for the common cold (Riley et al., 2018).

Infectious Disease: Acute Bronchitis and Cough

A 2016 systematic review of phytopharmaceutical treatments of acute respiratory syndrome found seven trials involving umckaloabo and other botanical formulations that met inclusion criteria. Risk of bias was heterogeneous. EPs 7630 appeared to be useful in the treatment of ARS. There was lower-level evidence for the other formulations. The authors concluded that herbal medicine might be effective for the treatment of acute respiratory syndrome but that further research was necessary (Koch et al., 2016).

A 2015 Cochrane review of herbs effective in treating cough found 34 RCTs ($n = 7083$) in total with 11 studies of umckaloabo that met inclusion criteria. Most studies had a low risk of bias. The meta-analysis revealed strong evidence for andrographis (SMD = -1.00; $P < 0.001$) and the combination ivy-primrose-thyme (RR = 1.40; $P < 0.001$) in treating cough; moderate evidence for umckaloabo (RR = 4.60; $P < 0.001$), and limited evidence for echinacea (SMD = -0.68; $P = 0.04$). The authors concluded that andrographis, ivy-primrose-thyme, and umckaloabo were significantly superior to placebo in alleviating the frequency and severity of cough symptoms (Wagner et al., 2015).

A 2013 systematic review of umckaloabo for the treatment of acute respiratory infections in children and adults found eight trials that met inclusion criteria. Three trials ($n = 746$) showed effectiveness for most outcomes with the liquid preparation but not with tablets. Three other trials ($n = 819$ children) showed similar results for acute bronchitis in children. One study in patients with sinusitis ($n = 103$ adults) showed significant treatment effects (complete resolution at day 21; RR = 0.43). One study of the common cold demonstrated efficacy after 10 days, but not 5 days. The study quality was rated as moderate for all studies. Adverse events were more common with umckaloabo, but none were serious. The authors concluded that umckaloabo may be effective in relieving symptoms of acute bronchitis in adults and children and sinusitis in adults (Timmer et al., 2013).

A 2008 Cochrane review to assess the efficacy of umckaloabo for treating acute bronchitis found six RCTs that met the inclusion criteria, four of which were suitable for statistical pooling. Methodological quality of most trials was good. One study compared EPs 7630 against acetylcysteine, and the other five studies tested EPs 7630 against placebo. All RCTs reported findings suggesting the effectiveness of umckaloabo in treating acute bronchitis. In the four RCTs that could be pooled, evidence suggested that EPs 7630 significantly reduced Bronchitis Severity Scale scores in patients with acute bronchitis by day 7. No serious adverse events were reported. The authors concluded there was encouraging evidence that umckaloabo was effective compared with placebo for patients with acute bronchitis (Agbabiaka et al., 2008).

A 7-day RCT in adults ($n = 217$) with acute bronchitis compared EPs 7630 30 drops TID with placebo drops. Individual change in Bronchitis Severity Scale scores over 7 days, individual symptoms, patient satisfaction, and adverse events were measured. After 7 days of treatment, the Bronchitis Severity Scale scores decreased by 7.6 points with umckaloabo and by 5.3 points with placebo ($P < 0.0001$). There were also marked improvements in the individual symptoms of cough, chest pain on coughing, sputum, rales/rhonchi, and dyspnea with umckaloabo relative to placebo. Patient satisfaction was "very good." Only minor and transitory adverse events were recorded. No serious adverse events occurred during the trial. The authors concluded that this umckaloabo formulation was well tolerated and effective for acute bronchitis in adults (Matthys et al., 2007).

Further analyses of the 2007 study noted above focused on both the most important features of acute bronchitis and pharmaco-economic aspects of the disease. Compared with placebo, a marked improvement had been shown for the umckaloabo extract for all disease symptoms (cough, sputum, rales, dyspnea, pain on coughing, hoarseness, headache, fatigue, fever, and limb pain). Especially strong antitussive and antifatigue effects with an early onset during treatment were observed. Patients given umckaloabo were confined to bed to a lesser extent and were sooner able to return to work. The authors concluded that EPs 7630 was superior to placebo in the treatment of acute bronchitis and led to faster remission of bronchitis related symptoms (Matthys and Funk, 2008).

A 7-day RCT in patients ($n = 406$) with acute bronchitis compared EPs 7630 10 mg, 20 mg, or 30 mg TID and with placebo. Bronchitis Severity Scale scores decreased from baseline by 4.3, 6.2, 6.3, and 2.7 with 10 mg, 20 mg, 30 mg, and placebo doses, respectively ($P < 0.0001$, for all doses compared with placebo). All documented adverse events were of mild-to-moderate intensity and their frequency was dose dependent. No serious adverse events were reported. The authors concluded that umckaloabo at all three doses tested was superior to placebo for acute bronchitis and that the 20 mg tablets of EPs 7630 taken TID constituted the optimal dose with respect to the benefit-risk ratio (Matthys et al., 2010).

A 7-day open-label trial in patients ($n = 205$) with acute bronchitis or acute exacerbation of chronic bronchitis measured the effects EPs 7630. The change in the total score of the five main symptoms typical for bronchitis (cough, expectoration, expiratory wheezing, chest pain during coughing, and dyspnea), and for additional symptoms (hoarseness, headache, aching limbs, and fatigue) were assessed. The total score of the bronchitis symptoms decreased from 6.1 to 2.8 by day 7. About 60% of the patients assessed their health condition at the end of the study as much improved or free from symptoms. The onset of action appeared after 2 days on average. Adverse events occurred in a total of 16 patients with no serious adverse events. Altogether, 78% of the patients were "satisfied" or "very satisfied" with the treatment (Matthys et al., 2007).

A 7-day RCT in patients ($n = 220$) with acute bronchitis investigated EPs 7630 10-30 drops TID based on ages (1-6 years/>6-12 years/>12-18 years) compared with placebo. The decrease in the Bronchitis Severity Scale total score was 4.4 and 2.9 with umckaloabo and placebo, respectively ($P < 0.0001$). Improvements were most pronounced for coughing and rales. Tolerability was similarly good in both groups. The authors concluded that this formulation was efficacious and well-tolerated for the treatment of acute bronchitis in children and adolescents who were not candidates for antibiotics (Kamin et al., 2012).

A 7-day RCT in adults ($n = 468$) with acute bronchitis present ≤ 48 h compared EPs 7630 with placebo 30 drops TID. The decrease in the Bronchitis Severity Scale score from baseline to day 7 was 5.9 with umckaloabo and 3.2 with placebo ($P < 0.0001$). Working inability decreased to 16% and 43% with umckaloabo and placebo, respectively ($P < 0.0001$). Within the first 4 days, onset of treatment effect was recognized in 54%

and 36% of patients treated with umckaloabo and placebo, respectively ($P < 0.0001$). Duration of illness was also significantly shorter with umckaloabo compared with placebo ($P < 0.001$). Adverse events occurred in 20/233 patients given umckaloabo and 16/235 patients given placebo. All events were assessed as non-serious. The authors concluded that the umckaloabo formulation was superior to placebo in adults with acute bronchitis, reducing severity of symptoms and reducing time away from work by 2 days (Matthys et al., 2003).

A 7-day dose-finding RCT in children ages 6 to 18 years ($n = 400$) compared EPs 7630 30 mg/day, 60 mg/day, 90 mg/day and placebo. The change in the Bronchitis Severity Scale score was significantly better in the 60 mg and 90 mg groups compared with placebo. Coughing, sputum, and rales improved with umckaloabo. Onset of effect was faster, time of bed rest shorter, and treatment outcome and satisfaction with treatment were rated better. Tolerability was comparable to placebo in all treatment groups. The authors concluded that this formulation of umckaloabo was effective in acute bronchitis in children and adolescents with a dose of 60 or 90 mg/day offering the best benefit/risk ratio (Kamin et al., 2010b).

A 7-day RCT in patients ($n = 200$) with bronchitis compared EPs 7630 10-30 drops TID based on age (1-6 years, >6-12 years, >12-18 years). The mean Bronchitis Severity Scale score improved by 3.4 and 1.2 points with umckaloabo and placebo, respectively ($P < 0.0001$). On day 7, outcome of treatment with EPs 7630 was significantly better than placebo ($P < 0.0001$), satisfaction with treatment more pronounced (77.6% vs 25.8%, respectively; $P < 0.0001$), onset of effect faster, and time of bed rest shorter. All adverse events were assessed as non-serious. The authors concluded that this umckaloabo formulation was effective and safe in the treatment of acute bronchitis in children and adolescents who were not candidates for antibiotics (Kamin et al., 2010a).

A 7-day RCT in adults ($n = 124$) with acute bronchitis ≤ 48 h compared EPs 7630 30 drops TID with placebo. The mean decreases in Bronchitis Severity Scale scores from baseline to day 7 was 7.2 points and 4.9 points with umckaloabo and placebo, respectively ($P < 0.0001$). Within the first 4 days, onset of treatment effect was recognized in 68.8% and 33.3% of patients with umckaloabo and placebo, respectively

($P < 0.0001$). Health-related QOL improved more in the umckaloabo group. Adverse events occurred 15/64 and 10/60 patients with umckaloabo and placebo, respectively, with all events being nonserious. The authors concluded that this umckaloabo formulation was better than placebo in treatment of adults with acute bronchitis (Chuchalin et al., 2005).

Immune Function

An RCT in athletes submitted to intense exercise compared umckaloabo with placebo to evaluate the action of umckaloabo on the immune response that tends to be suppressed with intense exercise. Umckaloabo was shown to modulate the production of secretory IgA in saliva, IL-15 and IL-6 in serum, and IL-15 in the nasal mucosa. Secretory Ig A levels were increased, while levels of IL-15 and IL-6 were decreased. The authors concluded that umckaloabo may exert a strong modulating influence on the immune response associated with the upper airway mucosa in athletes submitted to intense physical activity (Luna et al., 2011).

A 7-day RCT in patients ($n = 28$) with transient hypogammaglobulinemia of infancy compared umckaloabo with placebo during an episode of URI. Umckaloabo resulted in increased appetite, decreased nasal congestion and improvement in daily and nocturnal coughing. However, the difference from placebo did not reach statistical significance. The authors recommended larger studies on the subject (Patiroglu et al., 2012).

ACTIVE CONSTITUENTS

Root

- Carbohydrates
  - Organic acids: shikimic acid 3-O-gallate
- Phenolic compounds
  - Phenolic acids (antioxidant): gallic acid and gallic acid methyl ester (antiviral, antibacterial)
  - Coumarins (venotonic, lymphatotonic): umckalin (unique to this genus), fraxetin, artelin (antiviral, antibacterial)
    - Coumarin glycosides: magnolioside, isofraxoside, umckalin-7-β-D-glucoside
    - Coumarin sulfates
  - Flavonoids: gallocatechin, epigallocatechin
    - Anthocyanidins (antioxidant, antiinflammatory, antineoplastic): prodelphinidins

- Steroids
  - Phytosterols: β-Sitosterol (reduces GI cholesterol absorption, inhibits 5-α-reductase)

Aerial Parts

- Carbohydrates
  - Organic acids: glucogallin, shikimic acid 3-O-gallate
- Phenolic compounds
  - Phenolic acids (antioxidant): gallic acid (antiviral, antibacterial)
  - Coumarins: umckalin (antibacterial), fraxetin (anticancer, hepatoprotective, antifibrotic, antiosteoporotic), artelin (antiviral, antibacterial)
    - coumarin glycosides: magnolioside, isofraxoside, umckalin-7-β-D-glucoside
  - Flavonoids (antiviral, antibacterial): dihydrokaempferol 3-O-β-D-glucoside, taxifolin-3-O-β-D-glucoside, luteolin 7-O-β-D-glucoside, quercetin (anti-inflammatory, antioxidant, hypotensive, antidiabetic, antispasmodic, neuroprotective, XO inhibition, antibacterial, anticancer), vitexin (antioxidant, anti-inflammatory, hepatoprotective, estrogen-β agonism, antihyperalgesic, antiarthritis, neuroprotective, antidepressant, dopaminergic, serotonergic, anticancer), isovitexin (hepatoprotective, anticarcinogenic, apoptotic, antistapyholcoccal), orientin, isoorientin, epigallocatechin-3-O-gallate
    - Tannins

UMCKALOABO COMMONLY USED PREPARATIONS AND DOSAGE (FOR ADULTS UNLESS OTHERWISE SPECIFIED)

The following are examples of some available formulations and ranges of dosing for commercial herbal products. See Part III Introduction "How to prescribe medicinal herbs" for further guidance on herbal advising and prescribing.

Root

- Tincture of root (1:5, 50%): 1-1.5 mL BID-QID
- Homeopathic tincture of root (1:8-10, 11%), homeopathic 1X dilution: 1-1.5 mL TID based on age (homeopathic syrup and powder also available)

- Capsule or tablet of powdered (4:1) extract: 30-60 mg QD (for age > 12)
- 1X dilution chewable tablets for adults or children: 1 tablet BID-TID

SAFETY AND PRECAUTION

Side Effects

Allergic reactions including rash, urticaria, and respiratory reactions have been reported (34 reports from 2002 to 2006 in Germany). Possible GI disturbances including heartburn, nausea, gastric pain, and diarrhea have been reported. Most clinical trials showed that ADRs did not differ significantly between umckaloabo and placebo. Supplementation appears to be very well tolerated for periods of up to a month, and supplementation of double the standard dose for a single week has also been very well tolerated. Studies in children specifically (ages between 3 and 18 years) have failed to note any unique toxicological effects for their age group, and it appears to be equally well tolerated.

A proprietary database created from prescriptions and patient data of primary care CAM physicians who participated in the Evaluation of Anthroposophical Medicine Pharmacovigilance Network (formed in 2004 in Berlin) was analyzed for ADRs of both CAM and conventional drugs. The study period was January 2004 through June 2009. There were 1,018,626 drugs (54.8% CAM) prescribed by 38 anthroposophical physicians for 88,431 patients, and 412 ADRs reported in 389 patients; 30.1% of the ADRs were for CAM drugs. The majority were reported in children (69.2%, $n=285$) and females (56.3%, $n=232$). Of the four ADRs rated as being serious, all were associated with conventional drugs. In a subgroup of practices, of 327 total ADRs, 10 (3.1%) were serious. There were 4.4 per 10,000 ADRs for CAM prescriptions and 13.0 per 10,000 ADRs for conventional prescriptions. The CAM drug with the highest frequency of ADRs was *Pelargonium sidoides* root (0.21%). The most frequently reported ingredient in CAM was ivy leaves with an ADR frequency of 0.17%. The most reported drug connected with ADRs was amoxicillin (1.3%). The authors concluded that there were no serious ADRs reported for CAM drugs and in the subset of seven physicians who had agreed to report all nonserious and serious ADRs, 1.2% of patients experienced at least one ADR, with rates of ADRs per 10,000 prescriptions being 4.4 for CAM drugs and 13.0 for conventional drugs (Tabali et al., 2012).

Case Reports

The Drug Commission of the German Medical Association analyzed the hepatotoxic potential of umckaloabo used to treat the common cold and other respiratory tract infections. In a review of 15 case reports of hepatotoxicity, in no case was there a highly probable or probable causality for umckaloabo. Analysis revealed confounding variables including co-medication with synthetic drugs, major comorbidities, low data quality, lack of appropriate consideration of differential diagnoses, and multiple alternative diagnoses. The author concluded that convincing evidence was lacking that umckaloabo was a potential hepatotoxin in the analyzed cases (Teschke et al., 2012).

Toxicity

There have been sporadic reports of hepatotoxicity associated with supplementation of umckaloabo in Germany where it is prescribed as a medication, although it appears that causality is lacking in the majority of cases. (see *Case Reports*)

Pregnancy and Lactation

Insufficient human data.

Disease Interactions

There is theoretical concern for interaction with autoimmune disease due to enhanced immune mechanisms.

Caution advised with surgical procedures due to coumarins present in umckaloabo.

Drug Interactions

- Immunosuppressants: May theoretically reduce efficacy of azathioprine, basiliximab, cyclosporine, daclizumab, muromonab-CD3, mycophenolate, tacrolimus, sirolimus, corticosteroids and others
- Does not influence serum pharmacokinetics of warfarin nor does it influence the blood clotting potential of it, despite coumarin content

REFERENCES

Agbabiaka TB, Guo R, Ernst E. Pelargonium sidoides for acute bronchitis: a systematic review and meta-analysis. Phytomedicine 2008;15(5):378–85.

Anheyer D, Cramer H, Lauche R, Saha FJ, Dobos G. Herbal medicine in children with respiratory tract infection: systematic review and meta-analysis. Acad Pediatr 2018;18(1):8–19.

Bachert C, Schapowal A, Funk P, Kieser M. Treatment of acute rhinosinusitis with the preparation from Pelargonium sidoides EPs 7630: a randomized, double-blind, placebo-controlled trial. Rhinology 2009;47(1):51–8.

Bereznoy VV, Riley DS, Wassmer G, Heger M. Efficacy of extract of Pelargonium sidoides in children with acute non-group A β-hemolytic streptococcus tonsillopharyngitis: a randomized, double-blind, placebo-controlled trial. Altern Ther Health Med 2003;9(5):68–79.

Chuchalin AG, Berman B, Lehmacher W. Treatment of acute bronchitis in adults with a pelargonium sidoides preparation (EPs 7630): a randomized, double-blind, placebo-controlled trial. Explore (NY) 2005;1(6):437–45.

Kamin W, Maydannik V, Malek FA, Kieser M. Efficacy and tolerability of EPs 7630 in children and adolescents with acute bronchitis—a randomized, double-blind, placebo-controlled multicenter trial with a herbal drug preparation from Pelargonium sidoides roots. Int J Clin Pharmacol Ther 2010a;48(3):184–91.

Kamin W, Maydannik VG, Malek FA, Kieser M. Efficacy and tolerability of EPs 7630 in patients (aged 6-18 years old) with acute bronchitis. Acta Paediatr 2010b;99(4):537–43.

Kamin W, Ilyenko LI, Malek FA, Kieser M. Treatment of acute bronchitis with EPs 7630: randomized, controlled trial in children and adolescents. Pediatr Int 2012;54(2):219–26.

Koch AK, Klose P, Lauche R, et al. A systematic review of phytotherapy for acute rhinosinusitis. Forsch Komplementmed 2016;23(3):165–9.

Lizogub VG, Riley DS, Heger M. Efficacy of a pelargonium sidoides preparation in patients with the common cold: a randomized, double blind, placebo-controlled clinical trial. Explore (NY) 2007;3(6):573–84.

Luna Jr LA, Bachi AL, Novaes e Brito RR, et al. Immune responses induced by Pelargonium sidoides extract in serum and nasal mucosa of athletes after exhaustive exercise: modulation of secretory IgA, IL-6 and IL-15. Phytomedicine 2011;18(4):303–8.

Matthys H, Funk P. EPs 7630 improves acute bronchitic symptoms and shortens time to remission. Results of a randomised, double-blind, placebo-controlled, multicentre trial. Planta Med 2008;74(6):686–92.

Matthys H, Eisebitt R, Seith B, Heger M. Efficacy and safety of an extract of Pelargonium sidoides (EPs 7630) in adults with acute bronchitis. A randomised, double-blind, placebo-controlled trial. Phytomedicine 2003;10(Suppl 4):7–17.

Matthys H, Kamin W, Funk P, Heger M. Pelargonium sidoides preparation (EPs 7630) in the treatment of acute bronchitis in adults and children. Phytomedicine 2007;14(Suppl 6):69–73.

Matthys H, Lizogub VG, Malek FA, Kieser M. Efficacy and tolerability of EPs 7630 tablets in patients with acute bronchitis: a randomised, double-blind, placebo-controlled dose-finding study with a herbal drug preparation from Pelargonium sidoides. Curr Med Res Opin 2010;26(6):1413–22.

Matthys H, Pliskevich DA, Bondarchuk OM, Malek FA, Tribanek M, Kieser M. Randomised, double-blind, placebo-controlled trial of EPs 7630 in adults with COPD. Respir Med 2013;107(5):691–701.

Michaelis M, Doerr HW, Cinatl Jr J. Investigation of the influence of EPs® 7630, a herbal drug preparation from Pelargonium sidoides, on replication of a broad panel of respiratory viruses. Phytomedicine 2011;18(5):384–6.

Patiroglu T, Tunc A, Eke Gungor H, Unal E. The efficacy of Pelargonium sidoides in the treatment of upper respiratory tract infections in children with transient hypogammaglobulinemia of infancy. Phytomedicine 2012;19(11):958–61.

Pereira A, Bester M, Soundy P, Apostolides Z. Anti-proliferative properties of commercial Pelargonium sidoides tincture, with cell-cycle G0/G1 arrest and apoptosis in Jurkat leukaemia cells. Pharmaceutical Biology 2016;54(9):1831–40.

Riley DS, Lizogub VG, Zimmermann A, Funk P, Lehmacher W. Efficacy and tolerability of high-dose Pelargonium extract in patients with the common cold. Altern Ther Health Med 2018;24(2):16–26.

Tabali M, Ostermann T, Jeschke E, Witt CM, Matthes H. Adverse drug reactions for CAM and conventional drugs detected in a network of physicians certified to prescribe CAM drugs. J Manag Care Pharm 2012;18(6):427–38.

Tahan F, Yaman M. Can the Pelargonium sidoides root extract EPs® 7630 prevent asthma attacks during viral infections of the upper respiratory tract in children? Phytomedicine 2013;20(2):148–50.

Teschke R, Frenzel C, Schulze J, Eickhoff A. Spontaneous reports of primarily suspected herbal hepatotoxicity by Pelargonium sidoides: was causality adequately ascertained? Regul Toxicol Pharmacol 2012;63(1):1–9.

Timmer A, Günther J, Rücker G, Motschall E, Antes G, Kern WV. Pelargonium sidoides extract for acute respiratory tract infections. Cochrane Database Syst Rev 2008;3, CD006323.

Timmer A, Günther J, Motschall E, Rücker G, Antes G, Kern WV. Pelargonium sidoides extract for treating acute respiratory tract infections. Cochrane Database Syst Rev 2013;10, CD006323.

Wagner L, Cramer H, Klose P, et al. Herbal medicine for cough: a systematic review and meta-analysis. Forsch Komplementmed 2015;22(6):359–68.

75

UVA URSI/BEARBERRY/KINNIKINIC/ BEAR GRAPE (*ARCTOSTAPHYLOS UVA-URSI*)
Leaf

GENERAL OVERVIEW

Uva-ursi has been used traditionally as a urinary tract remedy, especially for urinary tract infection. Arbutin, the chief constituent found in the leaves of the herb, has been shown to have antibacterial properties via its metabolite hydroquinone glucuronide. The presence of hydroquinone glucuronide in the bladder prevents bacteria from adhering to the uroepithelium. Unfortunately, uva-ursi should not be used on a chronic preventive basis due to potential carcinogenicity of hydroquinone glucuronide.

Clinical trials are almost non-existent for this herb and indicate that uva-ursi may be beneficial for prevention of recurrent urinary tract infections but may not be effective for acute urinary tract infections. Additional research is needed.

IN VITRO AND ANIMAL RESEARCH

Uva-ursi has been reported to show antibacterial efficacy in more than 70 strains of bacteria known to exist in the urinary tract, partially due to reduction of bacterial adhesion to bladder epithelium (which is thought to be the mechanism by which cranberry also works). It has been shown that arbutin alone requires high doses for direct urinary antimicrobial effects against *Candida albicans*, *Staphylococcus aureus*, and *Escherichia coli*. Although it has been held that arbutin requires an alkaline environment for conversion to hydroquinone, hydroquinone glucuronide has been shown in vitro, regardless of pH, to be taken up by urinary bacteria and converted into hydroquinone, which is potently bactericidal.

An aqueous extraction of uva-ursi (leaf and berry) in vitro inhibited the growth of *S. aureus* less potently than vancomycin and tetracycline but more strongly than most other tested herbals. It also showed ability to inhibit quorum sensing which is essential for biofilm development. An aqueous extract of the uva-ursi leaves increased hydrophobicity *of E. coli* and *Acinetobacter baumannii*, leading to bacterial clumping and excretion, which may be a second mechanism for efficacy against urinary tract infections. Coralagin, another constituent of uva-ursi, appears to potentiate the efficacy of β-lactam antibiotics against MRSA.

The active constituent ursolic acid has been shown in mice to have beneficial effects on hematopoiesis and to protect the bone marrow against radiation damage. Ursolic acid has also been shown to have anti-HIV activity and to increase ceramide and collagen contents of cultured human epidermal and dermal cells. It has demonstrated potent AChE inhibiting activity as well.

In a mouse model of contact dermatitis, arbutin was shown to synergistically enhance the anti-inflammatory effects of prednisolone but required doses of 100 mg/kg to produce this effect when used as a single agent without prednisolone. Uva-ursi was shown in vitro to inhibit melanin production, suggesting depigmenting properties. A-arbutin has been shown to reduce melanin synthesis up to 76% of control values in vitro. In human cells, arbutin was shown to reduce melanin formation in melanocytes via inhibition of tyrosinase and DHICA polymerase. Application of 250 μg of arbutin to a human skin model has been shown to reduce melanin synthesis to 40% of control (Sugimoto et al., 2004).

Uva-ursi has demonstrated decreased urolithiasis in rats, likely due to presence of saponins. It has also demonstrated diuretic properties in rats. Arbutin has been shown to have antitussive properties in cats at a dose of 50 mg/kg similar to 10 mg/kg of codeine.

HUMAN RESEARCH

Genitourinary Disorders: Cystitis and Recurrent Urinary Tract Infection

An RCT in women ($n = 382$) with dysuria, urgency, or frequency of urination and suspected lower UTI studied the antibiotic-sparing effects of uva-ursi extract with or without ibuprofen compared with placebo. All women were provided with a back-up prescription for antibiotics. On days 2–4 there was no difference in urinary frequency between Uva-ursi and placebo or between ibuprofen and no ibuprofen. Eventual antibiotic consumption with uva-ursi was 39.9% and with placebo was 47.4%; (OR = 0.59, $P = 0.293$), and with ibuprofen antibiotic consumption was 34.9 (OR = 0.27, $P = 0.009$). The authors concluded that there was evidence that advice to take ibuprofen will reduce antibiotic consumption without increasing complications, with NNT = 7 (Moore et al., 2019).

In a double-blind trial of women ($n = 57$) who had experienced at least three episodes of cystitis over 1 year, uva-ursi tablets given over the course of 1 month resulted in no recurrences for the following year compared with recurrences in 23% of the placebo group. The authors concluded that uva-ursi extract exerted a prophylactic effect on recurrent cystitis (Larsson et al., 1993).

ACTIVE CONSTITUENTS

- Carbohydrates
  - Organic acids: malic acid, allantoin (wound healing)
- Phenolic compounds:
  - Simple phenols (antimicrobial, anti-adhesion, antimelanin, anti-inflammatory, antitussive): arbutin, methylarbutin
  - Phenolic acids (antioxidant): gallic acid
  - Flavonoids: hyperoside (antioxidant, antiinflammatory, antiproliferative, apoptotic, hepatoprotective, nephroprotective, anti-osteoporotic), myricetin, quercetin (anti-inflammatory, antioxidant, hypotensive, antidiabetic, antispasmodic, neuroprotective, XO inhibition, antibacterial, anticancer), hyperin, myricitrin, isoquercitrin, quercitrin
    - □ Tannins: ellagic and gallic tannins, corilagin (potentiates β-lactam efficacy against MRSA)
- Terpenes
  - Monoterpenes: picroside, linalool (sedative, antispasmodic)
  - Triterpenes: α-amyrin, uvaol
  - Triterpenoid saponins: ursolic acid (anti-lithic, anti-HIV, anti-EBV, antiviral, androgenic, AChEI, pro-collagen, pro-ceremide, antitumor)
- Aromatic compounds: linalool (sedative, antispasmodic), α-terpineol

UVA-URSI COMMONLY USED PREPARATIONS AND DOSAGES (FOR ADULTS UNLESS OTHERWISE SPECIFIED)

The following are examples of some available formulations and ranges of dosing for commercial herbal products. See Part III Introduction "How to prescribe medicinal herbs" for further guidance on herbal advising and prescribing.

Leaf

- Infusion of leaf: 1–2 tsp per cup TID.
- Fluid extract (1:1, 25%): 1–3 mL TID.
- Tincture (1:5, 25%–50%): 2–4 mL TID.
- Powdered leaf extract: 750 mg (1/3 tsp) QD-BID.
- Capsule or tablet of powdered leaf: 460–1440 mg BID-TID.
- Capsule or tablet of freeze-dried leaf: 350 mg TID.
- Capsule or tablet of standardized extract (standardized to 20% arbutin): 700–1000 mg TID (delivers approx. to 140–200 mg of arbutin TID).

The literature suggests limiting the course to 14 days due to theoretical carcinogenesis from hydroquinone. (See toxicity below.)

Controversial recommendation (see in vitro section) is to add 1.5 tsp baking soda daily to raise urinary pH or eat a high vegetable diet.

Pharmacokinetics: Tablet vs Aqueous Solution

A cross-over RCT in volunteers ($n = 16$) investigated a single oral dose of uva-ursi leaf dry extract tablets compared with the uva-ursi in aqueous solution for metabolites. The total amounts of hydroquinone equivalents excreted in the urine from the extracts were similar in both groups, with 65% and 67% excreted with tablets and liquid, respectively ($P = 0.61$). The maximum mean urinary concentration of hydroquinone equivalents was a little higher and peaked earlier with the aqueous solution than with the tablet ($P = 0.38$). The relative bioavailability of the tablet compared with the aqueous solution was 103.3% for total hydroquinone equivalents. The authors concluded there were no significant differences between the two groups in the metabolite patterns detected (hydroquinone, hydroquinone-glucuronide, and hydroquinone-sulfate) (Schindler et al., 2002).

SAFETY AND PRECAUTION

Side Effects

Cramping, nausea, and vomiting may occur. Uva-ursi may turn the urine green especially if exposed to air.

Case Reports

A healthy 56-year-old woman who continuously used uva-ursi tea for 3 years reported bilateral bull's-eye maculopathy. Since the herb has been shown to inhibit melanin production, it may have played a role.

Toxicity

Hydroquinone (from arbutin) may be carcinogenic, so long-term use should be avoided. However, evidence indicates that hydroquinone does not accumulate in the body following chronic exposure and is metabolized by P450 enzymes to hydroquinone sulfate or hydroquinone glucuronide, which do not appear to be carcinogenic. Extremely high doses would be required to reach the toxic levels as demonstrated in rat studies.

Pregnancy and Lactation

Has theoretical oxytocic effect. Avoid in pregnancy. Insufficient evidence for safety with breastfeeding.

Disease Interactions

Due to case report of bull's-eye maculopathy, avoid with macular degeneration.

Drug Interactions

- CYP: Inhibits CYP3A4.
- Caution with diuretics due to possible excess diuresis.

REFERENCES

Larsson B, Jonasson A, Fianu S. Prophylactic effect of UVA-E in women with recurrent cystitis: a preliminary report. Curr Ther Res 1993;53(4):441–3.

Moore M, Trill J, Simpson C, et al. Uva-ursi extract and ibuprofen as alternative treatments for uncomplicated urinary tract infection in women (ATAFUTI): a factorial randomized trial. Clin Microbiol Infect 2019;25(8):973–80.

Schindler G, Patzak U, Brinkhaus B, et al. Urinary excretion and metabolism of arbutin after oral administration of Arctostaphylos uvae ursi extract as film-coated tablets and aqueous solution in healthy humans. J Clin Pharmacol 2002.

Sugimoto K, et al. Inhibitory effects of α-arbutin on melanin synthesis in cultured human melanoma cells and a three-dimensional human skin model. Biol Pharm Bull 2004;27(4):510–4.

76

VALERIAN (*VALERIANA OFFICINALIS*)
Root

■ ■ ■ ■ ■ ■ ■ ■   ■ ■ ■ ■ ■ ■ ■ ■ ■

GENERAL OVERVIEW

It would be reasonable to assume that the pharmaceutical company that first marketed diazepam in the US selected the brand name in allusion to the herb valerian. However, there is no evidence of such a linkage even though the similarly named drug shares many of the effects of this medicinal herb. More likely, both the herbal and pharmaceutical names come from the Latin word "valere," which means "to be in health." Valerian is a sedating herb that has had widespread use for insomnia since 400 BCE. Although the evidence from human studies on insomnia is not as impressive as one might expect, this author can share an anecdotal experience after harvesting a bucketful of valerian root without wearing protective gloves as is generally advised. She found herself needing an uncharacteristic four-hour nap in the middle of the day. Valerian is also used for anxiety, often in combination with other herbal products with which it has the strongest evidence. Valerian also has evidence for benefits beyond the anxiolytic and soporific effects of diazepam.

Clinical research indicates that valerian, alone or in combination formulas, may be beneficial for premenstrual syndrome, dysmenorrhea, menopause, postoperative cognitive impairment, restless legs syndrome, anxiety, obsessive-compulsive disorder, and attention-deficit/hyperactivity disorder (with lemon balm). Trials with valerian alone for insomnia are mostly disappointing but consistently positive when combined with hops or lemon balm.

IN VITRO AND ANIMAL RESEARCH

In vitro, valerian shows antioxidant, cytoprotective, and neuroprotective effects. The valerian constituents hydroxypinoresinol and valerenic acid have been found to bind to GABA receptors similar to the activity of benzodiazepines. Valerian has activities that suggest potential benefit for cardiovascular, GI, and GU systems. It exhibits antispasmodic and hypotensive effects via potassium channel activation. It also demonstrates a protective effect against vasopressin-induced coronary spasm and pressor response. The antispasmodic effects of valeranone and didrovaltrate were studied ex vivo on guinea pig ileum and demonstrated equipotency to papaverine in inhibiting contractions, relaxing smooth muscle via direct musculotropic activity rather than via the autonomic nervous system.

In animal research valerian has shown antihypertensive, anxiolytic, antidepressant, and antispasmodic effects. The chief constituent valerenic acid has been shown in animal research to inhibit central catabolism of GABA, thereby increasing GABA concentration and decreasing CNS activity. The constituent valepotriate has been shown to increase norepinephrine and dopamine levels in rodents. Supplementation of 100 mg/kg valerian root or an equivalent amount of valerenic acid (340 mcg/kg) for 3 weeks in pre-aged rats appeared to improve memory and learning associated with decreases in serum corticosterone and lipid peroxidation in the hippocampus. Some valerian constituents have shown anticancer effects on ovarian, lung, prostate, colon, and liver cancer cell lines, but no clinical trials have yet been performed.

HUMAN RESEARCH

Women's Genitourinary Disorders: Premenstrual Syndrome and Dysmenorrhea

A three-cycle RCT in female students ($n = 100$) with PMS compared valerian BID with placebo during the last 7 days of each cycle for effect on PMS symptoms. A significant difference from baseline was seen in emotional, behavioral, and physical premenstrual symptom severity in the valerian group ($P < 0.001$) but not in the placebo group. The authors concluded that valerian may reduce emotional, physical, and behavioral symptoms of PMS (Behboodi Moghadam et al., 2016).

A two-cycle RCT in patients ($n = 100$) with dysmenorrhea compared valerian 255 mg TID with placebo for 3 days beginning at the onset of menstruation. The pain severity was significantly reduced with both valerian and placebo ($P < 0.001$), but the extent of the reduction was greater in the valerian group, with the difference between the two groups being statistically significant ($P < 0.05$). The total scores of the systemic manifestations associated with dysmenorrhea decreased similarly in the valerian and placebo groups, except for syncope ($P < 0.05$). The authors concluded that valerian seemed to be an effective treatment for dysmenorrhea, likely due to its antispasmodic effects (Mirabi et al., 2011).

Women's Genitourinary Disorders: Menopause

A 2017 review of clinical trials on herbal efficacy in menopausal symptoms used search terms menopause, climacteric, hot flushes, flashes, herb, and phytoestrogens. The authors found that valerian, passionflower, sage, lemon balm, black cohosh, fenugreek, black seed, chasteberry, fennel, evening primrose, ginkgo, alfalfa, St. John's wort, Asian ginseng, anise, licorice, red clover, and wild soybean were effective in the treatment of acute menopausal syndrome with different mechanisms. The authors concluded that medicinal plants could play a role in the treatment of acute menopausal syndrome and that further studies were warranted (Kargozar et al., 2017).

A 2016 systematic review to assess the effectiveness of herbal medicines in alleviating hot flushes found 19 RCTs that met inclusion criteria. Studies found that valerian, anise, licorice, soy, black cohosh, red clover, passionflower, chasteberry, avocado plus soybean oil, and St. John's wort could alleviate the side effects of hot flushes. The authors concluded that herbal medicine could be an alternative treatment for women experiencing hot flushes (Ghazanfarpour et al., 2016).

An 8-week RCT in menopausal women ($n = 68$) with hot flushes compared valerian 225 mg TID with placebo for effect on hot flushes. The severity of hot flushes decreased significantly from baseline with valerian ($P < 0.001$) but not with placebo. The difference in severity of hot flush at the end of treatment was significantly lower with valerian compared with placebo ($P < 0.001$). Valerian has also led to a reduction of hot flush frequencies after 4 and 8 weeks of treatment ($P < 0.001$). The authors concluded that valerian could be effective in treatment of menopausal hot flushes (Mirabi and Mojab, 2013).

A 2-month RCT in postmenopausal women ($n = 60$) compared valerian 530 mg BID with placebo for effect on hot flushes. The severity of hot flushes with valerian was significantly lower than with placebo after 1 and 2 months of intervention ($P = 0.048$ and $P = 0.020$, respectively). The mean frequency of hot flushes was also significantly reduced with valerian compared with placebo ($P = 0.033$). The authors concluded that healthcare providers should consider valerian to be effective for menopausal women with hot flushes (Jenabi et al., 2018).

A 4-week RCT in postmenopausal women ($n = 100$) with sleep disturbances compared valerian 530 mg BID with placebo. A statistically significant change was reported in the quality of sleep on the Pittsburgh Sleep Quality Index with valerian compared with placebo ($P < 0.001$). Improvement in quality of sleep occurred in 30% with valerian and 4% with placebo ($P < 0.001$). The authors concluded that valerian improved the quality of sleep in postmenopausal women with insomnia (Taavoni et al., 2011).

Neurological Disorders: Tension Headache

A 1-month RCT in patients ($n = 88$) with tension headaches compared valerian root extract 530 mg (Sedamin) with placebo, each given as two capsules after dinner. After 1 month, the mean scores of impact on ADLs with valerian and placebo were 51.2 and 57.0, respectively; $P<0.001$). The mean disability scores with valerian and placebo were 22.9 and 27.4, respectively ($P<0.001$). The severity scores showed greater reductions with valerian than with placebo (to 3.5 and 5.1, respectively; $P<0.001$). The authors concluded that valerian could reduce severity of tension headaches and impact on ADLs and disability (Azizi et al., 2020).

Neurological Disorders: Postoperative Cognitive Impairment

A 2-month RCT in patients ($n=61$) undergoing elective CABG using cardiopulmonary bypass compared valerian 530 mg BID with placebo starting 1 day before surgery and continuing for 60 days after surgery to assess effects on postoperative cognitive function. With valerian, mean MMSE score decreased from 27 preoperatively to 26.5 at the 10th postoperative day and then increased to 27.4 at the 60th postoperative day. With placebo mean MMSE score was 27.3 at baseline, 24 at day 10, and 24.8 at day 60. Valerian prophylaxis reduced odds of cognitive dysfunction compared with placebo (OR=0.108). The authors concluded that valerian may prevent early postoperative cognitive dysfunction after on-pump CABG (Hassani et al., 2015).

Neurological Disorders: Restless Legs Syndrome

An 8-week RCT in patients ($n=37$) with RLS compared valerian 800 mg QHS with placebo for effect on sleep quality and symptom severity. Both groups reported improvement in RLS symptom severity and sleep. When comparing sleepy and non-sleepy participants, significant differences before and after treatment were found in sleepiness ($P=0.01$) and RLS symptoms ($P=0.02$) in the valerian group, with a strong positive association between changes in sleepiness and RLS symptom severity ($P=0.006$). The authors concluded that valerian was associated with improved symptoms of RLS and decreased daytime sleepiness in the subjects who had baseline daytime sleepiness (Cuellar and Ratcliffe, 2009).

Psychiatric Disorders: Anxiety and Stress

A 2010 review to evaluate effectiveness of herbal medicines for GAD found that kava had an unequivocal anxiolytic effect. Isolated studies with valerian, ginkgo, chamomile, passionflower, and *Galphimia glauca*

showed a potential use for anxious diseases. Ginkgo and chamomile showed an effect size (Cohen's d=0.47 to 0.87) similar to or greater than standard anxiolytics drugs (benzodiazepines, buspirone and antidepressants) (Faustino et al., 2010).

A 2006 systematic review investigating the effectiveness and safety of valerian for treating anxiety disorders found only one RCT that met inclusion criteria. It was a 4-week pilot study of valerian, diazepam, and placebo. There were no significant differences between the valerian and placebo groups in HAM-A total scores, or in somatic and psychic factor scores. Similarly, there were no significant differences in HAM-A scores between the valerian and diazepam groups, although based on STAI-trait scores, significantly greater symptom improvement occurred in the diazepam group. There were no significant differences between the three groups in the number of patients reporting side effects or in dropout rates. The authors concluded that there was insufficient evidence to draw any conclusions about the efficacy or safety of valerian compared with placebo or diazepam for anxiety disorders (Miyasaka et al., 2006).

A single-dose RCT in women ($n=64$) with infertility undergoing hysterosalpingography studied valeric acid 1500 mg plus mefenamic acid 150 mg compared with mefenamic acid 150 mg alone given 30 min prior to the procedure for impact on anxiety. There was no difference between groups on baseline anxiety severity ($P=0.26$). After the intervention, a significant difference in anxiety severity was reported in both groups ($P<0.0001$), with the anxiety score in the valeric acid group compared with the control group reduced significantly. The authors concluded that valeric acid was effective in reducing anxiety in women undergoing hysterosalpingography (Gharib et al., 2015).

A single-dose RCT in patients ($n=20$) undergoing dental extractions compared valerian 100 mg with placebo 1 h before the surgical dental procedure to measure effect on anxiety. Based on reports from the surgeons and researchers, patients treated with valerian were calmer and more relaxed during surgery. Valerian had a greater effects on the maintenance of SBP and HR after surgery. The authors concluded that valerian was more effective than placebo at controlling anxiety when used for the conscious sedation in patients undergoing dental extractions (Pinheiro et al., 2014).

A 4-week RCT in patients ($n = 36$) with generalized anxiety disorder compared flexibly dosed valepotriates (mean daily dose: 81.3 mg) with diazepam (mean daily dose: 6.5 mg) and with placebo. No significant difference was observed in the change from baseline on HAM-A or STAI-trait scores. All three groups presented a significant reduction in the total HAM-A scores. However, only the diazepam and valepotriates groups showed a significant reduction in the psychic factor of HAM-A. The diazepam group also showed a significant reduction of the STAI-trait. The authors concluded that the valepotriates may have a potential anxiolytic effect on the psychic symptoms of anxiety (Andreatini et al., 2002).

A 28-day RCT in patients ($n = 182$) with adjustment disorder with anxious mood investigated Euphytose, a polyherbal product containing hawthorn, passionflower, valerian, *Ballota*, *Cola*, and *Paullinia* (the combination being theoretically both calming and stimulating), compared with placebo, two tablets TID for effects on anxiety. Comparing the two groups, 42.9% and 25.3% of the herbal and placebo groups, respectively, had a HAM-A score of less than 10 at day 28 ($P = 0.012$). The authors noted that from day 7 to day 28 there was a significant difference between the groups ($P = 0.042$), indicating that Euphytose was better than placebo in treatment of adjustment disorder with anxious mood (Bourin et al., 1997).

An acutely dosed RCT in healthy men ($n = 72$) investigated pre-dosing for 4 days with Ze 185, a fixed combination of valerian, passionflower, lemon balm, and butterbur, compared with pre-dosing with placebo and with a no-treatment control for effects on biological and affective responses to a standardized psychosocial stress paradigm. The stress paradigm induced significant and large cortisol and self-reported anxiety responses. Groups did not differ significantly in their salivary cortisol response to stress, but participants in the herbal group showed significantly attenuated responses in self-reported anxiety compared with placebo ($P = 0.03$) and with no treatment ($P = 0.05$). The authors suggested that the herbal combination reduced the self-reported anxiety response to stress without affecting the assumingly adaptive biological stress responses (Meier et al., 2018).

An acutely dosed crossover RCT with washout periods in healthy volunteers ($n = 24$) studied a combination of lemon balm plus valerian 600 mg, 1200 mg, and 1800 mg compared with placebo on separate days for effects on mood and anxiety under laboratory-induced stress. The results showed that the 600-mg dose of the combination ameliorated the negative effects of the Defined Intensity Stressor Simulation (DISS) battery on ratings of anxiety. However, the 1800-mg dose showed an increase in anxiety that was less marked, but which reached significance during one testing session. In addition, all three doses led to decrements in performance on the Stroop task module within the battery, and the two lower doses led to decrements on the overall score generated on the DISS battery. The authors concluded that the combination of valerian and lemon balm had anxiolytic properties that warranted further investigation (Kennedy et al., 2006).

An 8-day RCT in healthy volunteers ($n = 54$) compared kava with valerian and with controls for 7 days for moderation of laboratory-induced psychological stress. Compared with baseline, at the second stress-inducing testing session there was a significant decrease in SBP but not DBP responsivity with both kava and valerian. Subjects also reported less test-associated pressure after taking kava or valerian. Compared with baseline, the HR reaction to mental stress was found to decline in the valerian group but not in the kava group. There were no significant changes from baseline in BP, HR, or subjective reports of pressure in the control group. Test performance did not change between the groups over the two time points. The authors concluded that kava and valerian may be beneficial for reducing physiological reactivity during stressful situations (Cropley et al., 2002).

A 3.5-year retrospective case-control study of hospitalized psychiatric patients ($n = 3252$) evaluated an herbal extract combination of passionflower, valerian, lemon balm, and butterbur (Ze 185) compared with no additional herbal therapy to investigate whether the herbal combination would change the prescription pattern of benzodiazepines. Data showed that both treatment modalities had a comparable clinical effectiveness but there were significantly fewer prescriptions of benzodiazepines with the herbal combination ($P = 0.006$). The authors recommended that an RCT be performed (Keck et al., 2020).

A 2-week open-label trial in patients ($n = 777$) with complaints of nervousness or restlessness compared "valerian combination products" to the homeopathic preparation Neurexan (*Avena sativa* 4X, *Coffea arabica* 14X, *Passiflora incarnata* 4X, and *Zincum isovalerianicum* 6X) with dosing at the discretion of the physician. Subjects receiving the homeopathic tended to be female, to weigh less, to have fewer concomitant illnesses and slightly milder severity of nervousness or restlessness than the subjects receiving the valerian products. After 2 weeks, the score for nervousness or restlessness was reduced from 19 to 7.4 and from 21.4 to 12.6 with the homeopathic and valerian products, respectively. The changes from baseline and the differences between the groups were statistically significant. Similar significant differences in effects were seen on the subscores and on the subjects' assessments of effectiveness. Both study therapies were well tolerated. The authors concluded that Neurexan appeared to be an effective and well-tolerated alternative to valerian-based combination therapies for the treatment of nervousness or restlessness (Hubner et al., 2009).

Psychiatric Disorders: Insomnia

A 2015 systematic review to assess the safety and efficacy of herbal medicine for the treatment of insomnia found 14 RCTs ($n = 1602$) that met inclusion criteria. Four distinct herbs were identified (valerian, chamomile, kava, and *Xylaria nigripes*). There was no statistically significant difference between any herbal medicine and placebo or active control for any of the 13 measures of clinical efficacy. Adverse events with valerian were greater than placebo but were less than or equal to placebo with the other three herbs. The authors concluded that, although there was insufficient evidence to support the use of herbal medicine for insomnia, there was a clear need for further research in this area (Leach and Page, 2015).

A 2011 systematic review of CAM therapies for insomnia found 20 RCTs involving eight CAM interventions that met inclusion criteria. There was support for the treatment of chronic insomnia with acupressure ($d = 1.42$–2.12), tai chi ($d = 0.22$–2.15), and yoga ($d = 0.66$-1.20); mixed evidence for acupuncture and L-tryptophan; and weak and unsupportive evidence for herbal medicines such as valerian (Sarris and Byrne, 2011).

A 2010 meta-analysis evaluating the effects of valerian on sleep found 18 RCTs that met inclusion criteria. The mean differences in latency time between the valerian and placebo treatment groups was 0.70 min. The standardized mean differences between the groups for sleep quality VAS was -0.02. Valerian showed a relative risk of sleep quality improvement of 1.37 compared with placebo. There was heterogeneity in the three meta-analyses, but it diminished in the subgroup analysis. No publication bias was detected. The authors concluded that valerian could be effective for a subjective improvement of insomnia, although its effectiveness had not been demonstrated with quantitative or objective measurements (Fernández-San-Martín et al., 2010).

A 2007 systematic review that examined the evidence for valerian with insomnia, done with specific attention to the type of preparations tested and the characteristics of the subjects studied, found 37 RCTs that met inclusion criteria: 29 controlled trials investigated for both efficacy and safety, and 8 open-label trials investigated for safety only. Most studies found no significant differences between valerian and placebo either in healthy individuals or in persons with general sleep disturbance or insomnia. None of the most recent studies, which were also the most methodologically rigorous, found significant effects of valerian on sleep. The authors concluded that, while valerian is a safe herb associated with only rare adverse events, it does not appear to be effective as a sleep aid for insomnia (Taibi et al., 2009).

A 2006 systematic review to assess valerian for improving sleep quality found 16 RCTs ($n = 1093$) that met inclusion criteria. Most studies had significant methodologic problems, and the valerian doses, preparations, and length of treatment varied considerably. A dichotomous outcome of sleep quality (improved or not) was reported by six studies and showed a statistically significant benefit (RR = 1.8 for improved sleep), but there was evidence of publication bias. The authors concluded that valerian might improve sleep quality without producing side effects (Bent et al., 2006).

A 2005 review to evaluate the level of evidence regarding the safety and efficacy of nonprescription therapies used for insomnia found that rigorous scientific data supporting a beneficial effect was not found for most herbal supplements, dietary changes, and other nutritional supplements popularly used for treating insomnia symptoms. Studies were limited by small numbers of participants and, in some instances, inadequate design, lack of statistical analysis, and sparse use of objective measurements. There was preliminary but conflicting evidence suggesting valerian and first-generation H1-receptor antagonists had efficacy as mild hypnotics for short-term use. There were significant potential risks associated with the use of Jamaican dogwood, kava, alcohol, and L-tryptophan (Meolie et al., 2005).

A 2002 systematic review to evaluate efficacy of valerian as a sleeping aid found 18 RCTs that met inclusion criteria including two that compared valerian with pharmaceutical hypnotics. Most studies reported positive effects of valerian on subjective sleep parameters. Objective sleep measures yielded inconsistent results. All studies covered a short period of time. Few side effects were reported. The authors concluded that valerian may have some hypnotic effects (Pallesen et al., 2002).

A 2000 systematic review to assess the effects of valerian on insomnia found nine RCTs that met inclusion criteria. The findings of the studies were contradictory and there was great inconsistency between trials in terms of patients, experimental design and procedures, and methodological quality. The authors concluded that evidence for valerian as treatment for insomnia was inconclusive (Stevinson and Ernst, 2000).

An acutely dosed RCT in patients ($n = 128$) compared an aqueous valerian extract 400 mg with a proprietary valerian-containing preparation and with placebo for effect on sleep. The valerian extract produced a significant decrease in subjectively investigated sleep latency scores and a significant improvement in sleep quality that was most notable among people who considered themselves poor or irregular sleepers, smokers, and people who thought they normally had long sleep latencies. Valerian did not have significant effects on night awakenings, dream recall and somnolence the next morning. The proprietary valerian-containing preparation produced a significant increase only in reports of feeling more sleepy than normal the next morning (Leathwood et al., 1982).

A 2-week Phase II RCT in older women ($n = 16$) with insomnia compared valerian extract 300 mg with placebo 30 min before HS. There were no statistically significant differences between valerian and placebo after a single dose or after 2 weeks of nightly dosing on any measure of sleep latency, wake after sleep onset, sleep efficiency, and self-rated sleep quality. In fact, valerian increased wake after sleep onset significantly ($P = 0.02$) after 2 weeks of nightly valerian but not after placebo. Side effects were minor and did not differ significantly between valerian and placebo. The author concluded that valerian did not improve sleep in older women (Taibi et al., 2007).

A single-dose and 14-day multi-dose RCT in patients ($n = 16$) with psychopathological insomnia compared valerian with placebo for subjective and polysomnographic effects on sleep. After a single dose of valerian, no effects on sleep structure and subjective sleep assessment were observed. After multiple-dose treatment, sleep efficiency showed a significant polysomnographic improvement over baseline for both the placebo and valerian. Slow-wave sleep latency was reduced by 21.3 min and 13.5 min with valerian and placebo, respectively ($P < 0.05$). The slow wave sleep percentage of time in bed was increased with valerian compared with baseline (9.8% and 8.1% respectively; $P < 0.05$). Subjective assessment of sleep latency and a higher correlation coefficient between subjective and objective sleep latencies was noted with valerian. There was no difference between placebo and valerian with respect to increases in REM percentage and decreases in NREM1 percentage. Adverse events occurred in 3 and 18 patients with valerian and placebo, respectively (fewer with valerian). The authors concluded that valerian had positive effects on sleep structure and perception (Donath et al., 2000).

A 3-day study in elderly patients ($n = 14$) with poor sleep compared valerian extract 405 mg TID with placebo. Subjects in the valerian group showed an increase in slow-wave sleep and a decrease in stage 1 sleep. Density of K-complexes was increased with active treatment. There was no effect on sleep onset time or time awake after sleep onset. REM sleep was unaltered. There was also no effect on self-rated sleep quality. The authors hypothesized that valerian increased slow-wave sleep in subjects with low baseline values (Schulz et al., 1994).

A crossover study in volunteers ($n = 11$) looked at the effects of 60 and 120 mg valerian doses with a

1-week washout on computer analysis sleep stages and psychometric measures. Both dosages showed an increase in stages 1 and 2 sleep as well as wakefulness, and a decrease of stage 4 sleep and a slight reduction of REM-sleep. With 120 mg, the frequency of REM-phases declined during the first half of the night, whereas during the second part of the night, REM surplus occurred. Based on β-intensity of the EEG during REM-sleep, a stronger hypnotic effect was observed with 120 mg than with 60 mg. Maximum effect occurred 2–3 h after medication. Mood scales did not differ between groups (Gessner and Klasser, 1984).

A television-based recruitment RCT in participants ($n = 405$) compared valerian with placebo for effects on sleep. There was no significant difference between valerian and placebo in improvement of self-reported sleep quality (29% and 21%, respectively; $P = 0.08$). On the global self-assessment question at the end of the treatment period 5.5% more participants in the valerian group than in the placebo group perceived their sleep as better or much better ($P = 0.04$). Night awakenings occurred in 6% more patients in the valerian group than in the placebo group, and improved sleep duration occurred in 7.5% more patients in the valerian group than in the placebo group. There were no serious adverse events and no important or statistically significant differences in minor adverse events. The authors concluded that valerian appears to be safe and to have modest beneficial effects on insomnia (Oxman et al., 2007).

A sleep-lab based crossover RCT in patients ($n = 16$) with sleep disturbance compared valerian 300 mg with valerian 600 mg and with placebo given HS followed by a 6-day washout. Results showed no significant effect difference between valerian 300 mg, valerian 600 mg, or placebo on any EEG parameter or psychometric measure. The authors concluded that valerian at these two doses was ineffective when used acutely for sleep problems (Diaper and Hindmarch, 2004).

An 8-week RCT in children ($n = 5$) with intellectual deficits compared valerian with placebo for efficacy in disturbed sleep. Compared with baseline and placebo, valerian treatment led to significant reductions in sleep latencies and nocturnal time awake, lengthened total sleep time, and improved sleep quality. The treatment appeared to be most effective in children with deficits that involved hyperactivity. The authors concluded

that, pending confirmatory studies, valerian may be useful and safe in sleep disorders of children with intellectual deficits (Francis and Dempster, 2002).

Because valepotriates in valerian have cytotoxic effects, an RCT was undertaken to evaluate the sedative effects of Valerina Natt, a valerian compound that contains primarily sesquiterpenes. Of the subjects given the herbal product, 44% reported perfect sleep and 89% reported improved sleep, and these findings were significantly superior to placebo ($P < 0.001$) (Lindahl and Lindwall, 1989).

A 28-day RCT in patients ($n = 75$) with insomnia compared valerian 600 mg QHS with oxazepam 10 mg QHS for sleep improvement. In both groups sleep quality improved significantly ($P < 0.001$), and no statistically significant difference could be found between groups ($P = 0.70$). Effect sizes between groups varied between 0.02 and 0.25. Five persons withdrew due to possibly adverse drug reactions (two with valerian and three with oxazepam). No serious adverse events happened. The authors concluded that there were no differences in sleep efficacy between valerian and oxazepam (Dorn, 2000).

A 6-week RCT in patients ($n = 202$) with nonorganic insomnia compared valerian 600 mg QHS with oxazepam 10 mg QHS. Sleep quality, as measured by Sleep Questionnaire B (SF-B) was improved similarly with valerian and oxazepam. Both treatments markedly increased sleep quality compared with baseline ($P < 0.01$). Feeling of refreshment after sleep, psychic stability in the evening, psychic exhaustion in the evening, psychosomatic symptoms in the sleep phase, dream recall, and duration of sleep were similar between treatments. Clinical Global Impressions scale and Global Assessment of Efficacy by investigator and patient were similar between treatments. Adverse events occurred in 28.4% and 36% of patients receiving valerian and oxazepam, respectively, and were all rated mild to moderate. No serious adverse drug reactions were reported in either group. Most patients assessed their respective treatment as "very good" (82.8% in the valerian group and 73.4% in the oxazepam group). The authors concluded that valerian 600 mg was comparable to oxazepam 10 mg for non-organic insomnia (Ziegler et al., 2002).

A two-phase RCT in volunteers ($n = 102$) compared valerian root extract 600 mg with flunitrazepam 1 mg and with placebo on reaction time, alertness, and concentration. A single dose of each was followed by comparison the following morning. Then valerian was compared with placebo after given QHS for 2 weeks. With single and sustained administration of valerian, median reaction time was similar to placebo ($P = 0.448$). The authors concluded that neither single nor repeated evening administrations of 600 mg of valerian root extract had relevant negative impact on reaction time, alertness, and concentration the morning after intake (Kuhlmann et al., 1999).

A single-dosed RCT in healthy volunteers ($n = 80$) compared valerian plus hops tablets with valerian syrup, with flunitrazepam, and with placebo for residual sedative effects the following morning in addition to effects on quality of sleep. The subjective perception of sleep quality was improved in all three medication groups when compared with placebo. Subjective and objective impairment of performance on the morning after medication occurred only in the flunitrazepam group. Mild side effects were reported in 50% of the flunitrazepam group and 10% of the other groups. A very slight impairment of vigilance 1-2 hours after taking the valerian was statistically significant as was a retardation in the processing of complex information for the valerian plus hops group. The authors concluded that residual sedative effects observed in some earlier studies could not be confirmed for the recommended doses of the two herbal remedies but instead showed improved subjective reports of alertness, activity, and wellbeing. However, a slight impairment of performance during the first few hours after ingestion should be anticipated. The authors noted that impairment of vigilance on the morning after ingestion of benzodiazepines confirmed by this study constituted a potential hazard and that plant remedies such as those examined in this study should be considered as viable alternatives (Gerhard et al., 1996)

A 3-week RCT in patients with sleep disorders studied a combination of hops plus valerian compared with a benzodiazepine given for 2 weeks. The equivalence of both therapies according to sleep quality, fitness, and quality of life was proven by a Mann-Whitney-Statistic of 0.50. The patients' state of health (based on a four-point scale) improved during therapy while showing a deterioration after cessation with both

preparations. Withdrawal symptoms occurred only with the benzodiazepine. Abdominal complaints were reported with both the herbal product and the drug. The authors concluded that the hop-valerian preparation was a sensible alternative to a benzodiazepine for treatment of nonchronic and non-psychiatric sleep disorders (Schmitz and Jäckel, 1998).

A 14-week crossover pilot study in patients ($n = 24$) with stress-induced insomnia compared valerian 600 mg QD with kava 120 mg QD for 6 weeks each with a 2-week wash-out period. Total stress severity and insomnia were significantly reduced over baseline by both herbs ($P < 0.01$ for both parameters) with no significant differences between them. Side effects occurred in 42% of patients. The authors concluded that kava and valerian may be useful in the treatment of stress and insomnia (Wheatley, 2001).

An 8-week internet-based RCT in participants ($n = 1551$) with anxiety compared kava plus placebo with valerian plus placebo and with a double placebo for kava's effect on anxiety and valerian's effect on insomnia. Anxiety symptoms on the STAI-State questionnaire decreased by 11.7 and 14.4 points with kava and placebo, respectively. Insomnia based on Insomnia-Severity Index scored decreased by 7.9 and 8.3 points with valerian and placebo, respectively. The authors concluded that neither kava nor valerian relieved anxiety or insomnia more than placebo (Jacobs et al., 2005).

A 2-week pilot study in patients ($n = 30$) with mild-moderate non-organic insomnia investigated Ze 91019, a combination of valerian 250 mg plus hops 60 mg, two tablets HS for effects of polysomnography. A polysomnographic re-examination after 2 weeks of treatment revealed declines in the sleep latency and wake time. Stage 1 sleep was reduced, and slow-wave sleep was increased. In addition, the patients reported being more refreshed in the morning. No adverse events were observed (Fussel et al., 2000).

A 2-week RCT in patients ($n = 91$) with primary insomnia investigated NSF-3, an herbal combination containing valerian, hops, and passionflower, one tablet QHS compared with zolpidem 10 mg QHS. There was a significant improvement in total sleep time, sleep latency, number of nightly awakenings, and insomnia severity index scores in both groups. No statistically significant difference was observed between the groups. Epworth sleepiness scores did not change significantly over the study period. Mild adverse events were reported in 12 herbal subjects and 16 zolpidem subjects. The authors concluded that this combination of valerian, passionflower and hops was a safe and effective short-term alternative to zolpidem for primary insomnia (Maroo et al., 2013).

A 28-day RCT in patients ($n = 184$) with mild insomnia studied valerian 374 mg plus hops 84 mg QHS for 28 days compared with diphenhydramine 50 mg QHS for 14 days then placebo for 14 days and with placebo for 28 days for efficacy and safety in mild insomnia. At 14 days, patients in the valerian-hops and diphenhydramine groups rated their insomnia severity lower relative to placebo. The QOL component was significantly more improved in the valerian-hops group compared with the placebo group at the end of 28 days. Modest improvements of subjective sleep parameters were obtained with both the valerian-hops combination and diphenhydramine, but few group comparisons with placebo reached statistical significance. Valerian-hops produced slightly greater reductions of sleep latency relative to both placebo and diphenhydramine at the end of 14 days of treatment and greater reductions than placebo at the end of 28 days of treatment, but these changes did not reach statistical significance. Diphenhydramine produced significantly greater increases in sleep efficiency and a trend for increased total sleep time relative to placebo during the first 14 days of treatment. Polysomnography did not reveal any significant differences between groups for sleep continuity variables or for stages 3-4 sleep and REM sleep. There were no significant adverse events with either valerian or diphenhydramine and no rebound insomnia following their discontinuation. The authors concluded that there was a modest hypnotic effect for the valerian-hops combination and for diphenhydramine and that valerian-hops was associated with improved QOL (Morin et al., 2005).

A 4-week RCT in patients with non-organic insomnia studied Ze 91019, a combination of a fixed dose valerian 500 mg plus hops 120 mg compared with valerian 500 mg and with placebo each given QHS. The fixed combination was significantly superior to placebo in reducing the sleep latency. Valerian alone was not superior to placebo. The authors concluded that addition of hops to valerian for insomnia had merit (Koetter et al., 2007).

A 20-day RCT in patients ($n = 120$) with sleep disturbances investigated Vagonotte, a polyherbal compound of valerian, hops, and jujube, two pills QHS compared with placebo for effects on primary insomnia symptoms and sleep disturbances not related to medical or psychiatric causes. Sleep onset latency and nighttime awakenings were reduced, and total sleep time increased significantly with the herbal compound compared with placebo ($P < 0.001$ for all). Daily symptom improvement in subjects receiving the herbal compound showed significants reduction in tension and irritability, difficulty in concentration, and fatigue intensity compared with placebo ($P < 0.001$). None of the 60 subjects in the herbal group reported adverse reactions related to the herbal compound, and 98% of subjects judged the product as having from good to excellent safety and tolerability. The authors concluded that this polyherbal compound showed promise for primary insomnia (Palmieri et al., 2017).

An open-label study in children < 12 years ($n = 918$) with restlessness and dyssomnia assessed the efficacy and tolerability of Euvegal Forte, a combined valerian plus lemon balm preparation. The core symptoms of dyssomnia and restlessness were reduced from "moderate/severe" to "mild" or "absent" in most of the patients. Clear improvement occurred for dyssomnia in 81% and for restlessness in 70% of the patients. Both parents and investigators assessed efficacy as "very good" or "good" (60% and 68%, respectively). The tolerability of the product was "very good" or "good" in 97% of the patients. No adverse events occurred. The authors concluded that this herbal combination product was effective in the treatment of younger children with restlessness and dyssomnia and was very well tolerated (Müller and Klement, 2006).

An open-label 28-day study in patients ($n = 409$) with insomnia investigated the homeopathic preparation Neurexan (*Avena sativa* 4X, *Coffea arabica* 14X, *Passiflora incarnata* 4X, and *Zincum isovalerianicum* 6X) compared with valerian. Doses were at physicians' discretion. At day 14 sleep latency was reduced by 37 and 38 min with Neurexan and valerian, respectively, and sleep duration was increased by 2.2 and 2.0 h with Neurexan and valerian, respectively. On days 8, 12, and 14, sleep duration was significantly in favor of Neurexan. Lack of daytime fatigue was reported by 49% and 32% of the Neurexan and valerian groups, respectively ($P < 0.05$). Quality of sleep was not significantly different between groups by day 28. The authors concluded that Neurexan might be an effective and well-tolerated alternative to conventional valerian-based therapies for the treatment of mild-to-moderate insomnia (Waldschütz and Klein, 2008).

Psychiatric Disorders: Obsessive-Compulsive Disorder

An 8-week RCT in patients ($n = 31$) with OCD compared valerian 765 mg/day with placebo 30 mg/day for effects on OCD symptoms. The change in score on the Brief Obsessive-Compulsive Scale decreased from 31 to 17 with valerian and from 29 to 23 with placebo ($P = 0.000$). Somnolence was the only significant difference between the two groups in terms of observed side effects ($P = 0.02$). The authors concluded that valerian had some anti-obsessive and anti-compulsive effects and that further studies were warranted (Pakseresht et al., 2011).

Psychiatric Disorders: Somatoform Disorder

A 2-week RCT in patients ($n = 182$) with somatoform disorders investigated Ze185, a four-herb combination containing valerian, passionflower, lemon balm, and butterbur compared with a three-herb combination without the butterbur and with placebo. The combination containing butterbur was significantly superior to the combination without butterbur, which was superior to placebo for changes in VAS-Anxiety scale, Beck Depression Inventory, and Clinical Global Impression. In total nine non-serious adverse events were documented, but the distribution did not differ significantly between the treatment groups. The authors concluded that the herbal preparation Ze185 was an efficacious and safe short-term treatment in patients with somatoform disorders (Melzer et al., 2009).

Psychiatric Disorders: Attention-Deficit/Hyperactivity Disorder

A 2017 systematic review to assess efficacy of herbal therapies for ADHD in children found nine RCTs ($n = 464$) that met inclusion criteria. Seven different herbs were tested in the treatment of ADHD symptoms. Low level evidence could be found for lemon balm, valerian, and passionflower. Limited evidence could be found for pine bark extract and gingko. The other herbal preparations showed no efficacy in the treatment of ADHD symptoms (Anheyer et al., 2017).

A 7-week observational study in primary school children ($n = 169$) with hyperactivity and concentration difficulties but not meeting ADHD criteria received Sandrin, a standardized combination of valerian 640 mg plus lemon balm 320 mg daily. The fraction of children having "strong/very strong" symptoms of poor ability to focus decreased from 75% to 14%, hyperactivity decreased from 61% to 13%, and impulsiveness decreased from 59% to 22%. Parent rated social behavior, sleep, and symptom burden showed highly significant improvements. In two children mild transient adverse drug reactions were observed. The authors concluded that children with restlessness, concentration difficulties, and impulsiveness may benefit from this formulation of valerian and lemon balm (Gromball et al., 2014).

Infectious Disease: HIV Medication Psychiatric Side Effects

A 4-week pilot RCT in patients ($n = 51$) with HIV on efavirenz compared valerian 530 mg QHS with placebo for efficacy and safety in preventing neuropsychiatric adverse effects of efavirenz. Based on validated questionnaires, both sleep and anxiety significantly improved with valerian compared with placebo ($P \leq 0.001$ and $P = 0.001$, respectively). Dizziness was experienced by 92% and 84.6% of patients in valerian and placebo groups, respectively ($P = 0.35$). Nausea was experienced in 84% and 80% of patients in the valerian and placebo groups, respectively ($P = 0.39$). The authors concluded that in the first 4 weeks of ART including efavirenz, valerian significantly improved sleep and anxiety in HIV-positive patients (Ahmadi et al., 2017).

ACTIVE CONSTITUENTS

- Amino acid derivatives
  - Amino acids: GABA, tyrosine, arginine, glutamine
- Phenolic compounds
  - Phenylpropanoids (antioxidant, antimutagenic, antitumor, antimicrobial): chlorogenic acid

- Lignans: (neuroprotective) 8'-hydroxypin-oresinol, pinoresinol-4-O-β-glucoside
- Flavonoids: 6-methylapigenin, hesperidin, linarin
- Terpenes
  - Monoterpenes
    - Irioid valepotriates (autonomic nervous system regulation): acevaltrate (neuroprotective, antidepressant) valtrate, isovaltrate, dihydrovaltrate
  - Sesquiterpenes: valerenic acid (VA) (likely the main bioactive constituent), hydroxyvalerenic acid, acetoxyvalerenic acid, volvalerenone A (antidepressant), valeric acid, isovaleric acid (the "stinky foot" constituent), valerenal glycol, valeranone glycol, kessyl glycol (neuroprotective)
- Alkaloids
- Aromatic compounds: (sedative, antispasmodic) valeranone, valerenal, valerenic acids

VALERIAN COMMONLY USED PREPARATIONS AND DOSAGE (FOR ADULTS UNLESS OTHERWISE SPECIFIED)

The following are examples of some available formulations and ranges of dosing for commercial herbal products. See Part III Introduction "How to prescribe medicinal herbs" for further guidance on herbal advising and prescribing.

Dried Root

- Infusion: 2 tsp per cup HS (volatile oils may escape, so prepare at time of use and keep covered)
- Tincture (1:5, 40%–60%): 2.5–5 mL (up to 10 mL) HS prn insomnia
- Glycerite (1:4): 0.7 mL (175 mg) up to QID
- Powdered root (4:1) extract: 300–600 mg (1/8-1/4 tsp) HS for insomnia
- Capsule or tablet of powdered root: 500–2000 mg HS for insomnia
- Capsule or tablet of standardized extract (standardized to 80% dihydrovaltrate or to 0.8% valerenic acid or other volatile oils with additional 200–800 mg of whole root powder): 220–480 mg HS for insomnia

SAFETY AND PRECAUTION

Side Effects

There have been isolated reports of headache, diarrhea and other gastrointestinal complaints, daytime sedation/dullness, impaired alertness, depression, irritability, dizziness, sweating, heart palpitations, bitter taste, and benzodiazepine-like withdrawal symptoms with supplement cessation. However, one study showed that valerian did not impair ability to operate machinery and another study showed that 400 mg of valerian taken at night did not produce decreased alertness the following morning. However, another study showed that 900 mg did decrease alertness the next day. Higher doses may produce excess drowsiness.

Case Reports

One case report of possible withdrawal symptoms was noted after extremely high-dose and prolonged usage.

There have been two case reports of possible hepatotoxicity. It has also been linked to possible rare acute pancreatitis.

A psychiatric patient who consumed an excess (3.5 L) of valerian-containing beverages developed hyponatremia, more likely due to the excess water intake.

A man with GAD who self-medicated with valerian and passionflower while he was on lorazepam developed tremor, dizziness, throbbing, and muscular fatigue. An additive or synergistic effect was suspected to have produced these symptoms. The active principles of valerian and passionflower might increase the inhibitory activity of benzodiazepines binding to the GABA receptors, causing severe secondary effects.

Toxicity

One college student overdosed on 20,000 mg of valerian root with resultant fatigue, abdominal pain, and tremor of extremities.

Pregnancy and Lactation

In mice, valerian resulted in reduced zinc levels in fetal brains. A retrospective analysis of use during pregnancy in 630 mothers did not identify any adverse neonatal effects. However, there is insufficient human safety data for pregnancy and lactation.

Drug Interactions

- CYP: Inhibits CYP2D6 and CYP3A4
- Pgp: Inhibits P-glycoprotein transporters so can increase intracellular concentration of substrate drugs
- UGT: Modulates UGT enzymes in vitro so could increase SEs of drugs metabolized by them.
- May theoretically prolong barbiturate-induced sleep
- May be synergistic with other sedatives and anesthetics
- May cause hepatic damage when given in conjunction with haloperidol.
- May reduce symptoms of benzodiazepine withdrawal

REFERENCES

Ahmadi M, Khalili H, Abbasian L, Ghaeli P. Effect of valerian in preventing neuropsychiatric adverse effects of efavirenz in HIV-positive patients: a pilot randomized, placebo-controlled clinical trial. Ann Pharmacother 2017;51(6):457–64.

Andreatini R, Sartori VA, Seabra ML, Leite JR. Effect of valepotriates (valerian extract) in generalized anxiety disorder: a randomized placebo-controlled pilot study. Phytother Res 2002;16:650–654.18.

Anheyer D, Lauche R, Schumann D, Dobos G, Cramer H. Herbal medicines in children with attention deficit hyperactivity disorder (ADHD): a systematic review. Complement Ther Med 2017;30:14–23.

Azizi H, Shojaii A, Hashem-Dabaghian F, et al. Effects of Valeriana officinalis (Valerian) on tension-type headache: a randomized, placebo-controlled, double-blind clinical trial. Avicenna J Phytomed 2020;10(3):297–304.

Behboodi Moghadam Z, Rezaei E, Sirood Gholami R, Kheirkhah M, Haghani H. The effect of Valerian root extract on the severity of pre-menstrual syndrome symptoms. J Tradit Complement Med 2016;6(3):309–15.

Bent S, Padula A, Moore D, et al. Valerian for sleep: a systematic review and meta-analysis. Am J Med 2006;119(12):1005–12.

Bourin M, Bougerol T, Guitton B, Broutin E. A combination of plant extracts in the treatment of outpatients with adjustment disorder with anxious mood: controlled study vs placebo. Fundament Clin Pharmacol 1997;11:127–32.

Cropley M, Cave Z, Ellis J, Middleton RW. Effect of kava and valerian on human physiological and psychological responses to mental stress assessed under laboratory conditions. Phytother Res 2002;16(1):23–7.

Cuellar NG, Ratcliffe SJ. Does valerian improve sleepiness and symptom severity in people with restless legs syndrome? Altern Ther Health Med 2009;15(2):22–8.

Diaper A, Hindmarch I. A double-blind, placebo-controlled investigation of the effects of 2 doses of a valerian preparation on the sleep, cognitive and psychomotor function of sleep-disturbed older adults. Phytother Res 2004;18(10):831–6.

Donath F, Quispe S, Diefenbach K, Maurer A, Fietze I, Roots I. Critical evaluation of the effect of valerian extract on sleep structure and sleep quality. Pharmacopsychiatry 2000;33(2):47–53.

Dorn M. Efficacy and tolerability of Baldrian vs oxazepam in non-organic and non-psychiatric insomniacs: a randomised, double-blind, clinical, comparative study. Forsch Komplementarmed Klass Naturheilkd 2000;7(2):79–84.

Faustino TT, Almeida RB, Andreatini R. Medicinal plants for the treatment of generalized anxiety disorder: a review of controlled clinical studies. Braz J Psychiatry 2010;32(4):429–36.

Fernández-San-Martín MI, Masa-Font R, Palacios-Soler L, Sancho-Gómez P, Calbó-Caldentey C, Flores-Mateo G. Effectiveness of Valerian on insomnia: a meta-analysis of randomized placebo-controlled trials. Sleep Med 2010;11(6):505–11.

Francis AJ, Dempster RJ. Effect of valerian, Valeriana edulis, on sleep difficulties in children with intellectual deficits: randomised trial. Phytomedicine 2002;9(4):273–9.

Fussel A, Wolf A, Brattström A. Effect of a fixed valerian-hop extract combination (Ze 9109) on sleep polygraphy in patients with non-organic insomnia: a pilot study. Eur J Med Res 2000;5:385–90.

Gerhard U, Linnenbrink N, Georghiadou C, Hobi V. Vigilance-decreasing effects of 2 plant-derived sedatives. Praxis (Bern 1994) 1996;85(15):473–81.

Gessner B, Klasser M. Studies on the effect of Harmonicum much on sleep using polygraphic EEG recordings. EEG EMG Z Elektroenzephalogr Elektromyogr Verwandte Geb 1984;15(1):45–51.

Gharib M, Samani LN, Panah ZE, Naseri M, Bahrani N, Kiani K. The effect of valeric on anxiety severity in women undergoing hysterosalpingography. Glob J Health Sci 2015;7(3):358–63.

Ghazanfarpour M, Sadeghi R, Abdolahian S, Latifnejad RR. The efficacy of Iranian herbal medicines in alleviating hot flashes: a systematic review. Int J Reprod Biomed (Yazd) 2016;14(3):155–66.

Gromball J, Beschorner F, Wantzen C, Paulsen U, Burkart M. Hyperactivity, concentration difficulties and impulsiveness improve during seven weeks' treatment with valerian root and lemon balm extracts in primary school children. Phytomedicine 2014;21(8-9):1098–103.

Hassani S, Alipour A, Darvishi Khezri H, et al. Can Valeriana officinalis root extract prevent early postoperative cognitive dysfunction after CABG surgery? A randomized, double-blind, placebo-controlled trial. Psychopharmacology (Berl) 2015;232(5):843–50.

Hubner R, van Haselen R, Klein P. Effectiveness of the homeopathic preparation Neurexan compared with that of commonly used valerian-based preparations for the treatment of nervousness/restlessness—an observational study. Sci World J 2009;9:733–45.

Jacobs BP, Bent S, Tice JA, et al. An internet-based randomized, placebo-controlled trial of kava and valerian for anxiety and insomnia. Medicine (Baltimore) 2005;84(4):197–207.

Jenabi E, Shobeiri F, Hazavehei SMM, Roshanaei G. The effect of Valerian on the severity and frequency of hot flashes: a triple-blind randomized clinical trial. Women Health 2018;58(3):297–304.

Kargozar R, Azizi H, Salari R. A review of effective herbal medicines in controlling menopausal symptoms. Electron Phys 2017;9(11):5826–33.

Keck ME, Nicolussi S, Spura K, Blohm C, Zahner C, Drewe J. Effect of the fixed combination of valerian, lemon balm, passionflower, and butterbur extracts (Ze 185) on the prescription pattern of benzodiazepines in hospitalized psychiatric patients-A retrospective case-control investigation. Phytother Res 2020;34(6):1436–45.

Kennedy DO, Little W, Haskell CF, Scholey AB. Anxiolytic effects of a combination of Melissa officinalis and Valeriana officinalis during laboratory induced stress. Phytother Res 2006;20(2):96–102.

Koetter U, Schrader E, Käufeler R, Brattström A. A randomized, double blind, placebo-controlled, prospective clinical study to demonstrate clinical efficacy of a fixed valerian hops extract combination (Ze 91019) in patients suffering from non-organic sleep disorder. Phytother Res 2007;21(9):847–51.

Kuhlmann J, Berger W, Podzuweit H, Schmidt U. The influence of valerian treatment on "reaction time, alertness and concentration" in volunteers. Pharmacopsychiatry 1999;32(6):235–41.

Leach MJ, Page AT. Herbal medicine for insomnia: a systematic review and meta-analysis. Sleep Med Rev 2015;24:1–12.

Leathwood PD, Chauffard F, Heck E, Munoz-Box R. Aqueous extract of valerian root (Valeriana officinalis L.) improves sleep quality in man. Pharmacol Biochem Behav 1982;17(1):65–71.

Lindahl O, Lindwall L. Double blind study of a valerian preparation. Pharmacol Biochem Behav 1989;32:1065–6.

Maroo N, Hazra A, Das T. Efficacy and safety of a polyherbal sedative-hypnotic formulation NSF-3 in primary insomnia in comparison with zolpidem: a randomized controlled trial. Indian J Pharmacol 2013;45(1):34–9.

Meier S, Haschke M, Zahner C, et al. Effects of a fixed herbal drug combination (Ze 185) to an experimental acute stress setting in healthy men—an explorative randomized placebo-controlled double-blind study. Phytomedicine 2018;39:85–92.

Melzer J, et al. Fixed herbal drug combination with and without butterbur (Ze 185) for the treatment of patients with somatoform disorders: randomized, placebo-controlled pharmaco-clinical trial. Phytother Res 2009;23(9):1303–8.

Meolie AL, Rosen C, Kristo D, et al. Oral nonprescription treatment for insomnia: an evaluation of products with limited evidence. J Clin Sleep Med 2005;1(2):173–87.

Mirabi P, Mojab F. The effects of valerian root on hot flashes in menopausal women. Iran J Pharm Res 2013;12(1):217–22.

Mirabi P, Dolatian M, Mojab F, et al. Effects of valerian on the severity and systemic manifestations of dysmenorrhea. Int J Gynaecol Obstet 2011;115(3):285–8.

Miyasaka LS, Atallah AN, Soares BG. Valerian for anxiety disorders. Cochrane Database Syst Rev 2006;4, CD004515.

Morin CM, Koetter U, Bastien C, Ware JC, Wooten V. Valerian-hops combination and diphenhydramine for treating insomnia: a randomized placebo-controlled clinical trial. Sleep 2005;28(11):1465–71.

Müller SF, Klement S. A combination of valerian and lemon balm is effective in the treatment of restlessness and dyssomnia in children. Phytomedicine 2006;13(6):383–7.

Oxman AD, Flottorp S, Håvelsrud K, et al. A televised, web-based randomised trial of an herbal remedy (valerian) for insomnia. PLoS One 2007;2(10), e1040.

Pakseresht S, Boostani H, Sayyah M. Extract of valerian root (Valeriana officinalis L.) vs. placebo in treatment of obsessive-compulsive disorder: a randomized double-blind study. J Complement Integr Med 2011;8. pii: /j/jcim.2011.8. issue-1/1553-3840.1465/1553-3840.1465.xml.

Pallesen S, Bjorvatn B, Nordhus IH, Skjerve A. Valerian as a sleeping aid? Tidsskr Nor Laegeforen 2002;122(30):2857–9.

Palmieri G, Contaldi P, Fogliame G. Evaluation of effectiveness and safety of a herbal compound in primary insomnia symptoms and sleep disturbances not related to medical or psychiatric causes. Nat Sci Sleep 2017;9:163–9.

Pinheiro ML, Alcântara CE, de Moraes M, de Andrade ED. Valeriana officinalis L. for conscious sedation of patients submitted to impacted lower third molar surgery: a randomized, double-blind, placebo-controlled split-mouth study. J Pharm Bioallied Sci 2014;6(2):109–14.

Sarris J, Byrne GJ. A systematic review of insomnia and complementary medicine. Clin Rev 2011.

Schmitz M, Jäckel M. Comparative study for assessing quality of life of patients with exogenous sleep disorders (temporary sleep onset and sleep interruption disorders) treated with a hops-valarian preparation and a benzodiazepine drug. Wien Med Wochenschr 1998;148(13):291–8.

Schulz H, Stolz C, Müller J. The effect of valerian extract on sleep polygraphy in poor sleepers: a pilot study. Pharmacopsychiatry 1994;27(4):147–51.

Stevinson C, Ernst E. Valerian for insomnia: a systematic review of randomized clinical trials. Sleep Med 2000;1(2):91–9.

Taavoni S, Ekbatani N, Kashaniyan M, Haghani H. Effect of valerian on sleep quality in postmenopausal women: a randomized placebo-controlled clinical trial. Menopause 2011;18(9):951–5.

Taibi DM, et al. A systematic review of valerian as a sleep aid: safe but not effective. Sleep Med Rev 2007.

Taibi DM, et al. A randomized clinical trial of valerian fails to improve self-reported, polysomnographic, and actigraphic sleep in older women with insomnia. Sleep Med 2009.

Waldschütz R, Klein P. The homeopathic preparation Neurexan vs. valerian for the treatment of insomnia: an observational study. Sci World J 2008;8:411–20.

Wheatley D. Kava and valerian in the treatment of stress-induced insomnia. Phytother Res 2001;15(6):549–51.

Ziegler G, Ploch M, Miettinen-Baumann A, Collet W. Efficacy and tolerability of valerian extract LI 156 compared with oxazepam in the treatment of non-organic insomnia—a randomized, double-blind, comparative clinical study. Eur J Med Res 2002;7(11):480–6.

77

YARROW (*ACHILLEA MILLEFOLIUM*)
Flower, Leaf

GENERAL OVERVIEW

Herbalists have embraced yarrow for eons for its myriad beneficial properties. There is evidence that it was used medicinally by Neanderthals. It appears to hold promise for some challenging diseases such as multiple sclerosis. Despite a solid historical presence in herbal lore, human studies are remarkably lacking. Traditionally yarrow been used as an emmenagogue, a carminative to reduce flatulence, a diaphoretic to promote sweating as means to overcome viral infections, a bowel anti-inflammatory used for inflammatory bowel disease, a bitter to stimulate digestion, an antispasmodic for irritable bowel syndrome, a peripheral vasodilating hypotensive, a urinary antiseptic for urinary tract infections, a pelvic muscle tonifying relaxant (for dysmenorrhea), and an astringent styptic and vulnerary (wound healer).

It is used by modern herbalists for varicose veins, seasonal allergies, HTN, indigestion, dyspepsia, gastroparesis, anorexia, pelvic congestion, oligomenorrhea, dysmenorrhea, dysfunctional uterine bleeding, menorrhagia, uterine fibroids, and acute and chronic bronchitis.

Clinical research indicates that yarrow, alone or in combination formulas, may be beneficial for dysmenorrhea and multiple sclerosis.

IN VITRO AND ANIMAL RESEARCH

In vitro yarrow has been shown to have anti-inflammatory properties. In animal studies yarrow has been shown to reduce smooth muscle spasms, lower blood pressure, cause bronchodilation and stop bleeding. It is gastroprotective. Hot water extracts have been shown to inhibit basal acid secretion into the duodenal lumen. It has been shown to increase appetite and have anxiolytic effects.

A study in mice looked particularly at artemetin, a flavonoid in yarrow. The constituent reduced SBP in normotensive mice, and this was demonstrated to be at least partially due to ACE inhibition. A study to evaluate the hypotensive, cardio depressant, vasodilatory, and bronchodilatory activities of yarrow found that yarrow caused a dose-dependent decrease of BP in rats under anesthesia. When applied to spontaneously beating guinea pig atrial tissue, yarrow demonstrated negative inotropic and chronotropic effects. In isolated rabbit aortic rings, yarrow relaxed phenylephrine and hyperkalemic-induced contractions and exhibited calcium channel blocking activity similar to verapamil. In guinea pig tracheal strips, yarrow inhibited carbachol and hyperkalemic-induced contractions. The authors concluded that yarrow had hypotensive, cardiovascular inhibitory, and bronchodilatory effects supporting its traditional medicinal use for HTN and asthma (Khan and Gilani, 2011).

In a streptozotocin-induced diabetic mouse model, yarrow appeared to spare destruction of the pancreas and preserve normoglycemia through amelioration of IL-1β and iNOS gene over-expression, which can have a β-cell protective effect (Zolghadri et al., 2014).

A 28-day study in a streptozotocin diabetic model in rats, yarrow extract 25 mg/kg/day or 100 mg/kg/day was compared with metformin 25 mg/kg/day and with saline (control). There were significant reductions in blood glucose, serum liver enzymes, TG, TC, and LDL-C and inrceases in HDL-C with yarrow and metformin compared with control. With 100 mg/kg/day of yarrow these effects were comparable to metformin. The authors concluded that yarrow reduced lipid abnormalities, blood glucose, and liver enzymes in diabetic rats (Rezaei et al., 2020).

In a study to evaluate the efficacy of yarrow for gastroprotection rats were given ethanol-induced acute gastric lesions and acetic acid-induced chronic gastric ulcers. Yarrow given orally at 30 mg/kg, 100 mg/kg, and 300 mg/kg inhibited ethanol-induced gastric lesions by 35%, 56%, and 81%, respectively. Yarrow at 1 mg/kg and 10 mg/kg reduced the chronic gastric ulcers induced by acetic acid by 43% and 65%, respectively, and promoted significant regeneration of the gastric mucosa after ulcer induction. Yarrow demonstrated antioxidant activity in the face of the toxins, preventing reduction in GSH and SOD and inhibiting myeloperoxidase activity (Potrich et al., 2010).

A 7-day study was carried out in rats to evaluate the orexigenic effect of hydro-alcoholic extract yarrow 50 mg/kg, 100 mg/kg or 150 mg/kg compared with a control group given water. The change in energy intake after treatment by 50 mg/kg and 100 mg/kg of the extract was significantly higher than in other groups ($P < 0.001$). Administration of yarrow 100 mg/kg significantly ($P < 0.05$) decreased ghrelin level one hour after intervention, but there was no significant difference between the control and treated groups. The authors concluded that yarrow had a positive dose-related effect on appetite in rats, but the orexigenic activity was not related to changes in ghrelin levels (Nematy et al., 2017).

Estrogenic activity, albeit less than estradiol, has been demonstrated on MCF-7 cells and is attributed primarily to apigenin which stimulates α and β estrogen receptors and luteolin, which stimulates only the β estrogen receptors.

A study in mice with experimental autoimmune encephalomyelitis (EAE) investigated 1 mg, 5 mg, and 10 mg/day of yarrow aqueous extract. Treatment of mice with yarrow led to delays in the appearance of behavioral disabilities along with reduced severity of the behavioral disabilities. Yarrow also prevented weight loss, increased serum levels of TGF-β, and reduced cerebral infiltration of inflammatory cells. The results demonstrated that treatment with an aqueous extract of yarrow may attenuate disease severity, inflammatory responses, and demyelinating lesions in EAE-induced mice (Vazirinejad et al., 2014).

A study in mice subjected to stressful activities investigated the effects of yarrow on anxious behaviors. Yarrow exerted anxiolytic effects in the elevated plus-maze and marble-burying test after acute and chronic (25 days) administration similar to diazepam. The effects were likely not mediated by GABA-A neurotransmission and did not present tolerance after short-term, repeated administration (Baretta et al., 2012).

HUMAN RESEARCH

Cardiovascular Disorders: Hypertension and Dyslipidemia (*Achillea wilhelmsii*)

A 2010 systematic review looking at herbal medicine (including TCM formulations) for hyperlipidemia identified 53 RCTs that met criteria. There were significant decreases in TC and LDL-C after treatment with yarrow (*Achillia wilhelmsii*) as well as milk thistle, fenugreek, licorice, guggul, Daming capsule, chunghyul-dan, garlic powder, black tea, green tea, soy drink enriched with plant sterols, Went rice, C. Koch, Ningzhi capsule, cherry, composite salvia dropping pill (CSDP), shanzha xiaozhi capsule, Ba-wei-wan (hachimijiogan), rhubarb stalk, *Rheum ribes*, *Satureja khuzestanica*, *Monascus purpureus*, and primrose oil. Data were conflicting for red yeast rice, garlic, and guggul. No significant adverse effect or mortality were observed with licorice and several others. The authors concluded that 22 natural products were found effective in the treatment of hyperlipidemia and that further research was warranted (Hasani-Ranjbar).

A 6-month RCT in patients ($n = 120$) with hyperlipidemia and/or HTN studied *Achillea wilhelmsii* (a species of yarrow found in parts of the Middle East) 15-20 drops BID compared with placebo. At 2 months there was a significant decrease in TG with yarrow; at 4 months there were significant decreases in TG, TC, and LDL-C with yarrow. HDL-C increases reached significance at 6 months. A significant decrease was observed in SBP and DBP after 2 and 6 months, respectively ($P < 0.05$), with yarrow (Asgary et al., 2000).

Gastrointestinal Disorders: Cirrhosis

A 6-month RCT in patients ($n=36$) with hepatic cirrhosis investigated Liv-52, a polyherbal product containing yarrow, *Capparis spinosa*, *Cichorium intybus*, *Solanum nigrum*, *Terminalia arjuna*, *Mandur basma*, and *Tamarix gallica*, compared with placebo on liver cirrhosis outcomes. The patients treated with the polyherbal product had significantly better Child-Pugh scores, decreased ascites, and decreased serum ALT and AST. With placebo there was no significant change from baseline in any of the clinical parameters by 6 months. The authors concluded that this polyherbal product had hepatoprotective effects in cirrhotic patients attributed to the diuretic, anti-inflammatory, antioxidant, and immunomodulating properties of the component herbs (Huseini et al., 2005).

Nephrological Disorders: Chronic Kidney Disease

A 2-month RCT in patients ($n=31$) with CKD investigated powdered yarrow 1.5 g given 3 days per week compared with placebo for effects on NO levels as a marker for bleeding tendency. Although not statistically significant, plasma nitrite and nitrate concentrations decreased with yarrow from 0.82 μmol/L to 0.63 μmol/L and from 50.55 μmol/L to 44.09 μmol/L, respectively. These concentrations were slightly increased in the placebo group. The authors concluded that nitric oxide metabolites were marginally decreased with yarrow in patients with CKD and that higher doses or longer duration may produce significant results (Vahid et al., 2012).

Women's Disorders: Breastfeeding Nipple Fissures

A 7-day randomized trial in breastfeeding women ($n=150$) with cracked nipples compared topical yarrow, honey, and breast milk, each in addition to breastfeeding education, for efficacy in fissure healing. Yarrow, honey, and breast milk all led to significant reductions of nipple fissures ($P<0.001$ for all) with no significant difference between treatment modalities in the severity of fissure scores. The authors concluded that yarrow, honey, and breast milk could all be recommended to women with nipple fissures, and they suggested that honey and yarrow could be a good antifissure cream (Firouzabadi et al., 2020).

Women's Genitourinary Disorders: Vulvovaginal Candidiasis

A 7-day RCT in women ($n=80$) with vulvovaginal candidiasis compared clotrimazole 1% vaginal cream with a cream containing an aqueous extract of yarrow. The Dermatology Life Quality Index score showed significant reductions in both groups after treatment, but the reduction was significantly greater with clotrimazole ($P<0.05$). Improvement in vulvar erythema occurred in both groups with no significant difference between groups ($P=0.1$). Vaginal culture was negative for *Candida albicans* in 77% and 53% of patients applying clotrimazole and yarrow, respectively ($P<0.05$). The authors concluded that a vaginal cream containing yarrow could reduce complaints of vulvovaginal candidiasis and that further studies were warranted (Zakeri et al., 2020).

Women's Genitourinary Disorders: Dysmenorrhea

A two-cycle RCT in females with primary dysmenorrhea compared yarrow tea with placebo for 3 days during menses for severity of pain. The mean decrease in pain score with yarrow was significantly greater than with placebo at 1 month ($P=0.001$) and two months ($P<0.0001$). The authors concluded that yarrow was effective in minimizing pain severity in primary dysmenorrhea (Jenabi and Fereidoony, 2015).

Autoimmune Disorders: Multiple Sclerosis

A 1-year triple-blind RCT in patients ($n=75$) with MS compared yarrow 250 mg/day with yarrow 500 mg/day and with placebo as add-on to conventional therapy. The annual relapse rate decreased with both doses of yarrow. With placebo, 250 mg and 500 mg annual relapse occurred in 50%, 22.7%, and 33%, respectively ($P=0.003$ for 250 mg and $P=0.013$ for 500 mg). Mean time to first relapse was 230 days, 324 days, and 310 days with placebo, 250 mg, and 500 mg, respectively ($P=0.013$ for 250 mg, and $P=0.039$ for 500 mg). Greater than one relapse occurred in 36% of patients in the placebo group but no patients in the yarrow groups. Volume of gadolinium enhanced lesions was 232.74 mm^3, 222.35 mm^3, and 133.67 mm^3 with placebo, 250 mg, and 500 mg, respectively ($P=0.004$ for 500 mg compared with placebo). The multiple sclerosis functional composite MSFC z-score was increased with the 500 mg dose ($P = 0.003$ compared with placebo), and the expanded disability status scale was decreased more with 500 mg ($P = 0.030$ compared with 250 mg; $P = 0.001$ compared with placebo). Performance in word-pair learning, the Wisconsin card sorting test and paced auditory serial addition task were also improved significantly for both doses ($P = 0.025$ and $P = 0.009$ for 250 and 500 mg, respectively, for the latter task). The authors concluded that yarrow was beneficial as add-on therapy in MS patients (Ayoobi et al., 2019).

ACTIVE CONSTITUENTS

- Carbohydrates
  - Organic acids: succinic acid, ascorbic acid, folic acid
- Lipids
  - Alkamides (immunomodulatory, anti-inflammatory)
  - Polyacetylenes (immunomodulatory, anti-inflammatory)
- Amino acid derivatives
  - Bitters: achillein (choleretic, digestive stimulant)
- Phenolic compounds
  - Phenolic acids: salicylic acid
  - Phenylpropanoids: caffeic acid
  - Coumarins (venotonic, lymphatotonic, anticoagulant)
  - Flavonoids: rutin (antioxidant, anti-inflammatory, antidiabetic, nephroprotective, anti-osteoporotic, antispasmodic, neuroprotective, anti-anxiety), artemetin (hypotensive) apigenin (anti-inflammatory, antioxidant, antihistamine, hypotensive, anti-serotonin release, GABA agonism, antispasmodic, antibacterial, chemopreventive, antineoplastic, ERB), luteolin (anti-inflammatory, antispasmodic, antibacterial, hepatoprotective, anti-estrogenic, antiproliferative), kaempferol (anti-inflammatory, antidepressant, strengthens capillaries), quercitin, cynaroside I and cosmosiin II (antispasmodic)
    - Tannins (astringent and anti-hemorrhagic)

- Terpenes
  - Monoterpenes: linalool (sedative, antispasmodic), limonene (antineoplastic, detoxifying), cineole (antispasmodic, carminative and antiseptic, antimicrobial), thujone (antifungal, anti-microbial, emmenagogue, and immuno-stimulant)
  - Sesquiterpenes: achimillic acids A, B and C (active against mouse P-388 leukemia cells in-vivo), chamazulene (see "Aromatic compounds")
  - Sesquiterpene lactones: achillin, achillicin
  - Triterpenes
- Steroids: Phytosterols
- Alkaloids: achilletin (hemostatic, antispasmodic, choleretic, antimicrobial, tonifying), betonicine (hemostatic, antibacterial), stachydrine (anticancer, provascular, hypoglycemic), trigonelline (hypoglycemic, hypolipidemic, hypotensive, neuroprotective, antimigraine, sedative, memory-improving, antipyretic, antibacterial, antiviral, antitumor)
- Aromatic compounds (variable): borneol (antimicrobial), camphor, thujone (antifungal, anti-microbial, emmenagogue and immuno-stimulant), chamazulene (only present after distillation: increases cortisol release, reduces histamine, anti-inflammatory, hepatoregenerative, antifungal, antineoplastic), azulene, linalool (sedative, antispasmodic), limonene (antineoplastic, detoxifying), cineole (antispasmodic, carminative and antiseptic, antimicrobial), sesquiterpene lactones (anti-inflammatory, antimicrobial, cytotoxic), caryophyllene (anti-allergic, anti-inflammatory, and hepatic)

YARROW COMMONLY USED PREPARATIONS AND DOSAGE (FOR ADULTS UNLESS OTHERWISE SPECIFIED)

The following are examples of some available formulations and ranges of dosing for commercial herbal products. See Part III Introduction "How to prescribe medicinal herbs" for further guidance on herbal advising and prescribing.

Flower and leaf

- Infusion of dried flower: 1–2 teaspoons per cup; one cup TID or apply topically to wounds
- Infusion of dried leaf: 1–2 teaspoons per cup made into compress to stop bleeding
- Fluid extract (1:1, 25%): 1–2 mL TID
- Tincture (1:5, 25%–75%): 1–4 mL in water TID (before meals if for digestion)
- Capsule or tablet of powdered flowers with or without leaves: 320–650 mg BID-TID

SAFETY AND PRECAUTION

Side Effects

Long-term use may lead to photosensitivity. May cause atopic dermatitis in sensitive patients. Possible allergic reactions in those with ragweed allergies. Was shown in one study to cause sperm abnormalities in rats.

Toxicity

The volatile oil contains thujone, which is a neurotoxic compound. Do not exceed recommended doses.

Pregnancy and Lactation

Avoid during pregnancy due to mild uterine stimulant effect. Reduced fetal weight in rats in one study. Insufficient human evidence for lactation.

Drug Interactions

- Increases gut motility, so may theoretically decrease absorption of drugs
- Potential interactions with anticoagulants (increased bleeding), lithium (potential toxicity), acid blocking medications (may reduce efficacy), and antihypertensives (additive effects)

REFERENCES

Asgary S, Naderi GH, Sarrafzadegan N, Mohammadifard N, Mostafavi S, Vakili R. Antihypertensive and antihyperlipidemic effects of Achillea wilhelmsii. Drugs Exp Clin Res 2000;26(3):89–93.

Ayoobi F, Moghadam-Ahmadi A, Amiri H, et al. Achillea millefolium is beneficial as an add-on therapy in patients with multiple sclerosis: a randomized placebo-controlled clinical trial. Phytomedicine 2019;52:89–97.

Baretta IP, Felizardo RA, Bimbato VF, et al. Anxiolytic-like effects of acute and chronic treatment with Achillea millefolium L. extract. J Ethnopharmacol 2012;140(1):46–54.

Firouzabadi M, Pourramezani N, Balvardi M. Comparing the effects of yarrow, honey, and breast milk for healing nipple fissure. Iran J Nurs Midwifery Res 2020;25(4):282–5.

Hasani-Ranjbar S, Nayebi N, Moradi L, Mehri A, Larijani B, Abdollahi M. The efficacy and safety of herbal medicines used in the treatment of hyperlipidemia; a systematic review. Curr Pharm Des 2010;16(26):2935–47.

Huseini HF, Alavian SM, Heshmat R, Heydari MR, Abolmaali K. The efficacy of Liv-52 on liver cirrhotic patients: a randomized, double-blind, placebo-controlled first approach. Phytomedicine 2005;12(9):619–24.

Jenabi E, Fereidoony B. Effect of Achillea millefolium on relief of primary dysmenorrhea: a double-blind randomized clinical trial. J Pediatr Adolesc Gynecol 2015;28(5):402–4.

Khan AU, Gilani AH. BP lowering, cardiovascular inhibitory and bronchodilatory actions of Achillea millefolium. Phytother Res 2011;25(4):577–83.

Nematy M, Mazidi M, Jafari A, et al. The effect of hydro-alcoholic extract of Achillea millefolium on appetite hormone in rats. Avicenna J Phytomed 2017;7(1):10–5.

Potrich FB, Allemand A, da Silva LM, et al. Antiulcerogenic activity of hydroalcoholic extract of Achillea millefolium L.: involvement of the antioxidant system. J Ethnopharmacol 2010;130(1):85–92.

Rezaei S, Ashkar F, Koohpeyma F, Mahmoodi M, Gholamalizadeh M, Mazloom Z, Doaei S. Hydroalcoholic extract of Achillea millefolium improved blood glucose, liver enzymes and lipid profile compared to metformin in streptozotocin-induced diabetic rats. Lipids Health Dis 2020 Apr 27;19(1):81.

Vahid S, Dashti-Khavidaki S, Ahmadi F, Amini M, Salehi Surmaghi MH. Effect of herbal medicine achillea millefolium on plasma nitrite and nitrate levels in patients with chronic kidney disease: a preliminary study. Iran J Kidney Dis 2012;6(5):350–4.

Vazirinejad R, Ayoobi F, Arababadi MK, et al. Effect of aqueous extract of Achillea millefolium on the development of experimental autoimmune encephalomyelitis in C57BL/6 mice. Indian J Pharmacol 2014;46(3):303–8.

Zakeri S, Esmaeilzadeh S, Gorji N, Memariani Z, Moeini R, Bijani A. The effect of Achillea millefolium L. on vulvovaginal candidiasis compared with clotrimazole: a randomized controlled trial. Complement Ther Med 2020;52:102483.

Zolghadri Y, Fazeli M, Kooshki M, Shomali T, Karimaghayee N, Dehghani M. Achillea Millefolium L. Hydro- Alcoholic Extract Protects Pancreatic Cells by Down Regulating IL- 1β and iNOS Gene Expression in Diabetic Rats. Int J Mol Cell Med 2014;3(4):255–62.

APPENDIX I: MEDICAL AND RESEARCH ABBREVIATIONS

A1C: hemoglobin A1C glycated hemoglobin

Aβ: amyloid-β

AChEI: acetylcholinesterase inhibitor

ACR20: American College of Rheumatology arthritis scale; composite measure of 20% improvement for several parameters

ACS: acute coronary syndrome

ACT: Asthma Control Test

ACTH: adrenocorticotropic hormone

AD: Alzheimer's disease (sometimes also used for atopic dermatitis, but not in this text)

ADAS-Cog: Alzheimer's Disease Assessment Scale-Cognitive Subscale; ranges 0–70 with higher scores representing greater impairment

ADHD: attention-deficit/hyperactivity disorder

ADLs: activities of daily living

AE: adverse event

A-fib: atrial fibrillation

AHR: adjusted hazard ratio

AKI: acute kidney injury

AKT: phosphorylation activation of an oncogene

ALL: acute lymphocytic leukemia

ALP: alkaline phosphatase; enzyme especially from liver and bone

ALT: alanine transaminase (AKA SGPT); a liver enzyme

AMD (two meanings): (1) adjusted mean difference and (2) age-related macular degeneration (*also* ARMD)

AMPK: 5′ adenosine monophosphate-activated protein kinase; important for glucose and lipid metabolism

ANOVA: analysis of variance; reported as an F statistic, indicates statistical significance

ANOVA, RM: ANOVA, repeated measures

Anti-CCP: antibodies to cyclic citrullinated peptide

APAP: acetaminophen

Apo-A1: apolipoprotein A1; a constituent of HDL-C

Apo-B: apolipoprotein B; a constituent of LDL-C, VLDL-C

APTT: activated partial thromboplastin time; measure of blood coagulability

APOE−/−: apolipoprotein E-deficient strain; propensity toward atherosclerosis

ARMD: Age-related macular degeneration

ARR: absolute risk reduction; inverse of NNT

ASA: aspirin

ASCVD: Atherosclerotic cardiovascular disease

AST: aspartate transaminase or aspartate aminotransferase (AKA SGOT); a liver enzyme

AT-II: antithrombin II; together with heparin interferes with the interaction of thrombin and fibrinogen

ATP: adenosine triphosphate; provides energy to drive many processes in living cells

AUASI: American Urological Association Symptom Index or Score; seven questions, total scores range 0–35 with higher scores representing more severe BPH

AUC: area under the curve

B: type II error in statistical analysis

BAI: Beck Anxiety Inventory; 21 questions, total scores range from 0 to 63 with higher scores representing more severe anxiety

BAX: apoptosis regulating protein; Bcl-2 family

Bcl-2: B-cell lymphoma-2; antiapoptotic gene

BDNF: brain-derived neurotrophic factor; protein that promotes neuron growth

BG: blood glucose

BID: twice daily

BMD: bone mineral density

BMI: body mass index

BPH: benign prostatic hyperplasia (or hypertrophy)

BrdU: 5-bromo-2-deoxyuridine; a thymidine analogue, which is incorporated into the cells of the DNA synthetic phase

BT-20: breast cancer cell line; ER+

BUN: blood urea nitrogen; a measure of renal function and hydration

BW: body weight

Ca^{2+}: calcium ion

CAD: coronary artery disease (a.k.a. CHD: coronary heart disease and IHD: ischemic heart disease)

cAMP: $3',5'$-cyclic adenosine monophosphate; a second messenger used for intracellular transduction

CBP: chronic bacterial prostatitis

CCl4: carbon tetrachloride; experimental hepatic toxin

CCRF-CEM cells: a lymphoblastoid cell line

CD4+CD25+: regulatory T cells (Tregs); shut down completed immune response; prevent autoimmunity

CD8 cells: T cells; adaptive immunity

CDK1: cyclin-dependent kinase 1; a cell division protein homolog

CEE: conjugated equine estrogens

CETP: cholesteryl ester transfer protein; promotes the transfer of cholesteryl esters from antiatherogenic HDLs to proatherogenic apoB-containing lipoproteins

CGI: clinical global impression (of mood); three domains, each seven-point scale, rated by observer, with higher numbers indicating more severe illness

CGI-C: clinical global impression improvement or change (of mood) (*see CGI*)

CGI-S: clinical global impression severity (*see CGI*)

CHD: coronary heart disease (a.k.a. CAD: coronary artery disease and IHD: ischemic heart disease)

CINV: chemotherapy-induced nausea and vomiting

CIPN: chemotherapy-induced peripheral neuropathy

cGMP (two meanings): (1) guanosine $3',5'$-cyclic monophosphate; a second messenger molecule that activates intracellular protein kinases as secondary messenger and (2) current good manufacturing practices (FDA regulation); assure proper design, monitoring, and control of manufacturing processes and facilities

CMS: chronic mountain sickness

Chi-square test for homogeneity: tests to see if two populations come from the same unknown distribution. A low *P*-value for this test means that the heterogeneity in the data/results is significant

CK: creatine kinase; a muscle enzyme

CO: cardiac output

Coen's *d*: a measure of effect size. A *d* of 1 indicates the two groups differ by 1 standard deviation, a *d* of 2 indicates they differ by 2 standard deviations, etc. Large effect = 0.8; medium effect = 0.5, small effect = 0.2

COMT: catechol-*O*-methyltransferase; enzyme that degrades catecholamines

COPD: chronic obstructive pulmonary disease

COX: cyclooxygenase (prostaglandin-endoperoxide synthase); enzyme that forms thromboxane and prostaglandins from arachidonic acid

CREB or CREB-TF: (cAMP response element-binding protein); a cellular transcription factor that increases or decreases transcription of genes

CRH (CRF): corticotropin releasing hormone (factor); stimulates ACTH synthesis

C/S: caesarean section

CTS: carpal tunnel syndrome

CVA: Cerebrovascular accident or stroke

CVI: chronic venous insufficiency

Cyclin B1: regulatory protein involved in mitosis

Cyclin D1: a protein required for progression through the G1 phase of the cell cycle

CYP 450 (CYP 3A4, CYP 2C9, etc.): cytochrome P 450; superfamily of enzymes containing heme as a cofactor that function as monooxygenases; important for the clearance of various compounds, as well as for hormone synthesis and breakdown

Cysteinyl-LT: cysteinyl leukotrienes (LTC_4, LTD_4, LTE_4 LTF_4); slow-reacting substance of anaphylaxis

Cytokeratin-18 M30: a keratin protein commonly found in the intracytoplasmic cytoskeleton of epithelial tissue; an important component of intermediate filaments

D: standard difference between expected and obtained outcomes

DBP: diastolic blood pressure

df: degrees of freedom; the number of independent pieces of information that went into calculating the estimate; important for finding critical cutoff values for inferential statistical tests. A higher sample size translates to higher df and therefore gives more confidence that the findings are statistically significant

DHICA: 5,6-dihydroxyindole-2-carboxylic acid; an intermediate in the synthesis of melanin

DM: diabetes mellitus

DOT: directly observed therapy (usually for anti-TB drugs)

DXA: dual X-ray absorptiometry; measures bone density

EC50: half maximal effective concentration

ECG (EKG): electrocardiogram

EENT: eyes, ears, nose, and throat

EF: ejection fraction (cardiac)

ENT: ears, nose, and throat

eGFR: estimated glomerular filtration rate

EO: essential oil

ES: effect size; quantitative measure of the magnitude of a phenomenon

EGF: epidermal growth factor

eNOS: endothelial nitric oxide synthetase; responsible for most of the vascular NO produced

EPO: erythropoietin; stimulates red blood cell formation

ERα and ERβ: estrogen receptor-alpha and estrogen receptor-beta

ERB: estrogen receptor blocker

ERK1/2 (a.k.a. MAPK): extracellular signal-regulated kinases 1 and 2 (microtubule-associated protein kinase or mitogen-activated protein kinase); mediate cell proliferation and apoptosis

ES: effect size

ESCOP: European Scientific Cooperative on Phytotherapy

E-selectin: a cell adhesion molecule expressed only on endothelial cells activated by cytokines

ETOH: ethanol or alcohol

EULAR: European League Against Rheumatism arthritis scale; defines remission if each of four domains is ≤ 1

F score: a measure of a test's accuracy (range 0–1; perfect accuracy = 1)

FAST: functional analysis screening tool; Stages 1–7 with higher stages reflecting more severe decline in function

FBG: fasting blood glucose

FBS: fasting blood sugar

FEF: forced expiratory flow rate from lungs

FEV1: forced expiratory volume in one second from lungs

FMD: flow-mediated dilation

Friedman test: detects differences in treatments across multiple test attempts

FS: fractional shortening of cardiac left ventricle on 2D M-mode echocardiogram

FSFI: female sexual function index; 19 questions, 0–95 points, the lower the more severe dysfunction

FSH: follicle stimulating hormone

FT3: free T3 or triiodothyronine

FT4: free T4 or thyroxine

FVC: forced vital capacity of lungs

g (two meanings): (1) gram and (2) Hedges' g (a.k.a. "corrected effect size"); a measure of effect size utilized especially for small sample sizes

G2/M phase: the second growth phase followed by mitosis in the cell cycle

G6P: glucose 6-phosphate

GABA: gamma aminobutyric acid; inhibitory neurotransmitter with calming effect

GAD: generalized anxiety disorder

GAG: Glycosaminoglycan

GB: gallbladder

GFR: glomerular filtration rate; a measure of renal function

GI (two meanings): (1) gastrointestinal and (2) gingival index; measures gingivitis, scores 0–3 with higher scores indicating more severe gingival disease

GIV: generic inverse variance (in meta-analysis)

GLUT-4: glucose transporter type 4; insulin-regulated glucose transporter found primarily in adipose tissues and striated muscle

GM-CSF: granulocyte-macrophage colony-stimulating factor

GMP: good manufacturing practices; industry regulation

GRAS: Generally Recognized As Safe

GSH: glutathione; antioxidant

GSK3β: glycogen synthase kinase 3; abnormalities have been associated with bipolar disorder

5-HETE: 5-Hydroxyeicosatetraenoic acid; proinflammatory and proallergic eicosanoid

5-HT: 5-hydroxytryptamine or serotonin

5-HT 3A: one type of serotonin receptor

H1: histamine type 1

H_2O_2: hydrogen peroxide; an oxidizing compound

HA: hyaluronic acid; correlates with histological stages of liver fibrosis

HAM-A: Hamilton Anxiety Rating Scale; 14-items, scores range 0–56 with higher score reflecting more severe anxiety

HAM-D: Hamilton Depression Rating Scale; 17 items, scores range 0–52 with higher scores reflecting more severe depression

HBV: hepatitis B virus

HCV: hepatitis C virus

HDL-C: high-density lipoprotein cholesterol; antiatherogenic

HETE: hydroxyeicosatetraenoic acid; eicosanoid, metabolite of arachidonic acid

Hgb: hemoglobin

HIV: human immunodeficiency virus

HL-60 cells: human leukemia cell line used in research

HOMA-IR: Homeostatic Model Assessment of Insulin Resistance

HR (two meanings): (1) heart rate and (2) hazard ratio differs from RR and OR in that RRs and ORs are cumulative over an entire study, using a defined endpoint, while HRs represent instantaneous risk over the study time period and can indicate risks that happen before the endpoint

HRQL: Health-related quality of life

hs-CRP: high-sensitivity C-reactive protein; measure of inflammation

HSP (HSP60, HSP70, HSP90 and others): heat shock proteins; a family of proteins that facilitate cellular protein folding; help to protect cells from stress

HSV: herpes simplex virus

HTN: hypertension

I^2: measure of percentage of variation across studies due to heterogeneity rather than chance

IBD: inflammatory bowel disease (Crohn's disease, Ulcerative colitis, others)

IBS: irritable bowel syndrome

ICAM-1: intracellular adhesion molecule-1; a glycoprotein on endothelial and immune cells that binds to integrins of type CD11a/CD18, or CD11b/CD18; serves as an attachment site for rhinovirus as a receptor

ICS: inhaled corticosteroid

IFN (IFNα, IFNβ, IFNγ): interferon; antiviral proteins

IgG: immunoglobulin G; associated with long-term immunity

IgE: immunoglobulin E; associated with allergic response

IGF-1: insulin-like growth factor 1 (a.k.a. somatomedin C); is a growth hormone similar in molecular structure to insulin

IHD: ischemic heart disease (a.k.a. coronary artery disease and coronary heart disease)

IIEF: International Index of Erectile Function (15 questions, 4 domains; lower scores indicate more severe symptoms) of erectile dysfunction

IIEF-5: five-item version of the IIEF (severe, 1–7; moderate, 8–11; mild to moderate, 12–16; mild, 17–21; no ED, 22–25)

IκBα-kinase: enzyme complex upstream NF-κB signal transduction cascade

IL: interleukin (IL-1, IL-2, IL-4, IL-6, IL-10, etc.); cytokines, chemokines, and proteins expressed by helper CD4 lymphocytes and other cells, having an array of effects on various aspects of the immune system, some being proinflammatory and others antiinflammatory

IL-2: promotes regulatory T-cell production, reducing autoimmunity

IL-6: proinflammatory cytokine, antiinflammatory myokine

IL-10: antiinflammatory cytokine

IMT: intima-media thickness (of carotid arterial wall)

iNOS: inducible nitric oxide synthase

IOP: intraocular pressure

IP or i.p.: intraperitoneally

IPSS: International Prostate Symptom Score (mild symptoms, 0–7; moderate symptoms, 8–19; severe symptoms, 20–35)

IR: insulin resistance

IV: intravenous

JNK: c-Jun N-terminal kinase; a mitogen-activated protein kinase with a role in T-cell differentiation and apoptosis

KIM1: Kidney Injury Molecule-1, an upregulated protein in injured kidneys

KSI: Knee Swelling Index

LABA: long-acting beta-agonist

LAK: lymphokine activated killer cells

LDL-C: low-density lipoprotein cholesterol; atherogenic

LH: luteinizing hormone

LOX: lipoxygenases

LOX-1: lectin-like oxidized LDL receptor 1

LPS: lipopolysaccharides; endotoxins

LSIL: low-grade squamous intraepithelial lesion (precervical cancer)

LT-B4: leukotriene B4; inflammatory leukotriene; product of 5-LOX activity

LUTS: lower urinary tract symptoms

LVEDP: left ventricular end-diastolic pressure

LVM index: echocardiographic measure of left ventricular mass indexed to body surface area

M1G: byproduct of base excision repair (BER) of a specific type of DNA adduct called M_1dG

M: METs; a measure of energy expenditure, 1 kcal/kg/h

MAO: monoamine oxidase inhibitor (types A and B)

MAP: mean arterial blood pressure

MAPK: mitogen-activated protein kinase; kinase specific to serine and threonine, involved in directing cellular responses to mitogens, osmotic stress, heat shock and proinflammatory cytokines

MCF-7: breast cancer cell line (Michigan Cancer Foundation-7)

mcg: micrograms

MCI: mild cognitive impairment

MCP: metacarpophalangeal (hand joint)

MCP-1: monocyte chemoattractant protein-1; regulates migration and infiltration of monocytes/macrophages

MD: mean difference

MDA: malondialdehyde; marker for oxidative stress

MDI: metered dose inhaler

MEF: maximal expiratory flow from lungs

MENQOL: menopause-specific quality of life scale; 29-items, a total score and 4 domain scores (vasomotor, physical, psychosocial, sexual functioning) with higher scores reflective of worse QOL

MI: myocardial infarction

MIC: mean inhibitory concentration; to inhibit bacterial growth

MIG: monokine induced by interferon-gamma; chemoattractant for activated T cells

MMA: methylmalonic acid

MMEF: mid-maximal expiratory flow from lungs

MMP: matrix metallopeptidase (MMP-1, MMP-2, MMP-9, etc.); enzymes involved in degradation of extracellular matrix; markers of tissue inflammation and destruction

MMSE: Mini-Mental Status Exam; score range 0–30 with lower scores reflecting more severe dementia

MPTP: 1-methyl-4-phenyl-1,2,3,6-tetrahydropyridine; prodrug to the neurotoxin MPP +, which causes permanent symptoms of PD

mRNA: messenger ribonucleic acid; instrumental in protein synthesis

MS: multiple sclerosis

mTOR: mammalian target of rapamycin; a serine/threonine protein kinase that regulates cell growth and proliferation, insulin receptors, and IGF-1

MTX: methotrexate; rheumatologic and oncologic drug

NAFLD: nonalcoholic fatty liver disease

Nesfatin-1: neuropeptide causing diminished hunger

NF-κB: nuclear factor kappa-light-chain-enhancer of activated B cells; transcription factors that control DNA transcription, cytokine production, cell survival, regulation of the immune response to infection

NIH: National Institutes of Health

NIH-CPSI: National Institutes of Health Chronic Prostatitis Symptom Index; 13 items standardized onto a 0–100 scale, with higher scores representing greater disease severity

NK cells: natural killer cells; cytotoxic lymphocytes

NMDA: N-methyl-D-aspartate; the receptor for glutamate

NNT: number needed to treat (to achieve beneficial outcome)

NO: nitric oxide; pro-oxidant, vasodilator

NOAEL: no observed adverse effect level

Nordin index: X-ray of long bone measuring combined cortical index and total width

Notch signaling pathway: promotes proliferative signaling and neural differentiation during neurogenesis; coordinates angiogenesis

NOX: nitric oxide

NREM1: non-REM sleep stage 1

Nrf2: nuclear factor erythroid 2-related factor 2; regulates expression of antioxidant proteins

N.S.: not statistically significant

NSE: neuron-specific enolase; enzyme indicative of neuronal injury

N/V: nausea and vomiting

1,25OHD: 1,25-hydroxy vitamin D

25OHD: 25-hydroxy vitamin D

2OHE: 2-hydroxy estrone

2:16α-OHE: ratio of 2-hydorxyestrone to 16α-hydroxyestrone; lower ratio is a proposed risk for breast cancer

OA: osteoarthritis, osteoarthrosis

OAB: overactive bladder

OCD: obsessive-compulsive disorder

OGTT: oral glucose tolerance test

OHI: oral hygiene index; calculus and debris indexes, total score range 0–12 with higher scores reflecting poorer oral hygiene

OHI-S: oral hygiene plaque index—simplified

6-keto-PGF1α: a marker of PGI2 biosynthesis in vivo

P (*P*-value): a measure of the evidence against a null hypothesis; indicates statistical significance, lower number indicating greater significance

PI3K-Akt: intracellular signal transduction pathway that promotes metabolism, proliferation, cell survival, growth, and angiogenesis in response to extracellular signals

p21: cyclin-dependent kinase inhibitor 1; a major target of p53 activity, linking DNA damage to cell cycle arrest

p21WAF1 pathway: negative cell cycle regulator, blocks leukemogenesis

p53: tumor suppressor gene

p65 (a.k.a. RELA): one of the five components that form the NF-κB (enhancer of activated B cells) transcription factor family

PA: pyrrolizidine alkaloid, a class of potentially toxic herbal constituents

PAF: platelet-activating factor

PAH: pulmonary artery hypertension

PAI-1: plasminogen activator inhibitor 1; principal inhibitor of tissue plasminogen activator and urokinase; sustains blood clots)

PASI: Psoriasis Area and Severity Index; scores range 0–72 with higher scores reflecting more severe disease

PC-12 cells: neural crest cells, neuroblastic and eosinophilic

PCOS: polycystic ovary syndrome

PD: Parkinson's disease

PDE: phosphodiesterase; results in decreased cAMP and cGMP

PEF: peak expiratory flow rate from lungs

PEPCK: phosphoenolpyruvate carboxykinase; gluconeogenic enzyme

PEP/LVET: pre-ejection period/left ventricular ejection time ratio

PFT: pulmonary function tests

PGD2: prostaglandin D2; a major prostaglandin produced by mast cells—recruits Th2 cells, eosinophils, and basophils

PGE2: prostaglandin E2; causes cervical ripening, uterine contractions; vasodilating

PGF2-α: prostaglandin F2 alpha; a luteolytic and oxytocic prostaglandin

PGI2: prostaglandin I-2 or prostacyclin; vasodilator and platelet activation inhibitor

Pgp: P-glycoprotein aka multidrug resistance protein 1; an important protein of the cell membrane that pumps many foreign substances (including drugs and chemotherapy) out of cells

PI: plaque index; measurement of dental plaque, ranges 0–3 with higher scores indicating worse dental plaque

PIF: peak inspiratory flow from lungs

PMD: pooled mean differences

PMDD: premenstrual dysphoric disorder

PMN: polymorphonuclear leukocytes; acute inflammatory white blood cells

PMS: premenstrual syndrome

PPARγ: peroxisome proliferator-activated receptor gamma; increases hepatic synthesis and release of paraoxonase 1, reducing atherosclerosis

PPG: postprandial glucose (1hPPG = 1-h postprandial glucose, etc.)

PRA: plasma renin activity

PRL: prolactin

PRN: as needed

PRR: proportional reporting ratio

PSA: prostate-specific antigen

PSQI: Pittsburgh Sleep Quality Index; scores ≥5 indicate poor sleep

PSS: Perceived Stress Scale; score range 0–40 with higher scores indicating more stress

PT (two meanings): (1) protime; a measure of blood clotting and (2) physical therapy

PTT: partial thromboplastin time

PUD: peptic ulcer disease

PUPPP: pruritic urticarial papules and plaques of pregnancy

PVR: postvoid residual (urine volume)

PXR: the pregnane X receptor; a nuclear receptor, regulates the expression of drug-metabolizing enzymes and transporters

Q two meanings: (1) flow rate and (2) Cochran's Q: assesses whether the proportion of successes is the same between groups

Q_{max}: maximal flow rate

Q$_{avg}$: average flow rate

QD: daily

QID: four times daily

QOL: quality of life

r: the correlation coefficient; measures the strength and direction of a linear relationship between two variables on a scatterplot + 1 and –1

RA: rheumatoid arthritis

RBC: red blood cell

Rb protein: retinoblastoma protein; a tumor suppressor protein that is inactivated when phosphorylated

RCT: randomized controlled trial

RDS: respiratory distress syndrome

RLS: restless legs syndrome

ROS: reactive oxygen species

RR: relative risk, risk ratio, response ratio

RRR: relative risk reduction

s-100: protein marker of acute brain ischemia

SABA: short-acting beta agonist

SBI: sulcus bleeding index (in gingivitis)

SBP: systolic blood pressure

SCC: squamous cell carcinoma

SCORAD: SCORing Atopic Dermatitis; eight items, score range 0–103 with higher score indicating more severe disease

SEM: standard error of measurement; measures how much test scores are spread around a "true" score

SHGB: sex hormone binding globulin

SIBO: small intestinal bacterial overgrowth

SIRT-1: sirtuin 1 (a.k.a. NAD-dependent deacetylase sirtuin-1); an enzyme that deacetylates proteins that contribute to cellular regulation and insulin sensitivity

SLC transporters: solute carrier transporters; facilitate the transport of a wide array of substrates across biological membranes

SMD: standardized mean difference

SOD: superoxide dismutase; antioxidant enzyme

s/p: status-post; following procedure, e.g.

SREBP-1c: sterol regulatory element-binding protein; transcription factor

SSRI: selective serotonin reuptake inhibitor

STAI: State-Trait Anxiety Inventory; two sub-scales (state and trait), 20 items for each, score range 20–80 for each, higher scores indicating more severe anxiety

STAT-3: signal transducer and activator of transcription 3; transcription factor

SUI: stress urinary incontinence

SULT 2A1: gene that encodes bile salt sulfotransferase

SV: stroke volume (cardiac)

Sx: symptoms

T1DM: type 1 diabetes mellitus

T2DM: type 2 diabetes mellitus

T3: triiodothyronine

T4: thyroxine

TAC (two meanings): (1) total antioxidant capacity and (2) triamcinolone (corticosteroid)

TB: tuberculosis

TBARS: thiobarbituric acid reactive substances; formed as a byproduct of lipid peroxidation

Tbili: total bilirubin; a measure of liver function

TCM: traditional Chinese medicine

TD: tardive dyskinesia

TG: triglycerides

TGF-β: transforming growth factor beta; cytokine that leads to the activation of different downstream substrates and regulatory proteins, inducing transcription of different target genes that function in differentiation, chemotaxis, proliferation, and activation of many immune cells

Th-17: T-helper 17 cells; produce IL-17 and IL-17F which are proinflammatory, recruiting neutrophils and macrophages to infected tissues

Th-22: T-helper 22 cells; inflammatory to skin

TID: three times daily

TNF-α: tumor necrosis factor alpha; inflammatory cytokine

TNFR: tumor necrosis factor receptor (type 1 and type 2)

TPO: thyroid peroxidase; antibodies to this indicate Hashimoto's and other autoimmune thyroiditis

TPOAb: thyroid peroxidase antibodies

Treg: regulatory T cells; regulate or suppress other cells in the immune system

TRPA-1: transient receptor potential cation channel 1; sensor for environmental irritants

TSH: thyroid stimulating hormone

UACR: urinary albumin to creatinine ratio; microalbumin

UC: ulcerative colitis; an inflammatory bowel disease

UDP: uridine diphosphate

UGT: uridine 5′-diphospho-glucuronosyltransferase; catalyzes the transfer of the glucuronic acid component of UDP-glucuronic acid to a small hydrophobic molecule (glucuronidation)

UPDRS: Unified Parkinson's Disease Rating Scale

URI: upper respiratory infection

URTI: upper respiratory tract infection

UTI: urinary tract infection

UVA: ultraviolet A (light)

UVB: ultraviolet B (light)

VAS: visual analog scale; patient indicates on linear indicator the subjective status; scores range 0–100 mm with higher scores indicating worse condition

VCAM-1: serum soluble vascular adhesion molecule-1; mediates the adhesion of lymphocytes, monocytes, eosinophils, and basophils to vascular endothelium

VEGF: vascular endothelial growth factor; promotes the growth of new blood vessels

VEGFR: vascular endothelial growth factor receptor

VGF: (nonacronymic); neuropeptide; critical modulator of depression-like behaviors

WC: waist circumference

WHOQOL-BREF: World Health Organization quality of life brief version (26 questions vs 100 questions); higher scores denote higher QOL

WMD: weighted mean difference; the difference between two means, weighted by the precision of the study

WNT pathway: group of signal transduction pathways; involved in insulin signaling and development of cancer

WOMAC: Western Ontario and McMaster Universities Arthritis Index; three domains (pain 0–20, stiffness 0–8, physical function 0–68), higher scores indicate greater pain, stiffness, or physical function

APPENDIX II: BIBLIOGRAPHY AND ADDITIONAL RESOURCES

REFERENCES

Books

Blumenthal M. The ABC clinical guide to herbs. Austin, TX: American Botanical Council; 2003.

Bone K. A clinical guide to blending liquid herbs: herbal formulations for the individual patient. St. Louis, MO: Churchill Livingstone; 2003.

Cech R. Making plant medicine. Williams, OR: Horizon Herbs; 2000.

Hoffmann D. Medical herbalism: the science and practice of herbal medicine. Rochester, VT: Healing Arts Press; 2003.

Websites

American Botanical Council (herbal research database). http://cms.herbalgram.org/.

Association for Advancement of Restorative Medicine (restorative medicine monographs). https://restorativemedicine.org/library/monographs/.

Christopher Hobbs PhD (herbalism, botany, research). www.christopherhobbs.com/.

Drugs.com (MedFacts for natural products). www.drugs.com/npp/.

Examine.com (nutrition and herbal research database). https://examine.com.

Memorial Sloan Kettering Cancer Center (alternative cancer treatments). www.mskcc.org/cancer-care/diagnosis-treatment/symptom-management/integrative-medicine/herbs/search.

NCCIH (herb fact sheets). www.nccih.nih.gov/health/herbsataglance.

PubMed (extensive resource for preclinical and clinical research). https://pubmed.ncbi.nlm.nih.gov/?myncbishare=ihsl&holding=oboler_lib_fft_ndi.

Sigma Aldrich (plant chemistry). www.sigmaaldrich.com/life-science/nutrition-research/learning-center/plant-profiler.html.

ADDITIONAL RESOURCES

Books

Blumenthal M, Goldberg A, Brinckmann J. Herbal Medicine. Expanded commission E monographs. Newton, MA: Integrative Medicine Communications; 2000.

Duke J. The green pharmacy: the ultimate compendium of natural remedies from the world's foremost authority on healing herbs. New York, NY: St. martin's Paperbacks; 1998.

Hobbs C. Grow it, heal it: natural and effective herbal remedies from your garden or windowsill. New York, NY: Rodale Books; 2013.

Hobbs C. Christopher Hobbs's medicinal mushrooms: the essential guide: boost immunity, improve memory, fight cancer, stop infection, and expand your consciousness. North Adams, MA: Storey Publishing; 2021.

Natural Medicines Comprehensive Database. Stockton, CA: Therapeutic Research Faculty; 2007.

PDR for Herbal Medicines. Montvale, NJ: Thomson PDR; 2007.

Websites

Natural Standard (CAM database, subscription). https://naturalmedicines.therapeuticresearch.com/.

Natural Product Magnetic Resonance Database Project (open-access clearinghouse for all NMR data on natural products). http://www.np-mrd.org/.

Herbal Medicines Compendium (free-access herbal monographs). https://hmc.usp.org/monographs/final-authorized.

Apps

About Herbs (Memorial Sloan Kettering Cancer Center).

Herblist™ (National Center for Complementary and Integrative Health).

INDEX

Note: Page numbers followed by *t* indicate tables.

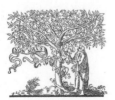

Printed and bound by CPI Group (UK) Ltd, Croydon, CR0 4YY

03/10/2024

01040305-0001